HANDBOOK OF DRUG THERAPY

HANDBOOK OF DRUG THERAPY

Edited by

Russell R. Miller, Pharm.D., Ph.D.
Division of Clinical Pharmacy
Department of Pharmacy
New England Medical Center Hospital
Boston, Massachusetts

David J. Greenblatt, M.D.
Clinical Pharmacology Unit
Department of Medicine
Massachusetts General Hospital
Boston, Massachusetts

ELSEVIER • NEW YORK
New York • Amsterdam

NOTICE The editors and the publisher of this work have made every effort to ensure that the drug dosage schedules herein are accurate and in accord with the standards accepted at the time of publication. Readers are advised, however, to check the product information sheet included in the package of each drug prior to administration to be certain that changes have not been made in either the recommended dose or contraindications. Such verification is especially important in regard to new or infrequently used drugs.

Elsevier North Holland
52 Vanderbilt Avenue, New York, New York 10017
Distributors outside the United States and Canada:

Elsevier/North-Holland Biomedical Press B.V.
Jan Van Galenstraat 335, P.O. Box 1527
Amsterdam, The Netherlands

Library of Congress Cataloging in Publication Data

Main entry under title:
Handbook of drug therapy.

Bibliography: p.
Includes index.
1. Chemotherapy—Handbooks, manuals, etc. 2. Drugs—Handbooks, manuals, etc. I. Miller, Russell R. II. Greenblatt, David J. [DNLM: 1. Drug therapy—Handbooks. WB330 H235]
RM262.H26 615'.58'0202 79-10559
ISBN 0-444-00329-0
ISBN 0-444-00253-7 pbk.

Manufactured in the United States of America

CONTENTS

CONTRIBUTORS

SALVADORE ALVAREZ, M.D.
Clinical Fellow, Infectious Diseases Section, Department of Medicine, Boston City Hospital, Boston, Massachusetts

GEORGE ARNOLD, M.D.
Clinical Instructor in Medicine, University of Pittsburgh School of Medicine, Pittsburgh, Pennsylvania

LLOYD AXELROD, M.D.
Assistant Professor of Medicine, Harvard Medical School; Assistant Physician, Massachusetts General Hospital; Chief, Medical Unit, Massachusetts Eye and Ear Infirmary, Boston, Massachusetts

JOHN G. BARTLETT, M.D.
Associate Professor of Medicine, Tufts University School of Medicine; Chief, Infectious Diseases Research Section, Veterans Administration Hospital, Boston, Massachusetts

MICHAEL BARZA, M.D.
Associate Professor of Medicine, Tufts University School of Medicine; Associate Physician, Infectious Disease Section, Department of Medicine, New England Medical Center Hospital, Boston, Massachusetts

ABBY S. BLOCH, M.S., R.D.
Head Clinical Diet/Nutrition Specialist, Memorial Sloan-Kettering Cancer Center, New York, New York

RONNI CHERNOFF, Ed.M., R.D.
Assistant Head Clinical Diet/Nutrition Specialist, Memorial Sloan-Kettering Cancer Center, New York, New York

WILLIAM CHIN, M.P.H., M.D.
Vector Biology and Control Division, Bureau of Tropical Diseases, Center for Disease Control, Atlanta, Georgia

G. ROBERT COATNEY, Ph.D., D.Sc.
Formerly Chief, Laboratory Parasite Chemotherapy, National Institute of Allergy and Infectious Diseases; Professor of Pharmacology, Louisiana State University Medical School; Consultant on Malaria, Center for Disease Control, Atlanta, Georgia

WILLIAM E. COBB, M.D.
Clinical Assistant Professor of Medicine, Tufts University School of Medicine; Assistant Physician, New England Medical Center Hospital, Boston, Massachusetts; Director of Medical Education, Quincy City Hospital, Quincy, Massachusetts

JAY D. COFFMAN, M.D.
Professor of Medicine, Boston University School of Medicine; Section Head, Peripheral Vascular Department, Robert Dawson Evans Memorial Department of Clinical Research, University Hospital, Boston, Massachusetts

MICHAEL M. COHEN, M.D.
Chief Neuro-Ophthalmologist, Episcopal Hospital, Philadelphia, Pennsylvania

DENIS CRADDOCK, M.D.
Honorary Librarian, Royal College of General Practitioners; Senior Partner, Group Practice, South Croydon, Surrey, England

CAROL M. CRONIN, B.S. Pharm.
Department of Pharmacy, Sidney Farber Cancer Institute, Boston, Massachusetts

WILLIAM F. CROWLEY, JR., M.D.
Instructor in Medicine, Harvard Medical School; Assistant in Medicine, Assistant in Gynecology, Massachusetts General Hospital, Boston, Massachusetts; Daland Fellow, American Philosophical Society

ROBERT A. CURTIS, Pharm.D.
Resident in Clinical Pharmacy, Department of Medicine, Truman Medical Center, University of Missouri–Kansas City, Kansas City, Missouri

GILBERT H. DANIELS, M.D.
Assistant Professor of Medicine, Harvard Medical School; Assistant Physician, Massachusetts General Hospital, Boston, Massachusetts

EVERETT M. DELABARRE, M.D.
Associate Professor of Rehabilitation Medicine, Tufts University School of Medicine; Department of Rehabilitation Medicine, New England Medical Center Hospital, Boston, Massachusetts

ZAREH DEMIRJIAN, M.D.
Instructor in Medicine, Harvard Medical School; Assistant in Medicine, Massachusetts General Hospital, Boston, Massachusetts

ROGER E. DIONNE, Pharm.D.
Resident in Clinical Pharmacy, Albert B. Chandler Medical Center, University of Kentucky, Lexington, Kentucky

VICTOR A. DRILL, M.D., Ph.D.
Professor of Pharmacology, University of Illinois School of Medicine, Chicago, Illinois

RONALD P. EVENS, Pharm.D.
Assistant Professor of Clinical Pharmacy, University of Texas at Austin College of Pharmacy; Director of Drug Information Service, University of Texas Health Science Center at San Antonio, San Antonio, Texas

MARTIN FARBER, M.D.
Associate Professor of Obstetrics and Gynecology, Director of Division of Reproductive Endocrinology, Tufts University School of Medicine; Physician, New England Medical Center Hospital, Boston, Massachusetts

KARMIN A. FAWAZ, M.D.
Assistant Professor of Medicine, Tufts University School of Medicine; Assistant Physician, New England Medical Center Hospital, Boston, Massachusetts

H. HARRIS FUNKENSTEIN, M.D.
Assistant Professor of Neurology, Harvard Medical School; Associate in Medicine (Neurology), Peter Bent Brigham Hospital, Boston, Massachusetts

RICHARD GLECKMAN, M.D.
Associate Professor of Medicine, Boston University School of Medicine; Physician, Infectious Diseases Section, Department of Medicine, Boston Veterans Administration Hospital, Boston, Massachusetts

STEPHEN GOLDFINGER, M.D.
Associate Professor of Medicine, Associate Dean for Continuing Education, Harvard Medical School; Physician, Massachusetts General Hospital, Boston, Massachusetts

DAVID J. GREENBLATT, M.D.
Assistant Professor of Medicine, Harvard Medical School; Director, Clinical Pharmacology Unit, Massachusetts General Hospital, Boston, Massachusetts

EDWARD S. GREENWALD, M.D.
Associate Clinical Professor of Medicine, Albert Einstein College of Medicine; Acting Director, Department of Oncology, Montefiore Hospital and Medical Center, Bronx, New York

PETER L. GROSS, M.D.
Instructor in Medicine, Harvard Medical School; Associate Chief, Emergency Medical Services, Assistant in Medicine, Massachusetts General Hospital, Boston, Massachusetts

SIGRID A. HAGG, M.D.
Instructor in Medicine, Harvard Medical School; Thorndike Laboratory, Beth Israel Hospital, Boston, Massachusetts

JOHN T. HARRINGTON, M.D.
Associate Professor of Medicine, Tufts University School of Medicine; Director, Hemodialysis Unit, Director, Medical Intensive Care Unit, New England Medical Center Hospital, Boston, Massachusetts

LESLIE HENDELES, Pharm.D.
Associate Professor of Pharmacy, University of Iowa College of Pharmacy; Clinical Pharmacist, Pediatric Allergy Clinic, University of Iowa Hospitals and Clinics, Iowa City, Iowa

DAVID A. HENRY, M.B.
Lecturer in Therapeutics, University of Nottingham School of Medicine; Physician, City Hospital, Nottingham, England

JOHN R. HILLS, M.D.
Associate Professor of Neurology, Tufts University School of Medicine; Neurologist, New England Medical Center Hospital, Boston, Massachusetts

DAVID H. HUFFMAN, M.D.
Associate Professor of Medicine and Pharmacology, University of Kansas School of Medicine, Kansas City, Kansas; Chief of Medicine, Veterans Administration Hospital, Kansas City, Missouri

IVOR M. D. JACKSON, M.D.
Associate Professor of Medicine, Tufts University School of Medicine; Physician, New England Medical Center Hospital, Boston, Massachusetts

DENNIS W. JOUBERT, B.S.
Supervisor, In-Patient Pharmacy Service, Boston Veterans Administration Hospital, Boston, Massachusetts

KERRISON JUNIPER, JR., M.D.
Professor of Medicine, Chief, Division of Gastroenterology, Southern Illinois University School of Medicine, Springfield, Illinois

DENNIS D. JURANEK, D.V.M., M.Sc.
Deputy Director, Parasitic Diseases Divison, Bureau of Epidemiology, Center for Disease Control, Atlanta, Georgia

MARSHALL M. KAPLAN, M.D.
Professor of Medicine, Tufts University School of Medicine; Chief, Gastroenterology Division, Department of Medicine, New England Medical Center Hospital, Boston, Massachusetts

COLLIN S. KARMODY, M.D.
Associate Professor of Otolaryngology, Tufts University School of Medicine; Physician, New England Medical Center Hospital, Boston, Massachusetts

CHARLES Y. KAWADA, M.D.
Assistant Professor of Obstetrics and Gynecology, Tufts University School of Medicine; Assistant Gynecologist, New England Medical Center Hospital, Boston, Massachusetts

MARTIN G. KISTIN, M.D.
Attending Consultant, University of New Mexico School of Medicine and Veterans Administration Hospital, Albuquerque, New Mexico

SPENCER K. KOERNER, M.D.
Professor of Medicine, University of California at Los Angeles School of Medicine; Director, Division of Pulmonary Medicine, Cedars-Sinai Medical Center, Los Angeles, California

DAVID H. LAWSON, M.D.
Visiting Professor, School of Pharmaceutical Sciences, University of Strathclyde; Consultant Physician, Glasgow Royal Infirmary, Glasgow, Scotland

ANN M. LEES, M.D.
Research Associate, Massachusetts Institute of Technology Arteriosclerosis Center, Cambridge, Massachusetts

ROBERT S. LEES, M.D.
Professor of Cardiovascular Disease and Director, Arteriosclerosis Center, Massachusetts Institute of Technology, Cambridge, Massachusetts; Director, Noninvasive Diagnostic Laboratory, Cardiac Unit, Massachusetts General Hospital, Boston, Massachusetts

GORDON D. O. LOWE, M.B.
Lecturer in Medicine, University of Glasgow; Honorary Senior Registrar, Glasgow Royal Infirmary, Glasgow, Scotland

NICOLAOS E. MADIAS, M.D.
Assistant Professor of Medicine, Tufts University School of Medicine; Assistant Physician, Renal Service, New England Medical Center Hospital, Boston, Massachusetts

PHILIP D. MARSDEN, M.D.
Professor of Medicine, University of Brasilia, Brasilia, Brazil

DANIEL S. MATLOFF, M.D.
Instructor in Medicine, Tufts University School of Medicine; Research Fellow in Gastroenterology, New England Medical Center Hospital, Boston, Massachusetts

SAMUEL J. MATTHEWS, Pharm.D.
Assistant Clinical Professor of Pharmacy, Northeastern University College of Pharmacy and Allied Health Professions, Boston, Massachusetts

CRAIG N. MATTSON, M.S.
Assistant Clinical Professor of Pharmacy, Northeastern University College of Pharmacy and Allied Health Professions; Clinical Pharmacist in Cardiology, New England Medical Center Hospital, Boston, Massachusetts

WILLIAM W. McCLOSKEY, Pharm.D.
Pharmacist, Division of Clinical Services, Department of Pharmacy, Rhode Island Hospital, Providence, Rhode Island

RICHARD H. MEADE, III, M.D.
Professor of Pediatrics, Tufts University School of Medicine; Chief, Pediatric Infectious Disease Service, Boston Floating Hospital; Service Physician, New England Medical Center Hospital, Boston, Massachusetts

PETER V. W. MIAO, M.D.
Research Fellow, Infectious Diseases Section, Department of Medicine, New England Medical Center Hospital, Boston, Massachusetts

RUSSELL R. MILLER, Pharm.D., Ph.D.
Assistant Professor of Pharmacology, Boston University School of Medicine; Senior Investigator, Boston Collaborative Drug Surveillance Program, Boston University Medical Center; Director, Division of Clinical Pharmacy, New England Medical Center Hospital, Boston, Massachusetts

LEO A. MILLETTE, Pharm.D.
Supervisor, Maine Poison Control Center and Regional Emergency Medicine Information Service, Maine Medical Center, Portland, Maine

RICHARD A. NORTON, M.D.
Associate Professor of Medicine, Tufts University School of Medicine; Physician, New England Medical Center Hospital, Boston, Massachusetts

EDWARD S. ORRIS, M.D.
Fellow in Gastroenterology, New England Medical Center Hospital, Boston, Massachusetts

JAMES F. PATTERSON, M.D.
Professor of Medicine, Tufts University School of Medicine; Chief, Ambulatory Internal Medicine, New England Medical Center Hospital, Boston, Massachusetts

DAVID S. PEARLMAN, M.D.
Clinical Professor of Pediatrics, University of Colorado Medical School; Senior Staff Physician, National Jewish Hospital and Research Center, Denver, Colorado

HENRY J. PFEIFER, B.S. Pharm.
Pharmacist, New England Medical Center Hospital, Boston, Massachusetts

KENNETH L. PINSKER, M.D.
Assistant Professor of Medicine, Albert Einstein College of Medicine; Acting Head, Division of Pulmonary Medicine, Montefiore Hospital and Medical Center, Bronx, New York

ANDREW G. PLAUT, M.D.
Professor of Medicine, Tufts University School of Medicine; Physician, New England Medical Center Hospital, Boston, Massachusetts

STEPHEN E. SALLAN, M.D.
Assistant Professor of Pediatrics, Harvard Medical School; Senior Clinical Associate, Sidney Farber Cancer Institute, Associate in Hematology/Oncology, Children's Hospital Medical Center, Boston, Massachusetts

JOSEPH M. SCEPPA, M.S.
Assistant Clinical Professor of Pharmacy, Northeastern University College of Pharmacy and Allied Health Professions; Assistant Director, Department of Pharmacy, New England Medical Center Hospital, Boston, Massachusetts

RICHARD T. SCHEIFE, Pharm.D.
Associate Clinical Professor of Pharmacy, Northeastern University College of Pharmacy and Allied Health Professions; Neuropharmacologist, Department of Neurology, Clinical Pharmacist in Neurology and Infectious Diseases, New England Medical Center Hospital, Boston, Massachusetts

RICHARD I. SHADER, M.D.
Associate Professor of Psychiatry, Director, Psychopharmacology Research Laboratory, Harvard Medical School; Director of Continuing Education, Massachusetts Mental Health Center, Boston, Massachusetts

MAURICE E. SHILS, M.D., Sc.D.
Associate Professor of Medicine, Cornell University Medical College; Attending Physician and Director of Nutrition, Memorial Sloan-Kettering Cancer Center, New York, New York

JAMES S. SINGER, M.D.
Fellow in Gastroenterology, New England Medical Center Hospital, Boston, Massachusetts

JOHN S. URBANETTI, M.D.
Assistant Professor of Pulmonary Medicine, Tufts University School of Medicine; Assistant Physician, Pulmonary Division, Department of Medicine, New England Medical Center Hospital, Boston, Massachusetts; Medical Emergency Supervisor, McGill University, Montréal, Québec, Canada

MILES WEINBERGER, M.D.
Associate Professor of Pediatrics and Pharmacology, University of Iowa College of Medicine; Chairman, Pediatric Allergy and Pulmonary Division, University of Iowa Hospitals and Clinics, Iowa City, Iowa

BRUCE WEINER, M.S.
Assistant Clinical Professor of Pharmacy, Northeastern University College of Pharmacy and Allied Health Professions; Clinical Instructor in Surgery, Tufts University School of Medicine; Clinical Pharmacist in Surgery, New England Medical Center Hospital, Boston, Massachusetts

PREFACE

The *Handbook of Drug Therapy* is intended to be a concise, authoritative, and scholarly guide to the clinical use of drugs. Indications, contraindications, adverse effects, interactions, dosage, preparations, and costs of nearly all drugs commonly used in medical practice are critically reviewed. Where clinically relevant, the pharmacologic properties, mechanism of action, and pharmacokinetics of individual drugs are discussed in considerable detail. The contributors have clearly identified what they believe to be the drugs of choice. Brief discussions of disease states are included, particularly in those chapters devoted to drugs used in the treatment of a specific disease (e.g., agents used in gout). Furthermore, each contributor has supported his or her observations with many citations to original research; these references should be useful for more detailed study.

All clinically useful drugs within the scope of each chapter are discussed, but not all marketed drugs are covered. Thus, nonessential drugs either may simply not be mentioned or may be given only brief coverage. Some categories of drug are not covered. For example, we have made no attempt to cover drugs that are used primarily by specialists (e.g., general anesthetics, oxytocics, antidiuretics). Certain other categories of drug that are used by both specialists and general practitioners (e.g., dermatologicals, ophthalmic drugs, otologic agents) are also not covered. Important investigational drugs, however, are covered. Similarly, investigational uses of marketed drugs are discussed if the contributors judged these indications valid.

Although a number of available reference books are devoted to the topic of clinical therapeutics, it is our judgment that none provides a sufficiently critical evaluation of the advantages and disadvantages of commonly used drugs within the context of clinical practice. Furthermore, no book has rigorously and comprehensively examined the published literature on drug therapy, and many sources provide only part of the information needed to use drugs wisely. This book attempts to bring all the pertinent information together in one place.

Russell R. Miller, Pharm.D., Ph.D.
David J. Greenblatt, M.D.

Boston, Massachusetts

ACKNOWLEDGMENTS

Many people and organizations have played important roles in making this book possible and bringing it to completion. Raymond Gosselin, president of the Massachusetts College of Pharmacy, enthusiastically supported the *Handbook* at its inception and helped us obtain a grant from the College to support some administrative costs. Roche Laboratories provided financial aid over a period of three years and made it possible for us to employ several editorial assistants. The Bingham Associates Fund provided salary support for Dr. Miller. Dr. Greenblatt was supported by Grant MH-12279 from the United States Public Health Service.

Our editorial assistants were Robert A. Curtis, Robert T. Groth, and Steven Surowitz. Without their diligent attention to numerous technical details, we could not have completed the book. Ann Werner, Corinne Murphy, and Kathleen McMahon prepared initial typescripts of the individual chapters. Ms. Werner coordinated all editorial work and manuscript preparation. She was responsible for final corrections to all chapters and also did meticulous copy editing. Since this book was prepared by an editor-controlled electronic phototypesetting system, Ms. Werner's role was critical. We are most grateful to her.

A panel of practitioners reviewed all chapters for clinical relevance as the final step in the editorial process. They were John K. Zawacki, M.D., Jonathan I. Morrison, M.D., Oscar M. Jankelson, M.D., and James D. C. Gowans, M.D. Their many useful comments immeasurably improved the book. Finally, we gratefully acknowledge the continuous help and support of Yale Altman, editor for Elsevier North Holland.

ORGANIZATION AND USE OF THE HANDBOOK

Most chapters are divided into two sections: a discussion of general principles and individual drug monographs. In those chapters that deal with drug therapy of a disease, the first section usually consists of a brief description of the disease and its appropriate treatment. In those chapters that are concerned with a category of drugs used to treat a symptom or several diseases, the principles section gives guidelines on the indications, contraindications, and adverse effects of the drugs as a group.

The drug monographs vary greatly in length and scope, depending on the organization of the chapter. They usually provide information on indications, contraindications, adverse reactions, interactions, and dosage. Only drug interactions that are clinically important in humans are discussed. Dosage recommendations are those of the author; they may not conform to those recommended in the official package insert. In most instances the title of a monograph is the official United States Adopted Name (generic name) of the drug. Commonly used trademark names are given in parentheses.

Nearly all chapters include a table describing available preparations and costs. Usually only those preparations that the author finds useful are listed; the tables are not complete listings of available preparations. The cost to the pharmacist is usually given for only one trademarked product if more than one is listed; other trademark names (not necessarily a complete list) are given in parentheses. Prices for generic products are given as ranges. All prices were taken from the 1978 Drug Topics Red Book (Medical Economics, Inc., Oradell, New Jersey); average wholesale prices were used when given.

ANTIMICROBIAL AGENTS

1. PENICILLINS

Michael Barza

The penicillins may be divided into three groups—'natural,' penicillinase-resistant, and 'broad-spectrum' (Table 1). The natural penicillins were the first to be derived and afforded definitive therapy for a number of previously lethal infections. With the increasing prevalence of penicillin-resistant strains of *Staphylococcus aureus* during the 1950s, the penicillinase-resistant congeners were developed. More recently two groups of 'broad-spectrum' penicillins have been marketed. The first comprises ampicillin and amoxicillin, as well as certain other agents which are broken down to ampicillin (eg, hetacillin and pivampicillin); these drugs are active against *Haemophilus influenzae* and *Escherichia coli*. The most recent additions to the class, carbenicillin and ticarcillin, exhibit a spectrum which includes many gram-negative bacilli, including Pseudomonas.

The penicillins are bactericidal antibiotics, that is, they do not simply interrupt the proliferation of bacteria but actually destroy them. They do so by interfering with the activity of enzymes (eg, transpeptidase) which crosslink the peptidoglycan molecule of the cell wall into a stable monomer.[1] Their activity, therefore, requires that the bacteria be growing. Gram-negative organisms, being endowed with a fairly strong lipopolysaccharide coat, are less dependent than gram-positive organisms upon the integrity of the peptidoglycan molecule for resistance to osmotic lysis; correspondingly, they are less susceptible to the action of penicillins than gram-positive bacteria.[2] Sensitive strains show different degrees of inhibition by the various analogs of penicillin; the reasons for this are not clear though a correlation can be shown with the lipid solubility of the particular antibiotic.[3]

Although it might seem that bactericidal antibiotics such as the penicillins should be therapeutically superior to bacteriostatic agents (eg, tetracyclines, chloramphenicol, sulfonamides), clinical proof of this is lacking except, perhaps, in the therapy of bacterial endocarditis.[4,5]

RESISTANCE

A 'resistant' organism is one that is not inhibited by levels of drug readily attainable in the serum. However, if massive doses of antibiotic are administered, or the infection lies in a site in which the agent is concentrated (eg, the urinary tract), ordinary susceptibility-testing may not be applicable. The level indicating resistance to carbenicillin and ticarcillin—drugs that are given parenterally in large doses—has been set at about 100-fold higher than that for other penicillins.

The mechanisms of bacterial resistance to the penicillins fall into three major groups:[1,6,7] (1) elaboration of substances (penicillinases) which inactivate the antibiotic; (2) alteration in the target site (cell-wall-forming enzymes) so that it no longer interacts with the drug; and (3) impermeability of the bacterium so that the antibiotic cannot reach its target.

Organisms that elaborate penicillinases tend to be resistant to very high levels of antibiotic. The production of penicillinase by staphylococci is controlled by an extra-chromosomal piece of deoxyribonucleic acid (DNA) which is passed 'horizontally' through the colony (phage transduction);[1] if a staphylococcus is not initially resistant to penicillin G, it will not become so in vivo unless another bacterial strain or a phage intrudes. Resistance to penicillin G connotes resistance to all of the congeners except the penicillinase-resistant ones. Methicillin-resistant staphylococci—widely prevalent in Europe but rare in North America at present—represent a special situation.[8–11] They are multiply drug-resistant organisms, often susceptible only to vancomycin. The mechanism of this resistance appears to be of the second kind noted above, in that these organisms exhibit a peculiarity of their cell wall structure.[10]

Resistance of gram-negative bacilli to penicillins is usually due to the production of penicillinases.[1] Among many of these organisms, including the recently recognized strains of ampicillin-resistant *Haemophilus influenzae,*[12–14] production of this enzyme is mediated by R-factors and is thus capable of being spread rapidly within a colony by sexual transfer (conjugation).[15,16] R-factors often carry the information for resistance to many antibiotics and may even be transmitted to different species of bacteria. Outbreaks of shigellosis due to strains resistant to various antibiotics are well documented, and multiply drug-resistant strains of Pseudomonas, Klebsiella, and other gram-negative bacilli have been isolated. The potential dangers of such R-factor-mediated resistance are clearly substantiated.[15,16]

The third mechanism is exemplified by the resistance of gonococci to penicillins. Though of low magnitude at present, the degree of resistance is rising progressively to the point where single-dose therapy for gonorrhea may no longer be possible. These organisms usually exhibit diminished susceptibility to a variety of antibiotics, presumably because they are relatively impermeable to these drugs.[17] Recently, there have been reports from various parts of the world documenting a rapid rise in the prevalence of moderately penicillin-resistant gonococci, as well as the appearance of some highly resistant strains that elaborate penicillinase.[18]

ANTIBACTERIAL SPECTRUM

The susceptibility patterns of various microorganisms to the penicillins are shown in Table 1.[19–32] Several 'axioms' regarding the therapeutic use of these agents may be stated:

1. Bacteria inhibited by the 'natural' penicillins (G and V) are usually more highly susceptible to these than to any other agent except possibly ampicillin or amoxicillin. Thus, penicillin G or V is the agent of choice for infection due to highly sensitive organisms.
2. The penicillinase-resistant penicillins are drugs of choice only for penicillin-resistant *Staphylococcus aureus*. At present, 60–80% of community staphylococci, and a higher proportion of hospital strains, exhibit such resistance.[33]
3. Sensitivity patterns among gram-negative bacilli vary from hospital to hospital and with time; thus, they are somewhat unpredictable.
4. Although most strains of *Staphylococcus epidermidis* (albus) are susceptible to penicillinase-resistant penicillins, about 10% are not.[31]

Most anaerobic bacteria pathogenic for man are highly susceptible to all penicillins except for the penicillinase-resistant analogs. One exception is *Bacteroides fragilis*, of which 90% of strains are inhibited

TABLE 1 Antimicrobial Spectrum of the Penicillins

Organism	"Natural" Penicillins	Penicillinase-Resistant	"Broad-Spectrum" Penicillins	
			Aminopenicillins	
	Penicillin G Penicillin V	Methicillin Nafcillin Oxacillin Cloxacillin Dicloxacillin	Ampicillin Amoxicillin	Carbenicillin Ticarcillin
Gram-Positive Cocci				
Staphylococcus aureus penicillin sensitive	+++[a]	+++	+++	+++
S. aureus penicillin resistant	Resistant	+++	Resistant	Resistant
S. epidermidis	Variable	90% susceptible	Variable	Variable
Streptococcus pyogenes	+++	++[b]	+++	+++
Pneumococcus	+++	++	+++	+++
Enterococcus	+[c]	± Weakly inhibited	+	+

Gram-negative cocci				
Meningococcus	+++	+	+++	+++ (Probably)
Gonococcus	+++	+	+++	++ (Probably)
Gram-Positive Rods				
Cor. diphtheriae	+++	?	+++	?
Listeria	++	?	++	++
Gram-Negative Rods				
Haemophilus influenzae	+	±	++ (occasionally resistant)	++
Escherichia coli	Resistant	Resistant	++ *(somewhat resistant)*	++
Klebsiella	Resistant	Resistant	Most resistant	Resistant
Enterobacter	Resistant	Resistant	Resistant	++
Proteus mirabilis	+/++	Resistant	+++ (somewhat resistant)	+++

TABLE 1 *(continued)*

Organism	"Natural" Penicillins	Penicillinase-Resistant	"Broad-Spectrum" Penicillins	
			Aminopenicillins	
	Penicllin G Penicillin V	Methicillin Nafcillin Oxacillin Cloxacillin Dicloxacillin	Ampicillin Amoxicillin	Carbenicillin Ticarcillin
Other proteus	Resistant	Resistant	Resistant	Variable
Pseudomonas	Resistant	Resistant	Resistant	++
Serratia	Resistant	Resistant	Resistant	Resistant
Anaerobes				
Bacteroides fragilis	90% inhibited at high concentration	Weakly inhibited	90% inhibited at high concentration	60% inhibited at high concentration
Clostridia	+++	++	+++	+++
Anaerobic cocci	+++	++	+++	+++

[a] +++ = highly susceptible.

[b] ++ = moderately susceptible.

[c] + = weakly susceptible.

only by high levels of penicillin G (32 μg/ml), and 60% by high levels of carbenicillin (128 μg/ml).[27]

The antibacterial activity of the two natural penicillins (G and V) is similar. In contrast, there are marked differences among the penicillinase-resistant penicillins, methicillin displaying the least, and dicloxacillin the greatest activity in vitro.[21,22] The spectrums of ampicillin and amoxicillin are similar, as are those of carbenicillin and ticarcillin; however, ticarcillin is severalfold more active against *Pseudomonas aeruginosa* than is carbenicillin.[28,29]

COMBINATION WITH OTHER DRUGS

The penicillins are often given together with other antimicrobial agents. There are disadvantages to the use of combinations of antibiotics.[30,34] These include: (1) increased risk of adverse drug reactions; (2) possibly greater susceptibility to suprainfection (not proven); and (3) drug antagonism. The last has been well demonstrated in vitro in a wide variety of settings,[30,34,35] and is most typically seen when a bactericidal agent is combined with a bacteriostatic one. In vivo evidence of such antagonism has been less clear cut, but several examples are persuasive.[33,36–38]

There are only a few instances in which a combination of a penicillin and another class of drugs have proven synergistic.[34] The most striking is in the therapy of enterococcal endocarditis with penicillin G and an aminoglycoside;[30] similar, though less impressive advantages of this combination have been claimed in endocarditis due to *Streptococcus viridans*.[39] The combination of carbenicillin and gentamicin exhibits synergism against the majority of strains of *Pseudomonas aeruginosa* in vitro and in animal studies;[40–42] whether this applies in man as well is not clear.[43–45] In vitro data support the value of a combination of nafcillin over oxacillin together with gentamicin for serious disseminated staphylococcal infections (eg, endocarditis),[46] and of penicillin G or ampicillin with gentamicin for Listeria infections;[47] however, in vivo data are lacking for these.[48]

CLINICAL PHARMACOLOGY

Absorption

Some pertinent characteristics of the pharmacology of the penicillins in man, summarized in a recent review,[49] are shown in Tables 2 and 3. Of all the congeners, only penicillin V and amoxicillin regularly exhibit >50% absorption by mouth.[19,49–51] For reasons that are not clear, the potassium salt of penicillin V is better absorbed than the sodium salt.[19] At least part of the relatively poor bioavailability of penicillin G, methicillin, carbenicillin and nafcillin is due to their acid-lability.[52–54] Although carbenicillin itself is minimally absorbed by mouth, the indanyl ester is moderately well assimilated; after absorption it is promptly broken down to the parent compound.[54] The presence of food in the stomach delays and impairs the absorption of most penicillins except penicillin V, ampicillin and amoxicillin; thus, patients should be advised to ingest penicillins 30–60 minutes before meals.

Serum Levels

The serum levels of various penicillins following a 500 mg oral dose are markedly dissimilar on account of differing degrees of absorption, metabolism and extent of serum protein-binding (Table 2).[23,25,51,55–65] Because antibiotic bound to serum protein is neither antibacterially active nor readily available for diffusion into tissues, it is of interest to examine the levels of free drug in the serum after this same oral dosage (Table 2).[53,54,58,59] The values are strikingly different from those for 'total' (bound plus unbound) antibiotic and tend to vitiate many of the apparent differences among closely related congeners (eg, oxacillin versus dicloxacillin).

Distribution

The penicillins are fairly well distributed into interstitial fluid, serosal cavities, synovial fluid and bone,[49] and the placenta.[66] Because they are relatively insoluble in lipid, they exhibit poor penetration into cells (including polymorphonuclear leukocytes) and across the blood-brain and blood-aqueous barriers.[49] Inflammation improves their traversal into the central nervous system and eye, both by reducing the normal barriers and by impairing the activity of the organic anion pumps in the choroid plexus (brain) and ciliary body (eye).[67,68] It has recently been reported that the intravenous administration of nafcillin in high doses (100 to 200 mg/kg/day) produces drug concentrations in the spinal fluid which should be more than adequate for the therapy of staphylococcal meningitis.[69] Similarly, it

TABLE 2 Pharmacology of the Penicillins in Man (Part 1)

Penicillin	Oral Absorption (%)	Peak Serum Level[a] (μg/mL)		Degree of Serum Protein-Binding[a] (%)	Percentage Penetration[b]		Metabolized (%)
		Total	Free		CSF Normal	CSF Inflamed	
Natural Penicillins							
Penicillin G	15–30	1.5–2.7	0.6–1.0	60	0.5–2	2–6	19
Penicillin V	60	3–5	0.8	80	—	—	56
Penicillinase-Resistant Penicillins							
Methicillin	Minimal	—	—	40	0.8–5	3–12	8
Nafcillin	Variable, low	–	—	90	—	9	—
Oxacillin	33	5–6	0.6	90	<6	—	49
Cloxacillin	49	7–14	0.6	93	—	—	22
Dicloxacillin	37	15–18	0.6	96	5[c]	2[c]	10

TABLE 2 *(continued)*

Penicillin	Oral Absorption (%)	Peak Serum Level[a] (μg/mL)		Degree of Serum Protein-Binding[a] (%)	Percentage Penetration[b]		Metabolized (%)
		Total	Free		CSF Normal	CSF Inflamed	
Broad-Spectrum Penicillins							
Ampicillin	30–50	2–6	1.6–5	20	4–5	36–40	12–20
Amoxacillin	74–80	7–8	6	20	—	—	28
Carbenicillin	Minimal	—	—	50	2–20	—	2
Indanyl carbenicillin	30	15	7.5	—	—	—	—

[a] After a 500-mg oral dose.

[b] Peak level in cerebrospinal fluid/Peak level in serum × 100.

[c] Data for one patient only.

has been shown that doses of penicillin G sufficient to produce peak serum concentrations of about 50 μg/ml (eg, 250,000 U/kg/day) in children will reliably generate levels in cerebrospinal fluid of about 1 μg/ml, sufficient for the therapy of most cases of streptococcal and meningococcal meningitis.[70] In treating meningitis, the dosage of penicillin should not be decreased as the disease improves because the permeability of the blood-brain barrier declines during convalescence. Although the issue is not firmly settled, the penicillins seem to penetrate young abscesses fairly well,[49,71,72] and it may well be that some phenomenon other than accessibility of drug is responsible for the failure of antimicrobial agents to sterilize such foci.

Elimination

The major route of elimination of most penicillins is in the urine as unchanged drug; thus, all of the congeners produce high urinary

TABLE 3 Pharmacology of the Penicillins in Man (Part 2)

	Half-Life (hour)		
Penicillin	Normal	Anuric	Hemodialysis
Natural Penicillins			
Penicillin G	0.7	6–10	3–5
Penicillinase-Resistant Penicillins			
Methicillin	0.43	4	Unchanged
Nafcillin	0.5–1.0	1.2	Unchanged
Oxacillin	0.4–0.7	0.5–1.0	Unchanged
Cloxacillin	0.5	0.8	Unchanged
Dicloxacillin	0.8	1–1.5	Unchanged
Broad-Spectrum Penicillins			
Ampicillin	0.5–1.0	8–20	2–5
Amoxicillin	1.0	5–7	3–5
Carbenicillin	1.0	10–20	5.5
Ticarcillin[48a]	1.2	15	3.5

concentrations if they are absorbed. A portion of each agent is metabolized (Table 2);[49,62] this is especially noteworthy with penicillin V and oxacillin and contributes to the minimal change in half-life of oxacillin in renal failure. Most penicillins are actively secreted into the bile, producing biliary concentrations that exceed those in serum; however, the transport mechanisms are easily saturated, particularly by oxacillin and carbenicillin. Levels of penicillin G and ampicillin in bile range up to 10 times those in serum, and the ratio is still higher for nafcillin (40:1 to 400:1).[49] Penetration into the bile is extremely poor in the presence of common duct obstruction. Despite the presence of active secretion, the only congener for which biliary secretion plays an important role in elimination is nafcillin.[73]

Because most penicillins are rapidly secreted into the urine, their half-lives in the serum are exceedingly short (Table 3).[61,74,75] Correspondingly, renal failure imposes a great hindrance upon elimination mechanisms, prolonging the half-life substantially.[52,74,76–81] Nafcillin, oxacillin, cloxacillin and dicloxacillin constitute exceptions to this general rule because of their more extensive metabolism, or biliary secretion, or both. Recently, a nomogram has been published for the adjustment of dosages of penicillin G in patients with renal impairment.[80] In the presence of complete anuria, it is generally inadvisable to exceed three million units of penicillin G per day; with coexisting advanced liver disease, this dosage should be halved. Those agents which exhibit the greatest prolongation of half-life in renal failure are (with the exception of methicillin) most easily hemodialyzed (Table 3).[76,77,79–83] None of the penicillins is readily removed by peritoneal dialysis.

The effects of combined hepatic and renal impairment on the elimination of the penicillins have not been well defined. In general, the superimposition of liver disease appears to prolong the half-life over that found in renal impairment by severalfold;[73,75–77,79,80] for nafcillin, the difference may be substantial. The effects of probenecid on the excretion and distribution of penicillins have been reviewed recently.[49]

Although not shown in the tables, the pharmacokinetics of flucloxacillin and ticarcillin resemble those of dicloxacillin and carbenicillin, respectively.[28,29,58,64,65,81] The repository forms of penicillin G include procaine penicillin G and benzathine penicillin G; these are absorbed from intramuscular sites much more slowly than are the sodium or potassium salts, but after absorption they exhibit the kinetics of penicillin G. Antibiotic is detectable in the serum for a prolonged period (12–24 hours) after intramuscular injection of procaine penicillin G, but the peak level following a dose of 600,000 units is only 1–3 μg/ml which is similar to the level produced by ingestion of potassium penicillin V 500 mg.[19,57,84]

ADVERSE REACTIONS

Hypersensitivity reactions, the major adverse effect of the penicillins, range in clinical severity from mild rash (± eosinophilia) through serum sickness to immediate anaphylaxis and death.[85–88] We have sometimes continued to treat patients with rash and eosinophilia when such therapy was warranted (eg, enterococcal endocarditis). Although all of the penicillins are capable of producing hypersensitivity reactions, rashes appear to be more common with ampicillin than with other congeners (7% versus 3%).[88] An ill-understood skin reaction to ampicillin is almost universal among patients who have infectious mononucleosis or cytomegalovirus infection.[86] Many individuals relate a history of penicillin allergy but manifest none on re-exposure to the drug years later. In some instances, this may be due to the development of blocking antibodies.[88]

Skin testing with penicillins is not an accurate way to predict anaphylaxis, apparently because conjugated metabolites, rather than the parent substance, are responsible for many of the reactions.[88] The use of penicillin derivatives (penicilloyl polylysine and minor determinant mixture) appears to correlate well with penicillin allergy,[87] and these preparations have recently become commercially available. It is preferable not to administer penicillins at all to individuals with a history of penicillin-related anaphylaxis or giant urticaria. Clinical cross-reactivity to cephalosporins occurs in only about 8–10% of penicillin-allergic individuals;[89] we have avoided cephalosporins in patients with penicillin-related anaphylaxis or giant hives but not in those with milder reactions.

Other reactions have been noted with the various penicillins. Although it seems reasonable to expect that any of the penicillins might produce these, some have been observed with only one or two agents. Examples are:

1. Coombs' positivity is noted in some recipients of penicillin; hemolytic anemia, however, is rarely seen.[89,90]

2. Selective or pancytopenia—various penicillins.[91]

3. Hepatitis—oxacillin, carbenicillin.[92]

4. Nephritis—appears to be most common with methicillin. Usually interstitial nephritis, often with fever, eosinophilia and an abnormal urinary sediment.[93–95] Glomerular and tubular damage have rarely been noted.

5. Systemic vasculitis.

6. Bleeding tendency because of platelet dysfunction[96]—carbenicillin.

7. Diarrhea—common with ampicillin and penicillinase-resistant congeners as well as indanyl carbenicillin in high dosage; questionably less frequent with amoxicillin than ampicillin.

8. Glossitis, stomatitis.

9. Convulsions—penicillin G or carbenicillin. Usually associated with high dosage in individuals with renal impairment; often some underlying seizure focus is present.[97]

10. Central nervous system reactions (other than seizures) have been noted in some recipients of procaine penicillin G, apparently due to rapid absorption of procaine.[98]

11. Pain and inflammation at injection sites (phlebitis, sterile intramuscular abscesses).

12. Suprainfection (1% of recipients).[84]

13. Hyperkalemia with potassium penicillin G (contains 1.7 mEq potassium ion per one million units) and an excessive sodium load with carbenicillin (contains 4.7 mEq sodium ion per gram of antibiotic).

14. Hypokalemia—penicillin G, carbenicillin,[99] ticarcillin.[100]

The first five reactions appear to be hypersensitivity reactions.

THERAPEUTIC USE

The penicillins are drugs of choice for infections due to organisms listed in Table 1 that are highly or moderately susceptible. They are also preferred therapy for anthrax, erysipeloid, salmonellosis, shigellosis, actinomycosis, rat-bite fever, syphilis, leptospirosis, one form of borreliosis and infections due to *Pasteurella multocida*. Because of the emergence of ampicillin-resistant *Haemophilus influenzae,*[101] it is now common practice to administer chloramphenicol together with penicillin G or ampicillin for meningitis in children until definitive identification and susceptibility testing of the infecting organism can

TABLE 4 Typical Dosages and Costs of Penicillins

Penicillin	Oral Dosage[a]	Cost of One Day's Oral Dosage[b] ($)	Intravenous Dosage[c]
Penicillin G	250 mg four times a day	0.05 to 0.34	Up to 40 million units/day (rarely may give more)
Penicillin V	250 mg four times a day	0.08 to 0.37	—
Methicillin	—	—	8–12 g/day (e.g., 2 g every 4 hours)
Nafcillin	250 mg four times a day	0.81	8–12 g/day (e.g., 2 g every 4 hours)
Oxacillin	250 mg four times a day	0.72 to 0.76	8–12 g/day (e.g., 2 g every 4 hours)
Cloxacillin	250 mg four times a day	0.87 to 0.92	—
Dicloxacillin	250 mg four times a day	0.89 to 1.21	—
Ampicillin	250 mg four times a day	0.19 to 0.66	8–12 g/day (e.g., 2 g every 4 hours)
Amoxicillin	250 mg three times a day	0.56 to 0.84	—
Carbenicillin	382 mg four times a day	1.28	24–36 g/day (e.g., 2–3 g every 2 hours)
Ticarcillin	—	—	16–20 g/day (e.g., 3 g every 4 hours)

[a]The lower end of the dosage range is given; higher doses are frequently indicated.

[b]Prices are taken from the 1978 Drug Topics Red Book and are for both generic and trademarked products.

[c]Dosage in adult patients with serious infections and normal renal function.

be done. Carbenicillin, which is relatively resistant to the beta-lactamase produced by these strains, is being studied as a therapeutic alternative.

Serious enterococcal infections such as endocarditis should be treated with penicillin G or ampicillin together with streptomycin or gentamicin. A penicillin alone should not be used for potentially dangerous illnesses due to gram-negative bacilli (enterobacteriaceae) until their susceptibility has been established. Pseudomonas bacteremia in the compromised host may best be treated with a combination of carbenicillin or ticarcillin plus gentamicin or tobramycin.[42,45,100]

The ideal chemotherapeutic approach to mixed aerobic and anaerobic infections of the abdomen (eg, peritonitis, chronic pelvic inflammatory disease) remains unsettled. In one randomized study, clindamycin and kanamycin were distinctly superior to cephalothin and kanamycin for penetrating abdominal trauma.[102] This is in keeping with the weak activity of cephalothin against anaerobes, particularly *Bacteroides fragilis*. The best-established regimens for infections involving *B. fragilis* have hitherto included clindamycin or chloramphenicol. There is accumulating evidence that the recently-released cephamycin, cefoxitin, is highly effective for this organism and metronidazole appears to be potent in this regard as well.

Recent data support the value of carbenicillin and ticarcillin as effective agents for intra-abdominal sepsis where *B. fragilis* is likely to be important. In one randomized comparison, carbenicillin alone (6 grams every 6 hours) was as effective as clindamycin plus gentamicin for penetrating abdominal trauma.[103] In another preliminary comparison, ticarcillin was as effective as clindamycin or chloramphenicol when each was combined with an aminoglycoside.[104] More extensive experience will be necessary to ascertain the relative merits of clindamycin, chloramphenicol, ticarcillin, carbenicillin, cefoxitin and metronidazole as anti-anaerobic agents. However, recent data suggest that ticarcillin combined with an aminoglycoside,[105] or cefoxitin alone,[106] may be equally effective.

Table 4 contains a list of suggested dosages of the penicillins for oral and intravenous administration, while regimens for the treatment of selected infections are shown in Table 5.[107–111] Although not widely tested, high doses of amoxicillin may be useful in the therapy of typhoid carriers.[112]

TABLE 5 Penicillin Therapy of Selected Infections

DISEASE	THERAPY WITH PENICILLINS[a]	ALTERNATIVE
Pneumococcal pneumonia	Penicillin G 2–4 million units i.v./day for 5–7 days[111]	Cephalosporin Erythromycin
Pneumococcal meningitis	Penicillin G 2 million units i.v. every 2 hours	Chloramphenicol Erythromycin
Streptococcal pharyngitis	Penicillin G or V 250 mg orally four times a day or procaine penicillin G 600,000 units i.m. daily for 10 days	Erythromycin Clindamycin
Streptococcus viridans endocarditis	Penicillin G 8–20 million units i.v./day for 4 weeks (some authors advocate addition of streptomycin for first 2 weeks[112])	Cephalosporin Erythromycin
Enterococcal endocarditis	Penicillin G 20–30 million units or ampicillin 12 g i.v./day *and streptomycin* (or if not synergistic, *gentamicin*) parenterally for 4 weeks	Vancomycin Erythromycin
Meningococcal meningitis or bacteremia	Penicillin G 2 million units i.m. every two hours for 10–14 days	Chloramphenicol Erythromycin
Gonorrhea[b]		
Uncomplicated genital	Aqueous procaine penicillin G 4.8 million units i.m. (two sites) + 1 g probenecid by mouth; or ampicillin 3.5 g by mouth + probenecid (for alternative drugs, dosage, and duration, see reference 113)	Tetracycline (not in pregnancy) Spectinomycin (? not in pregnancy) Erythromycin Cefazolin
Acute salpingitis Chronic pelvic inflammatory disease	See reference 113; requires higher doses than uncomplicated genital disease	
Arthritis-dermatitis syndrome	Various, including oral ampicillin (see reference 114)	
Diphtheria	Antitoxin therapy definitive; penicillin G 2–3 million units i.v. day or procaine penicillin G 600,000 units i.m. daily for 10–14 days to eliminate carriage of organism	Erythromycin Clindamycin

TABLE 5 *(continued)*

Disease	Therapy with Penicillins[a]	Alternative
Gas gangrene (clostridial)	Penicillin G 20–30 million units i.v./day	Cephalosporin Clindamycin
Listeria bacteremia and meningitis, or both	Penicillin G 2 million units i.v. every 2 hours for 2 weeks (an aminoglycoside may be synergistic)	
Shigellosis	Ampicillin 500 mg by mouth every 6 hours	Trimethoprim-sulfamethoxazole
Typhoid fever	Chloramphenicol is traditional drug of choice, though recent data indicate amoxicillin, 1 g by mouth every 6 hours, is equally good	Ampicillin (intravenous) Amoxicillin (oral) Trimethoprim-sulfamethoxazole
Aspiration pneumonia and lung abscess; oropharyngeal anaerobic infection	Penicillin G 4–8 million units/day for 2 weeks (pneumonia) to 6 weeks (lung abscess)[115]	Cephalosporin Clindamycin
Haemophilus influenzae meningitis	Treat with ampicillin (400 mg/kg parenterally/day) for 10–14 days; include chloramphenicol initially until susceptibility to ampicillin demonstrated	Cefamandole

[a]Penicillin G can be replaced by ampicillin, but not reliably by other penicillins.

[b]Some highly penicillin-resistant strains are beginning to appear; these seem to be susceptible to spectinomycin.[18]

PROPHYLACTIC USE

The efficacy of the penicillins in prevention of reoccurrences of rheumatic fever is indisputable; benzathine penicillin G (1.2 million units intramuscularly monthly) appears to be superior to oral regimens, possibly because some doses are omitted with the latter.[113] In contrast, the value of penicillin therapy in preventing glomerulonephritis[114] or rheumatic fever after streptococcal infection is established remains controversial.

For reliable prophylaxis against gonorrhea after sexual exposure, it is probably best to administer therapy in the same manner as for uncomplicated clinical disease (Table 5). This regimen is also adequate for the treatment of incubating syphilis if given within 24 hours after sexual contact; thereafter, 2.4 million units of intramuscular benzathine penicillin G provides more dependable therapy.

The problems of prophylaxis of bacterial endocarditis in patients with valvular heart disease have been reviewed recently by Kaye.[115] Although the value of such prophylaxis has not been proven, it is generally, and properly, advocated. Patients with a predisposing cardiac lesion should be informed of the kinds of procedures which carry a high risk, eg, dental manipulation, genitourinary instrumentation, and abdominal surgery. The current American Heart Association guidelines for prophylaxis, shown in Tables 6 and 7, are based on the assumption that *Streptococcus viridans* presents the major threat after oropharyngeal procedures, and the enterococcus after genitourinary and abdominal manipulations.

CHOICE OF A PENICILLIN

The efficacy of the penicillins in prevention of recurrence of from an initial perusal of the array of agents available. The physician must first consider which class of penicillin is indicated. For the treatment of infections susceptible to penicillin G, no other congener is more effective, although ampicillin and amoxicillin are as effective. (Carbenicillin in high dosages is likely to be successful as well.) If an oral drug is to be used, potassium penicillin V produces more reliable blood levels and is, therefore, slightly preferred over penicillin G.

The only indications for penicillinase-resistant penicillins are the suspected or demonstrated presence of *Staphylococcus aureas*. Since 60–80% of community, and a higher proportion of hospital strains of this organism currently produce penicillinase, a member of this group or a cephalosporin should be used in the initial therapy of staphylococcal infections until the sensitivity of the organism has been determined. The penicillinase-resistant penicillins will 'cover' mild to moderate streptococcal and pneumococcal infections as well as one due to anaerobes other than *Bacteroides fragilis* (intestinal) or clostridia. In high dosage, they also have some activity against *Haemophilus influenzae* and, combined with gentamicin, against enterococci.[116] This knowledge may help the physician to avoid adding a second penicillin pending identification of the infecting organism. In certain rare circumstances, however, it may be desirable to add another penicillin, usually penicillin G or ampicillin. There is

TABLE 6 Regimens Recommended by American Heart Association for Prophylaxis for Dental Procedures[a]

Penicillin

Intramuscular:

600,000 units of procaine penicillin G mixed with 200,000 units of crystalline penicillin G 1 hour before procedure and once daily for 2 days after procedure

or

Oral:

500 mg penicillin V or phenethicillin 1 hour before procedure and then 250 mg every 6 hours for remainder of that day and for 2 days after procedure

or

Oral:

1,200,000 units of penicillin G 1 hour before procedure and then 600,000 units every 6 hours for remainder of that day and for 2 days after procedure

In patients allergic to penicillin or receiving continual oral penicillin for prophylaxis against rheumatic fever, who may harbor penicillin-resistant viridans-type streptococci

Oral:

500 mg of erythromycin in adults (20 mg/kg in small children) 1.5–2 hours before procedure and then 250 mg every 6 hours (10 mg/kg in small children) for remainder of that day and for 2 days after procedure

[a]From reference 118.

little to choose among oxacillin, cloxacillin, dicloxacillin or flucloxacillin by the oral route, or among oxacillin, dicloxacillin, nafcillin or methicillin parenterally. Comparative studies have shown no important differences in therapeutic effect.[22,93,117] The marked acid-lability of methicillin could effect its stability in many intravenous solutions; in addition, this analog appears to produce interstitial nephritis more commonly than others.[93] For these reasons, we rarely use methicillin.

Ampicillin is especially useful for infections due to *Haemophilus influenzae* and *Escherichia coli,* and it may be more efficacious than penicillin G for serious disease due to the enterococcus and *Listeria monocytogenes.*[118] It is as useful as other agents in the treatment of uncomplicated *Escherichia coli* urinary tract infections, and for exacerbation of chronic bronchitis. It is generally effective for salmonellosis and shigellosis, though it should not be used for simple salmonella gastroenteritis.[119] Although amoxicillin produces twice the serum antibacterial activity of ampicillin after equivalent oral doses, the only evidence of an important therapeutic advantage is in the oral therapy of typhoid fever and possibly of typhoid carriers.[112,120,121] The

TABLE 7 Regimens Recommended by American Heart Association for Prophylaxis for Gastrointestinal and Genitourinary Tract Surgery and Instrumentation[a]

For most patients:

600,000 units of procaine penicillin G mixed with 200,000 units of crystalline penicillin G i.m. 1 hour before procedure and once daily for 2 days after procedure plus streptomycin, 1–2 g i.m., 1 hour before procedure and once daily for 2 days after procedure

In children, daily dose of streptomycin is 40 mg/kg (not to exceed 1 g/24 hours)

or

25–50 mg/kg ampicillin orally or i.v. 1 hour before procedure and then 25 mg/kg every 6 hours for that day and for next 2 days plus streptomycin as above

For patients allergic to penicillin:

Erythromycin as in Table 6 plus streptomycin as above

or

Vancomycin, 0.5–1.0 g i.v. (20 mg/kg in children) 1 hour before procedure and then 0.5 g i.v. (10 mg/kg in children) every 6 hours for 72 hours plus streptomycin as above

[a]From reference 118.

drug may be inferior to ampicillin for shigellosis[122] and is more expensive than the latter. Amoxicillin has been alleged to produce less diarrhea than ampicillin, especially as the pediatric suspension, but controlled data are not convincing.

Carbenicillin and ticarcillin exhibit activity unique among the penicillins. They are efficacious in the treatment of systemic infections due to gram-negative bacilli (except Klebsiella). The major advantage of ticarcillin over carbenicillin lies in its greater activity against Pseudomonas in vitro,[28,29] and this may be of clinical benefit.[100] The osmotic load of ticarcillin is substantially less than that of carbenicillin and this may be useful in patients with congestive failure or

TABLE 8 Preparations and Costs of Penicillins

Generic Name	Trademark Name(s)	Preparations and 1978 Costs
Penicillin G Potassium	generic	Tablets 100,000 units—$0.89–$1.50/100; 200,000 units—$1.45–$2.00/100; 250,000 units—$1.45–$2.50/100; 400,000 units—$1.70–2.80/100; 500,000 units—$2.10–$3.30/100 Powder for oral solution or suspension 200,000 units/5 ml—$0.96–$1.35/100 ml; 400,000 units/5 ml—$1.40–$2.10/100 ml Injection (powder) 1,000,000 units—$0.64–$0.98/vial; 5,000,000 units–$1.80–$1.86/vial
Penicillin G Benzathine	Bicillin (Permapen)	Oral suspension 150,000 units/5 ml—$1.93/2 oz; 300,000 units/5 ml—$3.69/2 oz Tablets 200,000 units—$7.56/36
Penicillin G Procaine	generic	Injection (suspension) 300,000 units/5 ml—$0.82/10 ml vial
Penicillin V Potassium	generic	Tablets 250 mg—$2.25–$4.60/100; 500 mg—$4.80–$12.80/100 Powder for solution 125 mg/5 ml—$1.35–$1.64/100 ml; 250 mg/5 ml—$2.17–$3.26/100 ml
Penicillin V Hydrabamine	Compocillin-V	Wafers (chewable) 250 mg—$10.63/100 Suspension 125 mg/5 ml—$1.73/100 ml
Phenethicillin Potassium	Maxipen (Syncillin)	Tablets 250 mg—$13.88/100
Ampicillin	generic	Capsules 250 mg—$4.75–$12.50/100; 500 mg—$9.45–$22.16/100 Powder for suspension 125 mg/5 ml—$1.15–$1.66/100 ml; 250 mg/5 ml—$1.80–$2.75/100 ml

TABLE 8 *(continued)*

GENERIC NAME	TRADEMARK NAME(S)	PREPARATIONS AND 1978 COSTS
Ampicillin Sodium	Polycillin-N (Amcill-S) (Alpen-N) (Omnipen-N) (Principen/N) (Penbritin-S)	Injection (powder) 125 mg—$0.95/vial; 250 mg—$1.12/vial; 500 mg—$1.48/vial; 1 g—$1.86/vial; 2 g—$3.28/vial
Hetacillin	Versapen	Powder for suspension (pediatric) 112.5 mg/ml—$3.38/15 ml Powder for suspension 112.5 mg/5 ml—$2.91/100 ml; 225 mg/5 ml—$4.38/100 ml
Hectacillin Potassium	Versapen-K	Capsules 225 mg—$20.32/100; 450 mg—$39.26/100
Amoxicillin Trihydrate	Larotid (Amoxil) (Polymox)	Capsules 250 mg—$31.33/100; 500 mg—$29.83/50 Drops for suspension (pediatric) 50 mg/ml—$2.75/15 ml Powder for suspension 125 mg/5 ml—$4.35/100 ml; 250 mg/5 ml—$7.69/100 ml
Methicillin Sodium	Staphcillin	Injection (powder) 1 g—$2.23/vial; 4 g—$8.13/vial; 6 g—$12.20/vial
Oxacillin Sodium	Prostaphlin	Capsules 250 mg—$21.80/100; 500 mg—$40.51/100 Solution 250 mg/5 ml—$4.59/100 ml Injection (powder) 250 mg—$0.12/vial; 500 mg—$0.23/vial; 1 g—$0.44/vial; 2 g—$0.85/vial; 4 g—$1.64/vial
Cloxacillin Sodium Monohydrate	Tegopen	Capsules 250 mg—$27.25/100; 500 mg—$54.32/100 Granules for solution 125 mg/5 ml—$3.75/100 ml
Dicloxacillin Sodium Monohydrate	Dynapen (Veracillin)	Capsules 125 mg—$19.97/100; 250 mg—$35.79/100 Powder for suspension 62.5 mg/5 ml—$2.54/80 ml

TABLE 8 *(continued)*

Generic Name	Trademark Name(s)	Preparations and 1978 Costs
Nafcillin Sodium	Unipen	Injection (powder) 500 mg—$2.10/vial; 1 g—$3.35/vial; 2 g—$7.64/vial Tablets 500 mg—$18.82/50 Capsules 250 mg—$20.31/100 Powder for solution 250 mg/5 ml—$4.45/100 ml
Carbenicillin Disodium	Geopen	Injection (powder equivalent to base) 1 g—$2.49/vial; 2 g—$4.54/vial; 5 g—$10.89/vial; 10 g—$21.36/vial
Carbenicillin Indanyl Sodium	Geocillin	Tablets equivalent to 382 mg of carbenicillin—38.00/100

other fluid and electrolyte problems. The oral preparation of carbenicillin (indanyl carbenicillin) produces relatively low serum levels of drug and is useful mainly in the treatment of urinary tract infections. Because sporadic urinary tract infections usually respond to much less expensive traditional agents, while complicated ones involving obstruction of indwelling catheters generally relapse promptly after (or during) therapy with indanyl carbenicillin, the number of instances in which this agent is of value is limited.

REFERENCES

1. Gale EF, Cundliffe E, Reynolds PE, et al: *The Molecular Basis of Antibiotic Action.* New York, John Wiley and Sons, 1972.
2. Lorian V: The mode of action of antibiotics on gram-negative bacilli. Arch Intern Med 128:623–632, 1971.
3. Biagi GL, Guerra MC, Barbaro AM, et al: Influence of lipophilic character on the antibacterial activity of cephalosporins and penicillins. J Med Chem 13:511–516, 1970.
4. Weinstein L, Dalton AC: Host determinants of response to antimicrobial agents. N Engl J Med 279:467–473, 524–531, 580–588, 1968.
5. Weinstein L, Schlesinger J: Treatment of infective endocarditis—1973. Prog Cardiovasc Dis 16:275–302, 1973.
6. Benveniste R, Davies J: Mechanisms of antibiotic resistance in bacteria. Annu Rev Biochem 42:471–506, 1973.
7. Smith JT, Hamilton-Miller JMT, Knox R: Bacterial resistance to penicillins and cephalosporins. J Pharm Pharmacol 21:337–358, 1969.
8. Jessen O, Rosendal K, Bulow P, et al: Changing staphylococci and staphylococcal infections. N Engl J Med 281:627–635, 1969.
9. Barrett FF, McGehee RF Jr, Finland M: Methicillin-resistant *Staphylococcus aureus* at Boston City Hospital. N Engl J Med 279:441–448, 1968.

10. Sabath LD, Leaf CD, Gerstein DA, et al: Cell walls of methicillin-resistant *Staphylococcus aureus*. Antimicrob Agents Chemother—1969, pp 73–77.
11. Blackwell CC, Feingold DS: Frequency and some properties of clinical isolates of methicillin-resistant *Staphylococcus aureus*. Am J Clin Pathol 64:372–377, 1975.
12. Elwell LP, DeGraff J, Seibert D, et al: Plasmid-linked ampicillin resistance in *Haemophilus influenzae* type b. Infect Immun 12:404–410, 1975.
13. Medeiros AA, O'Brien TF: Ampicillin-resistant Haemophilus influenzae type b possessing a TEM-type β-lactamase but little permeability barrier to ampicillin. Lancet 1:716–719, 1975.
14. Thornsberry C, Baker CN, Kirven LA, et al: Susceptibility of ampicillin-resistant *Haemophilus influenzae* to seven penicillins. Antimicrob Agents Chemother 9:70–73, 1976.
15. Sykes RB, Richmond MH: R factors, beta-lactamase, and carbenicillin-resistant *Pseudomonas aeruginosa*. Lancet 2:342–344, 1971.
16. Davies JE, Rownd R: Transmissible multiple drug resistance in Enterobacteriaceae. Science 176:758–768, 1972.
17. Sparling PF: Antibiotic resistance in Neisseria gonorrhoeae. Med Clin North Am 56:1133–1144, 1972.
18. Siegel MS, Thornsberry C, Biddle JW, et al: Penicillinase-producing *Neisseria gonorrhoeae:* results of surveillance in the United States. J Infect Dis 137:170–175, 1978.
19. Fishman LS, Hewitt WL: The natural penicillins. Med Clin North Am 54:1081–1099, 1970.
20. Sabath LD: Phenoxymethylpenicillin (penicillin V) and phenethicillin. Med Clin North Am 54:1101–1111, 1970.
21. Marcy SM, Kein JO: The isoxazolyl penicillins: oxacillin, cloxacillin and dicloxacillin. Med Clin North Am 54:1127–1143, 1970.
22. Gilbert DN, Sanford JP: Methicillin: critical appraisal after a decade of experience. Med Clin North Am 54:1113–1125, 1970.
23. Bear DM, Turck M, Petersdorf RC: Ampicillin. Med Clin North Am 54:1145–1159, 1970.
24. Smith CB, Wilfert JN, Dans PE, et al: In vitro activity of carbenicillin and results of treatment of infections due to Pseudomonas with carbenicillin singly and in combination with gentamicin. J Infect Dis 122(Suppl):S14–S25, 1970.
25. Neu HC: Antimicrobial activity and human pharmacology of amoxicillin. J Infect Dis 129(Suppl):S123–S131, 1974.
26. Finland M, McGowan JE Jr, Garner C, et al: Amoxicillin: in vitro susceptibility of 'blood culture strains' of gram-negative bacilli and comparisons with penicillin G, ampicillin, and carbenicillin. J Infect Dis 129(Suppl):S132–S138, 1974.
27. Tally FP, Jacobus NV, Bartlett JG, et al: In vitro activity of penicillins against anaerobes. Antimicrob Agents Chemother 7:413–414, 1975.
28. Klastersky J, Henri A, Daneau D: Ticarcillin, a new semisynthetic penicillin active on Pseudomonas aeruginosa: in vitro activity and blood levels in man. J Clin Pharmacol 14:172–175, 1974.
29. Ervin FR, Bullock WE: Clinical and pharmacological studies of ticarcillin in gram-negative infections. Antimicrob Agents Chemother 9:94–101, 1976.
30. Jawetz E: The use of antimicrobial combinations. Annu Rev Pharmacol 8:151–170, 1968.
31. Finland M: Changing patterns of susceptibility of common bacterial pathogens to antimicrobial agents. Ann Intern Med 76:1009–1036, 1972.
32. Kislak JW: The susceptibility of *Bacteroides fragilis* to 24 antibiotics. J Infect Dis 125:295–299, 1972.
33. Ross S, Rodriguez W, Controni G, et al: Staphylococcal susceptibility to penicillin G: the changing pattern among community strains. JAMA 229:1075–1077, 1974.
34. Rahal JJ Jr: Antibiotic combinations: the clinical relevance of synergy and antagonism. Medicine 57:179–195, 1978.
35. Acar JF, Sabath LD, Ruch PA: Antagonism of the antibacterial action of some penicillins by other penicillins and cephalosporins. J Clin Invest 55:446–453, 1975.
36. Lepper MH, Dowling HF: Treatment of pneumococcic meningitis with penicillin compared with penicillin plus aureomycin. Arch Intern Med 88:489–494, 1951.
37. Mathies AW Jr, Leedom JM, Ivler D, et al: Antibiotic antagonism in bacterial meningitis. Antimicrob Agents Chemother—1967, pp 218–224.
38. Carrizosa J, Kobasa WD, Kaye D: Antagonism between chloramphenicol and penicillin in streptococcal endocarditis in rabbits. J Lab Clin Med 85:307–311, 1975.

39. Wolfe JC, Johnson WD Jr: Penicillin-sensitive streptococcal endocarditis: in-vitro and clinical observations on penicillin-streptomycin therapy. Ann Intern Med 81:178–181, 1974.
40. Andriole VT: Synergy of carbenicillin and gentamicin in experimental infection with *Pseudomonas*. J Infect Dis 124(Suppl):S46–S55, 1971.
41. Kluge RM, Standiford HC, Tatem B, et al: The carbenicillin-gentamicin combination against *Pseudomonas aeruginosa:* correlation of effect with gentamicin sensitivity. Ann Intern Med 81:584–587, 1974.
42. Lumish RM, Norden CW: Therapy of neutropenic rats infected with *Pseudomonas aeruginosa*. J Infect Dis 133:538–547, 1976.
43. Klastersky J, Cappel R, Daneau D: Clinical significance of in vitro synergism between antibiotics in gram-negative infections. Antimicrob Agents Chemother 2:470–475, 1972.
44. Flick MR, Cluff LE: Pseudomonas bacteremia: review of 108 cases. Am J Med 60:501–508, 1976.
45. Anderson ET, Young LS, Hewitt WL: Antimicrobial synergism in the therapy of gram-negative rod bacteremia. Chemotherapy 24:45–54, 1978.
46. Watanakunakorn C, Glotzbecker C: Enhancement of the effects of anti-staphylococcal antibiotics by aminoglycosides. Antimicrob Agents Chemother 6:802–806, 1974.
47. Moellering RC Jr, Medoff G, Leech I, et al: Antibiotic synergism against *Listeria monocytogenes*. Antimicrob Agents Chemother 1:30–34, 1972.
48. Baird IM, Watanakunakorn C: Antimicrobial therapy of *Staphylococcus aureus* endocarditis. Clin Res 23:531A, 1975.
48a. Parry MF, Neu HC: Pharmacokinetics of ticarcillin in patients with abnormal renal function. J Infect Dis 133:46–49, 1976.
49. Barza M, Weinstein L: The pharmacology of penicillins in man. Clin Pharmacokinet 1:297–308, 1976.
50. Rolinson CN, Sutherland R: Semisynthetic penicillins. Adv Pharmacol Chemother 11:151–220, 1973.
51. Bergan T, Berdal BP, Holm V: Relative bioavailability of phenoxymethyl penicillin preparations in a cross-over study. Acta Pharmacol Toxicol 38:308–320, 1976.
52. Marcy SM, Klein JO: The isoxazolyl penicillins: oxacillin, cloxacillin, and dicloxacillin. Med Clin North Am 54:1127–1143, 1970.
53. Price KE: Structure-activity relationships of semisynthetic penicillins. Adv Appl Microbiol 11:17–75, 1969.
54. Butler K, English AR, Briggs B, et al: Indanyl carbenicillin: chemistry and laboratory studies with a new semisynthetic penicillin. J Infect Dis 127(Suppl):S97–S104, 1973.
55. Griffith RS: Comparison of antibiotic activity in sera after the administration of three different penicillins. Antibiot Med Clin Ther 7:129–135, 1960.
56. Sabath LD: Phenoxymethylpenicillin (penicillin V) and phenethicillin. Med Clin North Am 54:1101–1111, 1970.
57. Gower PE, Marshall MJ, Dash CH: Clinical, pharmacokinetic and laboratory study of penicillin V in the treatment of acute urinary infection. J Antimicrob Chemother 1:187–192, 1975.
58. Sutherland R, Croydon EAP, Rolinson GN: Flucloxacillin, a new isoazolyl penicillin, compared with oxacillin, cloxacillin, and dicloxacillin. Br Med J 4:455–460, 1970.
59. Brusch JL, Bergeron MG, Barza M, et al: An in vitro and pharmacological comparison of amoxicillin and ampicillin. Am J Med Sci 267:41–48, 1974.
60. Verbist L: Triple crossover study on absorption and excretion of ampicillin, pivampicillin, and amoxycillin. Antimicrob Agents Chemother 6:588–593, 1974.
61. Knirsch AK, Hobbs DC, Korst JJ: Pharmacokinetics, toleration and safety of indanyl carbenicillin in man. J Infect Dis 127(Suppl):S105–S110, 1973.
62. Cole M, Kenig MD, Hewitt W: Metabolism of penicillins to penicilloic acids and 6-aminopenicillanic acid in man and its significance in assessing penicillin absorption. Antimicrob Agents Chemother 3:463–468, 1973.
63. Gravenkemper CF, Bennett JV, Brodie JL, et al: Dicloxacillin: in vitro and pharmacologic comparisons with oxacillin and cloxacillin. Arch Intern Med 116:340–345, 1965.
64. Bodey GP, Vallejos C, Stewart D: Flucloxacillin: a new semisynthetic isoxazolyl penicillin. Clin Pharmacol Ther 13:512–515, 1972.
65. Bergeron MG, Brusch JL, Barza M, et al: Bactericidal activity and pharmacology of flucloxacillin. Am J Med Sci 271:13–20, 1976.

66. Sabath LD: Use of antibiotics in obstetrics. In *Obstetric and Perinatal Infections.* Edited by D Charles, M Finland. Philadelphia, Lea and Febiger, 1973, pp 564–565.
67. Thrupp LD, Leedom JM, Ivler D, et al: Ampicillin levels in the cerebrospinal fluid during treatment of bacterial meningitis. Antimicrob Agents Chemother—1965, pp 206–213.
68. Taber LH, Yow MD, Nieberg FG: The penetration of broad-spectrum antibiotics into the cerebrospinal fluid. Ann NY Acad Sci 145:473–481, 1967.
69. Kane JG, Parker RH, Jordan GW, et al: Nafcillin concentration in cerebrospinal fluid during treatment of staphylococcal infections. Ann Intern Med 87:309–311, 1977.
70. Hieber JP, Nelson JD: A pharmacologic evaluation of penicillin in children with purulent meningitis. N Engl J Med 297:410–413, 1977.
71. Barza M, Weinstein L: Penetration of antibiotics into fibrin loci in vivo, i: comparison of penetration of ampicillin into fibrin clots, abscesses, and interstitial fluid. J Infect Dis 129:59–65, 1974.
72. Greenwood D: Mucopeptide hydrolases and bacterial persisters. Lancet 2:465–466, 1972.
73. Nunes HL, Pecoro CC, Judy K, et al: Turnover and distribution of nafcillin in tissues and body fluids of surgical patients. Antimicrob Agents Chemother—1964, pp 237–249.
74. Standiford HC, Jordan MC, Kirby WMM: Clinical pharmacology of carbenicillin compared with other penicillins. J Infect Dis 122(Suppl):S9–S13, 1970.
75. Pagliaro LA, Benet LZ: Pharmacokinetic data: critical compilation of terminal half-lives, percent excreted unchanged, and changes of half-life in renal and hepatic dysfunction for studies in humans with references. J Pharmacokinet Biopharm 3:333–383, 1975.
76. Jackson EA, McLeod DC: Pharmacokinetics and dosing of antimicrobial agents in renal impairment, part I. Am J Hosp Pharm 31:36–52, 1974.
77. Hoffman TA, Cestero R, Bullick WE: Pharmacodynamics of carbenicillin in hepatic and renal failure. Ann Intern Med 73:173–178, 1970.
78. Dettli L: Individualization of drug dosage in patients with renal disease; symposium on individualization of drug therapy. Med Clin North Am 58:977–985, 1974.
79. Latos DL, Bryan CS, Stone WJ: Carbenicillin therapy in patients with normal and impaired renal function. Clin Pharmacol Ther 17:692–700, 1975.
80. Bryan CS, Stone WJ: 'Comparable massive' penicillin G therapy in renal failure. Ann Intern Med 82:189–195, 1975.
81. Parry MF, Neu HC: Pharmacokinetics of ticarcillin in patients with abnormal renal function. J Infect Dis 133:46–49, 1976.
82. Verhoef J, Oe PL, Simonian S: The clearance of antibiotics by the artificial kidney. Chemotherapy (Basel) 19:272–278, 1973.
83. Bennett WM, Singer I, Coggins CH: Guide to drug usage in adult patients with impaired renal function: a supplement. JAMA 223:991–997, 1973.
84. Weinstein L: Penicillins and cephalosporins. In *The Pharmacological Basis of Therapeutics,* 5th edition. Edited by LS Goodman, A Gilman. New York, Macmillan, 1975, pp 1130–1160.
85. Weinstein L, Weinstein AJ: The pathophysiology and pathoanatomy of reactions to antimicrobial agents. Adv Intern Med 19:109–134, 1974.
86. Levine BB: Skin rashes with penicillin therapy: current management. N Engl J Med 286:42–43, 1972.
87. Adkinson NF Jr, Thompson WL, Maddrey WC, et al: Routine use of penicillin skin testing on an inpatient service. N Engl J Med 285:22–24, 1971.
88. Isbister JP: Penicillin allergy: a review of the immunological and clinical aspects. Med J Aust 1:1067–1074, 1971.
89. Petz LD: Immunologic reactions of humans to cephalosporins. Postgrad Med J 47(Suppl):64–69, 1971.
90. Kerr RO, Cardamone J, Dalmasso AP, et al: Two mechanisms of erythrocyte destruction in penicillin-induced hemolytic anemia. N Engl J Med 287:1322–1325, 1972.
91. Reyes MP, Palutke M, Lerner AM: Granulocytopenia associated with carbenicillin: five episodes in two patients. Am J Med 54:413–418, 1973.
92. Wilson FM, Belamaric J, Lauter CB, et al: Anicteric carbenicillin hepatitis: eight episodes in four patients. JAMA 232:818–821, 1975.
93. Kancir LM, Tuazon CU, Cardella TA, et al: Comparison of methicillin and nafcillin in the treatment of staphylococcal endocarditis. Clin Res 24:25A, 1976.
94. Sanjad SA, Haddad GG, Nassar VH: Nephropathy, an underestimated complication of methicillin therapy. J Pediatr 84:873–877, 1974.

95. Border WA, Lehman DH, Egan JD, et al: Antitubular basement-membrane antibodies in methicillin-associated interstitial nephritis. N Engl J Med 291:381–384, 1974.
96. Brown CH, Natelson EA, Bradshaw W, et al: The hemostatic defect produced by carbenicillin. N Engl J Med 291:265–270, 1974.
97. Fossieck B Jr, Parker RH: Neurotoxicity during intravenous infusion of penicillin: a review. J Clin Pharmacol 14:504–512, 1974.
98. Green RL, Lewis JE, Kraus SJ, et al: Elevated plasma procaine concentrations after administration of procaine penicillin G. N Engl J Med 291:223–226, 1974.
99. Klastersky K, Vanderkelen B, Daneau D, et al: Carbenicillin and hypokalemia. Ann Intern Med 78:774–775, 1973.
100. Parry MF, Neu HC: A comparative study of ticarcillin plus tobramycin versus carbenicillin plus gentamicin for the treatment of serious infections due to gram-negative bacilli. Am J Med 64:961–966, 1978.
101. Smith AL: Current concepts: antibiotics and invasive *Haemophilus influenzae.* N Engl J Med 294:1329–1331, 1976.
102. Thadepalli H, Gorbach S, Broido PW, et al: Abdominal trauma, anaerobes, and antibiotics. Surg Gynecol Obstet 137:270–276, 1973.
103. O'Donnell V, Mandal AK, Lou MA, et al: Evaluations of carbenicillin and a comparison of clindamycin and gentamicin combined therapy in penetrating abdominal trauma. Surg Gynecol Obstet 147:525–528, 1978.
104. Harding GK, Marrie TJ, Buckwold F, et al: A controlled comparison of ticarcillin, clindamycin and chloramphenicol in the therapy of anaerobic infections. In *Program and Abstracts, 17th Interscience Conference on Antimicrobial Agents and Chemotherapy,* New York, October 1977, Abstract 178.
105. Swenson RM, Lorber B: Clindamycin and carbenicillin in treatment of patients with intraabdominal and female genital tract infections. J Infect Dis 135(Suppl):S40–S48, 1977.
106. Gorbach SL, Miao PV-W, O'Keefe JP, et al: Treatment of anaerobic infections with cefoxitin. In *Current Chemotherapy: Proceedings of the 10th International Congress of Chemotherapy,* Vol II. Washington, American Society for Microbiology, 1977, pp 300–302.
107. Brewin A, Arango L, Hadley WK, et al: High-dose penicillin therapy and pneumococcal pneumonia. JAMA 230:409–413, 1974.
108. Wolfe JC, Johnson WD Jr: Penicillin-sensitive streptococcal endocarditis: in vitro and clinical observations on penicillin-streptomycin therapy. Ann Intern Med 81:178–181, 1974.
109. Anon: Center for Disease Control: gonorrhea, recommended treatment schedules. Ann Intern Med 82:230–233, 1975.
110. Handsfield HH, Wiesner PJ, Holmes KK: Treatment of the gonococcal arthritis-dermatitis syndrome. Ann Intern Med 84:661–667, 1976.
111. Bartlett JG, Gorbach SL: Treatment of aspiration pneumonia and primary lung abscess: penicillin G vs clindamycin. JAMA 234:935–937, 1975.
112. Nolan CM, White PC Jr: Treatment of typhoid carriers with amoxicillin. JAMA 239:2352–2354, 1978.
113. Spagnuolo M, Pasternack B, Taranta A: Risk of rheumatic-fever recurrences after streptococcal infections: prospective study of clinical and social factors. N Engl J Med 285:641–647, 1971.
114. Weinstein L, LeFrock J: Does antimicrobial therapy of streptococcal pharyngitis or pyoderma alter the risk of glomerulonephritis? J Infect Dis 24:229–231, 1971.
115. Kaye D: Prophylaxis of endocarditis. In *Infective Endocarditis.* Edited by D Kaye. Baltimore, University Park Press, 1976, pp 245–265.
116. Marier RL, Joyce N, Andriole VT: Synergism of oxacillin and gentamicin against enterococci. Antimicrob Agents Chemother 8:571–573, 1975.
117. Martin CM, Kushnick TH, Nuccio PA, et al: Controlled double-blind efficacy trial of penicillin, methicillin and nafcillin in 346 adults and children, ii: comparative clinical efficacy. Antimicrob Agents Chemother—1963, pp 290–298.
118. Lavetter A, Leedom JM, Mathies AW Jr, et al: Meningitis due to *Listeria monocytogenes:* a review of 25 cases. N Engl J Med 285:598–603, 1971.
119. Aserkoff B, Bennett JV: Effect of antibiotic therapy in acute salmonellosis on the fecal excretion of Salmonellae. N Engl J Med 281:636–640, 1969.

120. Pillay N, Adams EB, North-Coombes D: Comparative trial of amoxicillin and chloramphenicol in treatment of typhoid fever in adults. Lancet 2:333–334, 1975.
121. Farid Z, Bassily S, Mikhail IA, et al: Treatment of chronic enteric fever with amoxicillin. J Infect Dis 132:698–701, 1975.
122. Nelson JD, Haltalin KC: Amoxicillin less effective than ampicillin against *Shigella* in vitro and in vivo: relationship of efficacy to activity in serum. J Infect Dis 129(Suppl):222–227, 1974.

2. CEPHALOSPORINS

Michael Barza and Peter V. W. Miao

The cephalosporins, which are derived from the fungus Cephalosporium, are closely related to some semisynthetic penicillins in structure, mechanism of action, antibacterial spectrum, pharmacological behavior and allergenicity. In the cephalosporins the beta-lactam moiety is adjacent to a six-membered ring, whereas in the penicillins, it is adjacent to a five-membered ring. This difference appears to enhance the resistance of the cephalosporins to penicillinase. Two recently marketed drugs, cefamandole and cefoxitin, possess antibacterial spectrums that differ importantly from those of available congeners (Table 1). (Strictly speaking, cefoxitin is not a cephalosporin but a cephamycin.) Several excellent reviews of various aspects of the cephalosporins have been published recently.[1–3]

MODE OF ACTION AND MECHANISMS OF BACTERIAL RESISTANCE

Cephalosporins, like penicillins, are 'bactericidal' antibiotics that act by inhibiting the enzymatic reaction(s) necessary for the production of a stable bacterial cell wall. Recent work suggests that the sites of action of the two groups of antibiotics may not be identical.[4–7] The mechanisms of resistance to cephalosporins and penicillins are similar, except that the cephalosporins are less readily inactivated by beta-lactamase enzymes of many gram-negative bacteria than are the penicillins.[1,8] The extended spectrums of cefamandole and cefoxitin correlate fairly well with their augmented resistance to beta-lactamase;[1,9] however, other factors, such as permeability barriers to the passage of antibiotic, also play a role.[10–12] Cephaloridine, cephapirin, and cefazolin are more susceptible to inactivation by staphylococcal penicillinase in vitro than is cephalothin,[13,14] but no clinical consequences of this phenomenon have been demonstrated.[15] Bacteria rarely become resistant to the cephalo-

TABLE 1 Preparations and Costs of Cephalosporins

Generic Name	Trademark Name(s)	Preparations and 1978 Costs
Cephalothin Sodium	Keflin	Injection (powder) 1 g—$2.81/vial; 2 g—$5.57/vial; 4 g—$11.02/vial
Cephaloridine	Loridine	Injection (powder) 500 mg—$2.61/vial; 1 g—$4.75/vial
Cefazolin Sodium	Ancef (Kefzol)	Injection (powder) 250 mg—$1.75/vial; 500 mg—$2.55/vial; 1 g—$5.05/vial; 5 g—$25.23/vial; 10 g—$50.47/vial
Cephapirin Sodium	Cefadyl	Injection (powder) 1 g—$2.96/vial
Cephalexin Monohydrate	Keflex	Capsules 250 mg—$30.52/100; 500 mg—$59.69/100 Pediatric drops 100 mg/ml—$1.51/10 ml Suspension 125 mg/5 ml—$3.54/100 ml; 250 mg/5 ml—$6.67/100 ml
Cephaloglycin Dihydrate	Kafocin	Capsules 250 mg—$33.83/100
Cephradine	Velosef (Anspor)	Capsules 250 mg—$33.73/100; 500 mg—$66.26/100 Suspension 125 mg/5 ml—$3.93/100 ml; 250 mg/5 ml—$7.36/100 ml Injection (powder) 250 mg—$1.05/vial; 500 mg—$1.86/vial; 1 g—$3.50/vial; 2 g—$6.94/vial; 4 g—$13.79/vial
Cefamandole Nafate	Mandol	Injection (powder) 1 g—$3.98/vial
Cefoxitin Sodium	Mefoxin	Injection (powder) 1 g—$6.19/vial

sporins in vivo unless another strain of the organism or bacteriophage intrudes, as may occur in superficial infections such as burns or wounds.

ANTIBACTERIAL ACTIVITY

Table 2 shows the antibacterial spectrum of the cephalosporins along with important differences among the congeners. In general, these compounds are highly inhibitory to gram-positive cocci except for enterococci and methicillin-resistant staphylococci; indeed, they are as active as oxacillin and nafcillin against *Staph. aureus* and *Staph. epidermidis,* though less effective than penicillin G against penicillin-susceptible strains.[16] Pneumococci and *Strep. pyogenes* are not as exquisitely sensitive to cephalosporins as to penicillin G or ampicillin but are still inhibited at concentrations below 2 μg/ml.[19] Cephalexin, cefoxitin, and cephradine are only one-tenth as active as other cephalosporins against gram-positive cocci.[1,16,17]

Meningococci are highly susceptible to cephalosporins,[18] and gonococci are moderately susceptible in vitro.[20,21] Based on a few isolates, *Listeria* appear to be inhibited by cephalothin but not cefoxitin.[22]

Among common gram-negative enteric bacilli, only *E. coli, Klebsiella, Proteus mirabilis, Salmonella,* and *Shigella* are regularly susceptible to cephalosporins; however, the two newly marketed drugs cefamandole and cefoxitin have extended the gram-negative spectrum to include *Enterobacter,* 'other proteus,' and even some strains of *Serratia.* In addition, *H. influenzae* are highly susceptible to cefamandole.

Cefoxitin exhibits activity against *Bacteroides fragilis,* which is unique among penicillins and cephalosporins; however, its prowess against other anaerobes is not exceptional.

Despite rare instances of antagonism in vitro,[28] the cephalosporins have been used in combination with penicillins (carbenicillin) or aminoglycosides with no evidence of interference; indeed, there is some suggestion of synergism with the aminoglycosides in vivo.[29] In contrast to the penicillins, including oxacillin[30] and nafcillin,[31] the cephalosporins are not reliably synergistic with aminoglycosides against enterococci.

CLINICAL PHARMACOLOGY

Pharmacological characteristics of the cephalosporins are summarized in Tables 3 and 4. Only cephalexin and cephradine are well absorbed by mouth.[37] The presence of food in the stomach delays, and reduces by about one-third, the peak serum level of cephalexin.[3,32]

Cefazolin and cephaloridine are well-tolerated intramuscularly.[2] All congeners, except cephalexin, are available as intravenous preparations.

Serum levels of cephalosporins are inversely related to the volume of distribution and the rate of elimination (metabolism and excretion) of the antibiotic. Considerable intra-subject variations are encountered in the serum levels recorded after a given dosage. Typical peak concentrations are shown in Table 3. Cefazolin produces higher serum levels than do other cephalosporins,[33] presumably on account of its smaller volume of distribution and longer half-life (slower elimination). Circulating cephalosporins are reversibly bound to serum albumin, cefazolin being the most highly bound (74–86%). Because protein-bound antibiotic is not antibacterially active nor readily available for diffusion to the periphery, it is useful to compare the peak serum levels of various cephalosporins in terms of free drug. When this is done, the differences among the various congeners are less striking (Table 3).

Cephalosporins, like penicillins, are relatively lipid-insoluble and do not penetrate cells (including polymorphonuclear leukocytes), ocular humors, or prostatic tissue well. However, they readily traverse interstitial[32,74,75] and synovial fluid[76] and limited data suggest fairly extensive passage across the placenta.[77–79] Penetration of cancellous bone is poor.[80] A major drawback to the use of cephalosporins is the low concentration achieved in spinal fluid (Table 3); this deficit appears to explain, at least in part, the disappointing results obtained with these agents in the therapy of meningitis.[18,81,82] There is some evidence that the newer congeners may offer an advantage in this respect (Table 3).

The cephalosporins are actively secreted into bile,[83] though this does not constitute a major route of their excretion. Cefazolin is more readily excreted than other commercially-available congeners into the common-duct bile.[83–87] For example, the following mean concentrations have been reported in choledochal bile after 1-gram parenteral dosages: cefazolin 31, cephalothin 4, and cephaloridine 9 μg/ml.[84] Cefazolin has been detected in concentrations as high as 50 μg/g of gallbladder tissue following the administration of 500 mg intramuscularly. However, cefamandole is excreted into common-duct bile in concentrations eight-fold those of cefazolin (ie, 350 μg/ml).[88] None of the cephalosporins passes readily into the common duct in the presence of choledochal obstruction or gallbladder bile in the presence of cystic duct obstruction.[84,86,87]

TABLE 2 Antibacterial Activity of the Cephalosporins

Species	Susceptibility to Cephalosporins	Differences among Cephalosporins
Gram-Positive Cocci		
Staphylococcus aureus *S. epidermidis* Streptococci Pneumococci	Highly sensitive	Cephalexin, cephradine, and cefoxitin one-tenth as active as cephalothin, cefazolin, cefamandole[1,16,17]
Enterococci	Most strains resistant	No important differences
Gram-Negative cocci		
Meningococci Gonococci	Moderately sensitive[18–21]	Not well studied (see text)
Gram-Positive Rods		
Listeria	Susceptible to cephalothin[22,23]	Not susceptible to cefoxitin[22]
Gram-Negative Rods (aerobic)		
Haemophilus influenzae	Most strains (80%) moderately sensitive[1,17,19,24]	Cefamandole by far the most active; cephalexin and cephradine very weakly active[24]
Escherichia coli	Moderately sensitive (90%)	Cefamandole, cefoxitin, and cefazolin most active[1,9,19,22,25]
Klebsiella	Moderately sensitive (80%)	Cefamandole, cefoxitin, and cefazolin most active[1,9,19,22,25]
Enterobacter	Most strains resistant except to cefamandole	Cefamandole most active[1,9,12,19,22,25]
Proteus mirabilis	Most strains weakly to moderately sensitive[1,19,22,25]	

Other *Proteus* *(vulgaris, morganii, rettgeri)*	Most strains resistant	Cefamandole and cefoxitin markedly more active than others[1,22,25]
Pseudomonas aeruginosa	Resistant	
Serratia	Resistant except 25–50% moderately sensitive to cefoxitin[1,17,22]	Only cefoxitin likely to be active
Salmonella	Most strains (90%) moderately sensitive[1,25]	
Shigella	Most strains moderately sensitive[1]	
Anaerobic Bacteria		
Bacteroides fragilis	Weakly susceptible (50% inhibited) except to cefoxitin	Most strains moderately to highly susceptible to cefoxitin[1,22,25–27]
Other anaerobes including clostridia	Moderately susceptible[25,26]	Cephalexin least active[26]

The terms highly, moderately, and weakly sensitive are used to indicate that the organisms are inhibited by low (usually <2 μg/ml), intermediate, or relatively high (e.g., 10–20 μg/ml) concentrations of the cephalosporin.

TABLE 3 Comparative Pharmacokinetics of Cephalosporins (Part 1)

	Peak Serum Levels (μg/ml)			
	500 mg Orally (Fasting)		1 g Intramuscularly	
Agent	Total	Free	Total	Free
Orally Absorbed				
Cephalexin[a]	18[2,32]	16	—	—
Cephradine	18[2,37]	15.5	10[37]	8.6
Parenteral				
Cephalothin			15–21[2,32,39–42]	5.3–7.4
Cephapirin			15–24[2,46]	7.5–12
Cefazolin			64[2,3,42]	12.8
Cephaloridine			38[2,32,42]	30.4
Cephradine			10[37]	8.6
Cefamandole			20–36[39,51]	6–10.8
Cefoxitin			22[40,41]	6.2

[a]Cephalexin not available commercially for parenteral use.

[b]Values inferred from data at different dosages.

[c]Absolute concentrations rather than percentage ratio.

[d]Unpublished data.

Elimination of the cephalosporins occurs mainly (50–100%) through the kidneys by a combination of glomerular filtration and active tubular secretion; active secretion of cephaloridine is negligible.[72,89] The transport pump is shared with the penicillins, probenecid, and paraaminohippuric acid;[71] all of these compete with the cephalosporins, resulting in a reduced rate of elimination and higher serum levels of antibiotic.[72,89] In addition, cephalothin and cephapirin undergo substantial (30–40%) biotransformation to products that are as much as three-fold less active against gram-positive cocci, and eight- to sixteen-fold less inhibitory to gram-negative bacilli, than the parent compounds.[58]

The mechanisms of renal excretion and biotransformation of the cephalosporins are so efficient that the serum half-lives of these drugs are short (Table 4); consequently, most of them must be administered

Peak Serum Levels (μg/ml)				
1 g Intravenously		Serum Protein	Penetration (Percentage of Peak Serum Level)	
Total	Free	Binding (%)	CSF Normal	CSF Inflamed
80[b,33]	70	12[2,33,34]	Not detectable[c,35]	1.7[36]
See below		8–20[2,37,38]	—	—
40–60[33,39,43]	14–21	65[2,33,34,39]	1.8[44]	1[45]
40–70[43,46]	20–35	44–45[2,38,47,48]	—	—
188[42]	38	74–86[3,33,34,48]	Not detectable[c,49]	0.4[49]
50–80[b,3,32]	40–64	10–30[2,33]	1.4[44]	0.4–5.6 μg/ml[c,50]
86[37]	74	8–20[2,37,38]	—	—
88[39]	26	67–74[39,52]	2[53]	4[54]
56–110[3,55]	15–30	65–79[2,55]	0.6[53]	10–25[d]

frequently (eg, every 2 to 4 hours) for effective therapy of serious infections. Cefazolin and cephaloridine exhibit a longer half-life on account of their slower excretion and minimal degradation; they may be administered less frequently.[a]

On the basis of limited data, it appears that the half-lives of the cephalosporins are only minimally altered by mild degrees of renal impairment but may be substantially prolonged by moderate or severe renal disease (Table 4). This increase is especially marked with cefazolin. Precise half-life values (and appropriate drug dosages) for a given degree of impairment are difficult to predict because of interindividual variations in the rates of nonrenal elimination and because of the accumulation of bioactive derivatives in the case of cephalothin and cephapirin. Thus, the dosage modifications provided

a Immediately after parenteral administration, there is a rapid decline in the serum levels of antibiotic due to the combination of distribution and elimination (alpha phase); thereafter, there is a slower decline attributable solely to elimination (beta phase). Strictly speaking, the beta phase provides a more accurate measurement of the biologic half-life; however, most of the half-life values in Table 4 apply to the alpha phase since this may be more clinically relevant with agents that are administered at such frequent intervals as are the cephalosporins.

TABLE 4 Comparative Pharmacokinetics of Cephalosporins (Part II)

Agent	Percentage Metabolized	Serum Half-Life (hours) Normal Renal Function	Moderate Renal Failure (Creatinine) Clearance (10–40 ml/min)	Severe Renal Failure
Orally Absorbed				
Cephalexin	Minimal	1.0[33]	3–6[56,57]	22[58]
Cephradine	Minimal	0.8[48]	—	—
Parenteral				
Cephalothin	33[58,61]	0.5[33,39,41,58]	1.1–1.8[61]	3–15[58,61]
Cephapirin	40[43,63,64]	0.5[43,46,48,63]	1–1.5[64]	1.8[64]
Cefazolin	Minimal	1.8[2,33,65]	10–14[34,65,66]	40–46[34,65,66]
Cephaloridine	Minimal	1.1–1.5[2,33,70,71]	4[70]	20–24[58,70]
Cefamandole	Minimal	0.6–0.8[39,51]	3[66]	8[66]
Cefoxitin	Minimal	0.8[2,40,41,48]	6[67]	13–18[66,67]

[a]Biphasic half-life; the larger number occurs after the 8th hour.

[b]First choice should be twice as great as subsequent ones (see text).

in Table 4 for various degrees of renal impairment are necessarily somewhat arbitrary. For situations in which the half-life of the drug becomes relatively long (eg, three hours or more), we have adopted the principle of administering a somewhat larger initial dose ('loading dose,' eg, 2 g cephalothin or cephapirin, 1 g cefazolin) followed by a 'half-dose' every half-life. Recently, an excellent nomogram has been published for the dosing of cephalexin; it permits the physician to select regimens that will produce a desired peak serum level in patients with varying degrees of renal impairment.[89a] Cephaloridine should be avoided in patients with renal impairment since it is inherently nephrotoxic when given in excessive amounts.[73,90,91] The

Serum Half-Life during Hemodialysis (hours)	Dosage in Adults with Normal Renal Function	Suggested Maintenance Dosage for Severe Infections	
		Moderate Renal Failure	Severe Renal Failure
2.5–6[57–60]	250–500 mg four times daily	250 mg every 6 hours[b]	250 mg every 24 hours[b]
—	250–500 mg four times daily		
3[57,61,62]	1 g every 3 hours or 2 g every 4 hours	1 g every 4–6 hours	1 g every 8 hours
1.8[3,64]	1 g every 3 hours or 2 g every 4 hours	1 g every 4–6 hours	1 g every 8 hours
9–14[34,65,66,68,69]	1 g every 4–6 hours	500 mg every 6–12 hours[b]	500 mg every 24–48 hours[b]
4[58,69,72,73]	1 g every 6 hours	Should not be given	Should not be given
6[66]	1 g every 2–6 hours	1 g every 6–8 hours	1 g every 12–24 hours
—	1 g every 2–6 hours	1 g every 8–12 hours	1 g every 24–36 hours

effects of coexisting renal and hepatic disease on the rates of elimination of cephalosporins have not been well studied; however, it would seem prudent to reduce the dosage of drugs such as cephalothin and cephapirin to a level below that which would be recommended for the renal dysfunction alone.

Peritoneal dialysis has little effect on the pharmacokinetics of cefazolin or cefamandole;[66] in contrast, all of the cephalosporins, with the possible exception of cefamandole, are moderately hemodialyzable.[66] Therefore, in treating serious infections, an additional maintenance dose (eg, 1 g cephalothin or cephapirin, 500 mg cefazolin) should be given at the end of each dialysis.

ADVERSE REACTIONS

Allergic Reactions

Up to 5% of individuals receiving cephalosporins experience allergic reactions.[2,42,92–94] These include maculopapular, morbilliform and urticarial rashes, eosinophilia, drug fever, serum sickness and, rarely, anaphylaxis. Occasional examples of reversible thrombocytopenia, neutropenia, and hemolytic anemia have been reported.[41,95–99]

Positive Coombs' tests are found in some 3% or more of patients treated with these antibiotics,[93,100] apparently for two reasons:[93,97,100] (1) nonspecific (nonimmune) adherence of cephalothin-protein complexes to the surface of erythrocytes; and (2) binding of specific anticephalothin antibody to drug-coated red blood cells. Rarely, hemolytic anemia has supervened due to the second mechanism.[97,98] There is a suggestion that cephalothin-related hemolysis may occur at lower dosages and earlier in the course of therapy than that associated with penicillin.[97,100] Hemolysis due to either antibiotic has clearly occurred in the absence of other manifestations of drug allergy. The hematologic abnormality may persist for weeks after discontinuation of the drugs.[97]

Despite the frequent presence of cross-reactive antibodies in the serum of recipients of either penicillins or cephalosporins,[71,101] clinically-evident allergic reactions to cephalosporins occur in only 8% (range 5 to 15%) of penicillin-allergic patients.[91] Individuals with a history of immediate hypersensitivity to penicillins (anaphylaxis, giant urticaria) should probably not be given cephalosporins because a cross-reaction could be life-threatening; however, milder, delayed reactions to penicillins do not constitute a contraindication to the administration of cephalosporins if there are other valid reasons for their use.

Non-Allergic Reactions

Local Effects. Other common adverse effects of the cephalosporins are related to the route of administration. Diarrhea and minor gastrointestinal upset sometimes accompany the ingestion of cephalexin or cephradine, with no difference between the drugs in this respect.[2,37,92] Pain on intramuscular injection appears to be less with cefazolin and cephaloridine than with the other congeners.[2] A number of controlled trials comparing the frequency of phlebitis with different cephalosporins have produced inconclusive results;[102,103]

however, cephapirin may be somewhat less irritating than other preparations when given intravenously in comparable dosage.[104]

Biochemical Abnormalities. Transient increases in SGOT, SGPT and alkaline phosphatase have rarely occurred after the administration of cephalosporins.[105] However, we are not aware of clinically-significant liver damage produced by these drugs.

Cephalothin in high concentrations has been reported to cause a number of defects in coagulation, including: (1) an abnormality of the second wave of platelet aggregation similar to that produced by carbenicillin;[106] (2) defective polymerization of fibrin with prolongation of the prothrombin and thrombin time;[106] and (3) inhibition of factor V activity in vitro.[107] These alterations appear to have little, if any, clinical significance.

Renal Toxicity. Cephaloridine, given in high dosages to experimental animals, injures the proximal tubular cells of the kidney; cefazolin produces a much lesser degree of damage, and cephalothin, a minimal one.[108,109] Acute renal failure has been well recognized in patients receiving cephaloridine, especially at dosages exceeding 6 g/day,[73,90,91] and has occasionally been observed with other cephalosporins.[110–112] However, interpretation of these reports is complicated by the frequent presence of other potentially nephrotoxic factors.[113] Pre-existing renal disease and the coadministration of furosemide may enhance the likelihood of nephrotoxicity due to the cephalosporins.[113,114] It has been stated that patients receiving gentamicin together with cephalothin have an increased risk of nephrotoxicity over that incurred from the aminoglycosides alone.[115–118] Although data from controlled studies in humans are conflicting,[113,119–122] it is our impression, based primarily on the results of prospective randomized trials,[118,119,122] that the combination is probably synergistically nephrotoxic in humans. (For reasons that are unclear, there is no evidence of such an adverse interaction in animals.[123]) We continue to use the combination without hesitation when clinical circumstances warrant; however, we monitor renal function daily (serum creatinine concentrations, BUN) in patients receiving these agents.

THERAPEUTIC USE

The therapeutic indications for the cephalosporins are somewhat difficult to define, and there is a widespread tendency to use these

TABLE 5 · Range of Costs to the Pharmacist of One Day's Therapy with Various Cephalosporins and Other Antibiotics

ANTIBIOTIC	TRADEMARK NAME(S)	DOSAGE	COST[a] ($)
Oral			
Cephalexin	Keflex	500 mg four times a day	2.39
Cephradine	Anspor	500 mg four times a day	2.23
	Velosef	500 mg four times a day	2.23
Oxacillin	Bactocill	500 mg four times a day	1.35
	Prostaphlin		1.42
Erythromycin (base and stearate)		500 mg four times a day	0.44 to 0.89
Penicillin V		500 mg four times a day	0.16 to 0.72
Ampicillin		500 mg four times a day	0.36 to 1.28
Parenteral			
Cephalothin	Keflin	12 g/day	33.72
Cefamandole	Mandol	8 g/day	31.84
Cefazolin	Ancef	6 g/day	30.30
	Kefzol		30.90
Cefoxitin	Mefoxin	6–8 g/day	37.14 to 49.52
Cephapirin	Cefadyl	12 g/day	29.88
Cephradine	Velosef	6 g/day	21.00
Oxacillin	Bactocill	12 g/day	43.08
	Prostaphlin		44.76

[a]Prices are taken from the 1978 Drug Topics Red Book and are for both generic and trademarked products when no trademark name is given.

drugs when penicillins would prove at least as effective. In terms of cost (Table 5) and rate of adverse reactions, the parenterally-administered cephalosporins do not differ substantially from anti-staphylococcal agents such as oxacillin or nafcillin; however, several criticisms can be levied against their use in infections known to be susceptible to penicillins: (1) penicillin G, penicillin V, or ampicillin are generally more active against susceptible organisms than any cephalosporin and are also considerably cheaper; (2) penicillins penetrate the central nervous system more readily than do cephalosporins;[18,71] and (3) penicillins, especially penicillin G and ampicillin, are much more active than commercially-available cephalosporins against enterococci[124] and *B. fragilis.*

Cephalosporins are drugs of choice in few circumstances (Table 6). These include infections due to *Staphylococcus aureus,* especially in the penicillin-allergic patient, and infections due to sensitive strains of *Klebsiella.* Hospital-acquired aspiration pneumonias often contain *Klebsiella,* staphylococci and pneumococci in addition to anaerobic mouth organisms; thus, cephalosporins may provide excellent therapy for this disease. These agents are also effective against most of the organisms found in biliary tract infections (*E. coli, Klebsiella,* clostridia and streptococci). Cefamandole may be particularly useful in this setting because of the relatively high concentrations it produces in the bile. However, enterococci are found with sufficient frequency in biliary tract infections that we prefer ampicillin together with an aminoglycoside. In the initial treatment of bacteremia of undetermined etiology, equally good results have been obtained with any pair of the following: a cephalosporin, an aminoglycoside (eg, gentamicin, tobramycin), or carbenicillin.[120,121] Cephalosporins should not be part of the combination when there is a substantial risk of central nervous system infection, enterococcal infection, or a high likelihood of *Pseudomonas* bacteremia.

Cephalosporins may provide a useful therapeutic alternative in patients allergic to penicillins (Table 6); however, they should not be given to individuals with a history of severe penicillin allergy (giant hives, anaphylaxis). Enterococcal infections respond poorly to cephalosporins and the alternative to penicillins should be erythromycin or vancomycin. Meningitis due to susceptible organisms has developed during therapy with the cephalosporins,[18] apparently due to poor penetration of the antibiotic into the meninges; therefore, these drugs should be avoided in patients with central nervous system infections, or those with a high risk of developing such a complication (for example, in meningococcal bacteremia). In the penicillin-allergic patient, chloramphenicol provides effective therapy of meningitis due to the pneumococcus, meningococcus, and *H. influenzae,* and erythromycin is also effective for the first two organisms. If it is decided to use a cephalosporin for some reason, the drug should be given in high dosage, and it may be prudent to administer intrathecal cephaloridine (12.5 to 50 mg/day) concomitantly.[18]

TABLE 6 Some Indications and Contraindications for Cephalosporins

A Reasonable Choice	A Good Alternative Drug (e.g. Penicillin Allergy: Where Indicated for Other Reasons)	Efficacy Not Proven	Generally Contraindicated
Penicillin-resistant *S. aureus* especially in penicillin-allergic patient[a]	Most gram-positive coccal infections except enterococcal	Diphtheria *Listeria*	Methicillin-resistant *S. aureus* (rare in USA)
Most *Klebsiella* infections[125,126] (80% sensitive)	Gonococcal—cefazolin may be used for penicillin-allergic pregnant patient[c]	Syphilis (cephaloridine may be be effective[127,128])	Enterococcal infections
Hospital-acquired aspiration pneumonia	Sensitive strains of *E. coli, P. mirabilis* and other gram-negatives (cefamandole and cefoxitin have extended gram-negative spectrum; cefamandole effective vs. *H. influenzae* (but probably not meningitis) and cefoxitin vs. *B. fragilis)*	Pelvic inflammatory disease Shigellosis	CNS infections
Combined with aminoglycoside (e.g., gentamicin, tobramycin) for initial therapy of undefined bacteremia[b]		*H. influenzae* (non-CNS)[d] Salmonellosis[129–131]	
Anaerobic infections (cefoxitin)	Infections due to "mouth anaerobes" (e.g., aspiration pneumonia)		

[a]Not in patients who have had anaphylactic reaction to penicillins.

[b]Other combinations equally effective (e.g., carbenicillin + gentamicin, carbenicillin + cephalosporin).

[c]Should probably be given for several days, not single dose.

[d]Cephalosporins effective in high dosage; cefamandole will probably prove more effective than other congeners.

Most commercially-available cephalosporins are only moderately inhibitory to *H. influenzae;* however, cefamandole appears more promising in this regard. Most of the cephalosporins currently on the market are only weakly active against *B. fragilis* and cannot be considered drugs of choice for peritonitis or chronic pelvic inflammatory disease; cefoxitin, however, appears to be effective for this kind of infection.[132,133] Cephalosporins are accepted therapy for gonorrhea only in the pregnant, penicillin-allergic individual with acute uncomplicated genital infection.[20,21,134] Although cefazolin 2 g intramuscularly together with probenecid 1 g by mouth is considered adequate in this instance,[134] failure rates as high as 20% have been reported[135] so that a course of treatment, rather than a single dose, may be preferable. Cephaloridine also is fairly effective as single-dose (2 g) therapy of acute gonorrhea. One cephalosporin (cephaloridine) has been used to treat syphilis, but its efficacy is not as well-documented as that of the penicillins. Although most strains of salmonella are relatively sensitive to cephalosporins in vitro, there is evidence that cephaloridine and cephalothin are ineffective in the treatment of typhoid fever.[129,130] In contrast, one recent study showed cefazolin in high dosage to be effective in the therapy of this disease.[131] This issue must be further evaluated before a conclusion can be reached. Data are insufficient to support the value of cephalosporins in the treatment of shigellosis.

The indications for oral cephalosporins are limited. Most urinary tract infections respond to much cheaper drugs (sulfisoxazole, ampicillin), and the majority of bacterial respiratory infections are due to organisms susceptible to ampicillin or erythromycin. Oxacillin or erythromycin are effective for soft-tissue infections due to gram-positive cocci.

The cephalosporins are frequently used for prophylaxis in patients undergoing replacement of heart valves, insertion of cardiac pacemakers, implantation of orthopedic protheses, vaginal hysterectomy and neurosurgical operations. The objective is to prevent bacterial colonization, especially by the staphylococcus. Short courses of parenteral drug given for this purpose appear to be reasonably efficacious and free of risk.[136]

CHOICE OF A CEPHALOSPORIN

There are no important differences between the two oral agents, cephalexin and cephradine.[137] For intramuscular injection, cephaloridine has largely been replaced by cefazolin which is equally well tolerated, not as nephrotoxic, and because of its relatively long half-life, may be administered three to four times daily.

The cephalosporins most commonly used intravenously are cephalothin, cefazolin and cephapirin. There are no substantial therapeutic differences among these three agents;[15,138] however, many physicians prefer cefazolin because it is administered in a lower dosage and somewhat less frequently.[3] A theoretical advantage of cephalothin over other cephalosporins for serious staphylococcal infections lies in its greater resistance to staphylococcal beta-lactamases.[14] There have been a few instances of failure of cefazolin in the therapy of staphylococcal endocarditis which could possibly be related to this observation.[139]

With the recent marketing of cefamandole, this antibiotic may become a drug of choice for the therapy of nosocomial and other non-pneumococcal bacterial pneumonias as well as for certain hepato-biliary infections. Cefoxitin may occupy a similar status for various anaerobic and mixed aerobic-anaerobic infections, especially those involving *Bacteroides fragilis* (eg, peritonitis, bowel perforation, prophylaxis of bowel surgery).

REFERENCES

1. Washington JA II: The in vitro spectrum of the cephalosporins. Mayo Clin Proc 51:237–250, 1976.
2. Moellering RC Jr, Swartz MN: The newer cephalosporins. N Engl J Med 294:24–28, 1976.
3. Nightingale CH, Greene DS, Quintiliani R: Pharmacokinetics and clinical use of cephalosporin antibiotics. J Pharm Sci 64:1899–1927, 1975.
4. Greenwood D, O'Grady F: Comparison of the responses of *Escherichia coli* and *Proteus mirabilis* to seven β-lactam antibiotics. J Infect Dis 128:211–222, 1973.
5. Greenwood D, O'Grady F: The two sites of penicillin action in *Escherichia coli*. J Infect Dis 128:791–794, 1973.
6. Lorian V, Sabath LD: Penicillins and cephalosporins: differences in morphologic effects on *Proteus mirabilis*. J Infect Dis 125:560–564, 1972.
7. Gale EF, Cundliffe E, Reynolds PE, et al: *The Molecular Basis of Antibiotic Action*. New York, John Wiley and Sons, 1972.
8. Smith JT, Hamilton-Miller JMT, Knox R: Bacterial resistance to penicillins and cephalosporins. J Pharm Pharmacol 21:337–358, 1969.
9. Neu HC: Cefamandole, a cephalosporin antibiotic with an unusually wide spectrum of activity. Antimicrob Agents Chemother 6:177–182, 1974.
10. Farrar WE Jr, Krause JM: Relationship between β-lactamase activity and resistance of *Enterobacter* to cephalothin. Infect Immun 2:610–616, 1970.
11. Weinrich AE, Del Bene VE: Characterization of β-lactamase activity in anaerobic bacteria. Clin Res 24:27A, 1976.
12. Findell CM, Sherris JC: Susceptibility of *Enterobacter* to cefamandole: evidence for a high mutation rate to resistance. Antimicrob Agents Chemother 9:970–974, 1976.
13. Regamey C, Libke RD, Engelking ER, et al: Inactivation of cefazolin, cephaloridine, and cephalothin by methicillin-sensitive and methicillin-resistant strains of *Staphylococcus aureus*. J Infect Dis 131:291–294, 1975.

14. Fong IW, Engelking ER, Kirby WMM: Relative inactivation by *Staphylococcus aureus* of eight cephalosporin antibiotics. Antimicrob Agents Chemother 9:939–944, 1976.
15. Saslaw S, Carlisle HN: Studies on therapy of staphylococcal infections in monkeys. VIII. Comparison of cephalothin, cephaloridine, cefazolin, cephacetrile, and cephanone. J Infect Dis 128(Suppl):S373–S378, 1973.
16. Sabath LD, Garner C, Wilcox C, et al: Susceptibility of *Staphylococcus aureus* and *Staphylococcus epidermidis* to 65 antibiotics. Antimicrob Agents Chemother 9:962–969, 1976.
17. Bergeron MG, Brusch JL, Barza M, et al: Bactericidal activity and pharmacology of cefazolin. Antimicrob Agents Chemother 4:396–401, 1973.
18. Fisher LS, Chow AW, Yoshikawa TT, et al: Cephalothin and cephaloridine therapy for bacterial meningitis. An Evaluation. Ann Intern Med 82:689–693, 1975.
19. Sabath LD, Wilcox C, Garner C, et al: In vitro activity of cefazolin against recent clinical bacterial isolates. J Infect Dis 128(Suppl):S320–S326, 1973.
20. Karney WW, Turck M, Holmes KK: Cefazolin in the treatment of gonorrhea. J Infect Dis 128(Suppl):S399–S403, 1973.
21. Nelson M: Cefazolin in the treatment of uncomplicated gonorrhea in men. J Infect Dis 128(Suppl):S404–S406, 1973.
22. Moellering RC Jr, Dray M, Kunz LJ: Susceptibility of clinical isolates of bacteria to cefoxitin and cephalothin. Antimicrob Agents Chemother 6:320–323, 1974.
23. Lavetter A, Leedom JM, Mathies AW, et al: Meningitis due to *Listeria monocytogenes*. A review of 25 cases. N Engl J Med 285:598–603, 1971.
24. Emerson BB, Smith AL, Harding AL, et al: Haemophilus influenzae type B susceptibility to 17 antibiotics. J Pediatr 86:617–620, 1975.
25. Ernst EC, Berger S, Barza M, et al: Activity of cefamandole and other cephalosporins against aerobic and anaerobic bacteria. Antimicrob Agents Chemother 9:852–855, 1976.
26. Tally FP, Jacobus NV, Bartlett JG, et al: Susceptibility of anaerobes to cefoxitin and other cephalosporins. Antimicrob Agents Chemother 7:128–132, 1975.
27. Kislak JW: The susceptibility of *Bacteroides fragilis* to 24 antibiotics. J Infect Dis 125:295–299, 1972.
28. Acar JF, Sabath LD, Ruch PA: Antagonism of the antibacterial action of some penicillins by other penicillins and cephalosporins. J Clin Invest 55:446–453, 1975.
29. Klastersky J, Cappel R, Daneau D: Clinical significance of in vitro synergism between antibiotics in gram-negative infections. Antimicrob Agents Chemother 2:470–475, 1972.
30. Marier RL, Joyce N, Andriole VT: Synergism of oxacillin and gentamicin against enterococci. Antimicrob Agents Chemother 8:571–573, 1975.
31. Musher D, Templeton G: Synergy between penicillins or cephalosporins and aminoglycosides against enterococci. Clin Res 24:26A, 1976.
32. Griffith RS, Black HR: Blood, urine and tissue concentrations of the cephalosporin antibiotics in normal subjects. Postgrad Med J 47(Feb Suppl):32–40, 1971.
33. Kirby WMM, Regamey C: Pharmacokinetics of cefazolin compared with four other cephalosporins. J Infect Dis 128(Suppl):S341–S346, 1973.
34. Craig WA, Welling PC, Jackson TC, et al: Pharmacology of cefazolin and other cephalosporins in patients with renal insufficiency. J Infect Dis 128(Suppl):S347–S353, 1973.
35. Davies JA, Strangeways JE, Holt JM: Absorption of cephalexin from the gastrointestinal tract in disease subjects. Postgrad Med J 46(Oct Suppl):16–19, 1970.
36. Ishiyama S, Nakayama I, Iwamoto H, et al: Absorption, tissue concentration, and organ distribution of cefazolin. Antimicrob Agents Chemother—1970, pp 476–480.
37. Neiss E: Cephradine—a summary of preclinical studies and clinical pharmacology. J Ir Med Assoc 66(Suppl):1–12, 1973.
38. Renzini G, Ravagnan G, Oliva B: In vitro and in vivo microbiological evaluation of cephapirin, a new antibiotic. Chemotherapy 21:289–296, 1975.
39. Fong I, Ralph E, Engelking E, et al: Clinical pharmacology of cefamandole as compared with cephalothin. Antimicrob Agents Chemother 9:65–69, 1976.
40. Brumfitt W, Kosmidis J, Miller J, et al: Cefoxitin and cephalothin—antimicrobial activity, human pharmacokinetics and toxicology. Antimicrob Agents Chemother 6:290–299, 1974.
41. Kosmidis J, Hamilton-Miller JMT, Gilchrist JNG, et al: Cefoxitin, a new semi-synthetic

cephamycin: an in vitro and in vivo comparison with cephalothin. Br Med J 3:653–655, 1973.

42. Gold J, McKee J, Ziv P: Experience with cefazolin: an overall summary of pharmacologic and clinical trials in man. J Infect Dis 128(Suppl):S415–S421, 1973.
43. Cabana B: Comparative metabolism of cephalothin and cephapirin in human volunteers. On file at Bristol Laboratories, August 1973.
44. Oppenheimer S, Beaty H, Petersdorf R: Pathogenesis of meningitis. VIII. Cerebrospinal fluid and blood conc. of methicillin, cephalothin and cephaloridine in experimental pneumococcal meningitis. J Lab Clin Med 73:535–543, 1969.
45. Vianna N, Kaye D: Penetration of cephalothin into spinal fluid. Am J Med Sci 254:216–220, 1967.
46. Axelrod J, Meyers BR, Hirschman SZ: Cephapirin: pharmacology in normal human volunteers. J Clin Pharmacol 12:84–88, 1972.
47. Chrisholm DR, Leitner F, Misiek M, et al: Laboratory studies with a new cephalosporanic acid derivative. Antimicrob Agents Chemother—1969, pp 244–246.
48. Thrupp L: Newer cephalosporins and 'expanded-spectrum' penicillins. Annu Rev Pharmacol 14:435–467, 1974.
49. Baker L, Hinthorn D, Romig D, et al: Penetration of cefazolin into CSF. In *Program and Abstracts, 14th Interscience Conference on Antimicrobial Agents and Chemotherapy,* San Francisco, September 1974, Abstract 410.
50. Lerner PI: Penetration of cephaloridine into cerebrospinal fluid. Am J Med Sci 262:321–326, 1971.
51. Meyers B, Ribner B, Yancovitz S, et al: Pharmacological studies with cefamandole in human volunteers. Antimicrob Agents Chemother 9:140–144, 1975.
52. Barza M, Melethil S, Berger S, et al: Comparative pharmacokinetics of cefamandole, cephapirin and cephalothin in healthy subjects and effects of repeated dosing. Antimicrob Agents Chemother 10:421–425, 1976.
53. Liu C, Hinthorn DR, Gerjarusak P, et al: Penetration of cefoxitin, cefamandole, ampicillin, and penicillin into human cerebrospinal fluids (CSF). In *Program and Abstracts, 17th Interscience Conference on Antimicrobial Agents and Chemotherapy,* New York, October 1977, Abstract 1.
54. Korzeniowski OM, Carvalho EM Jr, Rocha H, et al: Evaluation of cefamandole therapy of patients with bacterial meningitis. J Infect Dis 137(Suppl):S169–179, 1978.
55. Sonneville P, Kartodirdjo R, Skeggs H, et al: Comparative clinical pharmacology of intravenous cefoxitin and cephalothin. Eur J Clin Pharmacol 9:397–403, 1976.
56. Regamey C, Humair L: Pharmacokinetics of cephalexin in renal insufficiency. Postgrad Med J 47(Feb Suppl):69–78, 1971.
57. Linquist JA, Siddiqui JY, Smith IM: Cephalexin in patients with renal disease. N Engl J Med 283:720–723, 1970.
58. Kirby WM, DeMaine JB, Serrill WS: Pharmacokinetics of the cephalosporins in healthy volunteers and uremic patients. Postgrad Med J 47(Feb Suppl):41–46, 1971.
59. Reisberg B, Mandelbaum J: Cephalexin: absorption and excretion as related to renal function and hemodialysis. Infect Immun 3:540–543, 1971.
60. Brogard JM, Pinget M, Dorner M, et al: Determination of cefalexin pharmacokinetics and dosage adjustments in relation to renal function. J Clin Pharmacol 15:666–673, 1975.
61. Kabins S, Cohen S: Cephalothin serum levels in the azotemic patient. Antimicrob Agents Chemother—1964, pp 207–214.
62. Venuto R, Plaut M: Cephalothin handling in patients undergoing hemodialysis. Antimicrob Agents Chemother—1970, pp 50–52.
63. Cabana B, Hottendorf G, Van Harken D: Absorption and fate of cephapirin in man. In *Program and Abstracts, 12th Interscience Conference on Antimicrobial Agents and Chemotherapy,* Atlantic City, NJ, September 1972, Abstract 148.
64. McCloskey R, Terry E, McCracken A, et al: Effect of hemodialysis and renal failure on serum and urine concentrations of cephapirin sodium. Antimicrob Agents Chemother 1:90–93, 1972.
65. Levison ME, Levison S, Ries K, et al: Pharmacology of cefazolin in patients with normal and abnormal renal function. J Infect Dis 128(Suppl):S354–S357, 1973.
66. Andriole VT: Pharmacokinetics of cephalosporins in patients with normal or reduced renal function. J Infect Dis 137(Suppl):S88–S97, 1978.

67. Leroy A, Fillastre JP, Oksenhendler G, et al: Pharmacokinetics of cefoxitin in normal subjects and in uremic patients. In *Current Chemotherapy: Proceedings of the 10th International Congress of Chemotherapy,* Vol II. Washington, American Society for Microbiology, 1977, pp 763–764.
68. McCloskey R, Forland M, Sweeney M, et al: Hemodialysis of cefazolin. J Infect Dis 128(Suppl):S358–S360, 1973.
69. Welling PG, Craig WA, Amidon GL, et al: Pharmacokinetics of cefazolin in normal and uremic subjects. Clin Pharmacol Ther 15:344–353, 1974.
70. Pryor J, Joekes A, Foord R: Cephaloridine excretion in patients with normal and impaired renal function. Postgrad Med J 43(Aug Suppl):82–85, 1967.
71. Hewitt WL: The cephalosporins—1973. J Infect Dis 128(Suppl):S312–S319, 1973.
72. Foley T, Jones N, Barraclough M, et al: The renal excretion of cephaloridine in man. Postgrad Med J 43(Aug Suppl):85–87, 1967.
73. Kabins S, Cohen S: Cephaloridine therapy as related to renal function. Antimicrob Agents Chemother—1965, pp 922–932.
74. Bryant R: Distribution of cephapirin and cefazolin in tissue fluid. In *Program and Abstracts, 15th Interscience Conference on Antimicrobial Agents and Chemotherapy,* Washington, September 1975, Abstract 80.
75. Waterman NG, Kastan LB: Interstitial fluid and serum antibiotic concentrations. Arch Surg 105:192–196, 1972.
76. Nelson JD: Antibiotic concentration in septic joint effusion. N Engl J Med 284:349–353, 1971.
77. Hirsch HA: The use of cephalosporin antibiotics in pregnant women. Postgrad Med J 47(Feb Suppl):90–93, 1971.
78. Barr W, Graham R: Placental transmission of cephaloridine. Postgrad Med J 43(Aug Suppl):101–104, 1967.
79. Welles J: Pharmacology and toxicology of cephalosporins. In *Cephalosporins and Penicillins—Chemistry and Biology*. Edited by E Flynn. New York, Academic Press, 1972, pp 584–606.
80. Smilack J, Flittie W, Williams T Jr: Bone concentrations of antimicrobial agents after parenteral administration. Antimicrob Agents Chemother 9:169–171, 1976.
81. Love WC, McKenzie P, Lawson JH, et al: Treatment of pneumococcal meningitis with cephaloridine. Postgrad Med J 46(Oct Suppl):155–159, 1970.
82. McKenzie P, Love W, Lawson J, et al: Cephaloridine in pneumococcal and other forms of pyogenic meningitis. Postgrad Med J 43(Aug Suppl):142–145, 1976.
83. Nishida M, Murakawa T, Matsubara T, et al: Characteristics of biliary excretion of cefazolin and other cephalosporins with reference to the relationship between serum levels and administration conditions. Chemotherapy 22:30–36, 1976.
84. Ratzan K, Ruiz C, Irvin G III: Biliary tract excretion of cefazolin, cephalothin and cephaloridine in the presence of biliary tract disease. Antimicrob Agents Chemother 6:426–431, 1974.
85. Ram M, Watanatittan S: Levels of cefazolin in human bile. J Infect Dis 128(Suppl):S361–S363, 1973.
86. Ram M, Watanatittan S: Cephalothin levels in human bile. Arch Surg 108:187–189, 1974.
87. Mendelson J, Portnoy J, Sigman H, et al: Pharmacology of cephalothin in the biliary tract of humans. Antimicrob Agents Chemother 6:659–665, 1974.
88. Ratzan KR, Baker HB, Lauredo I: Excretion of cefamandole, cefazolin and cephalothin into T-tube bile. Antimicrob Agents Chemother 13:985–987, 1978.
89. Naumann P: Bacteriological and pharmacological properties of cephalothin and cephaloridine. Postgrad Med J 43(Aug Suppl):26–31, 1967.
89a. Spyker DA, Thomas BL, Sande MA, et al: Pharmacokinetics of cefaclor and cephalexin: dosage nomograms for impaired renal function. Antimicrob Agents Chemother 14:172–177, 1978.
90. Kleinknecht D, Jungers P, Fillastre J: Nephrotoxicity of cephaloridine. Ann Intern Med 80:421–422, 1974.
91. Mandell GL: Cephaloridine. Ann Intern Med 79:561–565, 1973.
92. Scheife RT, Levy M, Greenblatt DJ: Antimicrobial agents. In *Drug Effects in Hospitalized Patients.* Edited by RR Miller, DJ Greenblatt. New York, John Wiley and Sons, 1976, pp 227–264.

93. Petz LD: Immunologic reactions of humans to cephalosporins. Postgrad Med J 47(Feb Suppl):64–69, 1971.
94. Weinstein L, Kaplan K: The cephalosporins. Microbiological, chemical, and pharmacological properties and use in chemotherapy of infection. Ann Intern Med 72:729–739, 1970.
95. Bran J, Levison M, Kaye D: Clinical and in vitro evaluation of cephapirin, a new cephalosporin antibiotic. Antimicrob Agents Chemother 1:35–40, 1972.
96. Gralnick HR, McGinniss M, Halterman R: Thrombocytopenia with sodium cephalothin therapy. Ann Intern Med 77:401–404, 1972.
97. Gralnick HR, McGinniss M, Elton W, et al: Hemolytic anemia associated with cephalothin. JAMA 217:1193–1197, 1971.
98. Jeannet M, Bloch A, Dayer J, et al: Cephalothin-induced immune hemolytic anemia. Acta Haematol 55:109–117, 1976.
99. DiCato MA, Ellman L: Cephalothin-induced granulocytopenia. Ann Intern Med 83:671–672, 1975.
100. Garratty G, Petz LD: Drug-induced immune hemolytic anemia. Am J Med 58:398–407, 1975.
101. Levine B: Antigenicity and cross reactivity of penicillins and cephalosporins. J Infect Dis 128(Suppl):S364–S366, 1973.
102. Lane A, Taggart J, Iles R: Relative incidence of phlebitis caused by continuous intravenous infusion of cephapirin and cephalothin. Antimicrob Agents Chemother 2:234–235, 1972.
103. Inagaki J, Bodey G: Phlebitis associated with cephalosporins—cephapirin versus cephalothin. Curr Ther Res 15:37–43, 1973.
104. Berger S, Ernst E, Barza M: Comparative incidence of phlebitis due to buffered cephalothin, cephapirin and cefamandole. Antimicrob Agents Chemother 9:575–579, 1976.
105. Weinstein L: The cephalosporins. In *The Pharmacological Basis of Therapeutics,* 5th edition. Edited by LS Goodman, A Gilman. New York, Macmillan, 1975, pp 1158–1166.
106. Natelson EA, Brown CH III, Bradshaw W, et al: Influence of cephalosporin antibiotics on blood coagulation and platelet function. Antimicrob Agents Chemother 9:91–93, 1976.
107. Raccuglia G, Waterman NG: Anticoagulant effects of sodium cephalothin (Keflin). Am J Clin Pathol 52:245–247, 1969.
108. Silverblatt F, Harrison W, Turck M: Nephrotoxicity of cephalosporin antibiotics in experimental animals. J Infect Dis 128(Suppl):S367–S372, 1973.
109. Silverblatt F, Turck M, Bulger R: Nephrotoxicity due to cephaloridine: a light and electron-microscopic study in rabbits. J Infect Dis 122:33–44, 1970.
110. Pasternack DP, Stephens BG: Reversible nephrotoxicity associated with cephalothin therapy. Arch Intern Med 135:599–602, 1975.
111. Carling PC, Idelson BA, Casano AA, et al: Nephrotoxicity associated with cephalothin administration. Arch Intern Med 135:797–801, 1975.
112. Burton JR, Lichtenstein NS, Colvin RB, et al: Acute renal failure during cephalothin therapy. JAMA 229:679–682, 1974.
113. Barza M: The nephrotoxicity of cephalosporins: an overview. J Infect Dis 137(Suppl):S60–S73, 1978.
114. Linton AL, Bailey RR, Turnbull DI: Relative nephrotoxicity of cephalosporin antibiotics in an animal model. Can Med Assoc J 107:414–416, 1972.
115. Cabanillas F, Burgos RC, Rodriguez RC, et al: Nephrotoxicity of combined cephalothin-gentamicin regimen. Arch Intern Med 135:850–852, 1975.
116. Kleinknecht D, Ganeval D, Droz D: Acute renal failure after high doses of gentamicin and cephalothin. Lancet 1:1129, 1973.
117. Fillastre J, Laumonier R, Humbert G, et al: Acute renal failure associated with combined gentamicin and cephalothin therapy. Br Med J 2:396–397, 1973.
118. Bobrow SN, Jaffe E, Young RC: Anuria and acute tubular necrosis associated with gentamicin and cephalothin. JAMA 222:1546–1547, 1972.
119. Gaya H, Klastersky J, Schimpff SC: Nephrotoxicity during combined therapy with gentamicin and cephalothin. In *Program and Abstracts, 15th Interscience Conference on Antimicrobial Agents and Chemotherapy,* Washington, September 1975, Abstract 401.
120. Klastersky J, Hensgens C, Debusscher L: Empiric therapy for cancer patients: comparative study of ticarcillin-tobramycin, ticarcillin-cephalothin, and cephalothin-tobramycin. Antimicrob Agents Chemother 7:640–645, 1975.

121. Fanning WL, Gump D, Jick H: Gentamicin and cephalothin-associated rises in blood urea nitrogen. Antimicrob Agents Chemother 10:80–82, 1976.
122. Wade J, Smith C, Petty B, et al: Nephrotoxicity of gentamicin or tobramycin with methicillin or cephalothin. In *Current Chemotherapy: Proceedings of the 10th International Congress of Chemotherapy,* Vol II. Washington, American Society for Microbiology, 1977, pp 971–972.
123. Dellinger P, Murphy T, Pinn V, et al: Protective effects of cephalothin against gentamicin-induced nephrotoxicity in rats. Antimicrob Agents Chemother 9:172–178, 1976.
124. Rahal JJ, Meyers BR, Weinstein L: Treatment of bacterial endocarditis with cephalothin. N Engl J Med 279:1305–1309, 1968.
125. Gold JA, McKee JJ, Ziv DS: Experience with cefazolin: an overall summary of pharmacologic and clinical trials in man. J Infect Dis 128(Suppl):S415–S421, 1973.
126. Perkins RL, Saslaw S: Experience with cephalothin. Ann Intern Med 64:13–24, 1966.
127. Sparling PF: Diagnosis and treatment of syphilis. N Engl J Med 284:642–653, 1971.
128. Holder WR, Knox JM: Syphilis in pregnancy. Med Clin North Am 56:1151–1160, 1972.
129. Dawkins AT Jr, Hornick RB: Evaluation of antibiotics in a typhoid model. Antimicrob Agents Chemother—1966, pp 6–10.
130. Steinbrunn W, Haemmerli UP: Clinical trials of cephalothin, a new antibiotic. Ger Med Mon 12:170–174, 1967.
131. Uwaydah M: Cefazolin in the treatment of acute enteric fever. Antimicrob Agents Chemother 10:52–56, 1976.
132. McCloskey RV: Results of a clinical trial of cefoxitin, a new cephamycin antibiotic. Antimicrob Agents Chemother 12:636–641, 1977.
133. Gorbach SL, Miao PV-M, O'Keefe JP, et al: Treatment of anaerobic infections with cefoxitin. In *Current Chemotherapy: Proceedings of the 10th International Congress of Chemotherapy,* Vol II. Washington, American Society for Microbiology, 1977, pp 300–302.
134. Center for Disease Control: Gonorrhea: recommended treatment schedules. Ann Intern Med 82:230–233, 1975.
135. Duncan WC: Treatment of gonorrhea with cefazolin plus probenecid. J Infect Dis 130:398–401, 1974.
136. Tally FP, Gorbach SL: Antibiotics in surgery. Adv Surg 9:41–95, 1975.
137. Mogabgab WJ: Comparison of cephradine and cephalexin in the treatment of respiratory and urinary tract infections. Curr Ther Res 19:421–432, 1976.
138. Jackson GG, Riff LJ, Zimelis VM, et al: Double-blind comparison of cephacetrile with cephalothin/cephaloridine. Antimicrob Agents Chemother 5:247–254, 1974.
139. Bryant RE, Alford RH: Unsuccessful treatment of staphylococcal endocarditis with cefazolin. JAMA 237:569–570, 1977.

3. ERYTHROMYCIN

John G. Bartlett

Erythromycin is a macrolide antimicrobial, so named because of its large lactone ring containing one or more deoxy sugars. Although many macrolide antibiotics have been identified, erythromycin remains the only clinically important member of the group. It became available in 1952, and many derivatives were subsequently introduced in an attempt to improve oral absorption. Erythromycin is a relatively narrow spectrum agent with activity against most gram-positive bacteria, many anaerobes, *M. pneumoniae,* and Legionnaire's bacillus. Continued clinical efficacy and rare serious adverse effects may explain why erythromycin is currently the third most commonly prescribed antimicrobial in the United States (after tetracyclines and penicillins).[1]

MECHANISM OF ACTION AND RESISTANCE

Erythromycin inhibits protein synthesis by binding with the 50 S ribosomal subunit, thereby interfering with the site where amino acids are transferred from aminoacyl-soluble ribonucleic acid to protein.[2] The drug is bacteriostatic but may be bacteriocidal at high concentrations.

Resistance to erythromycin by gram-negative bacteria results from a barrier to cell wall penetration.[3] Resistance by gram-positive bacteria is due to a unique plasmid-mediated mechanism which may be constituative or inducible. This consists of an alteration of the target site by enzymatic methylation; the drug cannot bind methylated ribosomal RNA.[4]

SPECTRUM OF ACTIVITY

Erythromycin is active against most gram-positive bacteria including streptococci such as *S. pneumoniae,* Group A beta-hemolytic streptococci and most enterococci. Most strains are sensitive to concentrations of 0.5 μg/ml or less at neutral pH. The activity of erythromycin increases up to 300 fold at a pH of 8; the drug is inactivated in acid. Susceptibility of *S. aureus* is variable; most community-acquired strains are susceptible, but up to 50% of hospital-acquired strains are resistant in institutions where the drug is used extensively. *H. influenzae,* Neisseria, *C. diphtheriae, Pasteurella multocida,* listeria, brucella, rickettsia, mycoplasma, chlamydia and treponemes are usually sensitive. Activity versus anaerobic bacteria is erratic.[5] Less than half of *F. nucleatum* and *B. fragilis* are susceptible to 4 μg/ml; most anaerobic gram-positive cocci are susceptible. Aerobic and facultative gram-negative bacteria are resistant but may be susceptible to urinary levels in alkaline media. Some atypical mycobacteria, especially *M. kansasii* and *M. scrofulaceum,* are sensitive, but the clinical relevance of this observation is unknown because the experience with erythromycins for mycobacterial infections is sparse.[6]

INDICATIONS

The parenteral use of erythromycin is limited due to the frequency of thrombophlebitis. In most instances, the drug is given orally where the primary uses are for respiratory tract infections such as pharyngitis, otitis, sinusitis, dental infections, and pneumonitis. Penicillins (oral penicillin G, penicillin V, and ampicillin) are preferred for most of these infections, but erythromycin is a suitable alternative for patients who are penicillin sensitive. An exception is pneumonia caused by *Mycoplasma pneumoniae,* where penicillins are ineffective and erythromycin is regarded the agent of choice. Tetracyclines are also active against *Mycoplasma pneumoniae,* but erythromycin appears to be slightly superior in terms of duration of fever, pulmonary infiltrate, and duration of hospitalization.[7] Recent studies indicate that erythromycin is the preferred agent for pulmonary infections caused by Legionnaire's bacillus according to both in vitro susceptibility tests and limited clinical experience.[8]

The American Heart Association recommends erythromycin as an alternative to penicillin for both treatment and prevention of pharyngeal infections caused by Group A beta-hemolytic streptococci. The drug may also be used as a substitute for penicillin for pneumococcal pneumonia cases which can be treated with oral agents. Otitis media due to *S. pneumoniae* may be treated with erythromycin alone, but otitis due to *H. influenzae* is preferably treated with the combination of sulfonamides and erythromycin.[9] Again, these recommendations are generally restricted to patients with contraindications to penicillins.

Erythromycin base combined with neomycin has been found efficacious as an oral antimicrobial preparation for elective colon surgery.[10] This regimen substantially reduces both the aerobic and anaerobic flora of the colon, thus explaining the significant reduction in post-operative infections.

Erythromycin may be used in skin and soft tissue infections caused by *S. pyogenes* or susceptible strains of *S. aureus*. Many pediatricians regard this to be the preferred agent for impetigo. Erythromycin is considered ill-advised for staphylococcal infections subject to late relapse, such as osteomyelitis, because of the likelihood of resistance emerging during treatment.

For venereal diseases, erythromycin is advocated as an alternative agent for penicillin-allergic patients with syphilis, or pregnant females with uncomplicated gonorrhea. It may also be employed as an alternative to tetracyclines for genital infections due to *C. trachomatis;* these include some cases of non-specific urethritis, epididymitis and pelvic inflammatory disease. Although in vitro susceptibility data support the use of erythromycin in these conditions, clinical experience is limited. Cystitis and pyelonephritis caused by gram-negative bacilli may be treated with erythromycin by taking advantage of its increased activity at alkaline pH.[11] This is accomplished by giving the usual doses of erythromycin along with 12 to 15 g of sodium bicarbonate per day.

ABSORPTION AND METABOLISM

Absorption of erythromycin takes place primarily in the duodenum. The bioavailability of the oral preparations is dependent on formulation, gastric acidity, gastric emptying time, and the effect of multiple dosing.[12] Erythromycin base is acid-labile and commercially available as an enteric-coated tablet that is resistant to gastric acid. The stearate ester is less soluble in water and thus protected to some extent against acid. Erythromycin ethylsuccinate is partially dissociated in the intestine; both erythromycin and the undissociated ester are absorbed and, in the blood, the ester is hydrolyzed to release free erythromycin. Erythromycin estolate is acid-stable and dissociates in the small bowel releasing the propanoate ester; this ester is hydrolyzed in the blood to the free base over approximately 90 minutes.

Blood levels of biologically active drug achieved with enteric-coated erythromycin base and the various erythromycin esters generally range from 1.0 to 2.5 μg/ml with 500 mg oral doses.[13] Serum levels obtained with 500 mg intravenous infusions of erythromycin lactobionate are 8 to 12 μg/ml. Peak blood levels are seen 30 to 90 minutes after oral administration and the half-life is 1.5 to 2.5 hours.[14]

Erythromycin is distributed in the total body water, and tissue levels are generally good. Penetration into the central nervous system is poor except in the presence of meningeal inflammation where therapeutic levels in the cerebrospinal fluid are achieved. Erythromycin is one of the few antimicrobials which penetrates into prostatic fluid; however, unlike trimethoprim, it is not active against most bacteria which cause prostatitis. Levels in bronchial secretions exceed those of the serum.[12]

Excretion is primarily by the gastrointestinal tract and fecal levels are extremely high; this presumably accounts for its beneficial effect as a bowel preparation where a marked reduction of fecal anaerobes has been noted.[13] The high fecal level is due to both unabsorbed drug and enterohepatic circulation. Erythromycin is concentrated in the liver and bile levels are high. Only about 5 to 15% of the absorbed antimicrobial is excreted in the urine.[15]

ADVERSE REACTIONS

Erythromycin preparations are remarkably free of serious toxicity. The major adverse reactions with oral preparations are gastrointestinal complaints such as epigastric distress, nausea, and diarrhea. These are dose related and rarely are sufficiently severe to necessitate discontinuing the drug.

The most serious toxicity is cholestatic hepatitis, which occurs exclusively with the estolate derivative.[16] The essential factor for hepatotoxicity appears to be the propionyl ester linkage at the 2′ position.[17] Although hypersensitivity is thought to be responsible, efforts to detect tissue deposits of immunoglobulins and lymphoblastic transformation have failed. Symptoms include fever, abdominal pain, nausea, vomiting, jaundice, acholic stools and dark urine. The onset of symptoms usually occurs 10 to 20 days after initial exposure or immediately after re-exposure. Laboratory abnormalities

TABLE 1 Preparations and Costs of Erythromycin

GENERIC NAME	TRADEMARK NAME(S)	PREPARATIONS AND 1978 COSTS
Erythromycin	E-Mycin (Ilotycin) (Robimycin) (RP-Mycin)	Tablets (enteric-coated) 250 mg—$16.24/100
Erythromycin Estolate	Ilosone	Capsules 125 mg—$11.26/100; 250 mg—$20.79/100 Drops 100 mg/ml—$1.41/10 ml Granules for suspension 125 mg/5 ml—$2.20/60 ml; 250 mg/5 ml—$3.96/60 ml Tablets (chewable) 125 mg—$6.36/50; 250 mg—$10.40/50 Tablets 500 mg—$40.73/100
Erythromycin Ethylsuccinate	Pediamycin (EES 400)	Tablets (chewable) 200 mg—$10.69/50 Granules for drops (suspension) 100 mg/2.5 ml—$1.95/30 ml Granules for suspension 200 mg/5 ml—$2.84/60 ml, $3.72/90 ml, $6.13/150 ml Suspension 200 mg/5 ml—$4.46/100 ml; 400 mg/5 ml—$7.75/100 ml
	Erythrocin Ethylsuccinate	Injection (solution) 50 mg/ml—$0.96/2-ml ampul, $4.50/10-ml vial
Erythromycin Gluceptate	Ilotycin Gluceptate	Injection (powder) 250 mg—$2.21/vial; 500 mg—$3.64/vial; 1 g—$6.22/vial
Erythromycin Lactobionate	Erythrocin Lactobionate	Injection (powder) 500 mg—$4.00/vial; 1 g—$6.50/vial
Erythromycin Stearate	Erythrocin Stearate (Bristamycin) (Erypar) (Ethril) (Pfizer-E)	Tablets 125 mg—$5.21/50; 250 mg—$15.49/100; 500 mg—$23.16/100

are leukocytosis, eosinophilia, and liver function tests showing a cholestatic pattern with increased bilirubin, alkaline phosphatase and SGPT. Liver biopsy shows intrahepatic cholestasis and periportal inflammation with leukocytes, neutrophils, and eosinophils. Most patients improve promptly, with total resolution of hepatic abnormalities when the drug is discontinued.

Hypersensitivity reactions such as rash, drug fever, and eosinophilia are rare. Nephrotoxicity has not been described. Reversible hearing loss has been reported with large oral doses. Superinfections may occur, but the frequency is substantially less than with agents having a broader spectrum such as tetracycline.

Intramuscular administration of parenteral preparations are extremely painful. Intravenous administration may cause pain during the infusion and is associated with a high incidence of thrombophlebitis.

PREPARATIONS AND DOSES

Oral preparations include erythromycin base (with and without enteric coating), and erythromycin esters: estolate, stearate, and ethylsuccinate. Adult oral doses range from 0.25 g to 1.0 g every six hours; the usual dose is 500 mg every six hours. The usual pediatric dosage is 50 μg/kg/day. No dosage adjustment is necessary in renal failure.

Intravenous preparations include erythromycin lactobionate and erythromycin glucoheptonate. The usual dose is 1 to 4 g per day in 2 to 4 divided doses.

REFERENCES

1. Simmons HE, Stolley PD: This is medical progress? Trends and consequences of antimicrobial use in the U.S. JAMA 227:1023–1028, 1974.
2. Tardrew PH, Mao JC, Kenney D: Antibacterial activity of two esters of erythromycin. Appl Microbiol 18:159–163, 1969.
3. Taubeneck V: Susceptibility of *Proteus mirabilis* and its L-forms to erythromycin and other macrolides. Nature 196:195–198, 1962.
4. Lai CJ, Weisblum B: Altered methylation of ribosomal RNA in an erythromycin-resistant strain of *Staphylococcus aureus*. Proc Natl Acad Sci 68:856–861, 1971.
5. Sutter LV, Finegold SM: Susceptibility of anaerobic bacteria to 23 antimicrobial agents. Antimicrob Agents Chemother 10:736–752, 1976.
6. Molani A, Weinstein L: In vitro activity of erythromycin against atypical mycobacteria. J Infect Dis 123:216–218, 1971.
7. Rasch JR, Mogabgab WJ: Therapeutic effect of erythromycin on Mycoplasma pneumoniae pneumonia. Antimicrob Agents Chemother 5:693–697, 1965.
8. Fraser DW, Tsai TR, Orenstein W, et al: Legionnaire's disease. N Engl J Med 297:1189–1203, 1977.
9. Howie VM, Ploussard JH: Efficacy of fixed combination antibiotics versus separate components in otitis media. Pediatrics 44:940–946, 1969.
10. Clarke JS, Condon RE, Bartlett JG, et al: Preoperative oral antibiotics reduce septic complications of colo-rectal operations. Ann Surg 186:251–258, 1977.
11. Lorian V, Sabath LD: Effect of pH on the activity of erythromycin against 500 isolates of gram-negative bacilli. Appl Microbiol 20:754–756, 1970.

12. Nicholas P: Erythromycin: clinical review. NY State J Med 77:2088–2094, 1977.
13. Knothe H, Dette GA: Pharmacokinetics of erythromycin. Scott Med J 22:397–400, 1977.
14. Ochs HR, Greenblatt DJ, Dengler HJ: Absorption of oral tetracycline in patients with Billroth-II gastrectomy. J Pharmacokinet Biopharm 6:295–303, 1978.
15. Bartlett JG, Condon RE, Gorbach SL, et al: Veterans Administration cooperative study on bowel preparation for elective colon surgery. Ann Surg 188:126–131, 1978.
16. Braun P: Hepatotoxicity of erythromycin. J Infect Dis 119:300–305, 1969.
17. Tolman KG, Sannella JJ, Freston JW: Chemical structure of erythromycin and hepatotoxicity. Ann Intern Med 81:58–60, 1974.

4. CLINDAMYCIN AND LINCOMYCIN

John G. Bartlett

Lincomycin is a narrow spectrum antimicrobial produced by *Streptomyces lincolnesis,* originally found in a soil sample near Lincoln, Nebraska. Clindamycin differs from lincomycin by the presence of a chlorine atom in place of a hydroxyl group at the 7 position. Clindamycin has largely supplanted the parent compound in the United States because of its superior antimicrobial activity, although there continues to be extensive use of lincomycin in other countries. Early trials showed clindamycin to be effective in the treatment of a variety of infections outside the central nervous system, ranging from acne to intra-abdominal sepsis with *B. fragilis* bacteremia.[1] Subsequent investigations incriminated lincomycin and clindamycin as major causes of gastrointestinal illness, the most serious form being pseudomembranous colitis. This has resulted in a reassessment of the role of these agents, and most authorities now feel they should be reserved for restricted clinical settings. The primary indication is for serious infections in which *B. fragilis* is an established or suspected pathogen.

MECHANISM OF ACTION

Clindamycin inhibits the initiation of peptide chain synthesis. Its site of action is identical to that of chloramphenicol and erythromycin, although the mechanism of inhibiting protein synthesis with these agents is different. Clindamycin is bactericidal against some, but not all, susceptible bacteria. Resistance to clindamycin develops in *S. aureus* in slow stepwise fashion, probably by chromosomal mutation.[2] Enzymatic inactivation occurs only by *Streptomyces coelicolor,* which can phosphorylate both drugs. Plasmid-mediated resistance has been described but appears to be rare at the present time.

SPECTRUM OF ACTIVITY

Clindamycin is active against most gram-positive bacteria including streptococci (other than enterococci), and 95 to 97% of *Staphylococcus aureus*. Methicillin-resistant staphylococci are usually sensitive. Erythromycin-resistant *S. aureus* may initially be sensitive to clindamycin but these strains may rapidly develop resistance on exposure. The mechanism of this 'dissociated cross-resistance' with erythromycin is not known. Compared to lincomycin, clindamycin is 8 to 16 times more active against *S. pneumoniae* and *S. aureus*, and it is 2 to 4 times more active against *S. pyogenes* and viridans streptococci.[3]

Most anaerobic bacteria are susceptible to clindamycin at 0.5 μg/ml or less.[1] This includes *B. fragilis* which accounts for 70 to 80% of anaerobic bacteremias, is a major isolate in intra-abdominal or female genital tract infections, and is resistant to many other commonly used antimicrobials such as penicillins, cephalosporins and aminoglycosides.[4] Anaerobes which are often resistant include *F. varium*, some clostridia other than *C. perfringens*, (*C. ramosum*, *C. tertium*, *C. sporogenes*, and *C. difficile*) and peptococci. *In vitro* susceptibility has also been demonstrated for Nocardia, *Mycoplasma hominis*, *Plasmodium falciparum* (Chloroquine sensitive or resistant), *Plasmodium vivax*, and *Toxoplasma gondii*. Infections with these organisms are not approved indications for clindamycin, and clinical efficacy is not established.

INDICATIONS

In view of potential gastrointestinal complications clindamycin is generally recommended only for those infections in which alternative, less toxic agents are not readily available.

One indication for clindamycin is serious infection in which *B. fragilis* is an established or suspected pathogen. This includes intra-abdominal sepsis (other than biliary tract infections and spontaneous peritonitis), non-venereal infections of the female genital tract, and selected soft tissue infections. In most instances the drug is combined with another agent that is active against aerobic gram-negative bacilli, since these conditions are usually mixed aerobic-anaerobic infections. Clindamycin should not be used in central nervous infections due to its poor penetration across the blood-brain barrier. Clindamycin also is an alternative choice in patients with contraindications to penicillins and cephalosporins for infections involving aerobic gram-positive cocci other than enterococci. Special consideration may be given to staphylococcal osteomyelitis due to the high levels of clindamycin achieved in bone even with oral administration.

PHARMACOKINETICS

Clindamycin is an extremely stable compound that retains activity despite autoclave temperatures or exposure to gastric acid with a pH of 1. Oral preparations are readily absorbed, with less than 5% recoverable in stool.[5] Some of the biologic activity in stool is in the form of the metabolite N-demethyl clindamycin. This metabolite is a more active antimicrobial than the parent compound, and animal studies have shown that it can be detected in feces for eight days after a single oral dose. Peak serum levels of 3 to 5 μg/ml are achieved at 30 to 45 minutes after oral administration of 300 mg of clindamycin hydrochloride or clindamycin palmitate. Concurrent food administration has little effect on serum levels. There is only a modest increase in peak levels with repeated dosing at 6 to 8 hour intervals. Intramuscular injections of 300 mg also produce levels of 3 to 5 μg/ml, while 600 mg doses yield peak levels of approximately 8 μg/ml. Intravenous administration of 600 mg yields peak levels of 10 to 12 μg/ml.[6]

Clindamycin is extensively distributed to body tissues except for the eye and central nervous system.[7] Levels in bile are 2 to 5 times higher than those in serum. Less than 10% of biological activity is found in the urine. It is presumed that most of the drug is eliminated as biologically inactive metabolites. The serum half-life of 2 to 3 hours is only slightly increased in renal failure, but it increases fivefold in hepatic failure.

PREPARATIONS AND DOSAGE

Clindamycin preparations are the hydrochloride, the 2-palmitic acid ester and the 2-phosphoric acid ester. The two esters are not biologically active and must be hydrolyzed in the gastrointestinal tract or blood. Clindamycin hydrochloride is recommended for oral use in adults in doses of 150 to 450 mg every 6 to 8 hours, usually 300 mg every 6 hours. Flavored granules of clindamycin palmitate are made into an oral suspension for pediatric patients; the usual dose is 8 to 20 mg/kg/day. Clindamycin phosphate is the parenteral preparation, and it is given in doses of 300 to 900 mg every 6 to 8 hours for adults; the usual dose is 600 mg every eight hours. The usual parenteral dose in children is 20 to 40 mg/kg/day. No dose modification is necessary in renal failure. The usual parenteral dose in patients with severe liver disease is 300 mg every eight hours.

TABLE 1 Preparations and Costs of Clindamycin and Lincomycin

Generic Name	Trademark Name(s)	Preparations and 1978 Costs
Clindamycin Hydrochloride	Cleocin Hydrochloride	Capsules 75 mg—$19.69/100; 150 mg—$36.38/100
Clindamycin Palmitate Hydrochloride	Cleocin Pediatric	Granules for suspension 75 mg/5 ml—$5.31/100 ml
Clindamycin Phosphate	Cleocin Phosphate	Injection (solution) 150 mg/ml—$4.80/2-ml ampul, $8.66/4-ml ampul
Lincomycin Hydrochloride Monohydrate	Lincocin	Capsules 250 mg—$4.93/24; 500 mg—$9.06/24 Syrup 250 mg/5 ml—$2.84/60 ml Injection (solution) 300 mg/ml—$2.44/2-ml ampul, $11.03/10 ml vial

ADVERSE REACTIONS

The major adverse effects are gastrointestinal complications, and the most common of these is uncomplicated antibiotic-associated diarrhea; the most serious is pseudomembranous colitis. Surveys indicate that 4 to 20% of clindamycin recipients develop diarrhea.[8,9] This usually subsides when the drug is discontinued, although occasional patients have protracted diarrhea with electrolyte disturbances or hypoalbuminemia.

Incidence data for pseudomembranous colitis are poorly established. According to one prospective study, 20% of all patients treated with clindamycin developed diarrhea and fully half of these individuals had pseudomembranous colitis on sigmoidoscopic examination.[8] Two features of this study are noteworthy: first, all patients recovered without sequelae when the drug was discontinued; the high mortality rates for pseudomembranous colitis noted in the older literature were not verified. The second important factor is that this study was probably conducted during an epidemic of the disease at one institution. Subsequent studies have found a substantially lower incidence, and a more realistic figure is 0.01% rather than 10%.[10]

Antibiotic-associated colitis actually includes a spectrum of pathologic changes including mild inflammation ('nonspecific colitis'), ulcerative colitis or proctitis resembling inflammatory bowel disease, and the more classically-recognized pseudomembranous colitis with typical plaque-like lesions on gross inspection and the stalked or summit lesion on histologic study.[11] Colitis may occur with either oral or parenteral administration of clindamycin. The incidence appears to be lower in young persons, and no dose relationship has been noted.

The course of antibiotic-associated colitis is mediated by an enterotoxin produced by clindamycin-resistant strains of *C. difficile*.[12] These organisms reside in the colon of susceptible individuals; it is presumed that selective antimicrobial pressure favors the growth and toxin production by these organisms. The toxin is a protein which is cytopathic, can be neutralized by clostridial antitoxins, and reproduces the disease in experimental animals.[13] Tissue cultures showing cytotoxicity of stools with inactivation by clostridial antitoxin appears to be a relatively sensitive and specific test for detecting this toxin.[11]

Treatment of antibiotic-associated colitis consists of discontinuation of clindamycin, avoidance of antiperistaltic medications,[14] and supportive care. Preliminary data suggest that cholestyramine or vancomycin may be of value.[15,16]

Other side effects include a morbilliform rash in 3 to 5% of patients. Less common hypersentivity reactions are urticaria, Stevens-Johnson syndrome, exfoliative dermatitis, angioedema, and anaphylaxis. Transient abnormalities of liver function are rather common, are not dose-related, and return to normal when the drug is discontinued or treatment is continued.[17]

REFERENCES

1. Bartlett JG, Finegold SM: Treatment of anaerobic infections with lincomycin and clindamycin. N Engl J Med 287:1006–1010, 1972.
2. Benner EI, Adams AP Jr: Unusual resistance of Staphylococcus aureus in lincomycin and 7-chlorolincomycin. Antimicrob Agents Chemother, 1969, pp 100–103.
3. McGehee RF Jr, Smith CB, Wilcox C, et al: Comparative studies of antibacterial activity *in*

vitro and absorption and excretion of lincomycin and clindamycin. Am J Med Sci 256:279–292, 1968.
4. Gorbach S, Bartlett JG: Anaerobic infections. N Engl J Med 290:1177–1184, 1237–1245, 1289–1294, 1974.
5. Keusch GT, Present DH: Summary of workshop on clindamycin colitis. J Infect Dis 133:578–587, 1976.
6. DeHaan RM, Metzler CM, Schellenberg D, et al: Pharmacokinetic studies of clindamycin phosphate. J Clin Pharmacol 13:190–209, 1973.
7. Panzer JD, Brown DC, Epstein WL: Clindamycin levels in various body tissues and fluids. J Clin Pharmacol 12:259–262, 1972.
8. Friedman GD, Gerard MJ, Ury HK: Clindamycin and diarrhea. JAMA 236:2498–2500, 1976.
9. Tedesco FJ, Barton RW, Alpers DH: Clindamycin-associated colitis. A prospective study. Ann Intern Med 81:429–433, 1974.
10. Ramirez-Ronda CH: Incidence of clindamycin-associated colitis. Ann Intern Med 81:860, 1974.
11. Price AB, Davis PR: Pseudomembranous colitis. J Clin Pathol 30:1–12, 1977.
12. Bartlett JG, Chang TW, Gurwith M, et al: Antibiotic-associated pseudomembranous colitis due to toxin-producing clostridia. N Engl J Med 298:531–534, 1978.
13. Bartlett JG, Onderdonk AB, Cisneros RL, et al: Clindamycin-associated colitis in hamsters due to toxin producing clostridia. J Infect Dis 136:701–705, 1977.
14. Novak E, Lee JG, Seckman CE, et al: Unfavorable effect of atropine-diphenoxylate (Lomotil) therapy in lincomycin caused diarrhea. JAMA 235:1451–1454, 1976.
15. Bartlett JG, Onderdonk AB, Cisneros RL: Clindamycin associated colitis in hamsters: protection with vancomycin. Gastroenterology 73:772–776, 1977.
16. Burbige EJ, Milligan FD: Pseudomembranous colitis: association with antibiotics and therapy with cholestyramine. JAMA 231:1157–1158, 1975.
17. Elmore M, Rissing JP, Rink L, et al: Clindamycin-associated hepatotoxicity. Am J Med 57:627–630, 1974.

5. POLYMYXINS

John G. Bartlett

The polymyxins are a group of closely related polypeptides labeled A, B, C, D, and E. The least toxic and most frequently used forms are polymyxin B and colistin. The latter was discovered independently and subsequently was shown to be identical to polymyxin E.[1] These drugs were commonly employed during the 1950's and 1960's for infections caused by resistant gram-negative bacilli, especially *Pseudomonas aeruginosa*. Recently the polymyxins have been largely supplanted by other drugs which are less toxic and more effective clinically.

MECHANISM OF ACTION

The polymyxins are amino acids linked to form a decapeptide ring with a fatty acid side chain. Their detergent-like effect on the cell wall-cytoplasmic membrane complex of gram negative bacteria malorients the membrane and reduces its osmotic stability. The activity is rapid and irreversible. Resistance is due either to a lack of an appropriate phospholipid membrane receptor, or failure of the drug to penetrate the cell wall. Enzyme inactivation has not been described. There is cross-resistance among all polymyxins, but not between polymyxins and other antimicrobials.

SPECTRUM OF ACTIVITY

Nearly all aerobic gram-negative bacilli are susceptible *in vitro*. Notable exceptions are Proteus and Providencia which are usually resistant because of a failure of the drug to penetrate the cell wall. *In vitro* activity of polymyxins against *Pseudomonas aeruginosa* is antagonized by divalent cations.[2] The antagonism is specific for *P. aeruginosa,* applies at physiological concentrations (ie, serum inhibits activity), and may represent impaired binding of the drug to its receptor site.[3] Polymyxins are unique among antimicrobials in their ability to neutralize endotoxins and prevent the generalized Schwartzman reaction.[4] This may represent a potential use for these drugs that is independent of their antimicrobial activity.

INDICATIONS

The use of polymyxins is limited because of a high incidence of toxicity, poor clinical results in infections caused by *P. aeruginosa*,[5] relatively poor diffusion into tissues and body fluids, and the availability of alternative agents. For these reasons, polymyxins are seldom used for systemic infections. Topical polymyxin B is commonly employed for local infections involving susceptible bacteria, including otitis externa and keratitis. The activity of topical polymyxin against *P. aeruginosa* may be enhanced by combining the antibiotic with an agent that chelates divalent cations.[5]

PHARMACOKINETICS

Absorption with oral or topical application is minimal even when applied to large inflamed surfaces. Peak serum levels with intramuscular administration of colistin in recommended doses are 4 to 8 μg/ml.[6] Similar levels are achieved with intravenous administration of polymyxin B except for high initial peak levels. (Effective serum levels of colistin may not be accurate since the drug must be hydrolyzed from methanesulfonate for antimicrobial activity and this hydrolysis may occur during the biological assay). Penetration across the blood-brain barrier is poor and necessitates intrathecal administration when polymyxin B is used for central nervous system infections. Excretion is primarily by the renal route with both colistin and polymyxin B, but urine levels are higher with colistin.[7] Half-lives are 1.5 to 3 hours for colistin and 4 to 7 hours with polymyxin B. These half-lives increase to 3 days in severe renal disease.

PREPARATIONS AND DOSAGE

Polymyxin B is available as a sulfate and colistin is available as the methanesulfonate (colistimethate). The complexing with methanesulfonate reduces severe pain of polymyxin at injection sites so that colistin is the preferred preparation for intramuscular administration. However, the methanesulfonate also has no antimicrobial availability; the active drug is released by hydrolysis and this occurs at an uncertain rate.[8] The recommended dose of colistin for adults is 2.5 to

5 mg/kg/day in 2 to 4 divided doses; the recommended dose for children is 5 to 8 mg/kg/day. In renal insufficiency the adult dose is 2.5 mg/kg over 2 to 4 days with serum creatinine levels of 1.5 to 5, and half this dosage with serum creatinine levels exceeding 5 mg/100 ml.

TABLE 1 Preparations and Costs of Polymyxins

GENERIC NAME	TRADEMARK NAME(S)	PREPARATIONS AND 1978 COSTS
Colistimethate Sodium (Colistin Methanesulfonate)	Coly-Mycin M	Injection (powder equivalent to base) 20mg—$2.19/vial; 150 mg—$10.55/vial
Polymyxin B Sulfate	Aerosporin	Injection (powder) 500,000 units (equivalent to polymyxin B standard 50 mg)—$2.75/vial

Polymyxin B doses are frequently expressed in 'units,' with 10,000 units equal to 1 mg of polymyxin B base. Aqueous suspensions of polymyxin B sulfate are the preferred polymyxin preparations for intravenous and topical use. The usual intravenous dose is 2.5 mg/kg/day given every 12 hours for adults and 4 mg/kg/day for children. In renal insufficiency the adult dose is 1.5 mg/kg over 2 to 4 days with a creatinine of 1.5 to 5, and half this amount with creatinine levels exceeding 5.

ADVERSE REACTIONS

The adverse effects of polymyxin B and colistin are similar, although the incidence of nephrotoxicity is greater with colistin. Nephrotoxicity has been noted in 20% of patients receiving colistin despite the use of recommended doses.[9] The incidence increases with higher doses or preexisting renal disease. Manifestations are hematuria, proteinuria, casts, oliguria, and rising serum creatinine. Nephrotoxicity often progresses for one to two weeks after therapy is discontinued, but is usually reversible. Acute tubular necrosis has been noted in 2% of recipients of colistin.[9]

Neurotoxicity includes facial and peripheral paresthesias, dizziness, ataxia, weakness, visual disturbances, slurred speech, or hyporeflexia. These are reported in 7% of patients treated with systemic polymyxins, and are usually reversible.[9,10] Respiratory arrest due to neuromuscular blockade has been noted in 2% of patients and is most common with persons receiving anesthetics or muscle relaxants, or individuals with myesthenia gravis.[9,11] This reaction is not reversed with neostigmine but may respond to calcium gluconate.

Hypersensitivity reactions are rare, although rash, drug fever, and eosinophilia have been reported.

REFERENCES

1. Wilkinson S: Identity of colistin and polymyxin E. Lancet 1:922–923, 1963.
2. Davis SD, Iannetta A, Wedgwood RJ: Activity of colistin against Pseudomonas aeruginosa: inhibition by calcium. J Infect Dis 124:610–612, 1971.
3. Brown MRW, Melling J: Role of divalent cations in the action of polymyxin B and EDTA on *Pseudomonas aeruginosa*. J Gen Microbiol 59:263–274, 1969.
4. Corrigan JJ Jr, Bell BM: Endotoxin induced intravascular coagulation: prevention with polymyxin B sulfate. J Lab Clin Med 77:802–810, 1971.
5. Davis SD, Iannetta A, Wedgwood RJ: Antibiotics for *Pseudomonas aeruginosa* sepsis: inadequate proof of efficacy. J Infect Dis 124:104–105, 1971.
6. Froman J, Gross L, Curatola S: Serum and urine levels following parenteral administration of sodium colistimethate to normal individuals. J Urol 103:210–214, 1970.
7. Pederson MF, Pederson JF, Madsen PO: A clinical and experimental comparative study of sodium colistimethate and polymyxin B sulfate. Invest Urol 9:234–237, 1971.
8. McMillan FH, Pattison IC: Sodium colistimethate. I. Dissociations of aminomethanesulfonates in aqueous solution. J Pharm Sci 58:730–737, 1969.
9. Koch-Weser J, Sidel VW, Federman EB, et al: Adverse effects of sodium colistimethate. Ann Intern Med 72:857–868, 1970.
10. Fekety FR Jr, Norman PS, Cluff LE: The treatment of gram-negative bacillary infections with colistin. Ann Intern Med 57:214–229, 1962.
11. Decker DA Jr, Fincham R: Respiratory arrest in myasthenia gravis with colistimate therapy. Arch Neurol 25:141–144, 1971.

6. TETRACYCLINES

John G. Bartlett

The first tetracycline, chlortetracycline, was isolated from *Streptomyces aureofaciens* in 1948.[1] Tetracycline was subsequently produced by catalytic hydrogenation to remove the chlorine atom from the parent compound. This was the first chemical modification of an antibiotic produced by fermentation. Numerous other tetracycline analogs have followed.

Tetracyclines have a broad spectrum of antimicrobial activity, are well absorbed after oral administration, and are generally well tolerated with few serious side effects. In the United States, more prescriptions are written annually for these agents than any other class of antimicrobials including penicillins.[2] Nevertheless, tetracyclines are regarded as the drugs of choice for relatively few microbial pathogens; most authorities feel that widespread abuse of tetracyclines in both clinical and veterinary medicine is responsible for increasing rates of resistance.[3]

MECHANISM OF ACTION

Tetracyclines block the binding of the transfer RNA-amino acid complexes to the ribosome, thus making amino acids unavailable to messenger RNA for protein synthesis. These drugs may also interfere with mammalian protein synthesis, thus accounting for the catabolic state in renal failure.[4] Resistance is primarily due to widely prevalent plasmids which are inducible. The main biochemical mechanism of resistance is a block in drug penetration.[5]

SPECTRUM OF ACTIVITY

The tetracyclines are active against many gram positive and gram negative bacteria as well as rickettsia, mycoplasma, and chlamydia. The antibacterial spectrum, although broad, is often unpredictable.[6] Most gonococci, *H. influenzae* and *S. pneumoniae* are sensitive, but there is increasing resistance among each of these species. Resistance among gram positive bacteria include about 50% of *S. aureus,* 10 to 30% of beta-hemolytic streptococci, and virtually all enterococci. Susceptibility of *E. coli, Proteus mirabilis,* Klebsiella, Shigella, and Salmonella is quite variable. Most strains of indole-positive Proteus, Serratia, *Pseudomonas aeruginosa,* Providenceae and Enterobacter are resistant. Activity against anaerobes is erratic—as many as 40% of Peptostreptococci, 10 to 40% of *B. melaninogenicus,* and 30 to 60% of *B. fragilis* are resistant.

The analogs of tetracyclines show similar spectra of activity, and cross resistance is usually complete. Exceptions are: minocycline is more active against *S. aureus* and *Nocardia asteroides;* minocycline and doxycycline are somewhat more active against anaerobes and facultative gram negative bacilli; and oxytetracycline is sometimes effective against *P. aeruginosa* at concentrations which can be achieved in the urine.

INDICATIONS

Indications for tetracyclines may be considered according to microbial pathogen and by clinical entity.

1. Microbial Pathogens

Despite extraordinary utilization rates, the tetracyclines are regarded as drugs of choice for relatively few microbial pathogens commonly encountered in clinical practice.[7]

(a) *Mycoplasma pneumoniae* (equivalent to erythromycin)

(b) Chlamydia (psittacosis, lymphogranuloma venereum, inclusion conjunctivitis, trachoma, and nonspecific urethritis)

(c) Rickettsia (Rocky Mountain Spotted Fever, Q fever, typhus, rickettsialpox)

(d) *Vibrio cholerae* (cholera)

(e) *Borrelia recurrentis* (relapsing fever)

(f) *Pseudomonas pseudomallei* (melioidosis)

(g) Brucella

Tetracyclines are acceptable alternatives for most infections caused by *H. influenzae, S. pneumoniae, Pasteurella multocida,* and *N. gonorrhoeae;* syphilis; yaws; leptospirosis, actinomycosis, nocardiosis tularemia, plague, and pertussis.

2. Clinical Entities

(a) *Respiratory tract infections.* Tetracyclines or ampicillin are commonly used in respiratory tract infections where *H. influenzae* or *S. pneumoniae* are suspected pathogens. These include exacerbations of chronic bronchitis and pneumonitis that can be treated with an oral agent. Tetracyclines should not be used where group A beta-hemolytic streptococci are likely pathogens, as with pharyngitis.

(b) *Urinary tract infections.* Tetracyclines are favored drugs for uncomplicated urinary tract infections since they are easily administered, cause few serious side effects, and are active against most of the common urinary tract pathogens. Tetracyclines should not be used for empiric treatment of serious urinary tract infections in which the clinical setting suggests resistant pathogens, ie, renal stones, recent urologic surgery, multiple courses of antimicrobial therapy, indwelling catheters, etc.

(c) *Intra-abdominal infections.* Tropical sprue, blind loop syndrome, and Whipple's disease are indications for prolonged courses of tetracycline. These agents are not recommended for serious intra-abdominal sepsis because of their unpredictable activity against facultative gram negative bacilli and *B. fragilis.*

(d) *Venereal diseases.* Tetracyclines are agents of choice for nonspecific urethritis and other venereal diseases caused by chlamydia or mycoplasma. They are alternatives to penicillin for gonococcal infections and syphilis.

(e) *Skin and soft tissue infections.* Prolonged courses of tetracyclines (either topically or with low dose oral administration) are recommended for severe acne. Infections involving *S. aureus* or *Strep pyogenes* should not be treated with tetracycline.

PHARMACOKINETICS AND METABOLISM

The major difference in the various analogs of tetracyclines relate to pharmacokinetic properties (Table 1). The completeness of oral absorption when taken on an empty stomach generally ranges from 60 to nearly 100% with the different congeners. Food interferes with absorption but this effect is minimal with minocycline and doxycycline. Divalent metal ions, such as those found in antacids and dairy products, impair intestinal absorption of all tetracyclines.[8]

Peak serum levels with a 250 mg oral dose of tetracycline are 1 to 3 μg/ml at 1 to 2 hours, and up to 5 μg/ml with a 500 mg dose.[9]

TABLE 1 Pharmacokinetic Properties of Tetracyclines[a]

	Dosage		Completeness of Oral Absorption (%)	Elimination Half-life (hours)	Peak Serum Level (μg/ml)	Excretion	
	Oral	Intravenous				Renal	Other
Tetracycline	250–500 mg QID	250–500 mg q 12 h	80	10	2–4	60%	—
Chlortetracycline	250–500 mg QID	250–500 mg q 12 h	30	7	2–7	20%	Biliary tract
Oxytetracycline	250–500 mg QID	250–500 mg q 12 h	60	9	1–3	70%	—
Demeclocycline	150–300 mg QID	—	70	15	2–4	40%	—
Doxycycline	100 mg q 12 h first day then 100 to 200 mg/day in one or two doses	200 mg initially, then 100 mg q 12 h	90	15	2–6	35%	Intestinal lumen
Minocycline	200 mg initially, then 100 mg q 12 h	200 mg initially, then 100 mg q 12 h	100	17	2–4	10%	Metabolized

[a] Adapted from reference 6.

Intravenous therapy gives levels of 8 to 10 μg/ml depending on the rate of infusion and should not exceed 15 μg/ml. Recommended doses of the various tetracycline analogs give comparable peak blood levels, but dosing intervals are highly variable depending on half-life.

Tetracyclines penetrate tissue and body fluids well. Liver and bile levels are one to three times the serum levels. The most lipid-soluble forms are minocycline and doxycycline; these tetracyclines penetrate lipid barriers of the central nervous system, eye and prostate better than other congeners.[10] Protein binding ranges from 55 to 80% for all tetracyclines except oxytetracycline which is 30% bound.

Elimination of tetracyclines is primarily by the gastrointestinal tract (unabsorbed drug or excretion via the biliary tract or intestine) and the urinary tract. Tetracycline and oxytetracycline give the highest urinary levels and are, therefore, sometimes preferred for urinary tract infections. The primary mechanism of elimination for doxycycline is excretion into the intestinal lumen where it appears in a chelated form. Since the chelated form is not an active antimicrobial, doxycycline has minimal effect on the fecal flora.[11] With renal failure, the half-life of tetracycline and oxytetracycline increases to about 100 hours; the half-lives of chlortetracycline and doxycycline are not appreciably influenced by impaired renal function.

PREPARATIONS AND DOSAGE

Doses for tetracyclines are summarized in Table 1; preparations and costs are given in Table 2. Intramuscular administration is not recommended due to severe pain and poor absorption; intramuscular injections of 100 mg of tetracycline give peak serum levels of only 0.2 to 0.3 μg/ml—considerably lower than the levels achieved with oral administration. Tetracyclines should be avoided in children under 8 years of age (see Adverse Reactions). However, if a tetracycline is indicated, the pediatric dose of tetracycline hydrochloride is 25 to 50 mg/kg/day orally and 10 to 20 mg/kg/day intravenously.

In most clinical situations the various tetracycline analogs are considered equally efficacious if proper doses and dosing intervals are employed. The following considerations may dictate a preference for a particular agent from this class. 1) Tetracycline is the least expensive. 2) Tetracycline and oxytetracycline achieve the highest urinary levels and may be preferred for urinary tract infections. 3) Minocycline is more active than the other tetracyclines against *S.*

TABLE 2 Preparations and Costs of Tetracyclines

Generic Name	Trademark Name(s)	Preparations and 1978 Costs
Chlortetracycline Hydrochloride	Aureomycin	Capsules 250 mg—$19.82/100 Injection (powder) 500 mg—$4.01/vial
Demeclocycline	Declomycin	Drops (pediatric) 60 mg/ml—$2.58/60 ml Syrup 75 mg/5 ml—$18.60/pint
Demeclocycline Hydrochloride	Declomycin Hydrochloride	Capsules 150 mg—$30.80/100 Tablets 75 mg—$4.35/25; 150 mg—$30.80/100; 300 mg—$6.89/12
Doxycycline Calcium	Vibramycin Calcium	Syrup 50 mg/5 ml—$2.33/30 ml
Doxycycline Hyclate	Vibramycin Hyclate (Doxy II)	Capsules 50 mg—$21.36/50; 100 mg—$38.40/50 Injection (powder) 100 mg—$7.71/vial; 200 mg—$15.18/vial
Doxycycline Monohydrate	Vibramycin Monohydrate	Powder for suspension 25 mg/5 ml—$2.34/60 ml
Minocycline Hydrochloride	Minocin (Vectrin)	Capsules 50 mg—$32.49/100; 100 mg—$27.08/50 Syrup 50 mg/5 ml—$3.24/60 ml Injection (powder) 100 mg—$3.63/vial
Oxytetracycline	Terramycin	Tablets 250 mg—$18.92/100 Injection (solution, intramuscular) 50 mg/ml—$3.62/2 ml ampul, $14.13/10-ml vial
Oxytetracycline Calcium	Terramycin	Syrup 125 mg/5 ml—$14.56/pint
Oxytetracycline Hydrochloride	Terramycin	Capsules 125 mg—$12.41/100; 250 mg—$22.47/100 Injection (powder, intravenous) 250 mg—$1.83/vial; 500 mg—$3.23/vial
Tetracycline	Achromycin V (Panmycin) (Robitet) (SK-Tetracycline) (Sumycin) (Tetracyn) (Tetrex-S)	Syrup 125 mg/5 ml—$11.72/pint

TABLE 2 *(continued)*

Generic Name	Trademark Name(s)	Preparations and 1978 Costs
Tetracycline Hydrochloride	Achromycin (Panmycin) (Robitet) (SK-Tetracycline) (Tetracyn)	Capsules 100 mg—\$3.60/100; 250 mg—\$4.57/100; 500 mg—\$9.18/100 Injection (powder, intramuscular) 100 mg—\$0.99/vial; 250 mg—\$1.79/vial
	generic	Injection (powder, intravenous) 250 mg—\$1.79/vial; 500 mg—\$2.84/vial
Tetracycline Phosphate Complex	Tetrex bidCaps	Capsules 250 mg—\$26.46/100; 500 mg—\$25.96/50

aureus and *Nocardia asteroides*. However, in both instances, other antimicrobials are considered the agents of choice for infections involving these microbes. 4) Doxycycline and minocycline are more convenient for patients due to twice daily dosing regimens and the minimal effect of food on absorption. These may be particularly important considerations when patient compliance is questioned. 5) Minocycline causes high incidence of vertigo. 6) Doxycycline does not require a renal route of excretion, making this the tetracycline of choice for patients with renal failure.

ADVERSE REACTIONS

Gastrointestinal side effects are common and include nausea, vomiting, anorexia, unpleasant taste, and diarrhea. These complications are dose related and occur in approximately 10% of patients receiving 2 g of tetracycline per day. Tetracyclines were frequently responsible for cases of pseudomembranous colitis reported in the 1950's, but, for unexplained reasons, this side effect is now rarely encountered despite increasing recent usage.

Superinfections are common and include oral candidiasis and vulvovaginitis.

Hepatotoxicity ranges from mild abnormal liver function tests to severe hepatic failure with jaundice followed by azotemia, acidosis, shock, and death. Liver biopsy shows fatty degeneration with little necrosis or biliary stasis. Hepatotoxicity is usually related to excessive dosage, pregnancy, renal disease, or previous hepatic disease.[12,13]

Increases in blood urea nitrogen may occur due to inhibition of hepatic protein synthesis while catabolism continues, thus increasing the urea load.[4] Creatinine measurements more reliably reflect nephrotoxicity. In the presence of impaired renal function, there may be increasing acidosis, hyperphosphatemia, anorexia, nausea, vomiting, weight loss, and severe electrolyte disturbances. These effects are related to dose, duration of therapy, extent of previous renal function, and administration of diuretics or methoxyflurane anesthesia. They may be noted with any tetracycline other than doxycycline.

Intravenous administration frequently causes thrombophlebitis. Intramuscular injections may cause severe pain, and drug absorption is poor. This route of administration is rarely indicated.

Tetracyclines are deposited in teeth during early stages of calcification and cause yellow or brown discoloration.[14] The intensity of pigmentation is dose related. There may also be disturbances in fetal bone growth. These potential complications contraindicate use of tetracycline in children under eight years and in females more than five months pregnant, corresponding to times of formation of deciduous and permanent teeth.

Hypersensitivity reactions are uncommon and include rashes (morbilliform, urticaria or exfoliative dermatitis), fever, angioneurotic edema, eosinophilia, and anaphylaxis. Cross sensitivity between tetracyclines has been suggested.

Photosensitivity may occur with any tetracycline analog but is most common with demeclocycline. This reaction is presumably due to accumulation of these drugs in the skin, and it may be prevented with windowglass or a sunscreen preparation containing para-aminobenzoic acid.

Vestibular toxicity is unique to minocycline, and has been reported in up to 90% of persons receiving this agent.[15] The effect is dose related and reversible.

REFERENCES

1. Finland M: Twenty-fifth anniversary of the discovery of Aureomycin: the place of the tetracycline in antimicrobial therapy. Clin Pharmacol Ther 15:3–8, 1974.
2. Simmons HE, Stolley PD: This is medical progress? Trends and consequences of antibiotic use in the United States. JAMA 227:1023–1028, 1974.
3. Smith DH, Gardner P: The ecology of R factors. N Engl J Med 282:161–162, 1970.

4. Bread NS Jr, Armentrout SA, Weisberger AS: Inhibition of mammalian protein synthesis by antibiotics. Pharmacol Rev 21:213–245, 1969.
5. Benveniste R, Davis J: Mechanisms of antibiotic resistance in bacteria. Annu Rev Biochem 42:471–506, 1973.
6. Barza M, Scheife RT: Antimicrobial spectrum, pharmacology and therapeutic use of antibiotics. I. Tetracyclines. J Maine Med Assoc 67:368–376, 1976.
7. Anon: The choice of antimicrobial drugs. Med Lett Drugs Ther 20:1–8, 1978.
8. Neuvonen PJ: Interactions with the absorption of tetracyclines. Drugs 11:45–54, 1976.
9. Barr WH, Gerbracht LM, Letcher K, et al: Assessment of the biologic availability of tetracycline products in man. Clin Pharmacol Ther 13:97–108, 1972.
10. Barza M, Brown RB, Shanks C, et al: Relation between lipophilicity and pharmacological behavior of minocycline, doxycycline, tetracycline and oxytetracycline in dogs. Antimicrob Agents Chemother 8:713–720, 1975.
11. Bartlett JG, Bustetter LA, Gorbach SL, et al: Comparative effect of tetracycline and doxycycline on the occurrence of resistant *E. coli* in the fecal flora. Antimicrob Agents Chemother 7:55–57, 1975.
12. Schultz JC, Adamson JS Jr, Workman WW, et al: Fatal liver disease after intravenous administration of tetracyclines in high dosage. N Engl J Med 269:99–1004, 1963.
13. Dowling HF, Lepper MH: Hepatic reactions to tetracyclines. JAMA 188:307–309, 1964.
14. Grossman ER, Walchek A, Freedman H: Tetracyclines and permanent teeth: the relation between dose and tooth color. Pediatrics 47:567–570, 1971.
15. Fanning WL, Gump DW: Vestibular reactions to minocycline—follow-up. Morbid Mortal Weekly Report 24:55–56, 1975.

7. CHLORAMPHENICOL

John G. Bartlett

Chloramphenicol was first isolated in 1947 and became the first antibiotic to be synthesized in 1948. It was marketed in 1949 and quickly proved clinically effective in a number of serious infections caused by a variety of bacteria or rickettsia. However, the initial enthusiasm for chloramphenicol was quickly tempered by reports of serious blood dyscrasias. The *Journal of the American Medical Association* published stern warnings regarding these potential complications in 1952 and 1960. In each instance, sales plummeted temporarily, but annual production levels of 45 to 55 million grams were reached again. A survey of chloramphenicol usage by the American Medical Association Council on Drugs in 1967 showed the drug was prescribed for 'proper' indications in only 6 to 7% of patients. This was followed by the Nelson hearings which resulted in a precipitous drop in annual sales to the present levels of 5 to 10 million grams per year.[1] Despite the overall trends and repeated warnings, a survey of the Tennessee Medicaid program for 1973 to 1974 showed that half of the chloramphenicol prescribed for outpatients was for upper respiratory tract infections.[2]

Chloramphenicol has unique properties of lipid solubility and activity against a number of important infectious pathogens which are not easily treated by other antimicrobials. Unfortunately, the drug has been greatly overused for infections in which either no antimicrobial is indicated or where alternative agents are readily available. This abuse has resulted in numerous lethal cases of aplastic anemia as well as increasing rates of resistance.

MECHANISM OF ACTION

Chloramphenicol inhibits microbial protein production by suppressing peptidyl transferase activity on the 50S sub-unit of the ribosome. It is bacteriostatic.

The major mechanism of resistance in clinical isolates of gram negative bacilli is the R-factor mediated enzymatic acetylation.[3] These acetyltransferase proteins are synthesized constitutively and located intracellularly. Resistance in gram positive bacteria is similar except that the acetyltransferase is inducible.[4] Other less important mechanisms of resistance include inducible permeability block and reduction of the nitro group.[5,6]

SPECTRUM OF ACTIVITY

S. pneumoniae, S. pyogenes, H. influenzae and *Neisseria* are usually sensitive although there are occasional exceptions. *S. aureus* species are usually sensitive but this is highly variable, with as many as 50% being resistant at some hospitals, particularly where the drug has been used extensively. Activity against aerobic gram negative bacilli is erratic. *E. coli*, Shigella and *Proteus mirabilis* are generally sensitive. About 30 to 60% of Klebsiella, Citrobacter, indole-positive Proteus, Providencia and Serratia are susceptible.[7] *Pseudomonas aeruginosa* is almost always resistant. Salmonella are usually sensitive and chloramphenicol is regarded as the drug of choice for typhoid fever. However, chloramphenicol-resistant *S. typhosa* have recently been reported in Mexico, India, Thailand and Vietnam.[8] This is presumably due to worldwide abuse of the drug, resulting in intestinal bacteria which carry R factors for chloramphenicol resistance.

Anaerobic bacteria are virtually always susceptible. This includes *B. fragilis* which is generally resistant to other commonly used antimicrobials.

Chloramphenicol is also active against rickettsia, chlamydia and mycoplasma.

INDICATIONS

Chloramphenicol should be reserved for selected, serious infections because of the risk of aplastic anemia and the threat of widespread development of resistance.

(1) Typhoid fever—chloramphenicol is regarded as the drug of choice although susceptibilities of the organism should be confirmed with *in vitro* susceptibility tests. Chloramphenicol may also be used in cases of enteric fever due to species of Salmonella other than *S. typhosa,* although ampicillin is generally preferred if the organism is

susceptible. Chloramphenicol should not be used to treat the carrier state of salmonella.

(2) Anaerobic infections in which *B. fragilis* is an established or suspected pathogen—some authorities consider the drug inferior to clindamycin for *B. fragilis* due to clinical failures attributed to inactivation via nitroreduction, despite *in vitro* susceptibility.[9]

(3) Central nervous system infections—chloramphenicol penetrates the blood brain barrier well even in the absence of inflammation. It is regarded as a preferred agent for brain abscess in which *B. fragilis* is a common pathogen. Chloramphenicol is an alternative to penicillin or ampicillin for meningitis due to *S. pneumoniae, N. meningiditis,* or *H. influenzae.* It is used in central nervous system infections involving gram negative bacilli, providing these organisms are susceptible.

(4) Serious infections involving *H. influenzae* such as meningitis or epiglottitis—chloramphenicol is an alternative to ampicillin for penicillin-allergic patients or for ampicillin-resistant strains. Susceptibility to chloramphenicol should be confirmed because resistance has been reported.[10]

(5) Rickettsial diseases—efficacy of chloramphenicol is well established for epidemic, murine, and recrudescent typhus, Rocky Mountain spotted fever, and Q fever. Tetracycline is usually preferred except where parenteral treatment is required.

PHARMACOKINETICS AND METABOLISM

Chloramphenicol is well absorbed after oral administration, with peak blood levels of 3 to 6 μg/ml following a 500 mg dose and 8 to 15 μg/ml following a 1 g dose. Absorption from intramuscular injection sites is poor, and the intramuscular route should not be used. Peak serum levels with intravenous administration in the usual doses are 10 to 20 μg/ml, depending on the infusion rate.

Chloramphenicol penetrates well into tissues and body fluids, including the central nervous system. Most of the drug is inactivated by conjugation with glucuronide in the liver. The half-life of 2 to 3 hours in patients with normal hepatic function increases in the presence of severe liver disease with jaundice. Chloramphenicol increases the half-life of tolbutamide, diphenylhydantoin, and coumarin.[11] Most of the drug is excreted in the urinary tract as inactive metabolites. Only 5 to 10% of the biologically active form is found in urine. Renal failure results in accumulation of nontoxic metabolites with minimal influence on the half-life of the biologically active and potentially toxic form. By contrast, severe liver disease increases the potential for high levels of free chloramphenicol due to decreased glucuronide conjugation.

PREPARATIONS AND DOSAGE

Chloramphenicol is available for oral and intravenous use. The usual dose is 50 to 100 mg/kg/day in four divided doses. Premature and newborn infants should not receive more than 25 mg/kg/day.[12] Maximum doses for adults with severe renal disease are 2 to 3 g/day. Ascites or jaundice due to liver disease is a relative contraindication to chloramphenicol and, if required, daily dosage should not exceed 2 g/day.

TABLE 1 Preparations and Costs of Chloramphenicol

Generic Name	Trademark Name(s)	Preparations and 1978 Costs
Chloramphenicol	Chloromycetin	Capsules 50 mg—$9.99/100; 100 mg—$18.08/100; 250 mg—$6.75/16 Injection (solution) 250 mg/ml—$4.77/2-ml ampul
	Mychel	Capsules 250 mg—$10.00/100
Chloramphenicol Palmitate	Chloromycetin Palmitate	Suspension equivalent to chloramphenicol 150 mg/5 ml—$6.47/60 ml
Chloramphenicol Sodium Succinate	Chloromycetin Sodium Succinate	Injection (powder) 1 g—$5.19/vial
	Mychel-S	Injection (powder) 1 g—$1.80/vial

ADVERSE REACTIONS

The principle side effects are two types of bone marrow toxicity. One form is dose related and reversible.[13] It is characterized by anemia, low reticulocyte counts, increased serum iron, and a cellular marrow showing vacuolization and maturation arrest of erythroid and myeloid precursors. Leukopenia and/or granulocytopenia may also occur. These are regarded as pharmacologic effects of the drug due to mitochondrial injury, and correlate with high blood levels of free drug.[14] Monitoring of blood counts, reticulocyte counts, and serum iron at 2 to 3 day intervals permits early detection of this toxicity. The advisability of continuing the drug in the presence of this anemia depends on the clinical setting; transfusions may be required. Discontinuation of chloramphenicol is followed by bone marrow recovery in 1 to 3 weeks.

The most dreaded complication of chloramphenicol therapy is a non-dose-related, idiosyncratic aplastic anemia. The peripheral blood shows pancytopenia and the marrow may be aplastic or hypoplastic. This is generally irreversible and usually occurs several weeks after treatment has been discontinued, indicating that monitoring of blood counts during therapy is of no value. Most cases are fatal due to hemorrhage or infection. The risk of this complication is 1 per 25,000 to 50,000 courses of therapy, and it is somewhat more common in white, female children or with repeated use.[15] The reaction may result from inhibition of DNA synthesis in marrow stem cells due to the para-nitrosulfathiazole group. Support for this thesis is the observation that thiamphenicol, an analogue which lacks the para-nitrosulfathiazole group, may cause erythroid suppression but has not been known to cause acute aplastic anemia despite millions of courses of therapy in Europe.[16] Another relevant observation is that aplastic anemia has not been reported when chloramphenicol was administered exclusively by the parenteral route.[17] This may reflect toxicity due to a metabolic product from colonic bacteria acting on orally admininistered drug or simply that oral usage is far more common.

Other side effects include nausea, vomiting, glossitis, unpleasant taste, perineal irritation, stomatitis, diarrhea, and pseudomembranous colitis. Superinfections due to candida, *S. aureus, P. aeruginosa* and other resistant gram negative bacilli are relatively common. Hypersensitivity reactions are uncommon. Optic neuritis, peripheral neuritis, or delirium are rare, although optic neuritis is not infrequent in children with cystic fibrosis. The 'gray syndrome' (abdominal distension, cyanosis, and circulatory failure) is seen in premature infants and neonates who are unable to conjugate and excrete chloramphenicol. It is for this reason that low dosage is recommended for children less than one month of age.

REFERENCES

1. Silverman M, Lee PR: *Pills, Profits and Politics.* Berkeley, University of California Press, 1974, pp 283–292.
2. Ray WA, Federspiel CS, Schaffner W: Prescribing of chloramphenicol in ambulatory practice. An epidemiologic study among Tennessee Medicaid recipients. Ann Intern Med 84:266–270, 1976.
3. Benveniste R, Davies J: Mechanism of antibiotic resistance in bacteria. Annu Rev Biochem 42:471–506, 1973.
4. Miyamura S, Ochiai H, Nitahara Y, et al: Resistance mechanism of chloramphenicol in *Streptococcus haemolyticus, Streptococcus pneumoniae* and *Streptococcus faecalis.* Microbiol Immunol 21:69–97, 1977.
5. Smith GN, Worrel CS: Enzymatic reduction of chloramphenicol. J Bacteriol 65:216–223, 1953.
6. Kanazawa Y, Kuramata T, Miyamura S: Inactivation of chemotherapeutic agents by Clostridia. Jpn J Bacteriol 24:281–289, 1969.
7. Sabath LD: Drug resistance of bacteria. N Engl J Med 280:91–94, 1969.
8. Anderson ES: The problem and implications of chloramphenicol resistance in the typhoid bacillus. J Hygiene 74:289–299, 1975.
9. Thadepalli H, Gorbach SL, Bartlett JG: Apparent failure of chloramphenicol in anaerobic infections. Curr Ther Res (in press).
10. Anon: Chloramphenicol-resistant *Hemophilis influenzae.* Morbid Mortal Weekly Report 25:267, 1976.
11. Christensen LK, Skousted L: Inhibition of drug metabolism by chloramphenicol. Lancet 2:1397–1399, 1969.
12. Snyder MJ, Woodward TE: The clinical use of chloramphenicol. Med Clin North Am 54:1187–1197, 1970.
13. Scott JL, Finegold SM, Belkin GA, et al: A controlled double-blind study of the hematologic toxicity of chloramphenicol. N Engl J Med 272:1137–1142, 1965.
14. Yunis AA, Smith US, Restrepo A: Reversible marrow suppression from chloramphenicol. A consequence of mitochondrial injury. Arch Intern Med 126:272–275, 1970.
15. Best WR: Chloramphenicol-associated blood dyscrasias. A review of cases submitted to the American Medical Association Registry. JAMA 201:181–188, 1967.
16. Beck EA: Chloramphenicol-und thiamphenicolschäden des bluts. Schweiz Med Wochenschr 105:1078–1080, 1975.
17. Hans RJ: Letter. Parke, Davis and Co., Detroit, Mich., Oct. 6, 1975.

8. AMINOGLYCOSIDES

Richard T. Scheife and Michael Barza

The aminoglycoside antibiotics are amino sugars linked to another moiety by a glycoside bond.[1] Streptomycin was the first to be discovered (1944) and was followed by neomycin (1949), paromomycin (1956), kanamycin (1957), gentamicin (1963), tobramycin (1967) and amikacin (1972). Sisomicin and netilmicin are investigational compounds.

MECHANISM OF ACTION

The aminoglycosides accumulate within sensitive cells by a complex series of steps, one of which involves an aerobically-generated active transport system.[2] The antibiotics bind irreversibly to bacterial ribosomes, blocking the 'recognition' step in protein synthesis and causing 'misreading' of the genetic code.[3,4] The ribosomes separate from messenger ribonucleic acid (RNA) and cell death ensues.[3]

BACTERIAL RESISTANCE

Increasing resistance of meningococci, gonococci and enteric bacilli to streptomycin was recognized early,[5] and three general mechanisms for this phenomenon were defined: (1) alteration of the target (ribosome) so that its affinity for the antibiotic is lost; (2) reduced accumulation of the drugs within the bacterium; and (3) elaboration of an enzyme which inactivates the antibiotic.

The first mechanism is primarily a laboratory phenomenon, although instances of selection of such mutants have been reported in burn centers[4] and other situations.[6] The second mechanism relates to the intracellular accumulation of antibiotic in sensitive cells; an important part of the transport process depends upon aerobically-generated energy, and this may explain the resistance to aminoglycosides of bacteria growing under anaerobic conditions.[2]

Most of the resistance encountered clinically among aerobic bacteria is attributable to the formation of antibiotic-inactivating enzymes.[7,8] The genes controlling production of these enzymes are normally carried on extrachromosomal fragments of deoxyribonucleic acid (DNA) called plasmids. Certain large plasmids are capable of transferring copies of themselves, by conjugation, into other bacteria. Such plasmids are called 'R' factors, and frequently confer simultaneous resistance ('infectious drug resistance') to more than one antibiotic.[9]

Resistance to amikacin is usually accompanied by cross-resistance to the other aminoglycosides. However, the majority of gentamicin-resistant strains are presently susceptible to amikacin.[10–14] The emergence of aminoglycoside-resistance during therapy is uncommon; when it occurs, it has been attributed to the selection of a few colonies of resistant organisms by suboptimal therapy[6,15,16] or to mutations.[6] Unfortunately, the indiscriminate use of any one aminoglycoside seems to be capable of fostering resistance to that agent,[11,17] and, possibly to other members of the class.

ANTIMICROBIAL SPECTRUM

Bacterial susceptibility to the aminoglycosides varies with geography and time. The data shown in Table 1, therefore, may not be fully representative of the situation in a particular hospital at a given moment. In most institutions at present, amikacin is active against a higher proportion of gram-negative aerobic bacilli (eg, 98%) than is gentamicin, tobramycin or netilmicin (eg, 95%). Furthermore, the majority of gentamicin-resistant strains are susceptible to amikacin, but the reverse is not true. These data underline the value of amikacin, but also caution against its indiscriminate use.

For purposes of Table 1, we have considered organisms susceptible if they are inhibited by levels of the drug which are one-half the usual peak serum concentration.

The aminoglycosides have found their greatest usefulness in the therapy of infections owing to gram-negative aerobic bacilli. The majority of strains listed in Table 1 are susceptible to gentamicin, tobramycin and amikacin; a small percentage is resistant to kanamycin and a larger one to streptomycin. The comparative activity of the aminoglycosides is summarized in Table 2, with the principal emphasis on gram-negative bacilli.

TABLE 1 Activity of Systemically Administered Aminoglycosides against Common Bacterial Pathogens[a]

	Aminoglycosides (% inhibited)				
BACTERIUM	STREPTOMYCIN	KANAMYCIN	GENTAMICIN	TOBRAMYCIN	AMIKACIN
Gram-Negative Enteric Bacilli (aerobic)					
Eschierichia coli	50[18,22]	80[23,24]	95[19,21,24]	95[21,24]	98[21,23,24]
Klebsiella	40[18,22]	80[23,24]	98[21,23,24]	98[21,24]	~100[21,23,24]
Enterobacter	60[22]	95[23,24]	95[21,23,24]	~100[21,24]	~100[21,23]
Proteus mirabilis	88[22]	92[22–24]	92[21,23,24]	92[21,24]	92[21,23,24]
P. vulgaris, morganii, rettgeri	60[18,22]	Generally 70–90%; as low as 30% for *P. rettgeri*[19,21–25]			
Pseudomonas aeruginosa	5[22]	5[23,24]	80–90[21,23,24]	95[21,24]	95[21,23,24]
Salmonella	50[22]	85–100[22,23,25]	~100[22,23,24]	~100[22,25]	~100[23]
Shigella	80[22]	96[22,23]	96[22,23]	96[22]	~100[23]
Serratia	60[22]	≧65[22–24]	≧80[21,23,24]	Variable[21,24,26]	98[21,23,24]

Gram-Positive Cocci					
Staphylococcus aureus	80–95[5,22]	98[23,24]	~100[21,23,24,28]	~100[21,24,28]	100[21,23,24,28]
S. epidermidis	90[28]	90[23,28]	~100[23,28]	~100[28]	~100[28]
Group A beta-hemolytic streptococcus	Weakly sensitive[5]	Weakly sensitive[25]	Weakly sensitive[25,29,30]	Weakly sensitive[25,29,30]	50% resistant[23]
Pneumococcus		Weakly susceptible[5,31]			
Enterococcus		Very few susceptible[5,23,32]			
Other Bacteria					
Haemophilus influenzae			~100[33]	~100[33]	Moderately sensitive[23]
Bacteroides fragilis					
Clostridia		Not sensitive[34,35]			
Anaerobic cocci					

[a]Based on inhibition by the following concentrations, which are half of the usual therapeutic serum level: streptomycin 12μg/ml[18]; kanamycin 12μg/ml[18–20]; gentamicin 2–4 μg/ml[19,21]; tobramycin 2–4 μg/ml[21]; amikacin 10μg/ml[19,20].

Staphylococcus aureus and *epidermidis* are generally susceptible to parenterally-administered aminoglycosides. In contrast, β-hemolytic streptococci (group a), *Strep. viridans* and pneumococci are weakly inhibited[5,19,25,29–31,42] and enterococci are generally resistant.[5,19,32] Listeria are readily inhibited by aminoglycosides.[43] Although gonococci and meningococci have not been examined extensively, the former were found to be fairly resistant to gentamicin in one study[31] and moderately sensitive in another.[42] (The aminocyclitol antibiotic spectinomycin which is used for therapy of gonorrhea is discussed later.)

Anaerobic bacteria, including *Bacteroides fragilis,* clostridia and anaerobic cocci are generally not susceptible to aminoglycosides.[34,35]

Mycoplasma, including *Mycoplasma pneumoniae,* are inhibited by kanamycin, gentamicin and tobramycin.[25] *M. tuberculosis* is susceptible in vitro to streptomycin, gentamicin,[33] and amikacin.[44]

COMBINATIONS WITH OTHER AGENTS

A synergistic (greater than additive) antimicrobial effect has been observed in a number of instances when aminoglycosides are combined with beta-lactam antibiotics such as penicillins and cephalosporins (Table 3).[55] The mechanism of this phenomenon, as studied in enterococci, is due to enhanced penetration of the bacterium by the aminoglycoside because of cell wall damage induced by the penicillin.[56] Synergism is not evident among enterococci which are extremely resistant to the aminoglycoside; such high-level resistance is rare with gentamicin, but was found in 40% of strains with streptomycin, and 20% with kanamycin, when blood culture isolates in one hospital were studied.[32] A laboratory test is available to screen for extreme resistance to aminoglycoside antibiotics.

Carbenicillin (or ticarcillin) plus gentamicin are, as a rule, synergistic only against strains of *Pseudomonas* which are susceptible to the aminoglycoside (exhibit a zone of inhibition around a standard 10-μg disc).[52] In vitro synergism between carbenicillin, ticarcillin or cephalosporins, on the one hand, and gentamicin or tobramycin, on the other, can be demonstrated for a majority of gram-negative bacilli aside from those shown in Table 3.[54,57] Moreover, there is a suggestion that the outcome of therapy of infections in immunosuppressed patients is better when the combination of drugs used is synergistic than when it is not.[49,54]

TABLE 2 Clinically Important Differences among Aminoglycosides in Their Antibacterial Spectrum

ANTIBIOTIC	SPECTRUM	COMMENTS
Streptomycin	Many gram-negative bacilli resistant	The only aminoglycoside with demonstrated activity against *Mycobacterium tuberculosis* in vivo[33]
Kanamycin	Most *Pseudomonas* resistant; some *E. coli* and *Klebsiella* resistant	
Gentamicin	Most aerobic gram-negative bacteria sensitive	Resistance is still uncommon among gram-negative aerobes, but is increasing. Some strains of *Proteus, Klebsiella, Serratia,* and *P. aeruginosa* resistant
Tobramycin	Similar to gentamicin. Bacteria highly resistant to gentamicin usually also resistant to tobramycin[36]	Although most (90%) of strains of *Pseudomonas* are sensitive to tobramycin and gentamicin, tobramycin is inhibitory at ⅓ the concentration of gentamicin. *Serratia* may be less sensitive to tobramycin than to gentamicin[22,24,25,30]
Amikacin	Similar to gentamicin, but active against many isolates of *Proteus, Pseudomonas,* and *Serratia* which are resistant to gentamicin and tobramycin[37,38]	A semisynthetic derivative of kanamycin that is resistant to many bacterial enzymes which degrade gentamicin and tobramycin[20,37]
Netilmicin	Similar to gentamicin[39–41]	Considerable diversity exists in reports of various investigators comparing in vitro activity of netilmicin with other aminoglycosides.[39–41] Netilmicin is probably no more active than gentamicin against most *Enterobacteriaceae;* organisms resistant to gentamicin will probably be resistant to netilmicin
Neomycin	Activity lies between that of kanamycin and gentamicin[42]	
Sisomicin	Similar to tobramycin[21,25]	

Drug antagonism has been demonstrated in vitro between aminoglycosides and clindamycin, chloramphenicol or tetracycline.[42,58] However, contradictory data have also been reported.[59] Fortunately, in view of the frequency with which the combination is used, there is no evidence of antagonism in vivo between clindamycin and gentamicin.[58]

PHARMACOLOGY

The aminoglycosides are highly polar molecules and are relatively insoluble in lipids. As a result: (1) they are minimally absorbed from the gut; (2) they penetrate the blood-brain and blood-ocular barriers poorly; (3) their dosage is more accurately calculated on the basis of 'lean' rather than total body weight;[60,61] (4) elimination occurs almost entirely by the kidney; and (5) they are moderately hemodialyzable. The pharmacokinetics of gentamicin, tobramycin, netilmicin and sisomicin appear to be very similar;[62–68] therefore, a common dosage schedule has been applied. Because of the similarity in the kinetics of kanamycin and amikacin,[69–71] these drugs are considered together, while streptomycin has been treated separately in this discussion. Detailed reviews of the pharmacokinetics of the aminoglycosides have been published recently.[72–74]

Absorption

The antibiotics are well absorbed by intramuscular injection, producing peak serum levels after about one hour (30 to 90 minutes).[62,71,72,75–78] In contrast, less than 1% of an oral dose is absorbed, and the resultant serum levels are usually insignificant in individuals with normal renal function.[73,75,77,79–82]

Repeated oral or rectal dosing may result in the accumulation of toxic levels of antibiotic in patients with impaired renal function.[80,83,84] Intoxication may also occur when aminoglycosides are applied topically to large denuded areas such as wounds, burns and ulcers, or are used to irrigate joints. Occasionally, absorption from these sites may be so extensive as to cause oto- or nephrotoxicity in persons without antecedent renal impairment.[75,85–88]

Peak Serum Levels

The aminoglycosides have similar volumes of distribution,[70,71,75,78,89–91] are eliminated by the kidney at comparable rates[70,71,75,77,78,92,93]

TABLE 3 Synergism between Aminoglycosides and Various Antibiotics

Disease	Synergism in vitro	Synergism in vivo	Comments
Streptococcus viridans endocarditis[45]	Penicillin G + streptomycin	No controlled trials	Many authors feel results not significantly different from those with penicillin G alone
Enterococcal endocarditis[32]	Penicillin G or ampicillin + streptomycin or gentamicin	Yes[32]	Strains that are extremely resistant to the aminoglycoside do not show synergism
S. aureus endocarditis	Nafcillin or oxacillin + aminoglycoside[46]	Not evident in preliminary studies[47]	Studies of this combination in humans are underway
Klebsiella pneumonia or bacteremia	Cephalosporin + aminoglycoside[48]	Data suggestive, but not statistically significant[49]	Some authors have recommended such a combination, especially in the immunosuppressed host[50]; others rely on a single antibiotic (cephalosporin or aminoglycoside) to which the organism is sensitive
Serious *Pseudomonas* infections	Carbenicillin or ticarcillin + gentamicin,[38,51,52] tobramycin, or amikacin[38,48]	Well demonstrated in experimental animals with and without granulocytopenia,[51,53] and clinical evidence exists of synergism in man[49,54]	For synergism to occur, the organism must be sensitive to the aminoglycoside[52]
Listeria monocytogenes[43]	Penicillin G or ampicillin + streptomycin or gentamicin	Not studied	May be of value in patients with *Listeria* meningitis or bacteremia with adverse prognostic factors

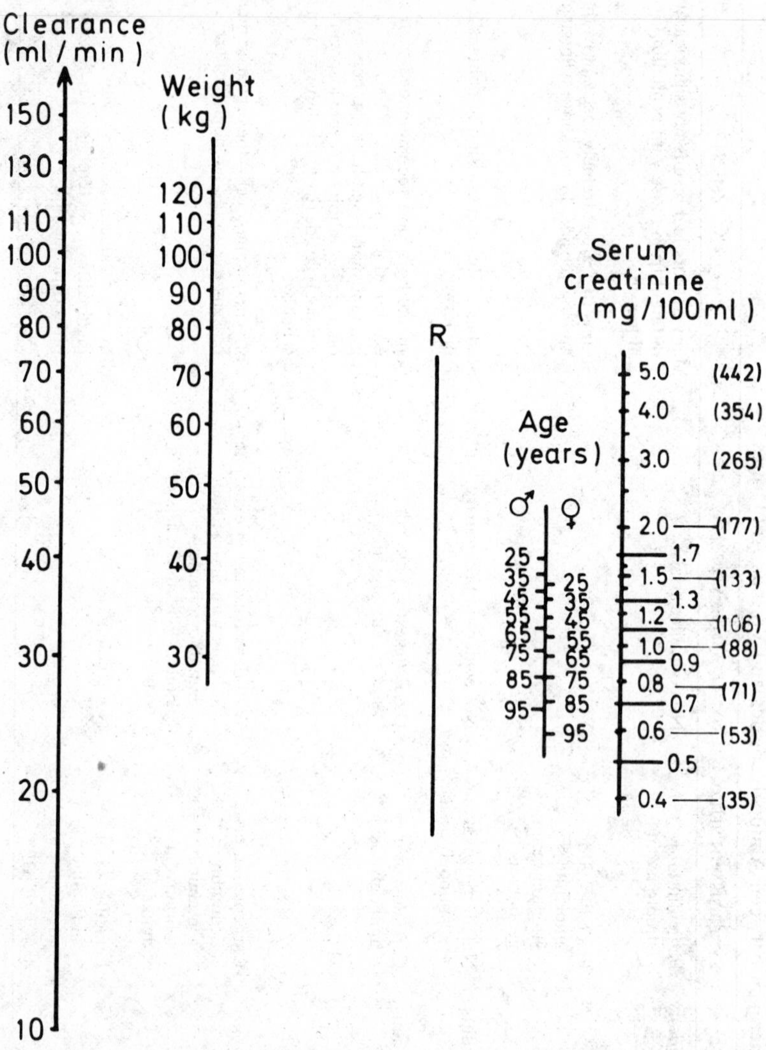

FIGURE 1. Nomogram for rapid evaluation of endogenous creatinine clearance. With a ruler, join weight to age. Keep ruler at crossing point of line marked R. Then move the right-hand side of the ruler to the appropriate serum-creatinine value read the patient's clearance from the left side of the nomogram. (Reproduced with permission from Siersbaek-Nielsen.[135])

TABLE 4 Serum Half-Life and Dialyzability of Systemically Administered Aminoglycosides in Patients with Normal and Impaired Renal Function

Antibiotic	Percent Protein Bound	Half-life (hours)		Renal Clearance (ml/min)	Dialysis Clearance (ml/min)	
		Normal Renal Function	Anephric		Hemodialysis	Peritoneal Dialysis
Gentamicin	0[65,73,94]	2[59,64,75]	30–60[64,72,73,89,96]	75–85[64,73]	26–48[64,96–98]	5–10[89,99]
Tobramycin	0[65,73,94]	2–3[62,65,89,93,95]	50–70[64,75,89,94,95]	80–90[63,73,93]	50–60[64,90]	15[89]
Kanamycin	0[65,77,94]	2–3[70,71,75,78]	40–80[72,75,83]	70–80[71,77,78]	30–40[96,100]	5–8[75,89,100–102]
Amikacin	0[70]	2–3[69–71, 76]	30–86[69,103]	75[70,71]	22[103]	6.4[103]
Streptomycin	30–35[72,75,94]	2–3[72,75,94]	100–110[72,73,75]	30–70[75]	17[100,104]	No data
Neomycin	?	3[72]	?	?	30–50[83,100,105]	10[100]

and are minimally protein-bound[65,72,73,75,87,94,95] (Table 4). Differences in their peak serum levels are chiefly a function of dosage; this is determined by a compromise between the therapeutic concentration and the level that can be achieved without substantial risk of toxicity (Table 5).

Distribution

Because they are insoluble in lipids, the aminoglycosides are essentially excluded from most body cells including adipose tissue, and from organs such as the central nervous system and the eye. They are distributed in an extracellular fluid volume which constitutes about 30% of lean body weight[61,91,109] (about 20 liters in an average adult); this fact can be used to predict the serum levels which will result from a particular dose, eg, 80 mg of gentamicin is distributed in 20 liters to yield a concentration of 4 μg/ml in serum and interstitial fluid.

Penetration of the blood-ocular barrier is so meager that effective therapy of bacterial endophthalmitis requires peri-ocular injections of the aminoglycosides.[71,110–115] Intrathecal or intraventricular administration is necessary to ensure adequate concentrations in the cerebrospinal fluid.[116–118] In contrast, levels in synovial fluid and placental tissue are approximately 25 to 50% of those in the serum.[72,75,79,119,120]

The aminoglycoside antibiotics have a marked affinity for renal cortical tissue, accumulating in concentrations which are 10 to 50 times those in serum.[77,119,121–123] There are pronounced differences among the various agents in this regard, those which show the greatest tendency to accumulate being the most nephrotoxic.[124] Much lower levels of drug are found in the renal medulla. The tissue:serum gradients in both cortex and medulla may be strikingly diminished in diseased kidneys,[112,121] although not all authors agree on this point.[122]

Elimination

The aminoglycosides are eliminated from the body by renal glomerular filtration. The half-lives are about two to three hours in patients with normal renal function, but are markedly longer in individuals with renal impairment (Table 4). Because the drugs are neither metabolized nor excreted in substantial quantities in the bile, hepatobiliary disease has little effect on their rates of elimina-

TABLE 5 Dosage of Aminoglycosides in Adults with Normal and Impaired Renal Function

Antibiotic[a]	Desirable Serum Level (μg/ml)		Toxic Range (μg/ml)[b]	Usual Dosage: Normal Renal Function (IM or IV)	Impaired Renal Function		Supplemental Dose after Each Hemodialysis[c]
	Peak	Trough			Initial (Loading) Dose	Maintenance Dose	
Gentamicin, Tobramycin, Sisomicin, Netilmicin[d]	5–8	1–2	>10–12	1.7 mg/kg every 8 hours	2 mg/kg	0.8–1 mg/kg at intervals (hours) = 3–4 times the serum creatinine (mg/dl)	½–¾ of the loading dose
Kanamycin, Amikacin	20–25	5–10	>30–35	5 mg/kg every 8 hours	7.5 mg/kg	3.5 mg/kg at intervals = 3–4 times the serum creatinine (mg/dl)	½–¾ of the loading dose
Streptomycin	5–20	<5	>40–50	7.5 mg/kg (~500 mg) every 12 hours	15 mg/kg (~1 g)	See Appendix	~¼ of the loading dose

[a] Antibiotics within each group show similar pharmacokinetics (see text). In obese individuals, an attempt should be made to calculate all dosages on the basis of "lean" or "ideal" body weight rather than total weight.

[b] References: 72, 73, 75, 85, 91, 95, 97, 106, 107 for gentamicin, tobramycin, sisomicin; 73, 79, 108 for kanamycin, amikacin.

[c] The higher value should be used where some renal function persists, the lower one in individuals who are anuric.

[d] Toxic range and desirable serum levels not yet established; values are extrapolated from those for gentamicin and are probably understimates.

tion. [72,75,77,119,122,125,126]One exception is streptomycin, which displays a longer half-life in individuals with combined renal and hepatic disease than in those with renal disease alone.[72]

DOSAGES IN PATIENTS WITH NORMAL AND IMPAIRED RENAL FUNCTION

Selecting an optimal dosage of the aminoglycosides is difficult for two reasons. First, the toxic dose in not much greater than the therapeutic one (Table 5); second, there is considerable variation among individuals both in the peak level of drug produced by a given dose and in the half-life of the antibiotic.[109,127] Therefore, it is advisable to measure the peak and trough concentrations every few days, especially in patients with impaired renal function.[128]

In order to saturate tissues and fluids with adequate concentrations of antibiotic, the initial (or 'loading') dose for patients *with serious infections* should not be less than that shown in Table 5, irrespective of the state of renal function.[61,129–131] The aminoglycosides are only sparingly distributed into fatty tissue; hence, the dose in obese individuals should be based on an approximation of the 'lean body mass' or 'ideal body weight.'[60]

Dosage in Renal Impairment

A variety of approaches has been suggested for dosage adjustments in patients with renal impairment.[74] Many of these consist of equations or nomograms based upon the serum creatinine concentration or the creatinine clearance (Appendix). We have been unable to duplicate the high degree of predictability of serum concentrations claimed by the proponents of these methods, and prefer to rely upon the following simple rule-of-thumb guided by frequent measurements of the serum concentrations of antibiotic.

Half Dose Every Half-life. The serum half-life is the time required for the serum concentration of a substance to fall by 50%. If half of the loading dose is administered every half-life, serum levels will fluctuate between the peak and half of that concentration. For gentamicin, tobramycin, sisomicin and probably netilmicin, the 'half-dose' is 0.8–1.0 mg/kg; for kanamycin and amikacin, it is 3.5 mg/kg (Table 5). It has been empirically observed that the half-life, in hours, can be estimated by multiplying the serum creatinine concentration (mg/dl) by 3 or 4.[129,130,138] The value 4 seems to be more

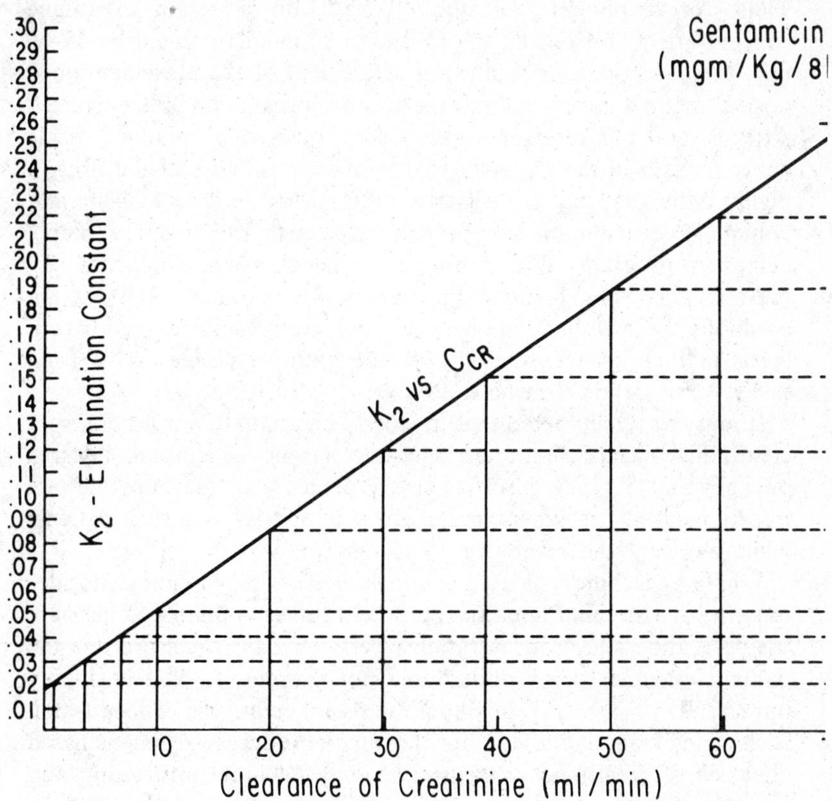

FIGURE 2. Gentamicin, tobramycin, and netilmicin nomogram for patients with renal failure. To use the nomogram regimen, a loading dose of gentamicin, 1.7 mg/kg body weight, is administered. The sustaining dose is determined by passing a line perpendicular from the patient's C_{cr} value to the point where it intercepts the sloping line (K_2 vs. C_{cr}) on the nomogram. From the point of intercept, a horizontal line intersects the dose schedule, on the right side. This dose should be given every 8 hours for steady-state therapy. (Reproduced with permission from Chan et al.[131])

applicable to patients with serum creatinine concentrations of $\geqq 6$ mg/dl, and the value 3 for those with less severe renal impairment.[130] Thus, for a patient weighing 60 kg, with a serum creatinine concentration of 4 mg/dl, the dosage of gentamicin would be 48–60 mg every 12 hours. A significant refinement of the aforementioned dosing method has been advanced by Sawchuk and associates.[139] After several measurements have been obtained of aminoglycoside concentration in the patient's serum following a dose of the drug, a highly individualized and accurate estimate of the drug half-life and volume of distribution can be calculated with the aid of a simple computer program. With these data, the clinician can accurately prescribe a dosing regimen that will result in blood levels of the antibiotic that will fluctuate between pre-determined peak and trough levels. Other dosage schemes for the aminoglycosides have been reviewed in detail elsewhere.[74,140]

It must be remembered that in elderly individuals, a normal serum creatinine concentration often belies the presence of a minimal degree of age-related renal insufficiency.[68] Except in the most severe infections, it is best to err on the low side of dosage in such patients while awaiting the results of serum assays.

Whatever technique is used to adjust the dosage of aminoglycosides in patients with renal impairment, it is extremely valuable to measure the peak and valley concentrations every few days to ensure that the patient is neither being underdosed nor overdosed. This is doubly important in individuals in whom the serum creatinine concentration is changing from day to day; for these patients dosage regimens based on a single creatinine concentration may be quite misleading and direct measurements of the serum level of antibiotic are indispensable. Blood for these determinations should be drawn just before, and approximately one hour after, the dose is given.

Carbenicillin and ticarcillin have been shown to inactivate gentamicin in vitro and in vivo.[141,142] This interaction is of no clinical significance in individuals with normal renal function if the drugs are not mixed and allowed to stand before they are administered;[143] however, the half-life of gentamicin may be shortened considerably in azotemic patients who are receiving ticarcillin or carbenicillin.[142] Measurements of the serum level of antibiotic are particularly useful in this situation.

The aminoglycosides are minimally removed by peritoneal dialysis, but are copiously hemodialyzable (Table 4). Thus, it is advisable to administer a supplemental dose after each hemodialysis. Because the

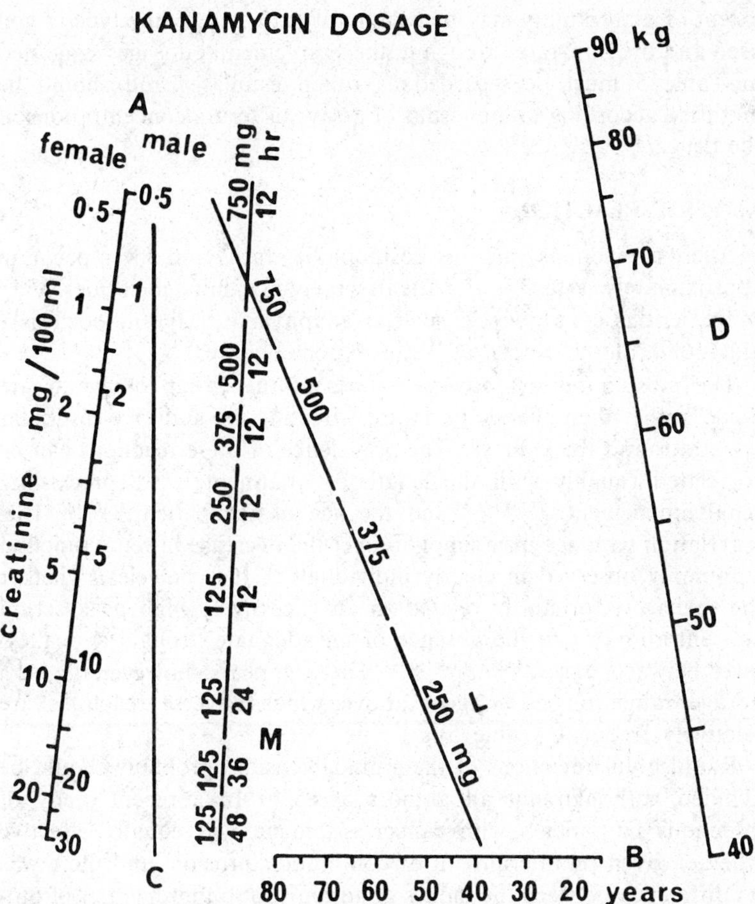

FIGURE 3. Kanamycin and amikacin nomogram for patients with renal failure. 1. Join with a straight line the serum-creatinine concentration appropriate to the sex on scale A and age on scale B. Mark the point at which the straight line cuts line C. 2. Join with a straight line the mark on line C and the body weight on scale D. Mark the points at which this line cuts the dosage lines L and M. 3. The loading dose (mg) is written against the marked part of line L. The maintenance dose (mg) and the appropriate interval (hours) between doses are written against the marked part of line M. 4. If the patient is severely oliguric, the dose schedule should be obtained by joining with a straight line the lowest point on line C to the body weight on scale D. 5. After a period of hemodialysis of 6 hours or more, a booster dose of half the loading dose is necessary in addition to the maintenance dose indicated by the nomogram. (Reproduced with permission from Mawer et al.[136])

extent of dialyzability may be profoundly affected by the type of coil used and the flow-rate through it, the supplemental dosages suggested in Table 5 must be regarded as rough estimates and should be modified according to the results of assays of serum concentrations of the drug.[89,90,96–99,102,128,131]

ADVERSE REACTIONS

Allergic reactions, such as eosinophilia, rash, and fever occur in approximately 1 to 3% of patients receiving aminoglycosides.[72,75,144] More serious consequences such as anaphylaxis,[87] agranulocytosis[145] and other blood dyscrasias,[75] are extremely rare.

The most important adverse effects of this group of agents are 'toxic' rather than allergic in nature, affecting the auditory-vestibular apparatus and the kidneys. The prevalence of these reactions can be correlated roughly with the length of treatment,[72,146,147] preexisting renal impairment, [72,144,147–149]and the age of the patient.[72,106,148] The correlation with age may simply reflect the decrease in renal function commonly observed in elderly individuals.[68] It is not clear whether the toxicity is primarily related to an excessively high peak serum concentration, or to the absence of an adequate 'trough' or 'valley' level between doses.[86,128,139,140,150,151] There appears, however, to be a dosage range for each agent above which adverse reactions are relatively frequent (Table 5).

Rapid bolus injections of the aminoglycosides probably should be avoided, although not all authors agree.[152] In a recent study of infections in patients with cancer, sisomicin was equally effective whether given by intermittent or continuous infusion, and there was no difference between the modes of administration in the rates of oto- or nephrotoxicity.[153]

Ototoxicity

Two types of ototoxicity have been observed. Cochlear damage, manifested by varying degrees of hearing loss, especially for high tones, is characteristic of kanamycin, amikacin, neomycin and paromomycin. Vestibular impairment, resulting in disequilibrium, nystagmus, nausea, vomiting, and vertigo, is more commonly associated with gentamicin, tobramycin and streptomycin. However, these distinctions are not absolute and any of the drugs can produce either or both forms of toxicity.

There is considerable disagreement as to the incidence of

TABLE 5 Dosage of Aminoglycosides in Adults with Normal and Impaired Renal Function

Antibiotic[a]	Desirable Serum Level (μg/ml)		Toxic Range	Usual Dosage: Normal Renal Function	Impaired Renal Function		Supplemental Dose after Each
	Peak	Trough	(2 g/ml)[b]	(IM or IV)	Initial (Loading) Dose	Maintenance Dose	Hemodialysis[c]
Gentamicin							
Tobramycin	5–8	1–2	>10–12	1.7 mg/kg every 8 hours	2 mg/kg	0.8–1 mg/kg at intervals (hours) = 3–4 times the serum creatinine (mg/dl)	½–¾ of the loading dose
Sisomicin							
Netilmicin[d]							
Kanamycin	20–25	5–10	>30–35	5 mg/kg every 8 hours	7.5 mg/kg	3.5 mg/kg at intervals = 3–4 times the serum creatinine (mg/dl)	½–¾ of the loading dose
Amikacin							
Streptomycin	5–20	<5	>40–50	7.5 mg/kg ≅ 500 mg) every 12 hours	15 mg/kg (≅ 1 g)	See Appendix	≅ ¼ of the loading dose

[a] Antibiotics within each group show similar pharmacokinetics (see text). In obese individuals, an attempt should be made to calculate all dosages on the basis of "lean" or "ideal" body weight rather than total weight.

[b] References: 72, 73, 75, 85, 91, 95, 97, 106, and 107 for gentamicin, tobramycin, sisomicin; 73, 79, and 108 for kanamycin and amikacin.

[c] The higher value should be used where some renal function persists, the lower one in individuals who are anuric.

[d] Toxic range and desirable serum levels are not yet established; values are extrapolated from those for gentamicin and are probably underestimates.

ototoxicity caused by the aminoglycosides. In part, this may be due to differences in the accuracy of monitoring of dosages in earlier studies, and to variable attention to the detection of subclinical damage by means of electronystagmography and audiometry. Overall, the incidence of *clinically-overt* ototoxicity in patients given usual dosages of antibiotics for not more than two weeks is approximately 2% for gentamicin[72,75,85,87,148] and 1% for kanamycin[77,144,149] and streptomycin.[75,144,154] Where less rigid criteria for dosage and duration of therapy were used, the incidence of this side effect has been found to be as high as 5 to 30% with kanamycin.[75] Although tobramycin appears to be less ototoxic than gentamicin in animals,[63,107,155] there is no basis for extending these impressions to humans.[156] Preliminary data suggest that the incidence of eighth nerve damage with amikacin is similar to that with gentamicin.[157] The ototoxicity of netilmicin appears to be strikingly less than that of gentamicin in experimental animals;[66] however, controlled comparisons in man are not yet available.[158] It must be emphasized that the frequency of subclinical ototoxicity is considerably higher than that of clinically-overt disease, approaching an incidence of 10–20% or higher with many of the congeners when these are given in high dosage for appreciable periods.[108,157]

There is also wide divergence of opinion as to the reversibility of aminoglycoside-related ototoxicity. Damage owing to gentamicin appears to be reversible in about half the cases,[148,150] while that owing to the other analogs may be less likely to improve with time.[75,122,144,159] Progressive eighth nerve damage after the drugs have been discontinued has been observed with many of the aminoglycosides with the possible exception of kanamycin.[72,108,149,160]

The ototoxic effects of the aminoglycosides are potentiated by coadministration of ethacrynic acid,[72,75,160–162] furosemide,[72,160] mannitol,[161] and possibly other diuretics.[75] Adverse effects are probably also increased by concomitant administration of other ototoxic antimicrobials, and perhaps by prior treatment with such agents.[72] It should be noted that vestibular dysfunction may be masked by the concurrent administration of drugs which suppress nausea and vomiting of vestibular origin and vertigo (eg, dimenhydrinate, meclizine).[162]

Patients receiving aminoglycosides should be observed carefully for signs and symptoms of ototoxicity. If possible, other drugs which may potentiate this effect should be avoided. Although they provide only a rough guide, it is often helpful to monitor the serum levels of an antibiotic.[128] If long-term therapy (eg, more than 10 to 14 days) is anticipated, it may be useful to obtain sequential tests of auditory and vestibular function.

Nephrotoxicity

Aminoglycosides damage the proximal tubular cells of the kidney, sparing the glomeruli. The resultant clinical picture is that of acute tubular necrosis of greater or less degree.[83,163] The mechanism of this phenomenon is not fully established, however, it is known that these antibiotics accumulate in renal cortical tissue in concentrations which greatly exceed those in the serum, and persist there for days following a single dose of drug.[121,122,163] Streptomycin, which is relatively free of nephrotoxicity, displays a much weaker affinity for renal tissue than do other aminoglycosides.[124] As is true of ototoxicity, the relative importance of the peak and trough serum levels is not clear.[128,140]

The incidence of clinically-significant renal damage varies widely among the congeners. As mentioned, streptomycin is essentially nontoxic in usual doses;[83,87] earlier reports suggesting a moderate incidence of renal dysfunction with streptomycin probably reflected the use of higher dosages and less pure preparations.[83] Gentamicin and tobramycin produce mild abnormalities of renal function in about 8% of the recipients[140] and more severe effects in about 2%.[72,85,87,95] However, recent data suggest that, in controlled comparisons, the rate of nephrotoxicity of tobramycin is less than that of gentamicin in humans.[72,85,87,95,156,164–166] For kanamycin, and probably amikacin, the corresponding rates of nephrotoxicity are approximately 6% and 3%, respectively.[70,72,75,144,157] Higher rates of nephrotoxicity have been reported with various aminoglycosides, especially in severely ill patients.[167] Data in animals suggest that netilmicin may be less nephrotoxic than gentamicin.[66] However, preliminary results in non-randomized patients do not support a major benefit for netilmicin in this regard.[158,a]

Absorption of neomycin and paromomycin from mucosal surfaces can result in damage to the ear and kidney; this phenomenon is usually, but not exclusively,[75,88] seen in patients with preexisting renal disease (see Absorption).[72,82,83,84,168]

In contrast to ototoxicity, renal damage is usually reversible if the aminoglycoside is discontinued at the first signs of renal dysfunction,[77,83,85,87,140,144] such as a rising blood urea nitrogen (BUN), serum

a Unpublished data.

creatinine or the presence of protein or tubular cells in the urine.[72,83,95] Oliguria may or may not be present. One of the earliest signs of nephrotoxicity is the finding of lysosomal hydrolase enzymes in the urine;[72,163,169] however, most laboratories are not able to perform such determinations.

Considerable controversy exists over the role of other factors in promoting the nephrotoxicity of the aminoglycosides. There is general agreement that dehydration (and, by extension, potent diuretics),[83] methoxyfluorane,[162] the polymyxins, amphotericin B and vancomycin[84] are capable of potentiating aminoglycoside-induced nephrotoxicity. Cephalothin was shown to have a similar effect in three studies,[166,170,171] but not in another.[168] A number of investigations have failed to show such an interaction between cephalosporins and aminoglycosides in laboratory animals; indeed, the former actually protected against aminoglycoside-induced nephrotoxicity when the two drugs were given simultaneously.[172,173] On the basis of available data, we conclude that there probably is an increased risk of nephrotoxicity with this pair of drugs in humans. Although we do not hesitate to use the combination where it is clinically warranted, we follow renal function carefully in such patients.

Other Adverse Reactions

Other potentially important adverse reactions that have been associated with aminoglycoside therapy include:

Neuromuscular blockade, qualitatively similar to that produced by conventional blocking agents (d-tubocurarine, pancuronium). Patients with myasthenia gravis or severe hypocalcemia as well as patients who have recently received other neuromuscular-blocking drugs appear to be particularly sensitive to this adverse effect,[72,162,174,175] although significant neuromuscular blockade has been reported in a rare patient with no such predisposing factors.[174,176] Peritoneal lavage with solutions of these drugs may precipitate apnea,[72,86,149] possibly because high concentrations of the antibiotic come into direct contact with the diaphragm.

The propensity of the various congeners to block neuromuscular transmission differs widely; the relative potency being, in decreasing order: neomycin > streptomycin > kanamycin and amikacin > gentamicin and tobramycin.[87,177,178] Studies in animals suggest that netilmicin may be among the more active paralysants.[66] Blockade induced by any of the aminoglycosides can be partially or completely reversed by the administration of calcium salts intravenously.[175,177–179] The efficacy of cholinomimetic agents (edrophonium, neostigmine) is highly variable. A detailed consideration of the mechanism underlying this adverse reaction is published elsewhere.[140,175,177,179]

Malabsorption of fat, protein, cholesterol, various sugars, iron, digitalis, and other substances has been observed following the oral administration of neomycin, kanamycin, and paromomycin.[72,75,81,180–184] The effect is trivial or absent when the drugs are administered parenterally.[75,184]

The following adverse effects have occasionally been attributed to aminoglycoside therapy, although the role of the antibiotic is often unclear: transient elevations of SGOT, SGPT, and alkaline phosphatase;[95] neurotoxicity manifested by pain and paresthesias,[75,87] blurring of vision, or an acute organic brain syndrome;[149] optic neuritis (scotomas and enlargement of the blind spot);[75,87,144] depression of cardiac function following rapid parenteral administration of streptomycin or kanamycin.[185]

Although bowel flora is altered in patients receiving oral aminoglycosides, suprainfection is infrequent and acute enterocolitis is exceedingly rare.[75,81]

Streptomycin and kanamycin rarely can cause ototoxicity to the fetus; the safety of the other aminoglycosides during pregnancy is not established.[186,187]

THERAPEUTIC USE (Table 6)

Gram-Negative Bacillary Infections

The aminoglycosides are highly effective for infections owing to a variety of aerobic gram-negative rods which are resistant to less toxic drugs (penicillins, cephalosporins). They are also valuable in combination with a penicillin, cephalosporin, and occasionally, chloramphenicol or clindamycin in the initial therapy of suspected bacteremia pending identification of the infecting organism. For empiric treatment of bacteremia in the immunosuppressed host, any pair of the following drugs provides equally effective therapy: a cephalosporin, carbenicillin or ticarcillin or an aminoglycoside.[170,171,188,189] It is useful to bear in mind some common pathogens which are not 'covered' by frequently-used combinations (Table 7).

TABLE 6 Therapeutic Use of Aminoglycosides[a]

Drugs of First Choice	Useful Alternative	Aminoglycosides "Cover"	Demonstrated Benefit in Combination	Ineffective or Weakly Effective
Infections due to aerobic gram-negative rods which are resistant to penicillins or cephalosporins (gentamicin or tobramycin)	Most gram-negative rod infections (gentamicin or tobramycin)	*Mycoplasma*	Enterococcal endocarditis (streptomycin or gentamicin)	Gonococcus, meningococcus
		Staphylococci		Anaerobic bacteria
	Gonorrhea (spectinomycin only)[b]	*Salmonella*	Tuberculosis (streptomycin)	CNS infection (unless administered intrathecally or intraventricularly)
Peritonitis (gentamicin or tobramycin)		*H. influenzae*	Serious *pseudomonas* infection (carbenicillin or ticarcillin with tobramycin, amikacin or gentamicin)	
Nongonococcal pelvic inflammatory disease (gentamicin or tobramycin)				Streptococci, pneumococci, enterococci
Most *Serratia* (gentamicin, amikacin)				
Most *pseudomonas* (tobramycin, gentamicin, or amikacin)				

[a]Although we have suggested specific congeners in parentheses, the choice may be altered by the results of in vitro susceptibility data or the pattern of sensitivity in the particular institution.

[b]See text.

TABLE 7 Common Pathogens Not Inhibited by Some Antimicrobial Combinations[a]

Combinations	Organisms Not Inhibited	Comments
Cephalothin + gentamicin	*B. fragilis* Enterococci Some strains of *Proteus*	Neither drug penetrates CNS well
Carbenicillin + gentamicin		May not be as effective as clindamycin vs. *B. fragilis*
Cephalothin + carbenicillin	*Serratia* Some strains of *Klebsiella*	Resistant pseudomonas may emerge
Clindamycin + gentamicin	Gonococci, meningococci Enterococci	Neither drug penetrates CNS well
Penicillin G or ampicillin + gentamicin	*B. fragilis* Some strains of *Proteus*	
Chloramphenicol + gentamicin		May not provide optimal coverage for staphylococcus and enterococcus

[a]In many instances (e.g., carbenicillin for *B. fragilis*, gentamicin for *S. aureus*), the combination does not provide the best therapy for a given pathogen, but will generally suffice as a "holding action" until the specific organism has been identified.

Combination Therapy for Defined Single Organisms

There are many examples of in vitro synergism involving aminoglycosides; however, only a few of these have been examined and shown to be of value in vivo (Table 3). The best known example is enterococcal endocarditis for which penicillin G or ampicillin should be combined with streptomycin or gentamicin.

Streptomycin, but not gentamicin,[33] is a first-line antituberculous drug. It should always be given in combination with other agents to forestall the development of antimicrobial resistance. It is important to note that while many isolates of *Mycobacterium tuberculosis* are sensitive in vitro to most of the aminoglycosides, all but streptomycin appear to be lacking in efficacy in the treatment of human and animal infections.[33,189a,189b]

Pseudomonas bacteremia remains a disease of high mortality despite the availability of potent anti-*Pseudomonas* antibiotics.[190] Because

TABLE 8 Preparations and Costs of Aminoglycosides

Generic Name	Trademark Name(s)	Preparations and 1978 Costs
Gentamicin Sulfate	Garamycin	Injection (solution) 10 mg/ml—$2.55/2-ml ampul; 40 mg/ml—$4.39/2-ml ampul
Kanamycin Sulfate	Kantrex	Injection (solution) 37.5 mg/ ml—$3.55/2-ml ampul; 250 mg/ml—$7.74/2-ml ampul; 333 mg/ ml—$13.93/3-ml ampul
Tobramycin Sulfate	Nebcin	Injection (solution) 10 mg/ ml—$2.20/2-ml ampul; 40 mg/ml—$4.42/2-ml ampul
Amikacin Sulfate	Amikin	Injection (solution) 50 mg/ ml—$4.97/2-ml ampul; 250 mg/ml—$8.33/2-ml ampul, $16.36/4-ml ampul
Neomycin Sulfate	Mycifradin Sulfate (Neobiotic)	Tablets 500 mg—$28.59/100 Solution 125 mg/5 ml—$1.46/2 oz Injection (powder) 500 mg—$3.73/vial
Streptomycin Sulfate	generic	Injection (powder) 1 g—$0.64–$0.68/vial; 5 g—$1.82–$2.20/vial

carbenicillin and aminoglycosides appear to exert a synergistic effect against this organism in vivo,[49,51,53,54] the combination should be strongly considered for the treatment of serious *Pseudomonas* infections, especially in immunosuppressed patients. There is recent evidence that ticarcillin plus tobramycin may be even more effective for serious pulmonary infection due to this organism.[191] In institutions with a substantial prevalence of gentamicin-resistant strains, amikacin will be the aminoglycoside of choice in this setting until the susceptibility of the infecting agent has been determined.

Mixed Infections

Peritonitis and suppurative pelvic disease in women are generally caused by a mixture of anaerobic and facultatively (optionally) aerobic organisms. These infections usually respond well to a combination of clindamycin and gentamicin; however, if there is any likelihood of the presence of the gonococcus, penicillin G or ampicillin should be added if there is persistent infection from which the enterococcus is cultured. Recent data suggest that ticarcillin plus an aminoglycoside may be as effective as clindamycin with an aminoglycoside for anaerobic sepsis[192] and ticarcillin should provide effective coverage for the enterococcus and gonococcus in situations in which these organisms may be present.

Aspiration pneumonia can generally be treated with penicillin G alone. This generalization does not apply to patients who are at high risk of nasopharyngeal colonization by gram-negative enteric bacilli because of residence for several days or more in the hospital, endotracheal or nasogastric intubation, or exposure to broad-spectrum antibiotics; when aspiration occurs in this setting, it is prudent to add an aminoglycoside until the bacteriology is defined.

Although aminoglycosides are not drugs of choice, they will generally 'cover' unsuspected *Staphylococcus aureus* and *epidermidis, Salmonella* and *H. influenzae* until more effective and safer therapy can be selected.

The aminoglycosides are *not effective* against anaerobic bacteria, meningococci, most strains of streptococci (including β-hemolytic streptococci and *Strep. viridans*), enterococci and pneumococci. Staphylococci are readily inhibited by aminoglycosides, but penicillins and cephalosporins provide much safer therapy for infections due to these organisms. Systemically-administered aminoglycosides do not penetrate the central nervous system (CNS) well; therefore, treatment of meningitis with these agents generally requires intrathecal or intraventricular injection (see below).

Spectinomycin, which is actually an aminocyclitol rather than an aminoglycoside, is given in a single intramuscular dose of 2 g for the treatment of uncomplicated anogenital gonorrhea in patients who cannot receive, or have failed on, penicillin G with probenecid.[193] Repeated doses of spectinomycin may be effective for more extensive gonococcal infections. Generally speaking, spectinomycin appears to be as effective as tetracycline.[194] It also appears to be active against penicillin-resistant gonococci. The drug does not provide reliable therapy for syphilis. Although other aminoglycosides may be effective for gonorrhea when given in high dosage,[195] they cannot be recommended for this purpose.

Intrathecal and Intraventricular Gentamicin

Gentamicin is useful in the therapy of meningitis due to aerobic enteric gram-negative rods.[187] Because of its poor penetration into the meninges even in the presence of inflammation, it should be given intrathecally for such infections.[196–199] A dosage of 4 mg produces peak cerebrospinal fluid concentrations of 20 to 40 μg/ml; this dosage should be repeated every 18 hours to maintain inhibitory concentrations.[196] The preferred vehicle is a relatively neutral solution such as normal saline without a bacteriostatic additive, or even cerebrospinal fluid itself. Adverse effects with this regimen are extremely uncommon.[200] For therapy of bacterial ventriculitis, it may be advisable to instill the drug into the ventricle through an Ommaya or Rickham reservoir because diffusion from the lumbar sac is inefficient.[117]

PROPHYLACTIC USE

Streptomycin or gentamicin in combination with penicillin G is useful for the prophylaxis of endocarditis in patients with valvular heart disease who are undergoing abdominal or pelvic surgery. Topical, and occasionally systemic, gentamicin has been effective in the short run in preventing *Pseudomonas* infections in burn patients;[201] but this therapy should be discouraged because of the risks of fostering gentamicin resistance. Controlled studies have demonstrated the efficacy of oral neomycin together with erythromycin or tetracycline in reducing the rate of postoperative wound infections in patients undergoing bowel surgery.[202] Oral antibiotic mixtures have been thought to be of value in 'sterilizing' the intestine of leukemic patients, thereby reducing the rate of infections.[92] Again, however, the risk of selecting resistant organisms poses a serious hazard.

SELECTION OF AN AMINOGLYCOSIDE

Clinical data support the value of streptomycin in the therapy of tuberculosis, brucellosis, tularemia and yersinia infections; several of these require the coadministration of another agent. The choice between streptomycin and gentamicin for combination therapy of enterococcal endocarditis may be simplified by knowledge of the prevalence of high-level streptomycin-resistant strains in the hospital, or by use of an in vitro screening test.[32] Neomycin is the agent used orally in the treatment of hepatic encephalopathy.[203] Paromomycin is presently indicated only for the treatment of amebic infections.

There appear to be few differences among gentamicin, tobramycin and amikacin in their efficacy against infections due to susceptible organisms[36,157,167,171,186] or in their relative safety. In general, tobramycin is somewhat more active than gentamicin against strains of *Pseudomonas aeruginosa* and somewhat less active against *Serratia*. However, the major difference among the congeners in terms of their antibacterial activity lies in the low but increasing prevalence of gram-negative bacilli which are resistant to gentamicin and tobramycin but susceptible to amikacin. As a result, in institutions in which gentamicin-resistant strains are of concern, amikacin is the aminoglycoside of choice for serious infections until the antibiotic susceptibility of the infecting bacterium has been determined. In terms of safety, there is a strong, but not statistically significant, suggestion that tobramycin is less nephrotoxic than gentamicin; where long-term therapy is indicated, the physician may wish to take advantage of the possibility of less nephrotoxicity with this agent. The relative safety of netilmicin remains to be determined.

APPENDIX: NOMOGRAMS AND EQUATIONS FOR DOSAGE ADJUSTMENTS IN RENAL FAILURE

1. Clearance from Serum Creatinine Concentration

The methods described in the body of this chapter for adjusting the dosage of aminoglycosides in patients with renal failure (half-dose every half-life, or full dose every two to three half-lives) are relatively imprecise. To some extent, this reflects the inexactness of the serum creatinine concentration as a measure of the glomerular filtration rate, and hence, of elimination of aminoglycoside antibiotics. Although the creatinine clearance is a more reliable guide to the rate of glomerular filtration than the serum creatinine concentration, it is subject to errors in the accuracy of the urine collection, and is also an imperfect measure of the rate of glomerular filtration.[132,133] Many authors favor the use of an *estimated creatinine clearance,* which is based upon the serum creatinine concentration, and corrected for age, sex, and (in some instances) body weight. The following formula[134] and nomogram (Figure 1) for the derivation of creatinine clearance are provided for the calculation of the half-life of gentamicin and related drugs:

Males:

$$\text{Estimated creatinine clearance (ml/min)} = \frac{98 - [0.8\,(\text{Age} - 20)]}{Cr_s}.$$

Females:

$$\text{Estimated creatinine clearance (ml/min)} = \text{0.9} \times \text{estimated creatinine clearance in males.}$$

Age is expressed in years, Cr_s is serum creatinine concentration (mg/dl).

2. Gentamicin, Tobramycin, Netilmicin, and Sisomicin in Renal Failure

a. Formula:[61]

$$t_{1/2} = \frac{3.5\ x\ \text{ideal body weight (kg)}}{\text{creatinine clearance (ml/min)}}.$$

A dose of 0.8–1.0 mg/kg is given every half-life.

b. Nomogram:[131] See Figure 2.

3. Amikacin in Renal Failure

Nomogram:[136] See Figure 3.

4. Streptomycin in Renal Failure [137]

Normal renal function: 7.5 mg/kg every 12 hours; creatinine clearance 50–80 ml/min: 7.5 mg/kg every 24 hours; creatinine clearance 10–50 ml/min: 7.5 mg/kg every 24–72 hours; and creatinine clearance <10 ml/min: 7.5 mg/kg every 72–96 hours.

In addition to these various regimens, it is possible to perform several sequential measurements of the serum levels of antibiotic after a dose and, by plotting the values on semilogarithmic coordinates, to determine the half-life of the drug directly. Despite the aura of precision and reliability that surrounds the various formulas and nomograms presented in this section, none of them has been shown to be substantially more accurate in the individual patient than the simple technique described in this paper (half-dose every half-life), and it is our belief that each of them should be monitored by assays of the peak and trough concentrations of antibiotic.

REFERENCES

1. Rinehart KL Jr: Comparative chemistry of the aminoglycoside and aminocyclitol antibiotics. J Infect Dis 119:345–350, 1969.
2. Bryan LE, van den Elzen HM: Streptomycin accumulation in susceptible and resistant strains of *Escherichia coli* and *Pseudomonas aeruginosa.* Antimicrob Agents Chemother 9:928–938, 1976.
3. Davis BD, Dulbecoo R, Eisen HN, et al: Protein synthesis. In *Microbiology,* 2nd edition. Hagerstown, Maryland, Harper and Row, 1973, pp 300–303.
4. Davis J: Bacterial resistance to aminoglycoside antibiotics. J Infect Dis 124(Suppl):S7–S10, 1971.
5. Finland M: Changing patterns of susceptibility of common bacterial pathogens to antimicrobial agents. Ann Intern Med 76:1009–1036, 1972.
6. Seal DV, Strangeways JEM: Aminoglycoside resistance due to mutation. Lancet 1:856–857, 1977.
7. Bryan LE, Shahrabadi MS, van den Elzen HM: Gentamicin resistance in *Pseudomonas aeruginosa:* R-factor-mediated resistance. Antimicrob Agents Chemother 6:191–199, 1974.
8. Dowding JE: Mechanisms of gentamicin resistance in *Staphylococcus aureus.* Antimicrob Agents Chemother 11:47–50, 1977.
9. Falkow S: *Infectious Multiple Drug Resistance.* London, Pion, Ltd., 1975.
10. Price KE, Casson K, DeRegis RG, et al: Amikacin: antimicrobial properties and resistance mechanisms affecting its activity. Am J Med (U.S. Amikacin Symposium) June, 1977, pp 14–24.
11. Davies J, Courvalin P: Mechanisms of resistance to aminoglycosides. Am J Med 62:868–872, 1977.
12. Seligman SJ: Frequency of resistance to kanamycin, tobramycin, netilmicin and amikacin in gentamicin-resistant gram-negative bacteria. Antimicrob Agents Chemother 13:70–73, 1978.
13. Acar JF, Witchitz JL, Goldstein F, et al: Susceptibility of aminoglycoside-resistant gram-negative bacilli to amikacin: delineation of individual resistance patterns. J Infect Dis 134(Suppl):S280–S285, 1976.
14. Reynolds AV, Hamilton-Miller JMT, Brumfitt W: In vitro activity of amikacin and ten other aminoglycoside antibiotics against gentamicin-resistant bacterial strains. J Infect Dis 134(Suppl):S291–S296, 1976.
15. Echeverria P, Lew MA, Smith AL: Apparent emergence of aminoglycoside-resistant *Escherichia coli* during neonatal meningitis. N Engl J Med 293:913–914, 1975.
16. Walker SH: Aminoglycoside-resistant *Esch. coli.* N Engl J Med 295:225–226, 1976.
17. Roberts NJ Jr, Douglas RG Jr: Gentamicin use and *Pseudomonas* and *Serratia* resistance: effect of a surgical prophylaxis regimen. Antimicrob Agents Chemother 13:214–220, 1978.
18. Geddes AM, Goodall JAD, Speirs CF, et al: Clinical and laboratory studies with tobramycin. Chemotherapy 20:245–256, 1974.
19. Price KE, Chisholm DR, Misiek M, et al: Microbiological evaluation of BB-K8, a new semisynthetic aminoglycoside. J Antibiot 25:709–731, 1972.
20. Tally FP, Louis TJ, Weinstein NM, et al: Amikacin therapy for severe gram-negative sepsis. Ann Intern Med 83:484–488, 1975.
21. Young LS, Hewitt WL: Activity of five aminoglycoside antibiotics in vitro against gram-negative bacilli and *Staphylococcus aureus.* Antimicrob Agents Chemother 4:133–139, 1973.
22. Burger LM, Sanford JP, Zweighaft T: Tobramycin: bacteriological evaluation. Am J Med Sci 265:135–142, 1973.
23. Yu PKW, Washington JA: Comparative in vitro activity of three aminoglycosidic antibiotics. II. BB-K8, kanamycin, and gentamicin. Antimicrob Agents Chemother 4:133–139, 1973.
24. Reynolds AV, Hamilton-Miller JMT, Brumfitt W: Newer aminoglycosides—amikacin and tobramycin: an in vitro comparison with kanamycin and gentamicin. Br Med J 3:778–780, 1974.
25. Waitz JA, Moss EL Jr, Drube CG, et al: Comparative activity of sisomicin, gentamicin, kanamycin and tobramycin. Antimicrob Agents Chemother 2:431–437, 1972.

26. Dienstag J, Neu HC: In vitro studies of tobramycin, an aminoglycoside antibiotic. Antimicrob Agents Chemother 1:41–45, 1972.
27. Duncan IBR, Penner JL: Comparative activity of tobramycin and gentamicin against *Pseudomonas, Proteus* and *Providencia* species. Can Med Assoc J 113:29–31, 1975.
28. Sabath LD, Garner C, Wilcox C, et al: Susceptibility of *Staphylococcus aureus* and *Staphylococcus epidermidis* to 65 antibiotics. Antimicrob Agents Chemother 9:962–969, 1976.
29. Black WA, van Buskirk F: Gentamicin as a selective agent for the isolation of beta haemolytic streptococci. J Clin Pathol 26:154–156, 1973.
30. Hyams PJ, Simberkoff MS, Rahal JJ Jr: In vitro bactericidal effectiveness of four aminoglycoside antibiotics. Antimicrob Agents Chemother 3:87–94, 1973.
31. Waitz JA, Weinstein MJ: Recent microbiological studies with gentamicin. J Infect Dis 119:355–360, 1969.
32. Moellering RC Jr, Wennersten C, Medrek T, et al: Prevalence of high-level resistance to aminoglycosides in clinical isolates of enterococci. Antimicrob Agents Chemother —1970, pp 335–340.
33. Sanders WE, Pejovic I, Cacciatore R, et al: Activity of gentamicin against *Mycobacteria* in vitro and against *Mycobacterium tuberculosis* in mice. J Infect Dis 124(Suppl):S33–S36, 1971.
34. Finegold SM, Sutter VL: Susceptibility of gram-negative anaerobic bacilli to gentamicin and other aminoglycosides. J Infect Dis 124(Suppl):S56–S58, 1971.
35. Gorbach SL, Bartlett JG: Anaerobic infections. N Engl J Med 290:1289–1294, 1974.
36. Klastersky J, Hensgens C, Henri A, et al: Comparative clinical study of tobramycin and gentamicin. Antimicrob Agents Chemother 5:133–138, 1974.
37. Price KE, Pursiano TA, DeFuria MD, et al: Activity of BB-K8 (amikacin) against clinical isolates resistant to one or more aminoglycoside antibiotics. Antimicrob Agents Chemother 5:143–152, 1974.
38. Kluge RM, Standiford HC, Tatem B, et al: Comparative activity of tobramycin, amikacin, and gentamicin alone and with carbenicillin against *Pseudomonas aeruginosa.* Antimicrob Agents Chemother 6:442–446, 1974.
39. Briedis DJ, Robson HG: Comparative activity of netilmicin, gentamicin, amikacin, and tobramycin against *Pseudomonas aeruginosa* and *Enterobacteriaceae*. Antimicrob Agents Chemother 10:592–597, 1976.
40. Meyer RD, Kraus LL, Pasiecznik KA: In vitro susceptibility of gentamicin-resistant *Enterobacteriaceae* and *Pseudomonas aeruginosa* to netilmicin and selected aminoglycoside antibiotics. Antimicrob Agents Chemother 10:677–681, 1976.
41. Brown KN, Benedictson J, Swanby S: In vitro comparison of gentamicin, tobramycin, sisomicin, and netilmicin. Antimicrob Agents Chemother 10:768–769, 1976.
42. Finland M, Garner C, Wilcox C, et al: Susceptibility of recently isolated bacteria to amikacin in vitro: comparisons with four other aminoglycoside antibiotics. J Infect Dis 134(Suppl):S297–S307, 1976.
43. Moellering RC Jr, Medoff G, Leech I, et al: Antibiotic synergism against *Listeria monocytogenes*. Antimicrob Agents Chemother 1:30–34, 1972.
44. Rodriguez JAG, Luengo F, Gonzales MCS: Activity of amikacin against *Mycobacterium tuberculosis*. J Antimicrob Chemother 4:293–294, 1978.
45. Wolfe JC, Johnson WD Jr: Penicillin-sensitive streptococcal endocarditis: in vitro and clinical observations on penicillin-streptomycin therapy. Ann Intern Med 81:178–181, 1974.
46. Watanakunakorn C, Glotzbecker C: Enhancement of the effects of anti-staphylococcal antibiotics by aminoglycosides. Antimicrob Agents Chemother 6:802–806, 1974.
47. Baird IM, Watanakunakorn C: Antimicrobial therapy of *Staphylococcus aureus* endocarditis. Clin Res 23:531A, 1975.
48. Klastersky J, Nyamubeya B, Vandenborre L: Antimicrobial effectiveness of kanamycin, aminosidin, BB-K8, sisomicin, gentamicin and tobramycin combined with carbenicillin or cephalothin against gram-negative rods. J Med Microbiol 7:465–472, 1974.
49. Anderson ET, Young LS, Hewitt WL: Antimicrobial synergism in the therapy of gram-negative rod bacteremia. Chemotherapy 24:45–54, 1978.
50. Young LS, Martin WJ, Meyer RD, et al: Gram-negative rod bacteremia: microbiologic, immunologic and therapeutic considerations. Ann Intern Med 86:456–471, 1977.

51. Andriole VT: Synergy of carbenicillin and gentamicin in experimental infection with *Pseudomonas.* J Infect Dis 124(Suppl):S46–S55, 1971.
52. Kluge RM, Standiford HC, Tatem B, et al: The carbenicillin-gentamicin combination against *Pseudomonas aeruginosa:* correlation of effect with gentamicin sensitivity. Ann Intern Med 81:584–587, 1974.
53. Lumish RM, Norden CW: Therapy of neutropenic rats infected with *Pseudomonas aeruginosa.* J Infect Dis 133:538–547, 1976.
54. Klastersky J, Cappel R, Daneau D: Clinical significance of in vitro synergism between antibiotics in gram-negative infections. Antimicrob Agents Chemother 2:470–475, 1972.
55. Rahal JJ Jr: Antibiotic combinations: the clinical relevance of synergy and antagonism. Medicine 57:179–195, 1978.
56. Moellering RC Jr, Weinberg AN: Studies on antibiotic synergism against enterococci. II. Effect of various antibiotics on the uptake of C^{14}-labeled streptomycin by enterococci. J Clin Invest 50:2580–2584, 1971.
57. Klastersky J, Henri A, Vandenborre L: Antimicrobial activity of tobramycin and gentamicin used in combination with cephalothin and carbenicillin. Am J Med Sci 266:13–21, 1973.
58. Ekwo E, Peter G: Effect of clindamycin on aminoglycoside activity in a murine model of invasive *Escherichia coli* infection. Antimicrob Agents Chemother 10:893–898, 1976.
59. Fass RJ, Rotilie CA, Prior RB: Interaction of clindamycin and gentamicin in vitro. Antimicrob Agents Chemother 6:582–587, 1974.
60. Devine BJ: Gentamicin therapy. Drug Intell Clin Pharm 8:650–655, 1974.
61. Hull JH, Sarubbi FA Jr: Gentamicin serum concentrations: pharmacokinetic predictions. Ann Intern Med 85:183–189, 1976.
62. Horikoshi N, Valdivieso M, Bodey GP: Clinical pharmacology of tobramycin. Am J Med Sci 266:453–458, 1974.
63. Simon VK, Mosinger EU, Malerczy V: Pharmacokinetic studies of tobramycin and gentamicin. Antimicrob Agents Chemother 3:445–450, 1973.
64. Lockwood WR, Bower JD: Tobramycin and gentamicin concentrations in the serum of normal and anephric patients. Antimicrob Agents Chemother 3:125–129, 1973.
65. Kirby WMM: The human pharmacology of tobramycin. Presented at a Symposium on the Management of Serious Gram-Negative Infections, San Diego, California, February 15, 1975.
66. Miller GH, Arcieri G, Weinstein MJ, et al: Biological activity of netilmicin, a broad-spectrum semisynthetic aminoglycoside antibiotic. Antimicrob Agents Chemother 10:827–836, 1976.
67. Kirby WMM, Clarke JT, Libke RD, et al: Clinical pharmacology and amikacin and kanamycin. J Infect Dis 134(Suppl):S312–S315, 1976.
68. Pijck J, Hallynck T, Soep H, et al: Pharmacokinetics of amikacin in patients with renal insufficiency: relation of half-life and creatinine clearance. J Infect Dis 134(Suppl):S331–S341, 1976.
69. Levy J, Klastersky J: Correlation of serum creatinine concentration and amikacin half-life. J Clin Pharmacol 15:705–707, 1975.
70. Anon: *Investigator's Manual—Amikacin (BB-K8).* Syracuse, New York, Bristol Laboratories, 1976.
71. Cabana BE, Taggart JG: Comparative pharmacokinetics of BB-K8 and kanamycin in dogs and humans. Antimicrob Agents Chemother 3:478–483, 1973.
72. Giusti DL: The clinical use of antimicrobial agents in patients with renal and hepatic insufficiency: the aminoglycosides. Drug Intell Clin Pharm 7:540–556, 1973.
73. Jackson EA, McLeod DC: Pharmacokinetics and dosing of antimicrobial agents in renal impairment. Part I. Am J Hosp Pharm 31:36–52, 1974.
74. Schumacher GE: Pharmacokinetic analysis of gentamicin dosage regimens recommended for renal impairment. J Clin Pharmacol 15:656–665, 1975.
75. Weinstein L: Streptomycin, gentamicin and other aminoglycosides. In *The Pharmacological Basis of Therapeutics,* 5th edition. Edited by LS Goodman, A Gilman. New York, MacMillan, 1975, pp 1167–1180.
76. Bodey GP, Valdivieso M, Feld R, et al: Pharmacology of amikacin in humans. Antimicrob Agents Chemother 5:508–512, 1974.
77. Kunin CM: Absorption, distribution, excretion and fate of kanamycin. Ann NY Acad Sci 132:811–818, 1966.

78. Doluisio JT, Dittert LW, LaPiana JC: Pharmacokinetics of kanamycin following intramuscular administration. J Pharmacokinet Biopharm 1:253–265, 1973.
79. Tally FP: Personal communication, June 17, 1976.
80. Kunin CM, Chalmers TC, Leevy CM, et al: Absorption of orally administered neomycin and kanamycin. N Engl J Med 262:380–385, 1960.
81. Weinstein L, Samet CA, Meade RH: Effect of paromomycin on the bacterial flora of the human intestine. JAMA 178:891–897, 1961.
82. Breen KJ, Bryant RE, Levinson JD, et al: Neomycin absorption in man. Ann Intern Med 76:211–218, 1972.
83. Kovnat P, Labovitz E, Levison SP: Antibiotics and the kidney. Med Clin North Am 57:1045–1063, 1973.
84. Last PM, Sherlock S: Systemic absorption of orally administered neomycin in liver disease. N Engl J Med 262:385–389, 1960.
85. Cox CE: Gentamicin. Med Clin North Am 54:1305–1315, 1970.
86. Davia JE, Siemsen AW, Anderson RW: Uremia, deafness, and paralysis due to irrigating antibiotic solutions. Arch Intern Med 125:135–139, 1970.
87. Johnson AH: Adverse effects of antibiotics. Semin Drug Treat 2:331–351, 1972.
88. Kelly DR, Nilo ER, Berggren RB: Deafness after topical neomycin wound irrigation. N Engl J Med 280:1338–1339, 1969.
89. Malacoff RF, Finkelstein FO, Andriole VT: Effect of peritoneal dialysis on serum levels of tobramycin and clindamycin. Antimicrob Agents Chemother 8:574–580, 1975.
90. Jaffe G, Meyers BR, Hirschman SZ: Pharmacokinetics of tobramycin in patients with stable renal impairment, patients undergoing peritoneal dialysis, and patients on chronic hemodialysis. Antimicrob Agents Chemother 5:611–616, 1974.
91. Gyselynck AM, Forrey A, Cutler R: Pharmacokinetics of gentamicin: distribution and plasma and renal clearance. J Infect Dis 124(Suppl):S70–S76, 1971.
92. Levin AS, Schimpff SC, Graw RF Jr, et al: Hematologic malignancies and other marrow failure states: progress in the management of complicating infections. Semin Hematol 11:141–202, 1974.
93. Naber KG, Westerfelder SR, Madsen PO: Pharmacokinetics of the aminoglycoside antibiotic tobramycin in humans. Antimicrob Agents Chemother 3:469–473, 1973.
94. Gordon RC, Regamey C, Kirby WMM: Serum protein binding of the aminoglycoside antibiotics. Antimicrob Agents Chemother 2:214–216, 1972.
95. Anon: *Investigator's Manual—Tobramycin Sulfate.* Indianapolis, Eli Lilly and Company, 1975.
96. Danish M, Schultz R, Jusko WJ: Pharmacokinetics of gentamicin and kanamycin during hemodialysis. Antimicrob Agents Chemother 6:841–847, 1976.
97. Christopher TG, Korn D, Blair AD, et al: Gentamicin pharmacokinetics during hemodialysis. Kidney Int 6:38–44, 1974.
98. Halpren BA, Axline SG, Coplon NS, et al: Clearance of gentamicin during hemodialysis: comparison of four artificial kidneys. J Infect Dis 133:627–636, 1976.
99. Smithivas T, Hyams PJ, Matalon R, et al: The use of gentamicin in peritoneal dialysis. I. Pharmacologic results. J Infect Dis 124(Suppl):S77–S83, 1971.
100. Schreiner GE, Teehan BP: Dialysis of poisons and drugs—annual review. Am Soc Artif Int Organs 17:513–544, 1971.
101. Greenberg PA, Sanford JP: Antibiotics and peritoneal dialysis. Ann Intern Med 66:465–479, 1967.
102. Atkins RC, Mion C, Despaux E, et al: Peritoneal transfer of kanamycin and its use in peritoneal dialysis. Kidney Int 3:391–396, 1973.
103. Regeur L, Colding H, Jensen H, et al: Pharmacokinetics of amikacin during hemodialysis and peritoneal dialysis. Antimicrob Agents Chemother 11:214–218, 1977.
104. Bailey GL, Vona JP: Pharmacodynamics and renal failure. In *Hemodialysis: Principles and Practice*. Edited by GL Bailey. New York, Academic Press, 1972, pp 172–174.
105. Krumlovsky FA, Emmerman J, Parker RH, et al: Dialysis in treatment of neomycin overdosage. Ann Intern Med 76:443–446, 1972.
106. Hewitt WL: Reflections on the clinical pharmacology of gentamicin. Acta Pathol Microbiol Scand Sect. B 81, Suppl 241:151–156, 1973.
107. Bechtol LD, Black HR: Tobramycin in renal impairment. Am J Med Sci 269:317–321, 1975.

108. Black RE, Lau WK, Weinstein RJ, et al: Ototoxicity of amikacin. Antimicrob Agents Chemother 9:956–961, 1976.
109. Barza M, Brown RB, Shen D, et al: Predictability of blood levels of gentamicin in man. J Infect Dis 132:165–174, 1975.
110. Barza M, Kane A, Baum JL: Regional differences in ocular concentration of gentamicin after subconjunctival and retrobulbar injection in the rabbit. Am J Ophthalmol 83:407–413, 1977.
111. Barza M, Kane A, Baum J: Intraocular penetration of gentamicin after subconjunctival and retrobulbar injection. Am J Ophthalmol 85:541–547, 1978.
112. Whelton A, Carter GG, Bryant HH, et al: Therapeutic implications of gentamicin accumulation in severely diseased kidneys. Arch Intern Med 136:172–176, 1976.
113. Golden B, Coppel SP: Ocular tissue absorption of gentamicin. Arch Ophthalmol 84:792–796, 1970.
114. Golden B: Subtenon injection of gentamicin for bacterial infections of the eye. J Infect Dis 124(Suppl):S271–S274, 1971.
115. Mathalone MBR, Harden A: Penetration and systemic absorption of gentamicin after subconjunctival injection. Br J Ophthalmol 56:609–612, 1972.
116. Spector R: The transport of gentamicin in the choroid plexus and cerebrospinal fluid. J Pharmacol Exp Ther 194:82–88, 1975.
117. Kaiser AB, McGree ZA: Aminoglycoside therapy of gram-negative bacillary meningitis. N Engl J Med 293:1215–1220, 1975.
118. Briedis DJ, Robson HG: Cerebrospinal fluid penetration of amikacin. Antimicrob Agents Chemother 13:1042–1043, 1978.
119. Rodriguez V, Stewart D, Bodey GP: Gentamicin sulfate distribution in body fluids. Clin Pharmacol Ther 11:275–281, 1970.
120. Riff LJ, Jackson GG: Pharmacology of gentamicin in man. J Infect Dis 124(Suppl):S98–S105, 1971.
121. Alfthan O, Rekonen OV, Sivonen A: Concentration of gentamicin in serum, urine and urogenital tissue in man. Acta Pathol Microbiol Scand Sect. B 81, Suppl 241:92–94, 1973.
122. Edwards CQ, Smith CR, Baughman KL, et al: Concentration of gentamicin and amikacin in human kidneys. Antimicrob Agents Chemother 9:925–927, 1976.
123. Chisholm GD, Calnan JS, Waterworth PM, et al: Distribution of gentamicin in body fluids. Br Med J 2:22–24, 1968.
124. Luft FC, Kleit SA: Renal parenchymal accumulation of aminoglycoside antibiotics in rats. J Infect Dis 130:656–659, 1974.
125. Smithivas T, Hyams PJ, Rahal JJ Jr: Gentamicin and ampicillin in human bile. J Infect Dis 124(Suppl):S106–S108, 1971.
126. Pitt HA, Roberts RB, Johnson WD Jr: Gentamicin levels in the human biliary tract. J Infect Dis 127:299–302, 1973.
127. Kaye D, Levison ME, Labovitz ED: The unpredictability of serum concentrations of gentamicin: pharmacokinetics of gentamicin in patients with normal and abnormal renal function. J Infect Dis 130:150–154, 1974.
128. Barza M, Lauermann M: Why monitor serum levels of gentamicin? Clin Pharmacokinet 3:202–215, 1978.
129. Cutler RE, Orme BM: Correlation of serum creatinine concentration and kanamycin half-life. JAMA 209:539–542, 1969.
130. Cutler RE, Gyselynck AM, Fleet WP, et al: Correlation of serum creatinine concentration and gentamicin half-life. JAMA 219:1037–1041, 1972.
131. Chan RA, Benner EJ, Hoeprich PD: Gentamicin therapy in renal failure: a nomogram for dosage. Ann Intern Med 76:773–778, 1972.
132. Brochner-Mortensen J, Rodbro P, Tougaard L: Measurements of glomerular filtration rate. N Engl J Med 295:513, 1976.
133. Ransil BJ, Greenblatt DJ, Koch-Weser J: Evidence for systematic temporal variation in 24-hour urinary creatinine excretion. J Clin Pharmacol 17:108–119, 1977.
134. Jelliffe RW: Creatinine clearance: bedside estimate. Ann Intern Med 79:604–605, 1971.
135. Siersbaek-Nielsen K: Rapid evaluation of creatinine clearance. Lancet 1:1133–1134, 1971.
136. Mawer GE, Lucas SB: Nomogram for kanamycin dosage. Lancet 2:45, 1972.
137. Bennett WM, Singer I, Coggins CJ: A guide to drug therapy in renal failure. JAMA 230:1544–1553, 1974.

138. McHenry MC, Gavan TL, Gifford RW Jr: Gentamicin dosages for renal insufficiency. Ann Intern Med 74:192–197, 1971.
139. Sawchuk RJ, Zaske DE, Cipolle RJ et al: Kinetic model for gentamicin dosing with the use of individual patient parameters. Clin Pharmacol Ther 21:362–369, 1977.
140. Barza M, Scheife RT: Antimicrobial spectrum, pharmacology, and therapeutic use of antibiotics: the aminoglycosides. Am J Hosp Pharm 34:723–737, 1977.
141. McLaughlin JE, Reeves DS: Clinical and laboratory evidence for inactivation of gentamicin by carbenicillin. Lancet 1:261–264, 1971.
142. Ervin FR, Bullock WE Jr, Nuttall CE: Inactivation of gentamicin by penicillins in patients with renal failure. Antimicrob Agents Chemother 9:1004–1011, 1976.
143. Winters RE, Chow AW, Hecht RH, et al: Combined use of gentamicin and carbenicillin. Ann Intern Med 75:925–927, 1971.
144. Scheife RT, Levy M, Greenblatt DJ: Antimicrobial agents. In *Drug Effects in Hospitalized Patients*. Edited by RR Miller, DJ Greenblatt. New York, John Wiley and Sons, 1976, pp 227–264.
145. Chang JC, Reyes B: Agranulocytosis associated with gentamicin. JAMA 232:1154–1155, 1975.
146. Wilfert JN, Burke JP, Bloomer A, et al: Renal insufficiency associated with gentamicin therapy. J Infect Dis 124(Suppl):S148–S153, 1971.
147. Nordstrom L, Banck G, Belfrage S, et al: Prospective study of the ototoxicity of gentamicin. Acta Pathol Microbiol Scand Sect. B 81, Suppl 241:58–61, 1973.
148. Jackson GG, Arcieri G: Ototoxicity of gentamicin in man: a survey and controlled analysis of clinical experience in the United States. J Infect Dis 124(Suppl):S130–S137, 1971.
149. Finegold SM: Toxicity of kanamycin in adults. Ann NY Acad Sci 132:942–956, 1966.
150. Tjernstrom O, Banck G, Belfrage S, et al: The ototoxicity of gentamicin. Acta Pathol Microbiol Scand Sect. B 81, Suppl 241:73–78, 1973.
151. Anon: Serum-gentamicin. Lancet 2:1185, 1974.
152. Meldelson J, Portnoy J, Dick V, et al: Safety of the bolus administration of gentamicin. Antimicrob Agents Chemother 9:633–638, 1976.
153. Feld R, Valdivieso M, Bodey GP, et al: A comparative trial of sisomicin therapy by intermittent versus continuous infusion. Am J Med Sci 274:179–188, 1977.
154. Caldwell JR, Cluff LE: Adverse reactions to antimicrobial agents. JAMA 230:77–80, 1974.
155. Brummett RE, Himes D, Saine B, et al: A comparative study of the ototoxicity of tobramycin and gentamicin. Arch Otolaryngol 96:505–512, 1972.
156. Fee WE Jr, Vierra V, Lathrop GR: Clinical evaluation of aminoglycoside toxicity: tobramycin versus gentamicin, a preliminary report. J Antimicrob Chemother 4(Suppl A):31–36, 1978.
157. Smith CR, Baughman KL, Edwards CQ, et al: Controlled comparison of amikacin and gentamicin. N Engl J Med 296:349–353, 1977.
158. Trestman I, Parsons J, Santoro J, et al: Pharmacology and efficacy of netilmicin. Antimicrob Agents Chemother 13:832–836, 1978.
159. Sheffield PA, Turner JS Jr: Ototoxic drugs: a review of clinical aspects, histopathologic changes and mechanism of action. South Med J 64:359–363, 1971.
160. Brummett RE, Traynor J, Brown R, et al: Cochlear damage resulting from kanamycin and furosemide. Acta Otolaryngol 80:86–92, 1975.
161. Johnson AH, Hamilton CH: Kanamycin ototoxicity—possible potentiation by other drugs. South Med J 63:511–513, 1970.
162. Hansten PD: *Drug Interactions,* 3rd edition. Philadelphia, Lea & Febiger, 1975, pp 86–89.
163. Luft FC, Patel V, Yum MN, et al: Nephrotoxicity of cephalosporin-gentamicin combinations in rats. Antimicrob Agents Chemother 9:831–839, 1976.
164. Kahlmeter G, Hallberg T, Kamme C: Gentamicin and tobramycin in patients with various infections—nephrotoxicity. J Antimicrob Chemother 4(Suppl A):47–52, 1978.
165. Mondorf AW, Zegelman M, Klose J, et al: Comparative studies on the action of aminoglycosides and cephalosporins on the proximal tubule of the human kidney. J Antimicrob Chemother 4(Suppl A):53–57, 1978.
166. Wade J, Smith C, Petty B, et al: Nephrotoxicity of gentamicin or tobramycin with methicillin or cephalothin. In *Current Chemotherapy: Proceedings of the 10th International Congress of Chemotherapy,* Vol. II. Washington, American Society for Microbiology, 1977, pp 971–972.

167. Feld R, Valdivieso M, Bodey GP, et al: Comparison of amikacin and tobramycin in the treatment of infection in patients with cancer. J Infect Dis 135:61–66, 1977.

168. Fanning WL, Gump D, Jick H: Gentamicin- and cephalothin-associated rises in blood urea nitrogen. Antimicrob Agents Chemother 10:80–82, 1976.

169. Patel V, Luft FC, Yum MN, et al: Enzymuria in gentamicin-induced kidney damage. Antimicrob Agents Chemother 7:364–369, 1975.

170. Klastersky J, Hensgens C, Debusscher L: Empiric therapy for cancer patients: comparative study of ticarcillin-tobramycin, ticarcillin-cephalothin, and cephalothin-tobramycin. Antimicrob Agents Chemother 7:640–645, 1975.

171. Gaya H, Klastersky J, Schimpff SC: Nephrotoxicity during combined therapy with gentamicin and cephalothin. *Program and Abstracts, 15th Interscience Conference on Antimicrobial Agents and Chemotherapy,* Washington, September 1975, Abstract 401.

172. Dellinger P, Murphy T, Barza M, et al: Effects of cephalothin on renal cortical concentrations of gentamicin in rats. Antimicrob Agents Chemother 9:587–588, 1976.

173. Dellinger P, Murphy T, Pinn V, et al: Protective effect of cephalothin against gentamicin-induced nephrotoxicity in rats. Antimicrob Agents Chemother 9:172–178, 1976.

174. Warner WA, Sanders E: Neuromuscular blockade associated with gentamicin therapy. JAMA 215:1153–1154, 1971.

175. Pittinger C, Adamson R: Antibiotic blockade of neuromuscular function. Annu Rev Pharmacol 12:169–184, 1972.

176. Holtzman JL: Gentamicin neuromuscular blockade. Ann Intern Med 84:55, 1976.

177. Kubikowski P, Szerniawski Z: The mechanism of the neuromuscular blockade by antibiotics. Arch Int Pharmacodyn Ther 146:549–560, 1963.

178. Pindell MH: The pharmacology of kanamycin. Ann NY Acad Sci 132:805–810, 1966.

179. Dunkley B, Sanghvi I, Goldstein G: Characterization of neuromuscular block produced by streptomycin. Arch Int Pharmacodyn Ther 201:213–223, 1973.

180. Thompson GR, Barrowman J, Gutierrez L, et al: Action of neomycin on the intraluminal phase of lipid absorption. J Clin Invest 50:319–323, 1971.

181. Cain GD, Reiner EB, Patterson M: Effects of neomycin on dissacharidase activity of the small bowel. Arch Intern Med 122:311–314, 1968.

182. Faloon WW, Paes IC, Woolfolk D, et al: Effect of neomycin and kanamycin upon intestinal absorption. Ann NY Acad Sci 132:879–887, 1966.

183. Keusch GT, Troncale FJ, Buchanan RD: Malabsorption due to paromomycin. Arch Intern Med 125:273–276, 1970.

184. Dobbins WO III: Drug-induced steatorrhea. Gastroenterology 54:1193–1195, 1968.

185. Cohen LS, Wechsler AS, Mitchell JH, et al: Depression of cardiac function by streptomycin and other antimicrobial agents. Am J Cardiol 26:505–511, 1970.

186. Saslaw S, Carlisle HN, Moheimani M: Comparison of tobramycin, gentamicin, colistin, and carbenicillin in *Pseudomonas* sepsis in monkeys. Antimicrob Agents Chemother 2:164–172, 1972.

187. Rahal JJ Jr: Treatment of gram-negative bacillary meningitis in adults. Ann Intern Med 77:295–302, 1972.

188. Schimpff SC, Landesman S, Hahn DM, et al: Ticarcillin in combination with cephalothin or gentamicin as empiric antibiotic therapy in granulocytopenic cancer patients. Antimicrob Agents Chemother 10:837–844, 1976.

189. Murillo J, Standiford HC, Schimpff SC, et al: Comparison of serum bactericidal activity among three antimicrobial combinations. Antimicrob Agents Chemother 13:992–996, 1978.

189a. Pejovic I, Cacciatore R, Vladez H, et al: Comparative activity of sisomicin against *Mycobacteria* in vitro and against *Mycobacterium tuberculosis* in mice. J Infect Dis 127:720–722, 1973.

189b. Kawamori Y, Nishizawa N: Studies on antituberculosis activity of amikacin. In *Chemotherapy,* Vol. 1. Edited by JD Williams, AM Geddes. New York, Plenum Press, 1975, pp 397–401.

190. Flick MR, Cluff LE: *Pseudomonas* bacteremia: review of 108 cases. Am J Med 60:501–508, 1976.

191. Parry MF, Neu HC: A comparative study of ticarcillin plus tobramycin versus carbenicillin plus gentamicin for the treatment of serious infections due to gram-negative bacilli. Am J Med 64:961–966, 1978.

192. Harding GK, Marrie TJ, Buckwold F, et al: A controlled comparison of ticarcillin, clindamycin and chloramphenicol in the therapy of anaerobic infections. In *Program and Abstracts, 17th Interscience Conference on Antimicrobial Agents and Chemotherapy,* New York, October 1977, Abstract 178.
193. McCormack WM, Finland M: Spectinomycin. Ann Intern Med 84:712–716, 1976.
194. Karney WW, Pedersen AHB, Nelson M, et al: Spectinomycin versus tetracycline for the treatment of gonorrhea. N Engl J Med 296:889–894, 1977.
195. Felarca AB, Laqui EM, Ibarra LM: Gentamicin in gonococcal urethritis of Filipino males: dosage and response. J Infect Dis 124(Suppl):S287–S292, 1971.
196. Rahal JJ Jr, Hyams PJ, Simberkoff MS, et al: Combined intrathecal and intramuscular gentamicin for gram-negative meningitis: pharmacologic study of 21 patients. N Engl J Med 290:1394–1398, 1974.
197. Saad AF, Farrar WE Jr: Intracisternal and intrathecal injections of gentamicin in *Enterobacter* meningitis. Arch Intern Med 134:738–740, 1974.
198. Moellering RC Jr, Fischer EG: Relationship of intraventricular gentamicin levels to cure of meningitis. J Pediatr 81:534–537, 1972.
199. Mangi RJ, Holstein LL, Andriole VT: Treatment of gram-negative bacillary meningitis with intrathecal gentamicin. Yale J Biol Med 50:31–41, 1977.
200. Hollifield JW, Kaiser AB, McGee ZA: Gram-negative bacillary meningitis therapy. Polyradiculitis following intralumbar aminoglycoside administration. JAMA 236:1264–1266, 1976.
201. MacMillan BG: Gentamicin in the management of thermal injuries. J Infect Dis 199:492–503, 1969.
202. Tally FP, Gorbach SL: Antibiotics in surgery. Adv Surg 9:41–95, 1975.
203. Dawson AM, McLaren J, Sherlock S: Neomycin in the treatment of hepatic coma. Lancet 2:1263–1268, 1957.

9. SULFONAMIDES

Richard Gleckman

Sulfonamides were the first chemical agents introduced into clinical practice for the management of systemic infections. 'Sulfonamide' is a general name for the thousands of derivatives of the compound para-aminobenzenesulfonamide, or sulfanilamide. The initially prominent therapeutic position of the sulfonamides was eroded by the emergence of bacteria resistant to these compounds and the subsequent development of other classes of antimicrobial agents. In contemporary practice the sulfonamides continue to occupy a position of importance, however, because they are relatively inexpensive, safe, and remain the drug of first choice for some infections.

The sulfonamides have been classified into six groups:[1] short-acting drugs (sulfisoxazole, sulfadiazine, and trisulfapyrimidines); intermediate-acting drugs (sulfamethoxazole); long-acting drugs (sulfamethoxypyridazine and sulfameter); poorly absorbed drugs (phthalylsulfathiazole) that are used for preoperative bowel preparation for elective colon surgery; sulfapyridines (sulfapyridine and sulfasalazine [salicylazosulfapyridine]) that are used specifically for the treatment of dermatitis herpetiformis and ulcerative colitis, respectively; topical drugs (mafenide acetate and silver sulfadiazine) that are used for the prevention and treatment of burn infections.

MECHANISM OF ACTION

Sulfonamides are of chemotherapeutic value because many micro-organisms cannot use exogenous folic acid (dihydrofolate) but must synthesize this essential compound by incorporating p-aminobenzoate. The folic acid that is formed from p-aminobenzoate is, in turn, converted to its functional form, folinic acid (tetrahydrofolate) by the enzume dihydrofolate reductase. Tetrahydrofolate cofactors are vital for the synthesis of methionine, purines, and thymine. Sulfonamides and p-anminobenzoate have a close structural similarity, and sulfonamides are thought to serve as competitive substrates for the enzyme that converts p-aminobenzoic acid to folic acid. Thus, sulfonamides block the production of folic acid and prevent the generation of the pool of tetrahydrofolate cofactors.

SPECTRUM OF ACTIVITY

Sulfonamides are bacteriostatic compounds that are generally ineffective in the presence of pus, hematoma and necrotic tissue. Those organisms that are usually susceptible to sulfonamides include *Escherichia coli* (isolated from community-acquired urinary tract infections), *Hemophilus influenzae, Hemophilus ducreyi, Streptococcus pneumoniae,* most group A beta hemolytic *Streptococcus pyogenes, Vibrio comma, Nocardia* sp. and *Chlamydia trachomatis.* Some strains of *Neisseria gonorrhoeae, Neisseria meningitidis, Shigella flexneri, Shigella sonnei, Bacillus anthracis, Corynebacterium diphtheriae, Pasteurella pestis, Pseudomonas pseudomallei, Brucella* sp., *Actinomyces* and *Donovania granulomatis* are resistant.

Sulfonamide resistance develops by several mechanisms. Some bacteria can synthesize enough p-aminobenzoic acid to antagonize sulfonamides. Other bacteria appear to alter the enzyme dihydropteric acid synthetase and effectively reduce its affinity for sulfonamides. R factor may mediate sulfonamide resistance by excluding sulfonamides from the susceptible cells, a mechanism that resembles tetracycline resistance.

ADVERSE REACTIONS

The list of untoward reactions attributed to the sulfonamides is substantial (Table 2). Which of the adverse reactions are actually caused by the sulfonamides and how often they develop is unknown. In prospective surveillance studies on hospitalized recipients of sulfisoxazole and sulfamethoxazole, the rate of untoward effects severe enough to require discontinuation of treatment was very low.[2] The most common untoward events were skin reactions (macular, maculopapular, urticarial), drug fever and gastrointestinal intolerance (anorexia, nausea, vomiting).

Cross-sensitization among the sulfonamides is incomplete, but these compounds should not be administered to patients with a suspected or known hypersensitivity to sulfonamides unless they are clearly the drugs of choice.

TABLE 1 Preparations and Costs of Sulfonamides

GENERIC NAME	TRADEMARK NAME(S)	PREPARATIONS AND 1978 COSTS
Short-Acting Sulfonamides		
Sulfachlorpyridazine	Nefrosul (Sonilyn)	Tablets 500 mg—$7.80/100
Sulfacytine	Renoquid	Tablets 500 mg—$7.99/100
Sulfadiazine	generic	Tablets 500 mg—$2.50–$4.80/100 Tablets (chewable) 300 mg—$6.28/100
Sulfadiazine Sodium	generic	Injection (solution) 250 mg/ml—$1.30/10-ml vial
Sulfamethizole	Thiosulfil	Tablets 250 mg—$3.42/100; 500 mg (Forte)—$6.22/100 Suspension 250 mg/5 ml—$5.16/16 oz
Sulfisoxazole	Gantrisin generic	Tablets 500 mg—$3.76/100 Tablets 500 mg—$1.85–$3.86/100
Sulfisoxazole Acetyl	Gantrisin	Liquid (timed-release) 1 g/5 ml (Lipo Gantrisin)—$13.38/16 oz Suspension (pediatric) 500 mg/5 ml—$1.85/4 oz Syrup 500 mg/5 ml—$6.58/16 oz
Sulfisoxazole Diolamine	Gantrisin	Injection (solution) 400 mg/ml—$0.54/5-ml vial; $0.98/10-ml vial
Trisulfapyrimidines	generic	Tablets 500 mg—$1.60–$5.10/100 Suspension 500 mg/5 ml—$2.90–$5.60/pint
Intermediate-Acting Sulfonamides		
Sulfamethoxazole	Gantanol	Tablets 500 mg—$8.16/100 Suspension 500 mg/5 ml—$11.75/16 oz
Long-Acting Sulfonamides		
Sulfameter	Sulla	Tablets 500 mg—$13.50/100
Sulfamethoxypyridazine	Midicel	Tablets 500 mg—$15.20/100

TABLE 1 *(continued)*

Generic Name	Trademark Name(s)	Preparations and 1978 Costs
Topical Sulfonamides		
Mafenide Acetate	Sulfamylon Acetate	Cream equivalent to 85 mg of base/g—$2.22/2 oz, $4.02/4 oz, $14.53/14.5 oz
Silver Sulfadiazine	Silvadene	Cream 10 mg/g—$3.25/50 g, $16.25/400 g
Miscellaneous Sulfonamides		
Phthalylsulfathizole	Sulfathalidine	Tablets 500 mg—$4.77/100
Sulfapyridine	generic	Tablets 500 mg—$3.34/100

The nephrotoxicity produced by the sulfonamides has been arbitrarily classified into obstructive uropathy (formation and deposition of crystalline aggregates in the renal pelvis, ureter or bladder; prevented or treated by alkalinization of the urine and hydration), precipitation of hemoglobin casts secondary to drug-induced hemolysis, and hypersensitivity nephritis (allergic interstitial nephritis, acute tubular necrosis and necrotizing angiitis).

The frequency of the Stevens-Johnson syndrome has been estimated to be one patient/metric ton of sulfonamide administered. Although the 'long-acting' sulfonamides have been singled out as causes of the Stevens-Johnson syndrome, sulfadiazine, a sulfonamide with a half-life of 17 hours, has not been incriminated.

There is good evidence that fever and skin eruptions caused by sulfonamides increase in direct proportion to the quantity of drug administered.

It has been advised that sulfonamides be avoided in the later stages of pregnancy because of the theoretical possibility that these compounds may cross the placenta and displace bilirubin from its conjugation with glucuronic acid. However, some authorities claim that it is unlikely that enough sulfonamide can cross the placenta to conjugate with sufficient binding sites to produce hyperbilirubinemia; they also point out that no cases of sulfonamide-induced kernicterus have been found.

The adverse reaction that may prove to be the most significant is accelerated vascular disease. One published study cites an increased

TABLE 2 Adverse Reactions Attributed to Sulfonamides

Gastrointestinal	Renal
Anorexia	Hematuria
Nausea	Crystalluria
Vomiting	Oliguria
Abdominal pain	Anuria
Diarrhea	Toxic nephrosis
Pancreatitis	Glomerulonephritis
Hepatitis	Interstitial nephritis
	Acute tubular necrosis
Neurologic	Necrotizing angiitis
Headache	
Lassitude	**Hematologic**
Confusion	Hemolytic anemia in patients with glutathione peroxidase deficiency, glucose-6-phosphate dehydrogenase deficiency, and unstable hemoglobins (hemoglobinopathy Zurich)
Depression	Granulocytopenia
Nightmares	Agranulocytosis
Insomnia	Aplastic anemia
Psychosis	Thrombocytopenia
Sterile meningitis	Methemoglobinemia
Ataxia	
Vertigo	**Miscellaneous Reactions**
Tinnitus	Fever
Benign intracranial hypertension	Behçet's syndrome
Convulsions	Serum sickness
Peripheral neuropathy	Anaphylaxis
Myalgia	Arthralgia
	Myocarditis
Skin Reactions	Conjunctivitis
Macular, papular, urticarial eruptions	Diffuse granuloma of organs
Phototoxic drug eruptions	Asthma
Erythema multiforme and Stevens–Johnson syndrome	Pulmonary infiltrates with eosinophilia
Erythema nodosum	Lupus erythematosus
Generalized exfoliative dermatitis	Periarteritis nodosa
Toxic epidermal necrolysis ("scalded skin syndrome")	Accelerated vascular disease

mortality occurring among patients who received prolonged therapy with a sulfonamide. The authors suggested that the sulfonamide accelerated vascular disease, and noted that their observations were similar to those reported in the University Group Diabetes Program. Until the significance of this observation is clarified, sulfonamides should not be considered the agents of choice for prolonged therapy of urinary tract infections.

DRUG INTERACTIONS

Sulfonamides have the potential to displace tolbutamide, methotrexate and warfarin from protein binding sites and this can result in transient hypoglycemia, methotrexate toxicity and bleeding. Phenylbutazone, acetylsalicylic acid and probenecid can displace sulfonamides from serum carrier sites and thereby cause increased sulfonamide toxicity. Sulfonamides inhibit hepatic biotransformation of tolbutamide, chlorpropamide and phenytoin with the potential for causing hypoglycemia and phenytoin toxicity. Sulfonamides compete with tolbutamide and methotrexate for renal tubular secretion, and this results in the potential for hypoglycemia and methotrexate toxicity. Sulfonamides given as intravenous infusions will crystallize in acidic polyionic solutions.

INTERFERENCE WITH LABORATORY TESTS

Sulfonamides will frequently cause an interference in the urinary glucose test performed by Benedict's method, resulting in a false positive result. Sulfonamides can also cause spuriously high serum amino acid concentrations. Rarely sulfonamides cause a positive LE cell test.

THERAPEUTIC USE

Short-acting sulfonamides are appropriate therapy for women and children with acute symptomatic or recurrent urinary tract infections caused by susceptible *Escherichia coli.*[3–5] These compounds are the drugs of choice for the treatment of nocardiosis and chancroid[6,7] *(Hemophilus ducreyi).* Short-acting sulfonamides are effective prophylactic agents for children who experience recurrent otitis media and penicillin-sensitive patients who require rheumatic fever prophylaxis.[8,9] Intimate contacts of patients with serious meningococcal disease caused by sulfonamide-susceptible strains are also candidates for preventive therapy with short-acting sulfonamides.[10]

Sulfapyridine is invaluable in the treatment of dermatitis herpetiformis, and sulfasalazine induces remissions and decreases the frequency of exacerbations of ulcerative colitis[11] (see Chapter 67).

SULFONAMIDES IN COMBINATION WITH OTHER DRUGS

Trisulfapyrimidines administered with erythromycin have proved to be effective therapy of otitis media caused by *Hemophilus influenzae.*[12] This combination appears to be an effective alternative to ampicillin or amoxicillin for the penicillin-sensitive patient.

Sulfadoxine (Fansidar), a long-acting sulfonamide, in combination with pyrimethamine, is the most effective prophylactic drug for the suppression of chloroquine-resistant *Plasmodium falciparum.* This drug is not available in the United States.

Sulfadiazine in combination with pyrimethamine is the recommended therapy for active chorioretinitis and disseminated disease caused by *Toxoplasma gondii.*

Sulfamethoxazole in combination with trimethoprim (Bactrim, Septra) is discussed in Chapter 13, Miscellaneous Antimicrobial Agents.

SELECTION OF A SULFONAMIDE

With a few exceptions (eg, sulfapyridine in dermatitis herpetiformis and sulfasalazine in ulcerative colitis), sulfisoxazole is the sulfonamide drug of choice.

Some authorities consider sulfadiazine the preferred short-acting sulfonamide for the treatment of systemic infections, because it has relatively low protein binding (55%). However, this compound is less soluble than sulfisoxazole in the urine and has a greater propensity to cause crystalluria. Although sulfadiazine is considered a short-acting sulfonamide, it has a half-life of 17 hours. Other single-entity short-acting sulfonamides (Table 1) have no advantage over sulfisoxazole.

Trisulfapyrimidines is a mixture of sulfonamides that is prescribed exclusively for the therapy of urinary tract infections.[13] Each component of the mixture maintains its individual solubility in the urine independently of the other. The theoretical advantage is additive antibacterial effectiveness with less risk of precipitation and obstruction.

The intermediate-acting and long-acting sulfonamides are no more effective than the short-acting sulfonamides for the treatment of systemic infections. Their main advantage is less frequent dosing. The long-acting compounds are rarely prescribed today as the sole drugs for the therapy of infectious diseases, because some investigators have incriminated them as a cause of the Stevens-Johnson syndrome (erythema multiforme skin lesions accompanied by bullous or vesicular lesions of the skin and mucous membranes). Other investigators have reviewed the data and raise some doubts about this indictment of 'long-acting' sulfonamides.[14]

DRUG MONOGRAPH

SULFISOXAZOLE (Gantrisin)

The prototype of the short-acting sulfonamides and the compound that is most widely used in the United States is sulfisoxazole.[15] For information on this drug's mechanism of action, spectrum of activity, adverse reactions, drug interactions, and therapeutic use, see the introductory section.

Pharmacology—Sulfisoxazole is rapidly and completely absorbed, mostly in the small intestine. Peak plasma levels, achieved 2 hours after administration of 2 g, range from 121 to 210 μg/ml of the intact drug. From 28 to 35% of sulfisoxazole is present in the blood in the acetylated form. The acetyl derivative is bacteriologically inactive but can contribute to toxicity.

The half-life of sulfisoxazole is 4.6 to 7.8 hours. Its calculated volume of distribution ranges from 13 to 20% of the body weight, a reflection of a high affinity for plasma protein. Sulfisoxazole is 85% protein bound. When it is administered to the patient with end-stage renal disease, protein binding decreases. The high degree of binding has several effects: restriction of tissue distribution, reduced penetration into inflammatory fluids, delayed renal excretion, and diminished antimicrobial activity.

Sulfisoxazole is eliminated exclusively by urinary excretion through the mechanisms of glomerular filtration and tubular secretion. Sulfisoxazole also undergoes tubular reabsorption. The urinary recovery of intact sulfonamide ranges from 40 to 65% of the administered dose. The remainder is excreted in the urine as the acetylated biotransformation product. The solubility of sulfisoxazole is enhanced with alkalinization of the urine.

In patients with renal insufficiency an accumulation of both intact and conjugated drug occurs, and elevated serum concentrations, enhanced toxicity, and reduced urinary concentrations of intact sulfisoxazole are observed.[12]

Sulfisoxazole penetrates into body fluids (pleural, peritoneal, synovial, cerebrospinal) and crosses the placenta.

Dosage—Oral: Adults. For severe infections the initial adult dose is 4 g, and the maintenance dose is 1 g administered every 4 hours. In children with severe infections the initial dose is 35 mg/lb, and the maintenance dose is 70 mg/lb/day, in divided doses given every 4 hours. The recommended adult dose for the treatment of urinary tract infections is 1 g every 6 hours. When the glomerular filtration rate is reduced to 10–50 ml/min, the dosage interval should be increased to every 8 to 12 hours if the patient is receiving sulfisoxazole for a serious systemic infection. When the glomerular filtration rate is less than 10 ml/min, the drug should be administered every 12 to 24 hours. If it is essential to achieve high urinary levels of free sulfonamide in the azotemic patient, the medication will have to be administered as frequently as every 6 hours. This strategy, however, increases the likelihood of drug toxicity due to increased serum levels of both the intact and acetylated derivative.

Hemodialysis and peritoneal dialysis extract enough sulfisoxazole to require a dosage supplement to insure adequate therapeutic blood levels.

Although hematuria and crystalluria are rare manifestations of sulfisoxazole therapy, adequate hydration should be maintained.

REFERENCES

1. Weinstein L, Madoff MA, Samet CM: The sulfonamides. N Engl J Med 263:793–800, 842–849, 900–907, 952–957, 1960.
2. Koch-weser J, Sidel VW, Dexter M, et al: Adverse reactions to sulfisoxazole, sulfamethoxazole, and nitrofurantoin: manifestations and specific reaction rates during 2,118 courses of therapy. Arch Intern Med 128:399–404, 1971.
3. Hughes J, Roberts LC, Coppridge AJ: Sulfacytine: a new sulfonamide: double blind comparison with sulfisoxazole in acute uncomplicated urinary tract infections. J Urol 114:912–914, 1975.
4. Ormonde NWH, Gray JA, McMurdoch J, et al: Chronic bacteriuria due to Escherichia coli. I. Assessment of the value of combined short- and long-term treatment with cycloserine, nitrofurantoin, and sulphadimidine. J Infect Dis 120:82–86, 1969.
5. Harding GKM, Ronald AR, Boutros P, et al: A comparison of trimethoprim-sulfamethoxazole with sulfamethoxazole alone in infections localized to the kidneys. Can Med Assoc J 112(Suppl):9–12, 1975.
6. Palmer DL, Harvey RL, Wheeler JK: Diagnostic and therapeutic considerations in Nocardia asteroides infection. Medicine 53:391–401, 1974.
7. Kerber RE, Rowe CE, Gilbert KR, et al: Treatment of chancroid: a comparison of tetracycline and sulfisoxazole. Arch Dermatol 100:604–607, 1969.
8. Perrin JM, Charney E, MacWhinney JB, et al: Sulfisoxazole as chemoprophylaxis for recurrent otitis media. N Engl J Med 291:664–667, 1974.
9. Feinstein AR, Wood HF, Spagnuolo M, et al: Oral prophylaxis of recurrent rheumatic fever. JAMA 188:489–492, 1964.

10. Jacobson JA, Fraser DW: A simplified approach to meningococcal disease prophylaxis. JAMA 236:1053–1054, 1976.
11. Dissanayake A, Truelove S: A controlled trial of long-term maintenance treatment of ulcerative colitis with sulphasalazine. Gut 14:818, 1973.
12. Sell SH, Wilson DA, Stamm JM, et al: Treatment of otitis media caused by Hemophilus influenzae: evaluation of three antimicrobial regimens. South Med J 71:1493–1497, 1978.
13. Lehr D: Lowered incidence of sensitization through use of sulphonamide combinations: new concept. Br Med J 2:543–548, 1948.
14. Bianchine JR, Macaraeg PVJ, Lassagna L, et al: Drugs as etiologic factors in the Stevens-Johnson syndrome. Am J Med 44:390–405, 1968.
15. Yow EM: Observation on use of sulfisoxazole (Gantrisin) in 1000 consecutive patients, with particular reference to frequency of undesirable side effects. Am Pract Digest Treat 4:521–525, 1953.
16. Adams WR, Dawborn JK: Urinary excretion and plasma levels of sulfonamides in patients with renal impairment. Aust Ann Med 3:250–254, 1970.

10. NITROFURANS

Richard Gleckman, Salvador Alvarez, and Dennis W. Joubert

The nitrofuran class of drugs includes nitrofurantoin (Cyantin, Furadantin, Macrodantin), furazolidone (Furoxone), and nitrofurazone (Furacin). Systemically-administered furazolidone has few, if any, acceptable uses and is not considered here. Nitrofurazone is used topically only and is not within the scope of this book.

DRUG MONOGRAPH

NITROFURANTOIN (Cyantin, Furadantin, Macrodantin)

Antimicrobial Spectrum—Nitrofurantoin is a bactericidal compound, and organisms do not readily develop resistance during therapy.[1–4] The vast majority of *Escherichia coli, Citrobacter* species, group B streptococci, enterococci, *Staphylococcus aureus* and *Staphylococcus epidermidis* are susceptible to nitrofurantoin. Most *Klebsiella pneumoniae* and *Enterobacter* species are susceptible. Virtually all *Pseudomonas aeruginosa* and *Pseudomonas cepacia* are highly resistant. Considerable disagreement exists in the literature as to the susceptibility of *Proteus* (mirabilis, morganii, vulgaris, rettgeri), *Providencia* species and *Serratia* species with the percentage of susceptible strains varying markedly in different laboratories. This phenomenon is somewhat explained by the fact that there had been a lack of standardization, with microbiologists using diverse discs, inoculum, and interpretations.[5] Most strains of *Acinetobacter* species, an organism associated with nosocomial urinary tract infections, are resistant.

Absorption, Distribution, and Metabolism—Oral suspension and tablets are well absorbed from the small intestine.[6] An oral dose of nitrofurantoin achieves insignificant serum levels in patients with normal renal function. In patients with impaired renal function repeated oral dosing results in the accumulation of toxic concentrations of nitrofurantoin.[7–9] Nitrofurantoin demonstrates enhanced bioavailability when taken with food.[10] Propantheline also augments nitrofurantoin bioavailability.[11]

Nitrofurantoin is excreted virtually exclusively in the urine and bile.[7] Urinary excretion results from glomerular filtration, tubular secretion, and tubular reabsorption.[6] Approximately 40% of ingested drug is recovered intact in the urine.

Nitrofurantoin does not appear to exert any untoward effects on the fetus when administered to the pregnant female.[12]

Excretion in Patients with Impaired Renal Function—The excretion of nitrofurantoin is directly related to the creatinine clearance.[9] Patients with mild reduction of glomerular filtration fail to excrete nitrofurantoin in therapeutic concentrations, and thus the drug is contraindicated for the azotemic patient.[7–9,13]

Interactions—Nitrofurantoin can cause an elevation of the urinary creatinine value, and the urine glucose determination using Benedict's reagent may yield a false positive result. Serum levels of glucose, bilirubin, alkaline phosphatase and blood urea nitrogen may be spuriously elevated. The values for carbon dioxide content and combining power may be altered.

Therapeutic Use—The conventional dosage for an established urinary tract infection is 50 or 100 mg four times a day. These doses produce comparable clinical and bacteriological response rates.

Treatment of acute symptomatic urinary tract infection. Cure rates of community acquired *E. coli* urinary tract infections in *adult women* who have received nitrofurantoin are approximately 75%.[14] The therapeutic response correlates directly with the tissue source of the infection, as women with acute cystitis are more frequently cured of the infection than women with pyelonephritis. Nitrofurantoin compares favorably with ampicillin.[14]

Nitrofurantoin has proven to be a very effective therapy of acute symptomatic urinary tract infections in *children* when the disease is caused by *E. coli.* The initial bacteriological response exceeds 90%. Ampicillin, sulfonamide and nitrofurantoin appear equally effective for this infection. For an established infection an appropriate amount is 5 to 10 mg/kg daily divided into four equal doses.

Recurrent urinary tract infections. Nitrofurantoin treatment results in an 80 to 100% immediate cure rate of urinary tract infections in *adult women* without obstructive uropathy who have asymptomatic bacteriuria and/or documented recurrent urinary tract infections caused by *E. coli*.[15–17] The results are not improved by extending the duration of therapy from 2 to 6 weeks.[16] The majority of the 'failures' of therapy are reinfections, a recurrent infection caused by an organism different from that producing the original infection and considered a reflection of defective host defenses rather than drug ineptitude. Therapeutic efficacy is not enhanced when alternative standard agents are prescribed for these women.[15–17]

Patients with what was formerly termed 'chronic urinary tract infections,' (currently termed 'recurrent' infections) due to *E. coli* and *Enterobacter* species experience immediate therapeutic response from nitrofurantoin, but they subsequently develop significant bacteriuria when chemotherapy is discontinued.

Approximately 90% of the nitrofurantoin treatment courses of *children* with recurrent urinary tract infections result in an immediate bacteriological cure. However, virtually all these patients subsequently develop another recurrence. Nitrofurantoin appears to be as effective as a sulfonamide or a tetracycline for the therapy of recurrent urinary tract infections in children.

Nitrofurantoin is not indicated for treatment of the patient with acute bacterial pyelonephritis or the man with recurrent urinary tract infection. The drug does not achieve therapeutic concentrations in the plasma following oral administration and it has not proved to be effective therapy for chronic bacterial prostatitis.

Prophylaxis of recurrent urinary tract infections. Recurrent urinary tract infections in women have been prevented by a single dose of nitrofurantoin administered post-intercourse and by continuous single nightly doses taken over a prolonged time.[17–20] The data are convincing that nitrofurantoin is a more effective prophylactic agent than a placebo and compares well with other chemotherapeutic agents used for this purpose.[17–20] Recurrent urinary tract infections occurring during therapy are usually caused by nitrofurantoin susceptible organisms.[20] When the continuous nitrofurantoin prophylaxis is discontinued, however, the recurrence rate over the ensuing six months is considerable.[17,19,21] This is not unique to nitrofurantoin, but characteristic of women with recurrent urinary tract infections.

Continuous prophylactic treatment with nitrofurantoin has resulted in a decreased incidence of recurrences in men with chronic urinary tract infections.[22]

For adult women a single nightly dose of 50 mg of nitrofurantoin is effective prophylaxis for recurrent urinary tract infections.[18,19] For adult men a dose of 50 mg of nitrofurantoin administered four times a day has been found to be effective prophylaxis,[22] but it is certainly possible that a reduced dose would be as effective.

Nitrofurantoin prophylaxis convincingly decreased the incidence of recurrent urinary tract infections in *children* who had no evidence of radiographically defined urinary tract abnormalities.[23,24] The incidence of recurrences was not diminished when prophylactic nitrofurantoin was administered to children with meningomyelocele. A single evening dose of 1 to 2 mg/kg has proven to be an effective amount of nitrofurantoin for the prevention of recurrent urinary tract infections in children.

Adverse Reactions—Adverse reactions to nitrofurantoin are infrequent. One study, a surveillance of untoward events experienced by hospitalized patients who had received nitrofurantoin, noted an incidence of 9.2%.[25] For a detailed review of adverse reactions to nitrofurantoin, readers are referred elsewhere.[26]

Gastrointestinal disturbances. Anorexia, nausea, and vomiting are the most common side effects.[17,25] Nausea and vomiting usually develop during the first week of therapy, are experienced more often by women than men or children, and appear to be related to the daily drug dose and the patient's weight.[25] A double-blind study has shown that patients are able to tolerate the macrocrystalline form better than crystalline nitrofurantoin.[21]

Skin eruptions. Macular, maculopapular or urticarial lesions are the second most common side effect of nitrofurantoin.[17,25] Allergic skin reactions attributable to nitrofurantoin were experienced by 1% of the hospitalized patients who received this chemotherapeutic agent.[27]

Hematologic toxicity. The best known and most intensively studied hematological abnormality associated with nitrofurantoin is the development of anemia in patients with red blood cells deficient in the enzyme glucose-6-phosphate dehydrogenase.[28]

Nitrofurantoin administration has also precipitated hemolytic anemia in patients who are deficient in other erythrocytic enzymes, namely enolase and glutathione-peroxidase. In addition hemolysis induced by nitrofurantoin has been reported in a patient who had no known erythrocyte enzymatic deficiency.

Rare reports exist in the literature which have associated nitrofurantoin therapy with the development of leukopenia, megaloblastic anemia, thrombocytopenia, agranulocytosis and aplastic anemia.

Some of these data are difficult to interpret or are subject to alternative interpretation, however.

Neurotoxicity. One of the more serious and frequent adverse reactions from nitrofurantoin is the development of peripheral polyneuropathy.[29] Nitrofurantoin-induced polyneuritis usually develops in a setting of azotemia. However, not only have electromyographic abnormalities been detected in non-azotemic patients receiving nitrofurantoin, but symptomatic polyneuritis has developed in patients with normal renal function.

The onset of the polyneuropathy is usually insidious and symmetrical, occurring after days to years of either continuous or intermittent nitrofurantoin therapy. The initial symptoms, paresthesias and dyesthesias, arise more often in the lower than the upper extremities. There is progression in a matter of days to include a number of sensory deficits, impairment of pain, light touch and vibration. All symptoms and physical findings begin distally and spread centripetally. Weakness and muscle wasting ensue, and result in a flaccid paresis. The severity of symptoms has not been related to the total amount of drug ingested.[29]

There may be incomplete, complete, or failure of resolution of the polyneuritis. There is no relationship between the amount of nitrofurantoin ingested and the degree of recovery, and resolution of the polyneuropathy varies inversely with the severity of the muscle weakness.[29] Complete recovery usually occurs within weeks, although it may happen within days to months. Sensation is restored faster than muscle strength.

Hepatotoxicity. Nitrofurantoin-induced hepatotoxicity is a rare event which is usually readily reversible with discontinuation of the medication.[30] However, persistent liver function abnormalities, life-threatening hemorrhage, and death have been reported. Hepatotoxicity does not appear to be dose-related, and jaundice is not invariably present. Some patients will experience fever, rash and arthralgia. Eosinophilia, elevated serum transaminase or alkaline phosphatase values are not consistently noted. Immunological abnormalities, including the development of antinuclear antibodies and antismooth muscle antibodies have been detected in an unspecified number of these patients. The pathology of the liver has been variable, including intrahepatic cholestasis, minimal cellular injury and chronic active hepatitis.

Pulmonary toxicity. The *acute* pulmonary reaction syndrome is characterized by the dramatic onset of fever, chills, cough, myalgia and dyspnea (with or without cyanosis); rales at the lung bases; lower lobe infiltrates on chest x-ray (with or without effusion); rapid resolution of clinical and radiological abnormalities following discontinuation of the medication; an elevated sedimentation rate; delayed onset of peripheral blood eosinophilia and recurrence of similar clinical manifestations, with a shortened incubation period, on subsequent exposure.[31,32] This reaction develops within hours to weeks of the ingestion of the drug and can be accompanied by headache, rash, generalized pruritis, chest discomfort, sputum production and shock. The syndrome has been mistaken for congestive heart failure, pulmonary embolism, bacterial pneumonia, asthmatic attack, anaphylaxis, myocardial infarction or pericarditis, influenza and Loffler's syndrome. On rare occasions the chest x-ray demonstrates no abnormalities. Physiological monitoring has demonstrated a restrictive lung pattern, ventilation/perfusion abnormalities and arterial-venous shunting, accompanied by hypocapnia and hypoxemia. Lung biopsy reveals alveolar exudation, interstitial inflammation and vasculitis.[32] The value of steroid therapy in accelerating the rate of resolution of this reaction is unproven. Acute nitrofurantoin pulmonary reaction virtually always completely resolves; however, death has been ascribed to this reaction.

Subacute pulmonary reactions from nitrofurantoin usually develop after one month of drug exposure and are characterized by persistent and progressive cough, dyspnea, orthopnea and fever.[32] Radiographically there is an interstitial pneumonitis. There may be an associated lupus-like syndrome consisting of arthralgia, pleural effusions, peripheral lymphadenopathy, impaired liver function, elevated sedimentation rate, polyclonal hypergammaglobulinemia, positive latex-agglutination test, antinuclear antibodies and antibodies to thyroid, glomeruli and smooth muscle. Discontinuation of nitrofurantoin therapy has been followed by complete resolution of the clinical, radiological, serological and immunological abnormalities.

Chronic nitrofurantoin pulmonary reaction is associated with the insidious development of non-productive cough and dyspnea. Physical examination reveals rales, but fever is not a consistent finding. The sedimentation rate is usually elevated, and there may be concomitant deranged liver function tests. There is no peripheral blood eosinophilia. Pulmonary function studies demonstrate a restrictive ventilatory pattern with impairment of carbon dioxide diffusing capacity. Histologically there is a nonspecific pattern of diffuse interstitial pneumonitis and fibrosis. Desquamative interstitial pneumonia has also followed prolonged therapy with nitrofurantoin. The chronic nitrofurantoin pulmonary reaction develops after six months of drug treatment and has occurred in children. Usually, but not always, regression of the syndrome follows discontinuation of nitrofurantoin therapy. Treatment with a steroid may improve the patient's symptoms, but there is no firm evidence that this medication favorably alters the pulmonary function or radiographs. Irreversible pulmonary fibrosis culminating in respiratory failure and death has resulted from long-term treatment with nitrofurantoin.

Preparations and 1978 Costs—Cyantin Tablets 50 mg—$2.74/100; 100 mg—$3.92/100. Furadantin Tablets 50 mg—$10.68/100; 100 mg—$21.54/100; Suspension 25 mg/5 ml—$2.00/60 ml. Macrodantin Capsules 25 mg—$11.16/100; 50 mg—$4.80/30, $15.06/100; 100 mg—$9.48/30, $29.82/100.

REFERENCES

1. Waisbren BA, Crowley W: Nitrofurantoin: clinical and laboratory evaluation. Arch Intern Med 95:653–661, 1955.
2. Richards WA, Riss E, Kass EH, et al: Nitrofurantoin: clinical laboratory studies in urinary tract infections. Arch Intern Med 96:437–450, 1955.
3. Turk M, Ronald AR, Petersdorf RG: Susceptibility of enterobacteriaceae to nitrofurantoin correlated with eradication of bacteriuria. Antimicrob Agents Chemother—1967, pp 446–452.
4. Rosenthal SL, Freundlich LF, Quraishi MAH, et al: Antibiotic sensitivity: Bronx municipal hospital-center 1976 report. NY State J Med 77:756–762, 1977.
5. Barry AL, Thrupp LD: Problems in evaluating nitrofurantoin susceptibility tests for Klebsiella-Enterobacter. Antimicrob Agents Chemother—1968, pp 415–422.
6. Conklin JD: Biopharmaceutics of nitrofurantoin. Pharmacology 8:178–181, 1972.
7. Goff JB, Schleger JV, O'Dell RM: Urinary excretion of naladixic acid, sulfa-methoxazole, and nitrofurantoin in patients with reduced renal function. J Urol 99:371–375, 1968.
8. Felts JH, Hayes DM, Gergen JA, et al: Neural, hematologic, and bacteriologic effects of nitrofurantoin in renal insufficiency. Am J Med 51:331–339, 1971.
9. Sachs J, Geer J, Noell P, et al: Effect of renal function on urinary recovery of orally administered nitrofurantoin. N Engl J Med 278:1032–1035, 1968.
10. Rosenberg HA, Bates TR: The influence of food on nitrofurantoin bioavailability. Clin Pharmacol Ther 20:227–232, 1976.
11. Jaffe JM: Effect of propantheline on nitrofurantoin absorption. J Pharm Sci 64:1729–1730, 1975.
12. Perry JE, Toney JD, LeBlanc AL: Effect of nitrofurantoin on the human fetus. Tex Rep Biol Med 25:270–272, 1967.
13. Kunin CM: Effect of renal failure on recovery of antimicrobial agents in the urine—nitrofurantoin, ampicillin and cephalexin. In *Renal Infection and Renal Scarring*. Edited by P Kincaid-Smith, KF Fairley. Melbourne, Australia, Mercedes Publishing Services, 1970, pp 181–194.
14. Brumfitt W, Percival A, Carter MJ: Treatment of urinary tract infections with ampicillin: a clinical trial. Lancet 1:130–133, 1962.

15. Asscher AW, Sussman M, Waters WE, et al: Asymptomatic significant bacteriuria in the non-pregnant woman. Br Med J 1:804–806, 1969.
16. Smith PK, Fairley KF: Controlled trial comparing effect of two and six weeks' treatment in recurrent urinary tract infection. Br Med J 2:145–146, 1969.
17. Ormonde NWH, Gray JA, Murdoch JMcC, et al: Chronic bacteriuria due to Escherichia coli. I. Assessment of the value of combined short and long-term treatment with cycloserine, nitrofurantoin, and sulphadimidine. J Infect Dis 120:82–86, 1969.
18. Bailey RR, Boberts AP, Gower PE, et al: Prevention of urinary tract infection with low-dose nitrofurantoin. Lancet 2:1112–1114, 1971.
19. Ronald AR, Harding GKM, Mathias R, et al: Prophylaxis of recurring urinary tract infection in females: a comparison of nitrofurantoin with trimethoprim-sulfamethoxazole. Can Med Assoc J 112:13S–16S, 1975.
20. Stamey TA, Condy M, Mihara GL: Prophylactic efficacy of nitrofurantoin macrocrystals and trimethoprim-sulfamethoxazole in urinary infections. N Engl J Med 296:780–783, 1977.
21. Kaslowski S, Radford N, Kincaid-Smith P: Crystalline and macrocrystalline nitrofurantoin in the treatment of urinary tract infection. N Engl J Med 280:385–387, 1974.
22. Freeman RB, Smith WMc, Richardson JA, et al: Long-term therapy for chronic bacteriuria in men: U.S. Public Health Service Cooperative Study. Ann Intern Med 83:133–147, 1975.
23. Lohr JA, Nonley DH, Howards SS, et al: Prevention of recurrent urinary tract infection in girls. Pediatrics 59:562–565, 1977.
24. Smellie JM, Katz G, Gruneberg RN: Controlled trial of prophylactic treatment in childhood urinary-tract infection. Lancet 2:175–178, 1978.
25. Koch-Weser J, Sidel VW, Dexter M, et al: Adverse reactions to sulfisoxazole, sulfamethoxazole, and nitrofurantoin. Arch Intern Med 128:399–404, 1971.
26. Gleckman R, Alvarez S, Joubert DW: Nitrofurantoin. Am J Hosp Pharm (in press).
27. Arndt KA, Jick H: Rates of cutaneous reactions to drugs. JAMA 235:918–922, 1976.
28. Tarlov AR, Brewer GJ, Carson PE, et al: Primaquine sensitivity: glucose-6-phosphate dehydrogenase deficiency: inborn error of metabolism of medical and biological significance. Arch Intern Med 109:209–234, 1962.
29. Toole JF, Parrish ML: Nitrofurantoin polyneuropathy. Neurology 23:554–559, 1973.
30. Stromberg A, Wengle B: Chronic active hepatitis induced by nitrofurantoin. Br Med J 2:174–175, 1976.
31. Kursh ED, Mostyn EM, Persky L: Nitrofurantoin pulmonary complications. J Urol 113:392–395, 1975.
32. Sovijarvi ARA, Lemola M, Stenius B, et al: Nitrofurantoin-induced acute, subacute and chronic pulmonary reactions. Scand J Respir Dis 58:41–50, 1977.

11. ANTITUBERCULOUS AGENTS

Kenneth L. Pinsker and Spencer K. Koerner

Mycobacterium tuberculosis is an obligate aerobe that preferentially flourishes in those tissues with high oxygen tensions, eg, the apices of the lung. It is characterized by a slow growth rate, ability to survive for long periods of time in a dormant state, and relative resistance to antibiotics. In addition, the tubercle bacillus is able to develop in vivo drug resistance, often in a matter of weeks, when exposed to a single antituberculous agent. Its slow growth rate necessitates treatment of tuberculosis for long periods of time. The presence of dormant phases also necessitates long treatment, so that all organisms will eventually be exposed to bacteriocidal drug levels when an active growth phase ensues.

The ability to develop drug resistance is the most important biologic characteristic of the acid-fast bacillus and the one which most influences the approach to chemotherapy. All natural populations of *Mycobacterium tuberculosis* contain varying numbers of drug-resistant organisms.[1] Fortunately, the occurrence of disease secondary to such organisms is rare, is limited to sporadic outbreaks, and has not appreciably increased in the past several years. The number of naturally-occurring, isoniazid-resistant organisms is about one in 100,000 bacilli, while the number of streptomycin-resistant organisms is about one in 1,000,000.[2] Naturally-occurring resistance to other drugs is observed with similar frequency. The probability of resistance to both of the above drugs or to any combination of drugs is the product of the resistances. Since most tuberculous lesions contain a minimum of 100,000 organisms, a minimum of two antituberculous agents should be used in order to avoid the emergence of resistant organisms.[3] It has been shown that administration of 1 g/day of streptomycin for four months will cause 80% of patients to excrete acid-fast bacilli resistant to therapeutic doses and that 50% of those bacilli are resistant to streptomycin levels of 1000 μg/ml.[4]

The pharmacologic properties of the antituberculous agents also play an important role in selecting a safe and efficient drug regimen. The ideal antituberculous agent should be: (a) non toxic; (b) easily absorbed; (c) orally administered; (d) able to penetrate into all tissues and into tuberculous lesions; (e) active against both extra- and intracellular acid-fast bacilli at both acid and basic pH levels; and (f) able to destroy dormant as well as reproducing organisms. None of the drugs in use today meets all of these criteria, but the most commonly used antituberculous agents closely approximate them.

ANTITUBERCULOUS REGIMENS IN PULMONARY TUBERCULOSIS

The physician today has many therapeutic options, and his primary concern should be with the ease and lack of toxicity with which bacteriologic cure is achieved. Cure rates approaching 100% should be the accepted norm, and any case not rapidly responding to therapy must be carefully re-examined.

Until recently the mainstay of antituberculous therapy has been the combination of isoniazid (INH), streptomycin (STM) and para-aminosalicylic acid (PAS). Many other regimens have been advocated, but two offer distinct advantages.

Isoniazid and Ethambutol

Because of low toxicity, ease of administration, patient acceptance, and excellent cure rates, most cases of pulmonary tuberculosis can be treated with a combination of isoniazid and ethambutol (EMB). INH is given in a single daily dose of 300 mg; EMB is given as a single daily dose of 25 mg/kg for three months and then continued at 15 mg/kg. The duration of treatment for both drugs is 24 months. In cases of far-advanced cavitary disease, the dose of INH may be increased to 450 mg/day. A small number of patients, whose disease may be complicated by coincident medical illness, do not respond adequately to the combination of INH and EMB.

In terms of greater efficacy and/or less toxicity, INH and initially-high dose EMB has been shown superior to the combination of (1) PAS 12 g/day and INH 300 mg/day in minimal and moderately advanced disease,[5] and (2) PAS 12 g/day, INH 300 mg/day, and STM 1 g/day for 90 days then 1 g three times a week for 90 days in far-advanced cavitary disease.[6] The addition of STM 1 g/day to the combination of EMB 25/15 and INH 450 mg/day in a study of far-advanced cavitary disease did not result in a higher frequency of sputum conversion but did result in a higher dropout rate, presumably because of greater adverse effects.[7]

Isoniazid and Rifampin

In studies of patients with advanced cavitary pulmonary tuberculosis the combination of rifampin 600 mg/day and INH 300 mg/day has been shown at least as effective as INH/EMB.[8–10] Sputum conversion rates of 100% at six months have been reported in some studies.[9] Toxicity due to rifampin has been low (see drug monograph). Liver enzymes are often mildly elevated, but few cases of clinical hepatitis have been reported.

The efficacy of rifampin in the treatment of pulmonary tuberculosis is well established, but its exact role is still unclear.[11] Some authorities advocate its use in the initial treatment of tuberculosis, while others feel it should be reserved for treatment of cases failing to respond to initial therapy.

Those who advocate initial use point to the ability of rifampin to sterilize large tuberculous lesions and thus avoid the development of resistant infections. They state that the resulting high proportion of initial cures will largely eliminate the problem of complex retreatment cases.

On the other hand, it is argued that the initial use of rifampin will only contribute to increasing rifampin resistance and to the elimination of the most potent agent used in the retreatment of tuberculosis. Authorities against initial use suggest the establishment of two separate regimens, one including INH that is used for initial therapy, and another containing rifampin that is used only for retreatment. Use of a rifampin regimen solely in retreatment, they argue, will still give a 95% sputum conversion rate for those patients initially treated with an INH regimen who fail to achieve bacteriologic cure. It is not yet clear which approach is correct, or if indeed there has to be rigid adherence to a single formula.

We feel at this time that the routine initial treatment of minimal and moderate pulmonary tuberculosis can be carried out with INH/EMB. However, in patients with far-advanced cavitary disease, INH/rifampin should be used. Other drug combinations do not offer any advantage over either of these regimens in initial therapy and their use is not recommended.

It is currently recommended that all patients receiving conventional antituberculous therapy be treated for a minimum of 18 to 24 months, depending on the severity of the disease and the rapidity of sputum and x-ray clearing. After two years of chemotherapy, relapse rates are extremely low (less than 2%). Outpatient follow-up need not continue, but patients should be advised to contact their physician for any new chest symptoms or constitutional problems.[12] Continuing chemotherapy for more than 24 months following successful initial therapy is not necessary.

SHORT-TERM THERAPY

With the introduction of rifampin and recognition of its unique antituberculous properties, there has been renewed interest in short-term therapy of pulmonary tuberculosis. Reduction in the total duration of therapy to one year or less without an accompanying decrease in cure rates would be of enormous value, especially in countries where financial or social conditions make 18 to 24 month therapy difficult. The advantages of short-term therapy are (1) a decrease in drug toxicity due to decreased drug exposure, (2) increased patient compliance, and (3) decreased need for extensive follow-up facilities.

Prior attempts at short-term therapy have been unsuccessful because of unacceptably high relapse rates, but recent work reported by Fox and Mitchison[13] suggests that with multiple drug regimens or with the use of INH/rifampin, the relapse problem is minimized. They report that a combination of INH, STM and rifampin daily for six months yielded virtually 100% sputum conversion; only two out of 112 patients had relapses, both of which occurred within 18 months after discontinuation of the therapy. The relapse patients were retreated and followed for a total of thirty months after the cessation of therapy and no further relapses were noted. A repeat study using the same regimen in 152 patients showed a comparable rate of relapse. All patients studied had moderately to far-advanced tuberculosis.

Other studies have assessed the use of INH/rifampin (without streptomycin) for six months. This was particularly important, as the elimination of an injectable drug increased patient acceptance and made self-administration of medications feasible. Unfortunately, the results were ambiguous. Only one patient failed to convert his sputum after six months of therapy, but after 12 months of follow-up there was a 5% (9/170) relapse rate, a figure which, if confirmed by larger studies, would be higher than one would accept after standard two-year therapy. INH and rifampin, while successfully converting sputum to negative within six months, does not appear to be satisfactory unless given for longer periods.

Other studies indicate that six to 12 months of therapy with the addition of ethambutol to INH and rifampin will result in an extremely low relapse rate. Pilheu reported on 136 patients from the Tuberculosis Clinic of Buenos Aires, 99 of whom received INH, rifampin and ethambutol for six months, and 37 of whom received the same three drugs for six months followed by seven months of intermittent therapy with INH.[14] All treatment was carried out on an ambulatory basis, and after six months all patients were bacteriologically negative. There was only one relapse, which occurred four months after stopping all chemotherapy. While these preliminary data suggest that short-term therapy for pulmonary tuberculosis is feasible, we feel it is presently suited only for situations in which conventional 18 to 24 month therapy cannot be carried out. Further investigation may, however, allow us to significantly reduce the duration of treatment in the near future.

INTERMITTENT THERAPY

For patients who cannot be relied upon to take daily medications, but who can be followed as outpatients in a clinic or at home two times a week, intermittent therapy should be considered as a substitute for long-term hospitalization. INH 15 mg/kg with either STM 25–30 mg/kg or EMB 50 mg/kg, given twice weekly, have been shown to produce acceptable cure rates. When INH is used in this type of regimen, pyridoxine 50 mg/day should be given with each dose to prevent peripheral neuritis. Optic neuritis has not been a problem with the increased dose of ethambutol, and reactions to STM are of the same type and frequency as those usually encountered. Such therapy is not currently recommended as a substitute for daily therapy by the American Thoracic Society and should only be given after an initial period of daily therapy for two to six months, depending on the extent of the disease; it should be continued for a total of 24 months. Acquired drug resistance is not a problem as long as a regular treatment schedule is followed.[15,16]

It would appear from the results of daily therapy with rifampin that it would be the ideal agent for intermittent therapy; however, this has not been proven. Biweekly use of rifampin has been associated with an adverse reaction rate as high as 20%, usually after six months of therapy.[17-19] These reactions fall into two categories. The most common is a systemic reaction, probably induced by the deposition of immune complexes in small blood vessels and producing fever, joint pain and abdominal and muscle cramps. The other is an antibody-induced thrombocytopenia. These reactions have also been described after the reinstitution of rifampin as long as several months after therapy has been discontinued.

In contrast to the above experience, the use of once-weekly rifampin at 30 mg/kg has, in one study, been shown to be extremely potent in producing sputum conversion when combined with EMB 100 mg/kg or INH 15 mg/kg, and not to be associated with any severe side effects.[20] The authors postulated that since the total duration of the intermittent therapy was less than six months (at that time, patients were switched to another regimen), the immunologic sensitization never developed.

It is our feeling that rifampin should not be used on an intermittent basis until more information is available about its immunologic effects.

RETREATMENT

Retreatment cases are among the most difficult problems in the therapy of pulmonary tuberculosis. Widespread lung destruction as sequelae of previous infections and multiple drug toxicities and drug resistances may be present. Cure rates in the past have been low, and the use of more toxic multiple drug regimens that rely on less efficient second line drugs has been necessary. The use of rifampin in combination with ethambutol appears to have markedly changed those statistics.[21] These two drugs have provided cure rates above 95% in retreatment cases, as demonstrated by numerous studies. As a result of the excellent cure rates with currently available initial and retreatment drug regimens, patients with persistently positive sputum will be rarely encountered.

SECOND-LINE DRUGS

Four other oral antituberculous agents are currently employed in the United States, but all are considered second-line drugs whose usefulness is limited by their toxicity and lack of demonstrated superiority over less toxic agents. These drugs are para-aminosalicylic acid (PAS), pyrazinamide, cycloserine, and ethionamide. In addition, kanamycin, viomycin and capreomycin, all of which are given only by injection, are rarely used in tuberculosis therapy because of their toxicities and their marginal effectiveness.

The dosage, route of administration, major adverse effects, and procedures for monitoring for adverse effects of first and second-line antituberculous drugs are presented in Tables 1 and 2, respectively.

HOSPITALIZATION OF TUBERCULOSIS PATIENTS

Routine long-term hospitalization of all tuberculosis patients is no longer necessary in view of the increased efficacy of modern chemotherapy.[22,23] Current recommendations as to the length of hospitalization or criteria for discharge of tuberculosis patients are not standardized, and wide variations in clinical practice occur. We feel that in most cases in which minimally to moderately advanced disease is present, brief hospitalization is sufficient for patient education and for observation for possible hypersensitivity or idiosyncratic drug reactions. More complex cases may require hospitalization for longer periods, but even far-advanced cases can often be discharged in a matter of weeks.

The traditional criteria of awaiting three negative smears and cultures before discharge was based on the impression that as long as acid-fast bacilli could be seen in the sputum or grown in culture medium, the patient was infectious. The limited infectivity of patients taking antituberculosis agents has been suspected for many years, and it has been shown that most cases of spread of tuberculosis occur from undiagnosed cases, not from patients undergoing active chemotherapy.[24,25]

Several recent studies suggest that after three to four weeks of antituberculous therapy, most of the acid-fast bacilli excreted are of low viability and consequently unlikely to cause infection in contacts. Examination of PPD (purified protein derivative of tuberculin diagnostic agent) conversion rates among household contacts of patients discharged with positive smears while on adequate chemotherapy has revealed an extremely low incidence of conversion.[26] Furthermore, continued clinical improvement, sputum conversion and x-ray improvement have been observed in patients discharged from the hospital after three to four weeks of therapy, provided a good outpatient program is initiated.[27] Early discharge of patients with positive sputa must always be considered in relation to the socio-economic nature of tuberculosis, and patients who are felt to be unreliable because of drug or alcohol abuse or because of character disorders must be hospitalized for longer periods of time. Consideration should be given to alternate forms of therapy, eg, short-term, intermittent, or supervised drug administration, but above all it should be emphasized that the best chance of cure for any patient lies in the initial course of therapy. Every effort must be made to achieve bacteriologic cure the first time the patient is treated.

CHEMOPROPHYLAXIS OF PULMONARY TUBERCULOSIS

Chemoprophylaxis of pulmonary tuberculosis is based on the demonstration that skin test conversion is caused by initial infection with *Mycobacterium tuberculosis* and that failure to treat the primary infection results in the appearance of active disease in a number of those infected.[28,29] Not all people with a positive skin test are equally at risk for the development of active disease, and the individual circumstances must always be evaluated so the risk of breakdown can be weighed against the possibility of serious drug reaction. For practical purposes, we must concern ourselves with the specific use of isoniazid as a chemoprophylactic agent and must examine in detail the possible hepatocellular damage resulting from its use.

The discovery of a positive skin test necessitates placing the patient into the correct risk category so that factors for and against chemotherapy can be evaluated. Generally, either a high, moderate or low risk is assigned.

High Risk

Household Contacts. The high-risk group includes all household contacts of patients with active tuberculosis. All such contacts should be screened with an intermediate PPD and with chest x-rays. It is estimated that approximately one in thirty household contacts will develop active tuberculosis if not treated. Any household contact with an abnormal chest x-ray should be fully evaluated for the presence of active tuberculosis, regardless of the status of his skin test. If a rapid determination of activity cannot be made, it is suggested that such patients be started on INH and EMB until the evaluation can be completed, and either continuation of therapy for active disease or chemoprophylaxis with INH alone is decided upon.

In the adult population, if a negative chest x-ray occurs together with a positive intermediate PPD, it is recommended that 300 mg of INH be given daily for one year. If a negative intermediate PPD coexists with a negative chest x-ray, no immediate therapy is necessary. If exposure was minimal, it is recommended that the skin test be repeated in three months and therapy initiated at that time if conversion has taken place. If the initial exposure was very heavy, chemoprophylaxis should be started and continued for three months, at which time the skin test should be repeated. If the skin test is still negative, INH prophylaxis can be discontinued, but if conversion has taken place, INH should be continued for a total of 12 months.

In the pediatric age group, it is recommended that all household contacts below the age of six who have a positive skin test be treated with INH 10–20 mg/kg up to 300 mg for one year. There are two possible approaches to the child who has a negative skin test and a history of household exposure. Certain authorities suggest that they should be treated for three months and the skin test repeated. If it remains negative, INH can be terminated; if conversion has taken place, treatment should be continued for one year. Other authorities advocate a mandatory one year of INH prophylaxis for pediatric household contacts regardless of skin test status. This is because of their increased risk of developing active tuberculosis and the almost nonexistent incidence of adverse effects of INH among children.[30]

Recent Converters. Also at high risk are those patients with a known recent conversion of their skin test within the prior 12 to 24 months. The risk of developing active disease is greatest (approximately 3%) in the first year of the conversion, and decreases each year therafter. Establishment of the exact time of conversion is of extreme importance to facilitate assignment of the correct risk category.

These patients should be screened with chest x-rays and, if no abnormality is found, prophylaxis with 300 mg INH a day for one year should be undertaken. Since there are great variations among reading procedures and techniques of administration of skin tests, rigid criteria for 'conversion' must be adhered to. They should include an increase in induration of at least 6 mm from a total of less than 10 mm to a total of greater than 10 mm, and must also include consideration of any so-called 'booster effect.' This effect is seen most frequently in patients over 50 years of age and occurs when delayed hypersensitivity wanes, so that the first of two tuberculin skin tests may serve to 'boost' the response to a second test given within a year or two. This may give rise to a false conversion when in fact the tests have been positive for many years.

Inadequately Treated Tuberculosis. In the remaining high-risk group we find patients with a definite past history of active tuberculosis who have never received adequate chemotherapy, and patients with positive skin tests who have radiologic evidence of inactive tuberculosis. The incidence of developing active disease in these patients is about 1 in 75 per year. These patients often are from the pre-antibiotic era and may have been treated with thoracoplasty or pneumothorax therapy or may have received STM and/or PAS, but never INH. It is recommended that these patients receive one year of INH 300 mg/day, with due consideration that this group of patients is often elderly and at higher risk for INH-induced hepatitis. Close follow-up is required and possible signs of INH toxicity must be carefully evaluated.

Moderate Risk

Patients found to have positive skin tests and normal chest x-rays, with no history of recent household contact and no evidence of recent conversion, are at moderate risk of developing active tuberculosis if they fall into several special clinical categories as outlined below. It is recommended by the American Thoracic Society that they receive one year of prophylaxis; life-long continuation of INH does not confer any added advantage.[29]

Patients on Corticosteroids or Immunosuppressive Agents. The exact incidence of breakdown of inactive tuberculosis lesions in patients receiving immunosuppressive drugs is not known, but there is sufficient clinical evidence to implicate these agents in the development of active disease if a previously inactive focus is present. It is currently recommended that patients in this category receive one year of INH prophylaxis. Intermittent INH 'coverage' of these patients while on immunosuppressives or corticosteroids is to be avoided, as it might foster the emergence of resistant organisms.

The Presence of Hematologic or Reticuloendothelial Diseases. It is difficult to separate these patients from the above groups, as they are often treated with immunosuppressive agents. They should be treated with one year of INH at the beginning of their disease process or upon institution of therapy. Accurate data regarding the past skin test status of such patients is essential so that current skin tests may be properly interpreted in view of the anergy these patients may exhibit. In all cases when such data are not reliable, the possibility of active tuberculosis must be exhaustively pursued.

The Presence of Diabetes Mellitus. The breakdown rate of primary lesions in patients with diabetes mellitus appears to be higher than in nondiabetic patients. Presentation of active tuberculosis may be atypical or modified by the diabetes and active disease must be excluded. If no indication of activity is present, these patients should receive one year of INH prophylaxis.

Silicosis. Patients with proven or suspected pulmonary silicosis should be given INH prophylaxis. The silicotic host is more susceptible to dissemination of tuberculosis, and the widespread parenchymal destruction often present makes any degree of active tuberculosis more of a threat.

Post-gastrectomy. For reasons which remain unclear, possibly related to nutritional status or some nonspecific decrease in host resistance, patients with subtotal or total gastrectomy have a high incidence of breakdown of their primary lesions. INH prophylaxis is recommended for patients with a gastrectomy who are found to have a positive skin test and a normal chest roentgenogram.

Low Risk

The last group of people to be considered for INH prophylaxis are those in the low-risk category where the incidence of developing active tuberculosis is about 1 in 1400 per year. These are people with a normal chest roentgenogram and a positive skin test of unknown duration who do not have any other indication for chemoprophylaxis. Under these circumstances, each case should be individualized, but prophylaxis is not indicated for patients above 35, at which time the risk of INH-associated hepatitis exceeds 1% and is therefore greater than the risk of breakdown.

FOLLOW-UP OF PATIENTS WITH INH PROPHYLAXIS

All patients placed on INH must have careful and frequent medical evaluation for the presence of INH-induced hepatocellular damage. There is no current agreement on the best method of monitoring these patients, or on the significance of the presence of mild elevations in transaminase, but certain precautions would seem indicated. All patients should be initially screened for the presence of liver dysfunction before prophylaxis is begun. Where mild or moderate chronic liver disease is not an absolute contraindication to the use of INH, patients with such damage have less reserve if INH toxicity should occur. Individuals who develop clinical hepatitis while on INH should have the medication discontinued. All patients with a continued significant elevation in transaminase (above 100 units) must be carefully monitored and if the rise continues to above 250 units, the INH should be discontinued. The presence of a mild rise in transaminase (between 100 and 250 units) as well as abnormality in another liver function test, eg, alkaline phosphatase, requires discontinuation of the drug.

CORTICOSTEROIDS

While not indicated in the routine treatment of pulmonary tuberculosis, corticosteroids have limited application in the therapy of severely toxic patients. They must never be given unless adequate antituberculous coverage is provided, and the occurrence of steroid-induced side effects must be evaluated in each individual case.

The benefits of corticosteroid therapy in the treatment of pulmonary tuberculosis are limited to the first one to three months during which a more rapid clinical improvement may occur. This is manifested by loss of fever, weight gain, and an increased feeling of well being. Long-term studies demonstrate, however, that at the end of six to twelve months of chemotherapy there is an equal degree of clinical improvement in patients treated with and without steroids.

Clinical or radiographic worsening after steroid withdrawal, and rapid progression of tuberculosis lesions while on steroids has been reported, so careful monitoring of these patients is mandatory. The currently recommended dose of corticosteroids is the equivalent of 40 mg/day of prednisone to be given for a maximum of six weeks and tapered gradually to avoid any rebound phenomena.

CHEMOTHERAPY OF MILIARY AND EXTRAPULMONARY TUBERCULOSIS

The diagnosis of disseminated tuberculosis presents a difficult clinical problem.[31] Physician recognition of miliary, gastrointestinal, genitourinary, or central nervous system disease, secondary to *M. tuberculosis,* is limited by: (1) failure to consider the diagnosis of disseminated tuberculosis; (2) the atypical clinical, roentgenographic and pathologic features that often characterize these forms of tuberculous infection; and (3) the presence of other disease entities, often related to alcohol abuse, which obscure the presence of tuberculous disease. It is beyond the scope of this chapter to completely review the chemotherapy of disseminated tuberculosis. However, several important points should be emphasized. There are few, if any, controlled studies that deal with this problem, especially since the introduction of ethambutol and rifampin. Most current studies include patients treated with various combinations of INH, ethambutol, streptomycin and rifampin and do not contain enough patients to permit statistical comparisons of the cure rates achieved by the various regimens. In addition, it should be noted that successful therapy of extrapulmonary disseminated tuberculosis may, in some instances, require surgical intervention. While no definite conclusions can be drawn from the current literature, it appears that the combination of INH and ethambutol is adequate for most cases. The use of INH and rifampin or perhaps the combination of all three agents should, in our opinion, be reserved for those patients who have overwhelming disease or who are markedly debilitated because of the presence of other disease processes. Treatment for two years appears advisable.[32–34]

DRUG MONOGRAPHS

Since the indications, contraindications, and dosage of the antituberculous drugs are covered above, the drug monographs are primarily concerned with the clinical toxicity of these drugs.

ISONIAZID

As INH is the most widely used antituberculous agent, its toxicity is perhaps the most frequently encountered and therefore its toxic manifestations should be well understood.[35]

The most important toxicity of isoniazid is its effect upon hepatocellular function. From 10 to 20% of patients taking 300 mg of INH daily, will show some transient or prolonged rise in SGOT and SGPT and a pathological picture resembling a mild viral hepatitis.[36,37] This change in liver function is usually benign, with enzymes returning to normal values or stabilizing after several months and with the patient showing no clinical signs of hepatitis. A more serious, idiosyncratic type of progressive hepatocellular damage occurs rarely. It is virtually never seen in patients below 20 years of age, and its frequency increases from approximately 0.3% in the age range of 20 to 34 to 2.3% at age 50 and above. Occasional cases of massive liver atrophy with death have been reported and, although other contributing factors (ie, alcohol or prior liver damage) may have been present in the initial reports, INH appears to be directly implicated.[38] Consideration of the above data is of extreme importance in the prophylaxis of tuberculosis with INH, but the benefits of INH as a therapeutic agent in active tuberculosis make its possible hepatic side effects of less concern in treating active disease.

The most common side effect of isoniazid is peripheral neuropathy. This is infrequent with dosage of 300 mg daily, except in alcoholic or severely malnourished patients and increases in frequency in high dosage INH therapy. Other potentially severe side effects and idiosyncratic reactions are: (1) central nervous system stimulation or depression, sometimes resulting in overt psychosis; (2) induction of lupus erythematosus or rheumatoid-like syndromes; (3) hematologic disturbances, including hemolytic anemia, pyridoxine responsive anemia, agranulocytosis, and red cell aplasia; and (4) hypersensitivity reactions consisting of fever, rash, eosinophilia, and arthralgias. Some of these reactions may be self-limited, while others may be progressive and require discontinuing INH and/or desensitization procedures. Routine use of pyridoxine is not recommended unless preexisting neuropathy, alcoholism, malnutrition, or pyridoxine-responsive anemia is present.

ETHAMBUTOL

This agent, now frequently used in combination with INH in initial therapy of pulmonary tuberculosis, has one major serious side effect: optic neuritis. The neuritis is dose-related and may manifest itself by loss in visual acuity or color discrimination. At currently employed

TABLE 1 First-Line Drugs in the Therapy of Tuberculosis

Drug	Daily Dose	Route of Administration	Major Adverse Effects	Monitoring
Isoniazid	300 mg (single dose)	Oral	Hepatitis Peripheral neuritis CNS disturbances Hematologic and rheumatoid disorders	Serum transaminase
Rifampin	600 mg (single dose)	Oral	Hepatitis Thrombocytopenia (with intermittent use)	Monthly serum transaminase
Ethambutol	25 mg/kg for 90 days, then 15 mg/kg (single doses)	Oral	Optic neuritis	Monthly visual acuity and color tests
Streptomycin	15 mg/kg up to 1.0 g daily for 90 days, then 1.0 g 3 times weekly (single doses)	Intramuscular	Vestibular toxicity Auditory toxicity Renal insufficiency	Monthly blood urea, nitrogen, and audiogram

dosages of either 15 mg/kg/day or 25 mg/kg/day, optic neuritis has rarely been described; it was primarily observed at doses of 50 mg/kg/day. In the Public Health Service trials using ethambutol at 15 mg/kg/day, there was no significant difference noted in the frequency of decreased visual acuity in the patients taking EMB, as compared to patients on other drug regimens. It is currently recommended that patients taking ethambutol have monthly monitoring of visual acuity and color discrimination, and that any significant change from baseline levels be evaluated fully.[39,40]

RIFAMPIN

The daily use of rifampin is associated with an occasional elevation of liver enzymes and bilirubin values; this is partially caused by false elevations due to interference of rifampin with bilirubin assay techniques. There are isolated occurrences of clinical hepatitis and, in addition, rare cases of generalized hypersensitivity reactions have been reported. In the Public Health Service cooperative trial using 600 mg/day of rifampin, approximately a 1% reaction rate was noted. Other studies have reported reaction rates in the 3 to 5% range, with the incidence of asymptomatic rises in transaminase as high as 18%. Rifampin is felt by most authors to be a reasonably benign drug, although the combination of rifampin/INH appears slightly more likely to induce hepatocellular damage than rifampin/EMB.[8]

An additional, recently-described side effect of rifampin is its interaction with oral contraceptives; contraceptive activity is diminished by increased estrogen metabolism.[41]

STREPTOMYCIN

The treatment-limiting toxicity of streptomycin is its effect on the vestibular branch of the eighth cranial nerve. Lesser effects on the auditory branch can sometimes be seen, but vestibular dysfunction usually precedes any decrease in hearing. Renal insufficiency can also be observed, but it is less common than with the other injectable aminoglycosides used in the treatment of tuberculosis, kanamycin, capreomycin and viomycin. Elderly patients are especially sensitive to the vestibular damage caused by streptomycin, and lower doses are often necessary to prevent the rapid onset of toxicity. Monthly

TABLE 2 Second-Line Drugs in the Therapy of Tuberculosis

Drug	Daily Dose	Route of Administration	Major Adverse Effects	Monitoring
p-Aminosalicylic acid	200 mg/kg up to 12 g (three divided doses)	Oral	Gastrointestinal disturbances Hepatitis Lupuslike syndrome	Monthly serum transaminase
Pyrazinamide	40–50 mg/kg up to 2–3 g (three divided doses)	Oral	Hepatitis Hyperuricemia	Monthly serum transaminase and uric acid
Cycloserine	15 mg/kg up to 1.0 g (four divided doses)	Oral	CNS disorders (seizures, psychosis)	Evaluation of neurologic status
Ethionamide	10–15 mg/kg up to 1.0 g (four divided doses)	Oral	Hepatitis Gastrointestinal upset	Monthly serum transaminase
Kanamycin	15 mg/kg up to 1.0 g five times weekly	Intramuscular	Renal insufficiency Auditory toxicity Vestibular toxicity	Same as for streptomycin
Viomycin	15 mg/kg up to 1.0 g five times weekly, or 2.0 g twice weekly	Intramuscular	Auditory toxicity Vestibular toxicity Renal insufficiency	Same as for streptomycin
Capreomycin	15 mg/kg up to 1.0 g five times weekly	Intramuscular	Auditory toxicity Vestibular toxicity Renal insufficiency	Same as for streptomycin

TABLE 3 Preparations and Costs of Antituberculous Agents

GENERIC NAME	TRADEMARK NAME(S)	PREPARATIONS AND 1978 COSTS
Isoniazid	generic	Tablets 100 mg—$0.80–$1.58/100; 300 mg—$0.96–$2.19/100
Ethambutol	Myambutol	Tablets 100 mg—$6.99/100; 400 mg—$22.81/100
Rifampin	Rifadin (Rimactane)	Capsules 300 mg—$75.00/100
Streptomycin Sulfate	generic	Injection (solution) 500 mg/ml—$0.68/2-ml ampul, $1.25–$1.82/10-ml vial
Aminosalicylate Calcium	Parasal Calcium	Tablets 500 mg—$10.80/1,000
Aminosalicylate Sodium	Parasal Sodium	Tablets 500 mg—$18.00/1,000
Capreomycin Sulfate	Capastat Sulfate	Injection (powder) 1 g—$4.88/5 ml
Cycloserine	Seromycin	Capsules 250 mg—$11.78/40
Ethionamide	Trecator-SC	Tablets 250 mg—$20.00/100
Kanamycin Sulfate	Kantrex	Injection (solution) 250 mg/ml—$0.77/2-ml ampul; 333 mg/ml—$1.39/3-ml ampul
Pyrazinamide	generic	Tablets 500 mg—$5.90/100
Viomycin Sulfate	Viocin	Injection (powder) 1 g—$1.75/vial

audiograms should be done on all patients receiving injectable aminoglycosides, and renal function should be carefully monitored, especially in patients with pre-existing renal damage. Because of the high percentage (up to 25%) of patients who demonstrate vestibular damage after long courses of streptomycin, the total dose should be limited to 1 g/day for 90 days, and then 1 g three times a week for an additional sixty days.

REFERENCES

1. Hobby GL, Johnson PM, Boytar-Papirnyik V: Primary drug resistance: a continuing study of tubercle bacilli in a veteran population within the United States, September 1970 to September 1973. Am Rev Resp Dis 110:95–98, 1974.
2. Canetti G: Host factors and chemotherapy of tuberculosis. In *Chemotherapy of Tuberculosis*. Edited by VC Barry. London, Butterworths, 1964, pp 175–191.
3. Rist N: Nature and development of resistance of tubercle bacilli to chemotherapeutic agents. In *Chemotherapy of Tuberculosis*. Edited by VC Barry. London, Butterworths, 1964, pp 192–227.
4. Weinstein L: Drugs used in the chemotherapy of tuberculosis and leprosy. In *The Pharmacological Basis of Therapeutics*, 5th edition. Edited by LS Goodman, A Gilman. New York, Macmillan, 1975, pp 1202–1223.
5. Bobrowitz ID, Robbins DL: Ethambutol-isoniazid vs PAS-isoniazid in the original treatment of pulmonary tuberculosis. Am Rev Resp Dis 96:428–438, 1967.
6. Bobrowitz ID: Ethambutol compared to streptomycin in original treatment of advanced pulmonary tuberculosis. Chest 60:14–21, 1971.
7. Bobrowitz ID: Ethambutol-isoniazid vs streptomycin-ethambutol-isoniazid in original treatment of cavitary tuberculosis. Am Rev Resp Dis 109:548–553, 1974.
8. Newman R, Doster B, Murray FJ, et al: Rifampin in initial treatment of pulmonary tuberculosis: a U.S. Public Health Service tuberculosis therapy trial. Am Rev Resp Dis 103:461–475, 1971.
9. Lees AW, Allen GW, Smith J, et al: Rifampin plus isoniazid in initial therapy of pulmonary tuberculosis, and rifampin and ethambutol in retreatment cases. Chest 61:579–582, 1972.
10. Corpe RF, Sanchez ES: Rifampin in initial treatment of advanced pulmonary tuberculosis. Chest 61:564–567, 1972.
11. London RG: The place of rifampin. Chest 61:524–525, 1972.
12. Reichman LB: Routine follow-up of inactive tuberculosis: a practice that has been abandoned. Am Rev Resp Dis 108:1442–1443, 1973.
13. Fox W, Mitchison DA: Short-course chemotherapy for pulmonary tuberculosis. Am Rev Resp Dis 111:325–353, 1975.
14. Pilheu JA: Short duration treatment of pulmonary tuberculosis. Chest 71:583–586, 1977.
15. Tuberculosis Chemotherapy Centre, Madras, India: Intermittent treatment of pulmonary tuberculosis. A concurrent comparison of twice-daily isoniazid plus streptomycin and daily isoniazid plus *p*-amino-salicylic acid in domiciliary treatment. Lancet 1:1078–1080, 1963.
16. Official ATS Statement: Intermittent chemotherapy for adults with tuberculosis. Am Rev Resp Dis 110:374–375, 1974.
17. Poole GW, Stradling P, Worlledge S: Potentially serious side effects of high dose twice weekly rifampin. Br Med J 3:343–346, 1971.
18. Blajchman MA, Lowry RC, Pettit JL, et al: Rifampin-induced immune thrombocytopenia. Br Med J 3:24–26, 1970.
19. Aquinas M, Allen WGL, Horsfoll PAL, et al: Adverse reactions to daily and intermittent rifampin regimen for pulmonary tuberculosis in Hong Kong. Br Med J 1:765–771, 1972.
20. Verbist L, Mbete S, Van Landry JH, et al: Intermittent therapy with rifampin once a week in advanced pulmonary tuberculosis. Chest 61:555–563, 1972.
21. Jeaves CWL, Jessamine AG, Eidus L: Treatment of chronic drug resistant pulmonary tuberculosis with rifampin and ethambutol. Can Med Assoc J 106:884–888, 1972.
22. Stead WW, Jurgens GH: Productivity of prolonged follow-up after chemotherapy for tuberculosis. Am Rev Resp Dis 108:314–319, 1973.
23. Curry FJ: The effect of acceptable and adequate outpatient treatment on the length of hospitalization and on readmission for relapse or retreatment of pulmonary tuberculosis. Chest 63:535–546, 1973.
24. Riley RL, Mills CC, O'Grady F, et al: Infectiousness of air from a tuberculosis ward. Am Rev Resp Dis 85:511–525, 1962.
25. Gunnels JJ, Bates JH, Swindoll H: Infectivity of sputum-positive tuberculosis patients in chemotherapy. Am Rev Resp Dis 109:323–330, 1974.

26. Brooks SM, Lassiter NL, Young EC: A pilot study concerning the infection risk of sputum positive tuberculosis patients on chemotherapy. Am Rev Resp Dis 108:799–803, 1973.
27. Abeles H: Early hospital discharge of tuberculosis patients with sputum containing acid-fast bacilli on microscopic examination. Am Rev Resp Dis 108:975–977, 1973.
28. Ferebee SH, Mount FW, Comstock GW: Use of chemotherapy as prophylactic measure in tuberculosis. Ann NY Acad Sci 106:151–156, 1963.
29. Official ATS Statement: Preventive therapy of tuberculosis infection. Am Rev Resp Dis 110:371–374, 1974.
30. American Thoracic Society: The treatment of tuberculosis in children. A statement by the Ad Hoc Committee on the Treatment of Tuberculosis in Children. Am Rev Resp Dis 99:304–307, 1969.
31. Grieco MH, Chmel H: Acute disseminated tuberculosis as a diagnostic problem. Am Rev Resp Dis 109:554–560, 1974.
32. Schultz K, Warner HA, Murray D: Intestinal tuberculosis, experience at a Canadian teaching institution. Am J Med 63:735–745, 1977.
33. Simon HB, Weinstein AJ, Pasternak MS, et al: Genitourinary tuberculosis, clinical features in a general hospital population. Am J Med 63:410–420, 1977.
34. Karney WW, O'Donoghue JM, Ostrow JH, et al: A spectrum of tuberculosis peritonitis. Chest 72:310–315, 1977.
35. Goldman AL, Braman SS: Isoniazid: a review with emphasis on adverse effects. Chest 62:71–77, 1972.
36. Bailey WC, Taylor SL, Dascomb HC, et al: Monitoring the hepatic function of 427 hospital employees receiving isoniazid chemoprophylaxis for tuberculosis. Am Rev Resp Dis 107:523–529, 1973.
37. Sharer L, Smith JP: Serum transaminase elevations and other hepatic abnormalities in patients receiving isoniazid. Ann Intern Med 71:1113–1120, 1969.
38. Anon: Possible INH-associated hepatitis (Report Number 2). US Pub Health Serv Letter, Dec 17, 1970.
39. Leibold JC: The ocular toxicity of ethambutol and its relation to dose. Ann NY Acad Sci 135:904–909, 1966.
40. Doster B, Murray FJ, Newman R, et al: Ethambutol in the initial treatment of pulmonary tuberculosis. Am Rev Resp Dis 107:177–189, 1973.
41. Bolt HM, Kappes H, Bolt M: Rifampin and oral contraception. Lancet 1:1280–1281, 1974.

12. ANTIFUNGAL AGENTS

Richard H. Meade, III

Both systemic and superficial infections due to fungi can now be treated with a variety of drugs, many of which have only recently become available. Barely 25 years ago the only agents useful in the treatment of systemic mycoses were the iodides for sporotrichosis and stilbamidine for blastomycosis. Amphotericin B, the first broad spectrum antifungal drug that could be given systemically, was introduced in 1956 and was the only agent available for a decade. It was followed in 1966 by 5-fluorocytosine, the first orally administered drug. In the last 5 years clotrimazole and miconazole, two imidazole derivatives, have been introduced. Rifampin, an antituberculosis drug, and minocycline, a tetracycline antibiotic, have been used experimentally in combination with amphotericin B and these combinations could become important therapeutic alternatives.[1,2]

Fungal infections involving the lungs, joints, skin, and meninges may resemble tuberculosis since they may be indolent while advancing relentlessly unless treated. They also could behave like acute bacterial infections and follow a fulminant course that requires the immediate use of large doses of an antifungal drug if life is to be saved. In most cases both the tuberculous-like and fulminant processes are curable if the cause of the disease is recognized and treated early.

Treatment of systemic fungal infections should be continued for a sufficient period to minimize the possibility of relapse. Patients should be observed for long periods after cessation of therapy to be sure that cure, and not simply remission, has been achieved.

DRUG MONOGRAPHS

AMPHOTERICIN B (Fungizone)

Amphotericin B is an antibiotic produced by *Streptomyces nodosus*.

Because of poor oral absorption, it is given parenterally for systemic infections and meningitis. It is also used topically to treat candidiasis of the skin, nails, or mucous membranes.

Indications—Amphotericin B is the single most effective drug for the treatment of the following systemic fungal infections: blastomycosis, histoplasmosis, cryptococcosis, candidiasis, sporotrichosis, aspergillosis, mycormycosis, and coccidiomycosis; however, the latter three infections do not always respond. Amphotericin B has been used with flucytosine in the treatment of cryptococcal meningitis, and the combination may be superior to amphotericin B alone.[3] It has also been used with rifampin to treat cryptococcal meningitis.[4]

Amphotericin B is of potential value in the treatment of infection caused by agents other than the fungi. It has in vitro effect upon the amoebae called Naegleria and could be of use in treating amoebic meningoencephalitis.[5] It is also of potential value in treating leishmaniasis.[6]

Pharmacology—Immediately after intravenous infusion of 50 to 75 mg of amphotericin B, peak serum concentrations of 1.9 μg/ml were achieved in one study; 24 hours later, concentrations of 0.6 μg/ml were observed.[7] Details of tissue distribution and possible pathways of metabolism of amphotericin have not been described. After distribution is complete, elimination proceeds with a half-life of about 15 days.[8] The concentration of amphotericin B in urine roughly parallels that in plasma. Since this represents only a small fraction of the given dose, no further accumulation of the drug occurs in the plasma of patients with impaired renal function.

Although amphotericin B reaches spinal fluid only in low concentrations after intravenous administration, meningeal infections caused by certain fungi have been cured with intravenous amphotericin B. Since some fungi are quite sensitive to amphotericin B, this could account for drug efficacy. On the other hand, coccidioidal meningitis is almost impossible to eradicate with intravenous therapy; successful treatment has been possible only with prolonged intrathecal or intraventricular therapy.

Mycotic infection of the eye caused by *Candida albicans* has been treated by intravitreal administration of 5 to 10 μg doses, without injury to the eye.[9]

Adverse Reactions—No other anti-infective drug causes toxic reactions as often as amphotericin B. However, the risks of adverse effects often are outweighed by the need for treatment in patients with potentially life-threatening, prolonged, and painful diseases.

Adverse effects are related both to the drug itself and its vehicle; the commercial product contains buffers and sodium deoxycholate (to permit colloidal dispersion of the insoluble antibiotic). Reactions that develop within minutes or hours (usually with doses greater than 0.25 mg/kg) include fever, chills, nausea and headache. Vomiting usually accompanies nausea as the dose is increased. These immediate effects occur in 20 to 90% of adult recipients. Phlebitis at the site of intravenous administration eventually develops in 70% of recipients; the time of onset and severity varies from patient to patient.[10] Aspirin, 0.9 g before and 3 hours after a dose of amphotericin B may prevent fever and chills. Addition of hydrocortisone acetate (25 to 50 mg) to intravenous infusions also reduces fever, nausea and vomiting; it may be more effective than aspirin. Heparin does not prevent phlebitis.

Renal toxicity is a more serious adverse effect of amphotericin B. Hypokalemia is common and requires monitoring of serum potassium and appropriate replacement to prevent both cardiac and neurological consequences. Calcium and magnesium may also be lost in sufficient quantities to cause major symptoms and require careful replacement. A reduction in inulin and creatinine clearance and impaired hydrogen ion excretion may occur.

The specific renal pathology involves the renal tubules sometimes accompanied by large deposits of calcium phosphate and calcification in the parenchyma surrounding the glomeruli. Glomerular filtration rate and creatinine clearance are reduced.

Mannitol in an adult dose of 25 g may prevent nephrotoxicity by increasing glomerular filtration and renal blood flow. It has been successfully used to prevent impairment of renal function in a small number of patients.[11]

Blood urea nitrogen and serum creatinine determinations should be made on alternate days while dosage is being increased and weekly thereafter during therapy. If tests of renal function reveal deterioration (ie, serum creatinine exceeding 3 mg/100 ml), amphotericin B should be discontinued until levels return to approximately normal values. Creatinine clearance is a better index of renal function than serum creatinine alone, but requires a complete 24-hour urine collection.

After 4 to 6 weeks of therapy, a normocytic, normochromic anemia often occurs. This has been attributed to suppression of hematopoeisis by amphotericin B.[12]

Liver damage following treatment with amphotericin B has been reported as a fatal adverse reaction.[13] A 32 year-old man had received a little more than a gram when anemia and renal toxicity developed. Amphotericin B was discontinued for a period of a month while recovery from these complications was observed. It was given twice more for varying periods and during the third exposure his bilirubin was elevated very slightly. He died with a large liver showing extensive fatty infiltration and metamorphosis attributed to a toxic reaction. This adverse effect is very rare.

Hypersensitivity reactions are considered rare[14] but do occur. A generalized papular rash occurred in one patient on each of several occasions when he received the drug.[15]

The toxic effects of intrathecally administered amphotericin include headache, nerve palsy (including foot drop), impaired bladder function, and pain along lumbar dermatomes.

Administration and Dosage—Amphotericin B is heat labile; therefore, the dry powder should be stored in a refrigerator. Solutions should be used promptly and are prepared by adding 10 ml of water for injection to 50 mg of amphotericin B and shaking the vial for at least three minutes to form a colloidal suspension. The suspension is then added to 500 ml of dextrose 5% injection (without preservatives) for intravenous infusion; the resulting solution has a concentration of 0.1 mg/ml. If given in an electrolyte solution, the colloidal suspension precipitates. Covering the bottle containing amphotericin B to prevent loss of potency, formerly thought essential, appears to be unnecessary.[16] The antifungal effects of amphotericin B are maximal between pH 6.0 and 7.5 and decrease at low pH.

Recommended adult doses are given in Table 1. The suspension should be administered intravenously over 8 hours for a full dose of 1 mg/kg. Smaller doses can be given in proportionately shorter periods. Some authorities recommend initiation of therapy with 0.25 mg/kg/day and increasing the amount given by 5 mg daily until a dose of 1 mg/kg is reached. This regimen reduces the possibility of sudden adverse effects such as tachycardia, hypotension, or tachypnea. Another method of initiating therapy is to begin with a total dose of only 1 mg. The dose is increased to 5 mg the next day, 10 mg the day after, etc., until 1 mg/kg is given. If the average effective serum concentration is 0.2 μg/ml, therapeutic levels are not attained until about the fifth day of therapy by this method.[8] While this delay is not important when treating patients with slowly progressive infection, it is clearly undesirable in those with fulminant disease.

TABLE 1 Drugs of Choice for Treatment of Mycotic Infections

	Nystatin	Flucytosine	Amphotericin B[a]	Clotrimazole	Miconazole[a]
Candida species					
Thrush	Suspension 200,000 U 3 times daily				
Vaginitis	Vaginal tablets (200,000 U)			Vaginal tablets 100 mg 2% cream	
Esophagitis	500,000 U suspension or tablets				
Chronic mucocutaneous infection			0.2–0.5 mg/kg IV		
Endocarditis and other visceral infection		100 mg/kg orally	0.3–1.0 mg/kg IV		
Aspergillus species					
Meningitis		100 mg/kg orally	0.6–1.0 mg/kg IV		
Pneumonia		100 mg/kg orally	0.6–1.0 mg/kg IV		

TABLE 1 *(continued)*

	Nystatin	Flucytosine	Amphotericin B[a]	Clotrimazole	Miconazole[a]
Other		100 mg/kg orally	0.6–1.0 mg/kg IV		
Histoplasma capsulatum			0.6–1.0 mg/kg IV		30–60 mg/kg IV
Coccidioides immitis			0.6–1.0 mg/kg IV		30–60 mg/kg IV
Blastomyces dermatidis			0.6–1.0 mg/kg IV		30–60 mg/kg IV
Sporothrichum schenckii			0.6–1.0 mg/kg IV		
Cryptococcus neoformans	100 mg/kg orally		0.6–1.0 mg/kg IV		30–60 mg/kg IV

[a]For meningeal infection by any of the fungi listed, intrathecal or intraventricular therapy is sometimes necessary. For amphothericin, the dose is 0.5 mg diluted in 5 ml of spinal fluid; this is given intraventricularly or intrathecally. Miconazole is given in 5% dextrose in water in a dose of 20 mg per intrathecal injection.

When intrathecal administration is indicated, the conventional approach is to dilute 50 mg of amphotericin B with at least 150 ml of 5% dextrose injection to make a solution with a concentration of about 0.3 mg/ml. Before injection the dose is mixed in the syringe with 10 to 30 ml of cerebrospinal fluid. However, this method frequently causes arachnoiditis and spinal nerve palsies. An alternative method involves giving the dose in hyperbaric dextrose solution and tilting the patient's head down. By allowing the drug to enter the cistern and ventricles the frequency of toxicity is reduced.[17]

The daily dose and the duration of therapy vary greatly and should be adjusted individually according to the severity of the disease and the tolerance of the patient. Small and nontoxic amounts can be used for some fungal infections.[18] Candidal vaginitis, esophagitis, and laryngitis are examples of infections for which 5 to 10 mg adult daily doses have been successful. Similarly, small amounts of amphotericin B have been used to treat severe forms of primary histoplasmosis.[19] A dose of 0.3 to 0.5 mg/kg every other day produced serum concentrations sufficient to cure patients with cryptococcal and histoplasma infections.[20]

Concern about amphotericin toxicity has also been a dominant factor in determining the total dose. One restriction that not more than 3 to 4 g be given over 10 to 12 weeks is based on the observation that larger amounts are associated with renal damage. While many patients exhibit marked susceptibility to the nephrotoxic effects of amphotericin and cannot be treated with it, many others have far greater tolerance and can be treated over a period of many months without such complications.

Duration of therapy varies with the disease. Superficial candida infection such as laryngitis requires no more than 4 to 7 days of treatment. Candidal and cryptococcal meningitis, on the other hand, respond more slowly and can require 6 to 10 weeks of treatment. Doses of 0.5 to 1 mg/kg every other day would require that a 70 kg adult receive only 0.5 to 1 g of drug at the end of six weeks. Thus, amphotericin B probably could be tolerated for longer periods if the infection persisted.

Installation of amphotericin B into the urinary bladder to treat candidal cystitis is an effective therapy that avoids the necessity of intravenous administration. Similarly, amphotericin B has been given intraperitoneally to treat postoperative infections caused by *Candida albicans*. The amount that can be given by this route is 0.1 to 0.2 mg on a daily basis or less frequently.

TABLE 2 Preparations and Costs of Antifungal Agents

GENERIC NAME	TRADEMARK NAME(S)	PREPARATIONS AND 1978 COSTS
Amphotericin B	Fungizone	Injection (powder) 50 mg—$5.17/vial Cream 3%—$4.44/20 g Lotion 3%—$6.08/30 ml Ointment 3%—$4.44/20 g
Clotrimazole	Lotrimin	Cream 1%—$2.73/15 g, $4.71/30 g Solution 1%—$2.39/10 ml, $5.07/30 ml
	Gyne-Lotrimin	Vaginal tablets 100 mg—$6.00/7
Flucytosine	Ancobon	Capsules 250 mg—$14.02/100; 500 mg—$26.87/100
Hydroxystilbamidine	generic	Injection (powder) 225 mg—$8.65/vial
Griseofulvin	Fulvicin-U/F (Grisfulvin V) (Grisactin) (Gris-PEG)	Tablets 125 mg—$9.50/100; 250 mg—$8.40/60; 500 mg—$15.99/60
Miconazole Nitrate	MicaTin	Cream 2%—2.25/15 g, $3.69/28 g, $5.34/85 g Lotion 2%—$2.10/12 ml, $4.25/30 ml
	Monistat	Injection (solution) 10 mg/ml—$4.22/10-ml ampul
Nystatin	Mycostatin (Nilstat)	Drops (suspension) 100,000 units/ml—$5.19/60 ml Tablets 500,000 units—$13.25/100 Vaginal tablets 100,000 units—$2.64/15, $4.79/30 Topical powder 100,000 units/g—$3.82/15 g Cream and ointment 100,000 units/g—$2.38/15 g, $4.07/30 g

CLOTRIMAZOLE (Gyne-Lotrimin, Lotrimin)

Clotrimazole is a chlorinated imidazole derivative that is used to treat topical fungal, dermatophyte, and yeast infections.[21]

Indications and Dosage—While clotrimazole has marked in vitro activity against many fungi, it is of little value in the treatment of systemic mycoses. It is useful for treating topical infections. *Vaginal:* One tablet (100 mg) is inserted daily for one week for candidal vaginitis. *Topical:* Sufficient cream or solution is applied twice daily to skin infected with *Candida albicans, Tricophyton,* or *Microsporum* species. Two weeks of therapy is usually sufficient. Clotrimazole has been used investigationally for the oral treatment of mucocutaneous candidiasis.[22–24]

Adverse Reactions—Side effects are few with topical use. Hypersensitivity reactions have not been reported.

FLUCYTOSINE (Ancobon)

Flucytosine (5-fluorocytosine) is an orally administered pyrimidine derivative that is soluble in water and is chemically related to fluorouracil and floxuridine.

Indications—Flucytosine has proven less effective in the treatment of human disease than the in vitro response of various organisms suggested. Some Candida species are sensitive to flucytosine, but the drug is only occasionally useful in the treatment of systemic candidal infections. In non-fulminant candidal infections, flucytosine may be preferable to amphotericin B because of its lesser toxicity; in the event of treatment failure, amphotericin B therapy can then be instituted. Flucytosine has been used successfully in treating candidal arthritis,[25] and occasional patients with cryptococcal meningitis have responded to it when used alone.[26] Combined therapy with flucytosine (100 to 200 mg/kg/day) and amphotericin B (0.3 to 0.5 mg/kg/every other day) is effective in cryptococcosis. Fewer and milder adverse reactions to amphotericin B occur, and the combination is more effective than larger doses of amphotericin B alone.[27]

While flucytosine may be effective in the treatment of Aspergillus pneumonia and meningitis,[28] flucytosine alone is not regarded as the best treatment for infections due to this fungus.

Mechanism of Action—In sensitive fungi, the enzyme cytosine deaminase cleaves flucytosine into fluorouracil. This antimetabolite is incorporated into fungal RNA, which may in turn alter protein synthesis. Flucytosine may inhibit DNA synthesis by conversion to fluorodesoxyuridine monophosphate.[29] Studies using tagged amino acids have shown decreased amounts of histidine in Candida species exposed to flucytosine, possibly due to interference with protein synthesis.[30]

Pharmacology—Flucytosine is eliminated largely by renal clearance of the intact drug; 90% of an oral dose appears in the urine unchanged.[29] It is minimally bound to plasma proteins and thus can be easily removed by hemodialysis; patients on hemodialysis should be given a dose of 37.5 mg/kg after each dialysis.

After a dose of 37.5 mg/kg in a person with normal renal function, therapeutic serum levels of 50 to 100 μg/ml are rapidly attained. Peak levels are reached in two hours, and the half-life is 6 hours. The dosage interval in patients with renal failure should be adjusted to maintain blood levels within the therapeutic range. Flucytosine is widely distributed throughout the body. Spinal fluid levels are about 70% of those achieved in serum, and similar concentrations are found in pleural, peritoneal and joint fluids.[31]

Adverse Reactions—Flucytosine may depress the bone marrow and cause leukopenia, neutropenia, and thrombocytopenia, together or as isolated events. Fatal aplastic anemia occurred in a 39 year-old diabetic patient who was treated on three occasions for recurrent cryptococcal meningitis.[32] Granulocytosis developed after the 17th day of therapy in a 9 year-old child with mucocutaneous candidiasis complicating thymic dysplasia and immunoglobulin deficiency.[33] Neither of these patients had renal failure, but both received large doses. Most hematologic complications have been reported in patients with renal failure, although many persons with renal disease have received flucytosine without complications.

Nausea, vomiting, diarrhea, and, less, frequently, confusion, hallucinations, headache, sedation, and vertigo have been reported. Hepatic toxicity is rare.[31,34]

Dosage—Oral: Adults, 100 to 200 mg/kg/day in patients with normal renal function.[29] The higher doses are used in treating life-threatening infections in which there is no time to adjust dosage according to serum concentration determinations. Such determinations should be done in patients with impaired renal function to prevent overdosage and reduce the likelihood of toxicity. The daily dose is usually given in 4 divided doses every 6 hours, unless creatinine clearance is reduced to 40 ml/min, in which case if such renal impairment is evident, then the divided dose is unchanged, but is given every 12 hours. If creatinine clearance is below 20 ml/min, a quarter of the daily dose is given every 24 hours.[29]

GRISEOFULVIN (Fulvicin-U/F, Grifulvin V, Grisactin, Gris-PEG)

Griseofulvin is an antibiotic produced by *Penicillium Janczewskii.* It is the only drug effective orally for dermatophytic infections.

Indications—Griseofulvin is most effective for tinea and ringworm infections caused by *Tricophyton* and *Microsporum* species. It is less effective for infection of the nails, and finger nail infections respond better than toe nail infections. It is not effective against other fungi, including *Candida* species. Griseofulvin is not recommended for infections that usually respond to a topical agent alone. Resistance to griseofulvin may be due to inadequate dosage or duration of therapy, the presence of complicating infection due to *Candida,* or to resistant strains of *Tricophyton* or *Microsporum* species.

Pharmacology—After an oral dose of 500 mg of microcrystalline griseofulvin, serum concentrations of 1 to 2 μg/ml are achieved in 4 hours. The serum half-life is about 36 hours. Most of the drug is excreted unchanged in the feces. Higher peak serum levels are attained if griseofulvin is taken after a high-fat meal because of more rapid absorption.[35] However, the total amount of drug absorbed is the same as when the drug is taken on an empty stomach. Griseofulvin is incorporated in keratin of the skin, hair, and nails. Cure of infection in these tissues occurs with outward movement of the drug-impregnated keratin and shedding of fungi from the replaced keratin.

Antifungal activity occurs at griseofulvin serum levels of 0.1 to 2 μg/ml. Fungal growth is inhibited by impairment of protein and nucleic acid synthesis.

Griseofulvin has anti-inflammatory activity accounting for its efficacy in acute gouty arthritis[36] and its capacity to reduce the size of a tuberculin reaction.[37] Increased coronary blood flow and an antianginal effect have been demonstrated.[38]

Product Formulations—Griseofulvin was originally marketed as a macrocrystalline product that required large doses and incurred a relatively high risk of toxicity. Subsequently, a microcrystalline form replaced the macrocrystalline preparation. Adequate blood levels are achieved with smaller doses and adverse reactions are less frequent. Recently, an ultramicrocrystalline product (Gris-PEG) has been marketed. Even lower doses are possible with this product, but there does not seem to be any therapeutic difference between the two crystalline forms.

Drug Interactions—Phenobarbital increases the demethylation of griseofulvin in the liver, and consequently may reduce griseofulvin serum levels. Griseofulvin induces hepatic enzymes responsible for the metabolism of warfarin and may decrease its hypoprothrombinemic effects.[39]

Adverse Reactions—Griseofulvin produces few adverse effects. Rare reports of toxicity include exacerbation of underlying porphyria, photodermatitis (similar to that seen with demeclomycin), headache,[37] severe angioneurotic edema, and generalized urticaria.[40]

Dosage—Microcrystalline form (Fulvicin-U/F, Grifulvin V, Grisactin). Oral: Adults, 500 mg daily in single or divided doses; for stubborn infections 1 g or more daily in divided doses may be necessary. *Children,* approximately 10 mg/kg daily in single or divided doses after meals. *Ultramicrocrystalline* form (Gris-PEG), one-half of the doses given above.

MICONAZOLE NITRATE (MicaTin, Monistat)

Miconazole is an imidazole derivative that closely resembles clotrimazole.

Indications and Dosage—Dermal Infections Caused by Candida, Tricophyton, and Microsporum Species. Topical: A sufficient amount of cream or lotion to cover the affected areas is applied twice daily. Two weeks of therapy is usually sufficient, but patients with tinea pedis should be treated for three to four weeks. *Vaginal:* One applicatorful of cream inserted high in the vagina each night for two weeks.

Systemic Infections. Miconazole has been used most often in the treatment of disease caused by *Coccidioides immitis,* including pulmonary, osseous and meningeal infections. The usual daily intravenous dose is 30 to 60 mg/kg. One-third of the daily dose is given by 1-hour infusion every 8 hours in 250 to 500 ml of 5% dextrose injection; less rapid infusions may result in subtherapeutic serum concentrations. For pulmonary and bone infections caused by *Coccidioides immitis,* good results have been achieved with 1 to 3 months of treatment. In some patients, regression in the size of pulmonary lesions occurs despite persistence of the organism in sputum or in resected pulmonary lesions. Some patients receive oral miconazole, 3 g daily, at the conclusion of intravenous therapy.

The efficacy of intravenous miconazole in cryptococcal meningitis, candidal osteomyelitis and candidal esophagitis is under investigation.

Pharmacology—After intravenous injection of 4 to 18 mg/kg miconazole, serum concentrations of up to 2 μg/ml are produced; a dose of 9 mg/kg provides blood levels of at least 1 μg/ml.[41] When given at intervals of 4 instead of 8 hours in the same daily dose, peak serum levels are lower but there is little elevation of trough concentrations. A rapid fall in serum levels occurs within 30 minutes of the dose due to distribution. The elimination half-life is 24 hours. Miconazole penetrates normal meninges to produce levels of 0.1 μg/ml when serum levels are 2 μg/ml; higher levels occur if there is meningeal inflammation. The drug does not penetrate into sputum.[41] The successful use of miconazole in the treatment of pulmonary, esophageal and osseous infections is evidence of penetration into these tissues although quantitative data are not available.

Adverse Reactions—Phlebitis often occurs after intravenous administration. This is of such severity that superficial veins frequently cannot be used, and catheterization of deep veins (eg, subclavian) is indicated. When administered by this means, some clinicians have reported few difficulties.[42] No kidney, liver, or bone marrow toxicity has been observed, even with 4 to 5 months of therapy. In some patients, elevated serum cholesterol and triglyceride values occur. This has been attributed to the solvent vehicle of polyethoxylated castor oil, methylparaben and propylparaben. When the vehicle was administered to animals, serum cholesterol and triglyceride values were elevated.[43]

After 1 to 2 weeks of miconazole therapy, three patients developed anemia and thrombocytosis.[44] While this is a very small number of patients, monitoring of hematocrit and platelet count seems prudent. Some clinicians report no particular difficulties with intrathecal therapy,[42] but fever, headache, transient hemiparesis, and pleocytosis can occur.

NYSTATIN (Mycostatin, Nilstat)

Nystatin is an insoluble polyene derived from *Streptomyces noursei*. It is not absorbed when taken by mouth and is too toxic for parenteral use.

Indications, Administration, and Dosage—Candidal Infection of the Oral Mucosa (Thrush). Oral: Children, for candidiasis involving the cheeks, palate or faucial tonsils, 1 ml of the oral suspension (100,000 units) is held in each of the affected sides of the mouth and then swallowed; this dose is given four times daily until the lesions clear (usually 3 to 4 days) and then for an additional 2 days. *Adults,* 2 ml of the oral suspension (200,000 units) is used.

Candidal Esophagitis. This infection does not always respond to treatment with topically-administered drug, but nystatin probably should be tried before resorting to intravenous amphotericin B. Patients with esophagitis usually have an underlying malignancy for which cytotoxic drug therapy, with or without corticosteroids, has been used. Thus, host defense mechanisms are undermined by both the underlying disease and its treatment. *Oral: Adults,* 500,000 units (suspension or tablets) four times daily.

Candidal Vaginitis. This infection occurs in women who have been treated with antibiotics (usually a tetracycline), in women who have taken oral contraceptives, and in mothers after delivery. It rarely occurs in prepubertal girls or postmenopausal women. *Vaginal:* 100,000 to 200,000 units as vaginal tablets once daily for 7 to 14 days. This dosage is ordinarily sufficient to eradicate candidal infection, especially if it developed as a consequence of antibiotic therapy. Persistent or recurrent infection, which is more common in women who have been pregnant or who have taken oral contraceptives, may require other therapy; clotrimazole may be more effective than nystatin. Low-dose intravenous amphotericin B therapy (eg, 10 mg every other day) has worked very well.[18]

Systemic Fungal Infections. Nystatin aerosols have been used to treat a small number of patients with pulmonary candidiasis or aspergillosis.[45,46] A child with both pulmonary and cutaneous *Aspergillus* lesions was successfully treated with 1,500,000 units of nystatin suspended in propylene glycol and given by aerosol during the night.[45] Others have used much smaller doses; eg, 25,000 units in 5 ml of normal saline by aerosol twice daily. Nystatin aerosol is not recommended as definitive therapy. Blood levels of only 3.7 units/ml have been achieved; this is less than the minimum inhibitory concentration for *Aspergillus* or *Candida.*[45] However, nystatin aerosol could be considered a temporary alternative to intravenous amphotericin B.

Adverse Reactions—Nystatin causes few adverse reactions, probably because systemic absorption is minimal. Nausea, vomiting, and diarrhea do not occur with usual doses, and hypersensitivity reactions have not been observed.

REFERENCES

1. Medoff G, Kobayashi GS, Kwan CN, et al: Potentiation of rifampicin and 5-fluorocytosine as antifungal antibiotics by amphotericin B. Proc Natl Acad Sci USA 69:196, 1972.
2. Lew MA, Beckett KM, Levin MJ: Combined activity of minocycline and amphotericin B in vitro against medically important yeasts. Antimicrob Agents Chemother 14:465–469, 1978.
3. Bennett JE, Dismukes W, Duma R, et al: Comparison of amphotericin B dose with amphotericin B and flucytosine in cryptococcal meningitis. 16th Interscience Conference on Antimicrobial Agents and Chemotherapy, Chicago, 1976. Abstract 308.
4. Ribner B, Keusch GT, Hanna BA, et al: Combination amphotericin B-rifampin therapy for pulmonary aspergillosis in a leukemic patient. Chest 70:681–683, 1976.
5. Duma RJ, Rosenblum WI, McGehee RF, et al: Primary amoebic meningoencephalitis caused by naegleria. Ann Intern Med 74:923–931, 1974.
6. Mahmoud AAF, Warren KS: Algorithms in the diagnosis and management of exotic diseases. XXIV Leishmaniasis J Infect Dis 136:160–163, 1977.
7. Bindschadler DD, Bennett JE: A pharmacologic guide to the clinical use of amphotericin B. J Infect Dis 120:427–436, 1969.
8. Atkinson AJ Jr, Bennett JE: Amphotericin B pharmacokinetics in humans. Antimicrob Agents Chemother 13:271–276, 1978.
9. Axelrod AJ, Peyman GA: Intravitreal amphotericin B treatment of experimental fungal endophthalmitis. Am J Ophthalmol 76:584–588, 1973.
10. Amphotericin B toxicity. Clinical Staff Conference. Ann Intern Med 61:334–354, 1964.
11. Rosch JM, Pazin GJ, Fireman P: Reduction of amphotericin B nephrotoxicity with mannitol. JAMA 235:1995–1996, 1976.
12. Brandriss MW, Wolff SM, Moores R, et al: Anemia induced by amphotericin B. JAMA 189:663–666, 1964.
13. Carnecchia BM, Kurtzke JF: Fatal toxic reaction to amphotericin B in cryptococcal meningo-encephalitis. Ann Intern Med 53:1027–1036, 1960.
14. Bennett JE: Chemotherapy of systemic mycoses. N Engl J Med 290:30–32, 320–323, 1974.
15. Lorber B, Cutler C, Barry WE: Allergic rash due to amphotericin B. Ann Intern Med 84:54, 1976.
16. Shadomy S, Brummer DL, Ingroff AV: Light sensitivity of prepared solutions of amphotericin B. Am Rev Respir Dis 107:303–304, 1973.
17. Alazraki NP, Fierer J, Halpern SE, et al: Use of a hyperbaric solution for administration of intrathecal amphotericin B. N Engl J Med 290:641–646, 1974.
18. Medoff G, Dismukes WE, Meade RH III, et al: A new therapeutic approach to Candida infections. Arch Intern Med 130:241–245, 1972.
19. Naylor BA: Low-dose amphotericin B therapy for acute pulmonary histoplasmosis. Chest 71:404–406, 1977.
20. Drutz DJ, Spickard A, Rogers DE, et al: Treatment of disseminated mycotic infection. Am J Med 45:408–418, 1968.
21. Plempel M, Buchel KH, Bartmann K, et al: Antimycotic properties of clotrimazole. Postgrad Med J 50:11–12, 1974.
22. Ipp MM, Boxall L, Gelfand E: Intermittent therapy in chronic mucocutaneous candidiasis. Am J Dis Child 181:305–307, 1977.
23. Meade RH III: Treatment of chronic mucocutaneous candidiasis. Ann Intern Med 86:314–315, 1977.
24. Montes LF, Soto TG, Parker JM, et al: Clotrimazole troches: a new therapeutic approach to oral candidiasis. Cutis 17:277–280, 1976.
25. Lindstrom FD, Lindholm T: *Candida albicans* arthritis treated with flucytosine. Ann Intern Med 79:131, 1973.
26. Tassel D, Madoff MA: Treatment of *Candida* sepsis and *Cryptococcus* meningitis with 5-fluorocytosine, a new antifungal agent. JAMA 206:830–832, 1968.
27. Utz JP, Garrigues IA, Sande MA, et al: Therapy of cryptococcosis with a combination of flucytosine and amphotericin B. J Infect Dis 132:368–373, 1975.
28. Atkinson GW, Israel HL: 5-Fluorocytosine treatment of meningeal and pulmonary aspergillosis. Am J Med 55:496–504, 1973.
29. Bennett JE: Flucytosine. Ann Intern Med 86:319–322, 1977.
30. Polack A: Effects of 5-fluorocytosine on protein synthesis and aminoacid pool in *Candida albicans*. Sabouraudia 12:309–319, 1974.

31. Steer PL, Marks MI, Klite PD, et al: 5-Fluorocytosine: an oral antifungal compound. Ann Intern Med 76:15–22, 1972.
32. Meyer R, Axelrod JL: Fatal aplastic anemia resulting from flucytosine. JAMA 224:1573, 1974.
33. Schlegel RJ, Bernier GM, Bellant JA, et al: Severe candidiasis with thymic dysplasia, IgA deficiency and plasma antilymphocyte effects. Pediatrics 45:526–536, 1970.
34. Record CO, Skinner JM, Sleight P, et al: Candida endocarditis treated with 5-fluorocytosine. Br Med J 1:262–264, 1971.
35. Crounse RG: Human pharmacology of griseofulvin: the effect of fat intake on gastrointestinal absorption. J Invest Dermatol 37:529–533, 1961.
36. Slonim RR, Howell DS, Brown HE Jr: Influence of griseofulvin upon acute gouty arthritis. Arthritis Rheumatol 5:397, 1962.
37. Blank H: Antifungal and other effects of griseofulvin. Am J Med 39:832–838, 1965.
38. Rubin AA: Coronary vascular effects of griseofulvin. JAMA 185:971–972, 1963.
39. Cullen SI, Catalano PM: Griseofulvin-warfarin antagonism. JAMA 199:582–583, 1967.
40. Goldblatt S: Severe reaction to griseofulvin. Arch Dermatol 83:936–937, 1961.
41. Stevens DA, Levine HB, Deresinski SC: Miconazole in coccidioidomycosis. Am J Med 60:191–202, 1976.
42. Sung JP, Grendahl JG, Levine HB: Intravenous and intrathecal miconazole therapy for systemic mycoses. West J Med 126:5–13, 1977.
43. Bagnarello AG, Lewis LA, McHenry MC, et al: Unusual serum lipoprotein abnormality induced by the vehicle of miconazole. N Engl J Med 296:497–499, 1977.
44. Marmlon LC, Desser KB, Lilly RB, et al: Miconazole induced thrombocytosis and anemia (abstract). Clin Res 24:93A, 1976.
45. Vedder JS, Schorr WF: Primary disseminated pulmonary aspergillosis with metastatic skin lesions. JAMA 209:1191–1195, 1969.
46. McKendrick GDW, Medlock JM: Pulmonary moniliasis treated with nystatin aerosol. Lancet 1:621–622, 1958.

13. MISCELLANEOUS ANTIMICROBIAL AGENTS

Richard Gleckman, Salvador Alvarez, Dennis W. Joubert, Samuel J. Matthews, and John G. Bartlett

DRUG MONOGRAPHS

METHENAMINE HIPPURATE (Hiprex, Urex)
METHENAMINE MANDELATE (Mandelamine)

Methenamine mandelate and methenamine hippurate are combinations of organic acids exerting antibacterial activity exclusively in the urine.[1] They are prescribed as prophylactic agents.

Mechanism of Action—The antimicrobial action of methenamine depends on its conversion in the urine to formaldehyde, a protein precipitant. Urinary concentration of formaldehyde must exceed 25 μg/ml to produce antimicrobial activity.[2,3]

Mandelic acid and hippuric acid by themselves possess modest bacteriostatic urinary activity. When combined with methenamine, mandelic and hippuric acids reduce the urinary pH and enhance the liberation of formaldehyde from methenamine.

Spectrum of Activity—Formaldehyde has activity against all bacteria that cause urinary tract infections.[4,5] When infection is caused by a urease-producing organism, such as *Proteus* sp., the alkalinity of the urine can reduce formaldehyde formation. Bacterial resistance to formaldehyde does not develop.[5]

Pharmacology—The mandelate and hippurate salts of methenamine undergo rapid and complete absorption following oral ingestion.[6,7] The rate and extent of absorption are reduced by enteric-coating;[8–10] methenamine mandelate is available as an enteric-coated tablet, whereas methenamine hippurate is marketed as a plain tablet. Measurements of serum concentrations of methenamine have no clinical relevance. Hydrolysis of methenamine in an acid medium releases formaldehyde in the urine.

The excretion of hippuric acid occurs by glomerular filtration and tubular secretion. Clearance is reduced only when renal function is greatly impaired.[11,12] Methenamine and mandelic acid are excreted in a similar fashion.[13]

Peak urinary levels of 'free' formaldehyde are generated approximately 2 hours after methenamine hippurate is ingested, and urinary concentrations range from 1 to 85 μg/ml.[7,9,10] When enteric-coated methenamine mandelate is administered, peak urine levels of 'free' formaldehyde do not occur before 3 to 8 hours.[8–10] Steady-state urinary formaldehyde concentrations are achieved 2 to 3 days after methenamine mandelate therapy is initiated.[7,14]

The marked variation in urinary concentrations of formaldehyde is partly explained by the pH-dependence of methenamine hydrolysis.[7,9,15] Formaldehyde formation increases as urinary pH decreases.[7,9] It is suggested that the degree of urinary acidity correlates with the therapeutic response to methenamine compounds,[7,15,16] but some investigators disagree.[2,9,17] This controversy led to a reassessment of the need to administer acidifying agents, such as ascorbic acid, when methenamine compounds are prescribed. In fact, recent reappraisal of the practice of 'acidifying' the urine with 2 to 6 g of ascorbic acid per day has revealed that these conventional doses of ascorbic acid fail to influence the urinary pH. Larger daily doses and more frequent administration of ascorbic acid can acidify the urine, but there is no documentation that therapeutic activity of the methenamine compounds is enhanced.

The concentration of 'free' formaldehyde in the urine also depends on urinary volume.[2,7] When urine flow rates increase from 25 to 40 ml per hour, the urinary concentrations of 'free' formaldehyde decrease from 39 to 46 μg/ml to 21 to 25 μg/ml. Patients who receive methenamine compounds should not be excessively hydrated, since urinary concentration of 'free' formaldehyde is associated with therapeutic response.

The influence of renal insufficiency on the pharmacology of methenamine compounds is unknown. In one report, therapeutic concentrations of formaldehyde were achieved in urine of the azotemic patient when methenamine hippurate was administered.[18]

Limited data suggest that methenamine compounds can be safely administered to pregnant women during the second and third trimester.

Indications—Methenamine mandelate and methenamine hippurate are safe and effective drugs for the prevention of recurrent urinary tract infections in children and adults who experience disabling symptomatic exacerbations.[19–24] These compounds are also indicated for the prevention of asymptomatic bacteriuria when this is a significant threat to health. Methenamine mandelate and methenamine hippurate appear to be equally effective and compare favorably with other standard prophylactic treatments (sulfonamides, nitrofurantoin, trimethoprim-sulfamethoxazole). Methenamine mandelate and methenamine hippurate are not indicated for the patient who has an indwelling Foley catheter or practices intermittent catheterization. Further, the drugs should not be prescribed for patients with bacterial cystitis, pyelonephritis, or prostatitis. The manufacturer of methenamine mandelate recommends the drug as appropriate therapy for an established bacterial urinary tract infection, but published data generally do not support this.[4,18]

Adverse Reactions—The actual incidence of adverse reactions produced by methenamine, methenamine mandelate and methenamine hippurate are not known since toxicity data are available only from reports of uncontrolled studies. Our review of published reports suggests that from 1 to 7% of patients who receive these compounds experience adverse reactions.[6,18,25–28]

Adverse effects are mild, reversible, and occur infrequently. Common untoward events are gastrointestinal intolerance (nausea, vomiting, abdominal cramps) and skin reactions (pruritus, urticaria, erythematous eruption).[6,18,29,30] One study implies that nausea occurs more frequently with the mandelate than with the hippurate.[29] Stomatitis, anorexia, headache, dyspnea and generalized edema are rare adverse events. Lipoid pneumonitis has also been reported.[31]

Very high doses of the methenamine compounds have produced urological abnormalities (dysuria, urgency, urinary frequency, hematuria) and intensified gastrointestinal symptomatology.[32] A recent article implicated methenamine as a cause of interstitial nephritis,[33] but a cause and effect relationship was not proven.

When urinary flow rates are reduced, methenamine mandelate can cause crystalluria.[34] In addition, the concurrent administration of methenamine mandelate with sulfathiazole has resulted in the asymptomatic precipitation of the sulfonamide in the urine.[35]

It is not established whether toxicity results from administration of the methenamine compounds to patients with renal insufficiency and metabolic acidosis. Methenamine drugs in theory could exacerbate the acidosis, but this is not proven. Until such information becomes available, it would appear wise to offer the azotemic patient an alternative to the methenamine compounds.

Drug and Laboratory Test Interactions—Methenamine compounds produce a significant decrease in the urinary concentration of estriol, which is attributed to the destruction of the hormone by formaldehyde. The enzymatic hydrolysis assay technique for estriol remains valid. Methenamine compounds cause a spurious elevation of urinary catecholamine and 17-hydroxycorticosteroid determinations and a decrease in urinary hydroxyindoleacetic acid measurements.

Dosage—Oral: Adults, for prophylaxis, 1 g twice daily of methenamine hippurate, or 1 g four times a day of methenamine mandelate.[29] *Children,* 2 g/m^2/day of methenamine mandelate divided into two or three equal doses.[36]

NALIDIXIC ACID (NegGram)

Nalidixic acid was introduced in 1964 for the oral therapy of bacterial urinary tract infections unassociated with bacteremia.[37]

Mechanism of Action—Nalidixic acid probably exerts bactericidal activity by interfering with deoxyribonucleic acid (DNA) polymerization.[38,39] Nalidixic acid does not bind to DNA, and does not affect those enzymes involved in DNA replication.[40,41] In susceptible bacteria the primary targets for nalidixic acid probably are the single stranded DNA precursors involved in late stages of chromosomal replication.[42] In addition to inhibiting DNA synthesis, nalidixic acid can also inhibit RNA synthesis.[43] However, this latter inhibition is only partial, and may not lead to important interference with bacterial growth.

Spectrum of Activity—The vast majority of *Escherichia coli, Citrobacter (diversus* and *freundii), Klebsiella* sp., *Enterobacter* sp., and *Proteus (mirabilis, morganii, vulgaris, rettgeri)* are susceptible to nalidixic acid. Additional gram-negative aerobic bacilli that are usually susceptible include *Providencia* sp., *Aeromonas hydrophilia, Pasteurella multicoda, Shigella* sp., and *Salmonella* sp. *Pseudomonas aeruginosa* isolates are invariably resistant.

Anaerobic organisms are uniformly resistant to nalidixic acid, and this compound is incorporated into selective media to enhance the growth and identification of anaerobes.

In general, gram-positive aerobic cocci (*Staphylococcus aureus, Staphylococcus epidermidis, Streptococcus viridans,* enterococci) are resistant to nalidixic acid. Gram-negative aerobic cocci *(Neisseria meningitidis, Neisseria gonorrheae)* are susceptible in vitro.

Pharmacology—Nalidixic acid is rapidly absorbed after oral administration and achieves peak blood concentrations in two to four hours.[44–50] Absorption from the gastrointestinal tract is nearly complete, resulting in minimal fecal excretion.[46–50] Serum concentrations range widely from 1.0 to 51.5 μg/ml, and this represents the unaltered parent compound plus the biologically active metabolite, hydroxynalidixic acid.[44–51] Steady-state serum concentrations are reached after three days of dosing.[50] Protein binding is approximately 93% for nalidixic acid and 63% for its hydroxylated metabolite.[47] Intact nalidixic acid accounts for approximately 2 to 3% of drug excreted in the urine, and the hydroxynalidixic acid component accounts for approximately 13%.[49,52] More than 80% of the dose is excreted as biologically inactive glucuronide and carboxylic acid metabolites.[49,52]

Following oral administration in man, wide distribution of nalidixic acid and hydroxynalidixic acid occurs.[46,47,51] Limited studies in humans suggest that the drug concentration in renal tissue and seminal fluid may exceed the simultaneous serum concentrations after repeated dosing.[53,54] Despite its lipid solubility, nalidixic acid does not penetrate biological membranes well, presumably because it is 95% ionized at the pH of the serum and is highly protein bound.[40,55]

Urinary concentrations of active nalidixic acid vary considerably and have been reported to range from 1.6 to 430 μg/ml.[45,49,50,56] The daily urinary recovery of administered drug is approximately 80% at steady-state.[44,50] Alkalinization of the urine will increase the overall excretion of nalidixic acid as well as the ratio of active drug to inactive metabolites.[44,57] This is not surprising since nalidixic acid, a weak acid with a pKa of 6.0, undergoes increased renal ion trapping and excretion as the pH is elevated.[55,57] However, an enhanced clinical effect from adjusting urinary pH has not been demonstrated.[58,59]

The plasma half-life of nalidixic acid in patients with normal renal function is 1.5 hours.[44,50] Renal insufficiency markedly prolongs the half-life, resulting in increased serum concentrations and decreased urine levels of the parent compound and its metabolites. The pattern of drug excretion does not absolutely parallel the creatinine clearance, possibly because of the role of liver metabolism. Both the urine and serum levels exceed the minimum inhibitory concentrations for most urinary tract pathogens despite the presence of severe kidney impairment. There are currently no guidelines for dosage modifications in patients with renal failure, and the potential toxic effects of retained nalidixic acid and its metabolites remain unknown.

There are insufficient data on the dialysis properties of nalidixic acid. Thus no firm recommendations can be offered for the management of the patient who undergoes peritoneal or hemodialysis.

The manufacturer states that nalidixic acid can be administered to pregnant women during the last two trimesters without fear of development of fetal abnormalities. The data that support this claim, however, have not been published.

Indications—Nalidixic acid can be considered an alternative form of therapy for the penicillin-sensitive or cephalosporin-sensitive adult who has a recurrent urinary tract infection caused by susceptible *Escherichia coli, Proteus* sp. and *Enterobacter* sp. that is not complicated by bacteremia. It should not be prescribed for patients with acute symptomatic urinary tract infection, patients experiencing bacteremia, or pregnant women, and it should not be used for prophylaxis.

A serious problem is the observation that rapid emergence of resistant mutants occurs during therapy with nalidixic acid.[60] More recent reports, however, suggest that inordinate selection of resistant mutants and treatment failure does not develop when a full therapeutic dosage of 4 g/day of nalidixic acid is administered.[61,62]

Nalixidic acid is also effective treatment of brucellosis[63] and shigellosis,[64] but these indiciations are not currently approved by the Food and Drug Administration.

Adverse Reactions—Adverse reactions to nalidixic acid appear to develop frequently, occur more readily with prolonged administration and have potentially serious consequences. The most common include gastrointestinal disturbances, skin lesions and neurological events. Unfortunately, the incidence of these side effects is not known.

Gastrointestinal reactions. Nausea is the most frequent adverse effect of nalidixic acid. Epigastric pain, abdominal discomfort, vomiting and diarrhea have also occurred.

Skin reactions. Skin reactions can include pruritus, urticaria, purpuric and maculopapular eruptions, exfoliative lesions and erythema multiforme. The most prevalent dermatologic reactions are the photosensitive bullous eruptions.[65,66] These bullous lesions have a predilection for the hands, feet and legs and tend to spare the face.[67–69] The bullae usually develop days to weeks after the start of nalidixic acid treatment, and have even occurred after more prolonged administration.[67,70] Although the lesions generally resolve within two weeks of discontinuation of therapy, blisters and increased skin friability can persist for months after nalidixic acid treatment ceases or sun exposure is avoided.[67,71] Reexposure to intense sunlight can cause a recurrence, and the hypersensitivity to sunlight can persist for as long as a year after the drug has been discontinued.[69,70] Nalidixic acid can be continued in patients who have experienced a photosensitivity skin reaction if direct sun exposure is avoided.[70]

Neurological reactions. Neurological reactions are among the most common and the most serious. These reactions are reversible and include tremulousness, confusion, drowsiness, headache and dizziness.[65] Visual disturbances (photophobia, halo formation, sensations of flashing lights, inability to focus, change in color perception, diplopia, blurring of outlines, visual hallucinations) have been reported in about 9 to 20% of patients, appear to be dose related, and may resolve despite continued treatment.[72–78] Toxic psychosis with confusion and hallucinations has occurred during nalidixic acid therapy, but a cause and effect relationship is not established.[79] Convulsions, with and without hyperglycemia, most commonly develop in patients who have taken an overdose or have a seizure disorder.[80] The relationship between hyperglycemia and nalidixic acid-induced seizures is controversial, since a metabolite of nalidixic acid can cause a 'false-positive' test reaction for serum and urinary glucose. A recent report, however, appears to confirm the association.[81] Seizures accompanied by hyperglycemia can also occur when appropriate ('conventional') dosage of nalidixic acid is administered to patients with no known seizure disorder.[81]

Nalidixic acid treatment has precipitated reversible intracranial hypertension in children.[82–84] This is manifested by bulging of the fontanelles, papilledema, headache and vomiting. These abnormalities may develop as early as 12 hours after the onset of therapy.[82] Intracranial hypertension recedes soon after discontinuation of the nalidixic acid, but papilledema can persist for months.[82,83]

Miscellaneous reactions. Rare and reversible untoward reactions attributed to nalixidic acid have included hematologic (hemolytic anemia in patients with erythrocytes deficient in the enzyme glucose-6-phosphate dehydrogenase,[79] leukopenia,[86] eosinophilia,[85,86] thrombocytopenia,[65] pancytopenia[87]), musculoskeletal (arthralgia, myalgia, polyarthritis)[65,74,77] and respiratory (depression of ventilation in patients with respiratory insufficiency)[88] events. Recently attention has been focused on a unique form of arthritis which develops in laboratory animals, but its relevance to clinical use is unknown.[89] Nalidixic acid may also cause fever,[74] anaphylaxis,[65] metabolic acidosis,[90] reduction in creatinine clearance and an increase in SGOT.[9]

Drug and Laboratory Test Interactions—Nalidixic acid decreases the binding of sodium warfarin to plasma proteins, thereby transiently potentiating its anticoagulant effects.[92]

Urinary metabolites of nalidixic acid can cause a false-positive test for urinary glucose when Benedict's Reagent or Clinitest tablets are used.[93] Using Clinistix or Testape will avoid this error.[93]

The determination of urinary levels of 17-ketosteroids and 17-ketogenic steroids may be falsely elevated when nalidixic acid has been prescribed.[94]

Dosage—Oral: Adults, 1 g four times a day for an established urinary tract infection. *Children,* 60 mg/kg/day divided into four equal doses.

OXOLINIC ACID (Utibid)

Oxolinic acid is a synthetic antimicrobial agent used to treat established bacterial urinary tract infections not associated with bacteremia in adults. The drug has a chemical structure, mechanism of action, spectrum of activity and potential for toxicity that resembles nalidixic acid.[95]

Mechanism of Action—As anticipated from the structural similarities of oxolinic and nalidixic acids, the mechanism of action of these chemotherapeutic agents appears to be identical, namely, interference with deoxyribonucleic acid (DNA) synthesis. Oxolinic acid, however, has demonstrated a ten-fold greater ability to inhibit DNA replication,[96] which is paralleled by its greater in vitro activity for enterobacteriaceae.[97,98]

Spectrum of Activity—Oxolinic acid exerts in vitro activity against most gram-negative aerobic bacilli that cause bacterial urinary tract infections. The majority of *Escherichia coli, Klebsiella* sp., *Enterobacter* sp. and *Proteus* sp. are susceptible. *Pseudomonas aeruginosa* and *Acinetobacter calcoaceticus* (var. livoffi and var. anitratus) are uniformly resistant, however.

Salmonella, Shigella and *Neisseria (meningitidis, gonorrheae)* are susceptible to oxolinic acid. Oxolinic acid possesses in vitro activity for *Staphylococcus aureus,* but no activity for other gram-positive aerobic cocci.

Pharmacology—After oral administration oxolinic acid is rapidly absorbed from the gastrointestinal tract.[50] Peak serum concentrations of the biologically active unconjugated drug are attained in 2 to 4 hours and range from 1.8 to 3.6 μg/ml.[50] Steady-state serum concentrations are achieved in 3 days, and drug accumulation does not occur after this time.[50,99] Lower serum levels of unconjugated drug occur during the first three days of dosing, suggesting a slow distribution of the chemical into the tissue pools. However, there are no published data to indicate the exact sites of oxolinic acid distribution in man. Protein binding of the drug is about 77 to 81%.[50]

The extent of oxolinic acid absorption from the gastrointestinal tract is unclear. Daily recovery of oxolinic acid and its metabolites in the urine account for only 43 to 49% of administered drug.[50] Fecal excretion is 16 to 20%; this relatively high figure could reflect either incomplete absorption or extensive biliary excretion.[50,100]

The half-life of oxolinic acid is not established. After repeated dosing, a biphasic excretion pattern has been observed. The initial phase is rapid with a half-life of about 1.5 hours, and is followed by a slow phase with a half-life of about 15 hours.[50] Urinary concentrations of unconjugated drug range from 15 to 155 μg/ml in patients with normal renal function.[50,99–101] There is apparently no significant pH dependence of urinary excretion.[102]

Unconjugated oxolinic acid represents only 1.4 to 21% of drug excreted in the urine.[99,103] Greater than 80% is in the form of glucuronide and non-glucuronide metabolites.

Renal insufficiency results in increased serum concentrations of unconjugated oxolinic acid (5.5 to 6.1 μg/ml), and only minimally decreased (35 to 76 μg/ml) urinary drug levels. Therapeutic urinary concentrations are achieved even in the presence of severe renal impairment, and excessive drug accumulation has not been observed when azotemia exists.[99]

Indications—Oxolinic acid is an alternative form of therapy for the penicillin-sensitive or cephalosporin-sensitive adult who has a recurrent urinary tract infection caused by susceptible *Escherichia coli* or *Proteus mirabilis* that is not complicated by bacteremia.[101,104] This medication should not be prescribed for patients with acute symptomatic urinary tract infection, patients experiencing bacteremia, pregnant women or children.

Oxolinic acid is no more effective or better tolerated than other drug treatments (trimethoprim-sulfamethoxazole, ampicillin, nalidixic acid) that are used in the treatment of bacterial urinary tract infections.[102,105,106] The therapeutic efficacy of oxolinic acid does not appear to be dose related.[106]

There is a marked propensity for oxolinic acid to evoke resistant mutants when the daily dose is less than 2 g.[104] When prescribed in the full therapeutic dose of 2 g/day, it does not evoke a greater incidence of resistant mutants than does nalidixic acid.

Oxolinic acid is an effective prophylactic agent for adult women who experience symptomatic recurrent urinary tract infections, and is an effective agent for children who experience acute symptomatic or recurrent bacterial urinary tract infections. However, oxolinic acid is not currently approved by the Food and Drug Administration for these indications.

Although oxolinic acid demonstrated in vitro activity for chloramphenicol-resistant strains of *Salmonella typhi,* this drug is not therapeutically effective for infections caused by this organism.[107] It has resulted in clinical and bacteriological response when administered to adult volunteers who developed shigellosis.[108] This is not an approved indication for oxolinic acid, however.

Adverse Reactions—Adverse reactions are experienced by 10 to 45% of patients who receive oxolinic acid. Untoward events are usually mild and resolve with the discontinuation of treatment,[101,102] but necessitate cessation of therapy in approximately 5% of patients.[100] The most common adverse effects include central nervous system and gastrointestinal reactions.

Central nervous system toxicity has included insomnia (the most frequent), restlessness, dizziness, headache, drowsiness, and visual disturbances. In contrast to nalidixic acid, oxolinic acid has not caused intracranial hypertension, and an association between oxolinic acid and convulsions has not been clearly established.[100] Oxolinic acid has a stimulatory effect on the central nervous system, and should not be prescribed for patients with known seizure disorders.

Gastrointestinal reactions include nausea (the most frequent), vomiting, abdominal discomfort and diarrhea.[101,102] These abnormalities can be minimized by concurrent administration of food or antacids.[102]

Less frequent miscellaneous reactions include fever,[109] skin eruptions,[110] photosensitivity,[100] palpitations,[111] dyspnea and a sense of chest tightness.[101] Transient elevations of the serum bilirubin, SGOT and alkaline phosphatase,[109,112] as well as leukopenia[112] and hemolytic anemia[109] have also been described.

Dosage—Oral: Adults, 750 mg twice daily for adults with established urinary tract infections.[99,101,102,111]

TRIMETHOPRIM-SULFAMETHOXAZOLE (Bactrim, Septra)

The trimethoprim-sulfamethoxazole combination (also known as co-trimoxazole) is the product of intensive pharmaceutical research to develop specific inhibitors of bacterial folate synthesis. Compared to its individual components, three advantages have been claimed for this combination: synergistic action, bacteriocidal action, and a lower rate of emergence of resistance to the individual components. The validity of these claims is controversial. At the present time trimethoprim-sulfamethoxazole has been approved by the Food and Drug Administration for the therapy of established recurrent bacterial urinary tract infections, *Pneumocystis carinii* pneumonitis, otitis media in children, and shigellosis.[113]

Mechanism of Action—The critical target of chemotherapy with trimethoprim-sulfamethoxazole is the microbial pool of tetrahydrofolate cofactors which are essential for bacterial growth and survival. Tetrahydrofolate cofactors are carriers of single carbon fragments, and are vital for the synthesis of purines, thymine, serine and methionine.

In contrast to humans, many microorganisms can synthesize dihydrofolate. (One of the substrates for this synthesis is para-aminobenzoic acid). Dihydrofolate is then reduced to its functional form, tetrahydrofolate, by the enzyme dihydrofolate reductase. Sulfonamides (such as sulfamethoxazole) compete with para-aminobenzoic acid, displace it, and block the biogenesis of dihydrofolate. Trimethoprim, a 2,4-diaminopyrimidine, inhibits dihydrofolate reductase by competing with dihydrofolate. The combination of sulfamethoxazole with trimethoprim produces a sequential blockade which will reduce the pools of tetrahydrofolate cofactors. The synergistic action of trimethoprim-sulfamethoxazole has been attributed to the impairment of tetrahydrofolate production at two different synthetic steps: sulfamethoxazole inhibits the production of dihydrofolate, and trimethoprim traps the cellular folates in the nonfunctional dihydro state.

Resistance to trimethoprim may occur among those organisms which, due to their loss of the enzyme thymidate synthetase, are dependent on exogenous thymine or thymidine, and thus no longer susceptible to the enzymatic blockade produced by trimethoprim.[114-117] The actual rate of occurrence of these metabolically altered strains as urinary tract pathogens is unknown, but probably is rare.[115] Infection with these mutants is more frequent in patients with renal calculi or chronic osteomyelitis who are receiving trimethoprim.[115,116,118,119] However, these organisms have been recovered from patients who have not received trimethoprim.[115] R-factor trimethoprim-mediated resistance has also been documented.[120,121] This form of resistance has been associated with minimum inhibitory concentrations that exceed 1,000 μg/ml.[120,121] Fortunately resistance to trimethoprim mediated by R-factors is rare.

The frequency of resistance to trimethoprim of urinary tract isolates (Enterobacteriacae) has remained low,[114] and apparently has not increased with the enhanced prescribing of trimethoprim-sulfamethoxazole.[114]

Spectrum of Activity—Performance of trimethoprim-sulfamethoxazole susceptibility determinations requires attention to detail, because the quantity and dispersal of the inoculum, as well as the constituents of the culture media, will markedly influence the test results. Undoubtedly this explains a number of discrepancies between various published reports.

In general, trimethoprim-sulfamethoxazole is inhibitory to most gram-positive aerobic cocci, including *Staphylococcus aureus, Staphylococcus epidermidis,* group A beta-hemolytic streptococci, *Streptococcus viridans, Streptococcus agalactiae* and *Streptococcus pneumoniae.* Resistant *Streptococcus pneumoniae* have, however, been isolated from the sputum of patients with acute bronchitis. Susceptibility of *Streptococcus faecalis* has been variable, probably because not all laboratories differentiate between *Streptococcus faecalis* and other group D streptococci (enterococci), such as *Streptococcus bovis.* Mutants of *Streptococcus faecalis* resistant to trimethoprim-sulfamethoxazole often emerge during or after therapy.

Meningococci are susceptible to trimethoprim-sulfamethoxazole, as are most strains of *Neisseria gonorrhoeae.*

Among the common gram-negative aerobic bacilli virtually all

Escherichia coli, Klebsiella, Citrobacter (diversus and freundii), Enterobacter (cloacae and agglomerans), Salmonellae, Shigella and Acinetobacter are susceptible to trimethoprim-sulfamethoxazole, as are the majority of strains of *Enterobacter aerogenes* and *Hemophilus influenzae.* Some salmonellae resistant to ampicillin and chloramphenicol are susceptible to trimethoprim-sulfamethoxazole. Trimethoprim-sulfamethoxazole has in vitro activity for some ampicillin-resistant *Hemophilus influenzae.* Approximately 50% of strains of Serratia, Providencia and Proteus are susceptible, but *Pseudomonas aeruginosa* are invariably resistant. Enterotoxigenic *E. coli,* a frequent cause of diarrhea in travellers, are susceptible to trimethoprim-sulfamethoxazole.

One report suggested that most *Bacteroides fragilis* were resistant to trimethoprim-sulfamethoxazole.[122] Others have not confirmed this and attribute the discrepancy to more careful sensitivity testing.[123,124]

Virtually all isolates of *Nocardia asteroides* are susceptible. Trimethoprim-sulfamethoxazole is also effective in the *Pneumocystis carinii* cortisone-treated rat model.

Resistant enterobacteriaceae do not emerge readily following exposure to trimethoprim-sulfamethoxazole, and the introduction of the drug has not been associated with the rapid appearance of resistant organisms.

In addition to its antimicrobial activity, trimethoprim-sulfamethoxazole has demonstrated immunosuppressive effects: prolongation of skin graft survival,[125] impairment of phytohaemagglutinin induced lymphocyte transformation[126] and suppression of antibody formation.[127] However, an altered immune response, as measured by lymphocyte blastogenesis of stimulated lymphocytes, did not occur in children who received trimethoprim-sulfamethoxazole for therapy of urinary tract infections.[128]

Pharmacology—Trimethoprim and sulfamethoxazole are rapidly absorbed after oral administration, achieving peak blood levels of trimethoprim of 0.6 to 1.8 μg/ml in one to four hours and 30 to 54 μg/ml of sulfamethoxazole in two to four hours (after 80/400-mg tablets).[129–136] Plasma concentrations of each component are directly related to the dose.[129,130] Steady-state serum levels in patients with normal renal function are attained in two to three days.[130–132] Trimethoprim and sulfamethoxazole are virtually completely absorbed from the gastrointestinal tract, as judged by the minimal fecal excretion.[133,137]

Trimethoprim exists in the plasma primarily as intact drug, 45% bound to protein.[133,134,138] Sulfamethoxazole exists as the intact, conjugated, and acetylated forms. Intact sulfamethoxazole accounts for 20% of excreted drug, while the remainder is excreted as the biologically inactive conjugated and acetylated metabolites.[138] Binding of sulfamethoxazole to plasma proteins is greater than 66%.[134,137]

Both trimethoprim and sulfamethoxazole are distributed throughout the body.[137] The apparent volume of distribution for trimethoprim has been calculated to be 47 to 133.3 liters, suggesting reasonably extensive tissue uptake.[134] Presumably, the wide distribution of trimethoprim is explained by its high lipid solubility, low protein binding, and minimal ionization in plasma.

Following oral administration, trimethoprim concentrations in prostatic secretions or tissues have equalled or exceeded those in serum.[139–142] Sulfamethoxazole, however, does not appear to penetrate the prostate in therapeutic concentrations.[141,142] Trimethoprim penetrates sputa, vaginal fluid, pleural effusions, and cerebrospinal fluid in therapeutic concentrations.[129,143,144] It is not known whether trimethoprim enters breast milk, the placenta, or the fetus, but the physicochemical properties of the compound certainly suggest that the risk of drug penetrance and potential for toxicity exist.

Plasma concentrations of trimethoprim and sulfamethoxazole do not exist in a fixed ratio.[129–131,134,135] One explanation is that the renal excretion, the major route of elimination of both compounds, is influenced by urinary pH,[145] which in turn determines the extent of ionization of each drug. Excretion of trimethoprim, a weak base with a pKa of 7.3, will be increased in an acid urine,[136,145] whereas that of sulfamethoxazole, a weak acid with a pKa of 5.7, is enhanced by alkalinization of the urine.[136,145]

Urinary concentrations of trimethoprim and sulfamethoxazole vary considerably, ranging from 10.9 to 206 μg/ml for trimethoprim and 27.0 to 125 μg/ml for intact sulfamethoxazole.[134,135,145] In patients with normal renal function, the ratio of trimethoprim to 'active sulfamethoxazole' approaches unity, and this relationship does not fluctuate with time.[131,134]

The half-life values of trimethoprim and sulfamethoxazole in patients with normal renal function are 8.6 to 11.6 hours and 8.7 to 14.5 hours, respectively.[130,131,133–135] This similarity in half-lives was one of the factors which influenced the manufacturers to select

TABLE 1 Dosage of Trimethoprim-Sulfamethoxazole in Patients with Renal Impairment

Creatinine Clearance (ml/min)	Serum Creatinine (mg/100 ml)	Dosage of 80/400 mg Tablets
25	Men 3 Women 2	2 tablets twice daily
15 –25	Men 3–7 Women 2–4.5	2 tablets twice daily for 3 days then 2 daily
15	Men 7 Women 4.5	2 tablets daily

sulfamethoxazole in preference to another sulfonamide for the development of a trimethoprim-sulfonamide combination.

Renal impairment prolongs of the half-life and reduces renal excretion of both sulfamethoxazole and trimethoprim.[135,136,145–149] Renal insufficiency does not cause higher plasma concentrations of intact (non-metabolically altered) sulfamethoxazole, but there is an elevation of the serum trimethoprim concentration. When creatinine clearance approaches 30 ml/min, metabolites of sulfamethoxazole are retained in the intravascular space.[147–149] Urinary excretion of trimethoprim declines when the creatinine clearance is reduced below 20 ml/min.[135] Even with severe renal disease, urinary concentrations of trimethoprim exceed the minimum inhibitory concentrations of most urinary pathogens.[136,145,146,149] Therapeutic urinary concentrations of sulfamethoxazole, however, are not invariably obtained in the presence of marked renal insufficiency. In order to prevent the accumulation of potentially toxic metabolites of sulfamethoxazole in patients with renal impairment, Reider and associates have devised a proposed dosage program (Table 1).[149]

Hemodialysis removes both trimethoprim and sulfamethoxazole,[136,147,148] but exact guidelines for dosage in patients undergoing hemodialysis are not available. The effect of peritoneal dialysis is not known.

Indications—Trimethoprim-sulfamethoxazole is the drug of first choice for the treatment of *Pneumocystis carinii* pneumonia[150–153] and shigellosis in areas where multiple antibiotic resistance is prominent.[154] Trimethoprim-sulfamethoxazole should also be given strong consideration as initial oral therapy for the management of recurrent urinary tract infections due to susceptible bacteria,[155,156] particularly for men who have concomitant chronic bacterial prostatitis.[157] Trimethoprim-sulfamethoxazole is an alternative to ampicillin and amoxicillin for the treatment of otitis media in children[158,159] and the preferred agent when the patient is penicillin-hypersensitive or has infection caused by beta-lactamase producing *Hemophilus influenzae.*[160]

Trimethoprim-sulfamethoxazole is effective in the treatment of acute urinary tract infections in adults, but is not recommended for a number of reasons. First, it is no more effective than its components[156,161–163] and conventional agents (eg, ampicillin, amoxicillin, cephalexin, tetracycline, nitrofurantoin).[161–164] Second, the vast majority of patients who experience this infection are young, otherwise healthy women who could be pregnant (and this information may not be known by the patient or her physician), and the safety of trimethoprim-sulfamethoxazole for pregnant women is not established. There is also the concern that extensive use of trimethoprim-sulfamethoxazole could encourage the emergence of resistant bacteria.

Ampicillin and trimethoprim-sulfamethoxazole are equally effective for the therapy of acute urinary tract infections in children,[165] but this is not an officially approved indication for trimethoprim-sulfamethoxazole.

Trimethoprim-sulfamethoxazole is extremely effective for many other infections, including acute exacerbations of chronic bronchitis,[166,167] brucellosis,[168] nocardiosis[169] and endocarditis caused by *Pseudomonas cepacia.*[170] Trimethoprim-sulfamethoxazole is also an invaluable treatment for the management of life-threatening salmonella infections (including those caused by ampicillin-resistant and chloramphenicol-resistant strains,[171,172] cholera when the disease is due to tetracycline-resistant *Vibrio cholerae,*[173] and gonorrhea produced by beta-lactamase-producing penicillin-resistant organisms.[174,175] Additional infections for which trimethoprim-sulfamethoxazole is effective are acute staphylococcal osteomyelitis,[176] neonatal *Escherichia coli* meningitis,[177] shigellosis,[178] toxoplasmosis[179] and *South American blastomycosis*. However, trimethoprim-sulfamethoxazole is currently considered as investigational for these miscellaneous infections.

Trimethoprim-sulfamethoxazole is an effective *prophylactic* agent for reduction of symptomatic reinfections in children and female adults who experience recurrent urinary tract infections.[180,181] Trimethoprim-sulfamethoxazole probably acts by interfering with colonization of the vaginal vestibule by fecal flora. Indeed, trimethoprim-sulfamethoxazole attains therapeutic concentrations in vaginal fluid following oral ingestion, and eradicates enterobacteriaceae (*E. coli, Proteus* sp., *Klebsiella* sp., *Enterobacter* sp.) from the fecal flora. Trimethoprim-sulfamethoxazole is a more effective form of prophylaxis (to prevent reinfections) than sulfamethoxazole alone, nitrofurantoin or methenamine compounds. Nonetheless, this is not an approved indication for this compound.

Adverse Reactions—An analysis of the adverse reactions ascribed to trimethoprim-sulfamethoxazole consistently reveals that gastrointestinal intolerance and skin eruptions are the most prevalent. Toxicity is virtually never life-threatening and is almost always completely reversible. The incidence of untoward events from this drug combination compares favorably with that of 'standard' agents administered for the same indications. One study suggests that the incidence of skin rashes and nausea are dose-related.[166] Most untoward events from trimethoprim-sulfamethoxazole develop within two weeks of the onset of therapy.[182]

Gastrointestinal. Gastrointestinal intolerance develops in about 3 to 8% of patients.[182] This is usually manifested as nausea, with or without vomiting, and frequently does not necessitate discontinuation of therapy. Diarrhea, glossitis and stomatitis occur more rarely. Pseudomembranous colitis has resulted from the administration of trimethoprim-sulfamethoxazole.[183,184] A toxin resembling that produced by *Clostridium sordellii* and incriminated as a cause of antibiotic-associated pseudomembranous colitis has been demonstrated in the feces of a patient who developed this disorder, presumably from trimethoprim-sulfamethoxazole therapy.[183] Trimethoprim-sulfamethoxazole induced pseudomembranous colitis has resulted in death.[184]

Skin reactions. Skin reactions develop in approximately 1 to 14% of patients. A more accurate incidence is probably 3%.[182,185] Skin reactions consist of erythema or urticaria or maculopapular, purpuric or morbilliform lesions. Rarely the Stevens-Johnson syndrome and toxic epidermal necrolysis have been ascribed to trimethoprim-sulfamethoxazole,[186] and fatalities have been reported.[187] Skin sensitivity can be limited to facial edema,[188] be associated with arthralgia[189] or comprise one component of a generalized reaction.[190] Reversible skin lesions, consisting of nodules, papules and pustules and attributed to a necrotizing vasculitis, have also been described.[190] Skin eruptions can develop on the first or during subsequent administration of trimethoprim-sulfamethoxazole and occasionally disappear during therapy. Skin reactions do not invariably recur on repeated drug exposure. Untoward skin reactions are not exclusively caused by the sulfonamide component of the combination.[161]

Hepatotoxicity. Hepatic injury is a very rare manifestation of trimethoprim-sulfamethoxazole toxicity.[191] This is not surprising since sulfonamides are a well recognized, although infrequent, cause of liver damage.[192] Hepatic necrosis with death has resulted from trimethoprim-sulfamethoxazole administration.[193]

Nephrotoxicity. Deterioration of renal function has developed in patients with normal or impaired renal function and is usually reversible.[194] The reduction in creatinine clearance does not appear to be due to an altered glomerular filtration rate.[195]

Hematologic toxicity. Life-threatening hematological reactions, including anemia[196] (hemolytic, macrocytic, aplastic, hypoplastic), thrombocytopenia,[197] granulocytopenia[198] and agranulocytosis[199] do occur and have, on rare occasion, resulted in death,[200] but these untoward events are extraordinarily rare.[201] Hemolysis in patients receiving trimethoprim-sulfamethoxazole who have erythrocytes deficient in glucose-6-phosphate dehydrogenase has virtually never been reported, and when it does occur probably is a manifestation of the infection rather than the drug.[202]

Miscellaneous reactions. One report suggests that trimethoprim-sulfamethoxazole caused a reversible polyneuropathy;[203] another report tends to refute this association.[204] Trimethoprim-sulfamethoxazole has reportedly produced multisystem organ toxicity and death.[205,206] and in some patients decreased sperm counts.[207] At present these relationships are very doubtful. One report suggested that diabetics who receive oral hypoglycemic agents and trimethoprim-sulfamethoxazole will manifest an increase in immunoreactive insulin and symptomatic hypoglycemia.[208] Urinary obstruction due to a stone consisting of metabolites of trimethoprim-sulfamethoxazole has been described.[209]

Limited data fail to demonstrate any relationship between trimethoprim-sulfamethoxazole administration and teratogenicity.[164,210] However, evidence is not sufficient to conclude that trimethoprim-sulfamethoxazole is safe for pregnant women.

Drug and Laboratory Test Interactions—Trimethoprim-sulfame-

sulfamethoxazole can potentiate the anticoagulant effect of coumadin and the hypoglycemic response to tolbutamide, as well as impede the renal excretion of methotrexate.[211–215] A proposed mechanism involves displacement of these drugs from their binding sites.

The clinical significance of a prolonged half-life of phenytoin when administered with trimethoprim-sulfamethoxazole is unclear.[212] Trimethoprim can interfere with the mechanism for the tubular secretion of creatinine, leading to spuriously elevated serum creatinine levels.[216] Trimethoprim-sulfamethoxazole can also produce 'falsely' elevated serum bilirubin and alkaline phosphatase concentrations.[217]

Dosage—Oral: Adults, for an established urinary tract infection, 160 mg trimethoprim and 800 mg of sulfamethoxazole twice daily for 10 to 14 days.[155,218] For *Pneumocystis carinii* pneumonia, 960 to 1200 mg trimethoprim and 4800 to 6000 mg sulfamethoxazole daily, divided into two or three equal portions.[219] For shigellosis, 160 mg trimethoprim and 800 mg sulfamethoxazole every 12 hours for five days. *Children,* for urinary tract infection and otitis media, 8 mg/kg trimethoprim and 40 mg/kg sulfamethoxazole every 24 hours in two divided doses for 10 to 14 days.[218] For *Pneumocystis carinii* pneumonia, 20 mg/kg trimethoprim and 100 mg/kg sulfamethoxazole daily, divided into four doses.[220] For shigellosis, 10 mg/kg trimethoprim and 50 mg/kg sulfamethoxazole daily, divided into two doses, for five days. For dosage in patients with renal failure, see Table 1.

VANCOMYCIN HYDROCHLORIDE (Vancocin Hydrochloride)

Vancomycin is a narrow spectrum antimicrobial that became available in 1958, primarily for the treatment of staphylococcal infections. With the introduction of penicillinase-resistant penicillins and cephalosporins in the 1960's, vancomycin was relegated to an alternative agent for patients who had contraindications to these primary choices. Although relatively nontoxic when therapy is properly monitored, vancomycin usage currently is quite limited.

Mechanism of Action and Spectrum of Activity—Vancomycin is readily absorbed by the cell walls of gram-positive bacteria. Antibacterial activity is based on interference with the biosynthesis of peptidoglycan.[221] Nearly all gram-positive bacteria are susceptible at levels of 0.3 to 5 μg/ml.[222] These include *S. aureus, S. epidermidis, Streptococcus viridans, S. pneumoniae,* enterococci, *S. pyogenes,*

TABLE 2 Preparations and Costs of Miscellaneous Antimicrobial Agents

Generic Name	Trademark Name(s)	Preparations and 1978 Costs
Methenamine Hippurate	Hiprex (Urex)	Tablets 1 g—$15.35/100
Methenamine Mandelate	Mandelamine	Tablets (enteric-coated) 250 mg—$2.70/100; 500 mg—$5.10/100; 1 g—$8.15/100 Suspension 250 mg/5 ml—$2.90/4 oz; 500 mg/5 ml—$7.80/8 oz Granules 500 mg—$7.60/56; 1 g—$11.95/56
Nalidixic Acid	NegGram	Tablets 250 mg—$6.91/56; 500 mg—$11.47/56 Suspension 250 mg/5 ml—$17.84/16 oz
Oxolinic Acid	Utibid	Tablets 750 mg—$18.50/50
Trimethoprim and Sulfamethoxazole (Co-trimoxazole)	Bactrim (Septra)	Tablets containing trimethoprim 80 mg and sulfamethoxazole 400 mg—$20.60/100 Tablets containing trimethoprim 160 mg and sulfamethoxazole 800 mg—$36.71/100 Suspension containing trimethoprim 40 mg and sulfamethoxazole 200 mg/5 ml—$10.95/16 oz
Vancomycin Hydrochloride	Vancocin Hydrochloride	Injection (powder) 500 mg—$8.95/vial Oral powder 10 g—$120.84/vial

Clostridia, peptococci, peptostreptococci, and anaerobic gram-positive bacilli. Minimum inhibitory and minimal bactericidal concentrations (MBCs) are usually the same with these organisms, indicating the drug is bactericidal. Exceptions are enterococci which show MBCs exceeding 10 μg/ml. These observations necessitate in vitro testing when vancomycin is used in patients with endocarditis. Neisseria are susceptible to vancomycin. Staphylococci which are methicillin-resistant are usually vancomycin-sensitive.[223] Gram-negative bacilli (aerobic and anaerobic), mycobacteria, fungi, mycoplasma, and cell wall-deficient bacteria are resistant. Resistance by gram-positive bacteria is unusual and seldom occurs during a course of treatment or even with sublethal concentration of vancomycin in vitro.

Indications—Systemic vancomycin is seldom used except for patients who have contraindications to the use of other antimicrobials active against gram-positive bacteria. The principal indications are as follows.

1. Staphylococcal shunt infections in renal dialysis patients—in this instance vancomycin is often regarded as the drug of choice since the prolonged levels in renal failure permit effective therapy with a single intravenous dose.

2. Staphyloccal endocarditis and other serious staphylococcal infections—vancomycin is usually the drug of choice for methicillin-resistant strains of *S. aureus* and *S. epidermidis*. It is an effective alternative to penicillins and cephalosporins in patients who have contraindications to these agents.[224]

3. Streptococcal endocarditis—vancomycin is an alternative to penicillin or ampicillin for enterococcal endocarditis in patients with a history of an immediate reaction to penicillins. Like the penicillins, vancomycin should be combined with an aminoglycoside for enterococcal endocarditis. Synergistic activity is more predictable with vancomycin plus gentamicin than with vancomycin plus streptomycin,[225] but this is optimally determined on an individual basis with in vitro testing. Vancomycin may have low MBCs for viridans streptococci and *Streptococcus bovis,* but this is variable and clinical experience with vancomycin as a single agent for endocarditis caused by these agents is sparse.

4. Oral vancomycin is used for staphylococcal enterocolitis,[226] and preliminary data suggest efficacy for antibiotic-associated pseudomembranous colitis due to *Cl. difficile.*[227] The oral form may also be used along with other antimicrobials for bowel sterilization.

Pharmacology—Vancomycin is not absorbed from the gastrointestinal tract and gives levels of up to 25,000 μg/g of stool with oral administration of 500 mg doses at 6 hour intervals. Intramuscular injection of vancomycin is extremely painful. The parenteral form is available only as an intravenous preparation for systemic infections.

Intravenous administration of 1 g provides peak serum levels of 25 to 40 μg/ml. Vancomycin is distributed to most tissues and body fluids, but bile and cerebrospinal fluid levels are low. Approximately

80% of the drug is excreted in biologically active form in the urine. The half-life of vancomycin averages six hours in patients with normal renal function and increases to nine days in anuric patients.

Adverse Reactions—The major toxicity is auditory nerve damage with deafness. This may progress after vancomycin is discontinued, and it is often irreversible. Ototoxicity is related to excessive dosage, prolonged courses of therapy, improper dose modification in renal insufficiency, concurrent use of other ototoxic drugs, old age, and previous hearing loss. This seldom happens when therapy is closely monitored and serum levels are maintained at 30 μg/ml or lower. Nephrotoxicity is unusual.

Thrombophlebitis is a common problem that may be minimized by administration in a volume of at least 200 ml and rotation of injection sites. Chills and fever may also occur. These local and systemic side effects may be minimized by adding small doses of hydrocortisone to the infusion.

Allergic reactions occur in 4 to 5% of patients, primarily in the form of skin rashes. Urticaria, eosinophilia, drug fever, and anaphylaxis are rare.

Preparations and Dosage—Vancomycin is a stable complex glycopolypeptide with a molecular weight of approximately 3,300. Activity is minimally affected with pH ranges of 6.5 to 8. The recommended intravenous dose of vancomycin for adult patients is 1 g every 12 hours. The appropriate dose is dissolved in 100 to 200 ml of 5% dextrose in water or saline and administered over 15 to 30 minutes. Doses of 3 g per day may be given to seriously ill individuals for the first 2 to 3 days of treatment. Somewhat lower doses (1.5 g/day) are recommended when vancomycin is given concurrently with an aminoglycoside. The pediatric dose is 25 to 40 mg/kg/day. Dose modification is required in renal insufficiency, and monitoring of blood levels is desirable. In general, patients with a serum creatinine of 1.5 to 5 should receive 1 to 2 g every four days; with a creatinine over 5 the usual dose is 1 g every 10 to 14 days. The usual dose of oral vancomycin is 500 mg every six hours.

REFERENCES

1. Gleckman R, Alvarez S, Joubert DW, et al: Methenamine mandelate and methenamine hippurate. Am J Hosp Pharm, in press (expected publication date: October, 1979).
2. Katul J, Frank IN: Antibacterial activity of methenamine hippurate. J Urol 104:320–324, 1970.
3. Musher DM, Griffith DP: Generation of formaldehyde from methionine: effect of pH and concentration, and antibacterial effect. Antimicrob Agents Chemother 6:708–711, 1974.

4. Knight V, Draper JW, Brady EA, et al: Methenamine mandelate: antimicrobial activity, absorption and excretion. Antibiot Chemother 2:615–635, 1952.
5. Scudi JV, Duca CJ: Some antibacterial properties of mandelamine (methenamine mandelate). J Urol 61:459–467, 1949.
6. Seneca H, Zinsser HH, Peer P: Chemotherapy of chronic urinary tract infections with methenamine hippurate. J Urol 97:1094–1098, 1967.
7. Miller H, Phillips E: Antibacterial correlates of urine drug levels of hexamethylenetetramine and formaldehyde. Invest Urol 8:21–23, 1970.
8. Scudi JV, Reinhard JF: Absorption, distribution, and renal excretion of mandelamine (methenamine mandelate). J Lab Clin Med 33:1304–1310, 1948.
9. Greenfield W, Berg R, Moore R: Determination of urine formaldehyde following administration of methenamine salts. Clin Chem 15:1180–1185, 1969.
10. Seneca H, Peer P: Clinical pharmacology and antibacterial action of methenamine and its salts (mandelate, hippurate, and sulfosalicylate). Med Times 97:243–251, 1969.
11. Knoefel PK, Huang KC: Biochemorphology of renal tubular transport: hippuric acid and related substances. J Pharmacol Exp Ther 126:296–303, 1959.
12. Corriere JN, Martin MM: Hippuric acid clearance in bacteriuric patients with degrees of renal impairment. Am J Med Sci 244:472–477, 1972.
13. Nagivekar JB: Kinetics of metabolism and urinary excretion of dextrorotatory and levorotatory mandelic acid in humans. Thesis, Temple Univ., 1965, p. 40.
14. McDonald DF, Murphy GP: Bacteriostatic and acidifying effects of methionine, hydrolyzed caseine and ascorbic acid on the urine. N Engl J Med 261:803–805, 1959.
15. Shohl A, Deming CL: Hexamethylenamine: its quantitative factors in therapy. J Urol 4:419–437, 1920.
16. Nilsson S: Long term treatment with methenamine hippurate in recurrent urinary tract infection. Acta Med Scand 198:81–85, 1975.
17. Kohler FP, Bodi T: Evaluation of methenamine sulfosalicylate as urinary tract antibacterial. Clin Med 76:27–29, (Aug) 1969.
18. Kasanen A, Mustakallio EK, Koskinen EH, et al: Methenamine hippurate in the treatment of urinary tract infections. Ann Clin Res 6:279–284, 1974.
19. Freeman RB, Smith WM, Richardson JA, et al: Long term therapy for chronic bacteriuria in men. Ann Intern Med 83:133–147, 1975.
20. Tanejo OP, Grover NK, Gulati SM, et al: Long term treatment of chronic urinary tract infections: a comparative study of four drugs. Indian J Med Sci 28:197–207, 1974.
21. Kincaid-Smith P, Friedman A, Nanra RS: Controlled trials of treatment in urinary tract infection. In *Renal Infection and Renal Scarring*. Edited by P Kincaid-Smith, KF Fairley. Melbourne, Mercedes Publishing Services, 1970, pp 165–174.
22. Kincaid-Smith P, Kalowski S: Co-trimoxazole in urinary tract infection. Med J Aust 1(Suppl):49–51, 1973.
23. Kasanen A, Kaarsalo E, Hiltunen R, et al: Comparison of long-term, low-dosage nitrofurantoin, methenamine-hippurate, trimethoprim and trimethoprim-sulphamethoxazole on the control of recurrent urinary tract infection. Ann Clin Res 6:285–289, 1974. 6:285–289, 1974.
24. Keswani RK, Chugh TD, Hooda RS, et al: Prevention of recurrent urinary tract infection with methenamine mandelate. Indian J Med Res 64:1168–1172, 1976.
25. Australian Drug Evaluation Committee: Adverse effects of drugs commonly used in the treatment of urinary tract infections. Med J Aust 1:435–438, 1972.
26. Bourque JP, Joyal J: The use of mandelamine in 100 unselected cases of various urinary tract infections. Can Med Assoc J 75:634–641, 1956.
27. Carroll G, Allen HN: The treatment of urinary tract infections with mandelamine (methenamine mandelate): a clinical study of 200 cases. J Urol 55:674–681, 1946.
28. Parvio S: Methenamine hippurate ('Hiprex') in the treatment of chronic urinary tract infections: a trial in a geriatric hospital. J Int Med Res 4:111–114, 1976.
29. Gow JG: A comparative trial of hexamine hippurate and hexamine mandelate in the prevention of recurrent infection of the urinary tract. Practitioner 213:97–101, 1974.
30. Freeman RB, Bromer L, Brancato F, et al: Prevention of recurrent bacteriuria with continuous chemotherapy. Ann Intern Med 69:655–672, 1968.
31. Timmerman RJ, Schroer JA: Lipoid pneumonia caused by methenamine mandelate suspension. JAMA 225:1524–1525, 1973.
32. Ross RR, Conway GF: Hemorrhagic cystitis following accidental overdose of methenamine mandelate. Am J Dis Child 119:86–87, 1970.

33. Tanaka T, Kitajima K, Naito T, et al: A necropsy case of interstitial nephritis probably related to cefazolin and methenamine. Acta Med Okayama 30:341–348, 1976.
34. Harvey SC: Antiseptics and disinfectants; fungicides; ectoparasiticides. In *The Pharmacological Basis of Therapeutics,* 5th edition. Edited by LS Goodman, A Gilman. New York, Macmillan, 1975, pp 987–1017.
35. Lipton JH: Incompatibility between sulfamethiazole and methenamine mandelate. N Engl J Med 268:92–93, 1963.
36. Holland NH, West CD: Prevention of recurrent urinary tract infection in girls. Am J Dis Child 105:560–567, 1963.
37. Gleckman R, Alvarez S, Joubert DW, et al: Nalidixic acid. Am J Hosp Pharm, in press (expected publication date: September 1979).
38. Bauerfeind A, Grummer G: Biochemical effects of nalidixic acid on Escherichia coli. Chemotherapia 10:95–102, 1965.
39. Gross WA, Deitz WH, Cook TM: Mechanism of action of nalidixic acid on Escherichia coli. II. Inhibition of deoxyribonucleic acid synthesis. J Bacteriol 89:1068–1074, 1965.
40. Bourguignon GJ, Levit JM, Sternglanz R: Studies on the mechanisms of action of nalidixic acid. Antimicrob Agents Chemother 4:479–486, 1973.
41. Boyle JV, Cook TM, Gross WA: Mechanism of action of nalidixic acid on Escherichia coli. VI. Cell free studies. J Bacteriol 97:230–236, 1969.
42. Crumpling GC, Smith JT: Nalidixic acid and bacterial chromosomal replication. Nature 260:643–645, 1976.
43. Crumpling GC, Smith JT: Nalidixic acid: an antibacterial paradox. Antimicrob Agents Chemother 8:251–261, 1975.
44. McChesney EW, Froelich EJ, Lesher GY, et al: Absorption, excretion, and metabolism of a new antibacterial agent, nalidixic acid. Toxicol Appl Pharmacol 6:292–309, 1964.
45. Gibbon NOK, Benstead JG, Misra GC: A comparative study of the levels of nalidixic acid in plasma and urine and its antibacterial activity in urinary infections of paraplegics. Postgrad Med J 41:501–508, 1965.
46. Moore WE, Portmann GA, Stander H, et al: Biopharmaceutical investigation of nalidixic acid in man. J Pharm Sci 54:36–41, 1965.
47. Portmann GA, McChesney EW, Moore WE: Pharmacokinetic model for nalidixic acid in man. II. Parameters for absorption, metabolism and excretion. J Pharm Sci 55:72–78, 1966.
48. Portmann GA, McChesney EW, Moore WE: Pharmacokinetic model for nalidixic acid in man. III. Effect of repeated oral dosage. J Pharm Sci 56:594–599, 1967.
49. Harrison LH, Cox C: Bacteriologic and pharmacodynamic aspects of nalidixic acid. J Urol 104:908–913, 1970.
50. Mannisto PT: Pharmacokinetics of nalidixic acid and oxolinic acid in healthy women. Clin Pharmacol Ther 19:38–46, 1976.
51. Portmann GA, McChesney EW, Moore WE: Pharmacokinetic model for nalidixic acid in man. I. Kinetic pathway for hydroxynalidixic acid. J Pharm Sci 55:59–62, 1966.
52. Hoeprick PD: New antimicrobics for the treatment of infections caused by gram-negative bacilli. Med Clin North Am 51:1127–1152, 1967.
53. Jameson RM: Tissue concentration of nalidixic acid in chronic pyelonephritis. Br Med J 2:621–622, 1965.
54. Armstrong J, Cook F, Robinson J: Concentration of antibiotic and chemotherapeutic agents in the ejaculum. J Urol 100:72–76, 1968.
55. Stamey TA, Mears EM, Winningham DG: Chronic bacterial prostatitis and diffusion of drugs in prostatic fluid. J Urol 103:187–194, 1970.
56. Newman RL, Holt RJ, Frankcombe CH: Nalidixic acid: microbiological and clinical studies of urinary infections in children. Arch Dis Child 41:389–394, 1966.
57. Santos-Martinez J, Diaz J: Nalidixic acid: intrarenal distribution and its effect upon para-aminohippurate excretion. J Urol 114:670–677, 1975.
58. Slade DA: A clinical trial of nalidixic acid (Negram, Win 18,320) in thirty-three patients with urinary tract infections in general practice. Br J Urol 35:125–128, 1963.
59. Murphy FJ, Zelman S, Mau W: Ascorbic acid as a urinary acidifying agent: 2. Its adjunctive role in chronic urinary tract infections. J Urol 94:300–303, 1965.
60. Ronald RR, Turck M, Petersdorf RG: A critical evaluation of nalidixic acid in urinary tract infections. N Engl J Med 275:1081–1089, 1966.

61. Cederberg A, Denneberg T, Ekberg M, et al: Nalidixic acid in urinary tract infections with particular reference to the emergence of resistance. Scand J Infect Dis 6:259–264, 1974.
62. Stamey TA, Bragonje J: Resistance to nalidixic acid: a misconception due to underdosage. JAMA 236:1857–1860, 1976.
63. Sharma B: Treatment of brucellosis by nalidixic acid. Lancet 1:1171–1173, 1965.
64. Moffat M, Hamilton N: Nalidixic acid (Wintomylon) in diarrhoeal disorders: a clinical trial. Med Proc 11:382–387, 1965.
65. Adverse effects of drugs commonly used in the treatment of urinary tract infections: A report from the Australian Drug Evaluation Committee. Med J Aust 1:435–438, 1972.
66. Alexander S, Forman L: Which of the drugs caused the rash? or the value of the lymphocyte transformation test in eruptions caused by nalidixic acid. Br J Dermatol 84:429–434, 1971.
67. Mathew TH: Nalidixic acid (letter). Med J Aust 2:243, 1966.
68. Brauner GJ: Bullous photoreaction to nalidixic acid. Am J Med 58:576–580, 1975.
69. Burry JN: Persistent phototoxicity due to nalidixic acid (letter). Arch Dermatol 109:263, 1974.
70. Ramsay CA, Obreshkova E: Photosensitivity from nalidixic acid. Br J Dermatol 91:523–528, 1974.
71. Ramsay CA: Photosensitivity from nalidixic acid (abstract). Proc R Soc Med 66:747, 1973.
72. Marshall BY: Visual side effects of nalidixic acid. Practitioner 199:222–224, 1967.
73. Navarro SS, Villegus LP, Garcia LJ: Relapsing salmonellosis and shigellosis treated with nalidixic acid: 30 cases. Sem Med Mex 48:215–220, 1966.
74. Bailey RR, Natale R, Linton AL: Nalidixic acid arthralgia. Can Med Assoc J 107:604–605, 1972.
75. Oller LZ: Treatment of gonorrhea with nalidixic acid. Br J Vener Dis 40:256–260, 1964.
76. Walker SH, Salanio I, Stand WE: Nalidixic acid in childhood urinary tract infection. Clinical and laboratory experience with patients. Clin Pediatr 5:718–721, 1966.
77. Pasquier CM Jr, St. Martin EC, Geissler WL: NegGram, a new urinary antiseptic. J La Med Soc 116:363–366, 1964.
78. Bailey RR: Nalidixic acid in 'full dosage' (letter). NZ Med J 80:226, 1974.
79. Kremer L, Walton M, Wardle EN: Nalidixic acid and intracranial hypertension (letter). Br Med J 4:488, 1967.
80. Islam MA, Sreedharan T: Convulsions, hyperglycemia, and glycosuria. JAMA 192:1100–1101, 1965.
81. Fraser AG, Harrower ADB: Convulsions and hyperglycemia associated with nalidixic acid (letter). Br Med J 2:1518, 1977.
82. Deonna T, Guignard JP: Acute intracranial hypertension after nalidixic acid administration (letter). Arch Dis Child 49:743, 1974.
83. Cohen DN: Intracranial hypertension and papilledema associated with nalidixic acid therapy. Am J Ophthalmol 76:680–682, 1973.
84. Anderson EE, Anderson B, Nashold S: Childhood complications of nalidixic acid. JAMA 216:1023–1024, 1971.
85. Beton EM, Jones RV: Haemolytic anaemia due to nalidixic acid (letter). Lancet 2:691, 1965.
86. Swinney J: Nalidixic acid. Practitioner 192:701–706, 1964.
87. Swanson M, Cook R: *Drugs, Chemicals and Blood Dyscrasias.* Hamilton, Illinois, Drug Intelligence Publications, 1977, pp 667–669.
88. Finegold SM, Ziment I: Sulfonamides, nitrofurans and nalidixic acid. Pediatr Clin North Am 15:95–105, 1968.
89. Eichenwald HF, McCracken GH: Antimicrobial therapy in infants and children. Part I. J Pediatr 93:337–356, 1978.
90. Kimball MI, Davies PA: Nalidixic acid for the newborn. Br Med J 2:310–311, 1967.
91. Zinsser HH: Nalidixic acid in acute and chronic urinary tract infections. Med Clin North Am 54:1347–1350, 1970.
92. Sellers EM, Koch-Weser J: Displacement of warfarin from human albumin by diazoxide and ethacrynic, mefanamic, and nalidixic acids. Clin Pharmacol Ther 11:524–529, 1970.
93. Klumpp TG: Nalidixic acid...false positive glycosuria and hyperglycemia (letter). JAMA 193:746, 1965.
94. Llerena O, Pearson OH: Interference of nalidixic acid in urinary 17-ketosteroid determinations. N Engl J Med 279:983–984, 1968.

95. Gleckman R, Alvarez S, Joubert DW, et al: Oxolinic acid. Am J Hosp Pharm, in press (expected publication date: September, 1979).
96. Staudenbauer WL: Replication of Escherichia coli DNA in vitro: inhibition by oxolinic acid. Eur J Biochem 62:491–497, 1976.
97. Kaminsky D, Von Strandtmann M: Synthetic antibacterial agents. Ann Rep Med Chem 5:87–100, 1969.
98. Pianotti RS, Mohan RR, Schwartz BS: Biochemical effects of oxolinic acid on Proteus vulgaris. J Bacteriol 95:1622–1628, 1968.
99. Mohring K, Madsen PO: Treatment of urinary tract infections with oxolinic acid in patients with normal and impaired renal function. Del Med J 43:376–380, 1971.
100. Guyer BM: Drug profile: prodoxal (oxolinic acid). J Int Med Res 2:458–460, 1974.
101. Pearson BS: Urinary tract infection treated with oxolinic acid. Med J Aust 1:140–141, 1975.
102. Ghatikar KN: A multicenter trial of a new synthetic antibacterial in urinary infections. Curr Ther Res 16:130–136, 1974.
103. Shapera RM, Matsen JM: Oxolinic acid therapy for urinary tract infections in children. Am J Dis Child 131:34–37, 1977.
104. Drummond M: A bacteriological and clinical assessment of a new drug—oxolinic acid. Br J Urol 47:233–234, 1975.
105. Guyer BM, Whitford GM: Oxolinic acid in urinary tract infection: a multi-centre trial. Curr Med Res Opin 2:636–640, 1975.
106. Truant JP, Katsampes C: Clinical effectiveness of oxolinic acid in the treatment of urinary tract infections. In *Progress in Antimicrobial and Anticancer Chemotherapy: Proceedings of the Sixth International Congress of Chemotherapy, Tokyo, 1969,* vol. 1. Edited by H Umezawa. Baltimore, University Park Press, 1970, pp 888–894.
107. Turner FJ, Ringel SM, Martin JF, et al: Oxolinic acid: a new semisynthetic antimicrobial agent: in vitro and in vivo activity. Antimicrob Agents Chemother—1967, pp 475–479.
108. DuPont HL, Hornick RB: Clinical approach to infectious diarrhea. Medicine 52:262–270, 1973.
109. D'Alessio DJ, Olexy VM, Jackson GG: Oxolinic acid treatment of urinary tract infections. Antimicrob Agents Chemother—1967, pp 490–496.
110. Clark H, Brown NK, Wallace JF, et al: Emergence of resistant organisms as a function of dose in oxolinic acid therapy. Am J Med Sci 261:145–148, 1971.
111. Lampe WT: Oxolinic acid treatment of urinary tract infections. Pa Med 74:59–62, (Jul) 1971.
112. Atlas E, Clark H, Silverblatt F, et al: Nalidixic acid and oxolinic acid in the treatment of chronic bacteriuria. Ann Intern Med 70:713–721, 1969.
113. Gleckman R, Alvarez S, Joubert DW: Trimethoprim-sulfamethoxazole. Am J Hosp Pharm, in press (expected publication date: July, 1979).
114. Wong CK, Harding GMK, Roland AR, et al: Trimethoprim-resistant Enterobacteriacea in urinary tract infection. Can Med Assoc J 112(Suppl):54S–58S, 1975.
115. Okubadejo OA, Maskell RM: Co-trimoxazole resistance (letter). Br Med J 2:227, 1974.
116. Barker J, Healing D, Hutchinson JGP: Characteristics of some co-trimoxazole resistant Enterobacteriacea from infected patients. J Clin Pathol 25:1086–1088, 1972.
117. Thomas M, Dzienjko M: Co-trimoxazole resistance (letter). Br Med J 1:328, 1974.
118. Lacey RW, Guillespie WA, Bruten DM, et al: Trimethoprim resistant coliforms. Lancet 1:409–410, 1972.
119. Okubadejo OA, Maskell RM: Thymine-requiring mutants of *Proteus mirabilis* selected by co-trimoxazole in vivo. J Gen Microbiol 77:533–535, 1973.
120. Fleming MP, Dalta N, Gruneberg RN: Trimethoprim resistance determined by R factors. Br Med J 1:726–728, 1972.
121. Dalta N, Hedges RW: Trimethoprim resistance confered by W plasmids in enterobacteriacea. J Gen Microbiol 72:349–355, 1972.
122. Rosenblatt JE, Stewart PR: Lack of activity of sulfamethoxazole and trimethoprim against anaerobic bacteria. Antimicrob Agents Chemother 6:93–97, 1974.
123. DeLouvois J, Gortvai P, Hurley R: Bacteriology of abscesses of the central nervous system: a multicenter prospective study. Br Med J 2:981–984, 1977.
124. Wust J, Wilkins TD: Susceptibility of anaerobic bacteria to sulfamethoxazole-trimethoprim and routine susceptibility testing. Antimicrob Agents Chemother 14:384–390, 1978.
125. Ghilchik MW, Morris AS, Reeves DS: Immunosuppressive powers of the antibacterial agent trimethoprim. Nature 227:393–394, 1970.

126. Gaylarde PM, Sarkany I: Suppression of thymidine uptake of human lymphocytes by co-trimoxazole. Br Med J 3:144–146, 1972.
127. Arvilommi H, Vuori M, Salmi A: Immunosuppression by co-trimoxazole. Br Med J 3:761–762, 1972.
128. Wolfish NM, Wassef NWG, Gonzalez H, et al: Immunologic parameters of children with urinary tract infection: effects of trimethoprim-sulfamethoxazole. Can Med Assoc J 112(Suppl):76S–79S, 1975.
129. Bach MS, Gold O, Finland M: Absorption and urinary excretion of trimethoprim, sulfamethoxazole, and trimethoprim-sulfamethoxazole: results with single doses in normal young adults and preliminary observations during therapy with trimethoprim-sulfamethoxazole. J Infect Dis 128(Suppl):S584–S599, 1973.
130. Kaplan SA, Weinfeld RE, Abruzzo CW, et al: Pharmacokinetic profile of trimethoprim-sulfamethoxazole in man. J Infect Dis 128(Suppl):S547–S555, 1973.
131. Kremers P, Duvivier J, Heusghem C: Pharmacokinetic studies of co-trimoxazole in man after single and repeated doses. J Clin Pharmacol 14:112–117, 1974.
132. Kaplan SA, Weinfeld RE, Cotler S, et al: Pharmacokinetic profile of trimethoprim in dog and man. J Pharm Sci 59:358–363, 1970.
133. Schwartz DE, Ziegler WH: Assay and pharmacokinetics of trimethoprim in man and animals. Postgrad Med J 45(Suppl):32–37, 1969.
134. Schwartz DE, Reider J: Pharmacokinetics of sulfamethoxazole and trimethoprim in man and their distribution in the rat. Chemotherapy 15:337–355, 1970.
135. Bergan T, Brodwall EK: Human pharmacokinetics of a sulfamethoxazole-trimethoprim combination. Acta Med Scand 192:483–492, 1972.
136. Craig W, Kunin C: Trimethoprim-sulfamethoxazole: pharmacodynamic effects of urinary pH and impaired renal function. Studies in humans. Ann Intern Med 79:491–497, 1973.
137. Brumfitt W, Hamilton-Miller JMT, Kosmidis J: Trimethoprim-sulfamethoxazole: the present position. J Infect Dis 128(Suppl):S778–S791, 1973.
138. Reider J: Metabolism and techniques for assay of trimethoprim and sulfamethoxazole. J Infect Dis 128(Suppl):S567–S573, 1973.
139. Nielsen ML, Hansen I: Trimethoprim in human prostatic tissue and prostatic fluid. Scand J Urol Nephrol 6:244–248, 1968.
140. Dabhoiwala NF, Bye A, Claridge M: A study of concentrations of trimethoprim-sulfamethoxazole in the human prostate gland. Br J Urol 48:78–81, 1976.
141. Madsen P, Kjaer T, Baumueller A: Prostatic tissue and fluid concentrations of trimethoprim and sulfamethoxazole. Urology 3:129–132, 1976.
142. Oosterlinck W, Defoort R, Renders G: The concentration of sulfamethoxazole and trimethoprim in human prostate gland. Br J Urol 47:301–304, 1975.
143. Stamey TA, Condy M: The diffusion and concentration of trimethoprim in human vaginal fluid. J Infect Dis 131:261–266, 1975.
144. Eatman FB, Maggio AC, Pecelinko R, et al: Blood and salivary concentrations of sulfamethoxazole and trimethoprim in man. J Pharmacokinet Biopharm 5:615–624, 1977.
145. Shapstone P: The renal handling of trimethoprim and sulfamethoxazole in man. Postgrad Med J 45(Suppl):38–42, 1969.
146. Bergan T, Brodwall EK: Kidney transport of sulfamethoxazole and trimethoprim. Chemotherapy 17:320–333, 1972.
147. Baetke R, Golde G, Gahl G: Sulphamethoxazole/trimethoprim: pharmacokinetic studies in patients with chronic renal failure. Eur J Clin Pharmacol 4:233–240, 1972.
148. Welling P, Craig W, Amidon G, et al: The pharmacokinetics of trimethoprim and sulfamethoxazole in normal subjects and in patients with renal failure. J Infect Dis 128(Suppl):S556–S566, 1973.
149. Reider J, Fernex M, Schwartz DE, et al: Pharmacokinetic data of the combination of sulfamethoxazole plus trimethoprim in patients with renal impairment. In *Proceedings of the Seventh International Congress of Chemotherapy, Prague, 1972,* vol. 1. Edited by H Ejzlar, N Semonsky, S Nasak. Baltimore, University Park Press, 1972, pp 79–82.
150. Kipson A, Marshall WC, Hayward AR: Treatment of Pneumocystis carinii pneumonia in children. Arch Dis Child 52:314–319, 1977.
151. Larter WE, John TJ, Sieber OF, et al: Trimethoprim-sulfamethoxazole treatment of Pneumocystis carinii pneumonitis. J Pediatr 92:826–828, 1978.
152. Lau WK, Young LS: Trimethoprim-sulfamethoxazole treatment of Pneumocystis carinii pneumonia in adults (abstract). Clin Res 24:113A, 1976.

153. Hughes WT, Feldman S, Chaudhary SC, et al: Comparison of pentamidine isethionate and trimethoprim-sulfamethoxazole in the treatment of Pneumocystis carinii pneumonia. J Pediatr 92:285–291, 1978.
154. Nelson JA, Kusmiesz H, Jackson LH, et al: Trimethoprim-sulfamethoxazole therapy for shigellosis. JAMA 235:1239–1243, 1976.
155. Gleckman RA: A cooperative controlled study of the use of trimethoprim-sulfamethoxazole in chronic urinary tract infections. J Infect Dis 128(Suppl):S647–S651, 1973.
156. Schnaars P, Escher J: Results obtained in the treatment of acute and chronic urinary tract infections with Bactrim or its components sulfamethoxazole and trimethoprim. Praxis 58:1279–1283, 1969.
157. Meares EM Jr: Observations on activity of trimethoprim-sulfamethoxazole in the prostate. J Infect Dis 128(Suppl):S679–S685, 1973.
158. Shurin PA, Pelton SI, Ingbe C, et al: Treatment of acute otitis media in children: trimethoprim-sulfamethoxazole compared to ampicillin in a randomized trial. 15th Interscience Conference on Antimicrobial Agents and Chemotherapy, Washington, 1975. Abstract 34.
159. Cooper J, Inman JS, Dowson AF: A comparison between co-trimoxazole and amoxicillin in the treatment of acute otitis media in general practice. Practitioner 217:804–809, 1976.
160. Anon: Trimethoprim-sulfamethoxazole for otitis media. Med Lett Drugs Ther 20:59–60, 1978.
161. Brumfitt W, Pursell R: Double-blind trial to compare ampicillin, cephalexin, co-trimoxazole, and trimethoprim in treatment of urinary infection. Br Med J 2:673–676, 1972.
162. Brumfitt W, Franklin I, Hayek LJ, et al: A comparative study of urinary tract infection in domiciliary practice with ampicillin, cephalexin, co-trimoxazole and trimethoprim. In *Urinary Tract Infection.* Edited by W Brumfitt, W Asscher. New York, Oxford University Press, 1973, pp 229–239.
163. Gruneberg RN, Kolbe R: Trimethoprim in the treatment of urinary tract infections in hospital. Br Med J 1:545–547, 1969.
164. Williams JD, Brumfitt W, Condie AP, et al: The treatment of bacteriuria in pregnant women with sulphamethoxazole and trimethoprim. Postgrad Med J 45:71–76, 1969.
165. Ellerstein NS, Sullivan TD, Balrah T, et al: Trimethoprim/sulfamethoxazole and ampicillin in the treatment of acute urinary tract infections in children. Pediatrics 60:245–247, 1977.
166. Pines A, Greenfield JSB, Raafat H, et al: Preliminary experience with trimethoprim and sulphamethoxazole in the treatment of purulent chronic bronchitis. Postgrad Med J 45(Suppl):89–94, 1969.
167. Hughes DTD, Drew CDM, Johnsson TBW, et al: Trimethoprim-sulfamethoxazole in the treatment of chronic chest infections. Chemotherapy 14:151–157, 1969.
168. Kontoyannis PA, Papapoulo SE, Mortoglon AA: Co-trimoxazole in chronic brucellosis: a two year follow-up study. Br Med J 2:480–481, 1975.
169. Maderazo EG, Quintiliani R: Treatment of nocordial infection with trimethoprim and sulfamethoxazole. Am J Med 57:671–675, 1974.
170. Speller DC: Pseudomonas cepacia endocarditis treated with co-trimoxazole and kanamycin. Br Heart J 35:47–48, 1973.
171. Ramachandran S, Godfrey JJ, Lyonel NDW: A comparative trial of co-trimoxazole and chloramphenicol in typhoid and paratyphoid fevers. J Trop Med Hyg 81:36–39, 1978.
172. Iwarson S: Long-term co-trimoxazole treatment of chronic salmonella carriers. Scand J Infect Dis 9:297–299, 1977.
173. Dutta JK, Santhanam S, Misra BS, et al: Effect of trimethoprim-sulfamethoxazole on vibrio clearance in cholera (El Tor): a comparative study. Trans R Soc Trop Med Hyg 72:40–42, 1978.
174. Hatos G, Tuza ILC: Treatment of gonorrhea with trimethoprim-sulfamethoxazole and rifampin. Med J Aust 1:1197–1199, 1972.
175. Ulman S, Niordson AM, Zacharie H: Trimethoprim-sulphamethoxazole in gonorrhea. Acta Derm Venereol 51:394–396, 1971.
176. Craven JL, Pugsly DJ, Blowers R: Trimethoprim-sulfamethoxazole in acute osteomyelitis due to penicillin-resistant staphylococci in Uganda. Br Med J 3:201–203, 1970.
177. Sabel KG, Brandberg A: Treatment of meningitis and septicemia in infancy with a sulfamethoxazole/trimethoprim combination. Acta Pediatr Scand 64:25–32, 1975.

178. Chang MJ, Dunkle LM, Van Reken D, et al: Trimethoprim/sulfamethoxazole compared to ampicillin in the treatment of shigellosis. Pediatrics 59:726–729, 1977.
179. Norrby R, Eilard T, Svedhem A, et al: Treatment of toxoplasmosis with trimethoprim-sulfamethoxazole. Scand J Infect Dis 7:72–75, 1975.
180. Kincaid-Smith P, Kalowski S, Nanra RS: Co-trimoxazole in urinary tract infections. Med J Aust 1(Suppl):49–51, 1973.
181. Smellie JM, Grüneberg RN, Leaky A, et al: Long-term low-dose co-trimoxazole in prophylaxis of childhood urinary tract infection. Br Med J 2:203–206, 1976.
182. Lawson DH, Jick H: Adverse reactions to co-trimoxazole in hospitalized medical patients. Am J Med Sci 275:53–57, 1978.
183. Larson HE, Price AB: Pseudomembranous colitis: presence of clostridial toxin. Lancet 2:1312–1314, 1977.
184. Cameron A, Thomas M: Pseudomembranous colitis and co-trimoxazole (letter). Br Med J 1:1321, 1977.
185. Lawson DH, MacDonald S: Antibacterial therapy in general medical wards. Postgrad Med J 53:306–309, 1977.
186. Salter AJ: The toxicity profile of trimethoprim-sulfamethoxazole after four years of widespread use. Med J Aust 1(Suppl):70–74, 1973.
187. Havas L, Fernex M, Lenox-Smith I: The clinical efficacy and tolerance of co-trimoxazole (Bactrim, Septrim). Clin Trials J 10:81–86, 1973.
188. Csonka GW: Therapeutic trial of some genital infections with trimethoprim-sulphamethoxazole. Postgrad Med J 45(Suppl):77–80, 1969.
189. Halpern GM: Unusual reaction to trimethoprim in combined therapy (letter). Br Med J 1:691, 1972.
190. Wåhlin A, Rosman W: Skin manifestations with vasculitis due to co-trimoxazole (letter). Lancet 2:1415, 1978.
191. Tonder M, Nordoy A, Elgjo K: Sulfonamide-induced chronic liver disease. Scand J Gastroenterol 9:93–96, 1974.
192. Fries J, Sirganian R: Sulfonamide hepatitis. N Engl J Med 274:95–97, 1966.
193. Colucci CF, Cicero ML: Hepatic necrosis and trimethoprim-sulfamethoxazole. JAMA 233:952–953, 1975.
194. Kalowski S, Nanra RS, Mathew TH, et al: Deterioration in renal function in association with co-trimoxazole therapy. Lancet 1:394–397, 1973.
195. Shouval D, Ligumsky M, Ben-Ishay D: Effect of co-trimoxazole on normal creatinine clearance. Lancet 1:244–245, 1978.
196. Jewkes RF, Edwards MS, Grant BJB: Haematological changes in a patient on long-term treatment with a trimethoprim-sulphonamide combination. Postgrad Med J 46:723–726, 1970.
197. Paulley JW: Drug neutropenia (letter). Br Med J 2:364, 1970.
198. McCarthy OR: Neutropenia after trimethoprim-sulphamethoxazole for bronchitis. Br Med J 3:113–114, 1969.
199. Evans DIK, Tell R: Agranulocytosis after trimethoprim and sulphamethoxazole (letter). Br Med J 1:578, 1969.
200. Frish JM: Clinical experience with adverse reactions to trimethoprim-sulfamethoxazole. J Infect Dis 128(Suppl):S607–S611, 1973.
201. Editorial: Co-trimoxazole and blood. Lancet 2:950–951, 1973.
202. Meyer HA: Acute haemolysis associated with typhoid fever and G-6-P.D. deficiency. Lancet 1:729–730, 1973.
203. Grossman AB, Braimbridge MV, Russell RWR, et al: Acute polyneuropathy possibly associated with co-trimoxazole. Lancet 2:616–617, 1977.
204. Vincent FM: Acute polyneuropathy possibly associated with co-trimoxazole (letter). Lancet 2:980, 1977.
205. Brockner J, Boisen E: Fatal multisystem toxicity after co-trimoxazole (letter). Lancet 1:831, 1978.
206. Finlayson WB, Johnson G: Multisystem toxicity after co-trimoxazole. Lancet 2:682–683, 1978.
207. Murdia A, Mathur V, Kothari LK, et al: Sulpha-trimethoprim combinations and male fertility. Lancet 2:375–376, 1978.

208. Mihic M, Mautner LS, Feness JZ: Effect of trimethoprim-sulfamethoxazole on blood insulin and glucose concentrations of diabetics. Can Med Assoc J 112:805–825, 1975.
209. Siegel WH: Unusual complication of therapy with sulfamethoxazole-trimethoprim. J Urol 117:397, 1977.
210. Ochoa AG: Trimethoprim and sulfamethoxazole in pregnancy (letter). JAMA 217:1244, 1971.
211. Hassal C, Feetam CL, Leach RH, et al: Potentiation of warfarin by co-trimoxazole. Lancet 2:1155–1156, 1975.
212. Hansen JM, Siersbaek-Nielsen K, Skovsted L, et al: Potentiation of warfarin by co-trimoxazole (letter). Br Med J 2:684, 1975.
213. Tilstone WJ, Nimmo-Smith RH, Gray JMB, et al: Interaction between warfarin and sulfamethoxazole. Postgrad Med J 53:388–390, 1977.
214. Liegler DG, Henderson ES, Hahn MA, et al: The effect of organic acid on renal clearance of methotrexate in man. Clin Pharmacol Ther 10:849–857, 1969.
215. Tucker HSG, Hirsch JI: Sulfonamide-sulfonylurea interaction (letter). N Engl J Med 286:110, 1972.
216. Berglund F, Killander J, Pompeius R: Effect of trimethoprim-sulfamethoxazole on the renal excretion of creatinine in man. J Urol 114:802–808, 1975.
217. Constantino NV, Kabat HF: Drug induced modifications of laboratory test values. Am J Hosp Pharm 30:24–71, 1973.
218. Fujii R, Ohkoshi M, Takasu T, et al: Trimethoprim-sulfamethoxazole in the treatment of bacterial infections: report of clinical trials in Japan. J Infect Dis 128(Suppl):S629–S635, 1973.
219. Lau WK, Young LS: Trimethoprim-sulfamethoxazole treatment of pneumocystis carinii pneumonia in adults. N Engl J Med 295:716–718, 1976.
220. Hughes WT: Pneumocystic carinii pneumonia. N Engl J Med 297:1381–1385, 1977.
221. Perkins HR, Nieto M: The chemical basis for the action of the vancomycin group of antimicrobials. Ann NY Acad Sci 235:348–363, 1974.
222. Geraci JE: Vancomycin. Mayo Clin Proc 52:631–634, 1977.
223. Geraci JF, Nichols DR, Wellman WE: Vancomycin in serious staphylococcal infections. Arch Intern Med 109:507–515, 1962.
224. Watanakunakorn C, Black C: Synergism of vancomycin—gentamicin and vancomycin—streptomycin against enterococci. Antimicrob Agents Chemother 4:120–124, 1973.
225. Benner EJ, Morthland V: Methicillin-resistant staphylococcus aureus. Antimicrobial susceptibility. N Engl J Med 277:678–680, 1967.
226. Khan MY, Hall WH: Staphylococcal enterocolitis treatment with oral vancomycin. Ann Intern Med 65:1–7, 1966.
227. Bartlett JG, Onderdonk AB, Cisneros RL: Clindamycin-associated colitis in hamsters: protection with vancomycin. Gastroenterology 73:772–776, 1977.

PARASITICIDAL AGENTS

14. ANTIMALARIAL AGENTS

William Chin and G. Robert Coatney

Human malaria is caused by one of four *Plasmodium* species: *P. vivax*, *P. ovale*, *P. falciparum*, and *P. malariae*. An infection due to *P. falciparum* is the most serious, and is the only malarial infection associated with a high fatality rate in untreated or inadequately treated non-immune patients.

No single antimalarial agent has a sufficiently broad range of activity to affect every stage of the malaria parasite's life cycle. The cycle begins with an inoculation of sporozoites by the bite of an infected female anopheline mosquito. The circulatory system carries the sporozoites to the liver where they enter parenchymal cells and begin their development into primary tissue schizonts. The time required for these schizonts to mature ranges from one to four weeks, depending on the species involved. This portion of the life cycle is clinically inapparent.

When mature, the tissue schizonts rupture, liberating hundreds of merozoites that invade red blood cells and initiate the clinical attack. At some point following the onset of illness, which may range from three to ten days, some of the asexual forms differentiate into sexual forms, the gametocytes. The gametocytes are clinically unimportant; however, they serve as a source of infection to susceptible mosquitoes, thereby completing the plasmodium's life cycle.

Some of the sporozoites or intermediate forms of the relapsing malarias (*P. vivax* and *P. ovale*) apparently remain dormant in liver cells. At various time intervals, depending on their genetic makeup, some of these latent forms mature into schizonts, release their merozoites, and thereby initiate a true relapse.[1] *Plasmodium falciparum* and *P. malariae* lack dormant forms and therefore relapse potential.[2] The recurrence of patent parasitemia following inadequate blood schizontocidal therapy is termed a recrudescence and should be distinguished from a true relapse.

Depending on the stage of the parasite most affected, antimalarials may be classified as

1. *Blood schizontocides*—Drugs such as 4-aminoquinolines and quinine that act against the asexual stages in the blood and are used to obtain clinical cure of the disease.
2. *Tissue schizontocides*—Drugs such as primaquine that prevent the normal development of the tissue schizonts in the liver. This class of drug is also known as 'causal prophylactics'; they are used to prevent relapses.
3. *Gametocytocides*—Drugs such as primaquine that render the gametocytes non-infectious to mosquitoes or eliminate gametocytes from the peripheral circulation. This class of drug prevents transmission of malaria by mosquitoes.

Resistance to the 4-aminoquinolines (chloroquine and amodiaquin) is associated only with falciparum malaria; other malarias are fully susceptible to these drugs. Resistant strains of *P. falciparum* are presently found in South America with Panama as the northern limit, Southeast Asia with India as the western limit, and certain Western-Pacific countries, including parts of Indonesia and the Philippines.[3,4] To date the presence of such strains has not been confirmed in Africa, the Middle East, Central America, or Haiti.

ANTIMALARIAL THERAPY

Clinical Attack

Since the symptoms of clinical malaria are due to the reproductive activities of the asexual stages, the disease is treated by administering blood schizontocides. Chloroquine and amodiaquin are the current drugs of choice, except for the treatment of drug-resistant falciparum malaria, which is discussed below. In cases of severe manifestations of malaria (eg, coma and protracted nausea and vomiting), parenteral administration of chloroquine hydrochloride may be required. Administration of 4-aminoquinolines to children and infants should be adjusted according to body weight.

In the treatment of falciparum malaria, monitoring the response to treatment by examining blood smears, at least on a daily basis, is essential. Since falciparum malaria has an asexual cycle of 48 hours, the parasite density 48 hours after commencement of treatment compared to pre-treatment density is extremely useful. (Normal clearance time for any of the malarias is 48 to 72 hours.) In falciparum malaria, if the parasite density remains unchanged or is higher 48 hours later, the presence of a resistant strain should be suspected and, depending on the patient's condition, alternative treatment should be considered.

Drug-Resistant Falciparum Malaria

The World Health Organization[3] has listed 16 different regimens for drug-resistant falciparum malaria utilizing 12 drugs in various combinations for periods of one to 14 days. This reflects the imperfect nature of available drugs against such resistant strains. Most of the regimens combine quinine, pyrimethamine, sulfonamides,[5] or tetracycline.[6]

Rational treatment of patients with resistant infections requires an understanding of the following basic facts:

(1) Sulfonamides and pyrimethamine potentiate the action of each other.[5]

(2) The type of sulfonamide used is not critical, provided that a sufficient blood level is maintained for at least five days.

(3) While combinations of a sulfonamide, pyrimethamine, and a tetracycline are effective as blood schizontocides, their rate of action is slow. Thus, quinine is important because it can rapidly reduce the parasite density to safe levels.

(4) Most of the regimens give rise to cure rates of 90% and sometimes higher, but cure rates seldom reach 100%. Thus, the patient should be advised of the possible recrudescence of infection, usually within one to two months after therapy.

The following are recommended regimens for the treatment of resistant falciparum malaria.

(1) Quinine sulfate, 650 mg three times a day for three days; pyrimethamine, 50 mg daily for three days; sulfadiazine, 0.5 g four times a day for five days. All drugs are administered concurrently.

(2) Quinine sulfate, 650 mg three times a day for three days; tetracycline, 250 mg four times a day for seven to ten days. Both drugs are administered concurrently.

Relapse

In cases of vivax[7] or ovale[8] malaria where the potential for relapse clearly exists, the treatment of the clinical attack should be followed by a course of primaquine, a tissue schizontocide.

Chemoprophylaxis

Weekly administration of a 4-aminoquinoline beginning approximately two weeks prior to exposure and continuing for at least four weeks after exposure is currently recommended. In areas with drug-resistant falciparum malaria, the use of amodiaquin may be preferred since this drug is somewhat more effective against resistant strains than chloroquine.[9,10]

DRUG MONOGRAPHS

CHLOROQUINE HYDROCHLORIDE (Aralen Hydrochloride)
CHLOROQUINE PHOSPHATE (Aralen Phosphate)

Chloroquine is a synthetic 4-aminoquinoline and must be considered as the blood schizontocide of choice, except in cases of drug-resistant falciparum malarias. It inhibits nucleic acid synthesis in the parasite. Chloroquine has anti-inflammatory properties and, accordingly, is especially useful in falciparum malaria.

Adverse Reactions—The ingestion of approximately 1 g of chloroquine has caused death in children, with cardiac arrest occurring as early as 30 minutes after the onset of intoxication symptoms.[11] Ocular damage resulting from high dosage levels given as treatment for collagen diseases over long periods has been reported. This effect is not seen, however, when chloroquine is used as an antimalarial for treatment of acute attacks, or for chemoprophylaxis over extended periods.[12] The most commonly reported transient side effects include headache, pruritis, nausea, vomiting, and diarrhea. Blurred vision or difficulty in focusing are reversible. Psychotic episodes or convulsions have been reported, but only rarely.

Dosage—Treatment of clinical malaria (all doses are expressed in terms of the free base content), Oral: Adults, a total dosage of 1.5 g is given as follows: 600 mg immediately, followed by 300 mg at 6, 24, and 48 hours after the first dose.

Children are treated on the basis of body weight with a total dosage of 25 mg/kg as follows: 10 mg/kg immediately, followed by 5 mg/kg at 6, 24, and 48 hours after the first dose.

Intramuscular: Adults, 200 mg (5 ml) is injected intramuscularly. If necessary, this dose may be repeated in 6 hours. The total parenteral dosage in the first 24 hours should not exceed 800 mg. Oral treatment should be started as soon as possible and continued until the total course of 1.5 g is completed.

In *children and infants*, parenteral administration must be undertaken with great caution since they are extremely susceptible to overdosage. The recommended single dose is 5 mg/kg. This may be repeated in 6 hours; however, the total dosage in any 24 hour period should not exceed 10 mg/kg. As in adults, parenteral administration should be terminated and oral therapy instituted as soon as possible.

Chemoprophylaxis: Oral: Adults, 300 mg (two tablets) once weekly beginning two weeks before exposure and continuing for at least four weeks after exposure.

Children, 5 mg/kg once weekly.

TABLE 1 Preparations and Costs of Antimalarial Drugs

GENERIC NAME	TRADEMARK NAME(S)	PREPARATIONS AND 1978 COSTS
Chloroquine Hydrochloride	Aralen Hydrochloride	Injection (solution) 50 mg/ml (equivalent to 40 mg of base)—$1.17/5-ml ampul
Chloroquine Phosphate	Aralen Phosphate	Tablets 500 mg (equivalent to 300 mg of base)—$7.41/25
	generic	Tablets 250 mg (equivalent to 150 mg of base)—$2.70–$6.65/100
Amodiaquine Hydrochloride	Camoquin Hydrochloride	Tablets 200 mg (base)—$5.46/36
Quinine Sulfate	generic	Capsules 130 mg—$6.98/100; 200 mg—$5.95–$15.33/100; 325 mg—$8.27–$15.63/100 Tablets 325 mg—$12.79–$15.33/100
Quinine Dihydrochloride	generic	Injection (solution) 488 mg/2 ml—$3.11/12 ampuls[a]
Pyrimethamine	Daraprim	Tablets 25 mg—$1.45/100
Primaquine Phosphate	generic	Tablets 26.3 mg (equivalent to 15 mg of base)—$6.68/100

[a]If unavailable locally, quinine dihydrochloride may be requested from the Parasitic Disease Drug Service Center for Disease Control, Atlanta, Georgia 30333; telephone (404) 329-3670, after regular hours: (404) 329-3644.

AMODIAQUINE HYDROCHLORIDE (Camoquin Hydrochloride)

Amodiaquine, another 4-aminoquinoline, parallels chloroquine in mode of action and adverse reactions. The degree of resistance against amodiaquine is somewhat less than against chloroquine in drug-resistant strains of falciparum malaria,[9,10] but amodiaquine appears to have no advantage over chloroquine against all other types of malarias.

Dosage—Treatment of clinical malaria (all doses are expressed as base content), Oral: Adults, 600 mg immediately, followed by 400 mg at 24 and 48 hours.

Chemoprophylaxis: 400 mg once weekly, beginning two weeks before exposure and continuing for at least four weeks after.

QUININE SULFATE
QUININE DIHYDROCHLORIDE

Quinine is an alkaloid from the bark of the cinchona tree. Its use for the treatment of malaria was first recorded in 1630, and it remains a useful antimalarial agent. Quinine is characterized by its potent action as a blood schizontocide, its rapid elimination, and its well-known toxic side effects. Quinine's mode of action is believed to be the intercalation of the quinoline moiety of the compound into the DNA of the parasite, thereby reducing the effectiveness of the DNA to act as a template. With the emergence of drug-resistant falciparum malaria, first documented in 1961,[13] quinine has regained its important position as an antimalarial agent.

Adverse Reactions—Quinine and related alkaloids give rise to a significant group of side effects collectively termed 'cinchonism', consisting of tinnitus, blurred vision, dizziness, and headache. Abdominal distress and occasional cutaneous reactions have also been reported. Though manifestations of cinchonism are always bothersome to the patient, their severity seldom warrants discontinuation of therapy.

Dosage—Oral: Adults, quinine sulfate 650 mg is given three times daily for 7 to 14 days. Quinine is currently used primarily as part of a combination treatment of two to three days duration (see treatment of drug-resistant falciparum malaria).

Intravenous: Adults, quinine dihydrochloride is the salt used for parenteral administration. This form of treatment should be reserved for urgent situations, such as a falciparum infection in a comatose patient. It may be given as 650 mg of quinine dihydrochloride in 500 ml of sterile normal saline solution administered as a slow intravenous infusion. If required, this dose may be repeated every eight hours. Patients should be switched to oral medication as soon as possible.

PYRIMETHAMINE (Daraprim)

This drug belongs to a class of compounds which affect the malaria parasite by inhibiting the enzyme dihydrofolate dehydrogenase. Pyrimethamine is one of very few drugs having a broad range of activity that affects every stage (except the sporozoite) of the parasite's life cycle. Its major drawback, which severely limits its usefulness, is the ease with which all the malarias develop resistance to it. Because of this limitation, current use of pyrimethamine is confined almost exclusively to combination treatment against drug-resistant falciparum malaria.

Adverse Reactions—When used as an antimalarial agent, pyrimethamine has relatively low toxicity and is well tolerated. When given in high doses, as required in the treatment of toxoplasmosis, side effects such as anorexia, vomiting, depression of marrow function with megaloblastic anemia, leukopenia, and thrombocytopenia may occur.

Dosage—See section on drug-resistant falciparum malaria in introduction.

PRIMAQUINE PHOSPHATE

Primaquine is a synthetic 8-aminoquinoline showing little activity against asexual parasites but pronounced activity against fixed tissue forms and against gametocytes. For this reason its use is confined to the prevention of relapses and to rendering gametocytes non-infective to mosquitoes. Studies of *P. fallax*, a bird malaria, indicate that primaquine causes damage to the parasite's mitochondria which, secondarily, leads to inhibition of protein synthesis.

Adverse Reactions—Primaquine has a toxic potential in about 10% of blacks and in a smaller percentage of whites who have an inherent deficiency of glucose-6-phosphate dehydrogenase (G-6-PD) in their red cells.[14] The toxic effect is manifested by intravascular hemolysis, but the hemolysis induced by primaquine is self-limiting since mainly older red cells are affected. The 14-day primaquine treatment regimen is well tolerated even in G-6-PD deficient individuals. Other side effects include mild to moderate abdominal cramps and occasional epigastric distress.

Dosage—Anti-relapse treatment (all doses are expressed in terms of free base content) Oral: Adults, primaquine phosphate, 15 mg daily for 14 days. *Children*, the daily dose for 14 days is as follows: nine to fourteen years, 10 mg; four to eight years, 5 mg; one to three years, 2.5 mg.

REFERENCES

1. Coatney GR: Relapse in malaria—an enigma. J Parasitol 62:3–9, 1976.
2. Collins WE, Contacos PG, Chin W: Experimental infection in man with *Plasmodium malariae*. Am J Trop Med Hyg 22:682–692, 1973.
3. Report of a WHO scientific group: Chemotherapy of malaria and resistance to antimalarials. WHO Tech Rep Ser No 529:39–47, 1973.
4. Sehgal PN, Sharma MID, Sharma SL, et al: Resistance to chloroquine in falciparum malaria in Assam state, India. J Com Dis 5:175–180, 1973.
5. Chin W, Contacos PG, Coatney GR, et al: The evaluation of sulfonamides, alone or in combination with pyrimethamine, in the treatment of multi-resistant falciparum malaria. Am J Trop Med Hyg 15:823–829, 1966.
6. Colwell EJ, Hickman LH, Intraprasert R, et al: Minocycline and tetracycline treatment of acute falciparum malaria in Thailand. Am J Trop Med Hyg 21:144–148, 1972.
7. Contacos PG, Collins WE, Jeffery GM, et al: Studies on the characterization of *Plasmodium vivax* strains from Central America. Am J Trop Med Hyg 21:707–712, 1972.
8. Chin W, Coatney GR: Relapse activity in sporozoite-induced infections with a West African strain of *Plasmodium ovale*. Am J Trop Med Hyg 20:825–827, 1971.
9. Rieckmann KH: Determination of the drug sensitivity of *Plasmodium falciparum*. JAMA 217:573–578, 1971.
10. Hall AP, Segal HE, Pearlman EJ, et al: Amodiaquine resistant falciparum malaria in Thailand. Am J Trop Med Hyg 24:575–580, 1975.
11. Cann HM, Verhulst HL: Fatal acute chloroquine poisoning in children. Pediatrics 27:95–102, 1961.
12. Appleton B, Wolfe MS, Mishtowt GI: Chloroquine as a malarial suppressive: absence of visual effects. Milit Med 138:225–226, 1973.
13. Moore DV, Lanier JE: Observations on two *Plasmodium falciparum* infections with an abnormal response to chloroquine. Am J Trop Med Hyg 10:5–9, 1961.
14. Kellermeyer RW, Tarlov AR, Brewer GJ, et al: Hemolytic effect of therapeutic drugs. JAMA 180:388–394, 1962.

15. AMEBICIDES

Kerrison Juniper, Jr.

The treatment of *Entamoeba histolytica* infections, or amebiasis, has been a recurring dilemma over the past 25 years.[1] Some effective drugs that were used for many years were removed from the United States market (eg, glycobiarsol [Milibis], chiniofon, iodochlorhydroxyquin [Entero-Vioform]) or are now used infrequently (eg, carbarsone) because of occasional serious toxic effects. Metronidazole, a highly effective amebicide, has carcinogenic effects in animals and mutagenic effects in bacteria. Despite demonstrated efficacy, newer agents that are widely used abroad (eg, diloxanide furoate) are not generally available in the United States. Widespread misdiagnosis and prophylactic use of amebicides have also contributed to the recurring problems in the treatment of amebiasis.

PHARMACOLOGIC PROPERTIES

Amebiasis has been successfully treated with six chemical classes of drugs—alkaloids, halogenated quinolines, arsenicals, chloracetamides, broad-spectrum antibiotics and imidazoles. These drugs may also be classified as either 'luminal' or 'tissue' amebicides. Luminal amebicides are used to treat infections of the intestinal wall. These drugs are usually poorly absorbed and achieve high luminal concentrations. Tissue amebicides are used to treat infections of internal organs, especially the liver. These drugs are well absorbed and their concentration in the gut is generally inadequate to kill amebae. The imidazoles seem to be an exception to this classification since metronidazole is effective both for intestinal and extraintestinal infections, provided sufficient doses are used.

The alkaloid amebicides include emetine, dehydroemetine, and emetine bismuth iodide. Dehydroemetine, a derivative of emetine, has the same amebicidal properties as emetine, but it is less toxic.

Emetine and dehydroemetine are effective against trophozoites, the active form of *E. histolytica*, within all body tissues except the nervous system, but their concentration within the gut lumen is inadequate to eradicate intestinal infections. Emetine bismuth iodide given orally is only partly absorbed, and its concentration within the gut lumen is sufficient to eradicate intestinal infections. However, emetine bismuth iodide is not used in the United States because of its adverse effects. The alkaloids are potentially more toxic than most other amebicides and have largely been supplanted by metronidazole for the treatment of invasive amebiasis. However, they remain effective alternative agents for invasive disease.

The halogenated quinoline amebicides include two subtypes: the iodohydroxyquinolines and chloroquinolines. Iodohydroxyquinolines useful as amebicides are chiniofon (Yatren), iodochlorhydroxyquin (Entero-Vioform), and diiodohydroxyquin (Yodoxin, formerly marketed as Diodoquin). Chiniofon, the least effective of the three drugs, was marketed only briefly before it was withdrawn because of its ability to cause liver damage. Iodochlorhydroxyquin (clioquinol) [Entero-Vioform] was widely used, especially for traveler's diarrhea, but was eventually withdrawn from the American market because it can cause optic nerve damage. Diiodohydroxyquin, the most effective of the three drugs, has become less popular recently because of the potential for halogenated quinoline drugs to occasionally cause neuromyelopathy. However, diiodohydroxyquin is an effective luminal amebicide which is still available in the United States.

Only one chloroquinoline drug, chloroquine (Aralen), has proved useful as an amebicide. Originally developed during World War II for treatment of malaria, it is concentrated in the liver and effective for treatment of amebic liver abscess. Chloroquine is completely absorbed and ineffective against intestinal infection. Like other halogenated quinolines, chloroquine can induce neuromyopathy, especially during prolonged use.

The arsenical drugs carbarsone and glycobiarsol are effective against invasive intestinal disease, although they often fail to eradicate luminal organisms. Therefore, they were commonly followed by diiodohydroxyquin. Once widely used, these arsenical drugs had a very low incidence of toxic effects when used in recommended dosage. Nevertheless, they were eventually discarded in favor of newer drugs.

The chloracetamide drug diloxanide furoate (Entamide furoate) is a luminal amebicide primarily used to treat nondysenteric amebiasis.[2] It has long been a popular amebicide abroad but is available in the United States only through the Parasitic Disease Drug Service at the Center for Disease Control.[3] Diloxanide furoate may eventually supplant diiodohydroxyquin as a luminal amebicide.

The broad-spectrum antibiotics most often used as amebicides include the tetracyclines and paromomycin sulfate (Humatin). The tetracyclines probably modify the intestinal flora necessary for amebic viability, they may also affect enzyme systems in trophozoites. Oxytetracycline (Terramycin), tetracycline (Achromycin), and chlortetracycline (Aureomycin) all are effective in amebiasis, but oxytetracycline is perhaps the most effective. When used in low doses for short periods of time, the tetracyclines are more likely to suppress rather than eliminate amebic infection. Their greatest value is for adjunctive control of invasive intestinal disease by antibacterial effects.

Two imidazole compounds are useful amebicides—metronidazole (Flagyl) and tinidazole (Fasigyn). Metronidazole, although well absorbed, is effective for both invasive amebiasis and luminal infection. Larger doses and more prolonged treatment are needed for luminal infections. Tinidazole, a newer agent, also is useful for luminal and tissue infections.[4]

CHOICE OF AN AMEBICIDAL DRUG

Amebiasis is readily curable and usually responds promptly and nearly always completely with appropriate management. The most common cause of treatment failure is incorrect diagnosis. When symptoms do not respond to treatment with an appropriate amebicide the diagnosis should be questioned. However, an apparent response to an amebicide is not diagnostic of amebiasis.[5]

General Principles

In some areas of the world, such as Great Britain, indigenously acquired amebic infection is uncommon (about 1%) and symptomatic disease is quite rare.[6] In such areas treatment of asymptomatic amebiasis often is not undertaken because infected persons are thought to be at low risk for development of clinically important tissue invasion.[5] In the southern United States, however, a high percentage of indigenously-acquired infections are associated with invasive amebic disease.[7–9] Treatment of all asymptomatic amebic infections is recommended unless the risk of reinfection is high.

When cysts are being excreted in feces, trophozoites are always present in the colon, and they are responsible for maintaining the amebic infection. The cystic stage, once formed, is incapable of excysting within the colon. Thus, all therapy is directed toward killing trophozoites—not cysts.

Critically Ill Patients with Invasive Amebic Colitis

Debilitated and severely malnourished individuals, especially custodial patients in mental institutions, seem to have an unusually high mortality due to amebiasis. Death often occurs between the third and fifth day of treatment, despite an apparent satisfactory symptomatic response. These patients should be considered critically ill, and treatment should be initiated with half-doses of metronidazole and oxytetracycline daily for three to five days; after which standard doses are used. If parenteral medication is necessary, half-doses of emetine or dehydroemetine and oxytetracycline should be given for three to five days. Subsequently, standard doses should be given, and oral medication instituted as soon as possible.

Acutely Symptomatic Amebic Colitis (Dysentery)

Acutely symptomatic intestinal disease should be treated with metronidazole, the tissue amebicide of choice. Since metronidazole is not available for parenteral administration in the United States, emetine or dehydroemetine should be used if oral medication cannot be taken. In most patients symptomatic response can be expected with 48 to 72 hours after initiation of therapy with one of these drugs. Initial drug therapy should be followed by treatment with a luminal amebicide—diiodohydroxyquin, diloxanide furoate, or paromomycin. Sometimes oxytetracycline is used conjointly with the tissue amebicide, but this is not usually necessary for patients with acutely symptomatic amebic colitis.

Mildly Symptomatic Amebic Colitis

Mildly symptomatic intestinal disease should be treated with metronidazole or paromomycin, followed by diiodohydroxyquin or diloxanide furoate.

Asymptomatic Intestinal Amebiasis

Metronidazole, diiodohydroxyquin, or diloxanide furoate are used for symptomatic intestinal disease. After the initial course of treatment, a second course of treatment can be given with a different drug, or further treatment may await demonstration of continued infection (see the section on Criteria for Cure).

Ameboma

Suspected ameboma should be treated with metronidazole, emetine, or dehydroemetine. The lesion should resolve within one to two weeks. Failure to resolve suggests that the lesion is a carcinoma, and further diagnostic procedures are indicated.

Amebic Abscess of the Liver

Metronidazole, emetine, dehydroemetine, and chloroquine are all effective for amebic liver abscess. Because treatment failures do occur, combined drug therapy has been used in the past. However, the cure rate with metronidazole used alone is equal to that of combined therapy. An alternative treatment is a combination of emetine or dehydroemetine with chloroquine. Emetine is probably the best first drug, then followed by chloroquine. When parenteral therapy is necessary, emetine or dehydroemetine will have to be used first.

A suspected amebic liver abscess probably should be aspirated prior to amebicidal therapy to permit demonstration of trophozoites in abscess fluid (50% of cases) and bacterial cultures. Amebicides are then started immediately if a clinical diagnosis of amebic abscess is made. Amebicides should not be instilled directly into the abscess. Surgical drainage of an amebic abscess is unnecessary unless secondary bacterial infection is present, in which case drainage is essential.

Small amebic liver abscesses heal rapidly without therapeutic aspiration. However, inadequate drainage is the most common reason for treatment failure and relapse.[5] Indications for needle aspiration include persistent local tenderness, findings suggesting impending rupture, and failure of drug therapy.

The effectiveness of treatment of a liver abscess is monitored by clinical response. The liver defect seen by various scanning methods commonly persists for many months, and does not indicate failure. Patients with extraintestinal amebic disease should be treated with a luminal amebicide since they may still have intestinal infection.

Other Extraintestinal Amebic Disease

Amebic lesions of the skin, lung and most other tissues respond rapidly to treatment with metronidazole, emetine, or dehydroemetine. Metronidazole generally is the drug of choice. Secondary bacterial infection should be treated with appropriate antibiotics. Surgical incisions sometimes are necessary to facilitate drainage of subcutaneous pockets, but no attempt should be made to excise cutaneous lesions since resolution usually is quite dramatic.

Amebic abscess of the brain is almost always fatal. Surgical drainage is mandatory. Emetine and chloroquine are not effective, presumably because of inadequate concentration of drug in brain tissue. The effectiveness of metronidazole is unknown, but it should be tried.

CRITERIA FOR CURE

An effective luminal amebicide should cause amebae to disappear from the feces in 3 to 5 days after treatment is initiated, but this does not necessarily indicate eradication of the infection. Effectiveness of treatment is assessed by examining three fecal specimens, examined by both stained film and concentration methods, at intervals of 1, 2, and 3 months after treatment is terminated. Specimens should be collected for examination only after the patient has received no interfering substances for two weeks. Interfering substances include non-absorbed antacids, barium sulfate and other heavy metal compounds, antibiotics, sulfonamides, and antidiarrheal products containing alkaline earths or heavy metals. Diphenoxylate hydrochloride (Lomotil) can be used to control diarrhea without interference.

PROPHYLACTIC TREATMENT

Traveler's diarrhea generally is due to pathogenic coliform or viral enteritis, and rarely from amebiasis. Prophylactic use of amebicides during travel is not recommended. The only indication for prophylactic treatment is for persons exposed to contaminated water which has caused a sudden outbreak of invasive amebiasis.[5] Prophylaxis also might be justified in custodial institutions where infection rates often are high and serious disease may be present.

TREATMENT FAILURE

No amebicide is 100% effective, especially in the lumen of the gut. Therefore, treatment failures occur occasionally and should be looked for by reassessment at appropriate intervals. Continued infection should be treated with another course of therapy with the same or another drug. Continued symptoms without demonstrable amebae usually indicates incorrect diagnosis rather than continuing infection. However, diagnostic methodology must be correct.

CONCLUSIONS

Amebiasis can be expected to respond completely to proper therapy in the majority of cases, especially when diagnosis is prompt. Metronidazole is the current drug of choice for treatment of symptomatic intestinal infection, although it probably should be followed by a luminal amebicide such as diiodohydroxyquin, diloxanide furoate, or paromomycin. Asymptomatic intestinal infection can be treated with metronidazole or one of the above luminal amebicides. Extraintestinal amebiasis, with the exception of brain abscess, responds well to metronidazole, emetine, or dehydroemetine. Amebic abscess of the brain usually is fatal. Potential mutagenic and carcinogenic effects of metronidazole may place some limitations on its use in the future. Tinidazole currently appears to be a promising 'broad-spectrum' amebicide.

DRUG MONOGRAPHS

CHLOROQUINE HYDROCHLORIDE (Aralen Hydrochloride)
CHLOROQUINE PHOSPHATE (Aralen Phosphate)[10–12]

Chloroquine is a tissue amebicide effective primarily in the liver, where it is concentrated 200 to 700 times above the plasma level. It is used only for the treatment of amebic liver abscess. Chloroquine is largely degraded in the body and excreted in the urine. Excretion is slow, especially in alkaline urine but can be increased by acidification.

Therapy should be initiated with a loading dose to achieve adequate plasma levels.

Adverse Reactions—Toxic effects are rare, dose-related, and usually reversible. They include mild headache, vomiting, abdominal distress, diarrhea, pruritus, central nervous system stimulation, and abnormality of visual accommodation. Long-term use of the drug has resulted in skin eruptions, bleaching of the hair, partial alopecia, localized discoloration of the skin, blood dyscrasias, toxic psychosis, neuromyopathy, vertigo, tinnitus, nerve-conduction deafness, and permanent damage to the cornea or retina. Children are particularly prone to acute overdosage, which causes cardiovascular collapse, convulsions, cardiac and respiratory arrest, and death.

Precautions—Chloroquine is contraindicated in patients with psoriasis and porphyria and should be used with caution in the presence of severe liver disease or glucose-6-phosphate dehydrogenase deficiency. Its use should be avoided in pregnancy since recent studies suggest that the drug can cause congenital defects. The drug should be discontinued if the patient develops muscular weakness, visual symptoms, or abnormalities in visual acuity, visual fields or retinal examination. Retinal changes and visual disturbance can progress even after cessation of therapy.

Dosage—Oral: Adults, the chloroquine phosphate loading dose is 250 mg four times daily for two days; the maintenance dose is 250 mg twice daily for 15 to 30 days. *Children,* 15 mg/kg (maximum 1 g) for 14 to 21 days. *Intramuscular: Adults,* chloroquine hydrochloride, 200 to 250 mg daily for up to ten to twelve days until oral medication can be used.

DIIODOHYDROXYQUIN (Yodoxin)[10,12–14]

Diiodohydroxyquin is a luminal amebicide often used to treat asymptomatic intestinal amebiasis, or as the second drug in treatment of symptomatic intestinal infection.

Adverse Reactions—Toxic reactions are infrequent but include ptyalism, headache, rash, furunculosis, chills, fever, nausea, vomiting, abdominal distress, diarrhea, anal itching, and slight enlargement of the thyroid gland. The drug can cause spurious elevations of the protein-bound iodine level.

Precautions—The drug is contraindicated in intolerance to iodine and in severe liver disease.

TABLE 1 Preparations and Costs of Amebicides

Generic Name	Trademark Name(s)	Preparations and 1978 Costs
Chloroquine Hydrochloride	Aralen Hydrochloride	Injection (solution) 50 mg/ml—$5.85/5-ml vial
Chloroquine Phosphate	Aralen Phosphate	Tablets 500 mg—$7.41/25
Diiodohydroxyquin	generic Yodoxin	Tablets 650 mg—$42.00/1000 Tablets 210 mg—$5.50/100
Diloxanide Furoate	Furamide Furoate	Tablets 500 mg[a]
Emetine Hydrochloride	generic	Injection (solution) 65 mg/ml—$1.04/1-ml ampul
Dehydroemetine Dihydrochloride	generic	Injection[a]
Metronidazole	Flagyl	Tablets 250 mg—$27.38/100
Oxytetracycline Hydrochloride	Terramycin	Capsules 250 mg—$22.47/100 Injection (powder) 250 mg—$1.83/vial; 500 mg—$3.23/vial
Paromomycin Sulfate	Humatin	Capsules 250 mg—$8.80/16 Syrup 125 mg/5 ml—$3.92/60 ml

[a]Not marketed in the United States, but available from the Parasitic Disease Drug Service, Center for Disease Control, Atlanta, Georgia 30333, telephone: (404) 329-3670; after regular hours: (404) 329-3644.

Dosage—Oral: Adults, 650 mg three times daily with food for 21 days. *Children,* 40 mg/kg (maximum 2 g) in divided doses for 21 days.

DILOXANIDE FUROATE (Furamide furoate)[2,14]

Diloxanide is a luminal amebicide that is hydrolyzed and mostly absorbed from the gut and excreted in the urine. In the United States it is not an approved drug and is available only from the Parasitic Disease Drug Service, Center for Disease Control, Atlanta, Georgia 30333, telephone 404–633–3311.

Adverse Reactions—Flatulence is common and other mild gastrointestinal symptoms can occur.

Precautions—This drug is not recommended during pregnancy

since there is little information concerning a possible teratogenic effect.

Dosage—Oral: Adults, 0.5 g three times daily for ten days. *Children,* 25 mg/kg daily in divided doses for ten days. A second course can be repeated immediately. It is not recommended for children under 2 years of age.

EMETINE HYDROCHLORIDE
DEHYDROEMETINE DIHYDROCHLORIDE[10,12–14]

Emetine is stored in most body tissues, especially the liver and lung, and excreted slowly by the kidney. It persists in some organs for several months. Emetine is a tissue amebicide which acts very rapidly. Dehydroemetine has a shorter biological half-life and appears to be less toxic; it is not approved for use in the United States but can be obtained from the Parasitic Disease Drug Service, Center for Disease Control, Atlanta, Georgia 30333, telephone 404–633–3311.

Adverse Reactions—Emetine is a local irritant and commonly produces aching and tenderness in the injection site, which presumably stems from myositis. Other reactions include eczema, urticaria and purpura. Diarrhea frequently is either aggravated or induced, and abdominal cramping occurs. Nausea is frequent, but vomiting is less common. Occasionally there is dizziness, fainting, and headaches, and the feces may contain mucus and blood. Skeletal muscles may manifest weakness, aching, tenderness and stiffness, especially in neck and limbs; significant muscle weakness is rare and reversible. There may be mild sensory disturbances and tremors, but the usual signs of neuritis do not develop. Weakness and muscular pain generally precede more serious symptoms and can signal overdosage.

Cardiovascular effects include hypotension, precordial pain, tachycardia and dyspnea. Electrocardiographic abnormalities occur in 50% of patients, usually T-wave changes and prolongation of the QT and PR intervals. Changes in rhythm are unusual. These electrocardiographic effects can persist for several months but eventually disappear with no evidence of permanent damage. They do not necessarily indicate a need to stop therapy.

Precautions—Emetine can precipitate impending heart failure or arrhythmias and should not be used in patients with organic heart disease unless absolutely necessary. Emetine is excreted by the kidneys and should be used with great caution in patients with renal disease.

Patients should be hospitalized and kept in bed during treatment, with frequent monitoring of vital signs and of the electrocardiogram. Treatment should be discontinued if the resting heart rate exceeds 110/min, if hypotension develops, or if significant neuromuscular symptoms or diarrhea develop. Electrocardiographic changes can progress for several days after the drug is stopped. The patient should be cautioned to avoid strenuous activity for a month after treatment.

Dosage—Emetine, Intramuscular: Adults, 1 mg/kg (maximum 65 mg) daily in two divided doses for ten days for extraintestinal disease, or for three to five days for initial control of dysentery. *Children,* 0.5 mg/kg twice daily (maximum daily dose, 65 mg) for five days. *Dehydroemetine, intramuscular: Adults,* 1.5 mg/kg (maximum 90 mg) daily in divided doses as above. *Children,* 1.5 mg/kg (maximum 90 mg) daily in two divided doses for five days.

Elderly or debilitated patients probably should receive half doses initially for several days. The total dose of emetine during a course of treatment should not exceed 10 mg/kg, or a total dose of 650 mg for adults. At least two months should elapse between courses of treatment. The possibility of a toxic reaction increases with repeated courses, and serious toxic effects occur with total doses of about 25 mg/kg in most species of animals.

METRONIDAZOLE (Flagyl)[10,11,13]

Metronidazole is the drug of choice for treatment of extraintestinal and symptomatic intestinal amebiasis, and is an alternative drug for asymptomatic intestinal infection. Recent evidence of carcinogenesis in rodents and mutagenesis in bacteria suggests that these choices may change in the near future, so the drug should be used with some caution. Generally the drug is well absorbed after oral administration with peak serum levels in one hour. Unchanged drug and several metabolites are excreted in the urine, and low concentrations of drug appear in saliva and breast milk.

Adverse Reactions—Nausea, headache, anorexia, a sharp unpleasant metallic taste and dark urine are common. Abdominal pain, constipation, glossitis, stomatitis and an overgrowth of *Monilia* in mouth or vagina are less common. The drug has a disulfiram-like effect after ingestion of alcohol, and it can potentiate the anticoagulant effect of warfarin drugs.

Precautions—The leukocyte count should be followed during therapy. Alcoholic beverages should be avoided during treatment. Appearance of abnormal neurological findings is an indication to stop therapy. Known or unrecognized monilial infections may become worse during treatment.

Contraindications—The drug should not be used during pregnancy, especially the first trimester, unless the risk can be justified. The drug appears in maternal milk, and its effect on the newborn is unknown.

Dosage—Oral: Adults, 750 mg three times daily for 10 days. *Children,* 35 to 50 mg/kg daily in three divided doses for 5 to 10 days.

OXYTETRACYCLINE HYDROCHLORIDE (Terramycin)[10–12,14]

Oxytetracycline is one of the most effective of the broad-spectrum antibiotics for amebic infection. It is often used to treat acutely symptomatic intestinal infections, and is an alternative drug for mildly symptomatic or asymptomatic intestinal infection.

Adverse Reactions—Oxytetracycline frequently causes diarrhea, abdominal pain, nausea, pruritus ani, fever, gastroenteritis, overgrowth of *Candida* or *Staphylococcus*, and occasionally a pseudomembranous enterocolitis. Impaired renal function can reduce the excretion of tetracyclines and cause toxic effects. Intravenous adult doses exceeding 1 g daily can cause acute hepatic and renal damage.

Precautions—Tetracycline drugs can cause permanent discoloration of the teeth and possibly hypoplasia of the enamel during tooth development. They should not be used for amebiasis during pregnancy or in children under the age of 8 years.

Dosage—Oral: Adults, 2 g daily in divided doses for 10 days. *Children* (8 years old or more), 20 to 40 mg/kg daily in divided doses for 10 days. *Intramuscular: Adults,* 1 g daily in divided doses for 10 days. *Children,* 12 mg/kg daily in divided doses for 10 days. Change to oral administration as soon as possible.

PAROMOMYCIN SULFATE (Humatin)[11,14]

This drug is both amebicidal and antibacterial. It is effective against many enteric bacteria, particularly species of *Salmonella* and *Shigella*, and is an alternative drug for treatment of acutely or mildly symptomatic intestinal amebiasis. It is not absorbed appreciably from the gut.

Adverse Reactions—The drug may cause diarrhea, cramping abdominal pain, heartburn and pruritus ani. Overgrowth of *Candida* can occur. Ingestion of alcohol may cause abdominal pain during treatment.

Dosage—Oral: Adults, 1.5 to 2.0 g daily in divided doses at mealtime for five days. *Children,* 25 mg/kg in divided doses at mealtime for five days.

REFERENCES

1. Kean BH: The treatment of amebiasis. A recurrent agony. JAMA 235:501, 1976.
2. Wolfe MS: Nondysenteric intestinal amebiasis. Treatment with diloxanide furoate. JAMA 224:1601–1604, 1973.
3. Memorandum: 'Parasitic Disease Drug Service', from the Director, Center for Disease Control, Department of Health, Education and Welfare, Public Health Service, Atlanta, Georgia, April 28, 1977.
4. Abiose PA, Olupitan SB, Yousuf M: Tinidazole in the treatment of amoebic liver abscess. Curr Ther Res 20:32–35, 1976.
5. Powell SJ: Therapy of amebiasis. Bull NY Acad Med 47:469–477, 1971.
6. Seaton DR: Amoebicides. Practitioner 206:16–19, 1971.
7. Juniper K Jr: Amebiasis in the U.S.A. Bull NY Acad Med 47:448–461, 1971.
8. Barbour GL, Juniper K Jr: A clinical comparison of amebic and pyogenic abscess of the liver in 66 patients. Am J Med 53:323–334, 1972.
9. Juniper K Jr, Worrell CL, Minshew C, et al: Serological diagnosis of amebiasis. Am J Trop Med Hyg 21:157–168, 1972.
10. Anon: Drugs for parasitic infections. In *Handbook of Antimicrobial Therapy*. New Rochelle, New York, The Medical Letter on Drugs and Therapeutics, 1976, pp 52–64.
11. *Physician's Desk Reference,* 31st edition. Oradell, New Jersey, Medical Economics Co., 1977.
12. Most H: Treatment of common parasitic infections of man encountered in the United States. N Engl J Med 287:495–498, 698–702, 1972.
13. Jung RC: Treatment of intestinal parasitic disease. South Med J 69:799–804, 1976.
14. Juniper K Jr: Parasitic diseases of the intestinal tract. In *Gastrointestinal Medicine*. Edited by M Paulson. Philadelphia, Lea & Febiger, 1969, pp 487–497.

16. ANTITRICHOMONAL AGENTS

Philip D. Marsden

Trichomonads that live in the mouth and the large bowel of man are commensals and require no treatment. *Trichomonas vaginalis* is frequently nonpathogenic but is also a common cause of vaginitis. What determines this change to a pathogenic role is not clear. However, it is known that *T. vaginalis* cannot survive at the normal acidic vaginal pH of 3.8 to 4.4, which is maintained by the conversion of glycogen in the epithelium to lactic acid by the normal bacterial flora and by the activity of sex hormones. Moréra[1] found trichomonal vulvovaginitis in 6.5% of 485 prepubertal girls; the vaginal pH was frequently neutral in the affected girls.

Apart from mucosal inflammation, a frothy yellow-white irritative discharge occurs in trichomonal vaginitis. Trichomonads with their characteristic morphology and motility can be demonstrated in this discharge or in swabs from the vaginal or vulval mucosa. The urinary meatus is often invaded and trichomonads are frequently found in routine urine specimens. Absence on direct microscopy in a patient with a suggestive clinical picture usually indicates that a culture should be done. In a study of 500 women, Kean and Day[2] found that cultures detected all clinically symptomatic patients, whereas direct microscopy detected only 75% of cases. Media such as CLPM (cysteine-peptone-liver-maltose) of Kupferberg's[3] are used with aqueous methylene blue as indicator to adjust the pH to 5.8–6.0.

Since the trichomonal parasite invades the periurethral glands and ducts in both sexes, infections in males are common. Male infections are usually asymptomatic, but a urethritis or balanitis may occur. Untreated male infections lead to frequent reinfection of the female partner—so-called ping-pong vaginitis.

Metronidazole (Flagyl) has dramatically changed the management of trichomoniasis. Before its introduction, a variety of powders, vaginal tablets, and jellies were used locally; they contained arsenicals, sulfonamides, antibiotics, and oxyquinoline derivatives. Measures to maintain vaginal acidity were also employed. Males usually went untreated and failure rates were high. Further, such local measures failed to reach trichomonads ensconced in glands and ducts. Metronidazole, a systemically acting compound, proved to be an effective antitrichomonal agent and made treatment of the carrier male practical for the first time.

DRUG MONOGRAPHS

METRONIDAZOLE (Flagyl)

Following the demonstration of the trichomonicidal action of 2-nitroimidazoles in 1956 a number of other nitroimadazole compounds were synthesized and tested.[4] Among these, metronidazole was found to be very effective, and it was subsequently marketed under the name of Flagyl. Metronidazole was later found to be of value in the treatment of amebiasis, giardiasis, anaerobic bacterial infections, and acute ulcerative gingivitis due to Vincent's organisms.

All of these infections occur in environments of low oxygen tension. Metronidazole is selectively taken up by anaerobes, and it kills them selectively. A major step in drug uptake is the reduction of the nitro group by ferredoxin or flavodoxin, compounds characteristic of the metabolism of anaerobes. The reduction generates a gradient that permits the uptake of the drug. A hydroxylamine derivative formed by reduction is cytotoxic, inhibiting some essential, but as yet unidentified, cellular process. Aerobic conditions markedly suppress the uptake of metronidazole by trichomonads.[5–7]

Metronidazole is quickly absorbed after oral administration and achieves a maximum serum concentration in one to two hours. Only traces are present in serum after 24 hours. Metabolites are recycled in the bile, and 50% of the drug or its metabolites are excreted in the urine. The unchanged drug is actively secreted by the mucosa and concentrated in the vagina where it is metabolized by microorganisms.[8] Some patients note a reddish-brown color in the urine due to water-soluble pigments. Metronidazole tablets should be protected from light by storage in a dark bottle. Syrups can be made by a pharmacist for treating children. Vaginal tablets are marketed in some countries (not in the United States), and some physicians recommend the insertion of one of these tablets as high as possible in the vagina in conjunction with oral therapy in resistant cases. However, there is no good evidence that the cure rate is higher with such vaginal inserts. Oral therapy will cure the great majority of patients.[9] In one study, 400 mg twice a day for seven days cured over 95% of 488 patients,[10] and the majority of resistant cases were cured by a further course. Other reports show that a repeat course of metronidazole at twice the above dose is frequently curative in apparently resistant cases.

A single dose of 2 g of metronidazole is effective and is the recommended treatment.[11,12] Ensuring that all contacts are treated continues to be a difficult problem.[13]

The reasons for apparent therapeutic failure are:

(1) An infected sexual partner initiates a fresh infection. Regular sexual partners should be treated at the same time as the patient if *Trichomonas* is present; otherwise, the patient will apparently recover only to relapse on being reinfected at intercourse. Also, it is naive to think that the physician will be told the whole situation about sexual contacts in one brief interview with a promiscuous patient. In resistant cases the patient's confidence must be won by an in-depth interview.

(2) When *T. vaginalis* has invaded periurethral glands or a breach of the mucosa, such as a cervical erosion, treatment of the erosion may be necessary before cure can be achieved.

(3) The integrity of vaginal mucosa may influence the chance of cure. In postmenopausal women, estrogen therapy before specific treatment may achieve success.

(4) Some patients fail to absorb the drug. In one study, cures occurred only in patients with serum levels greater than 6.0 μg/ml.[4]

(5) Intravaginal bacterial flora may inactivate metronidazole. Nichol, et al[14] suggested an organism of the genus *Mimac* was responsible for treatment failure. McFadzean, et al[15] found unchanged sensitivity in 25 strains of *T. vaginalis* isolated from women who failed to respond to metronidazole; this finding also suggests that bacteria may be responsible.

(6) Various workers have induced *in vitro* resistance (up to 24 fold) of *T. vaginalis* to metronidazole. *In vivo* resistance in mice may not correlate with *in vitro* resistance.[16] It is important to confirm and extend these studies. The isolation of resistant strains from man has rarely been reported and is not generally accepted.

TABLE 1 Preparations and Costs of Antitrichomonal Agents

GENERIC NAME	TRADEMARK NAME(S)	PREPARATIONS AND 1978 COSTS
Metronidazole	Flagyl	Tablets 250 mg—$27.38/100
Tinidazole	Fasigyn	—[a]

[a]Not marketed in the United States.

Adverse Reactions—Common adverse reactions are as follows:

(1) Gastrointestinal effects-nausea, anorexia, and, more rarely, vomiting and diarrhea.

(2) A sharp metallic taste, sometimes associated with a sore, furry tongue. Tobacco may become unpleasant. Therapy can be associated with an overgrowth of *Monilia.*

(3) Mild neurological symptoms such as dizziness, vertigo, and paresthesia.

(4) Urticarial rashes, pruritus, and flushing.

(5) Urinary symptoms, such as dysuria and a sense of pelvic pressure. The urine may be dark with an odd smell.

(6) Flattening of the T-wave on the electrocardiogram.

Usually these side effects are not severe enough to stop treatment although exceptions have been noted, especially with longer courses.[17] Serious blood dyscrasias with metronidazole have not been reported, but neutropenia occurs often. A selective depression of the hyperfunctioning suprarenal cortex has been noted.[18]

Metronidazole has a disulfiram-like action and has been tried in the treatment of alcoholism without much success.[19] Acute confusional states have been reported in alcoholics taking disulfiram (Antabuse) in conjunction with metronidazole.[20] Although many patients tolerate alcohol well while taking metronidazole, it is best to advise abstinence while taking the drug. Metronidazole also potentiates the hypoprothrombinemic action of warfarin due to its disulfiram-like effect.[21]

The carcinogenic effect of metronidazole in laboratory animals has led to the recommendation that it be used only for *Trichomonas* infections that cannot be treated by other means.[22] Unfortunately, this is not easy. Before the advent of metronidazole women's lives were made miserable by douches, vaginal insertions, etc., often only to relapse on stopping treatment.[8] The *Medical Letter* recommends tub baths twice daily or biweekly douches with a solution of a tablespoonful of white vinegar in a quart of warm water plus the avoidance of tight underclothing such as panty hose. A controlled trial of this scheme of therapy with metronidazole would be difficult but desirable.

The first paper suggesting a carcinogenic effect of metronidazole reported an increased incidence of bronchial adenomas and malignant lymphomas in mice.[23] Four other mouse studies and two in rats have confirmed this, but two in hamsters have been negative.[24] These animals were given high oral doses for long periods. Metronidazole increases the mutation rate in bacteria.[22,25] Whether such evidence really implies a cancer risk in man is debatable. With the advent of single-dose treatment, metronidazole therapy can be recommended until further evidence is available.

Long-term, high-dose metronidazole therapy has been associated with peripheral neuropathy, and a case of incomplete recovery after two years has been reported.[26] Neuropathy is unlikely to occur with the doses used to treat trichomonal vaginitis.

Contraindications—

Metronidazole therapy should be avoided or instituted with caution under the following circumstances:

(1) Although no teratogenic effects have been reported in man, metronidazole probably should not be used during the first three months of pregnancy.

(2) Lactating mothers should avoid metronidazole since it passes into breast milk.

(3) Patients with blood dyscrasias should avoid the drug.

(4) Patients with active neurological disease should avoid the drug.

(5) Alcoholism is a relative contraindication.

TINIDAZOLE (Fasigyn)

Tinidazole is another imidazole derivative, similar to metronidazole. It has a similar spectrum of activity, and its advantages over metronidazole seem to be limited. Tinidazole has a longer elimination half-life (12.5 hours versus 7.3 hours for metronidazole), and 20% of the drug is bound to plasma proteins.[27] Initially an oral dose of 15 mg twice a day for seven days was used with good results. Recently many studies report cure rates of over 90% with a single oral dose of 2 g.[28,29]

Information on the carcinogenic activity of tinidazole is not yet available. Tinidazole may have fewer side effects than metronidazole, but few comparative trials are available. In rare cases of sensitivity to metronidazole, tinidazole could be considered although it is clinically similar; a small test dose should be given initially. Tinidazole is an investigational drug in the United States.

REFERENCES

1. Moréra AJ: Tricomoniase vulvo vaginal na infancia. Thesis, Rio de Janeiro. 230 pages. 1976.
2. Kean BH, Day E: Trichomonas vaginalis infection. An evaluation of three diagnostic techniques with data on incidence. Am J Obstet Gynecol 168:1510–1518, 1954.
3. Kupferberg AB: Trichomonas vaginalis. Nutritional requirements and diagnostic procedures. Int Rec Med Gen Pract Clin 168:709–717, 1955.
4. Michaels RM: Chemotherapy of trichomoniasis. In *Advances in Chemotherapy*. Edited by A Goldin, F Hawking, RJ Schnitzer. New York, Academic Press, 1968, volume 3, pp 39–108.
5. Müller N, Lindmark DG, McLaughlin J: Mode of action of nitroimidazoles on *Trichomonas*. In *Biochemistry of Parasites and Host Parasite Relationships*. Edited by H Van Den Bossche. Amsterdam, Elsevier, 1976, pp 537–544.
6. Müller N, Lindmark DG: Uptake of metronidazole and its effect on viability in trichomonads and *Entamoeba invadens* under anaerobic and aerobic conditions. Antimicrob Agents Chemother 9:696–700, 1976.
7. Coombs GH: Studies on the activity of metronidazole. In *Biochemistry of Parasites and Host Parasite Relationships*. Edited by H Van Den Bossche. Amsterdam, Elsevier, 1976, pp 545–552.
8. Ings RMJ, McFadzean JA, Omcrod WE: The fate of metronidazole and its implications in chemotherapy. Xenobiotica 5:223–235, 1975.
9. Catterall RD: Trichomonal infections of the genital tract. Med Clin North Am 56:1203–1209, 1972.
10. Keighley EE: Trichomoniasis in a closed community. Efficacy of metronidazole. Br Med J 1:207–209, 1971.
11. Dykers JR Jr: Single-dose metronidazole for trichomonal vaginitis. N Engl J Med 293:23–24, 1975.
12. Fleury FJ, Van Bergen WS, Prentice RL, et al: Single dose of two grams of metronidazole for *Trichomonas vaginalis* infection. Am J Obstet Gynecol 128:320–322, 1977.
13. Dykers JR Jr: Single-dose metronidazole for trichomonal vaginitis: A follow up (letter). N Engl J Med 295:395–396, 1976.
14. Nichol CS, Evans AJ, McFadzean JA, et al: Inactivation of metronidazole (letter). Lancet 2:441, 1966.
15. McFadzean JA, Pugh IM, Squires SL, et al: Further observations on strain sensitivity of *Trichomonas vaginalis* to metronidazole. Br J Vener Dis 45:161–162, 1969.
16. De Carneri I, Achilli G, Monti G, et al: Induction of *in vivo* resistance of *Trichomonas vaginalis* to metronidazole. Lancet 2:1308–1309, 1969.
17. Scarpello JHB: Metronidazole and anaerobic sepsis (letter). Br Med J 1:104, 1977.
18. Taylor JAT: Modification of adrenocortical hyperfunction by imidazole derivative. JAMA 181:776, 1962.
19. Gelder MG, Edwards G: Metronidazole in the treatment of alcohol addiction: A controlled trial. Br J Psychiatry 114:473–475, 1968.
20. Robstein E, Clancy DD: Toxicity of disulfiram combined with metronidazole. N Engl J Med 280:1006–1007, 1969.
21. Kazmier FJ: A significent interaction between metronidazole and warfarin. Mayo Clin Proc 51:782–784, 1976.
22. Anon: Is Flagyl dangerous? Med Lett Drugs Ther 17:53–54, 1975.

23. Rustia M, Shubik P: Induction of lung tumours and malignant lymphomas in mice by metronidazole. J Natl Cancer Inst 48:721–729, 1972.
24. *Physicians' Desk Reference*. Oradell, New Jersey, Medical Economics, 1977, pp 1447–1448.
25. Lindmark DG, Müller N: Antitrichomonal action, mutagenicity and reduction of metronidazole and other nitroimidazoles. Antimicrob Agents Chemother 10:476–482, 1976.
26. Karlsson IJ, Hamlyn AN: Metronidazole neuropathy (letter). Br Med J 2:832, 1977.
27. Sawyer PR, Brogden RN, Pinder RM, et al: Tinidazole, a review of its antiprotozoal activity and therapeutic efficacy. Drugs 11:423–440, 1976.
28. Mati JKG, Wallace RJ: The treatment of trichomonal vaginitis using a single dose of tinidazole by mouth. East Afr Med J 51:883–888, 1974.
29. Schellen AMCM: Experiences with tinidazole in a single two gram dose in the treatment of *Trichomonas vaginalis*. Acta Ther 2:163–167, 1976.

17. ANTHELMINTICS

Richard H. Meade, III

Anthelmintics are like no other group of drugs used to treat infections. The differences between them and antifungal, antibacterial, and antiviral agents are not only in chemical configuration and mechanisms of action but, more importantly, in usage. Nothing used in the treatment of human illness in the United States is so little understood as anthelmintics. One reason is that only in some cities along the eastern seaboard and in some southeastern states are helminthic infections common. Another is that the marketing of these drugs is so limited that many are unavailable in this country despite decades of use in other parts of the world. Unlike the vast promotional and educational efforts for antibiotics, little effort has been expended on anthelmintics.

Because helminths are greatly more advanced than other infective agents and are far larger, they can be attacked in ways not possible in dealing with viruses, bacteria, rickettsia, or fungi. Though no longer commonly used, the simplest method was to kill parasites by direct assault on their cell walls with such irritant chemicals as hexylresorcinol. More sophisticated methods of attack are used now. Some parasites are rendered susceptible to phagocytic attack by diethylcarbamazine. Some are paralyzed by piperazine and bephenium and shed without resistance from the gastrointestinal tract. Other anthelmintics act by interfering with metabolic function, as in preventing glucose absorption or preventing the production of eggs. While one-dose therapies have been available against single species, current anthelmintics have both single-dose effectiveness as well as a wide spectrum of activity, thereby enabling treatment of patients infected with three or more different parasites.

While a great deal has been accomplished in providing relatively nontoxic drugs to treat many helminthic infections a number of problems remain. The largest therapeutic problems limiting the

TABLE 1 Drugs for Nematode (Roundworm) Infections

Parasite	Drug of Choice	Dose	Alternative Drugs	Dose
Ascaris lumbricoides (roundworm)	Mebendazole	100 mg BID for 3 days	Pyrantel pamoate	11 mg/kg, 1 dose
Trichuris trichiura (whipworm)	Mebendazole	100 mg BID for 3 days	Thiabendazole	50 mg/kg daily in 2 doses for 2 days
Necator americanus (New World or American hookworm)	Mebendazole	100 mg BID for 2 days	Pyrantel pamoate	11 mg/kg daily for 3 days
Ancylostoma duodenale (Old World, European, or common hookworm)	Mebendazole	100 mg BID for 2 days	Pyrantel pamoate *or* Thiabendazole	11 mg/kg, 1 dose 50 mg/kg daily in 2 doses for 2 days
Enterobius (Oxyuris) vermicularis (pinworm)	Mebendazole	100 mg BID for 1 day	Pyrantel pamoate *or* Pyrvinium pamoate	11 mg/kg, 1 dose 5 mg/kg, 1 dose
Trichostrongylus species	Thiabendazole	25 mg/kg/day in 2 doses for 2 days	Pyrantel pamoate	11 mg/kg, 1 dose (maximum dose 1 gram)
Strongyloides stercoralis (threadworm)	Thiabendazole	25 mg/kg/day in 2 doses for 2 days	Pyrvinium pamoate	5 mg/kg for 5 to 7 days (maximum dose 250 mg)
Trichinella spiralis (trichinae pork roundworm)	Prednisone	20–40 mg daily for 5–7 days for severe disease. Taper dose after 5th-7th day	Thiabendazole	20 mg/kg daily in 2 doses until clinical improvement occurs

Ascaris braziliense (cutaneous larva migrans)	Thiabendazole	25 mg/kg/day in 2 doses for 2 days or apply in ointment	Ethyl chloride spray	
Toxocara species (visceral larva migrans)	Prednisone for severe symptoms		Thiabendazole *or* Diethylcarbamazine	50 mg/kg daily in 2 doses until symptoms subside 6 mg/kg daily in 3 doses for 30 days
Wuchereria bancrofti Wuchereria (or Brugia) malayi Loa loa	Diethylcarbamazine	50 mg on day 1 50 mg 3 times a day on day 2 100 mg 3 times a day on day 3 3 mg/kg 3 times a day on days 4 through 21 (doses given in terms of base)		
Tropical eosinophilia	Diethylcarbamazine	Treat for 14 days (see above)		
Acanthocheilonema perstans	Diethylcarbamazine	Treat for 14 days (see above)		
Onchocerca volvulus	Diethylcarbamazine	Treat for 21 days (see above) *and*		
	Suramin	100 mg test dose IV Followed by 1.0 g IV weekly for 5 weeks		

effectiveness of any anthelmintic are those of delay in getting patients treated and of preventing reinfection. Mastery of these problems is considerably more difficult than finding new drugs and represents the largest barrier to control of helminthic infections.

SELECTION OF ANTHELMINTIC

The anthelmintics of first and second choice for 27 parasitic infections are listed in Tables 1, 2, and 3. Fourteen drugs cover the entire range of infections, and nine of these are commercially available in the United States. The remaining five can be obtained from the Parasitic Disease Drug Service of the Center for Disease Control, Atlanta, Georgia 30333 (see Table 4).

Five of the drugs used to treat helminthic infections (prednisone, ethyl chloride, chloroquine, paromomycin, and suramin sodium) are not classified as anthelmintics and, accordingly, are not described in the following drug monographs. In addition, anthelmintics that are no longer first or second choice drugs are not discussed. Bephenium hydroxynaphthoate (Alcopara) is effective in *Ancylostoma duodenale* and *Ascaris lumbricoides* infections and should be used if the drugs of choice are ineffective, not tolerated, or unavailable. Dichlorophen (Anthiphen) is effective against the tapeworms *Taenia saginata, Taenia solium, Hymenolepsis nana,* and *Diphyllobothrium latum* and may be used if needed. Piperazine citrate (Antepar, Multifuge) was, until recently, the most commonly used anthelmintic in oxyuriasis (pinworm) and ascariasis (roundworm) infections. Since mebendazole and pyrantel pameate have a wider anthelmintic spectrum and are less toxic, piperazine now has few indications. Stibophen (Fuadin) and antimony potassium tartrate (tartar emetic) were used in *Schistosoma mansoni* and *japonicum* infections, but they have been replaced by stibocaptate.

Despite the availability of new, broader spectrum anthelmintics (eg, mebendazole), accurate diagnosis of the specific helminth remains important. An appropriate specimen should be submitted to a parasitology laboratory for analysis. A drug that is effective against one helminth may only irritate another and cause it to migrate from the intestines to body tissues where it may become a grave danger to the patient.

TABLE 2 Drugs for Trematode (Fluke) Infection

Parasite	Drug of Choice	Dose	Alternative Drugs	Dose
Schistosoma haematobium	Niridazole	25 mg/kg/day in 3 divided doses for 5–7 days (max. is 1.5 g daily)	Stibocaptate	*Adults:* 8 mg/kg 1M once or twice a week for a total of 5 doses *Children:* 10 mg/kg 1M once or twice a week for a total of 5 doses
Schistosoma mansoni	Stibocaptate	Dose described above	Niridazole	Dose described above
Schistosoma japonicum	Stibocaptate	Dose described above	Niridazole	Dose described above
Clonorchis sinensis	Chloroquine phosphate	250 mg TID for 6 weeks		
Paragonimus westermani	Bithionol	30–50 mg/kg/day in 2 doses every other day for 10–15 doses		

TABLE 3 Drugs for Cestode (Tapeworm) Infection

Parasite	Drug of Choice	Dose	Alternative Drugs	Dose
Taenis saginata (beef tapeworm) Taenia Solium (pork tapeworm) Hymenolepsis nana (dwarf tapeworm) Diphyllobothrium latum (fish tapeworm) Echinococcus granulosus	Niclosamide	*Adults:* 4 tablets (2 g) chewed thoroughly in single dose after light meal. *Children 34 kg or more:* 3 tablets (1.5 g). *Children 10 to 34 kg:* 2 tablets (1 g)	Paromomycin	1 g ever 4 hours in adults. In children under 2, the individual dose is 250 mg; under 14, 500 mg

TABLE 4 Preparations and Costs of Anthelmintics

Generic Name	Trademark Name(s)	Preparations and 1978 Costs
Bephenium Hydroxynapthoate	Alcopara	Granules—$1.80/5 g
Bithionol	generic	Tablets 200 mg[a]
Dichlorophen	Antiphen	Tablets 500 mg[a]
Diethylcarbamazine Citrate	Hetrazan	Tablets 50 mg—$4.16/100
Mebendazole	Vermox	Tablets (chewable) 100 mg—$11.52/12
Niclosamide	Yomesan	Tablets 500 mg[a]
Niridazole	Ambilhar	Tablets 500 mg[a]
Piperazine Citrate	Antepar (Multifuge)	Syrup 500 mg/5 ml—$3.60/pt Tablets 500 mg—$3.15/100
Pyrantel Pamoate	Antiminth	Suspension 250 mg/5 ml—$7.94/60 ml
Pyrvinium Pamoate	Povan	Suspension 50 mg/5 ml—$3.74/2 oz
Stibocaptate	Astiban	Injection (solution) 0.5 g[a]
Thiabendazole	Mintezol	Suspension 500 mg/5 ml—$4.07/120 ml Tablets (chewable) 500 mg—$7.02/36

[a]Not marketed in the United States, but available from the Parasitic Disease Drug Service, Center for Disease Control, Atlanta, Georgia 30333; telephone (404) 633-3311, after regular hours (404) 633-2176.

DRUG MONOGRAPHS

BITHIONOL

This drug has been of great value in treating infections caused by the lung fluke *Paragonimus westermani*. It is less effective in the treatment of the liver fluke *Fasciola hepatica* but is much more effective than chloroquine or emetine, which require prolonged periods of administration and still allow recurrence in up to 80% of patients.[1] A 15-day course has been effective in the treatment of 90% of patients with pulmonary infection. Cerebral infection occurs in 0.8% of patients with pulmonary infection. In a group of 24 patients with cerebral infections, bithionol was effective in all in eliminating ova from the sputum and in terminating the production of rusty sputum. However, in only 9 patients was it effective in control of cerebral symptoms, including loss of vision, frank meningitis, and one case of intradural abscess. The last responded both to the drug and to surgical drainage.[2]

Adverse Reactions—Up to 40% of patients experience abdominal cramps, diarrhea, nausea and vomiting. Approximately 16% have skin eruptions, including pruritic urticarial or papular rashes.[3]

Dosage—Oral: Adults and children, see Table 2. The drug is given twice daily with meals to reduce the incidence of intensity of gastrointestinal symptoms.

DIETHYLCARBAMAZINE CITRATE (Hetrazan)

This piperazine derivative, available since 1947, is used to treat infections due to *Wuchereria bancrofti* and *malayi, Onchocerca volvulus, Loa loa,* and tropical eosinophilia.[4] It is available as both the citrate salt and the base for oral use.[5] The need for long-term treatment or repeated use and uncomfortable side effects make treatment with diethylcarbamazine unpleasant and unpopular. For visitors to endemic areas who acquire infection that can be recognized early, treatment can be reasonably well tolerated. For those with advanced disease due to large numbers of filaria, treatment can be almost unbearable.

Adverse Reactions—The rapid death of filariae causes fever, tachycardia, headache, and intense pruritis (sometimes with swelling, edema, and enlargement of the inguinal lymph nodes), about 16 hours after initiation of therapy. Symptoms can last for 3 to 7 days. Weakness, joint pains, loss of appetite, and nausea and vomiting may also occur. Patients with *Loa loa* have developed nodular swelling along the course of lymph channels due to the presence of dead worms. Conjunctivitis also can occur and may require topical or systemic corticosteroids.

Dosage—Oral: Adults and children, see Table 1. Inadvertant overdosage is possible since both the base and citrate salt are available. The dose of diethylcarbamazine citrate is 4 to 6 mg/kg, whereas the dose of the base is 2 to 3 mg/kg.[6] The drug should be given on a full stomach in three doses daily for a period of two to three weeks.

MEBENDAZOLE (Vermox)

Mebendazole, an imidazole derivative, is poorly absorbed after oral administration, although 10% of a dose appears in the urine within 24 to 48 hours.[7] It is the recommended treatment for *Ascaris lumbricoides* (roundworm), *Enterobius vermicularis* (pinworm), *Trichuris trichiura* (whipworm), *Ancylostoma duodenale* (common hookworm), and *Necator americanus* (American hookworm), and is useful in the treatment of patients infected simultaneously with several parasites. Mebendazole has a wider spectrum than pyrantel, pyrvinium, piperazine or bephenium, each of which is effective against two or more of these parasites. Mebendazole is lethal to susceptible parasites, although the worm is not immobilized and shed for several days. Eggs of *Trichuris* and of *Necator* fail to mature into larvae.

Trichuris infection is symptomatic only if large numbers of parasites are present. Treatment is not considered necessary for asymptomatic people having only ova in normal stools. For those with diarrhea and such additional problems as rectal prolapse, therapy is important and can be accomplished with mebendazole; thiabendazole is ineffective.[8] In a study of children with *Trichuris* infection, mebendazole caused egg reduction of 98% with a cure rate of 68%.[9] A cure rate of 99% was achieved in the treatment of ascariasis.[7] *Enterobius vermicularis* infections were cured in 96% of 74 patients treated with a single 100 mg dose of mebendazole; this is as good as the results for 5 mg/kg of pyrvinium pamoate, which cured 90% of 18 patients.[10]

While used in both children and adults, mebendazole is not considered safe for pregnant women due to reports of teratogenic effects in animals.

Adverse Reactions—Side effects of mebendazole are limited to local gastrointestinal disturbances. Symptoms of abdominal discomfort, including cramps, diarrhea, nausea, vomiting, headache, and vertigo, have been reported in small numbers of recipients.[11]

Dosage—Oral: Adults and children over 2 years, 100 mg twice a day for 2 to 4 days (Table 1). Good results against *Trichuris* infection, for example, have been obtained with 100 mg twice a day for three days.[11]

NICLOSAMIDE (Yomesan)

Niclosamide is the best available drug for the treatment of cestode (tapeworm) infections (Table 3). It has been in use for more than a decade in parts of the world where *Taenia saginata* and *Taenia solium* infections are common. The drug is also effective in infections with *Hymenolepsis nana* and *Diphyllobothrium latum*.[12–14] Since the parasite is not expelled, the effect of niclosamide treatment can be judged only by the disappearance of proglottid segments from the stool. Ova are not affected by the drug.

Adverse Reactions—Niclosamide is not absorbed and the dose used is small. It causes little or no abdominal discomfort. Hypersensitivity reactions in the form of a rash have been reported. It can be safely used in pregnant women.

Dosage—Oral: Adults, see Table 3. The patient should fast overnight before taking the drug. For the treatment of *Taenia saginata,* no further treatment is required. For *Taenia solium* infections in which ova released and not killed could produce cystocercosis, post-treatment purgation has been recommended. The results of therapy have been excellent. Only rarely has retreatment been required.

NIRIDAZOLE (Ambilhar)

Niridazole has been available for a number of years in Africa, South America, and Asia for treatment of schistosomal infections. It is at least partially effective against infections due to all three strains but of greatest value in the treatment of *S. haematobium* infection.[15] It has also been used for strongyloidiasis[16] and dracontiasis.[17]

Rapid binding of niridazole to albumin occurs in the liver. Its anthelmintic effects are not confined to inhabitants of the portal vein since the drug is widely distributed in body tissues and is effective in cases of dracontiasis. The parent compound as well as metabolic products appear to have pharmacologic activity.[18]

Niridazole is the best drug available for *S. haematobium* infection, but is less effective against *S. mansoni* or *japonicum*. It is effective against dracontiasis but less so than other drugs. Certain schistosomal infections, such as polyposis of the colon, have responded temporarily, but recurrence within 2 to 3 years has been observed.[19] Niridazole is more useful in treating patients who are not subject to reinfection than those in endemic areas.

Adverse Reactions—Minor side effects, in order of frequency, are diffuse abdominal pain, nausea and vomiting, diarrhea, and headache. In patients with severe liver disease due to schistosomiasis other side effects can preclude use of the drug. These include visual and auditory hallucinations, delirium, mental confusion, and local and generalized seizure activity.[20] Transient electroencephalographic abnormalities have been observed in these patients. In others, electrocardiographic changes, consisting of flattening or inversion of T-waves, have been seen. These changes are transient, lasting no more than 1 to 2 weeks after treatment has been concluded, and are associated with no clinical signs. Hemolysis has occurred in patients with G-6-PD deficiency.[21]

Dosage—Oral: Adults and children, see Tables 1 and 2.

PYRANTEL PAMOATE (Antiminth)

Pyrantel pamoate is used in the treatment of oxyuriasis (*Enterobius vermicularis*), as well as *Ascaris lumbricoides* (roundworm), *Necator americanus* (hookworm), and *Giardia lamblia* infections.[10] Though almost completely insoluble, the pamoate salt is absorbed slightly; 1% of the unchanged and 3% of the metabolized drug appear in the urine.[10] In a comparison of pyrantel, tetrachlorethylene, and bephenium hydroxynaphthoate, patients with *Necator americanus* infections in Ceylon were treated with varying dosage schedules of each. Pyrantel, 10 mg/kg/day for three days, was as effective as tetrachlorethylene in a single 5 ml dose. Because pyrantel was more expensive, the investigators preferred tetrachlorethylene. They also preferred to give tetrachlorethylene and piperazine together if there was coexistent ascaris infection.[22] Since pyrantel is active against both and is less toxic, it is the preferred drug.

The effect of pyrantel is prolonged and diminishes slowly, whereas acetylcholine effect is rapidly reversible. The effects of pyrantel are blocked by previous exposure of *Ascaris* muscle to piperazine.

Adverse Reactions—No serious toxic effects have occurred, but a number of minor symptoms have been observed. In one study, 65 of 1500 recipients had diarrhea, 53 had nausea, and 25 vomited. Abdominal cramps and headache also occurred in small numbers.[22] Pyrantel does not cause staining of the stool.

Dosage—Oral: Adults and children, see Table 1.

PYRVINIUM PAMOATE (Povan)

Pyrvinium pamoate is a deep red crystalline solid, insoluble in water, that has been used for the treatment of oxyuriasis (pinworm). Pyrvinium was once the drug of choice since single-dose therapy was possible and the drug had few adverse effects. Comparison of pyrvinium with pyrantel against *Enterobius* infection shows pyrantel to be more effective.[23]

Adverse Reactions—A single oral dose deposits enough of the drug in the bowel to result in bright red staining of the stool. The stain can get onto clothing and is difficult to remove. If there is vomiting this too can be vivid red, looking much like blood. Occasional gastrointestinal symptoms occur which consist of nausea, vomiting, abdominal cramps and diarrhea. Allergic reactions, consisting of fever, periorbital edema and an intensely pruritic rash have been described.[24]

Dosage—Oral: Adults and children, see Table 1. It is occasionally necessary to treat more than once.

STIBOCAPTATE (Astiban)

Although treatment with niridazole is effective against infection caused by *Schistosoma haematobium,* it is less effective against *S. mansoni* and *japonicum.* For these infections, two highly toxic antimony compounds, stibophen (Fuadin) and antimony potassium tartrate (tartar emetic), were formerly used. They have fallen into disfavor because of reports of fatal arrhythmias.[25] Stibocaptate (sodium antimony dimercaptosuccinate) is now considered the drug of choice in the treatment of *Schistosoma japonicum* and *Schistosoma mansoni* infections. It can be used as an alternative to niridazole for *Schistosoma haematobium* infection, but it is not as effective.

Stibocaptate is a trivalent compound that structurally resembles dimercaprol (BAL), which presumably restricts dissociation of the antimony ion. Treatment with stibocaptate is safer and easier for both physician and patient than with either stibophen or tartar emetic. Stibocaptate does, however, have a high frequency of adverse effects.

Stibocaptate was widely used in Africa, Egypt, Iraq, Brazil, and Israel in the 1960's and cure rates of 25 to 95% were reported.[26] Since then other schistosomicidal drugs, notably hycanthone, have been used. Hycanthone is highly effective and requires only one intramuscular injection or several oral doses.[27] Because of reports of sudden death following its administration, it has not been approved for use in the United States. A new preparation, oxamniquine, is undergoing trial and has proved effective after a single oral dose or intramuscular injection. It has a number of adverse effects, including pain at the injection site, but it may prove to be a useful drug.

Stibocaptate is contraindicated in patients with respiratory infections, untreated tuberculosis, acute febrile disorders, cardiac arrhythmias, coronary heart disease, renal insufficiency, compromised liver function, and anemia.[28] It also should not be given to pregnant women and children under the age of 6 years.

Adverse Reactions—Nausea, vomiting, and abdominal pain occur in 70 to 80% of recipients, while somewhat fewer have other symptoms such as a metallic taste and diarrhea. Smaller numbers exhibit cardiovascular, hepatic, dermatologic, and neurologic symptoms. Bradycardia resulting in Stokes-Adams attacks was reported in 2 of over 500 patients, while electrocardiographic abnormalities such as T-wave flattening were more common.[29] Other adverse effects include rare examples of hepatomegaly, transient eosinophilia, weakness, lassitude, and headache. Up to 63% of recipients have itching skin eruptions.

Dosage—See Table 2.

THIABENDAZOLE (Mintezol)

Thiabendazole is rapidly absorbed when taken by mouth and metabolized to the 5-hydroxy derivative. Both glucuronide and sulfate salts are excreted in the urine; 90% of the oral dose appears in the urine within 24 hours. Thiabendazole has a broad spectrum of activity against a number of nematodes (roundworms) and fungi[30] but is ineffective against trematodes (flukes) including the schistosomes, cestodes or protozoa such as *Giardia*. Thiabendazole is the drug of choice for *Strongyloides stercoralis, Trichostrongylus* species, cutaneous larva migrans and for *Dracunculus medinensis*.[31,32] It is ovicidal and larvicidal.

The effectiveness of thiabendazole in the treatment of trichinosis is debatable. Recent papers state that the drug has no effect on larvae that have reached muscles or other tissues,[33] although an early case report suggested that the drug might be effective against infection.[34]

Adverse Reactions—The most common problems are minor. Up to 13% of patients have nausea, loss of appetite, vomiting, and dizziness.

Urine may have an odor like that of asparagus. More serious but less common are reports of paresthesias, syncope, tinnitus, xanthopsia and enuresis. A case of transient, self-limited hematuria following a single oral dose of 1.5 g given to treat larvae cutaneous migrans has been reported.[35] Intrahepatic cholestasis was observed in one patient.[36] Angioneurotic edema, pruritis, urticaria, and fever are rare adverse effects.

Dosage—Oral: Adults and children, see Table 1. Doses should be taken after meals. A total of 3.0 grams can be given over a period of 3 days.[37]

REFERENCES

1. Yokogawa M, Iwasaki M, Shigeyasu M, et al: Chemotherapy of paragonimiasis with bithionol. V. Studies on the minimum effective doses and changes in abnormal x-ray shadows in the chest after treatment. Am J Trop Med Hyg 12:859–869, 1963.
2. Oh SJ: Bithionol treatment in cerebral paragonimiasis. Am J Trop Med Hyg 16:585–590, 1967.
3. Kim JS: Treatment of *Paragonimus westermani* infections with bithionol. Am J Trop Med Hyg 19:940–942, 1970.
4. Grone DI, Warren KS, Mahmoud AAF: Algorithms in the diagnosis and management of exotic diseases. VI. The filariases. J Infect Dis 132:340–352, 1975.
5. Brown HW: Anthelmintics, new and old. Clin Pharmacol Ther 10:5–21, 1969.
6. Del Castillo J: Pharmacology of nematoda in chemical zoology. *Volume III Echinodermata, Nematoda, and Acanthocephala.* Edited by M Florkin, BT Scheer. New York, Academic Press, 1969, pp. 521–552.
7. Vakil BJ, Dalal NJ, Enjetti E: Clinical trials with mebendazole, a new broad spectrum anthelmintic. J Trop Med Hyg 78:154–158, 1975.
8. Kotcher E, Chararria AP, Gamboa JA, et al: Community control of intestinal nematodes by thiabendazole treatment. Tex Rep Biol Med 27(Suppl 2):629–643, 1969.
9. Magbool S, Lawrence D, Katz M: Treatment of trichuriasis with a new drug, mebendazole. J Pediatr 86:463–465, 1975.
10. Pitts NE, Miglierdi JR: Antiminth, pyrantel pamoate. Clin Pediatr 13:87–94, 1974.
11. Chavarria AP, Swartzwelder JC, Villarejos VM, et al: Mebendazole, an effective broad spectrum anthelmintic. Am J Trop Med Hyg 22:592–595, 1973.
12. Nagaty HF, Rifant NA, Salem S: A trial of yomesan in Hymenolepsis nana infection. J Trop Med Hyg 65:128–129, 1962.
13. Kahra A, Veharanta T: Expulsion of tapeworms with yomesan. Suomen Laa Karilehti 18:325–327, 1963.
14. Keeling JED: The chemotherapy of cestode infections. Adv Chemother 3:110–152, 1968.
15. Clarke V deV, Blair DM: Dosage schemes and dosage responses of niridazole in schistosomiasis. Ann NY Acad Sci 160:645–649, 1969.
16. Raffier G: Activity of niridazole in strongyloidiasis. Ann NY Acad Sci 160:716–719, 1969.
17. Raffier G: Activity of niridazole in dracontiasis. Ann NY Acad Sci 160:720–728, 1969.
18. Bueding E, Fisher J: Biochemical effects of niridazole on *Schistosoma mansoni.* Mol Pharmacol 6:532–539, 1970.
19. Farid Z, El Masry NA, Young SW, et al: Treatment of schistosomal polyposis of the colon with niridazole (Ambilhar). J Trop Med Hyg 77:65–67, 1974.
20. Prata A: Clinical evaluation of niridazole in Schistosoma mansoni infections. Ann NY Acad Sci 160:660–669, 1969.
21. Sonnet J, Doyen A: Effects of niridazole on erythropoeisis of Congolese treated for schistosomiasis and amoebiasis. Ann NY Acad Sci 160:786–798, 1969.
22. Senewiratne B, Hettiarachchi K, Senewiratne K: A comparative study of the relative efficiency of pyrantel pamoate, bephenium hydroxynaphthoate and tetrachlorethylene in

the treatment of *Necator americanus* infection in Ceylon. Ann Trop Med Parasitol 69:233–239, 1975.

23. Nassif S, Bell WJ, Presscott JEG: Comparison of pyrantel pamoate syrup and pyrvinium pamoate syrup in the treatment of enterobiasis in Egypt. J Trop Med Hyg 77:270–271, 1974.
24. Desser KB, Baden M: Allergic reactions to pyrvinium pamoate. Am J Dis Child 117:589, 1969.
25. Shick RR, Ritterband AB, Lieberman AH: Fuadin therapy of schistosomiasis associated with ventricular tachycardia and death: A case report. Ann Intern Med 46:392–403, 1937.
26. Prata AR: TWSb in the treatment of schistosoma mansoni; observations of 42 cases. Hospital Rio 50:259–266, 1959.
27. Katz N: Chemotherapy of schistosomiasis mansoni. Adv Pharmacol Chemother 14:2–70, 1977.
28. Informational Material for Physicians: Sodium Antimony Dimercaptosuccinate (Astiban). Atlanta, Center for Disease Control, 1968.
29. Hsu J, Wu Y, Lu C, et al: Sodium antimony dimercaptosuccinate Sb58 in treatment of schistosomiosis japonicum. Chin Med J 80:530–537, 1960.
30. Robinson HJ, Silber RH, Graessle OE: Thiabendazole: toxicological, pharmacological and antifungal properties. Tex Rep Biol Med 27(Suppl 2):537–560, 1969.
31. Hennekeuser HH, Pabst K, Poeplau W, et al: Thiabendazole for the treatment of trichinosis in humans. Tex Rep Biol Med 27(Suppl 2):581–596, 1969.
32. Battistini F: Treatment of creeping eruption with topical thiabendazole. Tex Rep Biol Med 27(Suppl 2):645–658, 1969.
33. Katz M: Anthelmintics. Drugs 13:124–136, 1977.
34. Wilson R: Bearmeat trichinosis. Profound serum protein alterations, minor eosinophilia, and response to thiabendazole. Ann Intern Med 66:965–971, 1967.
35. Golden TA, McElveen FJ, Jupia JE: Hematuria following thiabendazole. Arch Dermatol 110:295, 1974.
36. Jalota R, Freston J: Severe intrahepatic cholestasis due to thiabendazole. Am J Trop Med Hyg 23:676–678, 1974.
37. Campbell WC, Cuckler AC: Thiabendazole in the treatment and control of parasitic infections in man. Tex Rep Biol Med 27(Suppl 2):665–692, 1969.

18. PEDICULICIDES AND SCABICIDES

Dennis D. Juranek

Louse infestations (pediculosis) and itch mite infestations (scabies) were rarely seen by physicians in the United States after World War II. However, in recent years these parasitic afflictions have become increasingly prevalent in the American population. Past epidemics of these diseases were attributed to poverty, poor sanitation, and crowding due to war and economic crises. But the recent wave of infestation in the United States has evolved in the absence of major social disturbance and has affected persons from all socioeconomic levels without regard for age, sex, or standards of personal hygiene. Fortunately, treatment of patients with these ectoparasites is not complicated. Successful therapy requires that a physician select an appropriate pediculicide or scabicide, ensure that the patient understands the method and frequency of application of the drug, and inform the patient about those measures necessary to prevent reinfestation.

Three types of lice infest man—head lice (*Pediculus humanus capitis*), body lice (*Pediculus humanus humanus*), and pubic or crab lice (*Phthirus pubis*).[1] Because treatment and preventive measures vary according to the type of louse involved, it is important to identify the infesting agent accurately. For practical purposes, head lice and body lice are morphologically identical. However, pubic lice have distinctly different morphologic characteristics (Figure 1). One commonly used method of identifying lice is through a knowledge of their preferred habitat on the human host. Head lice are adapted to life on the scalp and hair; they do not occur on eyebrows or eyelashes. Pubic lice most frequently infest pubic hair. However, they may also be found on coarse hair in other locations such as the axilla, eyelashes, eyebrows, mustache, or beard. In infants and young children, pubic lice are confined to the eyelashes and, occasionally, head hair. Body lice spend most of their time on clothing. They move to the skin to feed

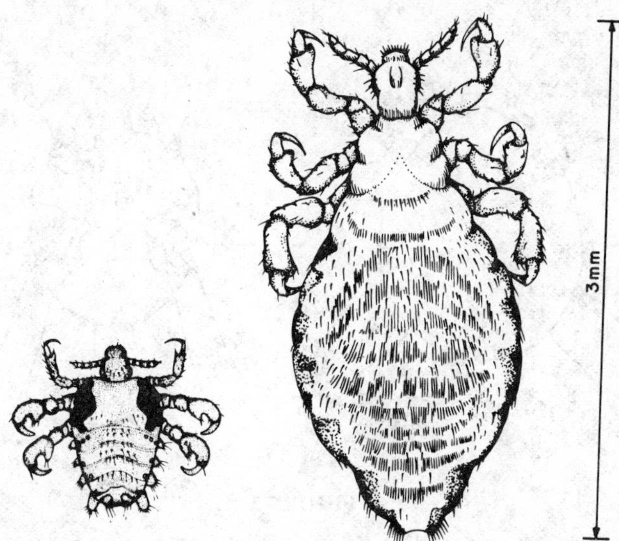

FIGURE 1.

and are more numerous where clothing is in continuous contact with the body, such as at the armpits and belt line.

Louse eggs (nits) are observed more often than nymphal or adult lice. The site of egg deposition is also a useful guide to the louse's identity. Head lice and pubic lice attach their eggs to hair in their respective habitats, whereas body lice attach their eggs to clothing fibers, principally in the seams of garments.

The etiologic agent of scabies is *Sarcoptes scabiei* var. *hominis* (Figure 2). This is the only species of mite transmissible from human to human. Other varieties of *S. scabiei* that infest animals are occasionally transmitted to humans, but these infestations are self-limited because the mites are unable to reproduce on the human host. Infestation with the human variety of *S. scabiei* is characterized by an intensely pruritic, follicular, papular rash. Pruritus is especially severe at night. Lesions predominantly occur around the finger webs, anterior surfaces of the wrists and elbows, anterior axillary fold, belt line, thighs, and external genitalia in men; nipples, abdomen, and lower portion of buttocks in women. Rash and itching are thought to be hypersensitivity reactions to the mites and may occur at sites quite

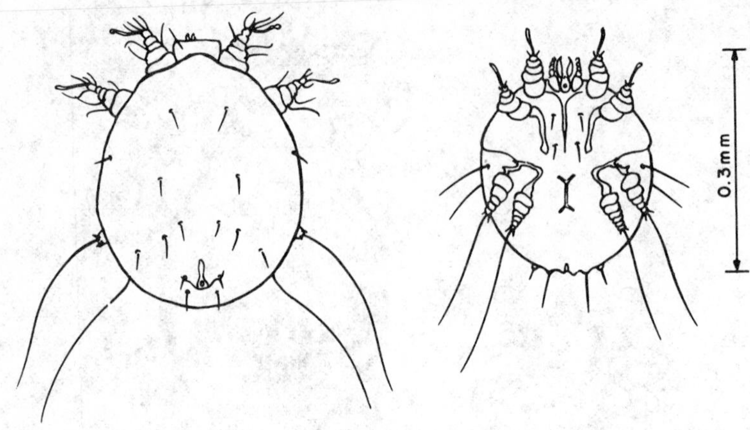

FIGURE 2.

distant from mite burrows. If scabies is suspected, skin scrapings or a cutaneous biopsy should be employed to confirm the diagnosis.

Additional biologic data of clinical importance for lice and mite infestations are summarized in Table 1. Therapeutic regimens and guidelines for preventing reinfestation are derived from these data.

MANAGEMENT OF PEDICULOSIS AND SCABIES

Body louse infestations need not be treated with pediculicides. Adults, nymphs, and eggs of this species can be eliminated by removing infested clothing, bathing the patient, and providing the patient with freshly laundered clothing and bedding. In contrast to head and pubic lice, body lice cannot become permanently established on a host who maintains good personal hygiene, including regular changes to clean clothing.

When only the eggs of head lice are found, it is important to determine whether the eggs have hatched (signifying past infestation) or are unhatched (indicating active infestation). Louse eggs can be examined microscopically to determine if the egg cap (operculum) is missing; absence of the operculum indicates the egg has hatched. An alternative method for differentiating active from inactive head louse infestations involves a search for eggs within 1/4 inch of the scalp.

TABLE 1 Clinically Useful Biologic Data on Lice and *S. scabiei*

BIOLOGICAL CHARACTERISTIC	BODY LOUSE	HEAD LOUSE	PUBIC LOUSE	*S. scabiei*
Most common habitat	Clothing	Head hair	Groin, eyelashes	Skin
Average number on host	10–15	10–15	10–15	10–15
Incubation period for eggs	7–10 days	7–10 days	7–10 days	4–6 days
Maturation period[a]	10 days	10 days	15 days	10–14 days
Life span of adults *on* host	35 days	30 days	30 days[10]	30 days
Life span of adults *off* host @ 22°C	4–7 days[9]	2 days[3,9]	1 day[10,19,20]	2 days[8]
Life span of eggs *off* host	30 days[9]	10 days[3,b]	No data	0 days
Temperatures lethal to adults and eggs	5 minutes at 51.5°C[9]	5 minutes at 51.5°C[9]	? assume same as other lice	10 minutes at 50.0°C[8]
Vector of disease	Yes[c]	No	No	No
Scabies incubation period	—	—	—	1–2 months

[a]Period of time required for a newly hatched larva or nymph to become an egg laying adult.
[b]Louse eggs will not hatch at room temperature (20–24°C).
[c]Typhus *(R. rickettsia)*, Trench fever *(R. quintana)*, Relapsing fever *(Treponema recurrentis)*.

Female lice attach their eggs to the base of the hair shaft at the scalp line. In one week (the incubation period for louse eggs), human hair grows about $^1/_4$ inch, carrying the egg with it. Therefore, eggs greater than $^1/_4$ to $^1/_2$ inch from the scalp have either hatched or are infertile and will never hatch; unless nymphal or adult lice are found on these patients, they should not be treated.

Selection of the safest and most efficacious drug(s) for scabies or pediculosis is encumbered by the absence of controlled clinical trials comparing various compounds and formulations with one another. Thus the drug most extensively used is not necessarily the drug of choice. Nor are prescription drugs necessarily superior to all 'over the counter' preparations. Selection of prescription drugs does allow the physician to limit the quantity of drug available to patients. This is important because patients with infestations tend to use topical preparations more frequently and over longer periods of time than prescribed by a physician.[2] Abuse of scabicides and pediculicides may cause a dermatitis or result in absorption of potentially toxic quantities of drug.

Drugs of choice for pediculosis and scabies are listed in Table 2. A number of other preparations, including DDT, are available in other countries, but not in the United States. Under most circumstances, these products offer no advantage over products available in this country. However, topical powders (gamma benzene hexachloride, malathion, and DDT) might be useful for controlling lice infestations in U.S. communities where the absence of running hot water and/or warm housing in the winter make shampooing undesirable.

Pediculicides and scabicides have not proved to be ovicidal when used according to the manufacturer's directions.[3,4] Therefore, it is generally recommended that infested patients be treated twice. The interval between treatments should approximate the incubation period for louse or mite eggs (1 week) so that any newly hatched parasites will be killed by the second application. Treatment intervals exceeding 10 days may allow some parasites to mature and lay more eggs.

Shaving hair infested by head or pubic lice does not facilitate treatment nor does it reduce the risk of transmission. The prevalence of head louse infestations is no different in children with long hair than in those with short hair.[5,6]

Supportive drugs that may be helpful in the treatment of scabies

TABLE 2 Pediculicides and Scabicides

INFESTATION	DRUG(S) OF CHOICE	ALTERNATIVE DRUGS
P. capitis and *P. pubis*	1% Gamma Benzene Hexachloride[a] *or* ≧0.165% pyrethrins with 2% piperonyl-butoxide	1. 0.03% copper oleate 2. Malathion (0.5% lotion *or* 1% powder)[b] 3. DDT (2–5% emulsion or 10% powder)[a,b]
P. pubis of eyelashes	Petrolatum Ophthalmic Ointment	1. Yellow oxide of mercury ophthalmic ointment 2. Physostigmine ophthalmic ointment
S. scabiei	1% Gamma Benzene Hexachloride *or* 10% Crotamiton	6% ointment of precipitated sulfur in petrolatum *or* Benzyl benzoate 12–15%[b]

[a]Resistance of head lice to these drugs has been demonstrated in Britain, but not in the United States.
[b]Drugs not readily available in the United States.

include antihistamines or salicylates to relieve itching, and systemic antibiotics when there is evidence of secondary bacterial infection.[2] Topical corticosteroid preparations may potentiate scabies infestation.[7]

PREVENTION OF REINFESTATION

Steps must be taken to prevent reinfestation from family members, sexual contacts, and fomites. Family members of patients with pediculosis should be examined, but they are treated only if found infested; one notable exception is sexual contacts of patients with *P. pubis* infestation who are often treated simultaneously without examination.[2] It is advisable to treat all asymptomatic as well as symptomatic household members and sexual contacts of patients with scabies because the incubation period for scabies may be 1 to 2 months. During the incubation period, infested contacts are capable of transmitting mites to previously treated or untreated persons.[2,8]

The potential for reinfestation via fomites is greatest for body lice because the parasite and its eggs can survive off the host longer than other lice and *S. scabiei* (see Table 1). Fomites play a lesser but still significant role in the transmission of head lice. They can survive on objects such as hair brushes, caps, scarves, coats, and towels for only a few days. If transmission is to occur, the head louse must become established on a new host within this time period. Head louse eggs that fall in an infested person's environment are of little importance in transmission because they do not hatch at room temperature (20°C). Only if head louse eggs are returned to their optimal incubation temperature (30°C) within 10 days will some of them hatch.[3,9] Eggs are most likely to be transferred from one person to another when combs or hair brushes are shared. While fomites have also been implicated in the transmission of pubic lice and *S. scabiei*, they are of far less importance than person-to-person transmission in the spread of these two parasites.[8,10]

Methods for disinfecting fomites include machine washing, machine drying, dry cleaning, ironing, and storage in plastic bags for a period of time that exceeds the life span of crawling forms and eggs off the host. Temperatures exceeding 52°C for 5–10 minutes are lethal to lice, mites, and their eggs. Most personal articles of clothing and bedding can be disinfected by machine washing in hot water and/or drying, using the hot cycle of a dryer. Boiling (100°C) of clothing or bedding is not necessary. Industrial hot water heaters maintain a water temperature of about 60°C, and most home hot water heaters can be adjusted to give this temperature. However, some household hot water heaters cannot sustain the 60°C water temperature when several loads of laundry are processed in succession or when other demands for hot water are made simultaneously. To maintain the laundry water at 60°C or higher in the home, time should be allowed between loads for water to be reheated to the disinfecting temperature. Personal articles of clothing or bedding that cannot be washed may be dry cleaned. Nonwashable fabrics may also be disinfected by sealing them in a plastic bag for a period of about 2 weeks (this method is not recommended for body lice whose eggs may remain dormant up to 30 days). Storage of clothing in plastic bags can be shortened by at least 1 week for *P. pubis* and *S. scabiei* infestations. Cleaning of houses, wards, and other rooms inhabited by infested patients should be limited to thorough vacuuming. Fumigation of rooms and use of insecticidal sprays on furniture and carpets to kill lice and mites are not recommended.[11]

DRUG MONOGRAPHS

SCABICIDES

GAMMA BENZENE HEXACHLORIDE (Gamene, Kwell)

Gamma benzene hexachloride (GBH, Lindane) is an easy-to-use scabicide and is considered by many authorities to be the drug of choice for the treatment of scabies in adults and older children. However, a good controlled clinical trial comparing GBH with alternative drugs is lacking. Rash and itching of scabies may persist for two to three weeks after treatment and should not be interpreted as a sign of drug resistance or reinfestation.

Adverse Reactions—GBH is irritating to the eyes, mucus membranes, and skin. Too frequent or prolonged use causes irritant dermatitis. Percutaneous absorption and urinary excretion of GBH

TABLE 3 Preparations and Costs of Pediculicides and Scabicides

Generic Name	Trademark Name(s)	Preparations and 1978 Costs
Crotamiton	Eurax	Cream 10%—$1.68/60 g
Gamma Benzene Hexachloride	Kwell	Cream 1%—$2.09/2 oz, $9.80/1 lb Lotion 1%—$2.01/2 oz, $9.44/pint Shampoo 1%—$2.04/2 oz, $9.57/pint
Petrolatum Ophthalmic Ointment	generic	$0.50—$1.45/⅛ oz
Pyrethrins and Piperonyl Butoxide	A-200 Pyrinate	Liquid (pyrethrins 0.165% and piperonyl butoxide 2.0%)—$1.99/2 oz, $3.32/4 oz
	A-200 Pyrinate Gel	Gel (pyrethrin 0.33% and piperonyl butoxide 4.0%)—$1.99/1 oz
	Rid	Liquid (pyrethrins 0.3% and piperonyl butoxide 3.0%)—$2.49/2 oz, $4.49/4 oz

have been documented.[12] Convulsions have been reported in children receiving excessive topical applications.[13]

Dosage—Topical: Following a warm bath or shower and towel drying, 20 to 30 g of cream or lotion is applied to all parts of the body from the neck down. The medication is washed off after 24 hours. Treatment is repeated in one week.

CROTAMITON (Eurax)

Crotamiton is an effective scabicide and a nonspecific antipruritic agent. It has been used in infants as well as older patients without important adverse effects.

Adverse Reactions—Crotamiton rarely causes contact or allergic dermatitis. It is irritating to acutely inflamed or denuded skin and should not be applied to raw, weeping lesions. Contact with the eyes and mucus membranes should be avoided.

Dosage—Topical: Crotamiton is applied to the entire body from the neck down. It is thoroughly massaged into the skin, paying particular attention to all folds and creases. Treatment is repeated in 24 hours. A cleansing bath is recommended 48 hours after the last treatment. The entire treatment is repeated one week later.

SULFUR

Sulfur is one of the oldest scabicides known to man. Some authorities still consider it the drug of choice for treating scabies in infants and young children.[2] The compound is messy, odoriferous, and stains clothing and bedding. No pharmaceutical preparations are available. Sulfur ointment must be compounded by a pharmacist. The usual formulation is a 6% ointment of precipitated sulfur in petrolatum.[2]

Adverse Reactions—Sulfur rarely causes irritation of the skin.

Interactions—Sulfur reacts with mercury compounds forming hydrogen sulfide which may be irritating and stain the skin black.

Dosage—Topical: After a warm soapy bath and towel drying, sulfur ointment is applied to the body from the neck down and left on for at least 24 hours. Treatment is repeated every night for three nights. Most patients prefer to take a bath before reapplying the drug and 24 hours after the final application.

PEDICULICIDES

GAMMA BENZENE HEXACHLORIDE (Gamene, Kwell)

Gamma benzene hexachloride (GBH, Lindane) is an effective pediculicide.

Adverse Reactions—See monograph above.

Dosage—Topical: One ounce or less of GBH shampoo is massaged into premoistened hair for four minutes. The hair is thoroughly rinsed with warm water and towel dried. Treatment is repeated in one week. For *P. pubis* infestations, GBH shampoo may be used as outlined above or GBH lotion may be substituted. When lotion is used, a thin layer is applied to infested and adjacent hairy areas, paying particular attention to the pubic mons and perianal areas. Application should be extended to the thighs, trunk, and axillary regions in persons having a large amount of body hair. GBH should not be used for *P. pubis* infestations of the eyelashes.

PYRETHRINS AND PIPERONYL BUTOXIDE (A-200 Pyrinate, Rid)

Pyrethrins are fast-acting insecticides extracted from flowers of the genus *Chrysanthemum.* Most preparations contain a synergist (piperonyl butoxide) that further potentiates insecticidal activity. This drug is commonly used in house and garden insect sprays. Synergized pyrethrins have also been shown to be effective against lice.[14]

Adverse Reactions—Experimental studies in laboratory animals indicate that pyrethrins are considerably less toxic than GBH.[14,15] Allergic dermatitis has been reported but is probably due to impurities in the flower extract rather than pyrethrin. Patients sensitive to ragweed are especially sensitive to impurities in pyrethrin preparations.[14] Commerical formulations are irritating to the eyes and mucus membranes.

Dosage—Topical: Formulations are applied to hair and scalp, or any other infested area, until the hair is thoroughly wet. After 10 minutes pyrethrin formulations are washed off using warm water and soap or shampoo. Treatment is repeated in one week.

PETROLATUM OPHTHALMIC OINTMENT

Yellow oxide of mercury and physostigmine ophthalmic ointments have been successfully used to treat *P. pubis* infestation of the eyelashes.[2,10,16] However, mercury oxide has practically no inherent insecticidal properties, and physostigmine (although closely related to carbamate insecticides) is ineffective as an insecticide.[17,18] Since petrolatum without other drug additives kills lice,[2,21] mechanical blockage of the insect's respiratory network is probably the principal mode of action of all of these products. Thus, the addition of yellow oxide of mercury or physostigmine to petrolatum appears to offer no chemotherapeutic advantage but does increase the potential for adverse reactions.

Dosage—Topical: Petrolatum is applied thickly to the eyelashes twice daily for 8 to 10 days. The remaining nits should be mechanically removed.[2]

REFERENCES

1. Keh B, Poorbaugh JH: Understanding and treating infestations of lice on humans. California Vector Views 18:23–31, 1971.
2. Orkin M, Epstein E Sr, Maibach HI: Treatment of today's scabies and pediculosis. JAMA 236:1136–1139, 1976.
3. Lang JD: Biology and control of the head louse, *Pediculus humanus capitus* (Anoplura: Pediculidae), in a semi-arid urban area. Doctoral thesis, University of Arizona, 1975.
4. Gordon RM, Lavoipierre MMJ: *Entomology for Students of Medicine*. Philadelphia, F.A. Davis, 1972.
5. Slonka GF, McKinley TW, McCroan JE, et al: Epidemiology of an outbreak of head lice in Georgia. Am J Trop Med Hyg 25:739–743, 1976.
6. Juranek DD: Epidemiology of pediculosis in school children. In *Scabies and Pediculosis*. Edited by M Orkin, HI Maibach, LC Parish, et al. Philadelphia, JB Lippincott, 1977, pp 168–173.
7. McMillan AL: Unusual features of scabies associated with topical fluorinated steroids. Br J Dermatol 87:496–497, 1972.
8. Mellanby K: *Scabies*. London, E.W. Classey, 1972.
9. International Symposium on the Control of Lice and Louseborne Diseases, Proceedings. Washington, Pan American Health Organization, Scientific Publication No. 263.
10. Ackerman AB: Crabs—the resurgence of *Phthirus pubis*. N Engl J Med 278:950–951, 1968.
11. Anon: Kwell and other drugs for treatment of lice and scabies. Med Lett Drugs Ther 19:18–19, 1977.
12. Feldmann RJ, Maibach HI: Percutaneous penetration of some pesticides and herbicides in man. Toxicol Appl Pharmacol 28:126–132, 1974.
13. Lee B, Groth R, Turner W: Suspected reactions to gamma benzene hexachloride. JAMA 236:2846, 1976.
14. Casida JE (ed): *Pyrethrum*. New York, Academic Press, 1973.
15. Ulmann E: *Lindane*. Freiburg Im Breisgau, Verlag K. Schillinger, 1972.
16. Epstein E: Pediculosis pubis. Med Aspects Human Sexuality. January, 1975, pp 8–27.
17. King WV: *Chemicals Evaluated as Insecticides and Repellants at Orlando, Florida*. Agriculture Handbook No. 69, U.S. Department of Agriculture, May 1954.
18. Matsumura F: *Carbamate Insecticides*. New York, Plenum Press, 1975.
19. Buxton PA: *Louse: An Account of Lice Which Infest Man, Their Medical Importance, and Control*. London, Arnold, 1939.

20. Nuttall GHF: Biology of *Phthirus pubis*. Parasitology 10:383–405, 1918.
21. Orkin M, Epstein E, Maibach HI: Treatment of today's pediculosis. In *Scabies and Pediculosis*. Edited by M Orkin, HI Maibach, LC Parish, et al. Philadelphia, JB Lippincott, 1977, pp 174–178.

ONCOLYTIC AGENTS

19. ANTINEOPLASTIC AGENTS

Edward S. Greenwald

The use of chemotherapeutic agents to treat disseminated cancer has increased markedly in the last few years. As recently as the late 1960's, the medical oncologist had to convince his colleagues of the occasional utility of anti-cancer drugs. The pendulum has now swung to the other extreme, so that most patients with metastatic cancer are given chemotherapy. It is doubtful, however, that more than 30% of those with advanced malignancy derive benefit from such treatment.

There are two major uses of anti-cancer drugs. One is to treat established metastatic disease, and the other is the so-called 'adjuvant chemotherapy.' The latter is used in those patients who are likely to have clinically inapparent 'micrometastases.' For example, patients who have radical amputation for what appears to be localized osteogenic sarcoma are cured less than one-fifth of the time. Most succumb to lung metastases within two years of diagnosis. Since few of these have local tumor recurrences, clinically inapparent lung metastases must have been present.

Anti-cancer drugs can cure several tumors such as Hodgkin's disease, childhood acute leukemia, uterine choriocarcinoma, Wilms' tumor, and testis cancer. Adjuvant chemotherapy increases cure rates in patients with osteogenic sarcoma, Ewing's sarcoma, and embryonal rhabdomyosarcoma of children. The use of adjuvant chemotherapy appears to delay recurrence of breast cancer after mastectomy if one or more axillary nodes contain cancer.

Chemotherapy is beneficial in patients with malignant lymphoma, breast cancer, chronic leukemia (myelogenous or lymphatic), multiple myeloma, Waldenström's macroglobulinemia, and ovarian cancer. The use of anti-cancer drugs is only marginally useful in colo-rectal and gastric cancer, lung cancer, and malignant melanoma. Table 1 lists drugs or regimens of choice for individual neoplasma.

Antineoplastic agents are classified as alkylating agents, anti-metabolites, plant alkaloids, antibiotics, or miscellaneous agents.

TABLE 1 Chemotherapeutic Drugs or Regimens of Choice

NEOPLASM	DRUG OR REGIMEN OF CHOICE
Chronic Myelogenous Leukemia	Busulfan
Chronic Lymphocytic Leukemia	Chlorambucil
Malignant Lymphoma other than Diffuse Histiocytic	In general, combinations of an alkylating agent, vincristine and prednisone
Diffuse Histiocytic Lymphoma	Intensive combination chemotherapy such as C-MOPP
Hodgkin's Disease	MOPP combination chemotherapy
Wilms' Tumor	Dactinomycin and/or vincristine plus radiotherapy
Embryonal Rhabdomyosarcoma	Combination chemotherapy: usually vincristine, cyclophosphamide and dactinomycin
Osteogenic Sarcoma	High dose methotrexate with citrovorum factor rescue
Ewing's Sarcoma	Adriamycin or various chemotherapy combinations
Multiple Myeloma	Melphalan or cyclophosphamide
Female Breast Cancer	Cyclophosphamide, methotrexate, fluorouracil combination, or cyclophosphamide, adriamycin, fluorouracil combination
Gastric Cancer	Fluourouracil or methyl CCNU, fluorouracil combination
Colon and Rectal Cancer	Same as gastric cancer
Ovarian Cancer	Cyclophosphamide, chlorambucil, or melphalan
Uterine Choriocarcinoma	Methotrexate or dactinomycin
Testicular Carcinoma	Various combinations of chemotherapeutic drugs. Most combinations utilize cis-platinum and bleomycin infusion with or without other drugs such as dactinomycin or vinblastine.
Malignant Melanoma	Dacarbazine
Small Cell Undifferentiated Lung Cancer	Intensive combination chemotherapy. Most regimens utilize cyclophosphamide plus methotrexate. Others add lomustine and/or adriamycin as well.

ADVERSE REACTIONS AND PRECAUTIONS

Anti-cancer drugs, with the exception of bleomycin and vincristine, are highly toxic to the bone marrow. Anemia is less common than leukopenia and thrombocytopenia. Since bone marrow depression is usually short-lived, death from infection is not very frequent. All patients with chemotherapy-induced leukocyte counts of less than 1000/mm^3 must be watched carefully for signs and symptoms of infection. If such a patient spikes a fever, cultures of appropriate body fluids must be taken and intensive antibiotic therapy started immediately without waiting for culture results.

Many cancer chemotherapeutic drugs cause ulceration of the mouth and small bowel mucosa. Mouth ulcers are very painful, while small bowel ulceration can lead to severe diarrhea, hemorrhage, or gram-negative sepsis. Alopecia is a common side effect of anti-cancer drugs, especially doxorubicin, vincristine, and cyclophosphamide. A number of cancer chemotherapeutic drugs, such as doxorubicin, vincristine, vinblastine, dactinomycin, and mechlorethamine, are extremely irritating to tissues, so that great care must be taken to ensure that there is no infiltration during intravenous administration. One method is to inject the drug into the sidearm of a running intravenous infusion. I prefer to use a 23 gauge butterfly needle and a saline filled syringe. When it is established that the injected saline is going only into the vein, the infusion syringe is changed to that containing the chemotherapeutic drug. After completion of the injection the butterfly needle is washed with more sterile solution and the needle removed from the vein.

DRUG MONOGRAPHS

ALKYLATING AGENTS

BUSULFAN (Myleran)

Busulfan, an alkylating agent, is the treatment of choice for chronic myelogenous leukemia.[1] No other therapy for this condition can be considered standard.

Adverse Reactions—As with other alkylating agents, the major toxicity of busulfan is bone marrow depression. Severe prolonged agranulocytosis may occur, and platelet count depression is a more

TABLE 2 Preparations and Costs of Antineoplastic Drugs

Generic Name	Trademark Name(s)	Preparations and 1978 Costs
Alkylating Agents		
Busulfan	Myleran	Tablets 2 mg—$1.50/25
Chlorambucil	Leukeran	Tablets 2 mg—$3.10/50
Cyclophosphamide	Cytoxan	Tablets 25 mg—$12.70/100; 50 mg—$23.32/100 Injection (powder) 100 mg—$2.84/vial; 200 mg—$4.09/vial; 500 mg—$7.50/vial
Mechlorethamine Hydrochloride (Nitrogen Mustard)	Mustargen Hydrochloride	Injection (powder) 10 mg—$2.06/vial
Melphalan	Alkeran	Tablets 2 mg—$5.20/50
Antimetabolites		
Cytarabine	Cytosar	Injection (freeze-dried powder) 100 mg—$4.30/vial; 500 mg—$19.11/vial
Fluorouracil (5-FU)	generic	Injection (solution) 50 mg/ml—$1.41/10-ml ampul
Mercaptopurine	Purinethol	Tablets 50 mg—$3.75/25
Methotrexate	generic	Tablets 2.5 mg—$20.21/100
Methotrexate Sodium	generic	Injection (solution) 2.5 mg/ml—$4.39/2-ml vial; 25 mg/ml—$11.49/2-ml vial
Plant Alkaloids		
Vinblastine Sulfate	Velban	Injection (lyophilized powder) 10 mg—$11.91/vial
Vincristine Sulfate	Oncovin	Injection (powder) 1 mg—$11.53/ampul; 5 mg—$51.14/ampul
Antibiotics		
Bleomycin Sulfate	Blenoxane	Injection (powder) 15 units—$44.73/ampul
Dactinomycin	Cosmegen	Injection (powder) 0.5 mg—$2.40/vial

TABLE 2 *(continued)*

GENERIC NAME	TRADEMARK NAME(S)	PREPARATIONS AND 1978 COSTS
Doxorubicin Hydrochloride	Adriamycin	Injection (powder) 10 mg—$15.66/vial; 50 mg—$74.28/vial
Miscellaneous Agent		
Procarbazine Hydrochloride	Matulane	Capsules 50 mg—$10.75/100

significant problem than with any other alkylating agent.[2] Other side effects, although less common, are of great practical and theoretic importance. Perhaps the most unusual is a syndrome resembling adrenal insufficiency, which is characterized by skin hyperpigmentation, severe weakness, fatigue, anorexia, and weight loss.[3] 'Busulfan lung,' a form of intra-alveolar fibrosis, is another serious although uncommon side effect of busulfan therapy;[4] it is characterized by severe and often irreversible dyspnea and hypoxia. Both syndromes are correlated with total cumulative busulfan dosage. Patients receiving busulfan therapy for several years have developed cytologic dysplasia in multiple organs, and there is a suggestion that carcinomas have occurred as a result of busulfan therapy.[5] Busulfan is teratogenic in animals and humans.

Dosage—Oral: Adults, initial therapy, 4 to 6 mg daily; maintenance, 2 mg twice a week to 2 mg daily.

CHLORAMBUCIL (Leukeran)

Chlorambucil, an orally administered alkylating agent, is the drug of choice for the treatment of chronic lymphatic leukemia[6] and Waldenström's macroglobulinemia.[7] It is also useful in the therapy of ovarian cancer[8] and malignant lymphoma of the lymphocytic type.[9] In all of the above conditions, except for ovarian cancer, oral corticosteroids are often used in conjunction with chlorambucil. The advantages of chlorambucil over other alkylating agents are oral administration, slower onset of action, and less prolonged duration of marrow suppression.

Adverse Reactions—Bone marrow suppression is practically the only toxicity and is rarely dangerous if the drug dose is adjusted according to the level of white blood cell and/or platelet count. The exact blood count at which the drug is stopped depends on such factors as the type of malignancy and the pre-treatment blood count.[10] Nausea is uncommon.

Interactions—Additive bone marrow suppression occurs when chlorambucil is given in conjunction with other cancer chemotherapeutic drugs. Chlorambucil is not commonly used in combination regimens.

Dosage—Oral: Adults, initial therapy, 6 to 12 mg daily on an empty stomach; maintenance dosage, 2 to 6 mg daily.

CYCLOPHOSPHAMIDE (Cytoxan)

Cyclophosphamide, the alkylating agent effective against the greatest variety of malignancies, is the agent of choice for treating oat cell lung cancer,[11]and the preferred alkylating agent for use in combination chemotherapy of non-Hodgkin's lymphomas.[12] Because of the rapid recovery from cyclophosphamide-induced bone marrow depression, this drug is the alkylating agent of choice for high-dose intermittent combination chemotherapy regimens used in oat cell lung cancer, non-Hodgkin's lymphoma, and childhood tumors such as embryonal rhabdomyosarcoma.[13] Cyclophosphamide is also one of the two preferred drugs for the treatment of multiple myeloma.[14] It is the only alkylating agent active against childhood acute lymphoblastic leukemia.[15]

Adverse Reactions—In addition to producing bone marrow depression, a side effect it shares with the other alkylating agents, cyclophosphamide produces cosmetically important but reversible alopecia in many patients. Long-term use or single, very high doses frequently cause cystitis, which may be severe enough to preclude further cyclophosphamide administration. Adequate hydration with production of dilute urine helps protect against the development of cystitis. High intravenous doses often produce hyponatremia due to inappropriate production of antidiuretic hormone. Nausea and vomiting are frequent when daily amounts exceed 200 mg, and are not uncommon with lower daily amounts. Single, very large intravenous cyclophosphamide injections can cause severe vomiting lasting for one to more than 24 hours.

Dosage—Many different cyclophosphamide regimens have been advocated. They can be generally grouped as follows:

(1) High-dose intermittent, 800 to 2,000 mg/m^2 body surface area, intravenously every three to four weeks. Marked, but transient, leukopenia often occurs with this regimen.

(2) Low-dose continuous, 50 to 150 mg/day by mouth.

(3) Intravenous loading, 2 to 6 mg/kg/day for four to ten days, followed by oral maintenance on a dose of 50 to 150 mg/day.

MECHLORETHAMINE HYDROCHLORIDE (Mustargen Hydrochloride)

Mechlorethamine, commonly known as nitrogen mustard, is an alkylating agent. While mechlorethamine was the first effective cancer chemotherapeutic agent, and the first alkylating agent available to the clinician, its present use is limited almost entirely to the treatment of Hodgkin's disease as part of the MOPP (mechlorethamine, Oncovin [vincristine], prednisone, procarbazine) combination chemotherapy regimen.[16] It also has minimal effectiveness in treating epidermoid carcinoma of the lung.[17] Mechlorethamine is frequently instilled directly into the pleural and peritoneal cavity to prevent the recurrence of malignant effusions. Unfortunately, this use is based on uncontrolled studies, and intraperitoneal administration probably induces more toxicity than benefit.[18]

The topical use of mechlorethamine for the treatment of the early stages of mycosis fungoides has been extensively investigated.[19] Whether this treatment is superior to the use of superficial radiotherapy is far from certain.

Adverse Reactions—Bone marrow depression may be severe and prolonged; the white blood cell count is frequently depressed to a greater extent than the platelet count, while red blood cell depression is usually of minor clinical significance.[20] Nausea and vomiting, which almost always occur within one to four hours of mechlorethamine administration, may last for several hours. Inadvertent extravascular extravasation of mechlorethamine will cause persistent painful induration and occasional sloughing of cutaneous and subcutaneous tissue.

Interactions—Administration of mechlorethamine in conjunction with other bone marrow suppressive anti-cancer drugs will lead to greater depression of formed elements in the peripheral blood. Appropriate dose adjustment is imperative.

Dosage—Intravenous: Adults, 0.4 mg/kg every 6 to 8 weeks. MOPP regimen: vincristine sulfate (Oncovin) 1.4 mg/m^2 on days 1 and 8 of each cycle; mechlorethamine 6 mg/m^2 on days 1 and 8 of each cycle. From days 1 through 14 of each cycle, oral procarbazine 100 mg/m^2 is administered, and in cycles 1 and 4, oral prednisone 40 mg/m^2 is administered from days 1 through 14. No therapy is then given for 14 days (days 15 through 28). The next cycle is then started on day 29. Six such cycles are given with appropriate dose modification dependent on the blood count.[16]

MELPHALAN (Alkeran)

Melphalan is the drug of choice for multiple myeloma,[21] and is also used in the therapy of ovarian cancer.[22,23] Recently melphalan has been tested an adjuvant therapy after radical mastectomy for breast cancer.[24]

Adverse Reactions—Bone marrow depression, occasionally of very long duration, is the major side effect. Mild nausea and vomiting are uncommon and dose-related.

Interactions—Additive bone marrow suppression can be expected when melphalan is administered with other cancer chemotherapeutic agents.

Dosage—Oral: Adults, either 0.15 to 0.25 mg/kg daily for four to five days every four to six weeks, or 2 to 4 mg daily. Sometimes daily administration is preceded by a loading dose of 60 to 70 mg given over a six to ten day period. If a loading dose is administered, it is customary to wait three to five weeks before starting daily maintenance therapy.

ANTIMETABOLITES

CYTARABINE (Cytosar)

Cytarabine is used almost exclusively in the treatment of adult acute leukemia, usually in combination with the antipurine compound, thioguanine.[25] Its mechanism of action appears to be by interference with DNA synthesis through its inhibition of DNA polymerase.

Adverse Reactions—Bone marrow depression occurs in approximately two-thirds of patients. Leukopenia and thrombocytopenia are the major manifestations. Nausea, vomiting, and diarrhea are uncommon.

Dosage—Intravenous: Adults and children, 100 mg/m^2 every 12 hours, along with thioguanine, 2.5 mg/kg given orally.

FLUOROURACIL (5-FU)

Fluorouracil is an antimetabolite which interferes with the methylation of uridylic acid to thymidylic acid, thus interfering with DNA synthesis. Its usefulness is limited to treating metastatic colo-rectal, gastric, and breast cancer. Fluorouracil is of no value as adjuvant therapy after resection of colo-rectal or gastric cancer, but, in combination with cyclophosphamide and methotrexate, it may prove useful for preventing recurrence after mastectomy for breast carcinoma in those women with positive axillary lymph nodes.[26]

Adverse Reactions—Bone marrow depression is one of the two major side effects of this drug. Although mild thrombocytopenia is frequent, it rarely leads to bleeding. Leukopenia, however, can be a serious complication, leading to major infections such as septicemia. Serious bone marrow depression is uncommon with newer regimens.

Gastrointestinal disturbances are the other major form of fluorouracil toxicity. Nausea and vomiting are common but rarely interfere with continued use of the drug. Severe stomatitis and ulcerative enteritis, formerly occurring in 10% to 25% of patients, are rare with newer dosage regimens.

Uncommon side effects include cerebellar ataxia[27] and mental confusion,[28] which are reversible on drug discontinuation, and dry, cracked skin on the palms of the hands and soles of the feet,[29] dermatitis in sun-exposed areas,[30] and alopecia.

Interactions—The dosage of fluorouracil must be lowered when it is given in conjunction with other anti-cancer agents.

Dosage—Oral administration is not standard therapy because of uncertain drug absorption. *Intravenous: Adults.* Two basic dosage regimens are used. The most popular and convenient is 15 mg/kg given intravenously once a week. Some chemotherapists prefer an initial loading dose of 12 mg/kg daily for five days before starting weekly maintenance treatment.

MERCAPTOPURINE (Purinethol)

Mercaptopurine, a purine antagonist which probably acts by inhibiting DNA synthesis, is one of the standard drugs for treating all varieties of acute leukemia.[31] It is also used as an 'immuno-suppressant' to treat a variety of non-neoplastic diseases.

Adverse Reactions—Bone marrow depression is common, but rarely lasts for more than seven days after stopping the drug. Leukocyte depression occurs more often than anemia or thrombocytopenia. Drug-induced obstructive jaundice due to intrahepatic cholestasis is seen occasionally, but almost all patients recover when the drug is stopped. Mouth ulcers occur in less than 20% of mercaptopurine-treated patients.

Interactions—Coadministration of other chemotherapeutic agents, although often necessary, can increase the likelihood of bone marrow depression. Since allopurinol (Zyloprim) inhibits the degradation of mercaptopurine, doses of mercaptopurine should be decreased to one-quarter of the usual amount when these two agents are used together.

Dosage—Oral: Adults, 2.5 to 3.0 mg/kg daily.

METHOTREXATE
METHOTREXATE SODIUM

Methotrexate inhibits DNA synthesis in both normal and neoplastic cells by preventing the reduction of folic acid to tetrahydrofolic acid. Approximately 50% of patients with uterine choriocarcinoma can be cured by methotrexate.[32] The drug is also very active against childhood acute lymphoblastic leukemia.[21] In addition to its systemic administration for remission maintenance in this disease, it is given by the intrathecal route to prevent central nervous system leukemic relapse.[33] Methotrexate is used in combination with cyclophosphamide and 5-fluorouracil as adjuvant[26] or palliative[34] therapy for breast cancer. This combination gives a 50% to 60% response rate, as opposed to 20% to 30% for each of the drugs administered alone. Response rates to methotrexate in epidermoid carcinoma of the head and neck as high as 50% have been reported,[35] but response duration averages only 6 to 8 weeks.

The use of high dose methotrexate infusions followed by citrovorum factor rescue must still be considered experimental, although in certain cancer centers, results with this technique for adjuvant therapy of osteogenic sarcoma have been excellent.[36]

Adverse Reactions—Bone marrow depression, a potentially fatal complication, is not rare. Leukopenia is more common and more serious than anemia or thrombocytopenia. While the duration of leukocyte suppression usually is less than one week, fatal infectious complications may occur. Superficial ulceration of the gastrointestinal tract mucosa is seen most commonly in the mouth and small bowel. When this occurs in combination with leukopenia, the dangers of gram-negative septicemia are greatly increased. Severe diarrhea and fluid loss are occasionally seen as a result of multiple small bowel ulcers.

Liver damage has occurred after long-term methotrexate administration, particularly in patients with psoriasis. Cirrhosis after methotrexate therapy appears to occur almost exclusively in patients with pre-existing liver disease.[37] Reversible pulmonary infiltrates have been described in leukemic children after methotrexate administration.[38]

Several varieties of neurotoxicity can follow intrathecal use of methotrexate.[27] Alopecia of mild degree is common. Methotrexate administered during the first trimester of pregnancy almost always leads to abortion or abnormalities in the fetus.[39]

Interactions—Drugs such as salicylates, sulfonamides, and diphenylhydantoin, reportedly can displace methotrexate from its binding to serum albumin and thus increase drug toxicity. This has not been investigated in animals or humans. Pre-treatment with folic acid will diminish methotrexate effectiveness and toxicity.

Dosage—Oral, Intramuscular, Intravenous, Intrathecal: Dosage regimens vary considerably. For the treatment of uterine choriocarcinoma, 15 to 25 mg daily for five days may be given as a single dose orally or parenterally. Such courses are repeated after one to two week rest periods, depending on toxicity. For acute leukemia maintenance, the usual dose is 30 mg/m^2 twice a week. Intrathecal dosage is 0.2 to 0.3 mg/kg every two to three days for approximately five doses. Such courses may be repeated every few months depending on the protocol.

PLANT ALKALOIDS

VINBLASTINE SULFATE (Velban)

Vinblastine is useful for treating only three neoplasms: Hodgkin's disease, testicular cancer, and Kaposi's sarcoma. Although vinblastine is probably the single most effective drug for treating Hodgkin's disease, the success of the MOPP combination chemotherapy regimen, which excludes vinblastine, has made this agent a second line chemotherapeutic drug in Hodgkin's disease patients. In Britain and the United States, however, vinblastine is used in combination chemotherapy regimens which appear to be just as effective as MOPP.[40] Vinblastine alone is not very effective in treating testicular cancer, but the most effective combination chemotherapy regimens for treating testicular cancer include vinblastine.[41,42] It appears that a significant number of patients with this tumor are cured by chemotherapy.[42]

Kaposi's sarcoma is a disease that is usually best managed by radiotherapy. Occasional patients, however, have such disseminated disease that systemic therapy is required. Although slightly less than half of patients respond, the long duration of response makes vinblastine the drug of choice in this disease.[43]

Adverse Reactions—As with most cancer chemotherapeutic agents, bone marrow depression is the major toxic effect. Leukopenia and thrombocytopenia may be severe, but rarely persist beyond four to six days. Minor neurotoxic effects are common, but rarely interfere with therapy. If vinblastine is inadvertently injected into soft tissue rather than directly into the vein, prolonged painful subcutaneous induration results.

Dosage—Intravenous: Adults, initial dose 0.1 mg/kg intravenously weekly. If peripheral white blood count permits, gradual dose elevation to 0.2 mg/kg once a week should be attempted. In Hodgkin's disease patients, response occurs in two to six weeks, but Kaposi's sarcoma patients may require several months of therapy before improvement occurs. In treating testicular cancer, it is strongly advised that original sources be consulted.[41,42]

VINCRISTINE SULFATE (Oncovin)

Vincristine administered with prednisone is the standard regimen for inducing remissions in childhood acute lymphoblastic leukemia. Complete responses are produced in up to 90% of patients.[44] Vincristine, prednisone, and cyclophosphamide are often used in combination to treat patients with non-Hodgkin's lymphoma.[12] Vincristine is also used in combination with other drugs to treat childhood tumors such as Wilms' tumor,[45] embyronal rhabdomyosarcoma,[13] and neuroblastoma.[46] It is also part of the MOPP combination chemotherapy regimen for the treatment of Hodgkin's disease.[16]

Adverse Reactions—Bone marrow suppressive effects of vincristine are minimal unless very high doses are given. A variety of neurotoxic side effects occur.[47] The earliest changes are paresthesias in the fingers and toes, followed by areflexia and muscular weakness in the extremities. Cranial nerve disturbances are less frequent, but autonomic disturbances are common, particularly bowel atony with resultant severe constipation. This complication may be life-threatening, and should be prevented by fecal softeners and other laxatives. The syndrome of inappropriate secretion of antidiuretic hormone has been reported after vincristine administration.[48] Extravasation of vincristine outside the vein leads to painful subcutaneous induration.

Dosage—Intravenous: Adults and children, 1 to 1.5 mg/m^2 weekly. Many authors recommend that no single dose exceed 2 mg.

ANTIBIOTICS

BLEOMYCIN SULFATE (Blenoxane)

Bleomycin, a mixture of chemically related antibiotics, is still a drug of limited usefulness. In combination with other agents for the treatment of metastatic testicular cancer, it appears to produce excellent results.[42,43] The actual cure rate is not yet established, but two- and three-year survival figures are far better than with earlier therapy. Bleomycin has definite activity against Hodgkin's disease, although remission duration is brief.[49] The use of bleomycin for the treatment of epidermoid carcinoma of the skin and head and neck region is usually futile. Although response rates are about 40%, remission duration averages three to six weeks.[49]

Adverse Reactions—Bleomycin alone has little bone marrow toxicity, but it may potentiate marrow-suppressive effects of other anti-cancer drugs. Pulmonary damage is the major side effect, and is in part related to cumulative dosage. The early change is edema of the alveolar wall and interstitial tissues accompanied by fibrinous edema of the alveolar space. This eventually leads to interstitial fibrosis, which is often fatal.[50] Mucocutaneous side effects are frequent but reversible.[49] Severe stomatitis is common, and may take several weeks to heal. Erythema, hyperpigmentation, and thickened skin in pressure areas and fingertips is common. Chills and fever may be seen when bleomycin is administered to patients with Hodgkin's disease or malignant lymphoma. These patients occasionally develop a shock-like state which sometimes leads to death.[49]

Interactions—Bleomycin may potentiate the bone marrow suppression induced by other anti-cancer drugs. These agents in turn may potentiate the pulmonary toxic effects of bleomycin.

Dosage—Intravenous or Subcutaneous: Adults and children, 10 to 20 unit/m^2 twice a week. Recent results indicate that constant intravenous infusion may be the best way to administer bleomycin when treating metastatic testicular cancer.[41,42] Maximum cumulative bleomycin dosage should not exceed 450 mg, so as to diminish the danger of developing pulmonary toxicity. A lower maximum dose should be observed in patients over age sixty-five.

DACTINOMYCIN (Cosmegen)

Dactinomycin, a specific inhibitor of messenger RNA synthesis, is an agent with a wide spectrum of anti-tumor activity. Approximately 50% of dactinomycin-treated women with choriocarcinoma are cured.[51] Dactinomycin is an effective agent for adjuvant therapy of Wilms' tumor,[45] and, administered in conjunction with low-dose irradiation, cures approxiamtely half of the children with lung metastases from this tumor. Dactinomycin is frequently used in combination with other anti-cancer drugs for treating soft tissue sarcomas,[52] childhood tumors such as embyronal rhabdomyosarcoma,[13] and metastatic testicular tumors.[41,42]

Adverse Reactions—Bone marrow suppression produced by dactinomycin occurs frequently and may be severe, but it rarely lasts more than a week. Both leukopenia and thrombocytopenia are common.[53] Nausea and vomiting of several hours duration is frequent. Stomatitis is uncommon, except when greater than average doses are given. Skin reactions are common, especially at the site of previous radiotherapy, where erythema or increased pigmentation resembling the usual radiation skin reaction may appear. Alopecia occurs frequently.[54] Infiltration of dactinomycin outside the vein leads to prolonged painful skin induration.

Interactions—Aggravation or reactivation of reactions to irradiation may occur. Radiotherapy dosage must be reduced when dactinomycin is administered concurrently. Other anti-cancer drugs will add to the bone marrow suppressive activity of dactinomycin.

Dosage—Intravenous: Adults, 0.010 to 0.015 mg/kg/day for five days, repeated when recovery from bone marrow suppression occurs. Some oncologists administer the drug in single doses of 1.5 to 3.0 mg every two to three weeks.

DOXORUBICIN HYDROCHLORIDE (Adriamycin)

Doxorubicin, an anti-tumor antibiotic which probably acts by interfering with both DNA and RNA synthesis, has the broadest anti-tumor spectrum of any chemotherapeutic drug. Doxorubicin is often used most effectively and safely in combination with other anti-cancer drugs. Doxorubicin alone[55] or with high dose methotrexate-citrovorum factor rescue[56] has been very successful as adjuvant therapy for osteogenic sarcoma. Doxorubicin combinations are being investigated for the treatment of metastatic soft tissue sarcomas. Preliminary results are impressive.[53] Doxorubicin alone produces 30 to 40% responses in metastatic breast cancer,[57] bladder cancer, and lymphomas, including Hodgkin's disease,[58] but remission duration averages only four months.

Adverse Reactions—Doxorubicin is an extremely dangerous drug, unless administered by an experienced chemotherapist. Given properly, its benefits far outweigh its side effects. Bone marrow depression, occurring within seven to fourteen days of administration, may be severe but usually lasts for less than a week.[59] Leukocytes and/or platelets may be affected. Nausea and vomiting occur, but severity is extremely variable from patient to patient, and is rarely troublesome enough to interfere with therapy. Mouth ulcers are seen in approximately 20% of patients, but usually heal within five days. The major toxic effect of doxorubicin is cardiac damage, which, when it occurs, is often irreversible, leading to death from cardiac arrest or congestive heart failure.[60] Clinically evident cardiac damage is uncommon with cumulative dosage of less than 550 mg/m^2. Patients who have had previous cardiac irradiation are more susceptible to doxorubicin-induced cardiomyopathy.[61] Reversible total alopecia occurs in most patients. Extravasation of doxorubicin outside the vein leads to severe prolonged painful induration of subcutaneous tissues.

Interactions—Increased bone marrow depression occurs when doxorubicin is administered concurrently with most other anti-cancer drugs.

Dosage—Intravenous: Adults and children, 40 to 60 mg/m^2 intravenously every three weeks. Some chemotherapists divide the dose over three consecutive days to minimize nausea and vomiting. Cumulative total dose should not exceed 550 mg/m^2. Lower doses are given when liver function is impaired.

MISCELLANEOUS AGENT

PROCARBAZINE HYDROCHLORIDE (Matulane)

The only standard use of procarbazine is in the MOPP combination used to treat Hodgkin's disease.

Adverse Reactions—As with most anti-cancer drugs, bone marrow depression is the major side effect. This is usually delayed for two to three weeks. Mild neurotoxicity has been described. The most disturbing form is a reversible psychotic reaction.

Interactions—Other chemotherapeutic drugs will potentiate the bone marrow depression. Procarbazine may potentiate the effects of phenothiazines and may lead to flushing if alcohol is consumed at the same time.

Dosage—Oral: Adults, in the MOPP regimen, 100 mg/m^2 daily for 14 days in each 28 day cycle.

REFERENCES

1. Stryckmans PA: Current concepts in chronic myelogenous leukemia. Semin Hematol 11:101–128, 1974.
2. Haut A, Abbott WS, Wintrobe MM: Busulfan in the treatment of chronic myelocytic leukemia. The effect of long term intermittent therapy. Blood 17:1–19, 1961.
3. Kyle RA, Schwartz RS, Oliner HL: A syndrome resembling adrenal cortical insufficiency associated with long term busulfan (Myleran) therapy. Blood 18:497–510, 1961.
4. Heard BE, Cooke RA: Busulfan lung. Thorax 23:187–199, 1968.
5. Feingold ML, Koss LG: Effects of long term administration of busulfan. Arch Intern Med 124:66–71, 1969.
6. Galton DAG, Wiltshaw E, Szur L: The use of chlorambucil and steroids in the treatment of chronic lymphocytic leukemia. Br J Haematol 7:73–98, 1961.
7. McCallister BD, Bayrd ED, Harrison EG: Primary macroglobulinemia. Review with a report on 31 cases and notes on the value of continuous chlorambucil therapy. Am J Med 43:394–434, 1967.
8. Masterson JG, Nelson JH Jr: The role of chemotherapy in the treatment of gynecologic malignancy. Am J Obstet Gynecol 93:1102–1111, 1965.
9. Ezdinli EZ, Stutzman L: Chlorambucil therapy for lymphomas and chronic lymphocytic leukemia. Br J Haematol 7:73–98, 1961.
10. Greenwald ES: Alkylating agents. In *Cancer Chemotherapy,* second edition. Edited by ES Greenwald. Flushing, New York, Medical Examination Publishing Company, 1973, pp 107–108.
11. Green RA, Humphrey E, Close H (Veterans Administration Lung Cancer Study Group): Alkylating agents in bronchogenic carcinoma. Am J Med 46:516–525, 1969.
12. Bagley CM Jr, DeVita VT Jr, Berard CW, et al: Advanced lymphosarcoma: intensive cyclical combination chemotherapy with cyclophosphamide, vincristine, and prednisone. Ann Intern Med 76:227–234, 1972.
13. Pratt CB, Hustu HO, Fleming ID: Coordinated treatment of childhood rhabdomyosarcoma with surgery, radiotherapy, and combination chemotherapy. Cancer Res 32:606–610, 1972.
14. Rivers SL, Patno ME: Cyclophosphamide versus melphalan in the treatment of plasma cell myeloma. JAMA 207:1328–1334, 1969.
15. Fernbach DJ, Sutow WW, Thurman WG: Clinical evaluation of cyclophosphamide: a new agent for the treatment of children with acute leukemia. JAMA 182:30–37, 1962.

16. DeVita VT Jr, Serpick AA, Carbone PP: Combination chemotherapy in the treatment of advanced Hodgkin's disease. Ann Intern Med 73:881–895, 1970.
17. Wolf J, Yesner R, Patno ME: Evaluation of nitrogen mustard in prolonging life of patients with bronchogenic carcinoma. Cancer Chemother Res 16:473–475, 1962.
18. Brown FE, Wright HK: Hypovolemia following intraperitoneal nitrogen mustard therapy. Surg Gynecol Obstet 121:528–530, 1965.
19. VanScott EJ, Kalmanson JD: Complete remission of mycosis fungoides lymphoma induced by topical nitrogen mustard (HN_2). Control of delayed hypersensitivity to HN_2 by desensitization and by induction of specific immunologic tolerance. Cancer 32:18–30, 1973.
20. Greenwald ES: Alkylating agents. In *Cancer Chemotherapy,* second edition. Edited by ES Greenwald. Flushing, New York, Medical Examination Publishing Company, 1973, pp 89–91.
21. Greenwald ES: Cancer chemotherapy. Part I. NY State J Med 72:2541–2556, 1972.
22. Smith JP, Rutledge F, Wharton JT: Chemotherapy of ovarian cancer. New approaches to treatment. Cancer 30:1565–1571, 1972.
23. Young RC, Hubbard SP, DeVita VT Jr: The chemotherapy of ovarian cancer. Cancer Treatment Rev 1:99–110, 1974.
24. Fisher B, Carbone P, Economu SG, et al: l-Phenylalanine mustard (L-PAM) in the management of primary breast cancer. A report of early findings. N Engl J Med 292:117–122, 1975.
25. Goldstein M: The management of acute leukemia. In *Cancer Chemotherapy,* second edition. Edited by ES Greenwald. Flushing, New York, Medical Examination Publishing Company, 1973, pp 378–394.
26. Bonadonna G, Brusamolino E, Valagussa P, et al: Combination chemotherapy as an adjuvant treatment in operable breast cancer. N Engl J Med 294:405–410, 1976.
27. Weiss HD, Walker MD, Wiernik PH: Neurotoxicity of commonly used antineoplastic agents. N Engl J Med 291:75–81, 1974.
28. Greenwald ES: Organic mental changes with fluorouracil therapy. JAMA 235:241–249, 1976.
29. Greenwald ES: Fluorouracil. JAMA 232:1126–1127, 1975.
30. Vaitkevicius VK, Brennan MJ, Beckett VL, et al: Clinical evaluation of cancer chemotherapy with 5-fluorouracil. Cancer 14:131–152, 1961.
31. Greenwald ES: Purine antagonists. In *Cancer Chemotherapy,* second edition. Edited by ES Greenwald. Flushing, New York, Medical Examination Publishing Company, 1973, pp 186–197.
32. Hertz R, Ross GT, Lipsett MB: Chemotherapy in woman with trophoblastic disease: choriocarcinoma, chorioadenoma destruens, and complicated hydatidiform mole. Ann NY Acad Sci 114:881–885, 1964.
33. Simone J: Acute lymphocytic leukemia in childhood. Semin Hematol 11:25–39, 1974.
34. Canellos GP, DeVita VT, Gold GL, et al: Combination chemotherapy for advanced breast cancer: response and effect on survival. Ann Intern Med 84:389–392, 1976.
35. Leone LA, Albala MM, Rege VB: Treatment of carcinoma of the head and neck with intravenous methotrexate. Cancer 21:828–837, 1968.
36. Frei E III, Jaffe N, Tattersall MHN, et al: New approaches to cancer chemotherapy with methotrexate. N Engl J Med 292:846–851, 1975.
37. Weinstein GD, Roenigk H, Maibach H: Psoriasis-liver-methotrexate interaction. Arch Dermatol 108:36–42, 1973.
38. Robbins KM, Gribetz I, Strauss L: Pneumonitis in acute lymphatic leukemia during methotrexate therapy. J Pediatr 82:84–88, 1973.
39. Nicholson HO: Cytotoxic drugs in pregnancy: review and reported cases. J Obstet Gynaecol Br Commonw 75:307–312, 1968.
40. Bloomfield CD, Weiss RB, Fortuny I, et al: Combined chemotherapy with cyclophosphamide, vinblastine, procarbazine, and prednisone (CVPP) for patients with advanced Hodgkin's disease—an alternative program to MOPP. Cancer 38:42–48, 1976.
41. Cvitkovic E, Hayes D, Golbey R: Primary combination chemotherapy (VAB III) for metastic or unresectable germ cell tumors. Am Soc Clin Oncol Abstracts, 1976, p 296.
42. Samuels ML, Johnson DE, Holyoye PY, et al: Large dose bleomycin therapy and pulmonary toxicity. A possible role of prior radiotherapy. JAMA 235:1117–1120, 1976.
43. Goldman J, Greenwald ES, Schulman PL: Vinblastine therapy of Kaposi's sarcoma. NY State J Med 74:1828–1831, 1974.

44. Henderson ES: Treatment of acute leukemia. Semin Hematol 6:271–319, 1969.
45. D'Angio GJ, Beckwith JB, Bishop HC, et al: Childhood cancer: the national Wilms' tumor study. A progress report. Urology 3:798–806, 1974.
46. James DH Jr, Hustu O, Wrenn EL: Combination chemotherapy of childhood neuroblastoma. JAMA 194:123–126, 1965.
47. Holland JF: Vincristine treatment of advanced cancer: a cooperative study of 392 cases. Cancer Res 33:1258–1264, 1973.
48. Cutting HO: Inappropriate secretion of antidiuretic hormone secondary to vincristine therapy. Am J Med Sci 5:269–271, 1971.
49. Blum RH, Carter SK, Agre K: A clinical review of bleomycin. A new antineoplastic agent. Cancer 31:903–914, 1973.
50. DeLena M, Guzzon A, Montardini S, et al: Clinical, radiologic, and histopathologic studies on pulmonary toxicity induced by treatment with bleomycin (NSC-125066). Cancer Chemother Rep Part I 56:343–356, 1972.
51. Goldstein DP, Facog PW, Shirley RL: Actinomycin D as initial therapy of gestational trophoblastic disease. Obstet Gynecol 39:341–345, 1972.
52. Gottlieb JA, Baker LH, O'Bryan RM, et al: Adriamycin (NSC-123127) used alone and in combination for soft tissue and bony sarcomas. Cancer Chemother Rep Part III 6:271–282, 1975.
53. Farber SF, Mitus AT: Role of actinomycin D (dactinomycin) in pediatric oncology. In *Actinomycin: Nature, Formation and Activities.* Edited by SA Waksman. New York, Interscience Publishers, 1968, pp 137–145.
54. Tan CTC, Dargeon HW, Burchenal JH: The effect of actinomycin D on cancer in childhood. Pediatrics 24:544–561, 1959.
55. Cortes EP, Holland JF, Wang JJ, et al: Adriamycin and amputation in primary osteogenic sarcoma. Am Soc Clin Oncol Abstracts, 1974, p 170.
56. Rosen G, Tan C, Sanmaneechai A, et al: The rationale for multiple drug chemotherapy in the treatment of osteogenic sarcoma. Cancer 35:936–945, 1975.
57. Torney DC: Adriamycin (NSC 123127) in breast cancer: an overview of studies. Cancer Chemother Rep Part III 6:319–328, 1975.
58. Gottlieb JA, Gutterman JU, McCreadie KB: Chemotherapy of malignant lymphoma with adriamycin. Cancer Res 33:3024–3028, 1973.
59. Wang JJ, Corest E, Sinks LF, et al: Therapeutic effect and toxicity of adriamycin in patients with neoplastic disease. Cancer 28:837–843, 1971.
60. Lefrak EA, Ditha J, Rosenbaum S: A clinicopathologic analysis of adriamycin cardiotoxicity. Cancer 32:302–314, 1973.
61. Merrill J, Greco FA, Zimbler H, et al: Synergistic cardiotoxicity. Ann Intern Med 82:122–123, 1975.

CARDIOVASCULAR—RENAL AGENTS

20. DIGITALIS GLYCOSIDES

David H. Huffman

The digitalis glycosides are the most useful and reliable of drugs for producing long-term increases in myocardial contractility. In addition, they are useful in the treatment of atrial tachyarrhythmias and for ventricular rate control in patients with atrial fibrillation or flutter. Because of these effects they have a deserved and well-recognized place in the treatment of patients with congestive heart failure and the above tachyarrhythmias.

It is no longer acceptable to place all patients with congestive heart failure (CHF) on a digitalis preparation and a diuretic without considering possible explanations for the clinical syndrome. These explanations include: (1) systemic hypertension; (2) pulmonary hypertension (due to chronic obstructive pulmonary disease, pulmonary emboli, etc.); (3) pericardial disease (eg, cardiac tamponade); (4) myocardial disease (eg, arteriosclerotic heart disease, myocardiopathy); (5) endocardial disease (eg, valvular heart disease, subacute bacterial endocarditis); (6) congenital abnormalities; (7) trauma; (8) mediastinal problems which restrict output; (9) excessive fluid overload; and (10) hypermetabolic conditions (eg, thyrotoxicosis, arterio-venous fistulae, Paget's disease, psoriasis, etc.). Failure to recognize and correct any of these factors may reduce the ability of the individual patient to respond to traditional methods of treatment of congestive heart failure. Additional factors which may make the patient with CHF refractory to conventional therapy include: (1) poor patient compliance; (2) inadequate therapeutic program; (3) iatrogenic factors (eg, overuse of digitalis and diuretics, hypokalemia or hyponatremia); (4) arrhythmias; (5) occurrence of a pulmonary embolus; (6) progression of the natural course, ie, the basic disease process; (7) development of a myocardiopathy; (8) development of a hypermetabolic state, such as fever or hyperthyroidism; (9) development of anemia, anoxia or other factors which increase cardiac output; and (10) development of a complicated disorder such as a neoplasm or an infectious disease process (eg, pneumonia). The approach to the patient should be to consider those factors which are reversible and to correct these abnormalities whenever possible.

The control of ventricular rate and atrial tachyarrhythmias is a well-established and long-recognized indication for the use of digitalis. In general, there is a successive decrease in ventricular rate as the dose of digitalis is increased. A plateau in ventricular rate control may be reached due to associated factors (fever, hypoxia, anemia, etc.) which increase cardiac rate. Care, therefore, should be exercised to avoid excessive doses of digitalis in these circumstances because of the possibility of toxicity.

PHARMACOLOGIC PROPERTIES

The basic pharmacologic properties of digitalis compounds are examined in recent reviews.[1–5] The various digitalis glycosides have few differences in their basic pharmacodynamic and toxicological properties. The major differences between the glycosides are in their pharmacokinetics (ie, absorption, distribution, metabolism, and routes of excretion). Digitalis increases the force of myocardial contraction. This inotropic effect makes digitalis useful in the management of congestive heart failure. In addition to this inotropic effect, digitalis has a number of electrophysiological effects on the heart including alterations in automaticity, excitability, conduction velocity, and refractory period. It is the latter effects, particularly the ability to decrease the rate of impulse propagation through the AV node, which makes digitalis useful in controlling ventricular rate in patients with atrial fibrillation. In addition, digitalis exerts a clinically important effect on myocardial oxygen consumption. This effect will depend upon the hemodynamic state of the patient. In the patient with CHF there is dilation of the ventricles with an increase in the left ventricular end-diastolic pressure and volume. At any given end-diastolic volume, the resulting stroke ejection fraction is decreased. Digitalis acts to reverse this process by increasing the work capacity at any given end-diastolic volume or pressure, thus reducing the residual systolic blood volume and dilated heart toward normal. Associated with these changes is an improvement in myocardial oxygen consumption, since the amount of cardiac work required to produce a certain cardiac output is less with the small ventricle than with a dilated filling chamber.

The pharmacokinetic differences for ouabain, digoxin and digitoxin, the three drugs for which good clinical pharmacokinetic data are available, are given in Table 1.[1-10] It is important to remember that the steady-state digitalis concentration and, correspondingly, the therapeutic effect of the drug is directly related to the maintenance digitalis dose, the fraction of the dose absorbed, and the half-life of the glycoside in that patient. The digitalis concentration is inversely related to the apparent distribution volume (which is related to lean body mass and is influenced by both renal[11,12] and thyroid function[13]) and the dosing interval.[14] Patients with ischemic heart disease tend to be more sensitive to digitalis and are more prone to develop toxicity at lower blood levels.[1] It is important, whenever possible, to determine the presence of other factors such as renal function, age, thyroid function, acidosis, hypokalemia, hypoxemia, hypomagnesemia, and hypercalcemia. All of these are important in determining the response of the individual patient to the digitalis compounds. These factors may alter the expected clinical response based on the serum digitalis concentration. Thus, clinical judgement remains the most important and essential factor in determining the appropriate therapy with digitalis compounds.

TABLE 1 Pharmacokinetic Parameters for the Useful Cardiac Glycosides

	Digitoxin	Digoxin	Ouabain
Oral absorption	90–100%	60–85%	Unreliable
Average half-life	7 days	1.7 days	0.9 day
Protein binding	86–95%	25%	?
Major route of elimination	1. Hepatic	1. Renal 2. Hepatic	1. Renal 2. Hepatic
Therapeutic level (6–8 hours after dose)	10–25 ng/ml	0.9–2.1 ng/ml	?
Toxic level	>35 ng/ml	>3 ng/ml	?

CHOICE OF A DIGITALIS DRUG

The choice of one preparation over another is generally based upon pharmacokinetic considerations, and how rapidly the digitalis effect is required. In recent years digoxin has been used with greater frequency than digitoxin or ouabain. Digoxin has a more rapid onset of action and a shorter half-life than does digitoxin. Although ouabain has rapid onset of action and a shorter half-life than digoxin, ouabain is not used for chronic digitalis therapy because of its erratic and poor oral absorption. Nonetheless, there are many clinical circumstances where digitoxin is a reasonable alternative to digoxin. Since digitoxin has a longer half-life, fluctuations in the serum digitoxin level will be less marked than they are with digoxin. Therefore, a missed dose will not result in a major change in the serum digitoxin. In addition, unlike digoxin, the pharmacokinetics of digitoxin are not greatly affected by renal failure.

The use of digitalis in acute myocardial infarction is controversial. Studies in animals[15,16] indicate that digitalis may increase the infarct size or increase the incidence of serious arrhythmias. No increase in ventricular tachyarrhythmias after intravenous digoxin was observed in patients.[17] This suggests that any increased sensitivity to digitalis during an acute myocardial infarction will be related to accompanying complications (eg, electrolyte imbalance, acidosis, hypoxia, or increased sympathetic tone) rather than the infarction itself.[18]

An additional controversial area is prophylatic digitalization. In one study,[19] however, the incidence of supraventricular arrhythmias decreased in patients who were given prophylactic digoxin prior to cardiac surgery.

ADVERSE REACTIONS

In a recent prospective study of 15% of patients taking digitalis on admission to a large hospital, 23% were found to have definite digitalis toxicity by serial electrocardiogram.[20] The importance of this problem is emphasized by the fact that the digitalis drugs are among the most frequently encountered drugs in toxicity surveys.[21,22] Therefore, the physician must be constantly aware of the possibility of digitalis toxicity and obtain the appropriate laboratory tests to substantiate the diagnosis. Although factors such as weight, dose and renal function are important in determining if the digitalis dose is too large, the most useful laboratory test for the diagnosis of digitalis intoxication appears to be digitalis radioimmunoassay.[20,23–27] Patients with atrial fibrillation can tolerate higher levels of digitalis without development of digitalis intoxication.[28] However, it is rarely necessary or advisable to increase the digitalis level to greater than that outlined in Table 1.

Criteria for clinical digitalis toxicity vary, but arrhythmias due to digitalis are the most important toxic manifestations. The patient should be questioned regarding gastrointestinal and visual symptoms, but these symptoms (with the exception of anorexia) correlate poorly with digitalis intoxication. Many different arrhythmias may occur in digitalis intoxication. They include ventricular premature beats; ventricular tachycardia; ventricular fibrillation; and various AV junctional problems, such as nonparoxysmal AV junction tachycardia and AV junctional escape rhythms. Atrial tachycardia with block as well as second and third degree heart blocks can occur. It is important when approaching a patient with suspected digitalis toxicity to consider the following questions:

(1) Are there predisposing factors, such as excessive dosage, reduced clearance, and other factors mentioned above, which increase myocardial susceptibility to digitalis?

(2) Are there extracardiac symptoms?

(3) Is there a cardiac arrhythmia and, most importantly, what happens to the arrhythmia with digitalis withheld?

(4) What is the serum digitalis concentration, keeping in mind the need to individualize interpretation of the digitalis blood level with respect to the individual patient?

The approach to the patient with digitalis toxicity is to monitor the patient carefully. If treatment is required, phenytoin and lidocaine are the agents of choice since these drugs do not decrease conduction velocity. Other forms include potassium replacement, propranolol, quinidine, and procainamide; however, these must be used with caution because they may potentiate the AV block produced by digitalis. If the patient is hypokalemic, however, replacement of potassium may be particularly helpful. Newer developments include the use of cholestyramine and activated charcoal to interrupt the enterohepatic cycle of digitoxin and possibly digoxin. The use of F_{ab} fragments of digoxin antibodies to treat massive overdose of digoxin has been described.[29]

DRUG AND DISEASE INTERACTIONS

The absorption of digoxin is incomplete and variable.[30-33] Clinically significant variations in the bioavailability of digoxin preparations have been demonstrated.[34] Although there is a correlation between the *in vivo* bioavailability of digoxin and the *in vitro* dissolution of the tablet[35,36] there are exceptions to this generalization.[37] The absorption of digoxin is impaired in some disease states with malabsorption[38,39] or alteration in gastrointestinal motility.[40] Neomycin and certain antacids (eg, aluminum hydroxide suspension) decrease the absorption of digoxin.[41,42] The extent of digoxin absorption, in contrast, is not affected by food,[43] partial gastrectomy[44] or jejunal-ileal bypass surgery.[45] The absorption and enterohepatic cycling of both digoxin and digitoxin is decreased by the oral administration of cholestyramine and presumably colestipol.[46,47] The absorption of digitoxin is nearly complete. The binding of digitoxin is decreased in patients with renal failure.[48,49] Despite this, no differences in the pharmacokinetics of digitoxin in renal failure were observed.[50] In contrast, both the distribution volume and the rate of clearance of digoxin are decreased in patients with renal failure. Therefore, the digoxin dose must be decreased in patients with renal failure regardless of the etiology. It is rarely necessary to exceed a digoxin maintenance dose of 2 to 3 μg/kg in patients with renal failure.

CONCLUSIONS

The digitalis glycosides remain the most useful and reliable drugs for producing a long-term increase in myocardial contractility. Accordingly, they have a deserved place in the treatment of CHF. It is important to consider the other factors involved in the development of CHF. The classical concept that heart failure is always an indication for digitalis therapy probably needs revision. In particular, patients with myocardiopathy, myocarditis, constrictive pericarditis, etc. are less responsive to digitalis and may be more prone to toxicity. Digoxin is used with greater frequency than the other digitalis preparations. However, in certain situations, digitoxin may be a more useful drug, particularly in the long-term management of a patient with chronic CHF. There are relatively few circumstances when the use of deslanoside and ouabain are indicated. Since it is a mixture of different substances, primarily digitoxin, digitalis leaf has no value. Most patients can be treated effectively with either digoxin or digitoxin. The choice of the two depends upon the rapidity with which the effect is desired and the chronicity of anticipated therapy. Finally, one should always assess the continued need for digitalis therapy. This is particularly important in the elderly patient who for various reasons may be more sensitive to the adverse effects of digitalis.[51,52]

DRUG MONOGRAPHS

DIGITALIS LEAF

This preparation is a mixture of various cardiac glycosides, the most important glycoside being digitoxin. Its potency is standardized biologically. Digitalis leaf lacks versatility, in that absorption is apparently incomplete and therefore variable from patient to patient. Digitalis leaf offers no advantages over digitoxin and for this reason is not recommended.

Adverse Reactions—See introduction.

Interactions—See introduction.

Dosage—Oral: Adults, loading dose of 100 to 150 mg three or four times daily for three days to a maximum of 1.5 grams. The maintenance dose is 150 mg (range 100 to 200 mg) daily for five to seven days each week. The dose must be reduced by 25 to 50 percent in elderly patients or in small patients with decreased lean body mass, or for those patients with ischemic heart disease or metabolic and electrolyte or impaired renal function disturbances.

DIGITOXIN

Digitoxin is the principal active glycoside and, on a weight basis, is 1000 times more active than digitalis leaf. Digitoxin has the advantage of a long (5 to 7 days) half-life and near-complete absorption. This makes it suitable for long-term maintenance therapy, since a patient may miss a dose and not have a significant decrease in clinical effect. Although digitoxin absorption is reportedly complete, bioavailability differences for different tablets do exist.[53] Digitoxin has a substantial enterohepatic recirculation, which can be interrupted by cholestyramine.[46] Although digitoxin is metabolized to a variety of compounds, including digoxin, these metabolites do not contribute appreciably to the pharmacokinetics of digitoxin.[9] It is

TABLE 2 Preparations and Costs of Digitalis Glycosides

GENERIC NAME	TRADEMARK NAME(S)	PREPARATIONS AND 1978 COSTS
Deslanoside	Cedilanid-D	Injection (solution) 0.2 mg/ml—$0.38/2-ml ampul, $0.61/4-ml ampul
Digitalis Leaf	generic	Capsules or tablets 100 mg—$1.80–$2.16/100
Digitoxin	Crystodigin (Purodigin)	Tablets 0.05 mg—$0.81/100; 0.1 mg—$1.14/100; 0.15 mg—$1.44/100; 0.2 mg—$1.73/100 Injection (solution) 0.2 mg/ml—$0.37/1-ml ampul
Digoxin	Lanoxin	Tablets 0.125 mg—$0.95/100; 0.25 mg—$1.03/100; 0.5 mg—$1.85/100 Elixir 0.05 mg/ml—$1.30/2 oz Injection (solution) 0.1 mg/ml—$0.22/1-ml ampul; 0.25 mg/ml—$0.21/2-ml ampul
Ouabain	generic	Injection (solution) 0.25 mg/ml—$0.55/2-ml ampul

highly protein bound, 93 to 95%, and this may present problems when there is concomitant administration of acidic drugs which might displace digitoxin from plasma protein binding sites. Patients with renal insufficiency have decreased binding of digitoxin. However, in a single dose study, digitoxin pharmacokinetics were not altered in renal insufficiency.[50] There is correlation between the serum digitoxin concentration (obtained 8 to 12 hours after a dose) and digitoxin intoxication.[27] A therapeutic concentration is from 10 to 25 ng/ml. Most patients with digitoxin concentration greater than 35 ng/ml will manifest signs or symptoms of toxicity.

Adverse Reactions—See introduction.

Interactions—See introduction.

Dosage—Oral, Intravenous: Adults, for treatment of patients with congestive heart failure who have not received digitoxin or other digitalis preparations for two to three weeks, the initial loading dose would be 1.2 mg (range: 1 to 1.5 mg), given in divided doses at six to eight hour intervals. The maintenance dose varies from 0.05 to 0.2 mg daily and depends upon lean body mass of the individual. Loading and maintenance doses should be reduced by 25 to 50% in elderly patients or in those with metabolic or electrolyte disturbances. It is probably not necessary to reduce the dose because of renal insufficiency *per se*, but these patients often have reduced body mass and accordingly may have a decreased digitoxin distribution volume. *Children,* for newborn infants, 0.075 mg/kg; infants under 2 years of age, 0.05 mg/kg; younger children 2 to 12 years of age, 0.025 mg/kg; in children over 12 years, the adult dose is satisfactory. Although the maintenance dose is approximately 10% of the loading dose, individualization of the dose on clinical grounds must be made. For patients with supraventricular tachycardia, atrial flutter, or atrial fibrillation, the dose and serum digitoxin concentration is usually based on the ventricular response rate of the individual patient, provided that excessive blood levels of greater than 35 ng/ml are not obtained.

DESLANOSIDE

This cardiac glycoside may be used if rapid initial loading is required, with the intention to substitute a longer-acting glycoside for maintenance therapy. The onset of action of deslanoside is 10 to 30 minutes following injection, with maximum effect at about 2 hours. Therefore, it is helpful in situations in which appreciable digitalis effect is required in a relatively short period of time. These include the management of supraventricular tachycardia and/or acute pulmonary edema.

Adverse Reactions—See introduction.

Interactions—See introduction.

Dosage—Intravenous: Adults, for patients with congestive heart failure who have not received digitalis for at least two weeks, the initial loading dose is 1.2 to 1.6 mg. One-half the loading dose is usually given immediately. This is followed by the remainder in divided doses at 30-minute intervals. The drug can be given on a maintenance basis with a daily dose of 0.4 to 0.5 mg in divided 12-hourly doses. The above dosages must be reduced 25 to 50% in small or elderly patients, or in those who have metabolic or electrolyte disturbances, ischemic heart disease and decreased renal function. *Children,* infants, 0.05 mg/kg; children 2 to 12, 0.025 mg/kg; children 12 and older, adult dose.

DIGOXIN

Digoxin is the most commonly used digitalis glycoside. It can be given orally or intravenously. Its onset of action is within 10 to 20 minutes after intravenous dosage with a maximal effect up to 5 hours. The drug is eliminated with a half-life of 37 to 40 hours. After the last dose, digoxin will be essentially completely eliminated from the body in approximately 6 to 10 days in patients with normal renal function. Digoxin is often used to achieve moderately rapid loading. It is also commonly used for maintenance therapy. The main disadvantages of digoxin are its incomplete and variable gastrointestinal absorption (see introductory comments) and the significant effects that renal insufficiency have on its clearance. Recent studies indicate that digoxin may undergo substantial enterohepatic recycling.[54] The simultaneous use of cholestyramine and orally administered digoxin reduces the absorption and interrupts the enterohepatic recycling of digoxin.[55] Digoxin is not appreciably bound to plasma proteins. It depends on glomerular infiltration for its elimination; consequently, reductions in glomerular filtration rate are associated with proportional reductions in the clearance of digoxin from the body. For example, the half-life of digoxin in a patient with chronic renal failure (creatinine clearance of less than 10 ml/min) is approximately 4.5 to 5.0 days. There is a correlation between the serum digoxin concentration, obtained 8 to 12 hours after a dose, and digoxin intoxication. A therapeutic concentration range is 0.9 to 2.1 ng/ml. Most patients with a serum digoxin concentration greater than 3 ng/ml will manifest symptoms or signs of toxicity.

Adverse Reactions—See introduction.

Interactions—See introduction.

Dosage—Oral or Intravenous: Adults, for patients with congestive heart failure who have not received digitalis for at least two weeks, the initial loading dose is 8 to 15 μg/kg intravenously. For rapid loading, one-half of the dose may be given at once, the remainder of the loading dose may be given in divided doses over the next 24 hours. The maintenance dose of digoxin is a function of lean body weight and the patient's renal function. The oral maintenance dose in the patient with normal renal function should be 2 to 6 μg/kg/day. The oral maintenance dose for the patient with renal insufficiency should be 1 to 3 μg/kg/day. The loading and maintenance doses should be reduced by 20 to 25 percent when digoxin is given intravenously because of its incomplete absorption. In addition, the oral dose should be reduced by 25 to 50% in small or elderly patients, or in those patients with certain metabolic or electrolyte abnormalities, impaired renal function or ischemic heart disease (see introductory comments). *Children,* initial loading dose for newborn infants, 0.04 to 0.06 mg/kg; infants to 2 years, 0.06 to 0.08 mg/kg; children 2 to 10 years, 0.04 to 0.06 mg/kg; maintenance dose, approximately 1/4 of the total loading dose given in single or divided doses. Intramuscular administration of digoxin is associated with considerable pain, elevation in CPK, and erratic and incomplete absorption.[47] Therefore, this mode of administration of digoxin is not recommended.

OUABAIN

This is the most rapidly effective digitalis glycoside available. After intravenous administration, its onset of action is 3 to 10 minutes with a maximum effect for one-half hour. It is eliminated from the body with a half-life of about 20 hours and therefore essentially complete elimination can be anticipated in 3 days. The drug is useful in the treatment of acute pulmonary edema or in the rapid management of atrial tachyarrhythmias where ventricular rate control is critical. Ouabain also is useful to determine the adequacy of digitalis loading since it can be given in small increments. It is usually only given in emergencies. A longer acting glycoside (digoxin or digitoxin) should be given for maintenance once clinical stablization is achieved.

Adverse Reactions—See introduction.

Interactions—See introduction.

Dosage—Intravenous: Adults, for treatment of patients with CHF who have not received digitalis therapy for two weeks the initial loading dose is 0.5 mg by infusion followed by 0.5 mg 8 hours later. No patient should receive a total of more than 1 mg. In the treatment of atrial tachyarrhythmias, it may be necessary to give a larger amount, and the dosage in this case should be titrated based upon the ventricular rate response and consideration of any potential adverse effect. In patients with decreased body mass, impaired renal function, or certain metabolic or electrolyte disturbances and ischemic heart disease, the dosage should be reduced by 25 to 50%, with particular attention to the individual patient's response. *Children,* the usual daily dose is 0.012 to 0.016 mg/kg in divided doses, but the amount can be modified by clinical factors. Occasionally patients are quite sensitive, responding in an excessive fashion to smaller doses.

REFERENCES

1. Smith TW, Haber E: Digitalis. N Engl J Med 289:945–952, 1010–1015, 1063–1072, and 1125–1129, 1973.
2. Lee KS, Klaus W: The subcellular basis for the mechanism of the inotropic action of cardiac glycosides. Pharmacol Rev 23:193–261, 1971.
3. Huffman DH: Clinical use of digitalis glycosides. Am J Hosp Pharm 33:179–185, 1976.
4. Doherty JE, Kane JJ: Clinical pharmacology of digitalis glycosides. Annu Rev Med 26:159–172, 1975.
5. Porter LK: Digitalis toxicity. Drug Intell Clin Pharm 8:700–708, 1974.
6. Marcus FI: Digitalis pharmacokinetics and metabolism. Am J Med 58:452–459, 1975.
7. Doherty JE: Digitalis glycosides. Pharmacokinetics and their clinical implications. Ann Intern Med 79:229–238, 1973.
8. Smith TW: Digitalis: contribution of quantitative assay techniques to the understanding of the clinical pharmacology of digitalis. Circulation 46:188–192, 1972.
9. Storstein L: Studies on digitalis. III. Biliary excretion and enterohepatic circulation of digitoxin and its cardioactive metabolites. Clin Pharmacol Ther 17:313–320, 1975.
10. Vohringer HF, Rietbrock N: Metabolism and excretion of digitoxin in man. Clin Pharmacol Ther 16:796–806, 1974.
11. Reuning RH, Sams RA, Notari RE: Role of pharmacokinetics in drug dosage adjustment. I. Pharmacologic effect of kinetics and apparent volume of distribution of digoxin. J Clin Pharmacol 13:127–141, 1973.
12. Jusko WJ, Weintraub M: Myocardial distribution of digoxin and renal function. Clin Pharmacol Ther 16:449–454, 1974.
13. Doherty JE, Perkins WH: Digoxin metabolism in hypo- and hyperthyroidism: studies with tritiated digoxin in thyroid disease. Ann Intern Med 64:489–507, 1966.
14. Wagner JG, Northam JI, Alway CD, et al: Blood levels of drug at equilibrium state after multiple dosing. Nature 207:1301–1304, 1965.
15. Beller GA, Smith TW, Hood WB Jr: Altered distribution of tritiated digoxin in the infarcted canine left ventricle. Circulation 46:572–579, 1972.
16. Thompson AJ, Hargis J, Murphy ML, et al: Tritiated digoxin XX: tissue distribution in experimental myocardial infarction. Am Heart J 88:319–324, 1974.
17. Reicansky I, Conradson TB, Holmberg S, et al: The effect of intravenous digoxin on the occurrence of ventricular tachyarrhythmias in acute myocardial infarction. Am Heart J 91:705–711, 1976.
18. Karliner JS, Braunwald E: Present status of digitalis treatment in acute myocardial infarction. Circulation 45:891–902, 1972.
19. Johnson LW, Dickstein RH, Fruehan CT, et al: Prophylactic digitalization for coronary artery bypass surgery. Circulation 53:819–822, 1976.
20. Beller GA, Smith TW, Abelmann WH, et al: Digitalis intoxication. A prospective clinical study with serum level correlations. N Engl J Med 284:989–997, 1971.
21. Ogilvie RI, Ruedy J: Adverse drug reactions during hospitalizations. Can Med Assoc J 97:1450–1456, 1971.
22. Miller RR: Hospital admissions due to adverse drug reactions: a report from the Boston Collaborative Drug Surveillance Program. Arch Intern Med 134:219–223, 1974.
23. Butler VP Jr, Chien JP: Digoxin-specific antibodies. Proc Natl Acad Sci 57:71–78, 1967.
24. Smith TW, Butler VP Jr, Haber E: Determinations of therapeutic and toxic serum digoxin concentrations by radioimmunoassay. N Engl J Med 281:1212–1216, 1969.
25. Grahame-Smith DG, Everett MD: Measurement of digoxin in plasma and its use in the diagnosis of digoxin intoxication. Br Med J 1:286–289, 1969.
26. Huffman DH, Crow J, Pentikainen P, et al: Association between clinical cardiac status, laboratory parameters and digoxin usage. Am Heart J 91:28–34, 1976.
27. Smith TW: Radioimmunoassay for serum digitoxin concentration: methodology and clinical experience. J Pharmacol Exp Ther 175:352–360, 1970.
28. Goldman S, Probst P, Selzer A, et al: Inefficacy of 'therapeutic' serum levels of digoxin in controlling ventricular rate in atrial fibrillation. Am J Cardiol 35:651–655, 1975.
29. Smith TW, Haber E, Yeatman L, et al: Reversal of advanced digoxin intoxication with F_{ab} fragments of digoxin specific antibodies. N Engl J Med 294:797–800, 1976.
30. Lindenbaum J, Mellow MH, Blackstone MD, et al: Variation in biologic availability of digoxin from four preparations. N Engl J Med 285:1344–1347, 1971.

31. Shaw TRD, Howard MR, Hamer J: Variation in the biologic availability of digoxin. Lancet 2:303–307, 1972.
32. Manninen V, Melin J, Hartel G: Serum digoxin concentrations during treatment with different preparations. Lancet 1:1215–1218, 1971.
33. Wagner JG, Christensen M, Sakmar E, et al: Equivalence lack in digoxin plasma levels. JAMA 224:199–204, 1973.
34. Shaw TRD: Clinical problems associated with variable biologic availability of digoxin. Am Heart J 87:399–401, 1974.
35. Lindenbaum J, Butler VP Jr, Murphy JE: Correlation of digoxin-tablet dissolution rate with biological availability. Lancet 1:1215–1218, 1973.
36. Johnson BF, Greer H, McCrerie J, et al: Rate of dissolution of digoxin as a predictor of absorption. Lancet 1:1473–1477, 1973.
37. Bochner F, Huffman DH, Shen DD, et al: Bioavailability of digoxin-hydroquinone complex: a new oral digoxin formulation. J Pharm Sci 66:644–647, 1976.
38. Heizer WD, Smith TW, Goldfinger SE: Absorption of digoxin in patients with malabsorption syndromes. N Engl J Med 285:257–259, 1971.
39. Jusko WJ, Conti DR, Molson A, et al: Digoxin absorption from tablets and elixir. The effect of radiation induced malabsorption syndromes. JAMA 230:1554–1555, 1974.
40. Manninen V, Apajalahti A, Melin J, et al: Altered absorption of digoxin in patients given propantheline and metoclopramide. Lancet 1:398–399, 1973.
41. Lindenbaum J, Maulitz RM, Butler VP Jr: Inhibition of digoxin absorption by neomycin. Gastroenterology 71:399–404, 1976.
42. Brown DD, Juhl RP: Decreased bioavailability of digoxin due to antacids and kaolin-pectin. N Engl J Med 295:1034–1037, 1976.
43. Greenblatt DJ, Duhme DW, Koch-Weser J, et al: Bioavailability of digoxin tablets and elixir in the fasting and postprandial states. Clin Pharmacol Ther 16:444–448, 1974.
44. Beermann B, Hellstrom K, Rosen A: The gastrointestinal absorption of digoxin in seven patients with gastric or small intestinal reconstructions. Acta Med Scand 193:293–297, 1973.
45. Marcus FI, Horton H, Jacogs S, et al: The effect of jejuno-ileal bypass in patients with morbid obesity on the pharmacokinetics of digoxin in man. Am J Cardiol 37:154, 1976.
46. Caldwell JH, Bush CA, Greenberger NJ: Interruption of the enterohepatic circulation of digitoxin by cholestyramine: effect on metabolic disposition of tritium labeled digitoxin and cardiac systolic intervals in man. J Clin Invest 50:2638–2644, 1971.
47. Greenblatt DJ, Duhme DW, Koch-Weser J: Evaluation of digoxin bioavailability in single dose studies. N Engl J Med 289:651–654, 1973.
48. Shoeman DW, Azarnoff DL: The alteration of plasma proteins in uremia as reflected in their ability to bind digitoxin and diphenylhydantoin. Pharmacology 7:169–177, 1972.
49. Kramer P, Kothe E, Saul J, et al: Uremic and normal plasma binding of various cardiac glycosides under 'in vivo' conditions. Eur J Clin Invest 4:53–58, 1974.
50. Vohringer HF, Rietbrock N, Spurney P, et al: Disposition of digitoxin in renal failure. Clin Pharmacol Ther 19:387–395, 1976.
51. Kelliher GJ, Roberts J: Effect of age on the cardiotoxic action of digitalis. J Pharmacol Exp Ther 197:10–18, 1976.
52. Fowvose HA: The efficacy of digitalis withdrawal in an institutionalized aged population. J Am Geriatr Soc 22:208–211, 1974.
53. Stoll RG, Christensen MS, Sakmar E, et al: Determination of bioavailability of digitoxin using the radioimmunoassay procedure. J Pharm Sci 62:1615–1620, 1973.
54. Caldwell JH, Cline HT: Biliary excretion of digoxin in man. Clin Pharmacol Ther 19:410–415, 1976.
55. Smith TW: New approaches to the management of digitalis intoxication. In *Symposium on Digitalis*. Edited by O Storstein. Oslo, Norway, Glydendal Norsk Forlag, 1974, p 312.

21. ANTIARRHYTHMIC AGENTS

David J. Greenblatt

Disorders of cardiac rhythm detected and classified by 'macro' methods such as electrocardiography actually represent a summation of actions and interactions of numerous cardiac muscle and nerve cells having specialized and complex functions. Much has been learned about the electrophysiological and mechanical functions of these cells, as well as the effects of various antiarrhythmic agents upon their functions.[1,2] However, cellular physiology still does not reliably predict the manifestations and time-course of clinical disorders of cardiac rhythm. Furthermore, the effects of various antiarrhythmic agents upon cellular physiology in vitro do not predict or correlate with their clinical efficacy or toxicity in the actual treatment of cardiac arrhythmias. Thus the clinical management of disorders of heart rhythm is largely an empirical science, based upon experience, epidemiology, and trial and error.

Antiarrhythmic therapy generally involves four sequential steps: (a) the diagnosis and classification of the rhythm disorder, (b) the decision as to whether pharmacotherapy is indicated, (c) the choice of one or more specific antiarrhythmic agents, and (d) the choice of dose, dosage schedule, and route of administration that will maximize the likelihood of therapeutic benefit while minimizing the probability of unwanted side effects.

DIAGNOSIS AND CLASSIFICATION OF CARDIAC ARRHYTHMIAS

Prompt and accurate identification of cardiac rhythm disturbances is a critical requisite for proper pharmacologic treatment.[3] Electrocardiography, the major diagnostic tool, accordingly receives high priority in all training programs in clinical medicine.

The two most important systems of arrhythmia classification focus on the mechanism of the arrhythmia and upon its anatomic correlates (Table 1).

TABLE 1 Classification of Cardiac Arrhythmias

Tachyarrhythmias and ectopic rhythm disorders

- Sinus tachycardia
- Paroxysmal atrial tachycardia
- Atrial premature contractions (APC)
- Paroxysmal atrial tachycardia (PAT)
- Multifocal atrial tachycardia
- Atrial fibrillation (AF)
- Atrial flutter

- Junctional premature contractions
- Accelerated junctional rhythm
- Junctional tachycardia

- Ventricular premature contraction (VPC)
- Ventricular tachycardia
- Ventricular fibrillation (VF)
- Parasystole

Conduction disturbances and bradyarrhythmias

- Atrioventricular (A-V) block
  - First degree
  - Second degree (including Wenckebach phenomenon)
  - Third degree (complete heart block)
- Bundle branch blocks
- Sinus bradycardia (including sick sinus syndrome)
- Slow junctional rhythm
- Asystole

Functional Classification of Arrhythmia Mechanisms

Functional schemes used to classify the mechanism of rhythm disturbances greatly oversimplify and in fact may bear no relation to molecular and electrophysiologic mechanisms. Nonetheless, understanding of arrhythmias in clinical practice can be enhanced by their categorization either as (a) disorders involving excessive or inappropriate activity of cardiac cells, or (b) disorders involving depressed automaticity or reduced velocity of impulse conduction.

Arrhythmias caused by excessive and inappropriate depolarization are often termed tachyarrhythmias or ectopic rhythm disturbances.[4] One subgroup of disorders involves relatively infrequent and random depolarization of single ectopic foci, as in the case of unifocal APC's or VPC's. A single ectopic focus may also depolarize at a relatively rapid and regular rate, as in the case of atrial flutter, PAT, or junctional tachycardia. Finally, depolarization from multiple ectopic foci may occur rapidly and chaotically, as in the case of AF, multifocal atrial tachycardia, or VF. Many clinical arrhythmias involve combinations of the above. The primary pharmacologic action of most antiarrhythmic agents used in clinical practice is the suppression of such tachyarrhythmias and ectopic rhythm disorders.

The second mechanistic class of rhythm disorders includes those with reduced automaticity and/or impaired impulse conduction, sometimes termed the bradyarrhythmias and conduction disturbances. Clinical consequences of these arrhythmias depend largely on the overall rate of ventricular contraction, which in turn is a major determinant of cardiac output. Rates of 30 to 40 contractions per minute or even less are occasionally observed in healthy, highly trained athletes. However, such slow rates generally indicate significant pathology, particularly when they occur in the setting of ischemic heart disease. Various degrees of atrioventricular (A-V) block may underlie ventricular bradyarrhythmias, inasmuch as proper transmission of sinus impulses via the A-V conduction system is an important determinant of ventricular rate. It is increasingly recognized that many tachyarrhythmias observed in clinical practice may actually result from impaired conduction in a segment of cardiac tissue. 'Reentry' of a delayed, slowly conducted impulse into normal cardiac tissue can depolarize the entire myocardium, causing what appears to be an ectopic beat.

Many drugs are available for the suppression of tachyarrhythmias, but few if any can be counted on to combat conduction disturbances and bradyarrhythmias—those that are available either are relatively ineffective or produce intolerable side effects. Persistent, clinically important bradyarrhythmias and conduction disturbances generally require placement of man-made electrical pacemakers for definitive control. An important problem associated with antiarrhythmic drug therapy is that iatrogenic bradyarrhythmias and/or conduction disturbances can result from excessive—or even seemingly appropriate—doses of most of the widely used antiarrhythmic agents. Thus, bradyarrhythmia may be an unwanted consequence of drug therapy of tachyarrhythmias. Finally, a perplexing group of cardiac rhythm disorders involve combinations of tachy- and bradyarrhythmias, or alternations from one to another. These hybrid disorders usually require a pacemaker since treatment with the usual antiarrhythmic agents may suppress ectopic activity at the expense of exacerbating the bradyarrhythmia.

Anatomic Classification of Rhythm Disorders

Identification of the apparent anatomic origin of cardiac arrhythmias may also be critical for the proper choice of antiarrhythmic agent. The three obvious sites are the atrium, the ventricle, or the intervening conduction system. Tachy- or bradyarrhythmias may develop at any of these sites. For reasons that are poorly understood, antiarrhythmic agents may be effective at suppressing ectopic rhythm disorders at one site, but essentially ineffective at another.

ASSESSING THE NEED FOR PHARMACOLOGIC THERAPY

Following correct identification and classification of a rhythm disturbance, the clinician's decision as to whether drug therapy is indicated depends in large part upon the possible consequences of the rhythm disorder (Table 2). At least three areas of concern can be

TABLE 2 Consequences of Cardiac Arrhythmias

I. Prognostic significance
   1. Definite precursor of life-threatening arrhythmia
   2. Possible precursor of life-threatening arrhythmia
   3. Not associated with subsequent life-threatening arrhythmia

II. Effects on cardiac output
   1. Zero cardiac output—incompatible with life
   2. Low cardiac output—not sufficient for maintained perfusion of vital organs (i.e., brain, heart, kidney)
   3. Low cardiac output—adequate perfusion of vital organs but not skeletal muscle
   4. Stress intolerance—cardiac output adequate under "normal" circumstances, but not under "stress" (i.e., exercise, intercurrent illness, etc.)
   5. Normal cardiac output under all conditions

III. Subjective effects
   1. Intolerable
   2. Tolerable but disquieting or inconvenient
   3. Asymptomatic

identified. One important consideration is the prognostic significance of the arrhythmia. Some arrhythmias are clear precursors of more serious or life-threatening disturbances, while others have no prognostic significance. In most cases, the prognostic importance is not known with certainty. The influence of the arrhythmia on cardiac output is a second important area of concern. Rhythm disorders can have a range of secondary effects on cardiac output, varying from complete cessation of cardiac function to negligible effects on cardiac output. Needless to say, the need for treatment becomes more urgent as cardiac function becomes more impaired. Finally, clinicians must consider the subjective effects of the rhythm disorder, which may range from the intolerable to the completely asymptomatic.

The need for treatment of a rhythm disorder must be weighed against the likelihood that drug therapy will be successful as well as the possible consequences and side effects of pharmacotherapy.[5,6] Adequate pharmacologic treatment is not available for every rhythm disorder. Furthermore, all antiarrhythmic agents have clinically important short- and long-term side effects. As the need for treatment becomes more urgent, physicians and patients must be more prepared to accept inevitable hazards and side effects of treatment, as well as a diminishing probability of success. Needless to say, life-threatening arrhythmias may require that such therapeutic decisions be made within a matter of seconds or minutes.

CHOICE OF A SPECIFIC ANTIARRHYTHMIC AGENT

Once the need for antiarrhythmic therapy is established, the clinician faces the choice of a specific antiarrhythmic agent. Again, numerous factors underlie the choice (Table 3). The probability that a given antiarrhythmic drug will be therapeutically effective in a specific clinical situation is only one such factor—other considerations may be at least as important. Procainamide, for example, is one of the most effective agents available to treat ventricular

TABLE 3 Factors Influencing the Choice of a Specific Antiarrhythmic Agent

Probability of therapeutic effectiveness
Short-term toxicity
Long-term toxicity
Cost
Drug interactions
Probability of compliance
Pharmacokinetic constraints:
Frequency of administration
Route of administration

tachyarrhythmias. The value of the drug in clinical practice, however, is greatly constrained by its intrinsic pharmacokinetic properties, leading to the need for frequent dosing (ie, every three to four hours around-the-clock) and the inevitable likelihood of noncompliance with such regimens. Furthermore, long-term use of procainamide is associated with an unacceptably high frequency of immune phenomena. A second example is that of lidocaine—a highly effective and relatively nontoxic antiarrhythmic. Its value as a long-term antiarrhythmic is minimal since the drug must be given by the parenteral route. Although phenytoin is generally less effective than the above two agents, it is sometimes an agent of choice since major side effects are dose-dependent and reversible, and since infrequent administration (ie, once- or twice-daily administration) is possible.

PHARMACOKINETIC APPROACH TO ANTIARRHYTHMIC THERAPY

Having chosen a specific antiarrhythmic agent, clinicians should then ensure that their therapeutic approach maximizes the likelihood of therapeutic benefit while minimizing the likelihood of toxicity.[7,8] This goal is generally most attainable when pharmacokinetic principles are used to guide the dosage, dosage interval, and route of administration.[9] Because the kinetic properties of a given drug can vary unpredictably from person to person, dosage schemes based on kinetic principles will not eliminate all problems with antiarrhythmic drug therapy, and must be supplemented by careful clinical monitoring and, if possible, determination of drug concentrations in serum or plasma.

The need for a loading dose generally is the first consideration. If therapy is initiated with a maintenance dose, a delay will ensue between the start of treatment and the attainment of 'steady-state' drug concentrations in serum or plasma. In general, attainment of the steady-state condition is more than 90% complete after a period of at least four times the drug's elimination half-life has elapsed since the start of treatment. In urgent or pressing clinical situations, this delay may be unacceptable, and a loading dose is required.[10,11] An appropriately chosen loading dose will immediately bring plasma drug concentrations to their steady-state level. This is a favorable outcome if the steady-state drug concentration is within the 'therapeutic' range for that patient; the outcome is unfavorable if the serum concentration is in the toxic range. Thus the rapid achievement of steady-state levels attained by the loading dose must always be weighed against the possibility that this level will be too high. Initiation of therapy with maintenance doses leads to slow attainment of steady-state, but the onset of toxicity, if it occurs, usually is gradual.

A number of schemes are available to guide the choice of maintenance dosage in clinical practice. These generally are based on identifiable factors such as body weight and renal function. However, many other factors can influence what constitutes an appropriate maintenance dosage—age, gender, serum albumin concentration, cardiovascular function, hepatic function, and concurrent use of other drugs. Unfortuantely, most of these factors either are not readily quantitated, or their precise effect upon pharmacokinetics is not clearly understood. Thus, rationally-chosen maintenance doses always are a first approximation. Clinicians must be prepared to titrate doses based upon clinical response and upon measurement of serum drug concentrations.

Schemes for choosing maintenance doses generally specify the 'average' dose per unit time—that is, milligrams per 24 hours. How often the daily dose should be subdivided is another important therapeutic consideration. Only when a drug is given by continuous intravenous infusion does the steady-state serum concentration fail to fluctuate over time. Dose-to-dose fluctuation is inevitable whenever a drug is given as individual, discrete doses. Minimal fluctuation between doses is a desirable therapeutic objective. The more the daily dose is subdivided and given with increased frequency, the less is the dose-to-dose fluctuation in serum concentration.[9] However, the requirement of very frequent dosing reduces the likelihood of compliance, and increases the inconvenience and disruption of the patient's life. The actual choice of dosage schedule in clinical practice results from weighing these two factors. For most drugs, the extent of interdose fluctuation in serum concentration is acceptable if the drug is administered at intervals equal to its elimination half-life. 'Sustained-release' oral preparations of antiarrhythmic agents may allow less frequent and more convenient dosing. However, clinicians should seek precise pharmacokinetic information on sustained-release preparations, inasmuch as the rate and extent of drug absorption may vary unpredictably within and between patients.

DRUG MONOGRAPHS

QUINIDINE SULFATE (Quinora, Quinidex Extentabs)
QUINIDINE GLUCONATE (Quinaglute Dura-Tabs)
QUINIDINE POLYGALACTURONATE (Cardioquin)

Quinidine derivatives are time-tested antiarrhythmic agents, and are effective against most tachyarrhythmias and ectopic rhythm disturbances encountered in clinical practice. Other advantages of quinidine derivatives include the option for both parenteral and oral dosage, as well as the possibility of relatively infrequent (ie, 2 or 3 times daily) dosing. Quinidine derivatives also have important disadvantages. The therapeutic index is intrinsically narrow, and individuals whose cardiac disease is marginally compensated may be particularly susceptible to the cardiac depressant effects of quinidine. In addition, some persons cannot tolerate the gastrointestinal irritant effects. Quinidine therapy should always be carefully monitored; dosage should be adjusted according to serum concentration determinations particularly early in the course of treatment.

When rapid achievement of therapeutic serum quinidine concentrations is required, the drug can be given by intravenous infusion. Traditional teaching dictates that intravenous quinidine is unacceptably hazardous, but recent studies clearly indicate that this route of administration is quite safe provided the infusions are slow and carefully monitored.[12–17] Quinidine can also be given by intramuscular injection, but the injections are painful and cause local muscle damage.[13] Furthermore, absorption of the drug from intramuscular injection sites is slow, erratic, and in many cases incomplete.

The elimination half-life of quinidine ranges from 4 to 10 hours in healthy persons, with a usual mean value of 6 to 7 hours.[13–15,17] The half-life is significantly prolonged in elderly persons, even when they are apparently healthy.[18] From 60 to 80% of a dose is metabolized by the liver; however, some of the biotransformation products may also have antiarrhythmic activity. Renal excretion of the intact drug comprises the remainder of total clearance.[13] Renal insufficiency has little overall effect upon the pharmacokinetics of quinidine, inasmuch as renal clearance comprises only a small proportion of total clearance. Quinidine is approximately 75% bound to serum proteins.[18,19]

TABLE 4 Preparations and Costs of Antiarrhythmic Drugs

GENERIC NAME	TRADEMARK NAME(S)	PREPARATIONS AND 1978 COSTS
Quinidine Gluconate	Quinaglute	Tablets (timed-release) 324 mg—$24.84/100
	generic	Injection (solution) 80 mg/ml—$3.71/10 ml vial
Quinidine Polygalacturonate	Cardioquin	Tablets 275 mg (equivalent to 200 mg of quinidine sulfate)—$14.56/50
Quinidine Sulfate	generic	Tablets 200 mg—$6.90–$14.10/100
	Quinidex	Tablets (timed-release) 300 mg—$21.80/100
Procainamide Hydrochloride	Pronestyl	Tablets 250 mg—$7.02/100; 375 mg—$9.78/100; 500 mg—$12.25/100 Injection (solution) 100 mg/ml—$3.12/10-ml vial; 500 mg/ml—$3.12/2-ml ampul
	generic	Capsules 250 mg—$2.60–5.82/100; 375 mg—$3.35–9.01/100; 500 mg—$4.20–$10.49/100
Lidocaine Hydrochloride	Xylocaine Hydrocloride	Injection (solution) 20 mg/ml—$0.40/2-ml vial; 100 mg/ml—$17.50/5-ml vial; 1 g/25 ml—$26.88/vial; 2 g/50 ml—$42.36/vial
Phenytoin Sodium	Dilantin Sodium	Capsules 30 mg—$2.61/100; 100 mg—$3.68/100 Injection (powder) 100 mg—$2.92/vial; 250 mg—$3.54/vial
Propranolol Hydrochloride	Inderal	Tablets 10 mg—$4.10/100; 40 mg—$7.08/100; 80 mg—$11.32/100 Injection (solution) 1 mg/ml—$0.53/1-ml ampul
Disopyramide Phosphate	Norpace	Capsules 100 mg—$11.42/100; 150 mg—$13.50/100
Bretylium Tosylate	Bretylol	Injection (solution) 50 mg/ml—$12.50/10-ml ampul

TABLE 4 *(continued)*

Generic Name	Trademark Name(s)	Preparations and 1978 Costs
Atropine Sulfate	generic	Injection (solution) 0.4 mg/ml—$0.10–$1.18/1-ml ampul or vial; 1 mg/ml—$0.18–$0.25/1-ml ampul or vial

Quinidine sulfate is the conventional oral quinidine preparation. When administered on an empty stomach, absorption is relatively rapid, with peak serum quinidine levels reached within 3 hours of the dose.[13] Absorption is approximately 80% complete. Because of its rapid absorption, maintenance doses of quinidine sulfate generally must be given every 6 to 8 hours to provide acceptable interdose fluctuation of serum concentrations.[20] The clinical value of 'sustained-release' quinidine preparations (ie, quinidine gluconate, quinidine polygalacturonate) is currently under investigation. The most data is available for sustained-release quinidine gluconate, from which absorption of quinidine is substantially slower than from quinidine sulfate. Acceptable interdose fluctuation is achieved with quinidine gluconate administered every 8 to 12 hours, thereby allowing more convenient dosing schedules.[20,21] The completeness of quinidine absorption from quinidine gluconate is about 70%—slightly lower (and possibly more variable) than from quinidine sulfate.[13] Clinicians should be aware that the sulfate and gluconate salts are not equivalent with respect to the amount of quinidine base provided per milligram. Quinidine sulfate contains 82% of quinidine base by weight, while quinidine gluconate contains only 62%. Appropriate dosage adjustments should be made when the particular quinidine preparation is changed.

Because of the narrow therapeutic index of quinidine, serum concentrations should be used to monitor therapy whenever possible. Although a 'therapeutic' range is not definitively established, therapeutic benefit is generally achieved with steady-state quinidine concentrations of 1.5 to 3.0 μg/ml. Higher concentrations increase the likelihood of toxicity. These estimates apply only to quinidine concentrations determined by relatively specific analytic techniques, such as extraction-fluorescence or chromatography. Older, less specific analytic methods quantitate quinidine metabolites as well as intact quinidine, thereby raising the therapeutic and toxic ranges.[22,23] Clinicians requesting serum quinidine determinations therefore should also ask that the method of analysis be specified.

Adverse Reactions—Gastrointestinal disturbances (nausea, vomiting, diarrhea, abdominal discomfort) are the most common side effects.[5,24–26] These occur with parenteral as well as oral dosage, suggesting that they may be of central origin (see below). In some sensitive individuals, gastrointestinal toxicity occurs without regard to dosage or serum concentrations. In most patients, however, gastrointestinal disturbances are dose- and concentration-dependent. Sometimes effective serum quinidine concentrations cannot be achieved without intolerable gastrointestinal side effects. The frequency and severity of gastrointestinal disturbances may be lower in patients taking sustained-release preparations, or in those who take conventional oral preparations together with meals.

Central nervous system (CNS) disturbances ('cinchonism') also are commonly associated with quinidine therapy. The usual manifestations are tinnitus, headache, and possibly visual disturbances. Gastrointestinal effects of quinidine may also be part of this syndrome. Again, some persons may experience untoward CNS effects without regard to dose or serum concentration; in most patients, effects are dose- and concentration-dependent.

Cardiovascular side effects of quinidine are controversial.[12] In healthy persons, therapeutic doses of quinidine produce tachycardia and prolongation of the QT interval, as well as slight prolongation of the QRS duration.[13] Hypotension or other evidence of impaired cardiac function generally is absent. However, in susceptible individuals such as those with marginally compensated cardiovascular disease, usual doses of quinidine may produce clinically important depression of cardiac function (hypotension, bradycardia, heart block, etc.). Thus quinidine therapy—particularly when initiated—should be carefully monitored in potentially susceptible individuals. Prolongation of the QRS duration beyond the usual 'upper' limit of 0.12 seconds, or an increase of 25% over the pre-quinidine QRS duration, are generally considered premonitory of more serious cardiac toxicity. These appear to be useful guidelines, although not firmly established as reliable.

Unusual side effects of quinidine include hepatotoxicity, hematologic toxicity, and skin reactions. 'Quinidine syncope'—a syndrome of unexpected syncope or even sudden death—has been anecdotally attributed to quinidine therapy. It is not established whether these incidents are due to quinidine-induced arrhythmias or to the underlying disease for which quinidine treatment was initiated.

Dosage—Intravenous: Adults, the usual single dose is 200 to 500 mg of quinidine base by continuous intravenous infusion at a rate of 0.2 to 0.3 mg/min/kg with monitoring of blood pressure and the electrocardiogram.

Oral Maintenance: Adults, quinidine sulfate, 600 to 1800 mg per day administered in divided doses every 6 to 8 hours. *Quinidine gluconate,* 660 to 1980 mg per day (ie, 2 to 6 tablets per day) in divided doses given every 8 to 12 hours.

Loading: Adults, a loading dose of twice the maintenance dose is usually appropriate. It can be given either intravenously or orally.

PROCAINAMIDE HYDROCHLORIDE (Pronestyl)

The efficacy of procainamide against ventricular tachyarrhythmias parallels that of quinidine.[27] However, procainamide is somewhat less effective against arrhythmias of atrial origin. The need for frequent dosing, together with immunologic phenomena commonly associated with long-term treatment, generally limits the use of procainamide to short-term treatment in the hospital setting.

As in the case of quinidine, procainamide can be given intravenously or by intramuscular injection if necessary, provided patients are monitored closely. Distribution of procainamide to body tissues is extensive. The elimination half-life in healthy persons is approximately 3 to 4 hours.[28–30] About 60% of the dose is excreted in the urine unchanged; the rest is biotransformed in the liver, predominantly by N-acetylation. Genetically-determined acetylator phenotype underlies the extent to which hepatic acetylation contributes to total clearance. As renal insufficiency supervenes, the total clearance of procainamide is reduced and the elimination half-life is prolonged, and hepatic biotransformation becomes the major route of clearance. The acetylated metabolite, N-acetylprocainamide (NAPA), appears to have pharmacologic activity similar to that of the parent compound.[31–34] Undoubtedly both contribute to the overall clinical activity during antiarrhythmic therapy with procainamide.

In healthy persons, oral procainamide is rapidly and nearly completely absorbed from the gastrointestinal tract. However, in those with compromised cardiovascular status, oral absorption can be unpredictably slow and incomplete.

The therapeutic serum concentration range for procainamide is commonly stated as 4 to 8 μg/ml.[30] Further studies are needed in which both procainamide and NAPA are simultaneously quantitated, so that therapeutic and toxic serum concentration ranges can be established for the combination of the two compounds.

Adverse Reactions—As with quinidine, gastrointestinal disturbances associated with procainamide can be idiosyncratic or unpredictable, as well as dependent on dose and serum concentration.[35] Manifestations of cardiovascular depression (hypotension, conduction disturbances, etc.) generally are dose- and concentration-dependent, and are more likely to occur in susceptible individuals with impaired cardiovascular status.

Long-term therapy with procainamide can be associated with immunologic phenomena manifested biochemically as an elevation in the antinuclear antibody (ANA) titer and clinically by such signs as fever and arthralgia.[36–38] The frequency of these effects appear to depend on dose, duration of therapy, and acetylator phenotype.[39] Immunologic side effects generally require discontinuation of procainamide treatment.

Dosage—Loading: 500 to 1000 mg. *Maintenance:* 250 to 500 mg every 3 to 4 hours (depending on body weight) in patients with normal renal function. In those with renal insufficiency, the dose should be reduced and/or the dosage interval increased. Loading and/or maintenance doses can be given either orally, by intramuscular injection, or by slow intravenous infusion (ie, no faster than 1.0 g per hour).

LIDOCAINE HYDROCHLORIDE (Xylocaine)

Lidocaine is an effective agent for the treatment of life-threatening ventricular tachyarrhythmias.[40,41] It is not very effective against arrhythmias of atrial origin. The widespread use of lidocaine is largely explained by its ability to suppress ventricular tachyarrhythmias with much less impairment of cardiac function than that associated with therapeutic concentrations of quinidine and procainamide.[40–42] The major drawback of lidocaine is the need for parenteral administration.

The usual mode of lidocaine dosage is continuous intravenous infusion. Since the elimination half-life in normal persons is approximately 90 minutes,[43,44] loading doses are almost always used to obviate the time necessary for attainment of the steady-state condition. The usual practice of single intravenous bolus loading doses often is clinically inadequate, since the short-lived effects of the bolus will terminate before drug accumulation attributable to the infusion is sufficient for continuous antiarrhythmic activity.[45–48] It is therefore recommended that therapy be initiated either with a succession of 2 to 3 bolus loading doses separated by 10 to 30 minutes, or by a relatively brief and rapid loading infusion. A maintenance infusion is begun either at the time of the first bolus or at the end of the loading infusion. Lidocaine can also be given by intramuscular injection—the usual dose is 300 mg.[41,49,50] The efficacy of intramuscular injection largely depends on whether effective serum concentrations (2 to 6 μg/ml) are achieved. The site of injection is an important variable—absorption is much more rapid from deltoid than from gluteal sites.[51] Oral administration of lidocaine is ineffective, since the drug is essentially completely cleared during the first-pass through the liver.

Hepatic biotransformation accounts for nearly all of lidocaine clearance.[41,43] The major metabolite appears to have pharmacologic activity.[33,52] Since hepatic clearance of lidocaine is partly dependent on hepatic blood flow, clearance may be reduced in patients with acute myocardial infarction or congestive heart failure.[41,43,53,54] Clearance is also reduced in patients with hepatic insufficiency. Dosage should be appropriately adjusted in such patients.

Adverse Reactions—Adverse effects of lidocaine generally involve the CNS and are dependent upon dose and serum concentration.[41,55] Initial manifestations include drowsiness, auditory disturbances, paresthesias, and reduction of level of consciousness. Appearance of such effects indicates that the infusion rate is too high. Failure to heed these warnings by slowing the infusion may result in more serious toxicity such as seizures and coma. Although lidocaine is much less likely to produce impairment of cardiac function than quinidine and procainamide, serious cardiac toxicity can result from lidocaine treatment in some susceptible individuals.[56–58]

Dosage—Loading: 50 to 200 mg as successive intravenous bolus doses or as a rapid loading infusion over 15 to 30 minutes. *Maintenance:* 2 to 4 mg per minute, depending on body weight and cardiovascular function. *Intramuscular:* 300 mg. Absorption is most rapid from deltoid injections, and least rapid from gluteal injections.

PHENYTOIN SODIUM (Dilantin)

Phenytoin is useful in the treatment of ventricular tachyarrhythmias in selected patients.[59,60] Its overall effectiveness is somewhat less than that of quinidine, procainamide, and lidocaine. However, in certain patients phenytoin is extremely effective. It may be particularly useful in the treatment of digitalis-induced arrhythmias. The major advantage of phenytoin is its long elimination half-life, making relatively infrequent (ie, twice daily) dosage schedules suitable for long-term antiarrhythmic therapy.

Considerable mythology surrounds the use of parenteral phenytoin. Rapid bolus injection can produce cardiac depression manifested by hypotension and bradycardia.[61,62] However, these effects are due largely to the irritating solvent vehicle, which is alkaline and contains high concentrations of propylene glycol.[63] Slow intravenous infusion is mandatory, but pharmaceutical sourcebooks caution against mixing phenytoin with intravenous fluids due to its poor solubility. Recent evidence suggests that dilute solutions of phenytoin (ie, 1 g mixed with 1 liter of 5% dextrose in water) can be prepared with negligible precipitation.[64–66] Such solutions can be infused safely over a suitably long period (ie, 2 to 4 hours). Phenytoin should not be given by intramuscular injection, since the injections are very painful and yield slow and erratic drug absorption.

The elimination half-life of phenytoin in healthy persons usually ranges from 20 to 24 hours. This kinetic pattern allows maintenance doses to be administered twice daily with acceptable interdose fluctuation in serum levels. Clearance of phenytoin is largely accomplished by hepatic biotransformation to pharmacologically inactive hydroxylated products.

Phenytoin possesses the relatively unusual pharmacokinetic property of saturable metabolism.[67–70] Its clearance and elimination half-life are dose-independent up to a point, after which clearance is reduced and elimination half-life prolonged as the dose and serum concentration increases. The implication for steady-state therapy is that an increase in dosage may produce a disproportionate increase in steady-state serum concentration. The 'saturation' point varies from person to person, but generally falls in the dose range of 300 to 500 mg per day. The saturability of phenytoin kinetics makes it essential that serum concentrations be used to monitor dosage, particularly as the higher dose range is being reached. At doses exceeding 300 mg per day, the effect of a dosage change upon steady-state serum concentration should be evaluated after no less than 1 week at the same daily dosage; in some cases, a longer delay may be advisable. The usual therapeutic serum concentration range is 10 to 20 μg/ml.[62,71] However, this is only an approximation since phenytoin is extensively bound to serum proteins. Only the unbound fraction is active, and small differences in binding could lead to large variations in clinical activity with relatively little change in total (bound plus unbound) serum concentration.

Oral phenytoin is reliably absorbed and is suitable for loading or maintenance therapy.

Adverse Reactions—Common side effects of phenytoin involve the CNS and include drowsiness, ataxia, dysarthria, nystagmus, and visual disturbances.[72–74] These are dependent on dose and serum concentration, and are reversible upon reduction of dosage. Cardiovascular toxicity of phenytoin is described above; such effects are generally attributable to excessively rapid intravenous infusions of the undiluted drug in its irritating solvent vehicle. Cardiovascular effects can generally be avoided by use of appropriately slow intravenous infusions.

Less common side effects of phenytoin[74] include various hematologic disturbances, gastrointestinal disturbances, and sensitivity reactions. In rare instances, the latter can be serious. Phenytoin has enzyme inducing properties and can stimulate the metabolism of other drugs. Chronic phenytoin therapy can produce vitamin D deficiency, osteomalacia, or rickets, presumably due to accelerated metabolism of vitamin D. Phenytoin has also been associated with folate-deficient megaloblastic anemia and peripheral neuropathy.

Dosage—Loading: Adults, 500 to 1000 mg by slow intravenous infusion or as divided oral doses over 12 to 24 hours. *Maintenance:* 200 to 500 mg per day in 2 or 3 divided doses. In some individuals, once-daily therapy is appropriate. Serum concentrations should be used to monitor and titrate dosage, particularly in the high dose range.

PROPRANOLOL HYDROCHLORIDE (Inderal)

The major pharmacologic property of propranolol is its ability to block peripheral beta-adrenergic receptors.[75] Effective beta blockade is achieved rapidly and with relatively low doses. Much has been made of a secondary pharmacologic property of propranolol, termed its ‘membrane-stabilizing’ or ‘quinidine-like’ effect. The clinical importance of these latter ‘direct antiarrhythmic’ properties, as well as of 'cardiac depressant' effects, are negligible at usual therapeutic doses, since they require blood and tissue concentrations greatly exceeding those encountered clinically.[76,77] The antiarrhythmic effects of propranolol undoubtedly result from beta-adrenergic blockade and approximately parallel the degree to which beta-adrenergic activity contributes to the formation or perpetuation of arrhythmic activity. As such, the drug has been used successfully in a variety of atrial and ventricular arrhythmias.[78]

Hepatic biotransformation accounts for essentially all of the total clearance of propranolol.[79] At least one metabolite—4-hydroxy-propranolol—is pharmacologically active.[80] The very high hepatic clearance of propranolol, and its short elimination half-life, render oral doses subject to extensive first-pass metabolism. Thus, oral doses must be 5 to 10 times higher than intravenous doses to produce equivalent clinical effects. Due to its short elimination half-life, propranolol generally must be administered every 6 to 8 hours. The clearance of propranolol appears to be reduced and its elimination half-life prolonged during multiple-dose therapy.[79] However, no clear clinical consequences of this are demonstrated, since a direct relation between plasma propranolol concentrations and clinical antiarrhythmic effect is not clearly established.

See Chapters 22 and 25 regarding the use of propranolol in angina pectoris and hypertension.

Adverse Reactions—In patients with normal cardiovascular status, propranolol is an extremely safe drug. However, the degree of compensation of some cardiac patients depends upon a high level of endogenous beta-adrenergic sympathetic activity. Such patients may have incompletely compensated congestive heart failure, acute myocardial infarction, valvular heart disease, etc. The degree of beta-adrenergic blockade produced by even a small dose of propranolol can lead to serious impairment of cardiac function, manifested by bradycardia, hypotension, or heart block.[81] Every effort should be made to identify individuals with heart disease that is not fully compensated (such as patients with resting tachycardia, exertional dyspnea, edema, etc.) who may develop this type of toxicity and probably should not receive propranolol. It is wise that all propranolol recipients receive an initial test dose in the presence of a physician.

Propranolol can induce bronchospasm and should not be administered to patients with a history of asthma or other bronchospastic disorders.[81] Propranolol impairs the subjective signs and symptoms associated with hypoglycemia, and caution should be observed during the use of this drug in diabetic patients, particularly those with insulin-dependent diabetes who are predisposed to hypoglycemia.

A variety of other nonspecific and generally minor side effects are associated with propranolol therapy.[81] The most common of these are gastrointestinal disturbances (loss of appetite, abdominal discomfort, nausea, vomiting, and diarrhea), and a variety of CNS disturbances (fatigue, lethargy, dizziness, depression, visual disturbances, etc.). Although a cause and effect relationship to propranolol therapy can seldom be established with certainty, the possible role of the drug should be considered in patients who develop such symptoms.

Dosage—Intravenous: 1 mg per minute to a total of 5 mg. *Oral:* 20 to 320 mg per day in 3 or 4 divided doses.

DISOPYRAMIDE PHOSPHATE (Norpace)

The spectrum of clinical activity of disopyramide resembles that of quinidine.[82–84] As with most new drugs, disopyramide has its proponents who claim that the drug has greater efficacy and less toxicity than other antiarrhythmics.

The elimination half-life of disopyramide is 4 to 8 hours in healthy subjects.[85,86] Renal excretion of the intact drug accounts for most of total clearance.[85–87] Thus, the elimination half-life is prolonged in patients with renal insufficiency, and appropriate dosage adjustments should be made. Biotransformation in the liver accounts for a smaller percentage of total clearance. The major metabolic product may have pharmacologic activity. Absorption of oral disopyramide is 80 to 90% complete.[85,86]

Therapeutic and toxic serum concentration ranges are not established.

Adverse Reactions—Cardiovascular toxicity associated with disopyramide, like those attributable to quinidine, probably are dependent on dose and serum concentration, and are more likely to occur in those with cardiovascular disease with borderline compensation. The usual effects of concern are hypotension, bradyarrhythmias, and conduction disturbances; appearance of any of these toxic manifestations indicates that dosage should be reduced or the drug discontinued.[82–84] Disopyramide has clinically important anticholinergic properties with usual therapeutic doses. A high percentage of patients experience dry mouth, blurred vision, tachycardia, and impairment of bowel and bladder motility.

Dosage—Oral: Adult, Loading, 200 to 300 mg. *Maintenance:* 400 to 800 mg per day. The usual dosage interval is every 6 hours. However, the dose and/or the dosage interval require adjustment in patients with renal insufficiency.

BRETYLIUM TOSYLATE (Bretylol)

Bretylium is an effective but potentially hazardous antiarrhythmic agent.[88–90] Currently it is recommended only for parenteral use in the treatment of life-threatening ventricular tachyarrhythmias that do not respond to usual therapeutic modalities. Bretylium appears to have both direct antiarrhythmic effects as well as indirect effects attributable to myocardial catecholamine depletion.

The catecholamine-releasing effects of bretylium can lead to transient hypertension as well as exacerbation of dysrhythmic activity. Initial doses of bretylium should be administered with careful monitoring. Postural hypotension attributable to catecholamine depletion is a common consequence of bretylium therapy.

Very little is known about the pharmacokinetics of bretylium. The duration of action of a single dose appears to be approximately 6 hours.

Adverse Reactions—Bretylium should be administered with continuous electrocardiographic monitoring. This is particularly true early in the course of therapy, when hypertension may occur and arrhythmias may be transiently exacerbated.

Following initial side effects attributable to catecholamine release, hypotension is the most common consequence of bretylium treatment.[88–90] Since it is largely postural, bretylium recipients should be kept supine with frequent monitoring of blood pressure.

The total duration of bretylium administration probably should not exceed several days, inasmuch as tolerance to its antiarrhythmic effects commonly develops.

Dosage—Loading: 5 to 10 mg per kilogram by slow intravenous infusion or intramuscular injection. *Maintenance:* approximately 5 mg per kilogram every 6 to 8 hours by intravenous infusion or intramuscular injection.

ATROPINE SULFATE

The anticholinergic agent atropine is one of the few potential pharmacologic treatments for bradyarrhythmias and/or conduction disturbances. Although the pharmacologic properties of atropine are reasonably well understood, specific guidelines as to when and in what dose it should be used are not firmly established. The major utility of atropine is in bradyarrhythmias complicating acute myocardial infarction, particularly those involving the inferior wall with concurrent ischemia to the sinoatrial or atrioventricular nodes leading to bradycardia and/or conduction disturbances. When these effects impair cardiac output enough to cause hypotension, administration of atropine or insertion of a transvenous pacemaker are frequently employed as therapeutic modalities.[91–93] The need for atropine therapy in patients with bradyarrhythmias having no hemodynamic consequences is not established.

The appropriate dosage of atropine is controversial. Due to its apparent central vagomimetic effect, low doses given slowly intravenously or by intramuscular injection may exacerbate bradyarrhythmias and/or conduction disturbances. On the other hand, excessively high doses can cause too much cardioacceleration, thereby increasing cardiac oxygen consumption, exacerbating ischemia, and possibly precipitating ventricular tachyarrhythmias.[94] A reasonable initial dose appears to be approximately 0.6 mg as a rapid intravenous injection.[95,96]

The usual duration of action of atropine is 3 to 4 hours. This approximately corresponds to its elimination half-life. However, some effects of atropine—such as mydriasis—may last considerably longer.

Adverse Reactions—Dose-dependent manifestations of cholinergic blockade are predictable consequences of atropine therapy. The usual initial signs, in addition to the desired tachycardia, are dry mouth, reduced sweating, mydriasis, and reduced bowel and bladder motility. Larger cumulative doses can lead to paralysis of accommodation (cycloplegia) and urinary retention. At even higher doses, CNS manifestations emerge. A variety of effects are possible ('atropine psychosis'), and usually include confusion, agitation, and delirium.[97,98]

Cardiovascular toxicity is usually secondary to increased cardiac work and myocardial ischemia resulting from excessive cardioacceleration.[99–102] Unfortunately, the development of such consequences is not readily predictable.

Dosage—Intravenous: Adults, the usual initial dose is 0.6 mg (range: 0.3 to 1.0 mg). This can be repeated in 2 to 4 hours if necessary.

DIGITALIS GLYCOSIDES

In patients with occult or overt congestive heart failure in whom increased myocardial oxygen consumption results from cardiac enlargement and high end-diastolic pressure, digitalis therapy can have secondary antiarrhythmic effects by improving the state of compensation and reducing myocardial oxygen demand.[103] On the other hand, arrhythmias are a well-known consequence of excessive concentrations of digitalis. Furthermore, the ischemic myocardium may be more sensitive to the arrhythmia-producing effects of digitalis. The net clinical outcome of the interaction of these factors is seldom predictable with certainty.

Digitalis glycosides appear to have therapeutic and prophylactic effects in certain supraventricular arrhythmias such as paroxysmal atrial tachycardia and possibly the atrial tachyarrhythmias associated with the Wolff-Parkinson-White syndrome.[103] Digitalis glycosides may be useful in the prevention and treatment of acute episodes.

High doses of digitalis glycosides are used to control ventricular rate in patients with atrial fibrillation. The presumed mechanism is digitalis-induced slowing of A-V nodal conduction, thereby reducing the ventricular response to the chaotic atrial activity.

Details of the approach to digitalis therapy, adverse reactions, and dosage can be found in Chapter 20.

REFERENCES

1. Sasyniuk BI, Ogilvie RI: Antiarrhythmic drugs: electrophysiological and pharmacokinetic considerations. Annu Rev Pharmacol 15:131–155, 1975.
2. Bigger JT Jr: Arrhythmias and antiarrhythmic drugs. Adv Intern Med 18:251–281, 1972.
3. Marriott HJL, Myerburg RJ: Recognition and treatment of cardiac arrhythmias and conduction disturbances. In *The Heart, Arteries and Veins,* 2nd edition. Edited by JW Hurst, RB Logue. New York, McGraw-Hill, 1970, pp 489–536.
4. Lown B, Temte JV, Arter WJ: Ventricular tachyarrhythmias. Circulation 47:1364–1381, 1973.
5. Bleifeld W: Side effects of antiarrhythmic drugs. Naunyn-Schmiedebergs Arch Pharmakol 269:282–297, 1971.
6. Mason DT, Spann JF Jr, Zelis R, et al: The clinical pharmacology and therapeutic applications of the antiarrhythmic drugs. Clin Pharmacol Ther 11:460–480, 1970.
7. Koch-Weser J: Pharmacokinetics of antiarrhythmic drugs. In *Innovations in the Diagnosis and Management of Myocardial Infarction.* Edited by AN Brest, L Wiener, EK Chung, et al. Philadelphia, F.A. Davis Co., 1975, pp 191–202.

8. Bigger JT Jr: Pharmacologic and clinical control of antiarrhythmic drugs. Am J Med 58:479–488, 1975.
9. Greenblatt DJ, Koch-Weser J: Clinical pharmacokinetics. N Engl J Med 293:702–705, 964–970, 1975.
10. Lemberg L, Castellanos A Jr, Arcebal AG, et al: The treatment of arrhythmias following acute myocardial infarction. Med Clin North Am 55:273–293, 1971.
11. Greenblatt DJ, Gross PL, Bolognini V: Pharmacotherapy of cardiopulmonary arrest. Am J Hosp Pharm 33:579–583, 1976.
12. Woo E, Greenblatt DJ: A reevaluation of intravenous quinidine. Am Heart J 96:829–832, 1978.
13. Greenblatt DJ, Pfeifer HJ, Ochs HR, et al: Pharmacokinetics of quinidine in humans after intravenous, intramuscular and oral administration. J Pharmacol Exp Ther 202:365–378, 1977.
14. Conrad KA, Molk BL, Chidsey CA: Pharmacokinetic studies of quinidine in patients with arrhythmias. Circulation 55:1–7, 1977.
15. Ueda CT, Hirschfeld DS, Scheinman MM, et al: Disposition kinetics of quinidine. Clin Pharmacol Ther 19:30–36, 1976.
16. Hirschfeld DS, Ueda CT, Rowland M, et al: Clinical and electrophysiological effects of intravenous quinidine in man. Br Heart J 39:309–316, 1977.
17. Ueda CT, Dzindzio BS: Quinidine kinetics in congestive heart failure. Clin Pharmacol Ther 23:158–164, 1978.
18. Ochs HR, Greenblatt DJ, Woo E, et al: Reduced quinidine clearance in elderly persons. Am J Cardiol 42:481–485, 1978.
19. Woo E, Greenblatt DJ: Pharmacokinetic and clinical implications of quinidine protein binding. J Pharm Sci (in press).
20. Ochs HR, Greenblatt DJ, Woo E, et al: Single- and multiple-dose pharmacokinetics of oral quinidine sulfate and gluconate. Am J Cardiol 41:770–777, 1978.
21. Woo E, Greenblatt DJ, Ochs HR: Short- and long-acting oral quinidine preparations: clinical implications of pharmacokinetic differences. Angiology 29:243–250, 1978.
22. Jones DT, Kostuk WJ, Gunton RW: Prophylactic quinidine for the prevention of arrhythmias after acute myocardial infarction. Am J Cardiol 33:655–660, 1974.
23. Bloomfield SS, Romhilt DW, Chou T-C, et al: Quinidine for prophylaxis of arrhythmias in acute myocardial infarction. N Engl J Med 285:979–986, 1971.
24. Abrams J: Quinidine toxicity: a review. Rocky Mt Med J 70:31–34, (Nov) 1973.
25. Cohen IS, Jick H, Cohen SI: Adverse reactions to quinidine in hospitalized patients: findings based on data from the Boston Collaborative Drug Surveillance Program. Prog Cardiovasc Dis 20:151–163, 1977.
26. Aviado DM, Salem H: Drug action, reaction, and interaction. I. Quinidine for cardiac arrhythmias. J Clin Pharmacol 15:477–485, 1975.
27. Bigger JT Jr, Heissenbuttel RH: The use of procaine amide and lidocaine in the treatment of cardiac arrhythmias. Prog Cardiovasc Dis 11:515–534, 1969.
28. Koch-Weser J: Pharmacokinetics of procainamide in man. Ann NY Acad Sci 179:370–382, 1971.
29. Karlsson E: Clinical pharmacokinetics of procainamide. Clin Pharmacokinet 3:97–107, 1978.
30. Koch-Weser J: Serum procainamide levels as therapeutic guides. Clin Pharmacokinet 2:389–402, 1977.
31. Elson J, Strong JM, Lee W-K, et al: Antiarrhythmic potency of N-acetylprocainamide. Clin Pharmacol Ther 17:134–140, 1975.
32. Drayer DE, Reidenberg MM, Sevy RW: N-acetylprocainamide: an active metabolite of procainamide. Proc Soc Exp Biol Med 146:358–363, 1974.
33. Drayer DE: Pharmacologically active metabolites. Clin Pharmacokinet 1:426–443, 1976.
34. Minchin RF, Ilett KF, Paterson JW: Antiarrhythmic potency of procainamide and N-acetylprocainamide in rabbits. Eur J Pharmacol 47:51–56, 1978.
35. Lawson DH, Jick H: Adverse reactions to procainamide. Br J Clin Pharmacol 4:507–511, 1977.
36. Kosowsky BD, Taylor J, Lown B, et al: Long-term use of procainamide following acute myocardial infarction. Circulation 42:1204–1210, 1973.
37. Henningsen NC, Cederberg Å, Hanson A, et al: Effects of long-term treatment with procaine amide. Acta Med Scand 198:475–482, 1975.

38. Davies DM, Beedie MA, Rawlins MD: Antinuclear antibodies during procainamide treatment and drug acetylation. Br Med J 3:682–684, 1975.
39. Lunde PKM, Frislid K, Hansteen V: Disease and acetylation polymorphism. Clin Pharmacokinet 2:182–197, 1977.
40. Harrison DC, Alderman EL: The pharmacology and clinical use of lidocaine as an antiarrhythmic drug—1972. Mod Treat 9:139–175, 1972.
41. Collinsworth KA, Kalman SM, Harrison DC: The clinical pharmacology of lidocaine as an antiarrhythmic drug. Circulation 50:1217–1230, 1974.
42. Rahimtoola SH, Sinno MZ, Loeb HS, et al: Lidocaine infusion in acute myocardial infarction. Arch Intern Med 128:416–418, 1971.
43. Benowitz NL: Clinical applications of the pharmacokinetics of lidocaine. In *Cardiovascular Drug Therapy*. Edited by KL Melmon. Philadelphia, F.A. Davis Co., 1974, pp 77–101.
44. Boyes RN, Scott DB, Jebson PJ, et al: Pharmacokinetics of lidocaine in man. Clin Pharmacol Ther 12:105–116, 1971.
45. Shen D, Gibaldi M: A hypothesis for the rapid attainment and maintenance of lidocaine plasma levels. J Clin Pharmacol 14:339–344, 1974.
46. Aps C, Bell JA, Jenkins BS, et al: Logical approach to lignocaine therapy. Br Med J 1:13–15, 1975.
47. Harrison DC: Practical guidelines for the use of lidocaine. JAMA 233:1202–1204, 1975.
48. Greenblatt DJ, Bolognini V, Koch-Weser J, et al: Pharmacokinetic approach to the clinical use of lidocaine intravenously. JAMA 236:273–277, 1976.
49. Sandler G, Dey N, Amonkar J: Prophylactic intramuscular lidocaine in myocardial infarction. Curr Ther Res 20:563–571, 1976.
50. Valentine PA, Frew JL, Mashford ML, et al: Lidocaine in the prevention of sudden death in the pre-hospital phase of acute infarction. N Engl J Med 291:1327–1331, 1974.
51. Schwartz M, Meyer MB, Covino BG, et al: Antiarrhythmic effectiveness of intramuscular lidocaine: influence of different injection sites. J Clin Pharmacol 14:77–83, 1974.
52. Burney RG, DiFazio CA, Peach MJ, et al: Anti-arrhythmic effects of lidocaine metabolites. Am Heart J 88:765–769, 1974.
53. LeLorier J, Grenon D, Latour Y, et al: Pharmacokinetics of lidocaine after prolonged intravenous infusions in uncomplicated myocardial infarction. Ann Intern Med 87:700–702, 1977.
54. Thomson PD, Melmon KL, Richardson JA, et al: Lidocaine pharmacokinetics in advanced heart failure, liver disease, and renal failure in humans. Ann Intern Med 78:499–508, 1973.
55. Pfeifer HJ, Greenblatt DJ, Koch-Weser J: Clinical use and toxicity of intravenous lidocaine: a report from the Boston Collaborative Drug Surveillance Program. Am Heart J 92:168–173, 1976.
56. Parameswaran R, Kahn D, Monheit R, et al: Sinus bradycardia due to lidocaine: clinical-electrophysiologic correlations. J Electrocardiol 7:75–78, 1974.
57. Klein HO, Jutrin I, Kaplinsky E: Cerebral and cardiac toxicity of a small dose of lignocaine. Br Heart J 37:775–778, 1975.
58. Marriott HJL, Phillips K: Profound hypotension and bradycardia after a single bolus of lidocaine. J Electrocardiol 7:79–82, 1974.
59. Mercer EN, Osborne JA: The current status of diphenylhydantoin in heart disease. Ann Intern Med 67:1084–1107, 1967.
60. Atkinson AJ Jr, Davison R: Diphenylhydantoin as an antiarrhythmic drug. Annu Rev Med 25:99–113, 1974.
61. Conn RD, Kennedy JW, Blackman JR: The hemodynamic effects of diphenylhydantoin. Am Heart J 73:500–505, 1967.
62. Bigger JT Jr, Schmidt DH, Kutt H: Relationship between the plasma level of diphenylhydantoin sodium and its cardiac antiarrhythmic effects. Circulation 38:363–374, 1968.
63. Louis S, Kutt H, McDowell F: The cardiocirculatory changes caused by intravenous Dilantin and its solvent. Am Heart J 74:523–529, 1967.
64. Greenblatt DJ, Shader RI: Intravenous phenytoin. N Engl J Med 295:1078, 1976.
65. Bauman JL, Siepler JK, Fitzloff J: Phenytoin crystallization in intravenous fluids. Drug Intell Clin Pharm 11:646–649, 1977.
66. Cloyd JC, Bosch DE, Sawchuk RJ: Concentration-time profile of phenytoin after admixture with small volumes of intravenous fluids. Am J Hosp Pharm 35:45–48, 1978.

67. Martin E, Tozer TN, Sheiner LB, et al: The clinical pharmacokinetics of phenytoin. J Pharmacokinet Biopharm 5:579–596, 1977.
68. Richens A, Dunlop A: Serum-phenytoin levels in management of epilepsy. Lancet 2:247–248, 1975.
69. Lambie DG, Johnson RH, Nanda RN, et al: Therapeutic and pharmacokinetic effects of increasing phenytoin in chronic epileptics on multiple drug therapy. Lancet 2:386–389, 1976.
70. Lund L, Alvan G, Berlin A, et al: Pharmacokinetics of single and multiple doses of phenytoin in man. Eur J Clin Pharmacol 7:81–86, 1974.
71. Vajda FJE, Prineas RJ, Lovell RRH, et al: The possible effect of long-term high plasma levels of phenytoin on mortality after acute myocardial infarction. Eur J Clin Pharmacol 5:138–144, 1973.
72. Greenblatt DJ: Antiarrhythmic agents. In *Drug Effects in Hospitalized Patients: Experiences of the Boston Collaborative Drug Surveillance Program, 1966–1975*. Edited by RR Miller, DJ Greenblatt. New York, John Wiley and Sons, 1976, pp 43–54.
73. Stone N, Klein MD, Lown B: Diphenylhydantoin in the prevention of recurring ventricular tachycardia. Circulation 43:420–427, 1971.
74. Eadie MJ, Tyrer JH: *Anticonvulsant Therapy*. Edinburgh, Churchill Livingstone, 1974.
75. Gibson DG: Pharmacodynamic properties of β-adrenergic receptor blocking drugs in man. Drugs 7:8–38, 1974.
76. Liang C-S, Hood WB Jr: The myocardial depressant effect of beta-receptor blocking agents. Circ Res 35:272–280, 1974.
77. Goldstein RE: A comparison of beta-blocking agents. Circulation 47:443–445, 1973.
78. Singh BN, Jewitt DE: β-Adrenergic receptor blocking drugs in cardiac arrhythmias. Drugs 7:426–461, 1974.
79. Johnsson G, Regardh C-G: Clinical pharmacokinetics of β-adrenoreceptor blocking drugs. Clin Pharmacokinet 1:233–263, 1976.
80. Fitzgerald JD, O'Donnell SR: Pharmacology of 4-hydroxypropranolol, a metabolite of propranolol. Br J Pharmacol 43:222–235, 1971.
81. Greenblatt DJ, Koch-Weser J: Clinical toxicity of propranolol and practolol: a report from the Boston Collaborative Drug Surveillance Program. In *Cardiovascular Drugs, Vol. 2: β-Adrenoreceptor Blocking Drugs*. Edited by GS Avery. New York, ADIS Press Australasia Pty Ltd, 1977, pp 179–195.
82. Zipes DP, Troup PJ: New antiarrhythmic agents: amiodarone, aprindine, disopyramide, ethmozin, mexiletine, tocainide, verapamil. Am J Cardiol 41:1005–1024, 1978.
83. Symposium on disopyramide. J Int Med Res 4(Suppl 1):1–108, 1976.
84. A seminar on Norpace (disopyramide phosphate): a new antiarrhythmic agent. Angiology 26:65–163, 1975.
85. Dubetz DK, Brown NN, Hooper WD, et al: Disopyramide pharmacokinetics and bioavailability. Br J Clin Pharmacol 6:279–281, 1978.
86. Hinderling PH, Garrett ER: Pharmacokinetics of the antiarrhythmic disopyramide in healthy humans. J Pharmacokinet Biopharm 4:199–230, 1976.
87. Cunningham JL, Shen DD, Shudo I, et al: The effects of urine pH and plasma protein binding on the renal clearance of disopyramide. Clin Pharmacokinet 2:373–383, 1977.
88. Bernstein JG, Koch-Weser J: Effectiveness of bretylium tosylate against refractory ventricular arrhythmias. Circulation 45:1024–1034, 1972.
89. Bacaner MB: Treatment of ventricular fibrillation and other acute arrhythmias with bretylium tosylate. Am J Cardiol 21:530–543, 1968.
90. Cooper JA, Frieden J: Bretylium tosylate. Am Heart J 82:703–706, 1971.
91. Cooper JA, Frieden J: Atropine in the treatment of cardiac disease. Am Heart J 78:124–127, 1969.
92. Epstein SE, Redwood DR, Smith ER: Atropine and acute myocardial infarction. Circulation 45:1273–1278, 1972.
93. Warren JV, Lewis RP: Beneficial effects of atropine in the pre-hospital phase of coronary care. Am J Cardiol 37:68–72, 1976.
94. Knoebel SB, McHenry PL, Phillips JF, et al: Atropine-induced cardioacceleration and myocardial blood flow in subjects with and without coronary artery disease. Am J Cardiol 33:327–332, 1974.
95. Klein MD, Barret J, Ryan TJ, et al: Atropine dose in acute myocardial infarction in man. Cardiology 60:193–205, 1975.

96. Chadda KD, Lichstein E, Gupta PK, et al: Effects of atropine in patients with bradyarrhythmias complicating myocardial infarction. Am J Med 63:503–510, 1977.
97. Shader RI, Greenblatt DJ: Uses and toxicity of belladonna alkaloids and synthetic anticholinergics. Semin Psychiatry 3:449–476, 1971.
98. Greenblatt DJ, Shader RI: Anticholinergics. N Engl J Med 288:1215–1219, 1973.
99. Zipes DP, Knoebel SB: Rapid rate-dependent ventricular ectopy. Chest 62:255–258, 1972.
100. Richman S: Adverse effect of atropine during myocardial infarction. JAMA 228:1414–1416, 1974.
101. Massumi RA, Mason DT, Amsterdam EA, et al: Ventricular fibrillation and tachycardia after intravenous atropine for treatment of bradycardias. N Engl J Med 287:336–338, 1972.
102. Horgan J: Atropine and ventricular tachyarrhythmia (letter). JAMA 223:693, 1973.
103. Smith TW, Haber E: Digitalis. N Engl J Med 289:945–952, 1010–1015, 1063–1072, 1125–1129, 1973.

22. ANTIANGINAL AGENTS

Craig N. Mattson

Angina pectoris is a frequent manifestation of ischemic heart disease and is due to an imbalance between myocardial oxygen requirements and delivery. Oxygen supply is insufficient because of decreased blood flow through the coronary vasculature. This imbalance leads to acute, reversible left ventricular failure and pain.[1] Although atherosclerotic changes in the coronary vessels appear primarily responsible, other unrecognized factors may also be involved.

Unfortunately, treatment of angina pectoris is only palliative, since there is no means of correcting the underlying pathophysiology. Relief of angina can theoretically be achieved by one or more therapeutic maneuvers. Increased oxygen extraction from hemoglobin is one possibility, but the heart has a limited ability to do this. Another alternative is to increase coronary blood flow by vasodilation. Although full dilation of the coronary vasculature in the ischemic area has probably been achieved in response to hypoxia, the vasculature in the nonischemic area can dilate further. In particular, it appears that dilation of collateral vessels can be sustained, more so than resistance vessels, and this action increases collateral flow and redistribution of blood towards the ischemic area.[2] The remaining alternative is to reduce the oxygen requirement of the whole heart or, more specifically, the ischemic area. The therapeutic effect of antianginal drugs is thought to be primarily mediated through reduction of the oxygen requirement of the whole heart (MVo_2) by peripheral vasodilation.

The three major determinants of MVo_2 are: (1) intramyocardial tension; (2) heart rate, and (3) myocardial contractility. Since intramyocardial tension depends on systolic intraventricular pressure and ventricular volume, the LaPlace relationship indicates that an increase in left ventricular pressure or volume would augment intramyocardial stress and thereby increase MVo_2. Likewise, the frequency of the stress also directly influences myocardial oxygen demand. Generally, a faster heart rate would predispose the patient to ischemic pain because of greater oxygen demand. Lastly, any event that increases contractility will ordinarily lead to higher myocardial oxygen consumption.[3] Thus, a complex interrelating series of mechanisms may play a part in the initiation and maintenance of myocardial ischemia. Drugs that diminish oxygen requirements in the failing heart by altering one or more of the above components of oxygen demand are the nitrates, propranolol, and digitalis glycosides.

EVALUATION OF ANTIANGINAL DRUGS

Because of the subjectivity and unpredictability of angina, differences in study design must be considered when evaluating the effectiveness of particular drug regimens. This point is clearly illustrated by Stipe and Fink[4] who reviewed 59 clinical studies to determine the relationship between the generally recognized elements of good experimental design and the stated conclusion of efficacy or non-efficacy of nitrates in immediate and prophylactic therapy of angina pectoris. Studies that included blinding procedures, appropriate controls, statistical analyses, and appropriate treatment allocation were considered well-designed. The authors showed that there were a significantly greater proportion of studies reporting effective therapy among the investigations that did not include one or more elements of good experimental design. Another important study criteria is the physiological matching of doses of the drugs involved.

NITROGLYCERIN

Nitroglycerin has been the mainstay of drug therapy in angina pectoris for almost a century. The exact mechanism of action of nitroglycerin and other organic nitrates is not clearly established. Dilation of the coronary arteries was previously considered the sole mechanism of action of nitroglycerin. Although such an effect cannot be dismissed, many authors[5–10] have concluded that the reduction in MVo_2 induced by nitroglycerin is primarily a result of peripheral venous dilation. Ganz and Marcus[11] attempted to substantiate this belief by demonstrating the ineffectiveness of intracoronary nitroglycerin and the effectiveness of intravenous nitroglycerin on pacing-induced angina. Unfortunately, the artificial conditions of the study prohibit a definite explanation of nitroglycerin's mechanism of action.

Venous dilation causes a decrease in venous return which leads to a diminution in ventricular size, stroke volume, and left ventricular end-diastolic pressure and thereby decreases MVo_2. Reductions in systolic intraventricular pressure and in systolic ejection further decrease myocardial oxygen demand. A decrease in arterial pressure, cardiac output, and stroke volume causes a reduction in external work performed by the left ventricle, leading to a decrease in myocardial oxygen consumption.

Sublingually-administered nitroglycerin is the drug of choice in an anginal attack. The dosage should be adjusted to achieve an optimal physiologic response. This can be estimated by decreasing the resting systolic blood presssure by 10 to 15 mmHg. This decrease may not always be attainable because of annoying side effects such as headache and postural hypotension, although tolerance may develop to these effects over time.

Sublingual nitroglycerin may also be used prophylactically and can be taken two to three minutes before beginning activities that characteristically induce angina. In such instances, angina probably will occur at the same threshold level, but nitroglycerin will increase the duration and intensity of exercise necessary to produce the same oxygen deficit.[12]

Oral nitroglycerin may also be effective in increasing exercise capacity,[13] but further studies are needed to assess the efficacy of this route of administration. Oral administration is reported to provide a more sustained effect than sublingual administration.

Another approach to prolonging the duration of action of nitroglycerin is the cutaneous administration of nitroglycerin ointment. Although Davis and Wiesel[14] introduced nitroglycerin ointment in 1955, it has received little use until recently. In 1976, Parker[15] demonstrated similar hemodynamic effects of nitroglycerin ointment and sublingual tablets during exercise. The beneficial effects of the ointment reportedly persist over three hours,[16] but the kinetics of transcutaneous nitrate absorption are unknown. To date, no nitrate tolerance or dependence has been demonstrated with the ointment, but further studies must be conducted before such phenomena can be discounted.

OTHER NITRATES

Although erythrityl tetranitrate, isosorbide dinitrate, and pentaerythrityl tetranitrate have become very popular, their use as 'long-acting' nitrates remains controversial. The mechanism of action of isosorbide dinitrate is probably similar to that of nitroglycerin,[12,17] and when given sublingually it is undoubtedly effective. Controversy centers around the oral use of these drugs. Because neither erythrityl tetranitrate nor pentaerythrityl tetranitrate have a documented advantage over isosorbide dinitrate, only the latter will be considered in detail.

Many parameters have been used to assess the duration of action of the 'long-acting' nitrates. The only clinically important therapeutic variables are increased exercise tolerance and decreased frequency of anginal attacks (more subjective).

Using physiologically matched doses of sublingual isosorbide dinitrate and nitroglycerin, Goldstein, et al[12] showed that the half-times for the exercise capacity improvement attributable to *both* drugs is approximately 20 minutes. Three other studies[18–20] document a prolonged therapeutic effect of sublingual isosorbide dinitrate in comparison to sublingual nitroglycerin in angina caused by exercise or atrial pacing. Each study found that sublingual isosorbide dinitrate (5 to 10 mg) had a protective effect for at least one hour, although there was a moderate amount of individual variation.

It is very difficult to make definitive statements on sublingual nitroglycerin versus the other sublingual nitrates, especially isosorbide dinitrate, since the peak effects of a drug and its duration of action are dependent on the particular dose of that drug. Thus, nitroglycerin may be equally effective if an appropriate dose were chosen.

Oral dosage forms of nitrate compounds were developed in an attempt to prolong activity. The animal study of Needleman, et al[21], showing a rapid and complete 'first-pass' hepatic degradation of oral isosorbide dinitrate, has been accepted as proof that oral isosorbide dinitrate is ineffective, but this route of administration is currently being reassessed in view of the demonstrated hemodynamic effects of larger doses (up to 20 mg) of oral isosorbide dinitrate.[17,22,23] Danahy, et al[24] demonstrated a significant increase in exercise tolerance persisting for three hours in most patients after a single dose of approximately 30 mg. They also found a good correlation ($r = 0.65$) between exercise response to sublingual nitroglycerin and response to oral isosorbide dinitrate.

Improved exercise tolerance following a single dose of isosorbide dinitrate does not establish long-term efficacy. Dependence[25,26] and tolerance[27] may occur during chronic use, and cross-tolerance with other nitrates has been suggested[28] but not clearly demonstrated. These possible consequences, as well as the large individual variations in clinical response, indicate that long-term therapy with high-dose isosorbide dinitrate requires considerable caution. Danahy and Aronow[29] demonstrated that partial hemodynamic tolerance developed after chronic use of high-dose oral isosorbide dinitrate, but that the acute antianginal efficacy of both sublingual nitroglycerin and oral isosorbide dinitrate was unimpaired.

PROPRANOLOL

If angina cannot be relieved by nitrate therapy and exercise training, then propranolol should be added unless a specific contraindication exists. Beta-adrenergic blockade is a logical approach, since increased sympathetic stimulation is the usual mechanism by which anginal attacks are precipitated.

Propranolol attenuates the sympathetically-mediated increase in heart rate and myocardial contractility. Arterial pressure is reduced secondary to a decrease in cardiac output and the antihypertensive effect of propranolol. Thus, propranolol may exert its beneficial effects in angina by reducing all three major determinants of MVo_2, ie, contractility, myocardial tension, and heart rate. On the other hand, propranolol may also have the undesirable effect of increasing MVo_2 by: (1) increasing ventricular size, (2) increasing left ventricular end-diastolic pressure, (3) prolonging the duration of the systolic ejection period, and (4) causing peripheral arteriolar vasoconstriction, secondary to unopposed alpha-adrenergic stimulation.[7] Despite the opposing effects on MVo_2, most patients receiving propranolol for angina are clinically improved, suggesting that the net effect is to decrease MVo_2. Those patients that fail to respond to propranolol may have occult congestive heart failure or are intolerant of effective doses.

Since the introduction of propranolol in 1964, 15 double-blind studies comparing oral propranolol therapy with placebo have been published. With one exception, they reported a reduction in frequency of anginal pain in 55 to 100% of propranolol recipients (average 78%; 280 of 359 patients). Propranolol was statistically superior to placebo in decreasing the frequency of anginal pain in all but two studies. The reduction in the duration and severity of anginal pain has been less easily quantified.[30] Unfortunately, several studies used fixed doses rather than individualized doses, and the results may underestimate propranolol's full therapeutic potential. The successful treatment of angina pectoris with propranolol has been observed with a broad dosage range (usually 80 to 400 mg/day). No study has been able to correlate propranolol dosage or serum level to increased exercise performance,[31–34] although Prichard and Gillam[31] showed a dose-dependent reduction of anginal attacks. Pine[32] found that maximum exercise performance occurred at less than complete beta blockade. Once the optimal dose of propranolol has been achieved by exercise testing, increasing the dose may result in decreased work capacity due to fatigue.[33] Thus, it may not be possible or desirable to completely eliminate all anginal attacks.

COMBINED NITRATE AND PROPRANOLOL THERAPY

Since propranolol and sublingual nitrates have complementary actions on some determinants of MVo_2, the combined administration of these drugs has been shown to increase exercise performance. Table 1 presents the pharmacologic actions of propranolol and nitrates and indicates the theoretical advantages of combined treatment.[7]

The early reports on the synergism of propranolol and sublingual nitrates were conflicting. Russek[35–37], in three separate studies, showed a 50% or greater reduction in frequency of anginal episodes and in nitroglycerin requirements, and a significant increase in exercise tolerance. However, Aronow and Kaplan[38], in 1969, found that 40% of their patients had a deterioration in their exercise performance after 90 minutes. Unfortunately, no recent clinical studies have examined this theoretical synergism.

Combination therapy should be tried in patients who are unresponsive to nitrates alone and who can tolerate beta blockade. The synergistic effect will last only as long as the shortest acting drug, which in most instances is isosorbide dinitrate. Maximal medical management of angina cannot be assured unless both nitrates and propranolol are administered.

There are numerous contraindications to propranolol therapy, including congestive heart failure, poor myocardial contractility, severe mitral or aortic valvular disease, sinus bradycardia, greater

TABLE 1 Theoretical Synergistic Action of Sublingual Nitrates and Propranolol in Angina Pectoris

Physiologic Effect	Nitrates	Propranolol	Combined
Heart rate	↑↑	↓↓	—
Myocardial inotropy and contractility	↑	↓↓	↓ or —[a]
Left ventricular size	↓	↑	—
Left ventricular end-diastolic pressure	↓	↑	—
Peripheral vascular tone	↓	↑	—
Systolic ejection time	↓	↑	—
Intramyocardial systolic tension	↓	↓↓	↓↓↓
Systemic blood pressure	↓↓	↓↓	↓↓↓
Venous return	↓↓	↓	↓↓↓
Peripheral venous pooling	↑↑	↑	↑↑↑
Myocardial oxygen consumption	↓	↓	↓↓

[a]The observed effect is dependent on the doses used.

than first-degree atrioventricular block, severe regional vascular insufficiency, chronic obstructive lung disease, or history of bronchial asthma.[39]

OTHER DRUGS

The role of other drugs in the prophylactic treatment of angina pectoris is questionable. Digoxin should be considered only in patients with abnormal ventricular function or a large heart.[40,41] Alcohol's previously benign role as an antianginal agent must be seriously questioned since it decreases the duration of exercise before angina and increases ischemic S-T segment depression after angina.[42] Perhexilene maleate is currently being investigated as an antianginal agent. It appears to have actions similar to both propranolol and nitroglycerin, but additional studies are needed to establish its efficacy and to assess its adverse effects.[43] No other currently available drugs have significant antianginal properties in well-designed studies.

DOSAGE

There is a great deal of interpatient variation on the same dose of an antianginal drug. Also, the duration of effectiveness for a specific antianginal drug is dose and route dependent. Therefore, it is difficult to derive meaningful dosing regimens. Perhaps the best guidelines are hemodynamic changes initially, followed by the ultimate clinical response, limited only by side efects.

DRUG MONOGRAPHS

NITROGLYCERIN

Sublingual nitroglycerin is the drug of choice for relief of anginal attacks and can be a very effective prophylactic agent if taken 2 or 3 minutes prior to the angina-provoking situation. It should not be taken on a scheduled basis because of its short duration of action (less than 1 hour).

The potency of nitroglycerin decreases over time because of its volatility. Therefore, nitroglycerin must be stored only in a tightly stoppered dark glass container. Nitroglycerin should be replaced every two to three months if the patient needs to use the medication frequently, hence exposing the contents of the bottle to the atmosphere frequently. If the tablets do not produce a slight stinging or burning sensation on the tongue or a characteristic fullness in the head they should be replaced.

Due to limited studies, the role of oral nitroglycerin cannot be fully appraised, therefore its use cannot be recommended at this time. Nitroglycerin 2% ointment may increase exercise capacity for 3 hours[16] and may be useful for scheduled prophylactic use.

Adverse Reactions—The most common adverse reaction is throbbing vascular headache, which is usually of relatively short duration. If headache accompanies the full therapeutic effect, analgesics may be helpful. Dizziness and syncopal episodes may occur occasionally and can be particularly troublesome in the elderly patient. Such patients should be instructed to sit or lie down when taking sublingual nitroglycerin.

Dosage—Sublingual: Adults, Nitroglycerin therapy should be started with low dosage, preferably 0.3 mg per tablet. During an anginal attack the patient should take one tablet every five minutes until relief is provided, but not more than three tablets. If anginal pain is not relieved in 20 minutes, the patient should be taken to the hospital for a suspected myocardial infarction. If no relief is attained and myocardial infarction has not occurred, the dose of nitroglycerin should be increased so that the maximum three tablets do cause improvement, with consideration for any associated adverse reactions. The optimal dose can also be titrated to produce a 10 mmHg fall in resting systolic blood pressure and/or a 10 beat per minute rise in resting heart rate.

Topical: Adults, Prophylactic therapy is begun with one-half inch of ointment as squeezed from the tube. The dose is increased by one-half inch increments in each successive application until the symptoms are relieved or until headache occurs, then the dose is decreased until headache no longer occurs. The dose may also be titrated by measuring the resting systolic blood pressure or resting heart rate as previously described. The ointment should be spread over a radius of approximately six inches and covered with plastic wrap. It can be applied anywhere on the body, but the chest affords some psychological benefit as well as convenience. Nitroglycerin ointment may be applied every three to four hours as required. In terminating treatment, both the dose and frequency of application should be gradually reduced to prevent possible withdrawal reactions.

ISOSORBIDE DINITRATE (Isordil, Sorbitrate)

Isosorbide dinitrate sublingual should be used only in prophylactic therapy. The sublingual tablet has a rapid onset of action (approximately 3 to 5 minutes). The duration of action is individual and dose dependent (5 mg has been reported to have antianginal effects of approximately 1 hour). Therefore, it can be used prior to an anginal-provoking situation, but because of its short duration of action fixed dosing schedules are irrational.

The oral tablet appears to have a longer duration of action (up to 3 hours has been reported), thus it can be put on a fixed dosage regimen. Because of large individual variation in clinical response, dosage must be accordingly individualized.

Either dosage form can be used with propranolol, remembering that

TABLE 2 Preparations and Costs of Antianginal Agents

GENERIC NAME	TRADEMARK NAME(S)	PREPARATIONS AND 1978 COSTS
Nitroglycerin	Nitrostat	Sublingual Tablets 0.3 mg—$1.75/100; 0.4 mg—$1.75/100;0.6 mg—$1.73/100
	generic	Sublingual Tablets 0.3 mg—$1.17/100; 0.4 mg—$0.75–$1.17/100; 0.6 mg—$0.75–$1.17/100
	Nitrol	Ointment 2%—$2.75/1 oz, $4.05/2 oz
Isosorbide Dinitrate	Isordil Sublingual	Sublingual Tablets 2.5 mg—$4.07/100; 5 mg—$4.38/100
	Isordil Chewable	Oral Tablets 10 mg—$5.03/100
	Isordil Titradose	Oral Tablets 5 mg—$4.38/100; 10 mg—$5.03/100; 20 mg—$9.17/100; 30 mg—$9.78/100
	Isordil Tembids	Timed-release Tablets 40 mg—$10.25/100 Timed-release Capsules 40 mg—$10.25/100
	Sorbitrate	Sublingual Tablets 2.5 mg—$4.07/100; 5 mg—$4.80/100 Chewable Oral Tablets 5 mg—$4.80/100; 10 mg—$5.50/100 Oral Tablets 5 mg—$4.80/100; 10 mg—$5.50/100; 20 mg—$9.44/100 Timed-release Tablets 40 mg—$10.25/100
Propranolol	Inderal	Tablets 10 mg—$4.10/100; 40 mg—$7.08/100; 80 mg—$11.32/100

the synergism lasts as long as the shortest acting drug. A lower dose of isosorbide dinitrate may be required when given concurrently with propranolol.

Adverse Reactions—See the monograph on nitroglycerin.

Dosage—Sublingual: Adults, Prophylactic therapy should begin with 5 mg sublingually as frequently as required for prophylaxis. If this dose produces undesirable side effects it may be decreased to 2.5 mg. Approximate dosage titrations may be accomplished hemodynamically, as with nitroglycerin. There is no maximum dose other than what the patient can tolerate for relief of angina.

Oral: Adults, Therapy should be initiated at the lowest dose, 5 mg, and adjusted until the smallest effective dose is determined. To maintain a therapeutic effect, the dosing interval may have to be approximately every 4 hours, but less frequent dosing may be tried in a more stable condition. The dosage range is usually 10 to 30 mg, but larger doses may be used if the patient tolerates it.

PROPRANOLOL

Propranolol is effective in reducing the frequency of anginal attacks and in increasing the exercise tolerance in most patients with uncomplicated angina. It is usually appropriate to add propranolol to maximum nitrate therapy rather than substitute propranolol for the nitrate. An exception would be the occasional patient who is totally intolerant of effective nitrate doses. For information regarding adverse reactions and interactions see Chapter 25, Antihypertensive Agents.

Dosage—Oral: Adults, Propranolol is usually started at 10 mg four times daily and is increased until the angina is controlled or intolerable side effects occur. If given without nitrates the dosage can be increased until a reduction in the pulse rate below 60 beats/minute is seen. When given concomitantly with nitrates the dosage requirements may be decreased. In either case the optimal response is usually very patient-specific, with maximal dosage frequently limited by side effects.

Abrupt discontinuance of propranolol may precipitate a rebound effect with serious exacerbations of cardiac ischemia; the severity may be proportionate to dosage. Therefore, propranolol withdrawal should be done gradually over 48 hours.

Intravenous: Propranolol should not be used by this route to control angina pectoris because of the careful monitoring required.

REFERENCES

1. Parker JD: Hemodynamic and metabolic changes during myocardial ischemia. Arch Intern Med 129:790–798, 1972.
2. Goldstein RE, Stinsin EB, Epstein SE: Effects of nitroglycerin on coronary collateral function in patients with coronary occlusive disease (abstract). Am J Cardiol 31:135, 1973.
3. Epstein SE, Redwood DR, Goldstein RE, et al: Angina pectoris: pathophysiology, evaluation and treatment. Ann Intern Med 75:263–296, 1971.
4. Stipe AA, Fink GB: Prophylactic therapy of angina pectoris with organic nitrates: relationship of drug efficacy and clinical experimental design. J Clin Pharmacol 13:244–250, 1973.

5. Nickerson M: Vasodilator drugs. In *The Pharmacological Basis of Therapeutics,* 5th edition. Edited by LS Goodman, A Gilman. New York, Macmillan, 1976, pp 727–743.
6. Goldstein RE, Epstein SE: Medical management of patients with angina pectoris. Prog Cardiovasc Dis 14:360–398, 1972.
7. Klein HO, Berger HJ: Synergistic actions of nitrite-β-adrenergic blocking agents in the therapy of angina pectoris: pharmacologic and therapeutic rationale. Cardiology 58:313–325, 1973.
8. Aronow WS: Medical treatment of angina pectoris. III. Pharmacology of sublingual nitrates as antianginal drugs. Am Heart J 84:273–275, 1972.
9. Greenberg H, Dwyer EM, Jameson AB, et al: Effects of nitroglycerin on the major determinants of myocardial oxygen consumption. An angiographic and hemodynamic assessment. Am J Cardiol 36:426–432, 1975.
10. Parratt JR: Pharmacological approaches to the therapy of angina. Adv Drug Res 9:103–134, 1974.
11. Ganz W, Marcus HS: Failure of intracoronary nitroglycerin to alleviate pacing-induced angina. Circulation 46:880–889, 1972.
12. Goldstein RE, Rosing DR, Redwood DR, et al: Clinical and circulatory effects of isosorbide dinitrate: comparison with nitroglycerin. Circulation 43:629–640, 1971.
13. Winsor T: Oral nitroglycerin as a prophylactic antianginal drug: clinical, physiologic and statistical evidence of efficacy based on a three phase experimental design. Am Heart J 90:611–626, 1975.
14. Davis JA, Wiesel BH: The treatment of angina pectoris with a nitroglycerin ointment. Am J Med Sci 230:259–263, 1955.
15. Parker JO: Effect of nitroglycerin ointment on the clinical and hemodynamic response to exercise. Am J Cardiol 38:162–166, 1976.
16. Reichek N, Goldstein RE, Redwood DR, et al: Sustained effects of nitroglycerin ointment in patients with angina pectoris. Circulation 50:348–352, 1974.
17. Willis WH, Russell RO, Mantle JA, et al: Hemodynamic effects of isosorbide dinitrate vs nitroglycerin in patients with unstable angina. Chest 69:15–22, 1976.
18. Klaus AP, Zaret BL, Pitt BL, et al: Comparative evaluation of sublingual long-acting nitrates. Circulation 48:519–525, 1973.
19. Steele RJ: Effects of isosorbide dinitrate on the response to atrial pacing in coronary heart disease. Am J Cardiol 36:206–210, 1975.
20. Bunn WH, Chremos AN: Clinical evaluation of sublingual nitrates: onset and duration of action of nitroglycerin and isosorbide dinitrate. Angiology 14:48–54, 1963.
21. Needleman P, Lang S, Johnson E: Organic nitrates: relationship between biotransformation and rational angina pectoris therapy. J Pharmacol Exp Ther 181:489–497, 1972.
22. Kasparian A, Wiener L, Duca P, et al: Comparative hemodynamic effects of placebo and oral isosorbide dinitrate in patients with significant coronary artery disease. Am Heart J 90:68–74, 1975.
23. Glancy DL, Richter MA, Ellis EV, et al: Effect of swallowed isosorbide dinitrate on blood pressure, heart rate and exercise capacity in patients with coronary artery disease. Am J Med 62:39–46, 1977.
24. Danahy DT, Burwell DT, Aronow WS, et al: Sustained hemodynamic and antianginal effect of high dose oral isosorbide dinitrate. Circulation 55:381–387, 1977.
25. Lange RL, Reid MS, Tresch DD, et al: Non-atheromatous ischemic heart disease following withdrawal from chronic industrial nitroglycerin exposure. Circulation 46:666–678, 1972.
26. Klock JC: Non-occlusive coronary disease after chronic exposure to nitrates: evidence for physiologic nitrate dependence. Am Heart J 89:510–513, 1975.
27. Shane SJ: High dose oral isosorbide and ischemic heart pain. Can Fam Phys 19:61–65, 1973.
28. Schelling JL, Lasagna L: A study of cross-tolerance to circulatory effects of organic nitrates. Clin Pharmacol Ther 8:256–260, 1967.
29. Danahy DT, Aronow WS: Hemodynamic and antianginal effects of high dose oral isosorbide dinitrate after chronic use. Circulation 56:205–212, 1977.
30. Warren SG, Brewer DL, Orgain ES: Long-term propranolol therapy for angina pectoris. Am J Cardiol 37:420–426, 1976.
31. Prichard BN, Gillam PM: Assessment of propranolol in angina pectoris. Clinical dose-response curve and effect on electrocardiogram at rest and in exercise. Br Heart J 33:473–480, 1971.

32. Pine M: Correlation of plasma propranolol concentrations with therapeutic responses in patients with angina pectoris. Circulation 52:886–893, 1975.
33. Frishman W, Smithen C, Befler B, et al: Noninvasive assessment of clinical response to oral propranolol therapy. Am J Cardiol 35:635–644, 1975.
34. Alderman FL: Dose reponse effectiveness of propranolol for the treatment of angina pectoris. Circulation 51:964–975, 1975.
35. Russek HI: Propranolol and isosorbide dinitrate synergism in angina pectoris. Am J Med Sci 254:406–415, 1967.
36. Russek HI: Propranolol and isosorbide dinitrate synergism in angina pectoris. Am J Cardiol 21:44–54, 1968.
37. Russek HI: The natural history of severe angina pectoris with intensive medical therapy alone: a five year prospective study of 133 patients. Chest 65:46–51, 1974.
38. Aronow WS, Kaplan MA: Propranolol combined with isosorbide dinitrate versus placebo in angina pectoris. N Engl J Med 280:847–850, 1969.
39. Aronow WS: Management of stable angina. N Engl J Med 289:516–519, 1973.
40. Harding PR, Aronow WS, Eisenman J: Digitalis as an antianginal agent. Chest 64:439–443, 1973.
41. Crawford MH, LeWinter MM, O'Rourke RA, et al: Combined propranolol and digoxin therapy in angina pectoris. Ann Intern Med 83:449–455, 1975.
42. Orlando J, Aronow WS, Cassidy J, et al: Effect of ethanol on angina pectoris. Ann Intern Med 84:652–655, 1976.
43. Masoni A, Tomasi AM, Oriani GA: Clinical evaluation of perhexiline maleate in the treatment of patients with chronic coronary insufficiency. Am Heart J 90:145–152, 1975.

23. VASODILATOR DRUGS USED IN PERIPHERAL VASCULAR DISEASE

Jay D. Coffman

Many drugs are advertised as useful in peripheral vascular disease. Adrenergically mediated vasoconstriction may be important in the pathogenesis or aggravation of peripheral ischemia through its normal activity in such vasospastic disorders as Raynaud's phenomenon, acrocyanosis and livedo reticularis. Most patients with vasospastic diseases need no therapy except reassurance and instructions to keep their extremities and bodies warm. In the more severe cases, agents which interfere with the action of the sympathetic nervous system may be useful.[1]

However, in patients with obstructive arterial disease, it is not established whether these drugs increase blood flow to the diseased limb.[2] Blood flow distal to a stenosed or obstructed blood vessel depends on the collateral blood vessels. Arterial blood pressure distal to the obstructing lesion is decreased due to the resistance to flow in small caliber collateral vasculature. During exercise this pressure falls even lower, due to vasodilation induced by the accumulation of metabolites. The tension of the contracting muscle then exceeds the low arterial pressure and markedly decreases or even stops blood flow.[3] Dilating the vessels distal to the obstruction may not increase blood flow, especially if the resistance of the collateral vessels remains fixed. To be effective, a vasodilator drug would have to dilate the collateral vessels or stimulate growth of new vessels. No drug has been demonstrated to do this.

PHARMACOLOGY

Vasodilator drugs act by interfering with sympathetic nervous system activity (reserpine, methyldopa, guanethidine, phenoxybenzamine, tolazoline), by stimulating beta receptors (nylidrin), or by direct vascular smooth muscle relaxation (isoxsuprine, niacin, papaverine, cyclandelate). Drugs that interfere with sympathetic nervous system activity would be expected to increase skin rather than muscle blood flow since there is little vasoconstrictor tone in skeletal muscle. Beta receptor stimulating drugs should increase muscle blood flow but not affect flow in cutaneous vessels where beta receptors are absent or sparse. Drugs that act directly on vascular smooth muscle would be expected to increase both cutaneous and muscle blood flow. Most of these drugs increase skin or muscle flow in animal preparations or in normal human subjects, but not in limbs with obstructive arterial disease except possibly after intra-arterial administration. Since these drugs induce a general vasodilation, an actual decrease in blood flow to the diseased limb has been demonstrated in some patients. If a vasodilator drug lowers systemic blood pressure, collateral vascular resistance will increase; in fact, raising the systemic pressure is a very effective means of increasing collateral blood flow.[4] Agents that interfere with sympathetic nerve transmitter activity have been shown to increase finger blood flow in patients with vasospastic disease.

ADVERSE EFFECTS

All vasodilator drugs can decrease systemic blood pressure. Postural hypotension and post-exercise hypotension are potentially serious side effects. Other frequent side effects include flushing, headache, palpitations, and gastrointestinal symptoms (many of the drugs increase gastric acid production). Drugs that interfere with the action of the sympathetic nervous system may cause nasal congestion, lethargy, depression, diarrhea, and male sexual dysfunction.

DRUG INTERACTIONS

Tricyclic antidepressants may block the action of guanethidine and related agents. Monoamine oxidase inhibitors should be discontinued at least one week before starting guanethidine or reserpine, since these drugs may initially increase extraneuronal norepinephrine and cause hypertensive episodes.

DRUG MONOGRAPHS

ISOXSUPRINE HYDROCHLORIDE (Vasodilan)

Isoxsuprine is advertised as a vasodilator for use in many conditions. Since beta-receptor blocking drugs do not antagonize its vascular effects, it must act directly on vascular smooth muscle.[5] In normal subjects, it increases muscle blood flow but does not influence skin flow.[6] In patients with arteriosclerosis obliterans, the drug had no effect on the systolic pressure gradient in the diseased limb, ankle systolic pressure after exercise, maximal treadmill walking time, or on muscle blood flow during exercise.[6-9] There is no adequate evidence that isoxsuprine is useful in peripheral vascular disorders.

Adverse Reactions—Frequent side effects include palpitations, flushing, and postural hypotension.

Dosage—Not of proven efficacy. Manufacturer recommends: *Oral:* 10 to 20 mg 3 to 4 times daily. *Intramuscular:* 5 to 10 mg 2 to 3 times daily.

PAPAVERINE HYDROCHLORIDE (Cerespan, Pavabid, Pavacen, Vasospan)
ETHAVERINE HYDROCHLORIDE (Ethaquin, Ethatab, Laverin)

Papaverine and its analogues are weak vasodilators which relax vascular smooth muscle by direct action when administered parenterally.[10] Uncontrolled studies of orally-administered papaverine have either reported no benefit[11] or good results[12] in patients with intermittent claudication. Variable results have also been reported in patients with Raynaud's phenomenon.[13,14]

Ethaverine has not been extensively studied in peripheral vascular disease; one study found an increase in resting calf blood flow and a decrease in digital blood flow in patients with arterial occlusive disease.[15]

Adverse Reactions—Flushing, malaise, gastrointestinal symptoms, and headache occur with papaverine and ethaverine preparations. Hepatotoxicity has been reported with papaverine.[16]

Dosage—Not of proven efficacy. Manufacturers recommend: *Oral:* timed-release capsules, 150 mg to 300 mg every 8 to 12 hours. *Intra-arterial:* 40 mg given slowly.

TABLE 1 Preparations and Costs of Vasodilator Drugs Used in Peripheral Vascular Disease

GENERIC NAME	TRADEMARK NAME(S)	PREPARATIONS AND 1978 COSTS
Cyclandelate	Cyclospasmol	Capsules 200 mg—$8.40/100; 400 mg— $9.11/60 Tablets 100 mg—$4.20/100
Dihydrogenated Ergot Alkaloids	Hydergine	Tablets (sublingual) 0.5 mg—$9.00/100; 1 mg—$17.10/100
Ethaverine Hydrochloride	Ethaquin	Tablets 100 mg—$10.50/100
	Ethatab	Tablets 100 mg—$8.90/100
	Laverin	Tablets 100 mg—$8.25/100
Guanethidine Sulfate	Ismelin Sulfate	Tablets 10 mg—$10.10/100; 25 mg $14.45/100
Isoxsuprine Hydrochloride	Vasodilan	Tablets 10 mg—$9.92/100; 20 mg—$15.86/100 Injection (solution) 5 mg/ml—$1.14/2-ml ampul
Methyldopa	Aldomet	Tablets 125 mg—$6.19/100; 250 mg—$8.74/100; 500 mg—$15.75/100
Niacin	NIAC	Capsules (timed-release) 300 mg—$6.50/100
	Nicobid	Capsules (timed-release) 125 mg—$6.60/100; 250 mg—$7.80/100
	Nicotinex	Elixir 50 mg/ml—$4.00/pint
	generic	Tablets 25 mg—$0.35–$0.90/100; 50 mg—$0.40–$1.20/100; 100 mg—$0.50–$2.10/100; 500 mg—$0.99–$3.85/100
Nicotinyl Alcohol	Roniacol	Elixir 50 mg/5 ml—$5.49/pint
Nicotinyl Alcohol Tartrate	Roniacol	Tablets 50 mg—$3.46/100
	Roniacol Timespan	Tablets (timed-release) 150 mg—$10.19/100
Nylidrin Hydrochloride	Arlidin	Tablets 6 mg—$8.58/100; 12 mg—$14.70/100

TABLE 1 *(continued)*

Generic Name	Trademark Name(s)	Preparations and 1978 Costs
Papaverine Hydrochloride	Cerespan	Capsules (timed-release) 150 mg—$11.63/100
	Pavabid	Capsules (timed-release) 150 mg—$10.38/100
	Pavacen	Capsules (timed-release) 150 mg—$8.25/100
	Vasospan	Capsules (timed-release) 150 mg—$9.75/100
	generic	Injection (solution) 30 mg/ml—$0.35/2-ml ampul; $0.82/10-ml vial
Phenoxybenzamine Hydrochloride	Dibenzyline	Capsules 10 mg—$4.10/100
Reserpine	Serpasil (Sandril)	Tablets 0.1 mg—$2.67/100; 0.25 mg—$4.50/100; 1 mg—$12.00/100 Elixir 0.2 mg/4 ml—$6.00/pt Injection (solution) 2.5 mg/ml—$1.20/2-ml ampul; $3.60/10-ml vial
Tolazoline Hydrochloride	Priscoline Hydrochloride	Tablets 25 mg—$5.60/100 Tablets (timed-release) 80 mg—$14.15/100 Injection 25 mg/ml—$5.85/10-ml vial

NIACIN (NIAC, Nicobid, Nicotinex) NICOTINYL ALCOHOL (Roniacol) NICOTINYL ALCOHOL TARTRATE (Roniacol Tartrate)

Niacin (nicotinic acid) and its derivatives directly relax blood vessels but produce more vasodilation of the blood vessels of the ears, face, and neck than of the extremities.[17] Clinical studies have failed to show a consistent increase in skin or muscle blood flow in patients with obstructive arterial disease. A decrease or no change in skin and muscle blood flow during exercise,[9,18] after exercise, and during reactive hyperemia[19] have been reported. Long-term studies describe either no benefit or symptomatic relief[20] in patients with intermittent claudication. One study[21] claimed symptomatic benefit in Raynaud's phenomenon.

Adverse Reactions—Intense flushing, gastrointestinal symptoms, rash, and postural hypotension may occur with niacin preparations or nicotinyl alcohol.

Dosage—Not of proven efficacy. Manufacturers recommend: *Oral:* Niacin or derivatives, timed-release capsules, 125 to 300 mg every 12 hours; Roniacol, elixir 50 to 100 mg or timed-release capsules 150 to 300 mg every 12 hours.

CYCLANDELATE (Cyclospasmol)

Cyclandelate acts directly to relax the smooth muscle of the blood vessels. Uncontrolled clinical trials report an increased walking distance in about 50 percent of patients with intermittent claudication and less benefit in patients with Raynaud's phenomenon.[22,23] No controlled studies or objective measurements have shown this drug to be of value in peripheral vascular disease. A single-blind, non-crossover study reported that patients with femoral artery arteriosclerosis obliterans appeared to improve while patients with iliac disease did not; oscillograph pulse volumes failed to correlate with the subjective responses.[24]

Adverse Reactions—Reported frequent side effects of cyclandelate include headache, flush, gastrointestinal symptoms, drowsiness, and dizziness.

Dosage—Not of proven efficacy. Manufacturer recommends: *Oral:* 200 to 400 mg 4 times daily.

NYLIDRIN (Arlidin)

Nylidrin stimulates beta receptors to increase muscle blood flow but probably also has a direct action on vascular smooth muscle.[5] Most studies have found no effect on skin blood flow.[6,25,26] Uncontrolled studies have reported symptomatic benefit in patients with intermittent claudication following oral administration,[27] and an increase in post-exercise calf blood flow with intravenous administration.[28] Well-controlled studies have found no effect on the clinical symptoms of intermittent claudication;[26,29] variable effects on calf blood flow have been reported.[26] Both muscle and skin blood flow may be decreased during exercise after intramuscular administration of nylidrin.[18] With oral use of large doses, exercise muscle blood flow is usually not increased in patients with femoral or aortoiliac arteriosclerosis obliterans.[9] There is no adequate evidence that nylidrin is useful in patients with peripheral vascular disease.

Adverse Reactions—Chills, flushing, palpitations, nausea, vomiting, and postural hypotension occur with nylidrin.

Dosage—Not of proven efficacy. Manufacturer recommends: *Oral:* 6 to 12 mg 3 or 4 times daily.

TOLAZOLINE HYDROCHLORIDE (Priscoline Hydrochloride)

Tolazoline, an alpha receptor blocking agent which also has a histamine-like effect,[30] increases skin blood flow in normal human subjects when given parenterally and orally.[6,31] Clinical studies of patients with peripheral vascular disease have reported variable results.[11,31,32] In one investigation,[32] intra-arterial or oral tolazoline produced relief of rest pain in patients with arteriosclerosis obliterans and healed finger ulcers in patients with Raynaud's disease; however, there was no increase in exercise tolerance. In another study,[33] foot blood flow responded favorably in patients with obstructive arterial disease, but only when rest pain was not present. Others report variable results with intra-arterial use and even a decrease in blood flow to ischemic feet in some patients.[19,31] Following large oral doses, no significant change occurred in resting foot or calf blood flow in patients with femoral or aortoiliac arteriosclerosis.[9] Tolazoline may be of some value in patients with Raynaud's phenomenon[1] but is of doubtful efficacy in obstructive arterial disease.

Adverse Reactions—Tolazoline often produces headache, paresthesias of the skin (especially the scalp), flushing, and palpitations. Nausea, chills, gastrointestinal disturbances, and postural hypotension also may occur.

Dosage—Oral: 25 mg every 4 to 6 hours or 80 mg (timed-release preparation) every 12 hours. *Intravenous, intramuscular, subcutaneous:* 10 to 50 mg every 6 hours. *Intra-arterial:* 25 to 75 mg injected slowly once or twice daily.

PHENOXYBENZAMINE HYDROCHLORIDE (Dibenzyline)

Phenoxybenzamine has been used in vasospastic peripheral vascular disorders; it dilates cutaneous blood vessels by blocking alpha-adrenergic receptors. No controlled studies are available.

Intra-arterial use failed to increase foot flow in patients with ischemia due to arterial occlusive disease.[31]

Adverse Reactions—Postural hypotension and palpitations often preclude use of phenoxybenzamine. Nasal congestion and gastrointestinal symptoms may also occur.

Dosage—Oral: Initial recommended dose is 10 mg with increments of 10 mg at 3 to 4 day intervals until relief of symptoms or adverse effects. The usual maintenance dose is 20 to 60 mg daily.

RESERPINE

Reserpine produces cutaneous vasodilation by depleting norepinephrine from the sympathetic nerves. Reserpine also produces brief vasodilation, unrelated to norepinephrine, when injected intra-arterially.[34] In Raynaud's phenomenon, reserpine may sometimes produce remarkable amelioration of symptoms,[1,35] evidently by an increase in nutritional blood flow to the digits.[1] A controlled study using saline placebo injections did not reveal long-term benefit from intra-arterial reserpine,[36] although others report more rapid healing of finger ulcers and improvement lasting months after single injections.[37,38]

Adverse Reactions—Reserpine should never be given to patients with depressive symptoms and/or a history of depression. Other frequent side effects include postural or post-exercise hypotension, lethargy, gastrointestinal symptoms, nightmares, and water retention. Nasal congestion and bradycardia are expected reactions from therapeutic doses. An increase in the frequency of breast cancer in hypertensive patients on long-term reserpine therapy has been reported,[39] but other studies have failed to confirm this carcinogenic effect.[40]

Interactions—Monoamine oxidase inhibitors should be discontinued at least a week before institution of reserpine therapy to avoid hypertension through norepinephrine release induced by initiating reserpine therapy. Tricyclic antidepressants could theoretically inhibit the action of reserpine.

Dosage—Oral: 0.25 mg to 1 mg daily. *Intra-arterial:* 0.5 mg.

GUANETHIDINE SULFATE (Ismelin Sulfate)

Guanethidine has been used in patients with Raynaud's phenomenon because it causes cutaneous vasodilation by interfering with the release of norepinephrine at the sympathetic neuroeffector junction. Guanethidine, in doses of 30 to 50 mg daily, has been demonstrated to increase digital capillary blood flow after cooling in patients with Raynaud's phenomenon due to scleroderma.[41]

Adverse Reactions—Postural or post-exercise hypotension limits the dose that can be used. Other frequent side effects include diarrhea, fatigue, and male sexual dysfunction.

Interactions—Tricyclic antidepressants block the action of guanethidine. Monoamine oxidase inhibitors should be discontinued at least one week before starting guanethidine, for hypertensive episodes may occur from the norepinephrine released by guanethidine.

Dosage—Oral: 10 to 60 mg daily.

METHYLDOPA (Aldomet)

Methyldopa dilates cutaneous blood vessels by interfering with the normal activity of the sympathetic nerves, and has been recommended for the treatment of Raynaud's phenomenon. Approximately 75 percent of patients ingesting 1 to 2 g of methyldopa a day reported subjective benefit; this was substantiated by an increased rate of rewarming of digits after cold exposure measured by skin temperature.[42]

Adverse Reactions—Methyldopa may cause drowsiness, headache, nasal congestion, postural hypotension, water retention, hemolytic anemia, and liver toxicity.

Dosage—Oral: 1 to 2 g daily.

DIHYDROGENATED ERGOT ALKALOIDS (Hydergine)

The dihydrogenated alkaloids of ergotoxine have an adrenergic blocking effect on the peripheral blood vessels. Dihydroergocornine increases blood flow to the extremities.[43,44] Hydergine (equal parts of dihydroergocornine, dihydroergocristine, and dihydroergokryptine mesylates) increases hand and foot blood flow significantly, but causes only small changes in calf blood flow when given intravenously to normal subjects.[45] Ischemic ulcers in patients with obstructive arterial disease reportedly healed somewhat faster during Hydergine oral administration.[46] Oral or intravenous administration of Hydergine or dihydroergotamine does not benefit patients with intermittent claudication.[11,46]

Dosage—Not of proven efficacy. Manufacturer recommends: *Sublingual:* 2 tablets 3 times daily.

REFERENCES

1. Coffman JD, Cohen AS: Total and capillary fingertip blood flow in Raynaud's phenomenon. N Engl J Med 285:259–263, 1971.
2. Coffman JD: Vasodilator drugs in peripheral vascular disease. J Maine Med Assoc 66:262–264, 266–269, 1975.
3. Coffman JD, Mannick JA: A simple, objective test for arteriosclerosis obliterans. N Engl J Med 273:1297–1301, 1965.
4. Coffman JD: Peripheral collateral blood flow and vascular reactivity in the dog. J Clin Invest 45:923–931, 1966.
5. Manley ES, Lawson JW: Effect of beta adrenergic receptor blockade on skeletal muscle vasodilatation produced by isoxsuprine and nylidrin. Arch Int Pharmacodyn Ther 175:239–250, 1968.
6. Coffman JD: Effect of vasodilator drugs in vasoconstricted normal subjects. J Clin Pharmacol 8:302–308, 1968.
7. Zsotér TT: Isoxsuprine as an oral vasodilator. Can Med Assoc J 110:1260–1261, 1974.
8. Strandness DE Jr: Ineffectiveness of isoxsuprine on intermittent claudication. JAMA 213:86–88, 1970.
9. Coffman JD, Mannick JA: Failure of vasodilator drugs in arteriosclerosis obliterans. Ann Intern Med 76:35–39, 1972.
10. Allen EV, Crisler GR: Result of intra-arterial injection of vasodilating drugs on the circulation: observations on vasomotor gradient. J Clin Invest 16:649–652, 1937.
11. Hamilton M, Wilson GM: The treatment of intermittent claudication. Q J Med 21:169–183, 1952.
12. Tibbs EE: Sustained release of papaverine in peripheral ischemia. South Med J 62:875–879, 1969.
13. Mulinos MG, Shulman I, Mufson I: On the treatment of Raynaud's disease with papaverine intravenously. Am J Med Sci 197:793–796, 1939.
14. Abramson DI, Zazeela J, Schkloven N: The vasodilating action of various therapeutic procedures which are used in the treatment of peripheral vascular disease. Am Heart J 21:756–766, 1941.
15. Asby GR Jr, Stein M, Conrad MC, et al: Hemodynamic effects of ethaverine hydrochloride in patients with peripheral vascular disease. Curr Ther Res 16:1096–1100, 1974.
16. Ronnor-Jessen V, Tjernlund A: Hepatotoxicity due to treatment with papaverine. N Engl J Med 281:1333–1335, 1969.
17. Spies TD, Bean WB, Stone RE: Treatment of subclinical and classic pellagra: use of nicotinic acid, nicotinic acid amide and sodium nicotinate, with special reference to the vasodilator action and the effect on mental symptoms. JAMA 111:584–592, 1938.
18. Zetterquist S: Muscle and skin clearance of antipyrine from exercising ischemic legs before and after vasodilating trials. Acta Med Scand 183:487–496, 1968.
19. Hansteen V, Lorentsen E: Vasodilator drugs in the treatment of peripheral arterial insufficiency. Acta Med Scand Suppl 556:1–62, (May) 1974.
20. Gillhespy RO: Nicotinyl alcohol tartrate in intermittent claudication. Br Med J 1:207–208, 1957.
21. Holti G, Newell DJ, Poole HG: Tetranicotinoylfructose in disorders of digital blood flow. Practitioner 207:654–658, 1971.
22. Van Wijk TW: The treatment of peripheral vascular diseases with Cyclospasmol. Angiology 4:103–113, 1953.
23. Gillhespy RO: Treatment of peripheral vascular disease with 'Cyclospasmol.' Angiology 7:27–31, 1956.
24. Fremont RE: Clinical and plethysmographic observations on the use of cyclandelate in arteriosclerosis obliterans. Am J Med Sci 247:182–194, 1964.
25. Hensel H, Ruef J, Golenhofen K: Human muscle and skin blood flow. Angiology 6:190–207, 1955.
26. Caliva FS, Eich R, Taylor HL, et al: Some cardiovascular effects of phenyl-2-butyl-norsuprifen hydrochloride (Arlidin). Am J Med Sci 238:174–179, 1959.
27. Stein ID: Arlidin: a clinical evaluation of a peripheral vasodilator with selective action on muscle vessels. Ann Intern Med 45:185–190, 1956.
28. DeCrinis K, Redisch W, Steele JM: Vascular effects of nylidrine hydrochloride during exercise. Proc Soc Exp Biol Med 102:29–31, 1959.

29. Karpman HL, Okun R: The effect of vasodilating drugs in peripheral vascular disease. Geriatrics 27:101–107, (Nov) 1972.
30. Ahlquist RP, Huggins RA, Woodbury RA: The pharmacology of benzylimidazoline (Priscol). J Pharmacol Exp Ther 89:271–288, 1947.
31. Gillespie JA: An evaluation of vasodilator drugs in occlusive vascular disease by measurement. Angiology 17:280–288, 1966.
32. Prandoni AG, Moser M: Clinical appraisal of intra-arterial priscoline therapy in the management of peripheral arterial diseases. Circulation 9:73–81, 1954.
33. Thomas M, Campbell H, Heard G: The effect of vasodilator drugs on skin blood-flow in peripheral vascular occlusion. Br J Surg 55:588–590, 1968.
34. Parks VJ, Sandison AG, Skinner SL, et al: The mechanism of the vasodilator action of reserpine in man. Clin Sci 20:289–295, 1961.
35. Kontos HA, Wasserman AJ: Effect of reserpine in Raynaud's phenomenon. Circulation 39:259–266, 1969.
36. McFadyen IJ, Housley E, MacPherson AIS: Intraarterial reserpine administration in Raynaud syndrome. Arch Intern Med 132:526–528, 1973.
37. Abboud FM, Eckstein JW, Lawrence MS, et al: Preliminary observations on the use of intra-arterial reserpine in Raynaud's phenomenon. Circulation 36(Suppl 2):49, 1967.
38. Willerson JT, Thompson RH, Hookman P, et al: Reserpine in Raynaud's disease and phenomenon: short term response to intra-arterial injection. Ann Intern Med 72:17–27, 1970.
39. Boston Collaborative Drug Surveillance Program: Reserpine and breast cancer. Lancet 2:669–671, 1974.
40. O'Fallon WM, Labarthe DR, Kurland LT: Rauwolfia derivatives and breast cancer. Lancet 2:292–296, 1975.
41. LeRoy EC, Downey JA, Cannon PJ: Skin capillary blood flow in scleroderma. J Clin Invest 50:930–939, 1971.
42. Varadi DP, Lawrence AM: Suppression of Raynaud's phenomenon by methyldopa. Arch Intern Med 124:13–18, 1969.
43. Goetz RH: The action of dihydroergocornine on the circulation with special reference to hypertension. Lancet 1:510–514, 1949.
44. Freis ED, Stanton JR, Litter J, et al: The hemodynamic effects of hypotensive drugs in man. II. Dihydroergocornine. J Clin Invest 28:1387–1402, 1949.
45. Barcroft H, Konzett H, Swan HJC: Observations on the action of the hydrogenated alkaloids of the ergotoxine group on the circulation in man. J Physiol 112:273–291, 1951.
46. Haeger K: Ischemic ulcers of the lower limb. Acta Chir Scand 130:584–592, 1965.

24. AGENTS USED IN HYPOTENSION AND SHOCK

Peter L. Gross

Shock is a clinical syndrome resulting from inadequate tissue perfusion. Manifestations depend on the degree of hemodynamic compromise at the tissue level in such vital organs as brain, heart, and kidney. The body's attempt to maintain homeostasis in the shock syndrome contributes to the clinical presentation. When physiologic defenses fail, inadequate tissue perfusion produces organ malfunction and the patient may develop oliguria, sensorium abnormalities, altered myocardial performance, and peripheral vascular changes.

CLASSIFICATION OF SHOCK

Numerous classification systems for shock have been devised, but none is adequate to explain all causes and mechanisms. Regardless of the etiology, several different mechanisms may be involved as the shock state develops.[1,2] Severe shock almost always involves derangement of cardiac pump function, intravascular volume status, and neurovascular balance. The following classification of shock is based on possible etiologies: 1) hypovolemic, 2) cardiogenic, 3) neurogenic, 4) septic, 5) anaphylactic, 6) mechanical, and 7) endocrine.

Hypovolemic shock results from exogenous or endogenous fluid losses. Blood loss due to hemorrhage or fluid and electrolyte loss from skin, gastrointestinal or renal sources are the principal causes of hypovolemic shock. Fluid shifts due to inflammation, trauma or allergic reactions can also produce intravascular volume changes and shock. *Cardiogenic shock* or pump failure arises from low output in the setting of severe congestive heart failure or myocardial infarction. *Neurogenic shock* refers principally to the failure of normal neurovascular function in spinal or general anesthesia or spinal cord injury. Drugs given in therapeutic doses (eg, ganglionic blockers and other antihypertensive agents) or in overdoses (eg, sedatives, hypnotics) may also affect neurovascular balance. *Septic shock* occurs in the setting of bacterial septicemia, most commonly with gram negative infections and endotoxemia. Antigen-antibody interaction with the release of humoral mediators can produce *anaphylactic shock* with smooth muscle and vascular consequences in target organs such as lung, skin, heart, and vessels. Several *mechanical* factors can interrupt blood flow and produce a shock state. These include cardiac tamponade, valvular disease, myxomatous cardiac obstruction, aortic dissection, tension pneumothorax, and massive pulmonary embolism. Finally, *endocrine failure* of pituitary, adrenal and/or thyroid function can result in a shock syndrome with or without stress.

PHYSIOLOGIC PRINCIPLES

While hypotension is often associated with shock, it is not always present, as in the previously hypertensive patient whose tissues are inadequately perfused with a blood pressure in the normal range. No single physiologic variable can fully characterize the shock state, and rational treatment requires attention to the interrelation of the physiologic variables that determine adequate blood flow at the tissue level.[3–5]

Blood flow is directly related to the driving pressure in blood vessels and inversely proportional to resistance to flow in those vessels (blood flow = pressure/resistance). Expressed in terms of cardiac output, this relationship states that cardiac output will vary directly with blood pressure and inversely with total peripheral resistance (cardiac output = blood pressure/total peripheral resistance). The contractile state of the myocardium and ventricular filling pressure also influence cardiac output. Therefore, the treatment of hypotension and shock requires appropriate attention to peripheral resistance, filling pressure, and the contractile state of the ventricle.

GENERAL THERAPEUTIC MEASURES

Pharmacologic therapy of shock with sympathomimetic agents is always secondary to general therapeutic measures. After attention to the patient's airway and oxygenation, the single most important non-pharmacologic maneuver is the establishment of adequate intravascular volume. Blood replacement must be accomplished if necessary and then fluids administered according to needs, preferably with central venous pressure (CVP) monitoring or Swan-Ganz catheter determinations of pulmonary capillary wedge (PCW) pressures.[6] The CVP is less reliable and may be elevated in situations of high output septic shock or in respiratory failure when the left atrial pressure, as reflected by PCW, is low indicating a need for more volume. When volume status is uncertain, a well-monitored fluid challenge is usually indicated.[7] Appropriate volume replacement may be the only therapy necessary in some patients with hypovolemic shock.[2]

Correction of metabolic abnormalities complicating the shock syndrome also has high priority for treatment. Correction of hypoxemia and reversal of acidosis will reduce the threshold for cardiac arrhythmias and will improve the performance of some sympathomimetic pressor amines.[8] Acidosis usually is secondary to increased lactate production in the setting of poor tissue perfusion.[9] Volume replacement may reverse this in part, but early treatment with sodium bicarbonate may be required. Treatment of electrolyte and other blood chemical abnormalities is also necessary.

Cardiac rhythm disturbances may precipitate or complicate shock. Both bradyarrhythmias and tachyarrhythmias should be controlled, especially if they contribute to poor tissue perfusion. However, some antiarrhythmic drugs may act as myocardial depressants and aggravate the shock syndrome.

Mechanical obstructions to blood flow in the heart, lungs, and great vessels can lead to shock. Where possible, the effect of vascular and valvular lesions on the therapeutic plan must be considered, tamponade must be relieved, and respirator effects on venous return minimized. Pneumothorax and tension pneumothorax must be looked for and treated.

When possible, any clear-cut primary cause of shock must be treated prior to or concurrently with sympathomimetic drugs or other pharmacologic agents. Thus, antibiotics are required in septic states, hormonal replacement is indicated in endocrine failure, and anesthetic agents should be eliminated, where possible, in spinal shock or in low tissue perfusion states that develop in the setting of general anesthesia. When hemodynamic compromise and shock is secondary to reversible coronary insufficiency, pharmacologic therapy must be first directed at the cause, with pressors or other agents used only adjunctively as necessary.

PHARMACOLOGIC THERAPY OF SHOCK

Adrenergic Agents

Sympathomimetic agents used in the treatment of shock stimulate adrenergic nervous system receptors, of which several subtypes exist[10] (Table 1). Sympathomimetic agents stimulate either alpha receptors, beta receptors, or both. Both direct and indirect mechanisms of action produce cardiac stimulation or peripheral vascular changes, depending on the drug.

Alpha adrenergic stimulation leads to vasoconstriction in peripheral, pulmonary, cerebral, skeletal, and abdominal blood vessels; mydriasis; and intestinal contraction. Phenylephrine and methoxamine are almost pure alpha receptor stimulators.[11] These drugs affect the peripheral vascular tree almost exclusively. They are sometimes used in combination with other sympathomimetic agents but also by themselves when depressed peripheral vascular tone is the principal problem. Cardiac effects of these agents are due to vagal reflexes secondary to increased peripheral vascular resistance.[12]

Beta adrenergic stimulation increases heart rate (chronotropic action) and the strength of ventricular contractions (inotropic action). Beta stimulation also increases ventricular automaticity and the likelihood of ectopic discharge, thereby increasing the risk of ventricular arrhythmias. In the periphery, beta stimulation produces

TABLE 1 Physiologic Effects of Stimulating Adrenergic Receptors

Receptor	Physiologic Effect
Alpha	Vasconstriction of peripheral, pulmonary, cerebral, skeletal, abdominal blood vessels Mydriasis Intestinal contraction (Essentially no direct cardiac effects but vagally mediated reflex bradycardia may occur)
$Beta_1$	Increase heart rate (chronotropic action) and strength of ventricular contractions (inotropic action) Increase ventricular automaticity and rate of idiopathic pacemakers, thereby increasing the risk of ventricular arrhythmias
$Beta_2$	Vasodilation of peripheral blood vessels Decrease of intestinal motility Relax smooth muscle in bronchi, bladder, and uterus

vasodilation, decreased intestinal motility and smooth muscle relaxation in bronchi, bladder, and uterus. Distinction is further made between $beta_1$ and $beta_2$ receptors.[13] The $beta_1$ receptors mediate cardiac inotropy and chronotropy, while the $beta_2$ receptors mediate the pulmonary bronchial response and the peripheral vascular changes. In contrast to the alpha adrenergic agents, such as phenylephrine and methoxamine, the beta agents have a direct effect on the heart in addition to a peripheral blood vessel effect producing vasodilation. Isoproterenol is an example of a relatively pure beta adrenergic agent.[14]

The advent of the drug dopamine raises the possibility of another kind of adrenergic receptor.[15] This drug, a biochemical precursor of norepinephrine, has adrenergic properties that are beta stimulatory on the heart at low doses and alpha stimulatory on the peripheral vascular bed when given in relatively high doses. However, at low doses dopamine has a vasodilating effect on the splanchnic and renal vascular beds that is not affected by any of the usual blocking agents.[16] These unique vascular ('dopaminergic') effects distinguish dopamine from other adrenergic drugs.

A number of drugs have mixed alpha and beta adrenergic properties, and dopamine has both alpha, beta and dopaminergic properties depending on the dose. Norepinephrine, epinephrine, and metaraminol have both alpha and beta stimulatory properties. The choice of adrenergic agents with mixed properties in the treatment of shock depends on the sum of physiologic effects of the agent and the pathophysiology of the shock state. In cardiogenic shock, mixed agents may improve tissue perfusion and blood pressure at a cost of increased myocardial work and decreased renal perfusion.

Sympathomimetic agents act directly or indirectly.[17] Phenylephrine, isoproterenol, and norepinephrine all act directly on alpha, beta, and mixed alpha and beta receptors, respectively.[18] In contrast, metaraminol, ephedrine, and dopamine may have some direct action on receptor sites, but also act indirectly by releasing norepinephrine from adrenergic nerve endings.[19,20] These indirect acting agents, in general, mimic norepinephrine in action but may have a slower onset and longer duration of action.[21] Extended use may lead to norepinephrine depletion and tachyphylaxis[22] while their use in patients having previously received norepinephrine depletors such as guanethidine or reserpine may result in diminished indirect effects.[23,24]

Steroids

Glucocorticoid replacement is specifically indicated for the treatment of shock due to adrenocortical insufficiency. In septic shock, pharmacologic doses of glucocorticoids may decrease mortality.[25] Physiologic and pharmacologic doses of steroids are also used to treat shock of other etiologies.[26,27] Despite possible benefits of steroids suggested by experimental studies,[28,29] the clinical efficacy of corticosteroids in shock due to causes other than adrenal insufficiency and possibly sepsis is not established.[30]

Glucagon

Glucagon is a polypeptide pancreatic hormone which produces hyperglycemia as its normal physiologic function. Glucagon also has positive inotropic and chronotropic effects in animals and man.[31,32] Its early popularity as a pressor agent has been considerably tempered by findings of clinical ineffectiveness in the setting of heart failure.[33] The role of this agent in shock syndromes is currently uncertain.

Vasodilators

In selected patients with cardiogenic shock, vasodilator agents that affect systemic vascular resistance are a potentially adjunctive measure.[34] Nitroprusside is commonly used and appears to directly affect vascular smooth muscle; it does not act through the adrenergic nervous system.[35]

Vasodilator agents reduce total peripheral resistance, but the effects on arterial blood pressure, heart rate and cardiac output depend on the pre-existing state of performance.[36] Patients in shock with low cardiac output in the setting of infarction or end stage heart failure may have increased peripheral resistance and only minimal or no response to sympathomimetic agents. After the usual general therapeutic measures have been instituted, cautious use of vasodilator drugs may decrease peripheral resistance and reduce filling pressure, thereby decreasing ventricular work and improving the overall contractile state of the myocardium. The net result may be an increased cardiac output without major adverse effects on heart rate or blood pressure.

These agents are generally rapid in action with quickly reversible hemodynamic effects. They require intensive, invasive physiologic monitoring, including arterial blood pressure lines, Swan-Ganz catheters for following pulmonary artery wedge pressures, and preferably cardiac output determinations. These agents may worsen hypotension with adverse effects on coronary perfusion and increased myocardial ischemia. Perfusion to other vital organs may also be adversely affected and the importance of hemodynamic monitoring in assessing the effect of this mode of therapy cannot be overemphasized.

Mechanical Circulatory Assistance. Mechanical circulatory assistance is a practical adjunctive measure in selected situations of cardiogenic shock. The most commonly used method is the intraaortic balloon timed to the electrocardiogram. Indications for the use of this device include shock complicating acute myocardial infarction, postoperative cardiogenic shock following coronary artery bypass surgery for main left coronary disease or in the setting of severe ventricular dysfunction.[37] General therapeutic measures remain the same and adrenergic agents may be required concurrently. Myocardial metabolism and systemic perfusion may improve,[38] but the effect on mortality has not been systematically studied.

The balloon is positioned in the upper descending aorta and inflates as the aortic valve closes. This action forces blood out of the central aorta increasing systemic pressure and coronary perfusion during diastole. Balloon deflation occurs at the beginning of systole decreasing impedance to ejection and decreasing ventricular work.[39] The procedure requires a femoral artery arteriotomy for balloon placement, an arterial line for pressure determinations, a Swan-Ganz catheter and preferably cardiac output determinations. Mechanical circulatory assistance may be utilized only temporarily, and inability to wean from the balloon after 48 to 72 hours is an ominous prognostic sign.

Choice of an Adrenergic Agent

With the exception of the use of epinephrine in anaphylactic shock, there are no absolute indications for the use of specific sympathomimetic agents in specific shock syndromes.[1] The choice of a specific agent must be based on specific clinical circumstances after primary therapy and general treatment measures have been instituted. Some guidelines, however, may be offered.

In hypovolemic shock, fluid replacement by itself sometimes does not improve tissue perfusion. In such cases a beta adrenergic agent may be tried for its inotropic and chronotropic action.[40,41] Isoproterenol is a reasonable choice but if the patient has tachycardia (greater than 120 beats/minute) or is severely hypoxemic (eg, chronic obstructive lung disease), this drug carries the risk of ventricular arrhythmias and decreased coronary perfusion.[4] In addition to its cardiac actions, the peripheral vascular vasodilating effects of isoproterenol may help to temporarily improve perfusion in the patient with severe peripheral vasoconstriction secondary to hypovolemia. There are, however, no good controlled studies proving the efficacy of beta adrenergic agents in hypovolemic shock, and myocardial ischemia is often a limiting factor.[42]

When shock is due to the loss of effective cardiac function secondary to infarction, congestive heart failure, and/or arrhythmias, pressor agents may be added to appropriate fluids, antiarrhythmic therapy, and attempts to reverse ischemia. Agents with mixed adrenergic effects have been most effective, although the likelihood of a successful outcome in advanced cardiogenic shock is limited.[43,44] Norepinephrine and metaraminol may be employed for their predominantly alpha adrenergic effects mediating peripheral vasoconstriction.[45–47] There is some beta adrenergic inotropic effect with these drugs, but the chronotropic action is largely counterbalanced by vagal reflexes so that cardiac output is unchanged or even decreased. Coronary flow may improve with these agents but at the expense of increased myocardial work and oxygen consumption.[38] Renal perfusion decreases, further complicating management.

Dopamine is a potentially useful agent in cardiogenic shock.[20,48] At low doses, actions on splanchnic and renal flow predominate, improving urine output.[49] Its beta adrenergic effects increase cardiac output due to effects on stroke volume and contractility.[50] The peripheral vascular changes depend on the dose of the drug; at infusion rates above 10 μg/kg/min, the drug largely resembles norepinephrine in action. Intermediate doses (2 to 5 μg/kg/min) may provide improved perfusion without the degree of peripheral vasoconstriction seen with high dose norepinephrine or the extent of increased cardiac work and arrhythmia potential seen with isoproterenol.[15] Dopamine must be used with care in the setting of acute coronary insufficiency, as the drug may cause increased ischemia if cardiac work increases.

A cautious trial of vasodilator agents may be utilized in selected cases of cardiogenic shock unresponsive to usual therapeutic measures or pressor agents. Extensive physiologic monitoring is necessary to assess beneficial or adverse effects on perfusion.

Neurogenic shock, occurring in the setting of spinal or general anesthesia, or as a drug side effect, is characterized by a loss of sympathetic tone and peripheral vascular resistance. Cardiac output and heart rate are usually depressed.[51] Volume replacement and elevation of the legs are immediate therapeutic possibilities. When a pressor agent is needed, a drug with mixed alpha and beta adrenergic actions is best.[1,21] Pure alpha agents, such as phenylephrine or methoxamine, will reverse the peripheral vascular loss of tone, but they reflexly slow heart rate and may further depress cardiac output.[52] Ephedrine is commonly used in anesthetic practice, but norepinephrine, metaraminol, or dopamine might also be used.[4] These agents will produce peripheral vasoconstriction but also increase cardiac inotropy.

Following overdosage with sedative-hypnotic agents or certain major tranquilizers, hypotension and shock often complicate clinical management. The causes of poor tissue perfusion in this situation may include hypovolemia due to unreplaced exogenous losses, relative hypovolemia due to venous pooling, myocardial depression, and peripheral vascular changes. As always, appropriate volume replacement is essential. General supportive measures are usually sufficient, but when pressor agents are necessary, the choice depends on the pathophysiology of the shock state. Beta adrenergic stimulators are useful if cardiac depression is the major problem, while an alpha adrenergic agent would be more appropriate if the patient in shock has warm extremities and other signs of peripheral vasodilation. A special situation may develop with phenothiazine ingestions since these drugs are alpha adrenergic blockers in high doses. The use of beta adrenergic drugs in this setting might exacerbate hypotension due to peripheral vasodilation.[53] If necessary, norepinephrine or methoxamine may be used cautiously. Sympathomimetic agents increase the likelihood of ventricular irritability in phenothiazine and tricyclic antidepressant overdoses.[54]

Complex mechanisms produce shock in sepsis. Vascular permeability, volume redistribution, vasodilation and disseminated intravascular coagulation may contribute.[55] Diagnosis and control of infection and volume adjustment are of major importance.[56] In early phases, there may be a 'warm' shock manifest by vasodilation, increased pulse pressure, and increased cardiac output, but this usually leads quickly to perfusion failure with hypotension, oliguria, peripheral vasoconstriction, and obtundation. Mixed alpha and beta adrenergic agents such as norepinephrine and metaraminol may exacerbate the peripheral vascular changes and, in general, beta adrenergic agents are preferred in septic shock when pressors are necessary.[57] Glucocorticoid treatment may reduce mortality.[28]

CONCLUSIONS

In summary, sympathomimetic agents are rarely the primary mode of therapy, except in anaphylactic shock. Their use usually follows any available primary therapy (volume, antibiotics, antiarrhythmics, etc.) and general therapeutic measures. Sympathomimetics should be used sparingly with constant attention to the patient's overall clinical status, level of alertness, urine output, acid-base balance, and other signs of adequate tissue perfusion. Adrenergic agents or vasodilator agents may be life-saving but they still are only temporizing measures while the primary causes of shock—hemorrhage, myocardial infarction, sepsis, anesthetic agents and other drugs, etc.—are reversed, if possible.

DRUG MONOGRAPHS

PHENYLEPHRINE HYDROCHLORIDE (Neo-Synephrine Hydrochloride)

Phenylephrine is a sympathomimetic amine with predominantly alpha adrenergic stimulatory properties.[11] It has significant direct effects on the vascular system and produces vasoconstriction and elevation of systolic and diastolic blood pressure. The drug has minimal central or direct cardiac effects, but increased peripheral vascular resistance produces vagally mediated reflex bradycardia.[12] The drug has little, if any, application to the treatment of shock states with the exception of its use in the conversion of paroxysmal atrial tachycardia associated with hypotension and poor perfusion.[1] Other therapeutic modalities, such as carotid sinus massage, digitalis, propranolol, edrophonium, and cardioversion, may be preferable in this setting.

Adverse Reactions—With high doses, potentially dangerous blood pressure elevations and headache may result. Reflex bradycardia and depression of cardiac output complicate its application to hypotension caused by spinal anesthesia and limit its use.[51]

Interactions—Cardiac arrhythmias have been reported with concomitant use of general anesthetic agents and phenylephrine. These arrhythmias seem to be more common with halogenated anesthetic agents.[58,59]

Dosage—In paroxysmal atrial tachycardia with associated hypotension, 0.15 to 0.8 mg is slowly injected intravenously, further doses being dependent on the blood pressure response. Assuming that tissue perfusion is adequate, the pressor response to 5 mg of intramuscular phenylephrine is approximately equal to 0.8 mg intravenously.[60] The drug is available in oral form, but absorption from this route is not reliable in the shock setting. Intravenous administration results in an immediate response with a duration of approximately 20 minutes.

METHOXAMINE HYDROCHLORIDE (Vasoxyl)

This sympathomimetic amine is similar to phenylephrine in action and application.[12] It is primarily a direct-acting alpha adrenergic agent producing vasoconstriction in vascular beds. Blood pressure is elevated due to marked peripheral vasoconstriction. Central or direct cardiac effects are minimal, but there is evidence in animals for antiarrhythmic and negative chronotropic cardiac action, perhaps secondary to weak cardiac beta blocking activity.[4] Like phenylephrine, this agent is limited to shock states of poor tissue perfusion produced by paroxysmal atrial tachycardia.[1] If other therapeutic modalities do not reverse the arrhythmia, methoxamine may be tried. Peripheral vasoconstriction produces vagally mediated reflex bradycardia that may lead to termination of the rhythm disturbance.[61]

Adverse Reactions—High doses may produce dangerous blood pressure elevations and headache. Urinary urgency, tingling in the extremities, and vomiting may occur. Reflex bradycardia and possible depression of cardiac output limit its application to neurovascular shock states induced by spinal anesthesia.[51]

Interactions—Like phenylephrine, methoxamine may produce cardiac arrhythmias when used with general anesthetic agents.[58,59]

Dosage—In paroxysmal atrial tachycardia, 3 to 5 mg of methoxamine may be given slowly, intravenously. Intramuscular injection can be used but is less reliable if there is poor tissue perfusion and peripheral vascular collapse.

TABLE 2 Preparations and Costs of Agents Used in Hypotension and Shock

GENERIC NAME	TRADEMARK NAME(S)	PREPARATIONS AND 1978 COSTS
Dopamine Hydrochloride	Intropin	Injection (solution) 40 mg/ml—$5.88/5-ml ampul
Ephedrine Sulfate	generic	Injection (solution) 25 mg/ml—$0.14–$0.34/1-ml ampul; 50 mg/ml—$0.14—$0.37/1-ml ampul
Epinephrine Hydrochloride	Adrenalin Chloride	Injection (solution) 1 mg/ml—$0.19/1-ml ampul; $1.16/30-ml vial
Isoproternol Hydrochloride	Isuprel Hydrochloride	Injection (solution) 0.2 mg/ml—$0.78/1-ml ampul; $2.66/5-ml ampul
Metaraminol Bitartrate	Aramine	Injection (solution) 10 mg/ml—$0.44/1-ml ampul; $2.27/10-ml vial
Methoxamine Hydrochloride	Vasoxyl	Injection (solution) 10 mg/ml—$1.16/10-ml vial; 20 mg/ml—$0.23/1-ml ampul
Nitroprusside Sodium	Nipride	Injection (powder) 50 mg—$5.64/vial
Norepinephrine (Levarterenol) Bitartrate	Levophed Bitartrate	Injection (solution) 1 mg of base/ml—$1.53/4-ml ampul
Phenylephrine Hydrochloride	Neo-Synephrine Hydrochloride	Injection (solution) 10 mg/ml—$0.74/1-ml ampul

ISOPROTERENOL HYDROCHLORIDE (Isuprel Hydrochloride)

This synthetic, direct-acting, sympathomimetic amine acts selectively on beta adrenergic receptors and accordingly produces cardiac stimulation, bronchial smooth muscle relaxation, and vasodilation in skeletal muscle vascular beds. There is little or no action on alpha adrenergic receptors. Because heart rate is increased and the strength of ventricular contraction is enhanced, cardiac output usually increases while systemic resistance decreases. Renal blood flow may change little or be decreased. Myocardial work, however, increases and coronary flow may be proportionally diminished compared to increased metabolic demands.[14,62] Excessive beta stimulation increases the risk of cardiac arrhythmias.[63]

Isoproterenol may be a useful adjunctive agent in shock states associated with hypovolemia, myocardial depression, bradyarrhythmias, pulmonary embolism, and possibly sepsis.[1,3,64–66] When complete heart block occurs due to disease above the bundle of His, isoproterenol will usually be effective in speeding ventricular response and reversing hypotension produced by this bradycardia.[67] However, its use for reflex bradycardia and coronary insufficiency, as in acute inferior myocardial infarction, is hazardous because of the risk of increased myocardial work and the potential of a relative decrease in coronary flow.[45,68]

Adverse Reactions—Tachycardia and the production of ventricular arrhythmias are the major adverse reactions.[63] Patients may complain of palpitations, nervousness, vertigo, headache or flushing. Angina pectoris may occur. Isoproterenol should generally be avoided in acute ischemic heart disease.[47]

Interactions—Like epinephrine, isoproterenol has been reported to produce cardiac arrhythmias during general anesthesia.[69] Its use in the setting of phenothiazine-induced alpha blockade is hazardous since peripheral vasodilation may predominate and hypotension may be enhanced.[53]

Dosage—For intravenous infusion, 0.05 to 0.3 μg/kg/min is given and titrated against the desired therapeutic response. A convenient mix is 2 mg in 250 ml of 5% dextrose in water.

EPINEPHRINE HYDROCHLORIDE (Adrenalin Chloride)

Epinephrine is a sympathomimetic amine with direct alpha and beta adrenergic actions. The beta effects predominate at lower doses and the drug has potent and rapid effects on blood pressure due to chronotropic and inotropic cardiac action and alpha adrenergic vasoconstrictive effects on vascular beds in the splanchnic circulation and skin.[19,21,64] Vasodilation occurs in skeletal muscle, and total peripheral resistance changes depend on the dose and the sum of effects on all vascular beds.[4]

Epinephrine has limited application to shock states in general, due to excessive cardiac stimulation, increased myocardial work and oxygen consumption, and a tendency toward ventricular irritability.[60] In addition, it reduces renal blood flow.[70] Epinephrine is, however, the treatment of choice for anaphylaxis.[1] It is also the drug of choice in cardiac standstill since its beta stimulation may help to reestablish electrical activity if external cardiac massage and attempts to reestablish ventilation and perfusion are used concomitantly.[71]

Adverse Reactions—Epinephrine can produce a state of restlessness and anxiety with headache, dizziness, tremor, and weakness. Nausea and vomiting can occur, and angina may be precipitated due to increased myocardial work.

Interactions—Cardiac rhythm disturbances have been reported with the simultaneous use of epinephrine and anesthetic agents, such as cyclopropane, halothane or other halogenated hydrocarbon anesthetics.[72,73] Ventricular arrhythmias, including ventricular fibrillation, have occurred. Arrhythmias may also develop with the use of parenteral epinephrine in patients receiving high doses of tricyclic antidepressants. Profound acidosis markedly diminishes the pressor effect of epinephrine while systemic alkalosis with a pH above 7.5 increases the likelihood of ventricular irritability.[3] Epinephrine should not be used to treat hypotension or shock associated with phenothiazine overdosage.

Dosage—In anaphylaxis, 100 to 500 μg or 0.1 to 0.5 ml of 1:1000 solution is slowly given intravenously. Alternatively 1 ml of 1:1000 solution may be given intramuscularly, but this route is not reliable if there is cardiovascular collapse. For intravenous infusions 0.025 to 0.3 μg/kg/min is given, depending on the desired response. A convenient infusion mix is 2 mg in 250 ml of 5% dextrose in water.

EPHEDRINE SULFATE

Ephedrine sulfate resembles epinephrine in its behavior, but it is less potent and has a longer duration of action.[18] It is principally a direct acting, mixed alpha and beta adrenergic stimulator, although some indirect action may occur due to the release of norepinephrine.[3,4] Cardiac effects predominate and result in an increased heart rate, stroke volume, and cardiac output. The peripheral vascular effects are directly and indirectly mediated vasoconstriction. These actions make the drug a reasonable choice for hypotension and myocardial depression of spinal anesthesia, but unpredictable responses and tachyphylaxis after repeated injection are occasional limiting factors.[4,74] The mechanism of tachyphylaxis is unclear. Ephedrine has little application to other shock states.

Adverse Reactions—Headaches, nervousness, palpitations and precipitation of angina and ventricular arrhythmias may occur, as with epinephrine. With continued use insomnia may occur.[60]

Interactions—During general anesthesia ephedrine may produce cardiac arrhythmias, although less commonly than with other sympathomimetic amines.[4,58,59] Indirect actions of ephedrine may precipitate excessive norepinephrine release when the drug is used in patients treated with monoamine oxidase (MAO) inhibitors, while cardiovascular effects may be lessened if the patients have previously received reserpine.[75]

Dosage—In hypotensive states associated with spinal anesthesia in adults, 20 to 30 mg of ephedrine may be given intravenously, or 30 to 40 mg may be given subcutaneously, although the latter route is less acceptable if hypotension and decreased tissue perfusion are present.

NOREPINEPHRINE BITARTRATE (Levophed Bitartrate)

Norepinephrine (Levarterenol) is a direct-acting agent stimulating both alpha and beta receptors.[3] It differs structurally from epinephrine in the absence of a methyl group, but in function the difference is considerable. Unlike epinephrine, alpha stimulation predominates with norepinephrine.[21]

Vasoconstriction of both capacitance and resistance vessels is produced in skin, skeletal muscle, and organs.[76] Increases in blood pressure are related to increased cardiac output and increased total peripheral resistance.[47] The vasoconstrictive alpha adrenergic-mediated effects far exceed the more mild beta effects on heart. While inotropic effects are produced, cardiac chronotropic changes are countered by reflex vagal stimulation due to peripheral vasoconstriction.[3] Increases in cardiac output can be limited or reversed as systemic vascular resistance increases.[77] Coronary blood flow may increase in relation to improved blood pressure.[38] Renal blood flow decreases and after prolonged administration intravascular volume may also decrease as transudation of fluid occurs secondary to vasoconstriction in post-capillary beds.[1,3]

Norepinephrine is a reasonable choice for the treatment of cardiogenic shock.[1,3,38,45,47] After general therapeutic measures have been directed at correction of volume, oxygenation and metabolic abnormalities, norepinephrine may help to improve blood pressure and coronary flow without the excessive increase in myocardial work of epinephrine or a pure beta adrenergic agent.[3,45] Increasing total peripheral resistance and decreasing renal blood flow may complicate the outcome if underlying ischemia, arrhythmias, or muscle pump failure are not reversed.

Norepinephrine is also used for shock caused by autonomic blockade, spinal or general anesthesia.[3,4] Its value in sedative-hypnotic overdoses associated with shock is questionable and often unnecessary, as most of these cases will respond to volume replacement and general supportive measures.[1,78] While norepinephrine has been used in septic shock states, there is data that its use is associated with decreased survival.[79] In shock caused by pericardial tamponade, norepinephrine may be used as a temporizing measure after volume replacement.[1] However, pericardicentesis or surgical relief of obstruction is the treatment of choice.

Adverse Reactions—Patients may complain of headache, tremor, dizziness and weakness, and angina pectoris may occur.[38] Bradycardia and hyperglycemia can occur while renal and cerebral hypoperfusion can alter mental status further. Extravasation of norepinephrine into tissues produces intense necrosis and sloughing.[3,47] Ideally, the drug is administered through a central venous catheter, but if a peripheral infusion is used, the addition of a small amount of phentolamine to the mix may minimize the risk of tissue necrosis.[1]

Interactions—Acidosis is a limiting factor in the effectiveness of norepinephrine as a pressor agent while systemic alkalosis (pH 7.5) may potentiate ventricular irritability.[3] Like epinephrine, norepinephrine interacts with anesthetic agents and produces cardiac arrhythmias.[69] This untoward effect has occurred with cyclopropane, halothane, and other halogenated agents.[80]

Dosage—Norepinephrine is given most conveniently by intravenous infusion at a rate of 0.03 to 0.1 μg/kg/min in an effort to establish a systemic arterial pressure of about 90 mmHg. A convenient mix is 4 mg in 250 ml of 5% dextrose in water. Phentolamine (5 to 10 mg) may be added to the infusion to minimize tissue injury if a peripheral vein is used.[3]

METARAMINOL BITARTRATE (Aramine)

Metaraminol is a synthetic sympathomimetic amine with both direct and indirect actions.[11] Its overall physiologic effects are similar to but less potent than norepinephrine; its duration of action is longer lasting. By direct action on alpha adrenergic receptors and indirect action through the release of norepinephrine from storage sites, the drug produces vasoconstriction, increased peripheral vascular resistance, and a resultant increased blood pressure. Reflex bradycardia usually occurs and as with norepinephrine, renal and cerebral blood flow decreases.[4] Cardiac inotropy increases, but less so than with norepinephrine and cardiac output remains unchanged or may slightly decrease if bradycardia occurs. Some beta adrenergic mediated vasodilation occurs with metaraminol, but alpha effects predominate. Tachyphylaxis may develop after prolonged administration, presumably secondary to norepinephrine depletion from storage sites.[22] A decrease in plasma volume may also occur as post-capillary vasoconstriction produces transudation of fluid into the extracellular space.[3,81]

The indications for the use of metaraminol are similar to those for norepinephrine. Shock states associated with myocardial infarction or failure, spinal or general anesthesia or pericardial tamponade may respond temporarily to the use of metaraminol.[1,4,45,46] There is no proven benefit to the application of this agent in septic shock states or in shock associated with sedative-hypnotic drug overdoses.[1]

In general, there is no major advantage to the use of a mixed indirect and direct-acting agent, such as metaraminol, compared to the use of norepinephrine. The slower onset of action may make for smoother control and subcutaneous tissue necrosis occurs only rarely, but the longer duration of action may be hazardous if overdosage and unintentional hypertension occurs. Furthermore, hypotension may recur after prolonged use, possibly secondary to norepinephrine depletion.[4]

Adverse Reactions—Adverse reactions with metaraminol are similar to those with norepinephrine. Increased myocardial oxygen consumption may precipitate angina, and cardiac arrhythmias may occur.[65] It is less likely to cause tissue necrosis after extravasation than norepinephrine, but this has been reported.[4]

Interactions—As with epinephrine and norepinephrine, acidosis and alkalosis have significant effects, with decreased potency noted under acidotic conditions and an increased tendency toward cardiac arrhythmias in alkalotic states.[3] General anesthetics, particularly the halogenated agents, can interact and cause ventricular arrhythmias.[69]

Metaraminol may also interact with antihypertensive drugs.

Guanethidine, reserpine, and methyldopa affect postganglionic nerve activity, either by decreasing norepinephrine stores or by effecting its release. Therefore, these drugs will interfere with the indirect norepinephrine-releasing actions of metaraminol and may limit its efficacy.[22–24]

MAO inhibitors also have the potential for drug interaction with metaraminol through inhibition of oxidative deamination of sympathomimetic amines.[75] The result may be an increased tissue store of norepinephrine, which will produce a heightened hypertensive response secondary to the indirect actions of metaraminol. Tyramine, amphetamine, levodopa and methyldopa could produce a similar response in MAO inhibitor treated patients.[82]

Dosage—Metaraminol 250 mg may be infused in 250 ml of 5% dextrose and water. The rate of infusion is titrated to obtain a mean arterial blood pressure of about 90 mmHg. Alternatively, the drug may be given by intermittent intramuscular or subcutaneous injections of 10 to 20 mg every 30 minutes to 2 hours.

DOPAMINE (Intropin)

Dopamine is a naturally occuring sympathomimetic amine, the immediate precursor of norepinephrine in the sympathetic nerve endings. Its action is unique among sympathomimetic agents in that it has direct alpha adrenergic stimulation and some indirect stimulation via norepinephrine release, beta stimulation, and so-called dopaminergic effects. These latter effects are in part dose-dependent.[15,16]

At infusion rates of 1 to 2 μg/kg/min, dopamine receptor stimulation predominates with selective vasodilation in splanchnic and renal vascular beds.[49] Peripheral resistance and blood pressure may fall slightly at this dose. At higher infusion rates of 2 to 10 μg/kg/min, cardiac beta inotropic and chronotropic stimulation are added to the dopamine receptor effects resulting in increased heart rate, increased cardiac output and increased blood pressure with a modest reduction in peripheral resistance.[50] As infusion rates exceed 10 μg/kg/min, peripheral alpha adrenergic effects begin to predominate producing peripheral vasoconstriction. Some beta cardiac effects remain but the dopamine (vasodilating) action on the splanchnic and renal circuits is overcome.[15]

Dopamine is becoming widely used in cardiogenic shock or after open heart surgery, and in some cases of severe congestive heart failure unresponsive to more traditional medications.[20,48] In contrast to other sympathomimetic agents, it is particularly useful in maintaining and improving renal perfusion (at moderate doses).[83] Dopamine may be used in combination with other adrenergic drugs such as isoproterenol, if there are signs of significantly elevated systemic resistance.[3] At high doses (above 10 to 15 μg/kg/min) the drug is similar to and has no advantage over norepinephrine.[15]

Adverse Reactions—Cardiac arrhythmias can occur and coronary insufficiency may be precipitated due to cardiac beta effects.[84] Patients may complain of headache, nausea, vomiting, and palpitations. Hypotension may actually be aggravated at low infusion rates due to vasodilation.[15]

Interactions—Like many sympathomimetic agents, there is a risk of ventricular arrhythmias when dopamine is employed in conjunction with general anesthetics.[85] The beta adrenergic cardiac effects may be reduced in patients receiving propranolol at beta-blocking doses, while alpha-blocking agents could limit the vasoconstricting response of dopamine.[15] MAO inhibitors may increase the hypertensive response to dopamine due to their effect on oxidative deamination of sympathomimetic amines.[86] Theoretically, drugs such as guanethidine and reserpine can interfere with the indirect acting effects due to norepinephrine depletion,[75] but the relative indirect and direct actions of dopamine are difficult to evaluate,[15] and the clinical significance of such interaction is unknown.

Dosage—Dopamine is infused in a 5% dextrose and water mix. The rate of infusion is titrated to obtain optimum blood pressure, urine output, and cardiac responses. As noted, dopamine receptor effects predominate at infusions of 1 to 2 μg/kg/min, while beta stimulation and some alpha adrenergic effects are added at rates of 2 to 10 μg/kg/min. Above 10 μg/kg/min, alpha adrenergic effects predominate.[15] The dosage range may be 140 to 2100 μg/min and a convenient mix is 500 mg in 500 ml of 5% dextrose solution.

SODIUM NITROPRUSSIDE

Sodium nitroprusside is a vasodilator agent with specific effects on vascular smooth muscle. It does not act through adrenergic receptors, nor does it affect other smooth muscle, cardiac muscle, or the central nervous system. Resistance arterial vessels and venous smooth muscle are both affected with a reduction in peripheral resistance producing changes in systemic blood pressure, cardiac output, and heart rate that depend on the pre-existing physiologic state.[36]

The drug may be tried with caution in selected situations of cardiogenic shock, especially those unresponsive to general therapeutic measures and sympathomimetic agents and associated with increased peripheral resistance. Extensive physiologic monitoring is necessary to assess the effect. Beneficial results have been reported in shock caused by acute myocardial infarction with pump failure and in states of poor perfusion associated with acute mitral regurgitation.[87–89] Concurrent use of a sympathomimetic pressor may be necessary to avoid hypotension.

Adverse Reactions—The major adverse effect of the use of vasodilator agents in shock states is worsened hypotension, and consequent organ and tissue hypoperfusion. Nausea, vomiting, diaphoresis, chest pain, and abdominal discomfort are reported to occur along with headache, tremor, respiratory distress, and seizures. Nitroprusside may combine with sulfhydryl groups in red cells and other tissues liberating cyanide which is converted to thiocyanate in the liver.[90] Thiocyanate is excreted by the kidney and will have an increased half-life when renal function is impaired. Thiocyanate toxicity occurs at plasma levels of 5 to 10 mg per 100 ml and is characterized by fatigue, nausea, confusion, psychosis, and muscle spasms. Levels of greater than 8 to 10 mg per 100 ml of thiocyanate require reduction in dose or discontinuation of the drug.[36,91]

Interactions—Hypotension may occur in the setting of concurrent use of oral antihypertensive medications and certain sympathomimetic agents. The drug is light sensitive and the solution should be protected by aluminum foil or other wrapping material. In the setting of renal disease or severe liver disease, nitroprusside infusions must be used with caution as thiocyanate may accumulate more rapidly. Daily determination of thiocyanate is necessary to avoid toxicity. Vitamin B_{12} metabolism may be altered by thiocyanate in the setting of nitroprusside therapy.

Dosage—Nitroprusside should be administered only by infusion pump and microdrip regulator to avoid changes in flow rate. The drug is supplied in 50 mg vials and is conveniently diluted in 500 ml of 5% dextrose and water. In hypotensive states the dose should be cautiously titrated, starting at approximately 0.5 μg/kg/min.

REFERENCES

1. Weil MH, Shubin H, Carlson R: Treatment of circulatory shock: use of sympathomimetic and related vasoactive agents. JAMA 231:1280–1286, 1975.
2. Moran NC: Evaluation of the pharmacologic basis for the therapy of circulatory shock. Am J Cardiol 26:570–577, 1970.
3. Tarazi RC: Sympathomimetic agents in the treatment of shock. Ann Intern Med 81:364–371, 1974.
4. Smith NT, Corbascio AN: The use and misuse of pressor agents. Anesthesiology 33:58–101, 1970.
5. Schumer W: Evolution of modern therapy of shock: science vs. empiricism. Surg Clin North Am 51:3–13, 1971.
6. Swan HJC, Ganz W, Forrester J, et al: Catheterization of the heart in man with use of a flow-directed balloon-tipped catheter. N Engl J Med 283:447–451, 1970.
7. Weil MH, Shubin H, Rosoff L: Fluid repletion in circulatory shock: central venous pressure and other practical guides. JAMA 192:668–674, 1965.
8. Trendelenburg U: Supersensitivity and subsensitivity to sympathomimetic amines. Pharmacol Rev 15:225–276, 1963.
9. MacLean LD, Duff JH, McLean APH: The patient in shock—part 1. Can Med Assoc J 105:78–83, 1971.
10. Ahlquist RP: A study of the adrenotropic receptors. Am J Physiol 153:586–600, 1948.
11. Moran NC: Adrenergic receptors within the cardiovascular system. Circulation 28:987–993, 1963.
12. Smith NT, Whitcher C: Acute hemodynamic effects of methoxamine in man. Anesthesiology 28:735–748, 1967.
13. Lands AM, Luduena FP, Buzzo HJ: Differentiation of receptors responsive to isoproterenol. Life Sci 6:2241–2245, 1967.
14. Krasnow N, Rolett EL, Yurchak PM, et al: Isoproterenol and cardiovascular performance. Am J Med 37:514–525, 1964.
15. Goldberg LI: Cardiovascular and renal actions of dopamine: potential clinical applications. Pharmacol Rev 24:1–29, 1972.
16. Allwood MJ, Ginsburg J: Peripheral vascular and other effects of dopamine infusions in man. Clin Sci 27:271–281, 1964.
17. Burn JH, Rand MJ: The action of sympathomimetic amines in animals treated with reserpine. J Physiol 144:314–336, 1958.
18. Aviado DM: *Sympathomimetic Drugs*. Springfield, Illinois, Charles Thomas, 1970.
19. Aviado DM: Pharmacologic approach to the treatment of shock. Ann Intern Med 62:1050–1059, 1965.
20. Goldberg LI, Talley RC, McNay JL: The potential role of dopamine in the treatment of shock. Prog Cardiovasc Dis 12:40–51, 1969.
21. Eckstein JW, Abboud FM: Circulatory effects of sympathomimetic amines. Am Heart J 63:119–135, 1962.
22. Watson LS: Current vasopressor drug armamentarium. In *Cardiovascular Drug Therapy,* The Eleventh Hahneman Symposium. Edited by AN Brest, JH Moyer. New York, Grune & Stratton, 1965, pp. 86–95.
23. Boura AL, Green AF: Adrenergic neuron blocking agents. Annu Rev Pharmacol 5:183–212, 1965.
24. Mashford MD, Mahon WA: Impairment of cardiovascular response to tyramine by reserpine administration in man. J Clin Invest 41:1382–1383, 1962.
25. Schumer W: Steroids in the treatment of clinical septic shock. Ann Surg 184:333–339, 1976.
26. Lefer AM, Verrier RL: Role of corticosteroids in the treatment of circulatory collapse states. Clin Pharmacol Ther 11:630–655, 1970.
27. Dietzman RH, Lillehei RC: The treatment of cardiogenic shock. V. The use of corticosteroids in the treatment of cardiogenic shock. Am Heart J 75:274–277, 1968.
28. Lillehei RC, MacLean LD: Physiological approach to successful treatment of endotoxin shock in the experimental animal. Arch Surg 78:464–470, 1959.
29. Sambhi MP, Weil MH, Udhoji VN: Acute pharmacologic effects of glucocorticoids: cardiac output and related hemodynamic changes in normal subjects and patients in shock. Circulation 31:523–530, 1965.

30. Nies AS: Cardiovascular disorders. I. Alteration of arterial pressure and regional blood flow. In *Clinical Pharmacology: Basic Principles in Therapeutics*. Edited by KL Melmon, HF Morrelli. New York, Macmillan, 1972, pp 176–179.
31. Kones RJ, Phillips JH: Glucagon: present status in cardiovascular disease. Clin Pharmacol Ther 12:427–444, 1971.
32. Glick G, Parmley WW, Wechsler AS, et al: Glucagon: its enhancement of cardiac performance in the cat and dog and persistence of its inotropic action despite beta receptor blockade with propranolol. Circ Res 22:789–799, 1968.
33. Gold HK, Prindle KH, Levey GS, et al: Effects of experimental heart failure on the capacity of glucagon to augment myocardial contractility and activate adenyl cyclase. J Clin Invest 49:999–1006, 1970.
34. Chatterjee K: Vasodilator therapy for heart failure. Ann Intern Med 83:421–423, 1975.
35. Rowe GG, Henderson RH: Systemic and coronary hemodynamic effects of sodium nitroprusside. Am Heart J 87:83–87, 1974.
36. Palmer RF, Lassiter KC: Sodium nitroprusside. N Engl J Med 292:294–297, 1975.
37. Gunnar RM, Loeb HS, Johnson SA, et al: Cardiovascular assist devices in cardiogenic shock. JAMA 236:1619–1621, 1976.
38. Mueller H, Ayres SM, Gianelli S, et al: Effect of isoproterenol, *l*-norepinephrine, and intraaortic counterpulsation on hemodynamics and myocardial metabolism in shock following acute myocardial infarction. Circulation 45:335–351, 1972.
39. Sanders CA, Buckley MJ, Leinbach RC, et al: Mechanical circulatory assistance—current status and experience with combining circulatory assistance, emergency coronary angiography, and acute myocardial revascularization. Circulation 45:1292–1313, 1972.
40. Morton AP: Shock. Med J Aust 1:920–923, 1972.
41. Weil MH, Shubin H: Isoproterenol for the treatment of circulatory shock. Ann Intern Med 70:638–641, 1969.
42. Kennedy JH, Bailas N: Support of the failing circulation: effects of isoproterenol in experimental left ventricular failure. Cardiologia 50:108–120, 1967.
43. Perlroth MG, Harrison DC: Cardiogenic shock: a review. Clin Pharmacol Ther 10:449–467, 1969.
44. Swan HJC, Forrester JS, Danzig R, et al: Power failure in acute myocardial infarction. Prog Cardiovasc Dis 12:568–600, 1970.
45. Kuhn LA: Shock in myocardial infarction—medical treatment. Am J Cardiol 26:578–587, 1970.
46. Shubin H, Weil MH: Practical considerations in the management of shock complicating acute myocardial infarction. Am J Cardiol 26:603–608, 1970.
47. Loeb HS, Rahimtoola SH, Gunnar RM: The failing myocardium: 1. Drug management. Med Clin North Am 57:167–185, 1973.
48. Loeb HS, Winslow EBJ, Rahimtoola SH, et al: Acute hemodynamic effects of dopamine in patients with shock. Circulation 44:163–173, 1971.
49. Breckenridge A, Orme M, Dollery CT: The effect of dopamine on renal blood flow in man. Eur J Clin Pharmacol 3:131–136, 1971.
50. Tsai TH, Langer SZ, Trendelenburg U: Effects of dopamine and α-methyl-dopamine on smooth muscle and on the cardiac pacemaker. J Pharmacol Exp Ther 156:310–324, 1967.
51. Greene NM: *Physiology of Spinal Anesthesia*, 2nd edition. Baltimore, Williams and Wilkins, 1969.
52. Li TH, Shimosato S, Etsten B: Methoxamine and cardiac output in non-anesthetized man and during spinal anesthesia. Anesthesiology 26:21–30, 1965.
53. Morrelli HF: Rational therapy of drug overdose. In *Clinical Pharmacology: Basic Principles of Therapeutics*. Edited by KL Melmon, HF Morrelli. New York, Macmillan, 1972, pp 617–618.
54. Fowler NO, McCall D, Chou T-C, et al: Electrocardiographic changes and cardiac arrhythmias in patients receiving psychotropic drugs. Am J Cardiol 37:223–230, 1976.
55. Robson HG: Pathophysiology and management of septic shock. Postgrad Med 50:149–154, (Nov) 1971.
56. Christy JH: Treatment of gram-negative shock. Am J Med 50:77–88, 1971.
57. Weil MH, Shubin H: Treatment of shock caused by bacterial infections (Medical Progress). Calif Med 119:7–13, (Nov) 1973.

58. Stephen CR, Margolis G, Fabian LW, et al: Laboratory observations with fluothane. Anesthesiology 19:770–781, 1958.
59. Catenacci AJ, DiPalma JR, Anderson JD, et al: Serious arrhythmias with vasopressors during halothane anesthesia in man. JAMA 183:662–665, 1963.
60. Innes IR, Nickerson M: Norepinephrine, epinephrine, and the sympathomimetic amines. In *The Pharmacological Basis of Therapeutics,* fifth edition. Edited by LS Goodman, A Gilman. New York, Macmillan, 1975, pp 477–513.
61. Aviado DM: Cardiovascular effects of some commonly used pressor amines. Anesthesiology 20:71–97, 1959.
62. Elliott WC, Gorlin R: Isoproterenol in treatment of heart disease. JAMA 197:315–320, 1966.
63. Trautwein W: Generation and conduction of impulses in the heart as effected by drugs. Pharmacol Rev 15:277–332, 1963.
64. Clauss RH, Ray JF: Pharmacologic assistance to the failing circulation. Surg Gynecol and Obstet 126:611–630, 1968.
65. Brown RS, Carey JS, Mohr PA, et al: Comparative evaluation of sympathomimetic amines in clinical shock. Circulation 34:260–271, 1966.
66. Kardos GG: Isoproterenol in the treatment of shock due to bacteremia with gram negative pathogens. N Engl J Med 274:868–873, 1966.
67. Criscitiello MG: Therapy of atrioventricular block. N Engl J Med 279:808–810, 1968.
68. Kuhn LA, Kline HJ, Goodman P, et al: Effects of isoproterenol on hemodynamic alterations, myocardial metabolism, and coronary flow in experimental acute myocardial infarction with shock. Am Heart J 77:772–783, 1969.
69. Katz RL, Epstein RA: The interaction of anesthetic agents and adrenergic drugs to produce cardiac arrhythmias. Anesthesiology 29:763–784, 1968.
70. Goldberg LI: Use of sympathomimetic amines in heart failure. Am J Cardiol 22:177–182, 1968.
71. Anon: Standards for cardiopulmonary resuscitation (CPR). JAMA 227(Suppl):833–860, 1974.
72. Dresel PE, MacCannell KL, Nickerson M: Cardiac arrhythmias induced by minimal doses of epinephrine in cyclopropane anesthetized dogs. Circ Res 8:948–955, 1960.
73. Matteo RS, Katz RL, Papper EM: The injection of epinephrine during general anesthesia with halogenated hydrocarbons and cyclopropane in man. Anesthesiology 23:360–364, 1962.
74. Patil PN, Tye A, LaPidus JB: A pharmacological study of the ephedrine isomers. J Pharmacol Exp Ther 148:158–168, 1965.
75. Anon: Adrenergic therapy. In *Evaluations of Drug Interactions,* second edition. Washington, American Pharmaceutical Association, 1976, pp 332–336.
76. Schmid PG, Eckstein JW, Abboud FM: Comparison of the effects of several sympathomimetic amines on resistance and capacitance vessels in the forearm of man. Circulation 34(Suppl. III):209–210, 1966.
77. Gunnar RM, Loeb HS: Use of drugs in cardiogenic shock due to acute myocardial infarction. Circulation 45:1111–1124, 1972.
78. Shubin H, Weil MH: Shock associated with barbiturate intoxication. JAMA 215:263–268, 1971.
79. Weil MH, Shubin H, Biddle M: Shock caused by gram negative microorganisms: analysis of 169 cases. Ann Intern Med 60:384–400, 1964.
80. Andersen N, Johansen SH: Incidence of catechol-amine-induced arrhythmias during halothane anesthesia. Anesthesiology 24:51–56, 1963.
81. Cohn JN: Relationship of plasma volume changes to resistance and capacitance vessel effect of sympathomimetic amines and angiotension in man. Clin Sci 30:267–278, 1966.
82. Goldberg LI, Whitsett TL: Cardiovascular effects of levodopa. JAMA 218:1921–1923, 1971.
83. Breckenridge A, Orme M, Dollery CT: The effect of dopamine on renal blood flow in man. Eur J Clin Pharmacol 3:131–136, 1971.
84. Allwood MJ, Cobbold AF, Ginsburg J: Peripheral vascular effects of noradrenaline, isopropylnoradrenaline and dopamine. Br Med Bull 19:132–136, 1963.
85. Katz RL, Lord CO, Eakins KE: Anesthetic-dopamine cardiac arrhythmias and their prevention by *beta* adrenergic blockade. J Pharmacol Exp Ther 158:40–45, 1967.

86. Goldberg LI, Sjoerdsma A: Effects of several monoamine oxidase inhibitors on the cardiovascular actions of naturally occuring amines in the dog. J Pharmacol Exp Ther 127:212–218, 1959.
87. Franciosa JA, Guiha NH, Limas CJ, et al: Improved left ventricular function during nitroprusside infusion in acute myocardial infarction. Lancet 1:650–654, 1972.
88. Chatterjee K, Parmley WW, Ganz W: Hemodynamic and metabolic responses to vasodilator therapy in acute myocardial infarction. Circulation 48:1183–1193, 1973.
89. Goodman DJ, Ronsen RM, Holloway D: Effect of nitroprusside on left ventricular dynamics in mitral regulation. Circulation 50:1025–1032, 1972.
90. Page IH, Corcoran AC, Dustan HP, et al: Cardiovascular actions of sodium nitroprusside in animals and hypertensive patients. Circulation 11:188–198, 1955.
91. Gifford RW Jr: Hypertensive emergencies and their treatment. Med Clin North Am 45:441–452, 1961.

25. ANTIHYPERTENSIVE AGENTS

David J. Greenblatt

Hypertension refers to at least two distinct entities. It can describe simply a reading on a cuff sphygmomanometer (or other recording device) indicating arterial blood pressure in excess of the usual range of 'normal.' Hypertension also refers to a pathophysiologic process —either disease or syndrome—associated with repeatedly elevated readings of arterial blood pressure. A single isolated observation of hypertension as a physical sign does not imply that the disease is present. Conversely, a normal reading on a blood pressure cuff on any one occasion does not exclude the presence of hypertensive disease. In general, the diagnosis of hypertensive disease should not be made until elevated blood pressure is observed repeatedly. Preferably, measurements should be taken at different times several days or weeks apart and at various times during the day. Whenever possible, efforts should be made to record the patient's blood pressure in the home and/or work environments, to ensure that the decision to treat is not based entirely upon readings taken in the physician's office.

Unfortunately, the criteria for 'high' or 'normal' arterial blood pressure are controversial, except in extreme cases. Readings consistently at or below 100/70 mmHg are not associated with any risk of morbidity and mortality, whereas readings consistently exceeding 160/100 mmHg almost certainly are. For the majority of the population, however, blood pressure readings usually fall within these limits, making it difficult to decide whether a person is 'hypertensive' or 'normotensive.' Most authorities would identify 140/90 mmHg as an arbitrary but generally reasonable division point, since individuals with blood pressure readings consistently higher than this have a clinically important increase in risk of cardiovascular morbidity and mortality. As with most arbitrary guidelines, the 140/90 mmHg division point cannot be considered rigid, and must be interpreted in light of the specific clinical situation. For example, most physicians would be considerably more aggressive in the evaluation and treatment of a blood pressure of 140/90 mmHg in a 15 year-old female than in an 80 year-old male.

Hypertensive disease is one of the few diseases of which early detection and treatment clearly reduces morbidity and mortality, and prolongs useful and actful life. Untreated hypertension is associated with an increased risk of morbidity, primarily from cerebrovascular disease, and secondarily from congestive heart failure, renal insufficiency, and accelerated ischemic cardiac and peripheral vascular disease.[1-4] The greater the degree and duration of hypertension —whether systolic, diastolic, or both—the greater the risk.[5] Partial or complete normalization of blood pressure via effective pharmacotherapy partially or completely nullifies the risk. The clear benefits of antihypertensive therapy should render the treatment of this disease a type of medical 'miracle.' Unfortunately, patients and physicians seldom view it as such. In the early stages of the disease—precisely when initiation of effective pharmacotherapy can have the greatest preventive benefit—most patients are active, productive, and entirely asymptomatic. They often resent and disbelieve the need for daily, life-long drug therapy of an invisible disease when they feel fine. This is reinforced by the continuous financial burden imposed by the medications, together with the inevitable array of annoying although usually minor medication side effects.[6] Therapeutic reluctance similarly infects many physicians, who realize that their only reward for undertaking effective drug therapy of hypertension may be ungrateful scowls and complaints. Finally, the lay press and popular media regrettably fuel the flames of medication paranoia in general, fostering and perpetuating the public's suspicions about the hazards of pill-taking. It is not surprising that even when hypertension is detected and clearly documented early in the course of the disease, effective long-term drug therapy is by no means the rule.

DIAGNOSTIC EVALUATION OF HYPERTENSION

In 95% or more of patients with elevated arterial blood pressure, no specific 'curable' cause or underlying disease can be found. This most common form of hypertensive disease ('essential' hypertension) is familial, asymptomatic, and of insidious onset during the 3rd, 4th, or 5th decades, is slowly and gradually progressive, and is characterized by normal cardiac output, increased peripheral vascular resistance, and normal values of extracellular fluid volume, plasma renin activity, aldosterone secretion, and plasma catecholamines.[1,2,7,8] The epidemiologic predominance of essential hypertension makes it unlikely that exhaustive diagnostic evaluation of any specific hypertensive patient will reveal one of the relatively unusual 'curable' causes (Table 1). On the other hand, overlooking of an underlying disease having hypertension as a secondary manifestation is an important error. Thus, health care professionals face conflicting objectives during evaluation of the hypertensive patient. Procedures required to identify treatable causes variously combine the undesirable characteristics of expense, inconvenience, discomfort, and hazard. Accordingly, the extent of diagnostic evaluation must be individualized based upon the specific characteristics and clinical findings in a given patient. A reasonable basic evaluation probably consists of medical history, physical examination, urinalysis, and measurement of serum concentrations of urea nitrogen (or creatinine), sodium, potassium, chloride, and bicarbonate. Selected patients, particularly those aged 40 and over, could have a chest x-ray, an electrocardiogram, and a plasma lipid profile. These objective tests will generally be normal in patients with 'essential' hypertension having no cardiovascular or renal sequelae. When screening procedures raise suspicion of a curable cause or end-organ disease is identified, more extensive testing can be undertaken. Further evaluation may also be appropriate for patients who are less than 25 to 30 years of age, those with very severe hypertension, or those in whom control of hypertension with usual therapies proves difficult or impossible.

TABLE 1 Curable Causes of Hypertension

Curable Causes of Hypertension
Pheochromocytoma
Renovascular disease
Renal parenchymal disease
Primary aldosteronism
Coarctation of the aorta
Urinary tract obstruction
Cushing's syndrome
Thyrotoxicosis
Hypertension of pregnancy
Drug-induced hypertension

APPROACH TO PHARMACOTHERAPY OF HYPERTENSION

The general objective of antihypertensive therapy should be normalization of arterial blood pressure. Implementation of this broad objective obviously must be individualized, since the definition of a 'normal' blood pressure, let alone how close to the norm a treated individual's blood pressure should be reduced, are not established. In general, the more the blood pressure is reduced, the better off is the patient from a cardiovascular risk status. However, there are limits to how low the blood pressure can be reduced. Excessive antihypertensive therapy will lead to symptomatic hypotension as well as increase the likelihood of medication side effects. In many individuals, particularly those with moderate to severe hypertension of long duration, no tolerable combination of drugs will completely 'normalize' blood pressure. This does not mean that therapy is of no value or should be abandoned; on the contrary, partial reduction of blood pressure partially reduces the associated cardiovascular risk, and is certainly far better than leaving the disease untreated.[9]

Diuretics

Many pharmacologic approaches can successfully reduce blood pressure. However, it is generally recognized that diuretic treatment should be the first step in all antihypertensive drug regimens. Adequate diuretic therapy will cause a 5 to 20% reduction in both systolic and diastolic blood pressure in nearly all hypertensive patients. Thus, diuretic therapy alone may be sufficient in many patients with mild hypertension. In others with more severe or atypical disease, a diuretic alone may not suffice; however, diuretic treatment should always be continued even when it is necessary to add other drugs.

Contrary to extensive promotional claims, a clear superiority of one diuretic agent or class of agents in antihypertensive therapy is not established.[10,11] Choice of a specific drug should be guided by what is least expensive and best tolerated. In the great majority of patients, thiazide diuretics meet both of these needs. The usual maximum effective dose is 100 mg of hydrochlorothiazide, 1 g of chlorothiazide, or the equivalent of another thiazide derivative. The daily dose may be given at once or subdivided. An initial choice of a more expensive diuretic (furosemide, chlorthalidone, metolazone, etc.) over a thiazide is seldom justified. The same can be said for potassium-sparing agents[12] (triamterene, spironolactone), or for diuretic combinations containing fixed quantities of thiazides and potassium-sparing agents (Dyazide, Aldactazide). Whatever diuretic is initially chosen, the effective dose should be continued for at least three to four weeks before it is decided whether diuretic therapy alone is sufficient.

Side effects of diuretics are a real problem, but should be placed in proper clinical perspective. With the exception of the potassium-sparing agents,[12] all diuretics have the potential to cause potassium depletion. Extensive investigation of potassium homeostasis during diuretic therapy[13–18] reveals the following facts: (a) some but not all patients receiving long-term diuretic therapy undergo net depletion of body stores of potassium; (b) since potassium is largely an intracellular ion, depletion of total body potassium may or may not be associated with hypokalemia; likewise, hypokalemia does not necessarily indicate a significant deficit of total body potassium; (c) the definition of clinically important hypokalemia (usually serum concentrations below 3.5 mEq/liter) is arbitrary; most patients tolerate a moderate degree of hypokalemia with no symptoms or untoward consequences whatsoever; (d) the need for intensive monitoring of serum potassium concentrations during long-term antihypertensive therapy, let alone the need for routine potassium supplementation, are not established. Thus, initiation of thiazide therapy without concurrent potassium supplementation and without intensive monitoring of serum potassium concentrations constitutes reasonable medical practice in the majority of patients.[19,20] Close monitoring of serum potassium, and/or institution of potassium supplementation, may be appropriate for patients who develop moderate to severe hypokalemia, for those concurrently receiving digitalis glycosides, or those in whom potassium loss is suspected as a possible cause of nonspecific symptoms of muscle weakness, fatigue, etc. Much the same can be said for the two other common metabolic consequences of diuretic therapy: hyperuricemia and hyperglycemia.[21,22] Most thiazide-treated patients experience some rise in serum urate levels, as well as some deterioration of glucose tolerance. Only rarely does hyperuricemia lead to acute gouty arthritis in patients not already so predisposed. Nor does diuretic-induced hyperglycemia necessarily lead to 'uncontrolled' diabetes or even to degrees of glucose intolerance that require intervention.

Individual diuretic agents are discussed in detail in Chapter 26.

Adjunctive Therapy

If a diuretic alone fails to produce adequate reduction in blood pressure, therapy with another antihypertensive agent is initiated concurrent with continuation of the diuretic. The general need for such combination therapy is well-established.[23] First, diuretics potentiate the hypotensive action of most other adjunctive drugs, usually making it possible to use lower doses of the adjunctive agent. Furthermore, nearly all adjunctive agents cause an increase in plasma renin activity, leading to retention of salt and water with partial nullification of antihypertensive effect. Diuretics offset this fluid-retaining property, allowing adjunctive agents to retain their effectiveness.

Several approaches to adjunctive antihypertensive treatment are in wide clinical use. The choice of a specific regimen depends upon evaluation of the relative cost, convenience, and potential side effects of each. Often the most appropriate regimen is selected only by trial and error. There is sound theoretical rationale for tailoring the choice of adjunctive antihypertensive therapy to fit specific pathophysiologic subtypes of hypertension (see below). However, since adequate confirmation of the clinical benefit of such schemes is lacking, attention is best focused upon control of blood pressure.

Alpha-Sympathoplegic Agents. One major class of adjunctive agents exert their blood pressure reducing activity at least in part by interfering with alpha-adrenergic transmission.[24] One subgroup (including rauwolfia alkaloids, methyldopa, and clonidine) appear to act largely via the central nervous system. The other drug in this class (guanethidine) has mainly a peripheral action.

With the exception of clonidine, the sympathoplegic agents are time-tested—they have been in wide clinical use for many years, the range and limits of their clinical efficacy are established, and their side effects are recognized. Some of these drugs (reserpine, guanethidine, and possibly methyldopa) can be given on a once-daily basis, thereby maximizing the convenience of therapy and enhancing the likelihood of compliance. In the case of reserpine, its availability as a generic drug substantially reduces the cost of long-term treatment. These benefits of sympathoplegic therapy must be weighed against their disadvantages. The frequency of side effects is high, and increases as the effective dose range is attained. In the case of guanethidine, troublesome side effects inevitably accompany effective dosage. With the centrally-acting agents, nonspecific central nervous system depression (ie, drowsiness, fatigue, lethargy) and impairment of intellectual function are common and very troublesome. Since the action of sympathoplegic agents mainly involves impairment of alpha-adrenergic transmission, their hypotensive effect is largely postural, making symptomatic postural hypotension another common therapeutic problem.

The outcome of the interaction of positive and negative aspects of sympathoplegic therapy in a given patient is unpredictable. In many patients, therapy with these drugs is highly effective and well-tolerated. In others, intolerable side effects prevent attainment of effective antihypertensive dosage regardless of how carefully a drug is chosen or the dose is titrated.

Vasodilator Agents. A second major class of adjunctive agents act mainly by a direct relaxant effect on arteriolar smooth muscle, thereby reducing peripheral resistance.[25,26] Their action appears unrelated to alpha-adrenergic transmission. Of the two drugs in this category available for clinical use, experience with hydralazine is by far the most extensive. Prazosin is more recently introduced, and its relative benefits and disadvantages are not fully established.

Hydralazine's relaxant effect upon resistance arterioles gives the drug a relatively 'specific' antihypertensive action and eliminates most of the troublesome side effects (ie, drowsiness, postural hypotension, impairment of male sexual function, nasal congestion, etc.) associated with the alpha-sympathoplegic agents.[25–27] As such, hydralazine is invariably better tolerated than the sympathoplegics. However, hydralazine is not without its disadvantages. A major problem is the need for multiple daily doses. Since the duration of action of each dose is short, three to four daily doses are generally required for 'smooth' antihypertensive action throughout the day. This reduces the convenience of therapy and works against patient compliance; it also increases the dollar cost of treatment with an already expensive drug.

Another major drawback of hydralazine therapy are the inevitable consequences of reflex sympathetic stimulation associated with peripheral vasodilation. These reflex effects can lead to tachycardia, palpitations, increased cardiac work, flushing and headache. As such, effective and tolerable therapy with hydralazine generally requires coadministration of another agent (such as propranolol) to antagonize reflex sympathetic stimulation.

Beta-Adrenergic Blockade. Propranolol and metoprolol are the two beta-adrenergic blockers approved for the treatment of hypertension. Experience with propranolol is by far the most extensive. Although the mechanism of its antihypertensive effect is not fully understood, propranolol is well-established as an effective hypotensive agent.[28-30] Many clinicians now recommend propranolol as the first adjunctive agent of choice if a diuretic alone does not adequately reduce blood pressure. Hydralazine is then added if the diuretic-propranolol combination is not sufficient.

Advantages of beta blockers include their non-interference with alpha-adrenergic function, thereby leaving postural blood pressure regulation intact. The antianginal and antiarrhythmic effects of propranolol make it particularly useful for hypertensive patients with coexisting ischemic heart disease or cardiac arrhythmias. Unfortunately, both propranolol and metoprolol are relatively high in dollar cost.

SPECIAL CATEGORIES OF ESSENTIAL HYPERTENSION

Recent studies of the biochemistry and circulatory physiology of essential hypertension have identified several apparent pathophysiologic subtypes. A convincing rationale suggests that specific pharmacologic treatment should match specific disease characteristics as closely as possible.[31,32] However, despite the theoretic appeal of this approach, there is no convincing evidence that it provides any clinical benefit beyond that derived from an effective lowering of blood pressure in general. Nonetheless, identification and characterization of these hypertensive subtypes may be of value to clinicians in understanding the disease process and the probable response to therapy.

Hypertension With Low or High Plasma Renin Activity (PRA)

Reliable biochemical determinations of PRA are available only in a limited number of medical centers, hence are unavailable to most practicing physicians. Characterization of PRA in essential hypertension has greatly enhanced understanding of the pathophysiology of the disease, but is not a requirement for effective clinical management.

Essential hypertension with high PRA can be identified in a relatively small proportion of hypertensive patients.[33,34] Epidemiologic studies suggesting that this disease type has a more ominous prognosis than hypertension with low or normal PRA[35–37] have been disputed.[33] In any case, the finding of high PRA associated with elevated blood pressure appropriately leads to the suspicion of renovascular disease, which is usually not found when further evaluation is undertaken. Because of its ability to reduce PRA, propranolol is suggested as a reasonable treatment of choice for these patients. However, a specific benefit of initial treatment with propranolol over the conventional diuretic-first approach is not clearly established.

Another group of hypertensive individuals have abnormally low levels of PRA, even after stimulation with a diuretic such as furosemide.[33–38] The findings suggest the presence of a mineralocorticoid secreting tumor, but further diagnostic evaluation (such as measurement of aldosterone secretion rates) usually does not document this. Treatment with the aldosterone antagonist spironolactone has been suggested as the most rational form of therapy, but it has no documented advantage over other diuretics. Furthermore, long-term therapy with spironolactone, particularly at high doses, commonly results in unacceptable endocrine side effects[12] (such as gynecomastia in male patients).

Labile (High-Output) Hypertension

A group of hypertensive patients have elevations in blood pressure which are very episodic and often largely systolic.[39,40] Such patients tend to be relatively young—in their 3rd and 4th decades. Peripheral vascular resistance is normal but cardiac output is elevated, particularly during episodes of high systolic blood pressure. The syndrome is probably similar or identical to a group of conditions characterized as 'hyperdynamic beta-adrenergic circulatory states.'[41] High-output labile hypertension in young individuals may be a precursor of 'sustained' essential hypertension with normal cardiac output.[42]

Since such individuals appear to have increased sensitivity of the cardiovascular system to beta-adrenergic stimulation, treatment with a beta blocker such as propranolol would appear to be the most logical approach to drug therapy. However, the need for any drug treatment of such individuals is not clearly established, nor has a short- or long-term clinical superiority of propranolol over diuretic treatment been confirmed.

Disproportionate Systolic Hypertension

Another group of hypertensive patients have systolic hypertension (ie, 200/90 mmHg) which is sustained rather than episodic in nature. Such patients generally are elderly, and have arteriosclerotic disease in normally distensible resistance arterioles and larger arteries. The stiffening and poor compliance of the diseased vessels leads to hypertension which is largely systolic.

Disproportionate systolic hypertension has always posed a therapeutic dilemma. In fact, many clinicians feel it should not be treated, in view of their belief (now known to be incorrect) that systolic hypertension is 'benign,' and that only diastolic hypertension requires drug therapy. Another therapeutic obstacle is the fact that partial or complete normalization of systolic pressure is usually accompanied by reduction of diastolic pressure to levels which may impair perfusion of vital organs.[43] Although these fears are probably exaggerated, the need for careful titration of antihypertensive therapy for patients with disproportionate systolic hypertension is very clear.

As with labile systolic hypertension, propranolol would appear to constitute a logical treatment for patients with sustained systolic hypertension. Whatever treatment is chosen, clinicians usually will have to settle for only partial normalization of systolic pressure, at the cost of reducing diastolic pressure to what may be uncomfortably low levels. Nonetheless, it appears that carefully monitored antihypertensive treatment is quite safe and probably associated with improvement of long-term prognosis.

HYPERTENSIVE EMERGENCIES

In the majority of patients with elevated blood pressure, the need for drug therapy is not urgent and can be undertaken over a period of weeks or months until adequate control is achieved. In unusual cases, rapid reduction of blood pressure is essential.[44-46] The availability of effective treatment of hypertension in its early (subacute) stages has greatly reduced the prevalence of hypertensive emergencies in clinical practice. Nonetheless, hypertensive emergencies may occur in patients with long-standing essential hypertension that has progressed to life-threatening levels, or in patients with moderate to severe essential hypertension under control with drug therapy which, for whatever reason, has been allowed to lapse. Hypertensive emergencies can also accompany pheochromocytoma, amphetamine poisoning, or may occur during treatment with a monoamine oxidase inhibitor in a patient who has ingested tyramine-containing foods.

Urgent treatment of hypertension is indicated when blood pressure reaches levels that are 'extremely elevated,' or when blood pressure is rising rapidly from minute-to-minute or hour-to-hour. Urgent treatment is also indicated when hypertension is associated with central nervous system disturbances (severe headache, impairment of consciousness, seizures, etc.), subjective visual disturbances or retinopathy (ie, exudates, papilledema), deteriorating renal function (proteinurea, hematuria, progressive azotemia), left ventricular failure, aortic dissection, or hemorrhage in the central nervous system or at peripheral sites.

Since hypertensive emergencies almost always are associated with excessive retention of sodium and water, and because other antihypertensive agents may exacerbate fluid retention, initial therapy should always consist of intravenous injection of a potent diuretic such as furosemide (40 to 80 mg). The dose is repeated or increased until an adequate diuresis ensues. Two choices of adjunctive therapy are possible, and in all cases therapy should be parenteral. One group of drugs (including reserpine, methyldopa, and diazoxide) are given in intermittent bolus doses. The time-course and magnitude of clinical response to these agents is not entirely predictable, but second-to-second monitoring and titration of clinical response is not essential. Two other drugs (trimethaphan and nitroprusside) are administered by continuous intravenous infusion. The response to these drugs is essentially instantaneous, and clinical effects can be closely titrated simply by adjusting the infusion rate. However, use of these two agents clearly requires continuous monitoring of blood pressure by medical personnel.

Control of blood pressure during the 'crisis' period is followed by gradual replacement of parenteral treatment with effective oral therapy, as well as investigation of underlying causes of the hypertensive emergency. Prognosis for recovery from such hypertensive episodes depends largely upon the reversibility of damage to kidney, heart, and brain.

DRUG MONOGRAPHS

This section considers only single-entity antihypertensive agents. Many fixed-combination preparations are commercially available, but these are not recommended for clinical use since doses of the components cannot be individually titrated.

ALPHA-SYMPATHOPLEGIC AGENTS

RAUWOLFIA ALKALOIDS

Reserpine and other rauwolfia alkaloids [alseroxylon (Rautensin, Rauwiloid), deserpidine (Harmonyl), rescinnamine (Moderil), and whole root rauwolfia (Raudixin)] are time-tested antihypertensive agents, all of which are therapeutically equivalent. Their blood pressure lowering effects generally are rather weak and only slightly greater than those of a diuretic alone. However, in many patients with mild to moderate essential hypertension, the combination of a diuretic plus a rauwolfia alkaloid is sufficient and satisfactory. Because the duration of action of rauwolfia alkaloids is long,[47] the drugs are usually administered in a single daily dose. This, together with the low cost of this class of drugs (particularly when dispensed as generic compounds), are important advantages of therapy.

Reserpine and its congeners deplete catecholamine neurotransmitters from the brain and from the peripheral sympathetic nervous system.[47] As such, their antihypertensive activity probably results from a combination of central and peripheral actions.

Intramuscular reserpine can be used in some hypertensive emergencies when instantaneous blood pressure control is not necessary. Since some patients are particularly sensitive to the effects of the drug, an intramuscular test dose of 0.25 mg is recommended. If the test dose is tolerated, the initial therapeutic dose is 1.0 mg, which is then doubled every 4 hours until blood pressure control is achieved or a total of 8.0 mg has been given. Unfortunately, the response to parenteral reserpine is not always predictable, and some patients do not respond at all.

Side Effects and Precautions—The most common side effects of treatment are nasal congestion, drowsiness, and gastrointestinal disturbances (such as diarrhea). These generally do not limit therapy. However, severe nonspecific central nervous system depression (reduction of the level of consciousness) may accompany administration of high-dose intramuscular reserpine during therapy of hypertensive emergencies; this may seriously impair evaluation of neurologic status.

TABLE 2 Preparations and Costs of Antihypertensive Agents

Generic Name	Trademark Name(s)	Preparations and 1978 Costs
Alpha-Sympathoplegic Agents		
Reserpine	Serpasil (Lemiserp) (Rau-Sed) (Reserpoid) (Sandril)	Tablets 0.1 mg—$2.67/100; 0.25 mg—$4.50/100; 1 mg—$12.00/100 Elixir 0.25 mg/5 ml—$6.00/pint Injection (solution) 2.5 mg/ml— $1.20/2-ml/ampul, $3.60/10-ml vial
	generic	Tablets 0.1 mg—$0.40–$0.80/100; 0.25 mg—$0.45–3.00/100; 0.5 mg—$0.85/100; 1 mg—$0.85–$1.40/100
Rauwolfia Serpentina (whole root)	Raudixin	Tablets 50 mg—$6.14/100; 100 mg—$10.22/100
Alseroxylon	Rauwiloid	Tablets 2 mg—$8.70/100
Deserpidine	Harmonyl	Tablets 0.1 mg—$3.89/100; 0.5 mg—$6.24/100
Rescinnamine	Moderil	Tablets 0.25 mg—$6.44/100; 0.5 mg—$9.01/100
Methyldopa	Aldomet	Tablets (enteric-coated) 125 mg—$6.19/100; 250 mg—$8.74/100; 500 mg—$15.75/100
Methyldopa Hydrochloride	Aldomet Ester Hydrochloride	Injection (solution) 50 mg/ml— $2.61/5-ml vial
Clonidine Hydrochloride	Catapres	Tablets 0.1 mg—$8.65/100; 0.2 mg—$11.84/100
Guanethidine Sulfate	Ismelin	Tablets 10 mg—$10.10/100; 25 mg—$14.45/100
Vasodilator Agents		
Hydralazine Hydrochloride	Apresoline Hydrochloride (Lopres)	Tablets 10 mg—$3.50/100; 25 mg—$5.00/100; 50 mg—$7.50/100; 100 mg—$10.50/100
Prazosin Hydrochloride	Minipress	Capsules 1 mg—$18.18/250; 2 mg—$25.30/250; 5 mg—$43.12/250

TABLE 2 *(continued)*

Generic Name	Trademark Name(s)	Preparations and 1978 Costs
Beta-Adrenergic Antagonists		
Metoprolol Tartrate	Lopressor	Tablets 50 mg—$8.50/100
Propanolol Hydrochloride	Inderal	Tablets 10 mg—$4.10/100; 40 mg—$7.08/100; 80 mg—$11.32/100
Agents Used Exclusively for Hypertensive Emergencies		
Diazoxide	Hyperstat	Injection (solution) 15 mg/ml—$9.32/20-ml vial
Trimethaphan Camsylate	Arfonad	Injection (solution) 50 mg/ml—$4.21/10-ml vial
Sodium Nitroprusside	Nipride	Injection (powder for solution) 50 mg—$5.64/vial

Reserpine is reportedly associated with depression of mood and affect (different from nonspecific central nervous system depression or reduced level of consciousness). Despite numerous anecdotal reports to this effect,[48–50] a cause and effect relationship between reserpine and depression is not established.[50] In any case, it is recommended that rauwolfia alkaloids be administered with caution, if at all, to patients with a history of depression, affective disorders, or suicide attempts. When a reserpine-treated individual develops manifestations of an affective disorder, the drug should be discontinued and another hypotensive agent substituted.

An association of reserpine with an increased incidence of peptic ulceration has also been suggested.[51] The drug should probably be avoided in patients with a history of this disease, and discontinued if an individual develops manifestations of peptic ulcer disease. A possible association of reserpine therapy with breast cancer[52–54] should be carefully weighed against the benefits of treatment in female patients.

Dosage—Oral: Adults, Whole Root Rauwolfia, 50 to 100 mg per day. *Alseroxylon,* 2 to 4 mg per day. *Deserpidine,* 0.1 to 0.25 mg per day. *Rescinnamine,* 0.25 to 0.5 mg per day. *Syrosingopine,* 1.0 to 2.0 mg per day. *Reserpine,* 0.1 to 0.25 mg per day.

Intramuscular: Adults, Reserpine, 0.1 to 0.25 mg test dose; if tolerated, the initial therapeutic dose is 1.0 mg, which is doubled every 4 hours until blood pressure control is achieved or a total dose of 8.0 mg is attained.

METHYLDOPA (Aldomet)
METHYLDOPATE HYDROCHLORIDE (Aldomet Ester Hydrochloride)

Methyldopa also is a time-tested antihypertensive agent. Its blood pressure lowering effect probably occurs predominantly in the central nervous system.

The elimination half-life of methyldopa is short and its hepatic clearance is high.[55–57] More than 50% of an oral dose fails to reach the systemic circulation, partly due to first-pass metabolism. Because systemic availability appears to vary from person to person, effective doses also vary considerably.

The clinical duration of action of methyldopa is not as short as predicted from its pharmacokinetic properties. The drug is traditionally given in three or four daily doses, but administration of a single dose at bedtime probably provides adequate blood pressure control throughout the day.[58]

Intravenous methyldopa (250 to 1000 mg) can be used to treat hypertensive emergencies. Unfortunately, its onset of action is slow, and the clinical response is very unpredictable. Furthermore, severe drowsiness and somnolence can be a major problem.

Side Effects and Precautions—Dose-dependent reversible drowsiness, fatigue, and impairment of intellectual function are the most common side effects of methyldopa therapy.[59–63] Individuals vary greatly in their sensitivity to these effects—in some cases even the smallest of doses (250 mg daily) causes intolerable drowsiness. The majority of patients receiving clinically effective antihypertensive doses of methyldopa perceive some degree of drowsiness or sedation which is usually acceptable provided doses are carefully titrated. Daytime drowsiness can usually be minimized by giving the majority of the day's dose at bedtime.

Additional common side effects include nasal congestion, mild postural hypotension, and impairment of male sexual function.[59–62,64]

Other side effects are much less common but potentially more serious. The development of Coombs' positivity during methyldopa therapy increases in frequency with the dosage and duration of therapy.[65–68] It is not necessarily associated with hemolytic anemia. A methyldopa-treated patient who develops a Coombs' positive test should be subsequently monitored, but need not discontinue treatment. Needless to say, evidence of hemolysis (such as falling hematocrit, jaundice, etc.) necessitates discontinuation of the drug.

Many reports have linked methyldopa treatment with the development of hepatocellular dysfunction.[68–72] Abnormal liver function tests arising during methyldopa treatment are an indication to discontinue therapy. Finally, a small percentage of methyldopa recipients develop fever, almost always within the first three weeks of treatment.[68] Unexplained fever is another indication for drug discontinuation.

Dosage—Oral: Adults, 250 to 4000 mg per day. When the total daily dose does not exceed 750 to 1000 mg, it can be given all at once at bedtime. For doses in the range of 1000 to 4000 mg, 1/2 to 2/3 can be administered at bedtime.

Intravenous: Adults, 250 to 1000 mg by slow infusion.

CLONIDINE HYDROCHLORIDE (Catapres)

The mechanism of action of clonidine appears to resemble that of methyldopa.[73] Promotional claims notwithstanding, there is no convincing evidence that clonidine is more effective or better tolerated than methyldopa. As with methyldopa, the effective dose of clonidine varies widely, and dosage must be carefully titrated and individualized.

Side Effects and Precautions—Many patients receiving effective doses of clonidine experience drowsiness and somnolence.[74,75] Dry mouth is another common side effect. Generally these do not limit therapy provided dosage is carefully titrated. As with other alpha-sympathoplegic agents, clonidine can cause postural hypotension, impairment of male sexual function, nasal congestion, and gastrointestinal disturbances. Depression has also been associated with clonidine therapy.

Abrupt discontinuation of clonidine therapy can lead to moderate to severe 'rebound' hypertension that in some ways resembles the hypertensive episodes occurring with pheochromocytoma.[76–79] Accordingly, discontinuation of clonidine therapy should always be done gradually rather than abruptly. Clonidine-treated patients should be instructed not to discontinue treatment for any reason without first consulting their physician.

Dosage—Oral: Adults, 0.2 to 0.8 mg per day in 2 or 3 divided doses.

GUANETHIDINE SULFATE (Ismelin)

Guanethidine produces dose-dependent partial or complete peripheral alpha-sympathetic blockade by preventing the uptake and storage of norepinephrine in presynaptic nerve terminals.[80,81] Guanethidine does not cross the blood-brain barrier, and consequently has no central nervous system effects.

Effective doses of guanethidine vary widely, ranging from 10 to 300 mg or more per day. Because the drug has a very long duration of action, dosage adjustment in clinical practice should be undertaken no more often than every three to five days.

Guanethidine is an unpopular antihypertensive agent. Although an appropriately adjusted dose will produce a satisfactory hypotensive effect in nearly all patients, adequate reduction of blood pressure almost always is accompanied by side effects attributable to sympathetic blockade.[59,60,80–83] In fact, the clinical efficacy and value of guanethidine in a given patient generally depends on his or her ability to adjust to and live with the inevitable side effects that accompany effective dosage. Because guanethidine's hypotensive effects are almost entirely postural in nature, it is essential that blood pressures taken in the sitting or standing position (preferably both) be used to adjust dosage.

Side Effects and Precautions—Symptomatic impairment of postural blood pressure regulation is a very common side effect. Patients should be cautioned regarding dizziness, lightheadedness, and even syncope that might accompany rapid changes in posture. Those who are not so warned will quickly learn. Postural effects are particularly pronounced following prolonged periods in the supine position—that is, upon first arising in the morning. It is sometimes helpful to advise patients to sleep with the head of their bed elevated 6 to 12 inches above the horizontal.

Impairment of sexual function is a common complaint of male patients receiving guanethidine, and it may limit therapy. The development of intractable diarrhea almost always indicates that an upper limit of dosage has been reached.

Tricyclic antidepressants and phenothiazines partially or completely nullify the antihypertensive effect of guanethidine, and such drug combinations are essentially contraindicated.[81] Hypertension attributable to pheochromocytoma should not be treated with guanethidine, inasmuch as paradoxical increases in blood pressure can occur.

Dosage—Oral: Adults, 10 to 300 mg per day in a single daily dose. Dosage adjustment should be undertaken no more often than every 3rd to 5th day.

VASODILATOR AGENTS

HYDRALAZINE HYDROCHLORIDE (Apresoline Hydrochloride, Lopres)

Hydralazine is an effective and well-tolerated antihypertensive agent. Because of its relatively specific action on peripheral resistance arterioles, attainment of effective dosage is generally possible with a minimum of side effects.[25–27] However, since 'unopposed' peripheral vasodilation may lead to reflex sympathetically-induced tachycardia and increased cardiac work, hydralazine therapy usually requires coadministration of a sympathoplegic agent, preferably propranolol.

Hydralazine is extensively biotransformed during the first-pass through the liver,[84,85] making parenteral doses much more effective than corresponding oral dosage. The major biotransformation pathway involves acetylation, implying that clinical efficacy at a given dosage level is greater in genetically-determined 'slow' acetylators than in rapid acetylators. The elimination half-life and duration of action of hydralazine is short, making multiple daily doses necessary for adequately 'smooth' antihypertensive action. However, recent studies suggest that less frequent hydralazine dosage is clinically effective and subjectively acceptable.[86,87]

Parenteral hydralazine has a reasonably prompt onset of action when used in hypertensive emergencies, although the overall clinical effect is unpredictable. The usual dose range is 5 to 50 mg by intramuscular injection or intravenous infusion.

Side Effects and Precautions—Tachycardia, palpitations, increased cardiac work, headache, and flushing accompany administration of hydralazine alone. Symptomatic myocardial ischemia may result from increased cardiac work in patients with coronary artery disease, indicating that hydralazine should be used with caution if at all in such patients. However, these untoward effects can be partly or completely eliminated by concurrent administration of propranolol.

An immune disorder can develop in patients receiving long-term hydralazine therapy.[88–91] Typical clinical manifestations are fever and joint pains; these are generally preceded by development of biochemical abnormalities that include the presence of antinuclear antibodies (ANA) and lupus erythematosus (LE) cells in the peripheral circulation. The disorder is related both to the dosage and the duration of therapy, and is most prevalent among patients receiving doses in the range of 200 to 400 mg per day. Manifestations are usually reversible upon discontinuation of the drug. Hydralazine-treated patients—particularly those getting high doses—should be periodically monitored for the appearance of ANA and/or LE cells. Most individuals developing these biochemical abnormalities remain asymptomatic; accordingly, biochemical changes do not necessarily warrant discontinuation of the drug. However, subjective symptoms clearly indicate that the drug should be stopped.

Dosage—Oral: Adults, 30 to 400 mg per day in three or four divided doses.

Intramuscular or intravenous: Adults, 5 to 50 mg.

PRAZOSIN HYDROCHLORIDE (Minipress)

The clinical action of prazosin appears to resemble that of hydralazine, and an advantage of prazosin over hydralazine is not clearly established. Early studies suggest that reflex sympathetic stimulation associated with prazosin may be somewhat less than that due to hydralazine.[92]

Side Effects and Precautions—Severe hypotension is sometimes associated with initial doses of prazosin, or with dosage increases.[93–95] It is recommended that the initial dose be taken at bedtime with the patient in the supine position. Physicians should be in close touch with patients during the first few days of prazosin therapy.

Dosage—Oral: Adults, 3 to 20 mg per day in three or four divided doses.

BETA-ADRENERGIC ANTAGONISTS

PROPRANOLOL HYDROCHLORIDE (Inderal)

The antihypertensive efficacy of propranolol is not well understood.[28–30] Propranolol reduces cardiac output and reduces plasma renin activity, but neither of these entirely account for its antihypertensive effect.[96–98] Propranolol is usually well-tolerated, since it does not interfere with postural blood pressure regulation or male sexual function. Many clinicians consider propranolol the drug of next choice if a diuretic alone is inadequate. The diuretic-propranolol combination is often successful; if not, hydralazine can be added.

The pharmacokinetic properties of propranolol are complex.[99] The drug is extensively transformed in the first-pass through the liver, accounting for the much greater activity of a given dose when administered parenterally rather than orally. However, transformation to at least one active metabolite (4-hydroxypropranolol) partly offsets the limitation of clinical activity associated with oral dosage. The drug is usually administered three or four times daily, but twice daily antihypertensive therapy appears to be satisfactory in many cases.[100]

Side Effects and Precautions—In patients with normal cardiovascular status, propranolol is an extremely safe drug. However, in patients with cardiovascular disease whose compensation depends upon sympathetic activity, the degree of beta-blockade produced by a small dose of propranolol can lead to cardiovascular collapse (bradycardia, hypotension, heart block).[101,102] Accordingly, patients with cardiac disease that is not fully compensated (such as those with resting tachycardia, exertional dyspnea, edema, etc.) should not receive propranolol. Most patients should receive a test dose in the presence of a physician.

Propranolol can induce bronchospasm and should not be administered to patients with a history of asthma or other bronchospastic diseases.

Propranolol impairs the subjective signs and symptoms associated with hypoglycemia. Caution should be observed during the use of propranolol in diabetic patients, particularly insulin-dependent diabetics who are predisposed to hypoglycemia.

A variety of other nonspecific and generally minor side effects have been associated with propranolol therapy.[101,102] The most common of these are gastrointestinal disturbances (loss of appetite, abdominal discomfort, nausea, vomiting, and diarrhea), and a variety of central nervous system disturbances (fatigue, lethargy, dizziness, depression, visual disturbances, etc.). Although a cause-and-effect relationship to propranolol therapy is seldom striking, the possible role of the drug should be considered in patients who develop such symptoms.

Dosage—Oral: Adults, 20 to 320 mg per day in two to four divided doses.

METOPROLOL TARTRATE (Lopressor)

Metoprolol is another beta-adrenergic blocker approved in 1978 for the treatment of hypertension.[103] Although metoprolol is claimed to have some selectivity for extrapulmonary beta-adrenergic receptors, this selectivity is only partial and relative. Metoprolol does produce some degree of blockade of pulmonary beta-receptors; this becomes increasingly evident at higher doses.

The clinical pharmacologic properties and antihypertensive efficacy of metoprolol are very similar to those of propranolol.[28] The elimination half-life of metoprolol is short, and its hepatic clearance is high.[99,104] Only about 40% of an oral dose reaches the systemic circulation because of first-pass metabolism.[104] Despite the short half-life of metoprolol, antihypertensive effects can be achieved with two or three daily doses. In one study, a single daily dose was effective.[105]

Side Effects and Precautions—See the monograph on propranolol. Metoprolol's cardioselectivity is only relative, and precautions regarding use in patients with bronchospastic disorders still hold.

Dosage—Oral: Adults, initial, 50 mg twice daily. Maintenance, 100 to 450 mg per day in 2 or 3 divided doses.

AGENTS USED EXCLUSIVELY FOR HYPERTENSIVE EMERGENCIES

DIAZOXIDE (Hyperstat)

Diazoxide is a direct peripheral vasodilator.[44–46] It is very powerful and can normalize blood pressure in most patients with severe hypertension. Because rapid protein binding of diazoxide results in substantial reduction of its clinical effect, the drug must be given by rapid intravenous bolus injection over 10 to 20 seconds.[106,107] A hypotensive effect is achieved almost immediately, following which the blood pressure gradually returns to its pretreatment level over a period of 2 to 12 hours. Repeated injections can be given as necessary. Coadministration of a diuretic is essential to prevent fluid retention associated with diazoxide therapy.

Side Effects and Precautions—Diazoxide impairs glucose tolerance, and can lead to moderate to severe degrees of hyperglycemia. Blood glucose levels should be monitored in patients receiving diazoxide; in some cases, short-term administration of insulin may be necessary. As with other vasodilator agents, coadministration of diuretics is essential to prevent salt and water retention. Reflex tachycardia and increased cardiac output associated with the vasodilating effects of diazoxide may require short-term administration of propranolol.

Dosage—Intravenous: Adults, 5 mg/kg (approximately 300 mg) by intravenous bolus injection over 10 to 20 seconds. The dose can be repeated in 4 to 12 hours. The usual duration of therapy does not exceed 3 days.

TRIMETHAPHAN CAMSYLATE (Arfonad)

Trimethaphan is a ganglionic blocking agent. Accordingly, its hypotensive effect is almost entirely postural, requiring that the drug be administered with the patient in the sitting position or with the head of the bed elevated. The drug is given by continuous intravenous infusion, and has an immediate hypotensive effect.[44–46] A nurse or physician must be in constant attendance during trimethaphan infusion; blood pressure must be monitored continuously, and frequent changes in the infusion rate are necessary.

Side Effects and Precautions—Unwanted effects of trimethaphan are predictably related to its ganglionic blocking properties, and include dry mouth, blurring of vision, urinary retention, and paralytic ileus. These inevitable effects, together with tachyphylaxis, generally limit the duration of trimethaphan therapy.

Dosage—Intravenous: Adults, 1 to 15 mg per minute by continuous intravenous infusion, with the exact infusion rate titrated according to repeated measurements of blood pressure. The infusion solution consists of 2 grams of trimethaphan camsylate per liter of 5% dextrose in water.

SODIUM NITROPRUSSIDE (Nipride)

Nitroprusside appears to be the most consistently effective drug for the treatment of hypertensive emergencies.[108–110] Like trimethaphan, it is administered by continuous intravenous infusion, and requires continuous monitoring and titration. However, its effects on resistance and capacitance vasculature make the antihypertensive effect relatively specific, and generally accompanied by few side effects. Coadministration of a diuretic is essential. The hypotensive effects of nitroprusside are not selectively postural, although some potentiation of effect may be gained by adjusting the patient to the head-up or seated position.

Side Effects and Precautions—Initial manifestations of toxicity include fatigue, anorexia, and nausea. Impairment of consciousness and muscular spasticity indicates more severe toxicity. Unwanted effects appear to be due to accumulation of thiocyanate, the major metabolite of nitroprusside. Since thiocyanate is largely cleared by the kidney, excessive accumulation will occur in patients with renal insufficiency or volume depletion. Because nitroprusside is light-sensitive, infusion solutions should be protected from light. All solutions should be freshly prepared, and discarded if more than 12 hours old.

Dosage—Oral: Adults, 0.03 to 0.5 mg/minute by continuous intravenous infusion, with continuous monitoring of clinical response. The infusion solution consists of 100 mg of sodium nitroprusside per liter of 5% dextrose in water.

REFERENCES

1. Duhme DW, Greenblatt DJ, Miller RR: Pharmacotherapy of essential hypertension. Am J Hosp Pharm 32:508–516, 1975.
2. Page LB, Sidd JJ: Medical management of primary hypertension. N Engl J Med 287:960–967, 1018–1023, 1074–1081, 1972.
3. AMA Committee on Hypertension: Drug treatment of ambulatory patients with hypertension. JAMA 225:1647–1653, 1973.
4. Smirk FH: The prognosis of untreated and of treated hypertension and advantages of early treatment. Am Heart J 83:825–840, 1970.
5. Kannel WB, Gordon T, Schwartz MJ: Systolic versus diastolic blood pressure and risk of coronary heart disease: the Framingham study. Am J Cardiol 27:335–346, 1971.
6. Anon: History of a hypertensive. Lancet 2:1243–1244, 1972.
7. Tobian L: A viewpoint concerning the enigma of hypertension. Am J Med 52:595–609, 1972.
8. Siegenthaler W, Werning C: The etiopathology of hypertension. Int J Clin Pharmacol 4:83–92, 1970.
9. Taguchi J, Freis ED: Partial reduction of blood pressure and prevention of complications in hypertension. N Engl J Med 291:329–331, 1974.
10. Anderson J, Godfrey BE, Hill DM, et al: A comparison of the effects of hydrochlorothiazide and of frusemide in the treatment of hypertensive patients. Q J Med 40:541–560, 1971.
11. Valmin K, Hansen T: Treatment of benign essential hypertension: comparison of furosemide and hydrochlorothiazide. Eur J Clin Pharmacol 8:393–401, 1975.
12. Ochs HR, Greenblatt DJ, Bodem G, et al: Spironolactone. Am Heart J 96:389–400, 1978.
13. Edmonds CJ, Josani B: Total-body potassium in hypertensive patients during prolonged diuretic therapy. Lancet 2:8–12, 1972.
14. Manner RJ, Brechbill DO, DeWitt K: Prevalence of hypokalemia in diuretic therapy. Clin Med 79:19–22, (Nov) 1972.
15. Leemhuis MP, Struyvenberg A: Significance of hypokalemia due to diuretics. Neth Med J 16:18–28, 1973.
16. Wilkinson PR, Issler H, Hesp R, et al: Total body and serum potassium during prolonged thiazide therapy for essential hypertension. Lancet 1:759–762, 1975.
17. Healy JJ, McKenna TJ, Canning BStJ, et al: Body composition changes in hypertensive subjects on long-term oral diuretic therapy. Br Med J 1:716–719, 1970.
18. Dargie HJ, Boddy K, Kennedy AC, et al: Total body potassium in long-term frusemide therapy: is potassium supplementation necessary? Br Med J 4:316–319, 1974.
19. Editorial: Who needs potassium? Br Med J 4:307–308, 1974.
20. Kosman ME: Management of potassium problems during long-term diuretic therapy. JAMA 230:743–748, 1974.
21. Weller JM, Malvin RL: Effects and side-effects of thiazide drugs. Med Clin North Am 53:1321–1330, 1969.
22. Schulz BW: Metabolic complications of hydrochlorothiazide therapy. Drug Intell Clin Pharm 7:501–510, 1973.

23. Gifford RW Jr: Drug combinations as rational antihypertensive therapy. Arch Intern Med 133:1053–1057, 1974.
24. Frolich ED: Inhibition of adrenergic function in the treatment of hypertension. Arch Intern Med 133:1033–1048, 1974.
25. Chidsey CA III, Gottlieb TB: The pharmacologic basis of antihypertensive therapy: the role of vasodilator drugs. Prog Cardiovasc Dis 17:99–113, 1974.
26. Koch-Weser J: Vasodilator drugs in the treatment of hypertension. Arch Intern Med 133:1017–1027, 1974.
27. Koch-Weser J: Hydralazine. N Engl J Med 295:320–323, 1976.
28. Waal-Manning HJ: Hypertension: which beta-blocker? Drugs 12:412–441, 1976.
29. Simpson FO: β-Adrenergic receptor blocking drugs in hypertension. Drugs 7:85–105, 1974.
30. Holland OB, Kaplan NM: Propranolol in the treatment of hypertension. N Engl J Med 294:930–936, 1976.
31. Koch-Weser J: Correlation of pathophysiology and pharmacotherapy in primary hypertension. Am J Cardiol 32:499–510, 1973.
32. Koch-Weser J: Individualization of antihypertensive drug therapy. Med Clin North Am 58:1027–1036, 1974.
33. Kaplan NM: The prognostic implications of plasma renin in essential hypertension. JAMA 231:167–170, 1975.
34. Brunner HR, Gavras H: Clinical implications of renin in the hypertensive patient. JAMA 233:1091–1093, 1975.
35. Laragh JH, Sealey J, Brunner HR: The control of aldosterone secretion in normal and hypertensive man: abnormal renin-aldosterone patterns in low renin hypertension. Am J Med 53:649–663, 1972.
36. Laragh JH: Modern system for treating high blood pressure based on renin profiling and vasoconstriction-volume analysis: a primary role for beta blocking drugs such as propranolol. Am J Med 61:797–810, 1976.
37. Bühler FR, Burkart F, Lütold BE, et al: Antihypertensive beta blocking action as related to renin and age: a pharmacologic tool to identify pathogenetic mechanisms in essential hypertension. Am J Cardiol 36:653–669, 1975.
38. Dunn MJ, Tannen RL: Low-renin hypertension. Kidney Int 5:317–325, 1974.
39. Frolich ED: Clinical significance of hemodynamic findings in hypertension. Chest 64:94–99, 1973.
40. Esler MD, Nestel PJ: Essential hypertension with symptoms of hyperkinetic circulation. Med J Aust 2:253–257, 1973.
41. Frohlich ED, Dustan HP, Page IH: Hyperdynamic beta-adrenergic circulatory state. Arch Intern Med 117:614–619, 1966.
42. Eich RH, Cuddy RP, Smulyan H, et al: Hemodynamics in labile hypertension: a follow-up study. Circulation 34:299–307, 1966.
43. Jackson G, Pierscianowski TA, Mahon W, et al: Inappropriate antihypertensive therapy in the elderly. Lancet 2:1317–1318, 1976.
44. AMA Committee on Hypertension: The treatment of malignant hypertension and hypertensive emergencies. JAMA 228:1673–1679, 1974.
45. Dranov J, Skyler JS, Gunnells JC: Malignant hypertension: current modes of therapy. Arch Intern Med 133:791–801, 1974.
46. Koch-Weser J: Hypertensive emergencies. N Engl J Med 290:211–214, 1974.
47. Stitzel RE: The biological fate of reserpine. Pharmacol Rev 28:179–205, 1977.
48. Lion JR, Millan C, Taylor RJ: Reserpine and the induction of depression: a case report. Dis Nerv Syst 36:321–322, 1975.
49. Ambrosino SV: Depressive reactions associated with reserpine. NY State J Med 74:860–864, 1974.
50. Goodwin FK, Bunney WE Jr: Depressions following reserpine: a reevaluation. Sem Psychiatry 3:435–448, 1971.
51. Bachrach WH: Reserpine, gastric secretion, and peptic ulcer. Am J Dig Dis 4:117–124, 1959.
52. Boston Collaborative Drug Surveillance Program: Reserpine and breast cancer. Lancet 2:669–671, 1974.
53. Armstrong B, Stevens N, Doll R: Retrospective study of the association between use of rauwolfia derivatives and breast cancer in English women. Lancet 2:672–675, 1974.

54. Heinonen OP, Shapiro S, Tuominen L, et al: Reserpine use in relation to breast cancer. Lancet 2:675–677, 1974.
55. Kwan KC, Foltz EL, Breault GO, et al: Pharmacokinetics of methyldopa in man. J Pharmacol Exp Ther 198:264–277, 1976.
56. Barnett AJ, Bobik A, Carson V, et al: Pharmacokinetics of methyldopa: plasma levels following single intravenous, oral and multiple oral dosages in normotensive and hypertensive subjects. Clin Exp Pharmacol Physiol 4:331–339, 1977.
57. Stenbaek O, Myhre E, Rugstad HE, et al: Pharmacokinetics of methyldopa in healthy man. Eur J Clin Pharmacol 12:117–123, 1977.
58. Wright JM, McLeod PJ, McCullough W: Antihypertensive efficacy of a single bedtime dose of methyldopa. Clin Pharmacol Ther 20:733–737, 1976.
59. Nies AS: Adverse reactions and interactions limiting the use of antihypertensive drugs. Am J Med 58:495–503, 1975.
60. Bulpitt CJ, Dollery CT: Side effects of hypotensive agents evaluated by a self-administered questionnaire. Br Med J 3:485–490, 1973.
61. Pillay VKG: Some side-effects of alpha-methyldopa. S Afr Med J 50:625–626, 1976.
62. Anon: Side effects of methyldopa. Br Med J 1:646–647, 1975.
63. Adler S: Methyldopa-induced decrease in mental activity. JAMA 230:1428–1429, 1974.
64. Newman RJ, Salerno HR: Sexual dysfunction due to methyldopa. Br Med J 4:106, 1974.
65. Marcus GJ, Stevenson M, Brown T: Alpha-methyldopa-induced immune thrombocytopenia. Am J Clin Pathol 64:113–115, 1975.
66. Perry HM Jr, Chaplin H Jr, Carmody S, et al: Immunologic findings in patients receiving methyldopa: a prospective study. J Lab Clin Med 78:905–917, 1971.
67. Hunter E, Raik E, Gordon E, et al: Incidence of positive Coombs' test, LE cells and antinuclear factor in patients on alpha-methyldopa ('Aldomet') therapy. Med J Aust 2:810–812, 1971.
68. Furhoff A-K: Adverse reactions with methyldopa—a decade's reports. Acta Med Scand 203:425–428, 1978.
69. Thomas E, Bhuta S, Rosenthal WS: Methyldopa-induced liver injury: rapid progression to fatal postnecrotic cirrhosis. Arch Pathol Lab Med 100:132–135, 1976.
70. Cacace LG, Cohen M: Alpha-methyldopa (Aldomet) hepatitis: report of a case and review of the literature. Drug Intell Clin Pharm 10:144–152, 1976.
71. Rodman JS, Deutsch DJ, Gutman SI: Methyldopa hepatitis: a report of six cases and review of the literature. Am J Med 60:941–948, 1976.
72. Toghill PJ, Smith PG, Benton P, et al: Methyldopa liver damage. Br Med J 3:545–548, 1974.
73. Pettinger WA: Clonidine, a new antihypertensive drug. N Engl J Med 293:1179–1180, 1975.
74. Mathew JY, Parker ML: The use of clonidine (Catapres) in the treatment of hypertension. Med J Aust 2:1120–1122, 1971.
75. Jain AK, Ryan JR, Vargas R, et al: Efficacy and acceptability of different dosage schedules of clonidine. Clin Pharmacol Ther 21:382–387, 1977.
76. Goldberg AD, Raftery EB, Wilkinson P: Blood pressure and heart rate and withdrawal of antihypertensive drugs. Br Med J 1:1243–1246, 1977.
77. Bailey RR, Neale TJ: Rapid clonidine withdrawal with blood pressure overshoot exaggerated by beta-blockade. Br Med J 2:942–943, 1976.
78. Hansson L, Hunyor SN, Julius S, et al: Blood pressure crisis following withdrawal of clonidine (Catapres, Catapresan), with special reference to arterial and urinary catecholamine levels, and suggestions for acute management. Am Heart J 85:605–610, 1973.
79. Husserl FE, deCarvalho JGR, Batson HM, et al: Hypertension after clonidine withdrawal. South Med J 71:496–497, 1978.
80. Freis ED: Guanethidine. Prog Cardiovasc Dis 8:183–193, 1965.
81. Woosley RL, Nies AS: Guanethidine. N Engl J Med 295:1053–1057, 1976.
82. Bauer GE, Hull RD, Stokes GS, et al: The reversibility of side effects of guanethidine therapy. Med J Aust 1:930–933, 1973.
83. Ferguson RK, Rothenberg RJ, Nies AS: Patient acceptance of guanethidine as therapy for mild to moderate hypertension: a comparison with reserpine. Circulation 54:32–37, 1976.
84. Talseth T: Kinetics of hydralazine elimination. Clin Pharmacol Ther 21:715–720, 1977.
85. Reidenberg MM, Drayer D, DeMarco AL, et al: Hydralazine elimination in man. Clin Pharmacol Ther 14:970–977, 1973.

86. Cooper I: Maintenance treatment of moderate hypertension with b.i.d. hydralazine. Curr Ther Res 10:579–588, 1976.
87. O'Malley K, Segal JL, Israili ZH, et al: Duration of hydralazine action in hypertension. Clin Pharmacol Ther 18:581–586, 1975.
88. Alarcon-Segovia D, Wakim KG, Worthington JW, et al: Clinical and experimental studies on the hydralazine syndrome and its relationship to systemic lupus erythematosus. Medicine 46:1–33, 1967.
89. Perry HM, Tan EM, Carmody S, et al: Relationship of acetyl transferase activity to antinuclear antibodies and toxic symptoms in hypertensive patients treated with hydralazine. J Lab Clin Med 76:114–125, 1970.
90. Perry HM: Late toxicity to hydralazine resembling systemic lupus erythematosus or rheumatoid arthritis. Am J Med 54:58–72, 1973.
91. Blumenkrantz N, Christiansen AH, Ullman S, et al: Hydralazine-induced lupoid syndrome. Acta Med Scand 195:443–449, 1974.
92. Kosman ME: Evaluation of a new antihypertensive agent: prazosin hydrochloride (Minipres). JAMA 237:157–159, 1977.
93. Bendall MJ, Baloch KH, Wilson PR: Side effects due to treatment of hypertension with prazosin. Br Med J 2:728–729, 1975.
94. Graham RM, Thornell IR, Gain JM, et al: Prazosin: the first-dose phenomenon. Br Med J 2:1293–1294, 1976.
95. Rosendorff C: Prazosin: severe side effects are dose-dependent. Br Med J 2:508, 1976.
96. Hollifield JW, Sherman K, Zwagg RV, et al: Proposed mechanisms of propranolol's antihypertensive effect in essential hypertension. N Engl J Med 295:68–73, 1976.
97. Bravo EL, Tarazi RC, Dustan HP: β-Adrenergic blockade in diuretic-treated patients with essential hypertension. N Engl J Med 292:66–70, 1975.
98. Stokes GS, Weber MA, Thornell IR: β-Blockers and plasma renin activity in hypertension. Br Med J 1:60–62, 1974.
99. Johnsson G, Regardh C-G: Clinical pharmacokinetics of β-adrenoreceptor blocking drugs. Clin Pharmacokinet 1:233–263, 1976.
100. Berglund G, Andersson O, Hansson L, et al: Propranolol given twice daily in hypertension. Acta Med Scand 194:513–515, 1973.
101. Greenblatt DJ, Koch-Weser J: Adverse reactions to β-adrenergic receptor blocking drugs: a report from the Boston Collaborative Drug Surveillance Program. Drugs 7:118–129, 1974.
102. Greenblatt DJ, Koch-Weser J: Clinical toxicity of propranolol and practolol: a report from the Boston Collaborative Drug Surveillance Program. In *Cardiovascular Drugs, Vol. 2:* β-Adrenoceptor Blocking Drugs. Edited by GS Avery. New York, ADIS Press Australasia Pty Ltd, 1977, pp 179–195.
103. Ablad B, Borg KO, Carlsson E, et al (eds): Animal and human pharmacological studies on metoprolol—a new selective adrenergic β_1-receptor antagonist. Acta Pharmacol Toxicol 36(Suppl 5):5–144, 1975.
104. Regardh CG, Borg KO, Johansson R, et al: Pharmacokinetic studies on the selective β_1-receptor antagonist metoprolol in man. Clin Pharmacokinet 2:347–364, 1974.
105. Reybrouck T, Amery A, Fagard R, et al: Beta-blockers: once or three times a day? Br Med J 1:1386–1388, 1975.
106. Mroczek WJ, Leibel BA, Davidov M, et al: The importance of the rapid administration of diazoxide in accelerated hypertension. N Engl J Med 285:603–606, 1971.
107. Sellers EM, Koch-Weser J: Protein binding and vascular activity of diazoxide. N Engl J Med 281:1141–1145, 1969.
108. Ahearn DJ, Grim CE: Treatment of malignant hypertension with sodium nitroprusside. Arch Intern Med 133:187–191, 1974.
109. Palmer RF, Lasseter KC: Sodium nitroprusside. N Engl J Med 292:294–297, 1975.
110. Tuzel IH: Sodium nitroprusside: a review of its clinical effectiveness as a hypotensive agent. J Clin Pharmacol 14:494–503, 1974.

26. DIURETICS

Nicolaos E. Madias and John T. Harrington

Diuretics increase the urinary excretion of sodium chloride by blocking its tubular reabsorption,[1,2] thereby producing a net loss of sodium from body fluids and a reduction in the extracellular (ECF) fluid volume. This largely accounts for the therapeutic effects of diuretics in edema and hypertension.

BASIC PHYSIOLOGY

Sodium chloride and bicarbonate are the major osmotically-active solutes in the extracellular compartment. More than 90% of exchangeable sodium is extracellular, and the ECF sodium concentration is tightly regulated. ECF volume (as a consequence of the regulation of the osmolality of body fluids) is determined primarily by the quantity of sodium it contains.

Since salt intake fluctuates with diet, ECF sodium content and volume are regulated by urinary sodium excretion.[3]

In a healthy person, approximately 25,000 mEq of sodium are filtered daily, of which more than 99% is reabsorbed. Thus, only some 0.5 to 1.0% of the filtered sodium load, equal to ingested sodium, normally escapes reabsorption.

Sixty to 70% of the filtered sodium and water is reabsorbed in the proximal tubule, accompanied mainly by chloride and bicarbonate anions (bicarbonate being preferentially reabsorbed). Approximately 90% of the filtered bicarbonate is reabsorbed proximally in exchange for sodium.

In the thick ascending limb of Henle's loop, approximately 25 to 30% of the filtered sodium is reabsorbed. Chloride, not sodium, is reabsorbed actively in this segment, but water is not reabsorbed. Hence the tubular fluid becomes hypotonic or dilute. The distal convoluted tubule and the collecting duct recapture virtually all of the remaining 5 to 10% of the filtered sodium, predominantly with chloride but also in exchange for hydrogen or potassium. Distal cation exchange is modulated by the rate of aldosterone secretion and by the rate of delivery of sodium to the exchange sites.

This pattern of sequential sodium reabsorption predicts the response to be anticipated when sodium chloride reabsorption is blocked in various segments of the nephron. First, despite the fact that the bulk of the filtered sodium is reabsorbed proximally, sole inhibition of proximal sodium reabsorption may not produce significant diuresis. The explanation for this unexpected outcome resides in the striking responsiveness of the reabsorptive rate of the Henle's loop to changes in the delivered load of salt. Second, since a substantial fraction of the filtered sodium is reabsorbed in the diluting segment of the Henle's loop and since the distal tubule and collecting duct have relatively limited reabsorptive capabilities, the inhibition of sodium transport in the loop of Henle may effect a profound diuresis. Third, potassium excretion may increase or decrease depending on the site of inhibition of sodium reabsorption. Lastly, simultaneous inhibition of sodium reabsorption at several segments along the nephron may produce a diuresis which would not occur if only one segment was inhibited.

INDICATIONS

Edematous States

Diuretics are used to treat edema associated with congestive heart failure, cirrhosis, and the nephrotic syndrome.[4] Diuretics, by inhibiting renal tubular sodium reabsorption, impair renal retention of sodium, producing a negative sodium balance and reduction of edema.

Edema is not an absolute indication for diuretic therapy. Evaluation and treatment of the underlying disease should take precedence over the use of diuretics. Since the goal of diuretic treatment is the achievement of negative sodium balance, dietary sodium intake should be restricted. Administration of diuretics that act simultaneously at different sites of the nephron, or use of diuretics following infusion of hyperoncotic colloid solutions, may lead to a more effective diuresis.

Essential Hypertension

Thiazide diuretics are the cornerstone of antihypertensive therapy. Although sodium depletion and ECF volume contraction are partly responsible for the hypotensive effect of diuretics, additional mechanisms such as lowered peripheral vascular resistance, have also been implicated. Diazoxide, a benzathiadiazine derivative, has no diuretic activity but produces a potent and prompt hypotensive effect; this lends support to the notion of a direct effect of thiazides on the vascular wall.

Diuretics alone may control mild hypertension. In moderate and severe hypertension, diuretics are usually used as adjuncts to other antihypertensive agents. Both adrenergic blockers and peripheral vasodilators may cause enough sodium retention and ECF volume expansion to blunt their hypotensive effect. Concomitant administration of a diuretic impairs sodium retention and renders hypertension more responsive.

Nephrogenic Diabetes Insipidus

Thiazide diuretics have been successfully used to treat nephrogenic diabetes insipidus. Diuretic-induced sodium depletion and ECF volume contraction increases proximal tubular sodium reabsorption, decreases delivery of filtrate to the loop of Henle, and allows the urine to be concentrated to an osmolality as high as 300 mOsm/kg. Thus, urine volume can be reduced by as much as two-thirds, relieving polyuria and polydipsia.

Hypercalcemia

Loop diuretics block sodium reabsorption in the loop of Henle, where a significant portion of the filtered calcium load is normally reabsorbed. Thus, a marked increase in calcium excretion can occur with these drugs, which may be useful in the acute treatment of hypercalcemia (in conjunction with saline infusions). Conversely, chronic administration of thiazide diuretics produces a sustained fall in urinary calcium excretion. Thiazides have also been used to treat calcium stones due either to absorptive or renal hypercalciuria.

Acute Tubular Necrosis

The effectiveness of loop diuretics as preventive, diagnostic, or therapeutic agents in the management of patients who are at risk of developing acute tubular necrosis or who already have established tubular necrosis remains controversial. We do not recommend diuretics in this condition.

TYPES OF DIURETICS

Diuretics That Act at the Proximal Tubule

Mannitol. Mannitol is a simple sugar (molecular weight = 182) widely used to initiate an osmotic diuresis, particularly in acute drug intoxications. Administration of large doses of mannitol (100 gm) to a normal, water-deprived adult can result in urine flow rates of up to 10 ml/min. The sodium concentration of the urine may rise to about 75 mEq/L, similar to that seen in a patient with diabetic ketoacidosis and heavy glycosuria.

Modest potassium loss occurs after mannitol diuresis. In patients with uncontrolled diabetes, up to 150 mEq of potassium may be lost in 24 hours. Other complications of mannitol therapy include an acute transient increase in extracellular fluid volume, hyponatremia with hyperosmolality, and overt volume depletion. Treatment of hypertonic volume depletion requires enough hypotonic fluid replacement (half normal saline) to restore extracellular fluid volume and tonicity to normal.

Mannitol can only be given intravenously. It is available as a 25% solution in 50 ml vials, or as a 20% solution in 500 ml bottles. To initiate osmotic diuresis in adults with drug intoxication, one can administer 25 g of mannitol, followed by 12.5 to 25 g in each liter of half normal saline containing 20 mEq potassium (assuming normal renal function).

Acetazolamide. Acetazolamide (Diamox) is a carbonic anhydrase inhibitor and blocks sodium bicarbonate reabsorption in the proximal tubule. The resultant alkaline diuresis causes mild systemic metabolic acidosis, which then inhibits the action of acetazolamide. The therapeutic value of acetazolamide is generally limited to patients requiring persistent alkalinization of urine (eg, those being treated with cytotoxic drugs in whom uric acid precipitation within the renal tubules is feared; sodium bicarbonate can be given during the day and acetazolamide 250 mg at night), and in those with glaucoma (in a dose of 250 mg four times a day).

Diuretics that Act at the Loop of Henle

Ethacrynic acid and furosemide. Ethacrynic acid (Edecrin) and furosemide (Lasix) can produce a fractional sodium excretion of approximately 25% or more of the filtered sodium load (approximately 3 to 5 times as potent as chlorothiazide). Although structurally unrelated, furosemide (40 mg) and ethacrynic acid (50 mg) can be considered interchangeable. The site of action of both is the ascending limb of Henle's loop. Both agents inhibit active chloride (not sodium) transport similarly to mercurial diuretics. Their oral effectiveness and low rates of adverse reactions led to greatly diminished use of organic mercurials.

The peak effect of furosemide and ethacrynic acid is at one to two hours when given orally, and 30 to 45 minutes when given intravenously. Since the duration of action seldom exceeds six to eight hours in adults who are resistant to diuretic agents, the oral dose can be doubled twice daily until a satisfactory response is observed, or until a maximum limit is reached (usually, the onset of gastrointestinal symptoms). For example: 40 mg of furosemide or 50 mg of ethacrynic acid can be given orally at 8:00 AM; if no response (no response measured in terms of urine output and weight loss) occurs after 8 hours, 2 tablets can be given at 4:00 PM; and if still no response, 4 tablets the following morning, etc. Although the usual maximum dose of both oral furosemide and ethacrynic acid is about 200 mg, under carefully controlled hospital conditions as much as 4.0 g of these drugs have been given daily. After patients receive these agents, their urine may contain as much as 150 mEq/L of sodium and chloride with little, if any, increase in bicarbonate. As a result, reduction of ECF volume and hypochloremic metabolic alkalosis are quite common. Kaliuresis, due to increased delivery of sodium to distal exchange sites, can increase fivefold. If a patient is receiving a maximum dose of one of these agents, there is no rationale for using the other since both block chloride reabsorption at the same site in the nephron.

Both of the loop diuretics, in contrast to thiazide diuretics, remain effective in patients whose glomerular filtration rate (GFR) is as low as 5 to 10 ml/min. However, when the GFR is this low, high doses (up to 500 to 1000 mg/day) are usually required.

Diuretics that Act at the Cortical Diluting Segment

Thiazides. Chlorothiazide (Diuril) was the first benzothiadiazide to be widely studied and is a model for all of the analogs (including the nonthiazide, chlorthalidone [Hygroton]) produced subsequently.

Chlorothiazide is readily absorbed from the gastrointestinal tract. Maximal diuretic activity occurs at 30 to 45 minutes after oral or intravenous administration, and its effect disappears in approximately 6 hours. The maximum fractional sodium excretion observed when thiazides are studied under standardized laboratory conditions is between 5 and 10% of the filtered load.

Since sodium reabsorption is blocked by thiazides 'upstream' from the site of distal Na^+—K^+ and Na^+—H^+ exchange, an accelerated rate of potassium and hydrogen ion secretion occurs following the administration of thiazides. Moreover, the loss of sodium and the concomitant reduction in plasma and ECF volume may lead to increased production of aldosterone via the renin-angiotensin mechanism, which will further accelerate distal cation exchange. The increase in Na^+—H^+ exchange and concomitant chloride depletion may produce metabolic alkalosis. Chlorothiazide 500 mg is equivalent to 50 mg of hydrochlorothiazide (HydroDiuril, Esidrix) 50 mg and to chlorthalidone 100 mg.

Agents that Act at the Distal Tubule

Spironolactone and triamterene. Spironolactone (Aldactone) competitively inhibits the action of aldosterone, while triamterene (Dyrenium), a pteridine derivative, blocks sodium reabsorption independently of aldosterone. For clinical purposes these two drugs are similar.

Spironolactone and triamterene are not potent diuretic agents; maximum fractional sodium excretion under standard laboratory conditions is approximately 2% (equal to or less than that of the carbonic anhydrase inhibitor—acetazolamide). The adult dose of spironolactone is 25 to 100 mg/day, of triamterene, 100 to 300 mg/day. Because of their limited diuretic effect, both drugs are usually employed in conjunction with a thiazide diuretic and/or a loop diuretic. Under these circumstances, there is a slight further increase in sodium excretion, but the major effect of distal blocking agents is inhibition of potassium excretion. Thus, the advantage of the combined use of spironolactone or triamterene with a thiazide or loop diuretic is a decreased incidence of hypokalemia; however, there is a much higher incidence of hyperkalemia.

ADVERSE REACTIONS

Diuretics may induce a number of metabolic abnormalities, including volume depletion, metabolic alkalosis, hypokalemia, hyponatremia, and hyperkalemia. Less commonly, hypercalcemia, carbohydrate intolerance, and hyperuricemia may occur.

Volume Depletion

Volume depletion is a common complication of diuretic therapy. Even with persistent edema or ascites, severe intravascular volume contraction and hypotension can occasionally occur if movement of interstitial fluid into the vascular compartment lags behind the rate of diuresis. Excessive volume depletion can usually be prevented by inducing a gradual (1 to 2 kg/day) diuresis. When clinically feasible, intermittent diuretic therapy may reduce the likelihood of volume depletion.

Metabolic Alkalosis

Metabolic alkalosis can occur with the administration of thiazides, furosemide, and ethacrynic acid. These agents produce chloride depletion and increase renal hydrogen ion excretion.[5] As long as chloride depletion and sodium avidity persist, the kidney maintains the induced alkalosis. Treatment consists of chloride administration, usually in the form of potassium chloride. Ordinarily, 40 mEq/day in 3 to 4 divided doses should suffice.

Hypokalemia and Potassium Deficits

Hypokalemia and potassium deficits commonly occur in patients receiving diuretics. Mannitol, acetazolamide, thiazides, and the loop diuretics all enhance renal potassium excretion.

Diuretics typically induce moderate to severe hypokalemia and marked potassium deficits in edematous patients maintained on severely salt restricted diets; however, hypertensive patients, free of cardiac edema and ingesting a normal salt diet, typically experience only mild degrees of hypokalemia (3.3 to 3.8 mEq/L) and potassium deficits in the range of no more than 5% of total body potassium stores, averaging approximately 200 mEq, after prolonged diuretic treatment.[6] Thus, it is not necessary to routinely prescribe potassium supplementation to non-edematous patients on diuretic treatment,[6] but significant potassium depletion and hypokalemia, once they occur, should be treated with potassium chloride, 40 to 60 mEq/day as 10% liquid potassium chloride (not potassium triplex, potassium bicarbonate [K-Lyte], or potassium gluconate [Kaon]). High potassium diets are unreliable. Digitalis recipients and cirrhotic patients being treated with diuretics should be closely monitored.

Hyponatremia

Although diuretic-induced hyponatremia is uncommon, diuretic therapy accounts for most cases of hyponatremia in clinical practice. Depending on the clinical findings, treatment involves cessation of the diuretic and appropriate water restriction or volume repletion.

Hyperkalemia

Hyperkalemia commonly develops during the use of the 'potassium-sparing' diuretics, particularly when oral potassium supplements are coadministered. A 9% incidence of hyperkalemia in hospitalized patients given spironolactone in a dose of 150 mg/day or less has been reported.[7] Hyperkalemia was more common in patients with azotemia or in those who were also receiving potassium chloride supplementation. Potassium-retaining diuretics should not be given in these two clinical settings; furthermore, even when renal function is normal, these diuretics should be avoided in diabetic patients since they appear to be unusually prone to the development of hyperkalemia.

Hypercalcemia

Long-term administration of thiazides or loop diuretics may induce hypercalcemia. This condition has been described in normal subjects, in hypertensive subjects, in patients with idiopathic hypercalciuria, in uremic patients on maintenance hemodialysis, in patients with hyperparathyroidism, and in patients receiving large doses of vitamin D. Thiazide-induced hypercalcemia requires withdrawal of the drug and should raise the possibility of primary hyperparathyroidism.

Carbohydrate Intolerance

Furosemide, ethacrynic acid, and more commonly, thiazide diuretics, may induce mild carbohydrate intolerance. These diuretics might worsen the carbohydrate intolerance of non-insulin dependent diabetics but ketoacidosis has not been described (see also the section on drug interactions below).

Hyperuricemia

Hyperuricemia has been most commonly observed with the administration of thiazides and furosemide. It appears to be a consequence of decreased urate clearance induced by volume depletion. However, since thiazides and loop diuretics are organic acids, they may also compete with uric acid for the organic acid secretory pathway. Although allopurinol will decrease the uric acid level in this setting, its administration is not routinely indicated (see the section on drug interactions).

Other Adverse Reactions

Thiazides and the loop diuretics have been implicated in several hypersensitivity reactions; purpura, dermatitis, necrotizing vasculitis, and allergic interstitial nephritis have been reported. Acute pancreatitis and cholestatic hepatitis have also been reported following treatment with thiazides. Large intravenous doses of both furosemide and ethacrynic acid may produce hearing loss which is usually reversible on cessation of drug administration, but permanent hearing loss has been described. An increased occurrence of gastrointestinal bleeding in patients receiving intravenous ethacrynic acid has been reported. Estrogen-like, dose-related side effects may occur with spironolactone therapy. The induction of overt gouty arthritis after institution of diuretic agents is very unusual; however, serum uric acid levels, frequently rise modestly. The uric acid level usually remains below 10 to 12 mg/100 ml. Xanthine oxidase inhibitors (allopurinol) are not required unless an attack of acute gout occurs.

DRUG INTERACTIONS

The commonly used diuretics—thiazides, ethacrynic acid, and furosemide—may interact with a number of other drugs. Clinically significant interactions occur with digitalis preparations, hypoglycemic agents, uricosuric agents, antihypertensive agents, lithium, and certain antibiotics.

Digitalis

Edematous cardiac patients receiving diuretics, have an increased risk of arrhythmias if they become hypokalemic. The likelihood of hypokalemia and potassium depletion is increased if dietary sodium chloride intake is restricted. While potassium depletion probably increases the risk of arrhythmias in patients receiving cardiac glycosides, the degree of depletion does not always correlate well with the frequency of toxicity.[8]

Potassium supplements probably should be given to edematous cardiac patients simply to maintain plasma potassium levels within normal limits.[9] The serum potassium concentration should be measured prior to administering digitalis and diuretics, and at frequent intervals thereafter, depending on the clinical situation. Supplemental potassium chloride (in the range of about 40 to 60 mEq/day as a liquid) should be given to those patients with low or low normal serum potassium levels. The risks of hypokalemia and potassium depletion in patients receiving diuretics are discussed in detail elsewhere.[6]

Hypoglycemic Agents

Diuretics, especially the thiazides, can elevate blood sugar and uric acid levels; however, data on the effect of diuretics on carbohydrate tolerance are conflicting.[6] Several studies have shown no alteration in blood glucose, while other studies have shown mild defects in glucose tolerance. It is recommended that blood sugar be measured prior to, and after, the institution of oral diuretic agents in any patient receiving hypoglycemic agents. If necessary, appropriate changes in dosage of the latter should be made.

Antihypertensive Agents

Since thiazide diuretics are in themselves hypotensive agents, addition of a diuretic to an antihypertensive drug regimen may further lower blood pressure. This is not really a drug interaction, but simply synergism.

Lithium

Lithium salts are widely used for treatment of manic-depressive states. Lithium is reabsorbed in the proximal nephron similarly to sodium. Under normal circumstances, 60 to 70% of the filtered load of either ion is actively reabsorbed proximally. More importantly, volume depletion increases proximal lithium reabsorption. Therefore, when a patient receiving lithium becomes volume-depleted due to the administration of diuretics, lithium reabsorption increases, the plasma lithium level rises, and signs and symptoms of lithium toxicity may occur.[10] Consequently, patients receiving lithium should not be given diuretics unless clearly indicated. If concomitant use is necessary, constant monitoring of lithium blood levels is mandatory to avoid clinical toxicity.

Antibiotics

Ototoxicity has been noted in patients receiving a number of different aminoglycoside antibiotics, including kanamycin and gentamicin. When administered intravenously, the loop diuretics —ethacrynic acid and furosemide—also cause either transient or permanent deafness in a small fraction of patients. The ototoxicity observed when a loop diuretic and an aminoglycoside antibiotic are given concurrently probably represents a summation of their separate ototoxic effects. Therefore, unless an emergency situation exists, patients receiving aminoglycoside antibiotics should not be given loop diuretics intravenously.

In one study, the concomitant administration of cephaloridine and loop diuretics was reported to result in an increased incidence of nephrotoxicity.[11]

DRUG MONOGRAPHS

ETHACRYNIC ACID (Edecrin)
ETHACRYNATE SODIUM (Sodium Edecrin)
FUROSEMIDE (Lasix)

Ethacrynic acid and furosemide provide the physician with very potent, orally effective, rapidly-acting diuretic agents. Their efficacy and relatively low rates of side effects,[12] have greatly reduced the need for injectable organomercurial preparations. Chemically, ethacrynic acid and furosemide are unrelated; ethacrynic acid is a derivative of phenoxyacetic acid, and furosemide is a sulfamylbenzene derivative of anthranilic acid. When administered orally, they are both absorbed within 10 to 20 minutes. When given intravenously, the onset of action is within 5 minutes. The peak effect occurs 30 to 45 minutes after intravenous dosage, and 1 to 2 hours following oral administration. The duration of action seldom exceeds 6 to 8 hours. Both drugs block chloride reabsorption in the ascending limb of Henle's loop, and can produce a fractional sodium chloride excretion of up to 20 to 30% of the filtered load. Urinary composition after the administration of these agents may contain as much as 150 mEq/L of sodium and chloride. Kaliuresis can reach levels five times that observed during the pre-drug control period. Both drugs effect a marked increase in urinary excretion of calcium and magnesium. Intravenous administration of large doses of either drug is uricosuric, but chronic oral administration leads to hyperuricemia. In usual diuretic dosages no consistent changes in glomerular filtration rate, effective renal plasma flow, or intrarenal distribution of blood flow occur, unless sodium depletion develops. An increase in venous capacitance has been described in patients treated with furosemide. This appears to account for the prompt symptomatic relief of pulmonary edema when furosemide is given intravenously. For practical purposes, furosemide (40 mg) and ethacrynic acid (50 mg) are interchangeable. In contrast to thiazide diuretics, both of the loop diuretics retain their efficacy even in patients with glomerular filtration rates as low as 5 to 10 ml/min.

Adverse Reactions—Marked volume depletion, hyponatremia, metabolic alkalosis, hypokalemia, and potassium deficits are common with either agent. The development of metabolic alkalosis does not impair pharmacologic efficacy. Prolonged administration may produce hypercalcemia and hyperuricemia. Both agents can also produce carbohydrate intolerance, but less commonly than thiazides. Gastrointestinal disturbances are common with either drug; an increased occurrence of gastrointestinal bleeding following intravenous administration of ethacrynic acid has been reported.[13] Acute pancreatitis, aplastic anemia, severe neutropenia, agranulocytosis, thrombocytopenia with purpura and Henoch-Schönlein purpura have, in a few cases, been associated with the use of these agents. Various forms of dermatitis (including urticaria, exfoliative dermatitis, and erythema multiforme) can be seen following furosemide administration. Large doses of either agent may produce transient hearing loss; however, permanent deafness has been described, more commonly following treatment with ethacrynic acid.

Dosage—Oral and Intravenous: Adults, the conventional oral dose of furosemide is 40 to 200 mg per day; and of ethacrynic acid, 50 to 200 mg per day. Much higher doses (up to 500 to 1000 mg per day) are often required in patients with severe renal insufficiency. Intravenous doses are comparable to oral doses. *Children,* the conventional oral and intravenous dose for both furosemide and ethacrynic acid is 0.5 to 2.0 mg/kg administered every 6 to 12 hours, as needed.

THIAZIDE DIURETICS

Thiazide diuretics were the mainstay of oral diuretic therapy until the introduction of the more potent loop diuretics. Thiazide diuretics continue to be effective therapeutic agents in patients with edema and hypertension. Many different congeners of chlorothiazide are now available but the mechanism of action, potency, and complications of all derivatives are similar to the parent compound. A choice of a particular thiazide derivative should therefore reflect personal experience and the relative cost of the available drugs.

Chlorothiazide is well absorbed orally. It achieves its maximal effect within 30 to 45 minutes after oral or intravenous administration, and its action is dissipated in 4 to 6 hours. Sodium balance initially is negative, but escape from negative balance occurs in normal or hypertensive subjects after 3 to 5 days. Chlorothiazide, 500 mg, is equivalent to hydrochlorthiazide, 50 mg, and to chlorthalidone, 100 mg.

Adverse Reactions—Reactions include hypersensitivity phenomena, interstitial nephritis, precipitation of hepatic coma in patients with advanced hepatic disease, and a variety of metabolic problems including metabolic alkalosis, hypokalemia, hyperuricemia, hyperglycemia, hyponatremia, and hypercalcemia (see Introduction).

Drug Interactions—See the Introduction.

Dosage—Oral: Adults, Chlorothiazide: 500 to 2000 mg in one or two divided doses per day; Hydrochlorothiazide: 50 to 200 mg in one or two divided doses per day; Chlorthalidone: 100 to 200 mg/day in one dose. There is no reason to use thiazide diuretics intravenously. *Children*, Chlorothiazide: 20 to 40 mg/kg/day in one or two divided

TABLE 1 Preparations and Costs of Diuretics

Generic Name	Trademark Name(s)	Prepartions and 1978 Costs
Thiazide Diuretics		
Chlorothiazide	Diuril	Tablets 250mg—$4.06/100; 500 mg—$6.42/100 Suspension 250 mg/5 ml—$2.91/237-ml vial
Hydroclorothiazide	HydroDiuril (Esidrix) (Oretic) (Thiuretic)	Tablets 25 mg—$4.06/100; 50 mg—$6.42/100; 100 mg—$11.55/100
Bendroflumethiazide	Naturetin	Tablets 2.5 mg—$6.54/100; 5 mg—$10.27/100; 10 mg—$15.84/100
Benzthiazide	Aquatag (Aquapres) (Exna)	Tablets 25mg—$4.20/100; 50 mg—$8.00/100
Cyclothiazide	Anhydron	Tablets 2 mg—$8.17/100
Hydroflumethiazide	Saluron (Diucardin)	Tablets 50 mg—$7.49/100; 50 mg—$4.66/100
Methyclothiazide	Enduron (Aquatensen)	Tablets 2.5mg—$6.96/100; 5 mg—$9.28/100
Polythiazide	Renese	Tablets 1 mg—$8.10/100; 2 mg—$10.60/100; 4 mg—$17.73/100
Trichlormethiazide	Naqua	Tablets 2 mg—$4.52/100; 4 mg—$7.06/100
Diuretics Related to Thiazides		
Chlorthalidone	Hygroton	Tablets 50 mg—$8.71/100; 100 mg—$10.85/100
Metolazone	Zaroxolyn	Tablets 2.5 mg—$7.76/100; 5 mg—$9.95/100; 10 mg—$11.47/100
Quinethazone	Hydromax	Tablets 50 mg—$11.00/100
Potassium-Sparing Diuretics		
Spironolactone	Aldactone	Tablets 25 mg—$12.05/100
Triamterene	Dyrenium	Capsules 50 mg—$7.25/100; 100 mg—$9.10/100

TABLE 1 *(continued)*

GENERIC NAME	TRADEMARK NAME(S)	PREPARTIONS AND 1978 COSTS
Loop Diuretics		
Ethacrynic Acid	Edecrin	Tablets 25 mg—$6.66/100; 50 mg—$9.51/100
Ethacrynate Sodium	Sodium Edecrin	Injection (powder) 50 mg—$3.98/vial
Furosemide	Lasix	Tablets 20 mg—$6.60/100; 40 mg—$9.25/100 Injection (solution) 10 mg/ml—$1.10/2-ml ampul, $5.23/10-ml ampul
Diuretic Combinations		
	Aldactazide	Tablets (hydrochlorothiazide 25 mg and spironolactone 25 mg)—$13.20/100
	Dyazide	Capsules (hydrochlorothiazide 25 mg and triamterene 50 mg)—$9.55/100

doses; Hydrochlorothiazide: 4 mg/kg/day in one or two divided doses; Chlorthalidone: 0.35 to 0.75 mg/kg/day in one dose.

SPRIRONOLACTONE (Aldactone)
TRIAMTERENE (Dyrenium)

These two agents block sodium reabsorption at distal exchange sites in conjunction with reducing potassium excretion. Spironolactone, a competitive inhibitor of aldosterone, inhibits the binding of aldosterone to receptor sites in the distal tubule. It is a relatively weak antagonist of aldosterone and must be given in high doses in order to exert an anti-aldosterone effect. As expected, spironolactone is ineffective in the absence of aldosterone. Triamterene is a pteridine derivative that blocks sodium reabsorption directly and, simultaneously, potassium secretion in the distal nephron. The effect of triamterene is independent of aldosterone.

Both agents are relatively weak diuretics; the maximum fractional sodium excretion is only 2% of the filtered load of sodium. Therefore, these drugs are usually administered in conjunction with a loop or thiazide diuretic. Fixed combinations of a thiazide diuretic and a distal-blocking agent are available and are widely employed by physicians. Such preparations have the advantage of increasing patient compliance but the disadvantage of a fixed drug ratio.

Adverse Reactions—The major and frequent hazard of both agents in hyperkalemia. Hyperkalemia is more common in patients with azotemia and in those receiving potassium supplements. Distal blocking agents should not be used in patients with renal insufficiency (serum creatinine greater than 2 mg/dl), and supplemental potassium therapy should be avoided. Furthermore, these diuretics should probably be avoided in diabetic patients, even when renal function is normal, since diabetics are unusually prone to the development of hyperkalemia. Dose-related, estrogen-like side effects such as decreased libido, impotence, and gynecomastia in men, and menstrual irregularity and painful breast englargement in women, may occur with spironolactone administration.

Dosage—Oral: Adults, 25 to 100 mg per day for spironolactone; 100 to 300 mg per day for triamterene. Much higher doses of spironolactone have been used in the treatment of primary hyperaldosteronism and 'low-renin' essential hypertension. *Children,* 1.5 to 3.0 mg/kg/day in two divided doses for spironolactone; 0.7 mg/kg/day in one dose for triamterene.

REFERENCES

1. Goldberg M: The renal physiology of diuretics. In *Handbook of Physiology*. Edited by J Orloff, RW Berliner. Washington, Williams and Wilkins Company, 1973, pp 1003–1031.
2. Burg MB: Mechanisms of action of diuretic drugs. In *The Kidney*. Edited by BM Brenner, FC Rector, Jr. Philadelphia, W.B. Saunders Company, 1976, pp 737–762.
3. Schrier RW, Humphreys MH, Ufferman RC: Role of cardiac output and the autonomic nervous system in the antinatriuretic response to acute constriction of the thoracic superior vena cava. Circ Res 29:490–498, 1971.
4. Dirks JH, Seely JF, Levy M: Control of extracellular fluid volume and the pathophysiology of edema formation. In *The Kidney*. Edited by BM Brenner, FC Rector, Jr. Philadelphia, W.B. Saunders Company, 1976, pp 495–552.
5. Schwartz WB, van Ypersele de Strihou C, Kassirer JP: Role of anions in metabolic alkalosis and potassium deficiency. N Engl J Med 279:630–639, 1968.
6. Kassirer JP, Harrington JT: Diuretics and potassium metabolism: a reassessment of the need, effectiveness and safety of potassium therapy. Kidney Int 11:505–515, 1977.
7. Greenblatt DJ, Koch-Weser J: Adverse reactions to spironolactone: a report from the Boston Collaborative Drug Surveillance Program. JAMA 225:40–43, 1973.
8. Beller GA, Smith TW, Abelmann WH, et al: Digitalis intoxication: a prospective clinical study with serum level correlations. N Engl J Med 284:989–997, 1971.
9. Davidson C, Burkinshaw L, McLachlan MSF, et al: Effect of long-term diuretic treatment on body-potassium in heart disease. Lancet 2:1044–1047, 1976.
10. Singer I, Rotenberg D: Mechanisms of lithium action. N Engl J Med 289:254–260, 1973.
11. Lawson DH, Macadam RF, Singh H, et al: Effect of furosemide on antibiotic-induced renal damage in rats. J Infect Dis 126:593–600, 1972.

12. Greenblatt DJ, Duhme DW, Allen MD, et al: Clinical toxicity of furosemide in hospitalized patients: A report from the Boston Collaborative Drug Surveillance Program. Am Heart J 94:6–13, 1977.
13. Slone D, Jick H, Lewis GP, et al: Intravenously given ethacrynic acid and gastrointestinal bleeding. JAMA 209:1668–1671, 1969.

ANALGESICS AND NARCOTIC ANTAGONISTS

27. STRONG ANALGESICS

Russell R. Miller

Analgesics can be divided into two groups—strong and mild. Characteristics of the two groups are compared in Table 1. The strong analgesics may, in turn, be divided into narcotic and non-narcotic subgroups. All narcotic analgesics can produce drug dependence of the morphine type and are included in Schedule II of the Comprehensive Drug Abuse Prevention and Control Act of 1970. Narcotic analgesics include opium preparations, purified alkaloids obtained from opium (eg, morphine), semisynthetic modifications of morphine (eg, hydromorphone), and synthetic compounds with many of the effects of morphine (eg, meperidine). Only two strong analgesics are classified as non-narcotic—pentazocine (Talwin) and methotrimeprazine (Levoprome); they are not subject to controls under the Controlled Substances Act.

INDICATIONS

Analgesic therapy should be directed toward elimination of the cause of pain wherever possible. When the cause of pain cannot be determined or quickly eliminated, symptomatic treatment with analgesics is indicated. Severe pain, such as that due to biliary, renal, or ureteral colic, or stemming from thoracic, upper abdominal, or bone surgery, requires a strong analgesic. These agents should not be used to treat mild or moderate pain that could be satisfactorily relieved by the safer mild analgesics. The pain relieving ability of the mild analgesics is frequently underrated, and for many patients with moderate pain aspirin or acetaminophen is as effective as strong analgesics.

Strong analgesics are often indicated for relief of the pain of myocardial infarction. Although the circulatory response to morphine is variable,[1] it is usually the analgesic of choice. Meperidine may cause an initial increase in arterial blood pressure, systemic vascular resistance, and heart rate followed by a fall in these parameters to below pretreatment levels.[2] Pentazocine has been associated with increases in pulmonary artery pressure and left ventricular minute work.[3,4] Thus, meperidine and pentazocine usually should be avoided in patients with acute myocardial infarction.

Strong analgesics have a number of special uses in obstetric analgesia, preoperative medication, and anesthesia that are not discussed in detail in this Handbook. Their use as antitussive agents and antidiarrheal agents are discussed in Chapters 58 and 64, respectively.

DEPENDENCE

Of all the characteristics of strong analgesics, dependence is probably foremost in the prescriber's mind. As a consequence, needless suffering often occurs because of inadequate dosage. The risk of making a hospitalized patient with a short-term painful condition into a physically dependent addict is infinitesimally small. But when treating patients suffering from chronic pain, dependence becomes a distinct possibility. Since close control of dosage and frequency of administration are not possible with outpatients, strong analgesics should be prescribed for self-use by non-hospitalized patients only under exceptional circumstances.

Dependence can be divided into two categories—psychic and physical. Psychic dependence, formerly referred to as habituation, is the repeated compulsive use of a drug because of a perceived need. Physical dependence, often referred to as addiction, is a physiological condition wherein tissues have adapted to the presence of a drug; continued administration of the drug is necessary for normal function. If the drug is abruptly withdrawn, the abstinence syndrome occurs.

Psychic dependence probably occurs fairly often in patients who receive strong analgesics over periods of greater than four or five days. Physical dependence develops only rarely and usually only after therapy with high doses for more than two weeks. Frequently the circumstances for such prolonged use involve terminal neoplastic disease, and there is little need for concern about dependence. In the relatively rare instance where long-term strong analgesic therapy is necessary in a patient without a terminal illness, a mild degree of physical dependence may occur; however, when the patient no longer

TABLE 1 Comparison of Strong and Mild Analgesics

	STRONG ANALGESICS	MILD ANALGESICS
1. Indications	Moderate to severe pain	Mild to moderate pain
2. Clinical Effects	Increase pain tolerance Alter psychological response to pain Suppress anxiety Some alteration in consciousness and behavior	Reduce sensitivity of pain receptors
3. Site of Action	Central	Primarily peripheral
4. Route of Administration	Usually parenteral	Usually oral
5. Narcotic Classification	With the exception of pentazocine and methotrimeprazine, all are subject to the Comprehensive Drug Abuse Prevention and Control Act of 1970	With the exception of codeine, none are subject to controls
6. Adverse Effects	About the same with all drugs and often of major importance	Varied and mostly minor
7. Recipients	Primarily hospitalized patients	Hospitalized and ambulatory patients

needs a strong analgesic the drug dosage can be slowly tapered and abstinence symptoms prevented. Subsequently the patient will not be dependent and will not have the psychic desire for the analgesic. This complete and uncomplicated withdrawal is possible because many of the behavioral attributes of 'street addiction' are usually absent in the hospitalized patient. Patients who have histories of drug dependence, especially to drugs obtained by illicit means, obviously require special consideration when prescribing strong analgesics.

TOLERANCE

When strong analgesics are used for prolonged periods, some patients seem to require an increasingly larger dose to provide the same degree of analgesia. The dose should be increased cautiously since tolerance does not develop to many of the adverse effects of strong analgesics which are dose-dependent (eg, respiratory depression).

To offset the development of tolerance, some clinicians give sedative agents, such as promethazine hydrochloride (Phenergan), concomitantly with strong analgesics. Sedative agents probably do not potentiate the analgesic action of strong analgesics, but a mixture of an analgesic and a sedative undoubtedly provides more sedation than either drug alone.

MECHANISM OF ACTION

Strong analgesics increase pain tolerance, alter the psychological response to the pain sensation, suppress anxiety, and have a general sedative effect; most of these effects appear to be centrally mediated. In contrast, mild analgesics appear to reduce the sensitivity of pain receptors, probably by inhibition of prostaglandin synthesis; few central effects are noted. Other differences between the strong and mild analgesics are summarized in Table 1.

Recent studies have demonstrated the existence of receptors in the brain that are specific for opiates. Binding of opiates to these receptors produces analgesia; binding of narcotic antagonists reverses the effects of analgesics. Since it is unlikely that there would exist in the brain receptors specific for compounds not normally found in the body, a search for naturally occurring opiates is underway. Substances called *endorphins* and *enkephalins* have been identified and shown to have extremely potent analgesic activity. Continuing research may yield new and more specific analgesic drugs without addictive qualities.[5]

METABOLISM

Most strong analgesics are metabolized in the liver. Biotransformation appears to be the chief process for terminating analgesic effects. Since the major metabolic pathway differs for each drug, there are differences in how impaired liver function affects drug metabolism and analgesic effects. Thus, since glucuronic acid synthesis is impaired early in hepatic disease, strong analgesics metabolized by glucuronide conjugation (eg, morphine) should be given in reduced dosage. Alternatively, analgesics that are metabolized by other means, such as demethylation and hydrolysis (eg, meperidine) could be used.

TABLE 2 Parenteral Strong Analgesics

Generic Name	Trademark Name(s)	Percentage of Total Hospital Usage[a]	Approximate Duration of Action (hours)	Approximate Intramuscular Adult Equianalgesic[b] Dose (mg)
Opium Alkaloids				
Morphine		24	4–6	10
Morphine Modifications				
Hydromorphone	Dilaudid	1	4	1.5
Oxymorphone	Numorphan	1	4	1.0–1.5
Synthetic Agents				
Meperidine	Demerol	53	3	100
Alphaprodine	Nisentil	1	1	40–60
Anileridine	Leritine	1	2	25–40
Levorphanol	Levo-Dromoran	1	4–6	2–3
Methadone	Dolophine	1	5–7	7.5–10.0
Narcotic Antagonists				
Pentazocine	Talwin	17	3	45–60
Phenothiazine Derivatives				
Methotrimeprazine	Levoprome	1	4	20

[a]Usage in selected medical wards of 22 hospitals monitored by the Boston Collaborative Drug Surveillance Program from July 1966 to May 1975. About 69% of the monitored patients were in hospitals in the United States, 6% in Canada, 13% in Israel, 4% in New Zealand, 6% in Scotland, 1% in Germany, and 1% in Italy.

[b]Morphine 10 mg is the reference drug.

DURATION OF ACTION

The average duration of satisfactory analgesic effect varies widely among the parenteral strong analgesics (Table 2). Morphine, hydromorphone, oxymorphone, levorphanol, methadone, and methotrimeprazine usually provide four or more hours of adequate analgesia. Alphaprodine and anileridine provide only one to two hours of analgesia and consequently are generally used where short-term analgesia is desired. Meperidine and pentazocine, the two most widely used drugs, have an average duration of action of only three hours. This fact does not seem to be well appreciated.

ANALGESIC EFFICACY

For moderate to moderately severe pain all of the parenteral strong analgesics are probably equally effective if given in equianalgesic dosage. However, for severe to very severe pain, some drugs are more effective than others, regardless of dosage (Table 3). Morphine, hydromorphone, oxymorphone, levorphanol, methadone, and methotrimeprazine appear to be the most effective. Meperidine, alphaprodine, anileridine, and pentazocine are less effective.

ADVERSE REACTIONS

Adverse reactions to strong analgesics are qualitatively and quantitatively similar with some exceptions (Table 3). The most common adverse effects are nausea and vomiting, respiratory depression, constipation, orthostatic hypotension, and sedation. Nausea and vomiting are probably caused, at least in part, by a disturbance of vestibular function since they are more common in ambulatory patients. They can be managed by either keeping the patient in bed or giving an antiemetic, such as prochlorperazine.

Respiratory depression is dose-related. Measurable depression occurs with small doses and increases with the dose.[6] It is ordinarily not of great clinical significance, but it can be life-threatening in elderly or debilitated patients, in patients having conditions characterized by hypoxia, and in patients receiving other respiratory depressants. Meperidine produces less respiratory depression than morphine in newborns delivered of mothers treated with these analgesics.[7]

Constipation is a frequent adverse effect but can be managed by adjustments in diet or the concurrent use of laxatives.

After administration of a strong analgesic the cardiovascular system has a decreased capacity to respond to gravitational shifts. On standing, peripheral vasodilation and pooling of blood occur.[6] Thus, patients receiving strong analgesics probably should remain in bed after injection of the drug and should ambulate cautiously.

Drowsiness is common and may outlast analgesia by many hours. Other adverse effects are described in the drug monographs.

PRECAUTIONS

Strong analgesics should be used cautiously and usually in reduced dosage in patients with hepatic disease or reduced respiratory reserve for reasons discussed in previous sections. Patients with reduced blood volume are considerably more susceptible to the hypotensive effects of strong analgesics. In hypovolemia, subcutaneous and intramuscular administration of an analgesic may not provide adequate analgesia due to poor absorption; if a strong analgesic is used at all, cautious intravenous administration may be preferable. Patients with head injuries may be subject to increased risk of respiratory depression and increased cerebrospinal fluid pressure; strong analgesics probably should be avoided. Strong analgesics have been reported to precipitate acute asthmatic symptoms in asthmatic patients, but the risk does not seem to be high. During attacks analgesics may be dangerous because they depress respiration, depress the cough reflex, dry secretions, and may release histamine.

DOSAGE

Strong analgesics usually should be given in the doses listed in Table 2 when patients are in severe pain. For patients experiencing moderate pain, smaller doses (usually about three-fourths that listed in Table 2) may be used. For patients receiving other respiratory or CNS depressants, patients with reduced respiratory reserve, or elderly patients, smaller doses should be used. If chronic pain persists either the dose should be increased or the interval between doses decreased. Another drug should be tried if relief is not achieved or if intolerable adverse effects occur.

When very rapid pain relief is required, a strong analgesic may be given intravenously. Morphine, for example, may be given as a 1 mg/ml solution at the rate of 1 ml/minute until relief is apparent. Slow administration avoids respiratory and cardiovascular depression.

TABLE 3 Comparison of Strong Analgesics: 10 Point Scale—Assuming Usual Analgesic Doses

Drug	Efficacy		Adverse Reactions				
	Parenteral	Oral[a]	Nausea and Vomiting	Respiratory Depression	Constipation	Orthostatic Hypotension	Sedation
Morphine	10	3	5	5	5	5	5
Hydromorphine	10	7	5	5	5	5	5
Oxymorphine	10	3	5	5	5	5	5
Meperidine	8	3	5	5	3	5	5
Alphaprodine	8	—	5	5	3	5	5
Anileridine	8	3	5	5	3	5	5
Levorphanol	10	8	5	5	5	5	4
Pentazocine	5	3	3	5	1	1	5
Methotrimeprazine	10	—	1	1	1	10	10
Methadone	10	10	3	5	5	3	5

[a]Comparative values for aspirin and codeine would be 6 and 4, respectively. Methadone's effectiveness is decreased by half when it is administered orally rather than parenterally.

Two to four times the usual dose may be necessary in very severe pain. The narcotic antagonist naloxone should be readily available if needed to reverse respiratory depression.

Children tolerate strong analgesics very well. The usual dose for morphine is 0.15 to 0.20 mg/kg.

When given for relief of acute pain, analgesics should be prescribed on an 'as needed' basis. Many types of pain, especially those due to trauma, rapidly subside in intensity and may vary at different times of the day. Analgesics should be given as soon as possible after the patient notes increasing pain intensity, since lower total dosage is required and the patient suffers less if pain is prevented rather than treated. Patients with chronic pain should be given analgesics on a regular, around-the-clock schedule.

Surveys of physician's attitudes on prescribing of narcotic analgesics have shown that many prescribe inadequate doses at too infrequent intervals because of irrational and unfounded fears of the risk of addiction.[8] The risk of addiction in hospitalized patients is very low and should not influence the prescribing of an effective dose of a narcotic analgesic.

CHOICE OF A PARENTERAL STRONG ANALGESIC

Morphine is the parenteral strong analgesic of choice in nearly all clinical situations where a strong analgesic is required. Its efficacy is unexcelled, its duration of action is relatively long, and its unwanted effects are no more serious than those of other analgesics. Morphine can be used for the entire spectrum of moderate to severe pain by adjusting the dose. There is no need to switch from morphine to a less powerful strong analgesic as pain subsides; the patients can be transferred directly to a mild analgesic, such as aspirin, when appropriate.

Hydromorphone, oxymorphone, levorphanol, and methadone appear to be as effective as morphine and have no major advantages over morphine. Oxymorphone has no antitussive effect, which may make it useful in some situations.

Meperidine, although the most widely used strong analgesic, is inferior to morphine. Meperidine has a shorter duration of action and is not as effective as morphine in many painful conditions. The meperidine congeners alphaprodine and anileridine have even shorter periods of effectiveness. Fentanyl, another meperidine congener, is almost exclusively used in neuroleptanesthesia; its action is too short and intense for the drug to be used outside the operating room.

Pentazocine has unpredictable efficacy, a relatively short duration of action, and no advantage over morphine with regard to adverse effects. It is relatively non-addicting, a useful characteristic in some patients.

Methotrimeprazine, a phenothiazine derivative, should only be used in bed-ridden patients because of its pronounced hypotensive and sedative effects. It appears to be as effective as morphine and has about the same duration of action. It causes little nausea, vomiting, and respiratory depression and has no addiction potential.

Codeine is often considered a strong analgesic. In 30 mg doses, it is considerably inferior to morphine 10 mg.[9] Even codeine 120 mg fails to equal morphine 10 mg. Codeine in doses of 60 mg or more has most of the disadvantages of morphine, including respiratory depression. Therefore, parenteral codeine has few indications; if a milder analgesic effect is desired, doses of morphine smaller than 10 mg can be used.

CHOICE OF AN ORAL STRONG ANALGESIC

Orally-administered strong analgesics are markedly less effective than parenterally-administered drugs. This may be due to poor or slow absorption from the gastrointestinal tract, rapid biotransformation in the liver ('first-pass effect'), or other factors.

While it is difficult to draw accurate conclusions on the comparative efficacy of the parenteral strong analgesics it is nearly impossible to do so with the oral drugs. This is because of a paucity of published well-designed comparative studies. Therefore, the comparative ranking of oral analgesics in Table 3 is more tentative than for parenteral drugs.

Methadone appears to be the most effective oral strong analgesic. However, methadone is not as effective orally as it is parenterally (see methadone monograph). On the basis of very limited evidence, levorphanol and hydromorphone appear to be the next most effective. All other strong analgesics are probably less effective than aspirin when given orally for most types of pain. However, aspirin may not always be effective, and codeine or oxycodone (Percodan) should be tried before prescribing methadone, levorphanol, or hydromorphone.

Although not considered a strong analgesic, codeine is often prescribed as one. In the published studies comparing codeine and aspirin, codeine 30 mg was either less effective than aspirin 600 mg or not significantly different from placebo. Codeine 60 mg has been shown to be as effective as aspirin 600 mg in some painful conditions and marginally effective or indistinguishable from placebo in others. For a more detailed discussion of the relative efficacy of codeine and other mild analgesics, see Chapter 28, Mild Analgesics.

In single oral doses, morphine 10 mg is less effective than aspirin 600 mg.[10] However, with repeated doses of 25 to 90 mg, serum levels may become high enough to provide satisfactory analgesia. This may account for the efficacy of Brompton's Mixture,[11] an extemporaneously prepared combination of morphine (5 to 90 mg/10 ml) and small amounts of cocaine sulfate (5 mg/10 ml) and alcohol (95%, 1.25 ml/10 ml); it is usually given with a phenothiazine (eg, prochlorperazine, [Compazine]). Controlled, double-blind studies of Brompton's Mixture are lacking. Since the stability of morphine in such a solution is unknown, Brompton's Mixture should be prepared locally and used within 25 to 30 days.

DRUG MONOGRAPHS

ALPHAPRODINE HYDROCHLORIDE (Nisentil) C-II

Alphaprodine is related chemically and pharmacologically to meperidine but has a more rapid onset of action and a shorter duration of effect.[12] It may be preferable to meperidine or morphine in clinical situations where a short duration of effect is desirable (eg, removing sutures). The adverse effects and interactions of alphaprodine are similar to those described for meperidine.

Dosage—Intravenous: Adults, 20 to 30 mg injected slowly over a three or four minute interval. *Subcutaneous: Adults,* 20 to 60 mg, dose may be repeated at two hour intervals.

ANILERIDINE HYDROCHLORIDE (Leritine Hydrochloride) C-II
ANILERIDINE PHOSPHATE (Leritine Phosphate) C-II

Anileridine is related chemically and pharmacologically to meperidine, but its duration of action is slightly shorter.[12] When given intravenously 40 mg of anileridine is equivalent to 100 mg of meperidine.[13,14] It is reasonably effective by the oral route.[15] However, it is not as effective by mouth as by injection.[16] The adverse

TABLE 4 Preparations and Costs of Strong Analgesics

GENERIC NAME	TRADEMARK NAME(S)	PREPARATIONS AND 1978 COSTS
Alphaprodine Hydrochloride	Nisentil	Injection (solution) 40 mg/ml—$0.51/1-ml ampul; 60 mg/ml—$0.66/1-ml ampul, $3.83/10-ml vial
Anileridine Hydrochloride	Leritine	Tablets 25 mg—$5.43/100
Anileridine Phosphate	Leritine	Injection (solution) 25 mg/ml—$0.28/1-ml ampul, $0.30/2-ml ampul, $2.68/30-ml vial
Hydromorphone Hydrochloride	Dilaudid	Tablets 1 mg—$7.13/100; 2 mg—$9.90/100; 3 mg—$11.18/100; 4 mg—$12.75/100 Injection (solution) 1 mg/ml—$0.28/1-ml ampul; 2mg/ml—$0.29/1-ml ampul; 3 mg/ml—$0.31/1-ml ampul; 4 mg/ml—$0.31/1-ml ampul
Levorphanol Tartrate	Levo-Dromoran	Tablets 2 mg—$7.98/100 Injection (solution) 2 mg/ml—$0.33/1-ml ampul, $2.16/10-ml vial
Meperidine Hydrochloride	Demerol	Tablets 50 mg—$7.61/100; 100 mg—$14.40/100 Elixir 50 mg/5 ml—$9.09/pt Injection (solution) 50 mg/ml—$0.25/0.5-ml ampul, $0.25/1-ml ampul, $0.26/1.5-ml ampul, $0.26/2-ml ampul, $3.31/30-ml vial
Methadone Hydrochloride	Dolophine	Tablets 5 mg—$1.74/100; 10 mg—$2.83/100 Injection (solution) 10 mg/ml—$0.41/1-ml ampul, $2.52/20-ml vial
Methotrimeprazine	Levoprome	Injection (solution) 20 mg/ml—$0.82/1-ml ampul, $5.45/10-ml vial
Morphine Sulfate	generic	Injection (solution) 8 mg/ml—$0.19–$0.32/1-ml ampul; 10 mg/ml—$0.20–$0.34/1-ml ampul; 15 mg/ml—$0.21–$0.36/1-ml ampul

TABLE 4 *(continued)*

Generic Name	Trademark Name(s)	Preparations and 1978 Costs
Opium Alkaloids	Pantopon	Injection (solution) 20 mg/ml—$0.30/1-ml ampul
Oxymorphone Hydrochloride	Numorphan Hydrochloride	Injection (solution) 1 mg/ml—$0.52/1-ml ampul, $0.46/1.5-ml ampul, $4.20/15-ml vial Suppositories 5 mg—$3.90/6
Pentazocine Hydrochloride	Talwin Hydrochlride	Tablets 50 mg—$12.22/100
Pentazocine Lactate	Talwin Lactate	Injection (solution) 30 mg/ml—$0.45/1-ml ampul, $0.52/1.5-ml ampul, $0.62/2-ml ampul, $3.23/10-ml vial

effects and interactions of anileridine are similar to those of meperidine.

Dosage—Oral, Intramuscular, Subcutaneous: Adults, 25 to 50 mg, dose may be repeated every 3 to 6 hours if necessary. For severe pain, 75 to 100 mg intramuscularly initially. *Intravenous (slow): Adults,* 5 to 10 mg of well-diluted solution, followed by 0.6 mg/minute until the desired amount is given.

HYDROMORPHONE HYDROCHLORIDE (Dilaudid) C-II

Hydromorphone (dihydromorphinone) is a semisynthetic modification of morphine. In equianalgesic parenteral doses hydromorphone does not differ significantly from morphine; 2 mg of hydromorphone is approximately equivalent to 10 mg of morphine.[17] After oral administration hydromorphone is better absorbed than is morphine, and it is one of the few strong analgesics that is reasonably effective orally;[18,19] however, it is much less effective orally than it is parenterally. The adverse effects of hydromorphone are similar to those of morphine.

Dosage—Oral, Intramuscular, Intravenous (slow), Subcutaneous: Adults, 2 mg as required; dose may be increased to 4 mg for severe pain.

LEVORPHANOL TARTRATE (Levo-Dromoran) C-II

Levorphanol is a synthetic analgesic related chemically and pharmacologically to morphine. It appears to be as effective as morphine when given in equianalgesic doses,[20] and its adverse effects are similar to those of morphine. Levorphanol is readily absorbed from the gastrointestinal tract.

Dosage—Oral, Subcutaneous: Adults, 2 to 3 mg.

MEPERIDINE HYDROCHLORIDE (Demerol) C-II

Meperidine (pethidine) is a synthetic narcotic analgesic which differs chemically from morphine but possesses many similar pharmacologic actions. It is not as effective as morphine in relieving some pain, regardless of dosage, and has few advantages over morphine with regard to adverse effects. Further, since the average duration of action of parenterally administered meperidine is 3 hours, more frequent injections are required than with morphine.[10] When given by mouth, meperidine is considerably less potent and reliable than when given by injection.[16,17,21] Because of its lesser spasmogenic effects, meperidine is preferable to morphine for relief of pain due to spasm (eg, biliary tract and colonic spasm).[16]

Adverse Reactions—Meperidine depresses respiration; in equianalgesic doses, it is not better than morphine in this respect.[16] Meperidine has more euphoriant side effects (hallucinations, bizarre feeling, etc.) than morphine.[21] The most common adverse effects of oral meperidine are nausea and vomiting and of parenteral meperidine, central nervous system depression (drowsiness, respiratory depression, etc.).[22] See the monograph on morphine for contraindications.

Drug Interactions—Administration of meperidine to patients on long-term monoamine oxidase (MAO) inhibitor therapy (eg, isocarboxazid, furazolidone, nialimide, phenelzine, tranylcypromine, pargyline, and procarbazine) may result in adverse effects characterized by excitation, convulsions, hypertension or hypotension, hallucinations, and impaired ventilation.[23–25] Phenobarbital enhances the metabolic conversion of meperidine to normeperidine which may lead to enhanced sedative effects.[26]

Dosage—Oral, Intramuscular, Intravenous (slow), Subcutaneous: Adults, 100 mg, higher doses are often indicated in patients with severe pain. 75 mg is effective for only two-thirds of patients with severe pain.[8] 50 mg is usually inadequate. Dose should be repeated at intervals of three to four hours if needed.

METHADONE HYDROCHLORIDE (Dolophine) C-II

Methadone, a synthetic narcotic analgesic, is equipotent to or slightly more potent than morphine when given parenterally.[27,28] In contrast to most other strong analgesics, it also provides considerable analgesia when given orally. In terms of total analgesic effect, it is approximately one-half as potent orally as parenterally.[28] In the past decade methadone has been widely used in the treatment of dependence to other narcotics.[29,30] Methadone, unlike other strong analgesics, has cumulative properties when administered repeatedly.[31,32]

Adverse Reactions—Nausea and vomiting occur less frequently than with equivalent doses of morphine.[33] After single doses, sedation is less marked with methadone than with morphine,[33] but after repeated doses sedation may be more common.[21] Orthostatic hypotension appears to occur less often with methadone.[21] Respiratory depression is rarely observed in most clinical situations. However, methadone and morphine have been shown to be equipotent as respiratory depressants.[34]

Dosage—Oral, Intramuscular, Subcutaneous: Adults, 5 to 10 mg, repeated every 4 to 5 hours as needed.

Note—Under current regulations of the Food and Drug Administration, methadone may be used as an analgesic for treating patients with severe pain only if a written statement stating the conditions of its intended use are sent to the pharmacy along with the customary narcotic prescription.

METHOTRIMEPRAZINE (Levoprome)

Methotrimeprazine is a phenothiazine drug with strong analgesic properties. It is as effective as morphine 10 mg when given by injection in doses of 10 to 15 mg.[35,36] Methotrimeprazine does not produce psychic or physical dependence and only partially suppresses the symptoms of narcotic withdrawal;[37] accordingly, it is not subject to narcotic controls.

Adverse Reactions—In comparison to morphine and meperidine, methotrimeprazine produces a higher incidence of sedation and orthostatic hypotension.[36,38] The latter effect greatly limits its therapeutic usefulness. Methotrimeprazine appears to cause little nausea and vomiting, respiratory depression.[39] and constipation; it apparently does not potentiate the respiratory depression of morphine but does add to morphine's sedative effect.[39]

Dosage—Intramuscular: Adults, 10 to 20 mg, repeated every four to six hours as needed.

MORPHINE SULFATE C-II

Morphine, a purified alkaloid extracted from opium, is the prototype of the strong analgesics. Small to moderate parenteral doses will relieve constant dull pain, and moderate to large doses will alleviate intermittent, sharp, lancinating pain of trauma or of visceral origin. Morphine is effective for relief of postoperative pain, as well as pain caused by vascular occlusion, neoplastic disease, biliary colic, renal colic, fractures, and burns. A recent study has shown that concomitant intramuscular administration of dextroamphetamine[40] potentiates the analgesic effect of intramuscular morphine and decreases the sedative effects.

After intramuscular or subcutaneous injection, morphine is rapidly absorbed and produces plasma levels of free drug from 15 minutes to 3 hours that are appreciably higher than levels after intravenous administration.[41] Intravenous morphine produces initially high plasma levels but undergoes more rapid tissue distribution, metabolism, and excretion as free drug. Morphine is well absorbed from the gastrointestinal tract but apparently is so rapidly conjugated with glucuronide in the intestinal mucosa and liver that appreciable levels of free morphine are not found in either the plasma or urine, whereas the levels of conjugated morphine are high. As a consequence, morphine is only one-sixth as potent when administered orally as when administered intramuscularly.[42]

Adverse Reactions—Vertigo, nausea, and vomiting are common untoward effects and can be minimized by confining recipients to bed after an injection; these effects occur in about 3% of recipients. The overall adverse reaction rate for morphine is about 6%.[21] Respiratory depression is the potentially most dangerous acute action of morphine; it develops most readily in elderly, debilitated patients and particularly in those having diseases characterized by hypoxia. Morphine should be given cautiously, or not at all, to patients in shock, since respiratory depression may further reduce the patient's circulating blood volume, cardiac output, and blood pressure. Morphine is contraindicated in patients with head injuries, delirium tremens, and conditions in which intracranial pressure is invariably increased. It should be used with caution in myxedema, Addison's disease, and hepatic cirrhosis, since even small doses may cause stupor or precipitate coma and respiratory failure.

Morphine increases intestinal tone different from normal coordinated propulsive activity. This, together with sphinteric spasm, causes a diminution in peristalsis with resultant constipation. The ability of morphine to produce spasm of smooth muscle also can cause increased pressure in the biliary system, sufficient at times to produce biliary colic. Hypotension due to morphine can occur, especially in patients who are sitting or standing.[16]

Dosage—Intravenous: Adults, 2.5 to 15 mg slowly injected. *Subcutaneous, Intramuscular: Adults,* optimal dose is 10 mg/70 kg of body weight,[43] depending on the use and individual patient; older patients require less drug. Repeat every four to five hours as needed. *Children,* 0.1 to 0.2 mg/kg; maximal dose 15 mg. Undertreatment with inadequate doses should be avoided (see introduction).

OPIUM ALKALOIDS (Pantopon) C-II

Pantopon is a mixture of purified opium alkaloids, including morphine. It has no advantage over morphine alone with regard to efficacy or adverse effects and thus has no special indications.[20]

Dosage—Intramuscular, Subcutaneous: Adults, 5 to 20 mg.

OXYMORPHONE HYDROCHLORIDE (Numorphan Hydrochloride) C-II

Oxymorphone is a semisynthetic derivative of morphine and is closely related chemically to hydromorphone. Its adverse effects are essentially those of morphine.[44,45] Respiratory depression is marked in older patients.[46] In terms of total analgesic effect, oral oxymorphone is one-sixth as potent as the intramuscular form.[44] Rectal administration of oxymorphone results in lower and more delayed peak analgesia and a longer duration of action than intramuscular administration. When both duration and intensity of analgesia are considered, rectal oxymorphone is one-tenth as potent as the intramuscular form. Thus, giving 5 to 10 mg oxymorphone by suppository provides analgesia comparable to 1 to 1.5 mg of intramuscular drug.[47]

Dosage—Intramuscular, Subcutaneous: Adults, 1 to 1.5 mg as required. *Intravenous: Adults,* 0.5 mg initially. *Rectal: Adults,* 5 to 10 mg as required.

PENTAZOCINE HYDROCHLORIDE (Talwin Hydrochloride) PENTAZOCINE LACTATE (Talwin Lactate)

Pentazocine, the N-allyl derivative of the narcotic analgesic phenazocine, is a strong analgesic with weak narcotic antagonist activity. Although it is chemically related to morphine and shares some of its pharmacologic action it reportedly has a much lower potential for dependence and abuse.[48] It is not subject to control under the Controlled Substances Act of 1970. Pentazocine's effects are antagonized by naloxone but not by nalorphine or levallorphan.

The optimal dose of parenteral pentazocine (lactate) in severe pain varies considerably. One well-controlled study in patients with post-operative pain has shown that about 35 mg of pentazocine will produce an effect equal to 10 mg of morphine over a four hour period.[49] Other studies in patients with chronic pain due to cancer have shown that 60 mg of pentazocine was necessary to provide total analgesia similar to that of morphine 10 mg.[50,51]

Pentazocine raises pulmonary artery pressure and increases myocardial work, potentially dangerous effects for patients with myocardial infarction.[52,53] Morphine remains the drug of choice for the pain of myocardial infarction.

Oral pentazocine (hydrochloride) 50 mg appears to be less effective than aspirin 650 mg and produces sufficient CNS and gastrointestinal adverse effects to make it of dubious value in ambulatory patients.[54]

In view of its relatively high frequency of adverse reactions and uncertain efficacy, pentazocine would appear to be less useful than morphine or meperidine when a parenteral strong analgesic is needed and less useful than aspirin as an oral analgesic. Parenteral pentazocine may have advantages when it is important to minimize the risk of compulsive drug use. However, physical dependence to pentazocine has been reported.[55–57]

Adverse Reactions—Sedation, nausea, and vomiting are the most common adverse effects of pentazocine. Hallucinations, bizarre feelings, agitation, disorientation, and nightmares are not uncommon.[58,59] In equianalgesic doses, pentazocine produces as much respiratory depression as morphine.[60] Injection site complications range from minor local reactions to more serious local and systemic changes; examples of the latter include a peculiar woody sclerosis, poorly healing ulcers, and myopathy.[61–65]

Dosage—Oral: Adults, 50 mg every three or four hours as necessary. *Intramuscular, Intravenous, Subcutaneous: Adults,* 30 mg every three to four hours as necessary. Oral and parenteral doses of one and a half to two times those given above may be indicated in some patients.

REFERENCES

1. Thomas M, Malmcrona R, Fillmore S, et al: Haemodynamic effects of morphine in patients with acute myocardial infarction. Br Heart J 27:863–875, 1965.
2. Rees HA, Muir AL, MacDonald HR, et al: Circulatory effects of pethidine in patients with acute myocardial infarction. Lancet 2:863–866, 1967.
3. Lal S, Savidge RS, Chabra GP: Cardiovascular and respiratory effects of morphine and pentazocine in patients with myocardial infarction. Lancet 1:379–381, 1969.
4. Jewitt DE, Maurer GJ, Hubner PJB: Increased pulmonary arterial pressures after pentazocine in myocardial infarction. Br Med J 1:795–796, 1970.
5. Snyder SH: Opiate receptors in the brain. N Engl J Med 296:266–271, 1977.
6. Eckenhoff JE, Oech SR: The effects of narcotics and antagonists upon respiration and circulation in man: a review. Clin Pharmacol Ther 1:483–524, 1960.
7. Way WL, Costley EC, Way EL: Respiratory sensitivity of the newborn infant to meperidine and morphine. Clin Pharmacol Ther 6:454–461, 1965.
8. Marks RM, Sachar EJ: Undertreatment of medical inpatients with narcotic analgesics. Ann Intern Med 78:173–181, 1973.
9. Lasagna L, Beecher HK: The analgesic effectiveness of codeine and meperidine (Demerol). J Pharmacol Exp Ther 112:306–311, 1954.
10. Beecher HK, Keats AS, Mosteller F, et al: The effectiveness of oral analgesics (morphine, codeine, acetylsalicylic acid) and the problem of placebo 'reactors' and 'non.reactors'. J Pharmacol Exp Ther 109:393–400, 1953.
11. Melzack R, Ofiesh JG, Mount EM: The Brompton mixture: effects on pain in cancer patients. Can Med Assoc J 115:125–129, 1976.
12. Miller RR: Dosage and choice of parenteral strong analgesics. Am J Hosp Pharm 31:780–782, 1974.
13. Keats AS, Telford J, Kurosu Y: Studies of analgesic drugs: anileridine dihydrochloride. Anesthesiology 18:690–697, 1957.
14. Chang FFC, Safar P, Lasagna L: Narcotic potency and side effects of anileridine and meperidine in man. J Pharmacol Exp Ther 122:370–378, 1958.
15. Kessling R, Keats AS: The efficacy of a placebo and several oral analgesics in the treatment of pain of alveolar osteitis. Oral Surg 11:736–741, 1958.
16. Lasagna L: The clinical evaluation of morphine and its substitutes as analgesics. Pharmacol Rev 16:47–83, 1964.
17. Eddy NB, Halbach H, Braeden OJ: Synthetic substances with morphine-like effect. Bull WHO 17:705–709, 1957.
18. Goldberg RL, Shuman FI: Oral hydromorphone in trauma. Curr Ther Res 7:284–287, 1965.
19. Cass LJ, Frederik WS: A controlled clinical evaluation of the analgesic effect of oral hydromorphone. Curr Ther Res 7:275–283, 1965.
20. Morrison JD, Loan WB, Dundee JW: Controlled comparison of the efficacy of fourteen preparations in the relief of postoperative pain. Br Med J 3:287–290, 1971.
21. Miller RR: Analgesics. In *Drug Effects in Hospitalized Patients.* Edited by RR Miller, DJ Greenblatt. New York, John Wiley and Sons, 1976, pp 133–164.
22. Miller RR, Jick H: Acute toxicity of meperidine in hospitalized medical patients. J Clin Pharmacol 18:180-189, 1978
23. Vigran IM: Dangerous potentiation of meperidine hydrochloride by pargyline hydrochloride. JAMA 187:953–954, 1964.

24. Taylor DC: Alarming reaction to pethidine in patients on phenelzine. Lancet 2:401–402, 1962.
25. Cocks DP, Passamore.Rowe A: Dangers of monoamine oxidase inhibitors (letter). Br Med J 2:1545–1546, 1962.
26. Stambaugh JE, Wainer IW, Hemphill DM, et al: A potentially toxic drug interaction between pethidine (meperidine) and phenobarbitone. Lancet 1:398–399, 1977.
27. Denton JE, Beecher HK: New analgesics. II. A clinical appraisal of the narcotic power of methadone and its isomers. JAMA 141:1146–1148, 1949.
28. Beaver WT, Wallenstein SL, Houde RW, et al: A clinical comparison of the analgesic effects of methadone and morphine administered intramuscularly, and of orally and parenterally administered methadone. Clin Pharmacol Ther 8:415–526, 1967.
29. Dole VP, Nyswander M: A medical treatment for diacetylmorphone (heroin) addiction: a clinical trial with methadone hydrochloride. JAMA 193:646–650, 1965.
30. Chappel JN: Methadone and chemotherapy in drug addiction: genocidal or life-saving? JAMA 228:725–728, 1974.
31. Vogel VH, Isbell H, Chapman KW: Present status of narcotic addiction, with particular reference to medical indications and comparative addiction liability of the newer and older analgesic drugs. JAMA 138:1019–1026, 1948.
32. Olsen GD, Wendel HA, Livermore JD, et al: Clinical effects and pharmacokinetics of racemic methadone and its optical isomers. Clin Pharmacol Ther 21:147–157, 1977.
33. Dundee JW, Clarke RSJ, Loan WB: Comparative toxicity of dimorphine, morphine, and methadone. Lancet 3:221–224, 1967.
34. Prescott F, Ransom SJ, Thorp RH, et al: Effect of analgesics on respiratory response to carbon dioxide in man. Lancet 1:340–344, 1949.
35. Lasagna L, DeKornfeld TJ: Methotrimeprazine: a new phenothiazine derivative with analgesic properties. JAMA 178:887–890, 1961.
36. Montilla E, Frederik WS, Cass LJ: Analgesic effect of methotrimeprazine and morphine: a clinical comparison. Arch Intern Med 111:725–728, 1963.
37. Fraser HF, Rosenberg DE: Observations on the human pharmacology and addictiveness of methotrimeprazine. Clin Pharmacol Ther 4:596–601, 1963.
38. Callaghan PE, Zelenik JS: Methotrimeprazine for obstetric analgesia. Am J Obstet Gynecol 95:636–639, 1966.
39. Pearson JW, DeKornfeld TJ: Effect of methotrimeprazine on respiration. Anesthesiology 24:38–40, 1963.
40. Forrest WH Jr, Brown BW Jr, Brown CR, et al: Dextroamphetamine with morphine for the treatment of postoperative pain. N Engl J Med 296:712–715, 1977.
41. Brunk SF, Delle M: Morphine metabolism in man. Clin Pharmacol Ther 16:51–57, 1974.
42. Houde RW, Wallenstein SL, Beaver WT: Clinical measurement of pain. In *Analgesics*. Edited by G deStevens. New York, Academic Press, 1965, pp 75–122.
43. Lasagna L, Beecher HK: The optimal dose of morphine. JAMA 156:230–234, 1954.
44. Beaver WT, Wallenstein SL, Houde RW, et al: Comparisons of the analgesic effects of oral and intramuscular oxymorphone and of intramuscular oxymorphone and morphine in patients with cancer. J Clin Pharmacol 17:186–198, 1977.
45. Eddy NB, Lee LE Jr: The analgesic equivalence to morphine and relative side action liability of oxymorphone (4.hydroxydihydromorphinone). J Pharmacol Exp Ther 125:116–121, 1959.
46. Resnick ME, Berkowitz RD, Rodman T, et al: Effect of 14-hydroxydihydromorphinone on respiration. JAMA 173:1649–1653, 1960.
47. Beaver WT, Feise GA: A comparison of the analgesic effect of oxymorphone by rectal suppository and intramuscular injection in patients with postoperative pain. J Clin Pharmacol 17:276–291, 1977.
48. Brogden RN, Speight TM, Avery GS: Pentazocine: a review of its pharmacological properties, therapeutic efficacy and dependence liability. Drugs 5:6–91, 1973.
49. Paddock R, et al: Analgesic and side-effects of pentazocine and morphine in a large population of postoperative patients. Clin Pharmacol Ther 10:355–365, 1969.
50. Beaver WT, Wallenstein SL, Houde RW, et al: A comparison of the analgesic effects of pentazocine and morphine in patients with cancer. Clin Pharmacol Ther 7:740–751, 1966.
51. Frankendal B, Kjellgren O: Severe pain in gynecologic cancer. Trial of pentazocine, morphine and placebo. Cancer 27:842–847, 1971.

52. Jewitt DE, Maurer BJ, Hubner PJB: Increased pulmonary arterial pressure after pentazocine in myocardial infarction. Br Med J 1:795–796, 1977.
53. Alderman EL, Barry WH, Graham AF, et al: Hemodynamic effects of morphine and pentazocine differ in cardiac patients. N Engl J Med 287:623–627, 1972.
54. Moertel CG, Ahmann DL, Taylor WF, et al: A comparative evaluation of marketed analgesic drugs. N Engl J Med 286:813–815, 1972.
55. Swanson DW, Weddige RL, Morse RM: Hospitalized pentazocine abusers. Mayo Clin Proc 48:85–93, 1973.
56. Parwatikar S, Gomez H, Knowles RR: Pentazocine dependency. Int J Addict 8:87–98, 1973.
57. Goetz RL, Bain RV: Neonatal withdrawal symptoms associated with maternal use of pentazocine. J Pediatr 84:887–888, 1974.
58. Miller RR: Clinical effects of pentazocine in hospitalized medical patients: a report from the Boston Collaborative Drug Surveillance Program. J Clin Pharmacol 15:198–215, 1975.
59. Wood AJJ, Moir DC, Campbell C, et al: Central nervous system effects of pentazocine. Br Med J 1:305–307, 1974.
60. Bellville JW, Green J: The respiratory and subjective effects of pentazocine. Clin Pharmacol 6:152–159, 1965.
61. Parks DL, Perry HO, Muller SA: Cutaneous complications of pentazocine injections. Arch Dermatol 104:231–235, 1971.
62. Swanson DW, Weddige RL, Morse RM: Hospitalized pentazocine abusers. Mayo Clin Proc 48:85–93, 1973.
63. Schlicher JE, Zuehlke RL, Lynch PJ: Local changes at the site of pentazocine injection. Arch Dermatol 104:90–91, 1971.
64. Winfield JB, Greer K: Cutaneous complications of parenterally administered pentazocine. JAMA 226:189–190, 1973.
65. Steiner JC, Winkelman AC, deJesus PV: Pentazocine-induced myopathy. Arch Neurol 28:408–409, 1973.

28. MILD ANALGESICS

Russell R. Miller and Robert A. Curtis

Most mild analgesics differ substantially, both chemically and pharmacologically, from the strong analgesics. Accordingly, they are largely used for the relief of different painful disorders. However, both strong and mild analgesics are useful for the treatment of postoperative, postpartum, and posttraumatic pain. When mild analgesics provide satisfactory relief they should be used in preference to strong analgesics because of a lower frequency of serious adverse effects. On the other hand, none of the mild analgesics, even in large doses, are useful in severe pain. A comparison of the strong and mild analgesics is provided in Table 1 of Chapter 27, Strong Analgesics.

The mild analgesics can be divided into two groups: (1) agents chemically related to the strong analgesics (codeine, ethoheptazine, oxycodone, and propoxyphene) and (2) analgesic-antipyretic agents. The latter group can be subdivided into salicylates, para-aminophenol derivatives, pyrazolone derivatives, and miscellaneous agents.

ANALGESIC EFFICACY

Strong Analgesic Derivatives

Codeine, a derivative of morphine, probably is the most effective of the mild analgesics that are chemically related to the strong analgesics. Propoxyphene, a methadone congener, is inferior to codeine in usual therapeutic doses.[1] Ethoheptazine, a meperidine congener, has not been compared to codeine but is probably less effective. The relative efficacy of oxycodone is unknown since clinical trials of this drug have not been published. Oxycodone is available only in Percodan and Percocet, combination products.

Contrary to popular belief, codeine is usually less effective than aspirin, and it has a higher frequency of adverse reactions (see codeine monograph). Propoxyphene 65 mg is clearly less effective than aspirin 650 mg but has fewer adverse effects (see propoxyphene monograph).

Ethoheptazine is less effective than aspirin (see ethoheptazine monograph).

Salicylates

The salicylates include aspirin, aluminum aspirin, choline salicylate, and sodium salicylate. Aspirin is the most effective salicylate and is not surpassed by any other mild analgesic in proven analgesic efficacy. Aluminum aspirin is slowly and incompletely absorbed from the gastrointestinal tract;[2,3] therefore, effective blood levels may not be achieved. No studies have shown aluminum aspirin to be as effective as aspirin.

Published clinical trials comparing choline salicylate (Arthropan) and aspirin are lacking. Choline salicylate is unlikely to be as effective as aspirin since salicylate is less effective than acetylsalicylate (see below). However, choline salicylate causes less gastrointestinal irritation than aspirin and, for this reason, it may be useful for treating rheumatoid arthritis (see Chapter 32).

Sodium salicylate is less effective than equal doses of aspirin in relieving pain and reducing fever.[4]

Salicylamide is not a salicylate but is usually considered with this group. It is less effective than aspirin as an analgesic and antipyretic.[4,5]

Since aluminum aspirin, choline salicylate, sodium salicylate, and salicylamide are probably less efficacious than aspirin, they are not recommended for use as simple analgesics and monographs on these drugs are not included in this chapter.

Para-Aminophenol Derivatives

Acetaminophen and phenacetin are members of this class. Since phenacetin is seldom prescribed as a single-entity product, its use as a sole analgesic is not considered here.

In a small number of studies, acetaminophen has been shown to be as effective as aspirin in relieving pain and reducing fever (see monograph on acetaminophen). However, unlike aspirin, acetaminophen has little anti-inflammatory activity (at usual daily doses of 2.4 g or less), and since inflammation is thought to be a component of many types of pain, aspirin may be more effective in some clinical conditions. This possible advantage of aspirin should be weighed against its higher frequency of adverse reactions. However, when acetaminophen is taken for long periods at doses above approximately 3.5 g or is taken in overdose amounts, hepatotoxicity is a distinct possibility.

Pyrazolone Derivatives

This group includes aminopyrine and dipyrone. Aminopyrine and dipyrone have analgesic and antipyretic properties but are without acceptable uses because of their potential to produce agranulocytosis.[6] They have been removed from the U.S. market.

Miscellaneous Agents

Mefenamic acid (Ponstel), an anthranilic acid derivative, is unrelated chemically to other analgesics. Since it has not been shown to be superior to aspirin or acetaminophen and can produce hemolytic anemia,[7–9] it is not recommended.

Although indomethacin (Indocin) is primarily used as an antirheumatic agent, it does possess analgesic and antipyretic properties. It should not be used as a simple analgesic since it may cause serious adverse reactions (eg, gastrointestinal bleeding and ulceration, hematological disturbances). Indomethacin has been found useful in controlling the pain of certain bony metastases, particularly those in which hypercalcemia is also a factor.

MIXTURES

A very large number of mixtures of analgesics and of analgesics with other drugs are available. They are exceedingly popular, both among prescribing physicians and lay consumers. Yet the efficacy of most of these preparations has not been established in well-designed clinical trials. Indeed, some mixtures have been shown to be inferior to single analgesics.[10]

Many analgesic mixtures are clearly irrational since they either include drugs of questionable analgesic efficacy, combine short and long-acting agents, or include miniscule doses of some ingredients.

In the relatively uncommon situation where the possibly greater analgesic effect of a combination product might be of value, a combination of codeine 65 mg and aspirin 650 mg could be tried. This combination has been shown to be slightly superior to aspirin 650 mg alone and probably has a lower dependence potential than oxycodone with aspirin, phenacetin, and caffeine (Percodan), which also has been shown to be slightly superior to plain aspirin[10] (see individual monographs on these mixtures). The combination of acetaminophen 600 mg and codeine 60 mg has been shown superior to either drug alone in some studies (see monograph). The greater analgesic efficacy of these combinations must be weighed against a possibly higher frequency of adverse reactions.

ADVERSE REACTIONS

In contrast to the strong analgesics, the mild analgesics cause relatively few serious adverse reactions. The character and frequency of adverse reactions among the various drugs differ greatly. Some analgesics, such as acetaminophen and propoxyphene, produce adverse reactions in less than 1% of recipients while others, such as aspirin and codeine, produce unwanted effects in 5 to 10% of recipients.[11] Most adverse effects appear to be dose-related. Specific untoward effects are discussed in the individual drug monographs.

Chronic use of mild analgesic mixtures has been associated with renal damage. The composition of these mixtures varies, but phenacetin is a common component. Thus, it has been singled out as the most likely causative agent. The evidence for this conclusion is indirect since a prospective controlled study of phenacetin alone has not been done and kidney damage due to phenacetin alone has not been observed; phenacetin is seldom used alone. However, the available data on analgesic nephropathy strongly implicate phenacetin. Thousands of cases of kidney disease associated with use of phenacetin-containing mixtures have been reported, while probably no more than ten well-documented cases of kidney disease associated with all other single-entity analgesics and mixtures not containing phenacetin have been reported.[12] Phenacetin has been removed from nonprescription drug products by government order in some countries. After a lag period of six to eight years, the incidence of analgesic nephropathy or death due to uremia has declined in Sweden,[13,14] Scotland,[15] and Finland.[16] Additional confirmatory evidence is provided by studies that show a correlation between the degree of phenacetin consumption and the probability of serious kidney damage.[17-20] In summary the available evidence overwhelmingly indicates that phenacetin causes analgesic nephropathy. Accordingly, phenacetin-containing products should be avoided.

CHOICE OF A MILD ANALGESIC

When a mild analgesic is indicated, most patients can be satisfactorily treated with aspirin. It has unsurpassed efficacy and is inexpensive. These advantages must be balanced against its adverse reactions, particularly in certain patients.

In many patients acetaminophen is a satisfactory alternative to aspirin for relief of mild pain and reduction of fever. It produces a remarkably low frequency of adverse reactions and is also inexpensive, although more expensive than aspirin. Codeine or propoxyphene may be useful in some patients but are generally less effective than aspirin. Other mild analgesics, including the many mixtures that are available, are seldom indicated.

DRUG MONOGRAPHS

ACETAMINOPHEN (Tylenol)

Acetaminophen (paracetamol) is a mild analgesic and antipyretic agent with little anti-inflammatory activity. Its analgesic and antipyretic effects are similar to those of aspirin. Since acetaminophen has a relatively low frequency of adverse effects, it is utilized as an alternative to aspirin in non-inflammatory conditions.[21,22]

Acetaminophen is rapidly absorbed from the gastrointestinal tract with peak plasma levels occurring within 1 to 2 hours after ingestion.[23] Following the administration of 1 g, total serum concentrations of acetaminophen range from 5 to 20 μg/ml; however, a relationship between serum concentrations and degree of analgesia is lacking.[24] The drug is not appreciably bound to plasma proteins[25] and is distributed throughout most body fluids.

Acetaminophen is metabolized in the liver, primarily by conjugation with glucuronic acid and to a lesser extent with sulfuric acid.[26–28] A small portion of the drug is metabolized by the P-450 oxidase enzyme system in liver microsomes, and it is believed the resulting metabolites play a prominent role in hepatotoxicity associated with acetaminophen overdose.[29] Acetaminophen metabolites are excreted by the kidney; however, in renal impairment, the half-life is unchanged.[26]

The analgesic efficacy of acetaminophen is well established[21,22] but,

TABLE 1 Preparations and Costs of Mild Analgesics

Generic Name	Trademark Name(s)	Preparations and 1978 Costs
Single-Entity Drugs		
Acetaminophen	Tylenol	Tablets 325 mg—$1.56/100 Chewable tablets 80 mg—$0.95/30 Capsules 500 mg—$1.49/50 Elixir 120 mg/5 ml—$0.84/2 oz, $1.56/4 oz, $5.31/pint
	generic	Suppositories 125 mg—$0.65–$3.60/12; 325 mg—$0.70–$4.00/12; 625 mg—$0.75–$4.30/12
Aspirin	generic	Tablets 75 mg—$0.39/36; 325 mg—$0.18–$4.00/100 Suppositories 60 mg—$0.67–$1.40/12; 120 mg—$0.61–$1.75/12; 300 mg—$0.61–$1.75/12; 600 mg—$0.72–$1.75/12
Codeine Phosphate or Sulfate	generic	Tablets 15 mg—$4.65–$5.31/100; 30 mg—$6.24–$9.68/100; 60 mg—$17.25–$18.49/100 Injection (solution) 30 mg/ml—$0.30–$0.45/1-ml ampul; 60 mg/ml—$0.33–$0.53/1-ml ampul
Ethoheptazine Citrate	Zactane	Tablets 75 mg—$7.01/100
Propoxphene Hydrochloride	Darvon (Dolene)	Capsules 32 mg—$3.91/100; 65 mg—$9.37/100
Propoxyphene Napsylate	Darvon-N	Tablets 100 mg—$8.31/100 Suspension 50 mg/5 ml—$5.67/16 oz
Mixtures		
Aspirin 230 mg, Phenactin 150 mg, Caffeine 30 mg	Empirin Compound	Tablets—$1.10/100
Aspirin 325 mg, Codeine phosphate 30 mg	Ascodeen-30	Tablets—$7.95/100
Aspirin 230 mg, Phenacetin 150 mg, Caffeine 30 mg, Codeine Phosphate 30 mg	Empirin Compound with Codeine No. 3	Tablets—$8.10/100

TABLE 1 *(continued)*

GENERIC NAME	TRADEMARK NAME(S)	PREPARATIONS AND 1978 COSTS
Propoxyphene Napsylate 50 mg, Acetaminophen 325 mg	Darvocet-N	Tablets—$4.85/100
Propoxyphene Napsylate 100 mg, Acetaminophen 650 mg	Darvocet-N 100	Tablets—$10.40/100
Propoxyphene Hydrochloride 65 mg, Aspirin 227 mg, Phenacetin, 162 mg, Caffeine 32 mg	Darvon Compound-65	Capsules—$7.69/100
Propoxyphene Hydrochloride 65 mg, Aspirin 325 mg	Darvon with A.S.A.	Capsules—$7.47.100
Butalbital 50 mg, Aspirin 200 mg, Phenacetin 130 mg, Caffeine 40 mg	Fiorinal	Tablets—$4.62/100
Oxycodone Hydrochloride 4.5 mg, Oxycodone Terephthalate 0.38 mg, Aspirin 224 mg, Phenacetin 160 mg, Caffeine 32 mg	Percodan	Tablets—$8.70/100
Oxycodone Hydrochloride 5 mg, Acetaminophen 325 mg	Percocet-5	Tablets—$9.10/100
Acetaminophen 300 mg, Codeine Phosphate 30 mg	Tylenol with Codeine	Tablets—$9.20/100
Ethoheptazine Citrate 75 mg, Aspirin 300 mg	Zactirin	Tablets—$3.90/48
Ethoheptazine Citrate 100 mg, Aspirin 227 mg, Phenacetin 152 mg, Caffeine 32.4 mg	Zactirin Compound-100	Tablets—$10.85/100

probably because of its limited anti-inflammatory effect, acetaminophen is not uniformly as effective as aspirin in all types of mild to moderate pain. For example, in patients with rheumatoid arthritis, aspirin is far superior to acetaminophen.[30,31] On the other hand, acetaminophen is equally as effective as aspirin in relieving pain due to oral surgery,[32] cancer,[33] and postpartum trauma.[34] In general, acetaminophen is an effective drug in the treatment of mild to moderate pain associated with headache, dysmenorrhea, trauma, and operative procedures.[22]

Acetaminophen 650 mg has been shown to be more effective than propoxyphene 65 mg in cancer patients,[33] and acetaminophen 1000 mg has been shown to be superior to the combination of propoxyphene hydrochloride 65 mg with aspirin, phenacetin and caffeine.[35]

Acetaminophen exerts its antipyretic effect centrally by causing the hypothalamic heat regulating center to increase the dissipation of body heat.[22] It inhibits prostaglandin synthetase found in the central nervous system and this action appears responsible for increased heat dissipation.[36]

Acetaminophen demonstrates antipyretic effects[37] equal to that of aspirin[38,39] and superior to salicylamide[40] and tepid sponging.[41] The duration of antipyretic effects of acetaminophen and aspirin also appear to be equal—both drugs exhibiting peak activity three hours after ingestion with a total duration of six hours.[38]

When equal amounts of acetaminophen (650 mg) were administered orally as a tablet and rectally as a suppository, no significant difference in antipyretic effect was observed. However, the relative potency of the suppositories was noted to be 0.6 times that of the tablet form when comparing reduction in degrees per minute.[42]

Toxicity—Because of dramatically increased usage, serious toxicity due to acetaminophen overdosage has become increasingly common in the United Kingdom and the United States.[29,43–45] Patients who ingest doses exceeding 13 to 15 g appear to undergo varying degrees of liver damage.[43,45]

As stated earlier, acetaminophen is primarily metabolized by conjugation with glucuronic and sulfuric acid, with the remaining drug being metabolized by the P-450 oxidase system.[26–28] Drug metabolized by the latter system produces a toxic intermediary metabolite, which is normally rendered harmless by either cysteine or glutathione.[46] It is believed that liver damage occurs when these two substances are depleted due to excessive quantities of the toxic metabolite present.[29] These toxic intermediaries bind with sulfhydryl groups in the liver, producing necrosis localized in the centrilobular region.[47–50] Patients who have been taking medication that induce P-450 hepatic microsomal enzymes (eg, phenobarbital) are predisposed to a higher propensity for liver damage, due to the increased rate of conversion to the toxic metabolite and the depletion of glutathione.[29]

Therapy of overdosage includes inducing emesis, gastric lavage and administration of activated charcoal.[51,52] Due to the rapid absorption of acetaminophen this therapy must be administered within a maximum of 60 minutes after ingestion.

A relatively new treatment for acetaminophen toxicity is the administration of a variety of sulfhydryl compounds—cysteamine, methionine, and acetylcysteine.[53–57] If administered within the critical time period of 10 hours postingestion, these agents appear to replenish or substitute for glutathione which then combines with the toxic intermediary metabolite from the P-450 oxidase system.[58] All of these agents have been reported effective in man; acetylcysteine is used most often in the United States. When administered orally, acetylcysteine is rapidly hydrolyzed to cysteine and replenishes body cysteine stores. It appears to have less side effects than the other agents and may prove to be very effective in the treatment of acetaminophen overdosage.[57,59,60]

Hemodialysis has been attempted in acetaminophen overdosage, but it appears to be of little value.[61]

Adverse Reactions—Since acetaminophen is a metabolite of phenacetin, it has been suspected as a cause of renal damage. This is a controversial subject.[62] At best, the evidence for renal toxicity at usual dosage is very limited. Renal failure has been reported in patients who have consumed toxic doses of the drug.[52,63,64]

One case of acetaminophen-induced pancreatitis has been noted; however, the patient had ingested a dose of 60 g.[65] In contrast to aspirin, acetaminophen exhibits few adverse effects. It does not produce gastric irritation or bleeding in therapeutic doses and does not alter platelet adhesiveness[66,67] nor potentiate oral anticoagulants.[68] Reports of thrombocytopenia, rash, methhemoglobinemia and hypersensitivity have been rare.[69–71]

Dosage—Oral, Rectal: Adults, 300 to 600 mg at 4 hour intervals. *Children 6 to 12 years,* 150 to 300 mg; *1 to 6 years,* 60 to 120 mg; *under*

1 year, 60 mg. These amounts are given as single doses every 4 to 6 hours.

ASPIRIN

Aspirin is the drug of choice when a mild analgesic or antipyretic is indicated; its efficacy has been documented in numerous studies.[4] Since it also has anti-inflammatory properties, aspirin is useful in the treatment of rheumatic diseases (see Chapter 32). When used as an analgesic, aspirin is most effective for relief of headache, neuralgia, myalgia, arthralgias, and other musculoskeletal pain. It is less useful in acute pain of visceral origin, but it may be effective in less severe postoperative and postpartum pain or in pain secondary to trauma and cancer. In these types of pain, aspirin may provide adequate relief and should be tried prior to use of strong analgesics.

Aspirin is one of the most effective and safe antipyretics. However, antipyretic therapy is only symptomatic; the cause of fever should be sought and treated whenever possible.

Chronic use of aspirin should be avoided in pregnancy since it has been associated with an increased incidence of anemia, antepartum and postpartum hemorrhage, prolonged gestation, longer spontaneous labor, and perinatal mortality.[72,73]

Aspirin is commonly used for symptomatic relief of the common cold and other respiratory viral infections. It provides some relief but probably not as much as alluded to by folklore. Further, aspirin increases the rate of virus shedding, and this may lead to increased spread of virus to contacts.[74]

After oral administration, aspirin is rapidly absorbed, primarily in the stomach and upper portion of the small intestine.[75–77] Prior to systemic distribution about 30% of the drug is metabolized to the active metabolite salicyluric acid by enzymes in the gastrointestinal tract and liver.[78,79] The enzyme system that metabolizes aspirin can easily be overloaded. Thus, in doses over 4 g daily, the usual metabolic pathways can be saturated and small increments of aspirin may raise the blood salicylate level to the point of toxicity. Small decrements may have a correspondingly greater effect than expected in lowering salicylate levels.

Salicylate blood levels do not correlate with analgesic activity, but blood level determinations are useful in the management of overdosage.

Aspirin has been shown to influence the synthesis and metabolism of prostaglandins, but the clinical application of these findings is presently unclear.

Dosage Forms—Aspirin is available in a number of oral dosage forms that are designed to alleviate gastric irritation and provide faster absorption, higher blood levels, and more prolonged analgesia. Experimental buffered aspirin tablets have been shown to dissolve more rapidly, have a higher absorption rate, and cause less gastric irritation than plain tablets.[80] However, these characteristics have not been convincingly demonstrated for Bufferin, Ascriptin, and other commercially available buffered aspirin tablets. Furthermore, Bufferin does not provide more pain relief than aspirin.[81] These preparations cannot be recommended since they are more expensive than plain aspirin.

Buffered effervescent aspirin products (eg, Alka-Seltzer) are absorbed more rapidly and provide higher plasma salicylate concentrations than regular aspirin tablets, primarily because the aspirin is in solution;[82] more rapid gastric emptying may also facilitate more rapid absorption. However, the total amount of aspirin absorbed is the same for both buffered effervescent and regular tablet preparations. When used repeatedly, the absorbable antacid in Alka-Seltzer alkalinizes the urine which leads to faster excretion and decreased blood levels of salicylate.[83] Another disadvantage of Alka-Seltzer is its relatively high sodium content. Thus, Alka-Seltzer can be recommended only for occasional use.

The disintegration, dissolution, and absorption characteristics of enteric-coated tablets of aspirin vary markedly depending on how they are manufactured. Further, inter- and intra-subject variations in absorption are marked.[84] Thus, enteric-coated aspirin tablets are not recommended.

Prolonged-release aspirin dosage forms (eg, Measurin and Bayer Timed Release Aspirin) offer no advantage over regular tablets. In a study of equal doses of Measurin and regular aspirin tablets, the regular tablets provided higher plasma salicylate concentrations than Measurin for the first four hours then slightly (but statistically significant) lower levels at six and eight hours; at 12 and 16 hours the differences were not statistically significant.[85] The total amount of salicylate absorbed (as measured by urinary excretion studies) was lower for Measurin. Prolonged-release aspirin caused bleeding gastritis in two patients who did not bleed with regular aspirin.[86]

When given as suppositories, aspirin is slowly, erratically, and incompletely absorbed. If suppositories are retained for two hours, even the better formulated preparations provide only about 40% absorption; most brands provide only about 20%.[87] Accordingly, rectal administration is generally not advisable.

Adverse Reactions—The most common adverse effects of aspirin are minor gastrointestinal (GI) disturbances (eg, heartburn, nausea, cramps, indigestion, vomiting).[88] Most of these effects probably stem from direct irritation of the stomach and can be diminished by taking aspirin with sufficient quantities of milk, food, antacid, or water.

Central nervous system effects are the second most common category of adverse reactions and include tinnitus, deafness, headache, and dizziness.[88] They occur most often at high doses (ie, more than 3 g/day) and usually disappear when dosage is reduced.

Occult GI bleeding is present in nearly all aspirin recipients, but is usually clinically insignificant. Occult bleeding is detected only occasionally, primarily when it leads to anemia.[88] Serious overt bleeding is rare. In one study of patients with no previous history of GI bleeding, the frequency of hospitalization for upper GI bleeding attributed to regular aspirin use (at least four days a week) was about 15 per 100,000 users per year.[89] Aspirin probably should be avoided by patients predisposed to peptic ulcer; acetaminophen is usually a logical alternative. Aspirin-induced ultrastructural changes in human gastric mucosa have recently been demonstrated.[90] The gastric mucosa does not adapt to continued aspirin exposure and remains in an injured state until aspirin is discontinued, but patients have symptoms infrequently.[91]

Aspirin may cause gastric ulcers in some patients, but this untoward effect also appears to be rare. The best available estimate on its incidence is 10 cases of newly diagnosed and uncomplicated benign gastric ulcer per 100,000 users per year among hospitalized patients who had taken aspirin regularly for four or more days a week.[89]

Hypersensitivity reactions occur infrequently and are seen most often in asthmatic patients. About 3 to 5% of asthmatics will have bronchospasm, urticaria, or other sensitivity reactions when they take aspirin. About 1.5% of patients with rhinorrhea and 0.9% of normal, non-allergic subjects have sensitivity reactions.[92] No analgesic can be unequivocally recommended for aspirin-sensitive patients since wheezing and airflow obstruction has been observed with most analgesics.[93]

Aspirin alone has been shown to cause an increase in prothrombin time, particularly when taken in relatively high doses and for prolonged periods.[94-96] In patients whose synthesis of the prothrombin complex is already depressed by oral anticoagulants, aspirin would be expected to cause a greater prolongation of the prothrombin time. However, present evidence indicates that usual doses (1.95 to 3.00 g/day) of aspirin have no major effect on the hypoprothrombinemic action of the coumarins.[97-99] Thus, the small increased risk of bleeding in coumarin recipients is not primarily due to a drug interaction but rather from the effect of aspirin on platelet function and other components of primary hemostasis and from its hemorrhagic action on the gastric mucosa. High doses (greater than 3 g/day) of aspirin augment the hypoprothrombinemia of oral anticoagulants; hemorrhage may occur in a previously controlled patient.[98] Persons with blood coagulation defects or severe anemia should avoid aspirin.

Renal damage has been associated with the use of analgesic mixtures, but it appears that phenacetin rather than aspirin is the most likely etiologic agent. Three studies have shown no association between renal damage and aspirin use.[100-102] However, in patients taking anti-inflammatory doses of aspirin, renal function may be reversibly impaired. The rate of aspirin-induced alterations in renal function is higher in systemic lupus erythematosus patients than in arthritis patients.[103]

Aspirin may cause reversible hepatic injury when it is taken in high doses.[104] Fortunately, the event appears to be rare.

Interactions—Small or large doses of aspirin inhibit the uricosuric action of sulfinpyrazone and other uricosuric agents.[105] In recipients of coumarin anticoagulants there is an increased risk of bleeding if aspirin is also taken (see adverse reactions section above).

Substances that lower urine pH (eg, ascorbic acid) may decrease excretion of salicylate and raise plasma salicylate concentrations; substances that raise urine pH (eg, sodium bicarbonate) may increase excretion and lower plasma salicylate concentrations.

Aspirin may influence laboratory tests of renal function since relatively high doses may cause a reversible elevation in serum creatinine and blood urea nitrogen and a decrease in creatinine clearance.[103]

Although salicylates may potentiate the hypoglycemic effect of chlorpropamide, tolbutamide, and possibly other sulfonylurea hypoglycemic agents,[106,107] documentation for this interaction is weak.

Concurrent use of aspirin and alcohol may enhance occult gastrointestinal bleeding and gastric damage caused by aspirin.[108]

Long-term (greater than a week) administration of aspirin (greater than 600 mg/day) results in decreased plasma and leucocyte levels and increased urinary excretion of ascorbic acid.[109] Although this interaction has not been shown to cause clinical evidence of ascorbic acid deficiency (bleeding gums, petechial tongue lesions, drowsiness, lethargy, and skin pigmentation), aspirin recipients with these symptoms should be evaluated for this deficiency.

Aspirin may decrease the serum levels of indomethacin when these drugs are given together.[110] The clinical significance of decreased serum indomethacin levels is unknown.

Limited clinical data suggest that the concurrent administration of methotrexate and aspirin may result in elevated or prolonged serum levels of free methotrexate;[111] this could lead to greater methotrexate toxicity.

In one study aspirin (3 g/day) increased the serum half-life of penicillin G.[112] The clinical significance of this interaction is unknown.

In a study of normal subjects, aspirin reduced the diuretic effect of spironolactone.[113] This interaction has not been reported in clinical practice. Aspirin absorption is reduced by cholestyramine when these drugs are given together, but this interaction can be avoided by giving the drugs at least one-half hour apart.[114]

Serum concentrations of naproxen are reduced by concurrent administration of aspirin.[115] The small magnitude of the decreased serum concentrations suggests that the likelihood of a meaningful interaction is small.

Dosage—Oral, Rectal: Adults, 600 mg every four hours; higher doses may be used. *Children,* 65 mg/kg daily divided into four or six doses.

CODEINE PHOSPHATE C-II
CODEINE SULFATE C-II

Codeine has variable analgesic efficacy that appears to be dependent on the nature of the painful condition. In a study of oral surgery patients, codeine 30 mg was indistinguishable from placebo while aspirin 650 mg and acetaminophen 600 mg were highly effective; codeine 60 mg was only marginally better than placebo.[32] In patients with episiotomy pain, codeine 60 mg was marginally effective while aspirin 600 mg and 1200 mg were effective; in patients with postpartum uterine pain codeine was indistinguishable from placebo while aspirin 650 mg was effective.[116] In postoperative patients, acetaminophen 600 mg and codeine 60 mg were approximately equieffective.[117] In patients with cancer pain, codeine 32 mg was slightly less effective than aspirin 600 mg.[5] In summary, codeine may be useful in some painful disorders when prescribed in a 60 mg dose, but it probably seldom surpasses the analgesic efficacy of aspirin 600 to 650 mg.[118–120] Since codeine has no anti-inflammatory activity and does not inhibit prostaglandin synthesis, whereas aspirin does, these differences in action may account for codeine's ineffectiveness in some types of pain. Parenterally administered codeine has few indications because it is inferior to parenteral morphine in relieving severe pain.[121]

Codeine has a low propensity to produce tolerance and physical dependence when given in usual therapeutic doses. Further, it is not a particularly attractive drug for abuse because it does not elicit psychic effects considered desirable by addicts.[4]

Adverse Reactions—Nausea, vomiting, constipation, sedation, and dizziness are the most common adverse effects and occur more frequently at higher doses and in ambulatory patients.[11]

ETHOHEPTAZINE CITRATE (Zactane)

Ethoheptazine is chemically related to meperidine. In three studies, it has been shown superior to placebo,[122–124] but in a recent well-designed trial ethoheptazine could not be distinguished from placebo.[31] In another study, ethoheptazine 75 or 150 mg was less effective than aspirin 600 mg.[125] Because of these equivocal credentials, ethoheptazine is not recommended.

PROPOXYPHENE HYDROCHLORIDE (Darvon, Dolene)
PROPOXYPHENE NAPSYLATE (Darvon-N)

Propoxyphene is a mild analgesic with no anti-inflammatory or antipyretic properties. It is chemically related to methadone. Propoxyphene hydrochloride 65 mg or propoxyphene napsylate 100 mg is less effective than 650 mg of aspirin and 30 to 65 mg of codeine.[1,126] The napsylate salt is no more or less effective than the hydrochloride when given in equimolar doses.

Overdosage—When taken in overdoses, propoxyphene can cause serious toxicity; propoxyphene-related deaths appear to be increasing.[127,128] The most frequently reported major overdose symptoms are coma, convulsions, and respiratory depression. Intravenous naloxone and supportive therapy are the preferred treatments.[126]

Dependence—Psychological dependence to propoxyphene has been frequently reported; it is substantially less than that seen with codeine, morphine, or heroin. Physical dependence with withdrawal symptoms has been documented in only a few case reports.[129,130]

Abuse and Misuse—The abuse potential of propoxyphene appears to be substantial. Large numbers of civilians and military personnel have used high doses of propoxyphene for its pleasurable subjective properties.[126] Propoxyphene is also misused by many people who have no abuse intentions. Patients may, for example, take higher than normal doses in an effort to obtain greater pain relief.

Adverse Reactions—Propoxyphene has a very low frequency of adverse reactions in hospitalized patients; the most common adverse reactions are minor gastrointestinal complaints.[11] Central nervous system symptoms (vertigo, lightheadedness, drowsiness, headaches, etc.) and rash also occur. Hepatotoxicity has been reported[131,132] but appears to be a rare untoward effect.

Dosage—Oral: Adults, 65 mg three or four times daily.

MIXTURES

As noted in the introduction, analgesic mixtures are seldom indicated. Those described below are among the most popular and are briefly discussed primarily to discourage their use.

ASPIRIN, PHENACETIN, AND CAFFEINE (APC, Empirin Compound)

This traditional analgesic mixture is widely used, presumably because it is thought to have some advantage over plain aspirin. However, numerous studies have failed to show that APC provides greater analgesia than aspirin alone.[81,133–135] Further, since phenacetin has little anti-inflammatory action, the combination is less effective than an equivalent amount of aspirin alone in treating inflammatory conditions. The prolonged use of large doses of phenacetin-containing mixtures has been associated with renal damage.

ASPIRIN AND CODEINE (Ascodeen-30) C-III
ASPIRIN, PHENACETIN, CAFFEINE, AND CODEINE (Empirin Compound with Codeine) C-III

The combination of aspirin 650 mg and codeine 60 mg may be more effective than two tablets of plain aspirin (650 mg) in some patients,[10] but this possible advantage should be weighed against a higher frequency of adverse reactions than with aspirin alone, especially with multiple doses.

Empirin Compound with Codeine has no advantage over the simple combination of codeine and aspirin; thus, the latter is preferred.

DARVOCET-N

This combination of propoxyphene napsylate and acetaminophen has been compared with its individual components in only one study.[136] The combination was not superior to acetaminophen alone, but it was superior to propoxyphene alone because propoxyphene could not be distinguished from placebo.

DARVON COMPOUND

This combination of propoxyphene and APC has not been compared to propoxyphene (Darvon) alone; two studies have compared Darvon Compound with APC. In one investigation[137] propoxyphene with APC was superior to APC, while in another[138] there was no difference. In a third study,[139] one capsule of Darvon Compound-65 provided less analgesia than 650 mg of aspirin.

DARVON WITH A.S.A.

This combination of propoxyphene with aspirin has been compared with its components in only one study.[10] This investigation showed no difference in efficacy between plain aspirin 650 mg and propoxyphene hydrochloride 65 mg with aspirin 650 mg.

FIORINAL

This is an irrational mixture of relatively short-acting analgesics and a relatively long-acting barbiturate sedative. If used repeatedly, the barbiturate will accumulate and cause excessive sedation. If a sedative effect is desired, a sedative drug, preferably a benzodiazepine (eg, diazepam), should be prescribed separately.

PERCOCET-5
PERCODAN

Clinical trials comparing Percodan, a combination of oxycodone with APC, or Percocet-5, a combination of oxycodone and acetaminophen, with aspirin are lacking. However, Moertel et al[10] compared a combination of oxycodone 9.76 mg and aspirin 650 mg (roughly comparable to two tablets of Percodan) with aspirin 650 mg and found that the combination provided somewhat more analgesia. A combination of codeine 65 mg and aspirin 650 mg was also superior to plain aspirin. If a combination is indicated, codeine and aspirin (eg. Ascodeen—30) would be a better choice than Percodan or Percocet-5 because oxycodone appears to have a higher addiction potential than codeine (roughly the same as morphine)[140,141] and may cause more adverse effects (eg, nausea, vomiting, dizziness).[142]

TYLENOL WITH CODEINE

It is not known if this mixture is more effective than aspirin alone. In a well-designed study of oral surgery outpatients, a combination of acetaminophen 600 mg and codeine 60 mg was no more effective than acetaminophen 600 mg alone; codeine was indistinguishable from placebo.[32] In a study of patients with episiotomy pain, a combination of acetaminophen 600 mg with codeine 30 mg provided greater pain relief than either acetaminophen 600 mg or codeine 30 mg alone.[143] In a study of postoperative pain, a combination of acetaminophen 600 mg and codeine 60 mg was superior to either drug alone.[117] In aspirin-intolerant patients who do not achieve adequate analgesia with acetaminophen alone this combination may be worth trying.

ZACTIRIN
ZACTIRIN COMPOUND—100

These mixtures contain ethoheptazine and aspirin or APC. While two studies[122,144] have shown that the combination of aspirin and ethoheptazine is more effective than aspirin alone, three other investigations[10,145,146] did not demonstrate any superiority. Thus, Zactirin preparations are probably little more than expensive aspirin.

REFERENCES

1. Miller RR, Feingold A, Paxinos J: Propoxyphene hydrochloride, a critical review. JAMA 213:996–1006, 1970.

2. Levy G, Sahli BA: Comparison of the gastrointestinal absorption of aluminum acetylsalicylate and acetylsalicylic acid in man. J Pharm Sci 51:58–62, 1962.
3. Levy G, Procknal JA: Unusual dissolution behavior due to film formation. J Pharm Sci 51:294, 1962.
4. Beaver WT: Mild analgesics: a review of their clinical pharmacology. Am J Med Sci 250:577–604, 1965; 251:576–599, 1966.
5. Houde RW, Wallenstein SL, Beaver WT: Clinical measurement of pain. In *Analgetics,* edited by G deStevens. New York, Academic Press, 1965, pp. 75–122.
6. Huguley CM: Agranulocytosis induced by dipyrone, a hazardous antipyretic and analgesic. JAMA 189:938–941, 1964.
7. Scott GL, Myles AB, Bacon PA: Autoimmune haemolytic anaemia and mefenamic acid therapy. Br Med J 3:534–535, 1968.
8. Farid NR, Johnson JR, Low WT: Haemolytic reaction to mefenamic acid (letter). Lancet 2:382, 1971.
9. Robertson JH, Kennedy CC, Hill CM: Haemolytic anaemia associated with mefenamic acid. Irish J Med Sci 140:226–229, 1971.
10. Moertel CG, Ahmann DL, Taylor WF, et al: Relief of pain by oral medications: a controlled evaluation of analgesic combinations. JAMA 229:55–59, 1974.
11. Miller RR: Analgesics. In *Drug Effects in Hospitalized Patients,* edited by RR Miller, DJ Greenblatt. New York, John Wiley and Sons, 1976, pp. 133–164.
12. Food and Drug Administration: Over-the-counter drugs: establishment of a monograph for OTC internal analgesic, antipyretic and antirheumatic products. Federal Register Vol. 42, No. 131, p. 35425, July 8, 1977.
13. Bengtsson U: A comparative study of chronic non-obstructive pyelonephritis and renal papillary necrosis. Acta Med Scand 388:5–71, 1962.
14. Nordenfelt O: Deaths from renal failure in abusers of phenacetin-containing drugs. Acta Med Scand 191:11–16, 1972.
15. Murray RM: Analgesic nephropathy: removal of phenacetin from proprietary analgesics. Br Med J 4:131–132, 1972.
16. Kasanen A: The effect of the restriction of the sale of phenacetin on the incidence of papillary necrosis established at autopsy. Ann Clin Res 5:369–374, 1973.
17. Burry AF, de Jersey P, Weedon D: Phenacetin and renal papillary necrosis: results of a prospective autopsy investigation. Med J Aust 1:873–879, 1966.
18. Bell D, Kerr DNS, Swinney J, et al: Analgesic nephropathy. Clinical course after withdrawal of phenacetin. Br Med J 3:378–382, 1969.
19. Murray RM, Lawson DH, Lington AL: Analgesic nephropathy: clinical syndrome and prognosis. Br Med J 1:479–482, 1971.
20. Grimlund K: Phenacetin and renal damage at a Swedish factory. Acta Med Scand 174:3–26, 1963.
21. Ameer B, Greenblatt DJ: Acetaminophen. Ann Intern Med 87:202–209, 1977.
22. Koch.Weser J: Acetaminophen. N Engl J Med 295:1297–1300, 1976.
23. Rumack BH, Matthew H: Acetaminophen poisoning and toxicity. Pediatrics 55:871–876, 1975.
24. Gwilt JR, Robertson A, McChesney EW: Determination of blood and other tissue concentrations of paracetamol in dog and man. J Pharm Pharmacol 15:440–444, 1963.
25. Gazzard BG, Ford-Hutchinson AW, Smith MJH, et al: The binding of paracetamol to plasma proteins of man and pig. J Pharm Pharmacol 25:964–967, 1973.
26. Prescott LF: The metabolism of phenacetin in patients with renal disease. Clin Pharmacol Ther 19:383–394, 1969.
27. Miller RP, Roberts RJ, Fischer LJ: Acetaminophen elimination kinetics in neonates, children and adults. Clin Pharmacol Ther 19:284–294, 1976.
28. Albert KS, Sedman AJ, Wagner JG: Pharmacokinetics of orally administered acetaminophen in man. J Pharmacokin Biopharm 2:381–393, 1974.
29. Mitchell JR, Jollow DJ, Potter WZ, et al: Acetaminophen-induced hepatic necrosis: I. Role of drug metabolism. J Pharmacol Exp Ther 187:185–194, 1973.
30. Huskisson EC: Simple analgesics in arthritis. Br Med J 4:196–200, 1974.
31. Hajnal J, Sharp J, Popert AJ: A method for testing analgesics in rheumatoid arthritis using a sequential procedure. Ann Rheum Dis 18:189–206, 1959.
32. Cooper SA, Beaver WT: A model to evaluate mild analgesics in oral surgery out-patients. Clin Pharmacol Ther 20:241–250, 1976.

33. Moertel CG, Ahmann DL, Taylor WF, et al: A comparative evaluation of marketed analgesic drugs. N Engl J Med 286:813–815, 1972.
34. Kantor TG, Meisner M, Laska E, et al: A computer program for the clinical study of analgesic compounds (abstract). Fed Proc 23:176, 1964.
35. Smith MT, Levin HM, Bare WW, et al: Acetaminophen extra strength capsules versus propoxyphene compound-65 versus placebo: a double-blind study of effectiveness and safety. Curr Ther Res 17:452–459, 1975.
36. Flower RJ, Vane JR: Inhibition of prostaglandin synthetase in brain explains the anti-pyretic activity of paracetamol (4-acetaminophenal). Nature 240:410–411, 1972.
37. Cornely DA, Ritter JA: N-acetyl-p-aminophenol (Tylenol Elixir) as a pediatric antipyretic-analgesic. JAMA 160:1219–1221, 1956.
38. Colgan MT, Mintz AA: The comparative antipyretic effect of N-acetyl-p-aminophenol and acetylsalicylic acid. J Pediatr 50:552–555, 1957.
39. Tarlin L, Landrigan P: A comparison of three antipyretic effects of acetaminophen and aspirin. Am J Dis Child 124:880–882, 1972.
40. Eden AN, Kaufman A: Clinical comparison of three antipyretic agents. Am J Dis Child 114:284–287, 1967.
41. Hunter J: Study of antipyretic therapy in current use. Arch Dis Child 48:313–315, 1973.
42. Maron JJ, Ickes AC: The antipyretic effectiveness of acetaminophen suppositories versus tablets: a double-blind study. Curr Ther Res 20:45–52, 1976.
43. McJunkin B, Barwick KW, Little WC: Fatal massive hepatic necrosis following acetaminophen overdose. JAMA 236:1874–1875, 1976.
44. Boyer TD, Rouff SL: Acetaminophen-induced hepatic necrosis and renal failure. JAMA 218:440–441, 1971.
45. Clark R, Borirakchan YV, Davidson AR: Hepatic damage and death from overdose of paracetamol. Lancet 1:66–69, 1973.
46. Mitchell JR, Thorgeirsson SS, Potter WZ, et al: Acetaminophen-induced hepatic injury: protective role of glutathione in man and rationale for therapy. Clin Pharmacol Ther 18:676–684, 1974.
47. James O. Roberts SH, Douglas A, et al: Liver damage after paracetamol overdosage. Lancet 2:579–58w, 1975.
48. Prescott LF, Roscoe P, Wright N, et al: Plasma-paracetamol half-life and hepatic necrosis in patients with paracetamol overdosage. Lancet 1:519–522, 1971.
49. Goulding R, Volans GN, Prome P, et al: Paracetamol toxicity (letter). Lancet 1:358, 1976.
50. Krenzelok EP, Best L, Manoguerra AS: Acetaminophen toxicity. Am J Hosp Pharm 34:391–394, 1977.
51. Dordoni B, Willson RA, Thompson RPH: Reduction of absorption of paracetamol by activated charcoal and cholestyramine. Br Med J 3:86–87, 1973.
52. Levy G, Houston JB: Effect of activated charcoal on acetaminophen absorption. Pediatrics 58:432–435, 1976.
53. Prescott LF, Swanson CP, Forrest ARW, et al: Successful treatment of severe paracetamol overdose with cysteamine. Lancet 1:588–592, 1974.
54. Prescott LF, Park J, Proudfoot AT: Cysteamine for paracetamol poisoning (letter). Lancet 1:357, 1976.
55. Prescott LF, Sutherland GR, Park J, et al: Cysteamine, methionine and penicillamine in the treatment of paracetamol poisoning. Lancet 2:109–113, 1976.
56. Crome P, Vale JA, Volans GN, et al: Methionine in the treatment of acetaminophen poisoning (letter). N Engl J Med 296:824, 1977.
57. Peterson RG, Rumack BH: Treating acetaminophen poisoning with acetylcysteine. JAMA 237:2406–2407, 1977.
58. Harvey F, Goulding R: Action of cysteamine in paracetamol poisoning (letter). Lancet 2:1082, 1974.
59. Peterson RG, Rumack BH: N-acetylcysteine for acetaminophen overdosage (letter). N Engl J Med 296:515, 1977.
60. Lyons L, Studdiford JS, Somumakipa AM: Treatment of acetaminophen overdosage with N-acetylcysteine (letter). N Engl J Med 296:174, 1977.
61. Farid NR, Glynn JP, Kerr DNS: Haemodialysis in paracetamol self poisoning. Lancet 2:396–398, 1972.
62. Edwards OM, Edwards P, Juskisson EC, et al: Paracetamol and renal damage. Br Med J 2:87–89, 1971.

63. Maclean D, Peters TJ, Brown RAG, et al: Treatment of acute paracetamol poisoning. Lancet 2:849–852, 1968.
64. Rose PG: Paracetamol overdose and liver damage (letter). Br Med J 1:381–382, 1969.
65. Gilmore IT, Tourvas E: Paracetamol-induced acute pancreatitis. Br Med J 1:753–754, 1977.
66. Mielke CH, Heiden D, Britten AF, et al: Hemostasis, antipyretics, and mild analgesics. JAMA 235:613–615, 1976.
67. Mielke CH, Britten A: Use of aspirin or acetaminophen in hemophilia (letter). N Engl J Med 282:1270, 1970.
68. Antlitz AM, Awalt LF: A double-blind study of acetaminophen used in conjunction with oral anticoagulant therapy. Curr Ther Res 11:360–361, 1969.
69. Skokan JD, Hewlett JS, Hoffman GC, et al: Thrombocytopenia purpura associated with ingestion of acetaminophen (Tylenol). Cleve Clin Q 40:89–91, 1973.
70. Maclean D, Robertson PGG, Bain S: Methaemoglobinaemia and paracetamol (letter). Br Med J 4:390, 1968.
71. Michelson PA: Rash, weakness and acetaminophen (letter). Ann Intern Med 83:374, 1975.
72. Lewis RB, Schulman JD: Influence of acetylsalicylic acid, an inhibitor of prostaglandin synthesis, on the duration of human gestation and labor. Lancet 2:1159–1161, 1973.
73. Collins E, Turner G: Maternal effects of regular salicylate ingestion in pregnancy. Lancet 2:335–338, 1975.
74. Stanley ED, Jackson GG, Panusarn C, et al: Increased virus shedding with aspirin treatment of rhinovirus infection. JAMA 231:1248–1251, 1975.
75. Hogben CAM, Schanker LS, Tocco DJ, et al: Absorption of drugs from the stomach. II. The human. J Pharmacol Exp Ther 120:540–545, 1957.
76. Truitt EB Jr, Morgan AM: Absorption of aspirin from the stomach in man. Toxicol Appl Pharmacol 2:237–241, 1960.
77. Truitt EB Jr, Morgan AM: Gastrointestinal factors in aspirin absorption: a quantitative study. J Pharm Sci 53:129–134, 1964.
78. Rowland M, Riegelman S, Harris PA, et al: Kinetics of acetylsalicylic acid disposition in man. Nature 215:413–414, 1967.
79. Rowland M, Riegelman S, Harris PA, et al: Absorption kinetics of aspirin in man following oral administration of an aqueous solution. J Pharm Sci 61:379–385, 1972.
80. Leonards JR, Levy G: Effect of pharmaceutical formulation on gastrointestinal bleeding from aspirin tablets. Arch Intern Med 129:457–460, 1972.
81. DeKornfeld TJ, Lasagna L, Frazier TM: A comparative study of five proprietary analgesic compounds. JAMA 182:1315–1318, 1962.
82. Ekenved G, Elofsson R, Solvell L: Bioavailability studies on a buffered acetylsalicylic acid preparation. Acta Pharm Suec 12:323–332, 1975.
83. Caravati CM, Cosgrove EF: Salicylate toxicity: the probable mechanism of its action. Ann Intern Med 24:638–642, 1946.
84. Mayersohn M: Aspirin (bioavailability monograph). J Am Pharm Assoc NS17:107–112, 1977.
85. Hollister LE: Measuring Measurin: problems of oral prolonged action medications. Clin Pharmacol Ther 13:1–5, 1972.
86. Hoon JR: Bleeding gastritis induced by long-term release aspirin. JAMA 229:841–842, 1974.
87. Gibaldi M. Grundhofer B: Bioavailability of aspirin from commercial suppositories. J Pharm Sci 64:1064–1066, 1975.
88. Miller RR, Jick H: Acute toxicity of aspirin in hospitalized medical patients. Am J Med Sci 227:271–279, 1977.
89. Levy M: Aspirin use in patients with major upper gastrointestinal bleeding and peptic-ulcer disease: a report from the Boston Collaborative Drug Surveillance Program. N Engl J Med 290:1158–1162, 1974.
90. Baskin WN, Ivey KJ, Krause WJ, et al: Aspirin-induced ultrastructural changes in human gastric mucosa: Correlation with potential difference. Ann Intern Med 85:299–303, 1976.
91. Metzger WH, McAdam L, Bluestone R, et al: Acute gastric mucosal injury during continuous or interrupted aspirin ingestion in humans. Am J Dig Dis 21:963–968, 1976.
92. Settipane GA, Chafee FH, Klein DE: Aspirin intolerance: II. Prospective study in an atopic and normal population. J Allergy Clin Immunol 53:200–204, 1974.
93. Anon: Analgesics and asthma. Br Med J 3:419–420, 1973.

94. Meyer OO, Howard B: Production of hypoprothrombinemia and hypocoagulability of the blood with salicylates. Proc Soc Exp Biol Med 53:234–237, 1943.
95. Shapiro S, Redish MH, Campbell HA: Studies on prothrombin: IV. The prothrombinopenic effect of salicylate in man. Proc Soc Exp Biol Med 53:251–254, 1943.
96. Quick AJ, Clesceri L: Influence of acetylsalicylic acid and salicylamide on the coagulation of blood. J Pharmacol Exp Ther 128:95–98, 1960.
97. Koch.Weser J, Sellers EM: Drug interactions with coumarin anticoagulants (second of two parts). N Engl J Med 285:547–558, 1971.
98. O'Reilly RA, Sahud MA, Aggeler PM: Impact of aspirin and chlorthalidone on the pharmacodynamics of oral anticoagulant drugs in man. Ann NY Acad Sci 79:173–186, 1971.
99. Udall JA: Drug interference with warfarin therapy. Clin Med 77:20–25, 1970.
100. New Zealand Rheumatism Association: Aspirin and the kidney. Br Med J 1:593–596, 1974.
101. Macklon AF, Craft AW, Thompson M, et al: Aspirin and analgesic nephropathy. Br Med J 1:597–600, 1974.
102. Burry HC: Reduced glomerular function in rheumatoid arthritis. Ann Rheum Dis 31:65–68, 1972.
103. Kimberly RP, Plotz PH: Aspirin-induced depression of renal function. N Engl J Med 296:418–424, 1977.
104. Zimmerman HJ: Aspirin-induced hepatic injury (editorial). Ann Intern Med 80:103–105, 1974.
105. Yu TF, Dayton PG, Gutman AB: Mutual suppression of the uricosuric effects of sulfinpyrazone and salicylate: a study on interactions between drugs. J Clin Invest 42:1330–1339, 1963.
106. Stowers JM, Constable LW, Hunter RB: A clinical and pharmacological comparison of chlorpropamide and other sulfonylureas. Ann NY Acad Sci 74:689–695, 1959.
107. Schulz E: (Severe hypoglycemic reactions after tolbutamide, carbutamide, and chlorpropamide). Arch Klin Med 214:135–162, 1968.
108. Goulston K, Cooke AR: Alcohol, aspirin, and gastrointestinal bleeding. Br Med J 4:664–665, 1968.
109. Loh HS, Watters K, Wilson CWM: The effects of aspirin on the metabolic availability of ascorbic acid in human beings. J Clin Pharmacol 13:480–486, 1973.
110. Jeremy R, Towson J: Interaction between aspirin and indomethacin in the treatment of rheumatoid arthritis. Med J Aust 2:127–129, 1970.
111. Liegler DG, Henderson ES, Hahn MA, et al: The effect of organic acids on renal clearance of methotrexate in man. Clin Pharmacol Ther 10:849–857, 1969.
112. Kampmann J, Hansen JM, Siersback.Nielsen K, et al: Effect of some drugs on penicillin half-life in blood. Clin Pharmacol Ther 13:516–519, 1972.
113. Tweeddale MG, Ogilvie RI: Antagonism of spironolactone-induced natriuresis by aspirin in man. N Engl J Med 289:198–200, 1973.
114. Brunk SF, Kuentzel WP, Delle M: Cholestyramine-salicylate interaction in man (abstract). Clin Res 19:648, 1971.
115. Segre EJ, Chaplin M, Forchielli E, et al: Naproxen-aspirin interactions in man. Clin Pharmacol Ther 15:374–379, 1974.
116. Bloomfield SS, Barden TP, Mitchell J: Aspirin and codeine in two postpartum pain models. Clin Pharmacol Ther 20:499–503, 1976.
117. Beaver WT, Feise G: Comparison of the analgesic effect of acetaminophen and codeine and their combination in patients with postoperative pain (abstract). Clin Pharmacol Ther 23:108, 1978.
118. Boyle RW, Solomonson CE, Petersen JR: Analgesic effect of dextropropoxyphene hydrochloride in elderly patients with chronic pain syndromes. Ann Intern Med 52:195–200, 1960.
119. Corgill DA, Ligon WCW, DeFelice EA: Double-blind comparison of namoxyrate, codeine, aspirin and placebo. Curr Ther Res 7:263–274, 1965.
120. Moertel CG, Ahmann DL, Taylor WF, et al: Aspirin and pancreatic cancer pain. Gastroenterology 60:552–553, 1971.
121. Lasagna L, Beecher HK: The analgesic effectiveness of codeine and meperidine (Demerol). J Pharmacol Exp Ther 112:306–311, 1954.
122. Cass LJ, Frederik WS, Bartholomay AF: Methods in evaluating ethoheptazine and ethoheptazine combined with aspirin. JAMA 166:1829–1833, 1958.

123. Wang RIH: A controlled clinical comparison of the analgesic efficacy of ethoheptazine, propoxyphene and placebo. Eur J Clin Pharmacol 7:183–185, 1974.
124. Winter L, Calman HI, Caruso WA, et al: A double-blind comparison of ethoheptazine citrate, propoxyphene hydrochloride, and placebo. Curr Ther Res 15:383–390, 1973.
125. DeKornfeld TJ, Lasagna L: Clinical trial of two analgesics: WIN 14,098 and ethoheptazine (abstract). Fed Proc 18:382, 1959.
126. Miller RR: Propoxyphene: a review. Am J Hosp Pharm 34:413–423, 1977.
127. McBay AJ, Hudson P: Propoxyphene overdose deaths (letter). JAMA 233:1257, 1975.
128. Bennett IF: Misuse of propoxyphene (letter). JAMA 235:1686, 1976.
129. Elson A, Domino EF: Dextropropoxyphene addiction: observations of a case. JAMA 183:482–485, 1963.
130. Wolfe RC, Reidenberg M, Vispo RH: Propoxyphene (Darvon) addiction and withdrawal syndrome. Ann Intern Med 70:773–776, 1969.
131. Klein NC, Magida MG: Propoxyphene (Darvon) hepatotoxicity. Dig Dis 16:467–469, 1971.
132. Daikos GK, Kosmidis JC: Propoxyphene jaundice. JAMA 232:835, 1975.
133. Currier RD, Westerberg MR: Evaluation of a salicylamide compound in the treatment of headache. University Michigan Med Bull 24:415–418, 1958.
134. Frey GH: The role of placebo response in clinical headache evaluations. Headache 1:31–38, 1961.
135. Marrs JW, Glas WW, Silvani J: Report of an investigation of D-propoxyphene hydrochloride. Am J Pharm 131:271–276, 1959.
136. Hopkinson JH III, Bartlett FH Jr, Steffens AO, et al: Acetaminophen versus propoxyphene hydrochloride for relief of pain in episiotomy patients. J Clin Pharmacol 13:251–263, 1973.
137. Bauer RO, Baptisti A Jr, Gruber CM Jr: Evaluation of propoxyphene napsylate compound in *post partum* uterine cramping. J Med 5:317–328, 1974.
138. Gruber CM Jr, Doss J, Baptisti A Jr, et al: The use of postpartum patients in evaluating analgesic drugs: the effectiveness of dextropropoxyphene, codeine, and meperidine when administered orally with acetylsalicylic acid compound and alone. Clin Pharmacol Ther 2:429–440, 1961.
139. Getter L, Levin MP, Ayer WA: Comparative effectiveness of some commonly prescribed drugs for the relief of post-surgical discomfort. Anesth Progress 20:137–140, 1973.
140. Eddy NB, Halbach H, Braenden OJ: Synthetic substances with morphine-like effect. Bull WHO 17:705–709, 1957.
141. Bloomquist ER: The addiction potential of oxycodone (Percodan). Calif Med 99:127–130, 1963.
142. Popkes DL, Folsom TC Jr: Comparative study of three analgesic agents used in oral surgical procedures. J Oral Surg 27:950–954, 1969.
143. Levin HM, Bare WM, Berry FN, et al: Acetaminophen with codeine for the relief of severe pain in postpartum patients. Curr Ther Res 14:921–927, 1974.
144. Cass LJ, Frederik WS: Experimental and statistical problems in the study of new drugs. Can Med Assoc J 83:831–836, 1960.
145. Brenman HS: Oral analgesics: preoperative vs postoperative use. J Am Dent Assoc 67:23–27, 1963.
146. Bruni JR, Holt RE: Controlled double-blind evaluation of three analgesic medications for postpartum discomfort. Obstet Gynecol 25:76–81, 1965.

29. NARCOTIC ANTAGONISTS

Russell R. Miller and Roger E. Dionne

Narcotic antagonists are principally used to counteract excessive respiratory depression in hospitalized recipients of narcotic analgesics. They are also used to treat acute overdosage stemming from illicit use of opiates and to diagnose possible narcotic dependence. Some experimental antagonists are being investigated for the long-term management of narcotic addicts.

Narcotic antagonists can be divided into three groups: (1) pure antagonists (naloxone), (2) partial antagonists (nalorphine and levallorphan), and (3) weak antagonists (pentazocine).

PHARMACOLOGY

Pure antagonists block the actions of narcotics but elicit no pharmacologic response of their own in either recipients or non-recipients of narcotics. Naloxone is the only pure antagonist marketed in the United States.

Partial antagonists, when given in usual doses to narcotic recipients, have predominantly antagonistic actions but exert some agonist (narcotic) effects. Because of this agonist-antagonist activity, partial antagonists reverse most of the effects of large doses of narcotics, but they only partially reverse the effects of usual analgesic doses and may actually potentiate the effects of small doses of narcotics.[1,2] When partial antagonists are given in usual therapeutic doses (5 to 10 mg of nalorphine) to patients who have not been pretreated with narcotics, they cause dose-dependent respiratory depression and other side effects comparable to those produced by narcotics.[3,4] When nalorphine is given in larger doses (10 to 15 mg), it provides analgesia equivalent to usual therapeutic doses of morphine.[4] However, nalorphine is not useful as an analgesic because of a high incidence of psychotomimetic and other side effects.[4–6] Levallorphan and naloxone, on the other hand, in doses capable of antagonizing narcotic-induced respiratory depression, have little or no analgesic activity.[1] Tolerance and dependence develop to the partial antagonists[7] and have been shown to be due to their agonist properties.

Weak antagonists are used clinically for their agonist properties. Pentazocine and butorphanol are the only weak antagonists currently available in the United States. For information on pentazocine see Chapter 27, Strong Analgesics.

INDICATIONS

Excessive Respiratory Depression in Hospitalized Narcotic Recipients

Narcotic antagonists are used to reverse the effects of narcotics (morphine, fentanyl, meperidine) when they are used with nitrous oxide for general anesthesia. Narcotic antagonists may also be used to reverse respiratory depression associated with the use of narcotic analgesics as preoperative medications. The respiratory depression that occasionally occurs in hospitalized narcotic recipients is most common in the elderly, debilitated, or those who have received other respiratory depressants. Patients should be titrated to a level of antagonism wherein respiratory depression is decreased but some analgesia is retained.

Acute Narcotic Overdosage

The degree of antagonism produced by a narcotic antagonist is dependent upon the specific narcotic involved, its total dose, the times of administration of narcotic and antagonist, and the degree of physical dependence and tolerance present. Profound respiratory depression, coma, and convulsions due to acute narcotic overdosage are life-threatening, and treatment with a narcotic antagonist is essential. The partial antagonists nalorphine and levallorphan are effective in severe narcotic poisoning but may not counteract mild respiratory depression and may even add to it. Naloxone is the drug of choice.

Narcotic Depression of the Newborn

Narcotic antagonists are used to reverse neonatal respiratory depression induced by narcotics given to the mother prior to or during labor.

Management of Narcotic Addiction

Narcotic antagonists may be useful in treating highly motivated narcotic addicts. Unfortunately, presently available antagonists are relatively ineffective when given orally. Futhermore, their short duration of action necessitates frequent dosage. Naloxone is the only currently available antagonist that has any application since nalorphine and levallorphan have too many agonist-type adverse effects. Naloxone is rapidly absorbed after oral administration but a large proportion of a dose appears to be metabolized on the first pass through the liver.[8] Naltrexone, a congener of naloxone, is currently under investigation. It is a pure antagonist and is several times more potent and more effective orally than naloxone; it also has a longer duration of action.[9,10]

PRECAUTIONS

Acute abstinence syndromes may be produced by administration of a narcotic antagonist to patients who are physically dependent to narcotics. The dose required to induce withdrawal symptoms is inversely proportional to the degree of physical dependence.[6] Therefore, the more severe the dependence the smaller the dose required to produce the abstinence syndrome. Usual subcutaneous doses of an antagonist may precipitate moderate to severe withdrawal symptoms. These begin with personality changes and generalized malaise and progress to rhinorrhea, tearing, sweating, goosepimples, yawning, chills, hyperpnea, hyperpyrexia, muscle hyperactivity, vomiting, and diarrhea.[6,9,11] Although these symptoms may be severe in strongly dependent addicts, they will last only as long as the antagonist is effective and are generally not felt to be medically dangerous.[11]

CHOICE OF A NARCOTIC ANTAGONIST

Naloxone is the drug of choice in most clinical situations where a reversal of narcotic action is desired. It has no agonist properties and can be used in treating coma and respiratory depression of unknown or mixed etiology without fear of adding to the depressant effects of non-narcotic drugs. Naloxone is the only agent available for reversing the agonist effects of pentazocine.[12,13]

TABLE 1 Preparations and Costs of Narcotic Antagonists

Generic Name	Trademark Name(s)	Preparations and 1978 Costs
Levallorphan Tartrate	Lorfan	Injection (solution) 1 mg/ml—$0.68/1-ml ampul, $3.45/10-ml vial
Nalorphine Hydrochloride	Nalline	Injection (solution) 5 mg/ml—$2.21/1-ml ampul, $3.95/2-ml ampul, $10.76/10-ml vial; 0.2 mg/ml—$1.64/1-ml ampul
Naloxone	Narcan	Injection (solution) 0.4 mg/ml—$2.49/1-ml ampul; 0.02 mg/ml—$2.16/2-ml ampul

DRUG MONOGRAPHS

NALOXONE (Narcan)

Naloxone is the narcotic antagonist of choice in most clinical applications. It is a pure antagonist and, as such, has no agonist properties (see introduction).[14] Unlike nalorphine and levallorphan, naloxone is effective in reversing both mild and severe narcotic-induced central nervous system depression, yet is incapable of worsening the depression of non-narcotic agents.

The mechanism of action of naloxone is thought to be a competitive antagonism of agonistic opiates at several receptors in the brain. In contrast, nalorphine and other partial antagonists block only one or two types of opiate receptors and act as agonists at others.[14]

Adverse Reactions—When naloxone is used to reverse the effects of large doses of narcotics administered for anesthesia, life-threatening adverse events may occur. Patients may suddenly awake with severe pain which causes activation of the sympathetic nervous system. This, in turn, may lead to hypertension,[15] acute pulmonary edema,[16] and ventricular arrhythmias.[17] Therefore, naloxone (or any other antagonist) should be given cautiously when it is used to reverse narcotic anesthesia.

Dosage—In using naloxone the goal is to achieve a distribution of the antagonist that is sufficient to displace the intoxicating narcotic from its attachment to narcotic receptors. The beneficial effects of naloxone will continue only if sufficient levels of the antagonist are maintained relative to the amount of narcotic present.[13,18,19] Since naloxone is metabolized more rapidly than most narcotics, naloxone concentrations may fall to subtherapeutic levels while narcotic concentrations remain at toxic levels. Thus, symptoms of narcotic depression may recur within minutes of a naloxone dose. The requirement for additional naloxone should be determined by continued monitoring of pulse, respiratory rate, mental status, and pupil size. Arterial pCO_2 may also be monitored, when indicated and available.

For acute narcotic overdosage, the usual initial adult dose of naloxone is 0.4 mg[13] or 5 μg/kg[20] intravenously. If no change in vital signs is observed within two to three minutes a second dose is given. If no change is noted after a third dose alternative treatment for non-narcotic depression is indicated. Relatively large doses may be needed to reverse the narcotic depression caused by pentazocine or nalorphine.

If physical dependence is suspected and the patient is not in imminent danger of respiratory failure or circulatory collapse, smaller doses (eg, 0.1 to 0.2 mg) may be given intravenously at 10-minute intervals until the desired degree of reversal is attained. The airway should be protected in case vomiting should occur.

The dosage of naloxone in postoperative patients depends on the degree of respiratory depression. Longnecker[18] has suggested using 15 μg/kg, one-third given initially by the intravenous route and two-thirds given intramuscularly 15 minutes later; this dosage satisfactorily antagonized 1.5 mg/kg of morphine for up to 6 hours. Johnstone et al[21] have reported that naloxone 40 μg/kg infused slowly over 10 hours (3.66 μg/kg loading dose given over 15 minutes followed by 3.66 μg/kg/hr given as a 50 ml solution by a constant-rate syringe pump) effectively antagonizes 2 mg/kg of morphine.

For prevention of neonatal respiratory depression, intramuscular naloxone in doses of 18 to 40 μg/kg of maternal weight prevents narcotic depression in both mother and infant when given 10 to 15 minutes prior to delivery.[22] Naloxone appears in the fetal blood as early as two minutes after intravenous injection into the mother, with a gradual rise over the next 10 to 30 minutes.[22] After delivery, naloxone may also be given to the infant. The preferred route of administration for infants is intramuscular injection.[23] In one study, a single 200 μg dose reversed all effects of meperidine (given to the mother during labor) for up to 48 hours. Intravenous administration of 40 μg reverses depression for only about 30 minutes.[23]

NALORPHINE HYDROCHLORIDE (Nalline Hydrochloride) LEVALLORPHAN TARTRATE (Lorfan)

Nalorphine and levallorphan are partial antagonists and reverse respiratory depression caused by large doses of narcotics. They have the potential for worsening the depression caused by non-narcotic agents or by low doses of narcotics. For example, nalorphine 10 mg does not antagonize the respiratory depression of morphine 10 mg and may even cause a mild additional sedative effect.[2] However, smaller doses of nalorphine are capable of antagonizing the respiratory depression caused by morphine 60 mg.[6] Neither agent is effective in reversing pentazocine overdosage.

Adverse Reactions—The partial antagonists have many of the actions of narcotics (agonists) and these will often become evident in patients who have overdosed with non-narcotic drugs or who have received usual therapeutic doses of narcotics.

Dosage—Intravenous: For treatment of respiratory depression, *adults,* 5 to 10 mg of nalorphine or 1 to 2 mg of levallorphan initially; *children,* 0.1 mg/kg of nalorphine or 0.02 mg/kg of levallorphan initially. The dose may be repeated at 10 to 15 minute intervals if necessary, but not more than three doses should be given; *neonates,* 0.2 mg of nalorphine or 0.05 to 0.1 mg of levallorphan is directly injected into the umbilical vein and repeated as necessary. Respiration should be supported by mechanical ventilation until the antagonist becomes effective. If available, oxygen should be administered.

REFERENCES

1. Foldes FF: The human pharmacology and clinical use of narcotic antagonists. Med Clin North Am 42:421–442, 1964.
2. Keats AS, Teleford J: Subjective effects of nalorphine in hospitalized patients. J Pharmacol Exp Ther 119:370–377, 1957.
3. Foldes FF, Duncalf D, Kuwabara S: The respiratory, circulatory, and narcotic antagonistic effects of nalorphine, levallorphan, and naloxone in anaesthetized subjects. Can Anaesth Soc J 16:151–160, 1969.
4. Lasagna L, Beecher HK: The analgesic effectiveness of nalorphine and nalorphine-morphine combinations in man. J Pharmacol Exp Ther 112:356–363, 1954.
5. Jasinski DR, Martin WR, Haertzen CA: The human pharmacology and abuse potential of N-allylnoroxymorphone (naloxone). J Pharmacol Exp Ther 157:420–425, 1967.
6. Wikler A, Hovelock FF, Isbell H: N-allylnormorphine: effects of single doses and

precipitation of acute 'abstinence syndromes' during addiction to morphine, methadone or heroin in man (post-addicts). J Pharmacol Exp Ther 109:8–20, 1953.
7. Martin WR, Gorodetzky CW: Demonstration of tolerance to and physical dependence on n-allylnormorphine (nalorphine). J Pharmacol Exp Ther 150:437–442, 1965.
8. Weinstein SH, Pfeffer M, Schor M, et al: Absorption and distribution of naloxone in rats after oral and intravenous administration. J Pharm Sci 62:1416–1419, 1973.
9. Tornabene VW: Narcotic withdrawal syndrome caused by naltrexone. Ann Intern Med 81:785–787, 1974.
10. Gritz ER, Shiffman SM, Jarvik ME, et al: Naltrexone: physiological and psychological effects of single doses. Clin Pharmacol Ther 19:773–776, 1976.
11. Blachly PH: Naloxone for diagnosis in methadone programs. JAMA 224:334–335, 1973.
12. Kallos T: Naloxone reversal of pentazocine-induced respiratory depression (letter). JAMA 204:932, 1965.
13. Evans LEJ, Roscoe P, Swainson CP, et al: Treatment of drug overdosage with naloxone, a specific narcotic antagonist. Lancet 1:452–455, 1973.
14. Martin WR: Naloxone. Ann Intern Med 85:765–768, 1976.
15. Tanaka GY: Hypertensive reactions to naloxone (letter). JAMA 228:25–26, 1974.
16. Flacke JW, Flacke WE, Williams GD: Acute pulmonary edema following naloxone reversal of high-dose morphine anesthesia. Anesthesiology 47:376–378, 1977.
17. Michaelis LL, Hickey PR, Clark TA, et al: Ventricular irritability associated with the use of naloxone hydrochloride. Ann Thorac Surg 18:608–614, 1974.
18. Longnecker DE, Grazis PA, Eggers GWN Jr: Naloxone for antagonism of morphine-induced respiratory depression. Anesth Analg 52:447–453, 1973.
19. Evans JM, Hogg MIJ, Lunn JN, et al: Degree and duration of reversal by naloxone of effects of morphine in conscious subjects. Br Med J 2:589–591, 1974.
20. Fischer CG, Cook DR: The respiratory and narcotic antagonistic effects of naloxone in infants. Anesth Analg 53:849–852, 1974.
21. Johnstone RE, Jobes DR, Kennell EM, et al: Reversal of morphine anesthesia with naloxone. Anesthesiology 41:361-367, 1974.
22. Clark RB, Beard AG, Greifenstein FE, et al: Naloxone in the parturient and her infant. South Med J 69:570–575, 1976.
23. Wiener PC, Hogg MIJ, Rosen M: Effects of naloxone on pethidine-induced neonatal depression. Part I—Intravenous naloxone. Part II—Intramuscular naloxone. Br Med J 2:228–231, 1977.

30. AGENTS USED TO TREAT MIGRAINE AND CLUSTER HEADACHE

John R. Hills and Richard T. Scheife

Although migraine and cluster headache are both vascular headaches and share some symptomatology, they are two distinct entities and should be managed differently. Some of the drugs that are useful in the treatment of migraine are also useful in cluster headache, but the appropriate use of these drugs in each condition differs.

MIGRAINE

Migraine is a type of vascular headache that usually begins as a unilateral dull ache in the supra-orbital, retro-orbital, or fronto-temporal areas. As the pain increases in intensity, it assumes a throbbing or pulsating character. The pain rises to a crescendo and tends to become more diffuse and constant. Often the pupils are dilated and the patient experiences nausea and vomiting for two or more hours; some patients have a diuresis. Most patients experience photophobia and prefer to lie in a quiet, dark room.[1,2] The headaches are of variable duration but not uncommonly continue for a full day.

In 'classic' migraine, which represents about 10% of the migrainous population, the headache is preceded by an 'aura' or prodrome of 5 to 40 minutes duration. Most commonly, the prodrome is visual and includes scintillating scotomata, often bordered by streaks of light. These effects most often occur in the visual field opposite the ensuing headache. The prodrome sometimes includes overt visual field deficits. Much less common prodromal symptoms are sensory changes such as numbness and tingling of the fingertips of one hand and of the lips. Transient aphasia or thickness of speech may also occur. Other prodromata include transient hemiparesis (hemiplegic migraine),[3] drop attacks, transient vertigo, dysarthria (basilar migraine), and transient bouts of severe abdominal pain (abdominal migraine).[4] Prodromal symptoms are usually consistent from attack to attack in a given patient. They usually develop to a maximum just prior to the onset of the headache and then characteristically recede.[5]

In 'common' or 'vulgar' migraine, which represents about 90% of migraineurs, the headache is not preceded by prodromata. It may be unilateral or generalized at onset and may or may not be accompanied by nausea and vomiting.

Other conditions such as temporal arteritis, cerebral arteriovenous malformation, aneurysm, and occipital neuralgia should be considered in the differential diagnosis.

The pathogenesis of migraine is not established. It is postulated that during the prodromal phase, serotonin is spontaneously released from platelets and histamine and proteolytic enzymes are released from mast cells.[6,7] The transiently high plasma levels of serotonin cause a profound vasoconstriction of intra- and extracranial vessels and a decrease in cerebral blood flow, which may give rise to prodromal symptoms.[8] Serotonin and histamine also increase capillary permeability, allowing transudation of the serotonin as well as plasma kinins into the vessel wall. As a result, the local pain threshold is lowered.[6,9] At this point, there is a rapid reuptake of serotonin by the platelets and the spleen, and the kidney rapidly excretes the excess serotonin. This produces a precipitous fall in plasma serotonin levels.[6,10] In an environment of relative serotonin depletion, the involved vessels dilate and passively distend, resulting in the classic pulsatile headache. The perception of this pain is augmented by the presence of serotonin and plasma kinins in the vessel walls.[6,9]

A second theory accepts all of the above mechanisms as participatory but not primary in the pathogenesis of migraine pain. This theory proposes that the primary flaw is a relative deficiency of central serotonin leading to a 'disinhibition' of central pain centers. This leads to a heightened sensitivity to afferent pain impulses and increased perception of pain.

Treatment

Drug therapy of migraine consists of symptomatic treatment of acute attacks and prophylactic therapy to reduce the frequency and severity of headaches. Treatment also involves careful consideration of precipitating factors, such as coffee, tea, and cola beverages, chocolate, cheese, alcohol, estrogens and progestogens (including oral contraceptives), and fasting.

Symptomatic Therapy of Acute Attacks. In mild migraine attacks, a mild analgesic (eg, aspirin, acetaminophen, Fiorinal) may provide symptomatic relief. For severe attacks ergotamine tartrate is the most effective drug. For most patients, oral administration is the preferred route, but administration by the parenteral, rectal, inhalation, or sublingual route may be indicated in some patients. Cafergot, a combination of ergotamine tartrate and caffeine, is better absorbed than ergotamine alone (Ergomar, Gynergen). The importance of early administration of adequate doses of ergotamine cannot be overstated.

Ergonovine is only mildly effective in migraine, but it has the advantage of better oral absorption and fewer gastrointestinal adverse effects. Dihydroergotamine mesylate (D.H.E. 45) has a less pronounced vasoconstrictor effect and fewer patients respond to it than to ergotamine; it has the further disadvantage of being available only for injection. Midrin, a combination of isometheptene mucate, dichloralphenazone, and acetaminophen, is less effective than ergotamine, but it may be useful when ergotamine is ineffective or causes intolerable adverse effects.

Recent evidence suggests that flufenamic acid, a potent inhibitor of prostaglandin activity and synthesis, may be effective in the symptomatic treatment of migraine.[11] Further clinical trials are needed to determine the role of this and related drugs.[12]

In addition to Cafergot and Midrin, a number of other combination products are available for the treatment of acute attacks (eg, Bellergal, Cafergot P-B, Migral, Wigraine). We are not convinced that these fixed combinations are better than Cafergot. Antianxiety agents (eg, diazepam [Valium]), and sedatives (eg, phenobarbital) may be useful in reducing apprehension and reaction to pain and in permitting sleep. Antiemetics may alleviate nausea and vomiting.

In migraine that is particularly resistant to therapy with other drugs, systemic adrenal corticosteroid therapy has occasionally been beneficial.

Prophylactic Therapy. Prophylactic therapy should be considered in patients with headaches occurring with intolerable frequency and in patients who cannot tolerate or who are unresponsive to symptomatic therapy. Amitriptyline (Elavil) and pizotyline (Pizotifen), an investigational drug in the United States, are the prophylactic drugs of choice. They are as effective as methysergide (Sansert) but have far fewer adverse effects and often can be discontinued without recurrence of migraine.

Methysergide is an effective prophylactic agent but frequently causes minor adverse effects and some life-threatening reactions.

Propranolol (Inderal) may be effective in preventing migraine attacks, but more controlled studies are needed to establish its efficacy. It prevents vasodilation of cerebral arteries by its beta-adrenergic blocking action, and this may be its mode of action in migraine.[13–15]

The monoamine oxidase inhibitors (phenelzine [Nardil], isocarboxazid [Marplan], and tranylcypromine [Parnate]) are effective prophylactic agents, but they have an unacceptably high frequency of serious adverse effects.

Clonidine (Catapres), an antihypertensive agent, was no more effective than placebo in controlled trials.[16,17] Similarly, bromocriptine is of little value in migraine.[18] Studies of cyproheptadine (Periactin) and reserpine[19,20] are conflicting. Metoclopramide has been shown effective[7,13,16] in some studies,[21,22] but further investigations are needed.

Ergotamine should not be used prophylactically, since continuous therapy may increase the frequency of migraine attacks.[23,24] Prophylactic use is also inadvisable because of ergotamine's ability to accumulate, its potent peripheral vasoconstrictive action, and because a certain form of dependence may occur, wherein the patient must take increasingly frequent doses to avoid 'rebound' headache.

CLUSTER HEADACHE

Of all the headache syndromes, cluster headache (histamine headache, histaminic cephalgia, Horton's headache, periodic migrainous neuralgia, Sluder's syndrome, sphenopalatine neuralgia) is probably the most distressing to the patient, the most spectacular to the observer, and the most difficult to treat.[25] Cluster headache differs from migraine in several respects. Attacks tend to occur in clusters with as many as four headaches a day. These 'clusters' often last several weeks and are characteristically followed by a headache-free period of weeks, months, or even years.[2,25–27] A headache episode typically begins as an intense, sometimes throbbing, rather sharply localized pain somewhere about the cheek or eye on one side. It increases in intensity more quickly than migraine, usually over three to five minutes, and usually lasts from 15 to 45 minutes. Unlike migraine, cluster headaches are often associated with numerous ipsilateral autonomic phenomena, such as nasal and conjunctival congestion, increased lacrimation, an increase in skin temperature, sweating, and Horner's syndrome. The latter may persist for weeks or months after the end of the cluster and, in some cases, may be permanent.[25,26]

The pain of cluster headache is characteristically intolerable and incapacitating. In contrast to the migraineur who often seeks a quiet, dark room to rest, the patient with cluster headache usually paces about restlessly. Epigastric discomfort frequently accompanies headaches, but vomiting is uncommon.[2,25,26] After a variable period of time, the headache subsides as rapidly as it began. Postictal fatigue or somnolence is rare and most patients resume their previous activities.[26] During periods of 'clustering,' patients will regularly report that headaches are induced by exogenous vasodilating substances (eg, alcohol, nitroglycerin).

Attacks usually occur regularly at about the same time each day and usually affect the same side of the head, unlike migraine.[25,26] The duration and intensity of the headache is remarkably constant from attack to attack, whether it be spontaneous or drug-induced.[26,27] Early morning attacks are common and often awake the patient; cluster headache is the only functional headache that commonly arouses patients from sleep.[26]

In contrast to migraine, cluster headache occurs predominantly in males,[27] has no prodromal symptoms, and usually occurs in persons who have no family history of vascular headaches.

Treatment

As with migraine, precipitating factors should be identified and then avoided where possible. While provocative stimuli vary from patient to patient, the most common ones are ethanol and nitroglycerin.[10,25,27] The value of symptomatic and preventive drug therapy is not well established.

Symptomatic Therapy of Acute Attack. Mild analgesics, narcotics, antianxiety agents, sedatives, and conventional antihistamines are of little or no benefit in cluster headache. Ergotamine may be beneficial if used properly. Since cluster headaches have no prodrome and are relatively brief, orally administered ergotamine is often of marginal value.[26] However, since headaches often occur at the same time each day, oral administration of ergotamine an hour before the anticipated time of the attack is often effective. Patients who experience nocturnal attacks may respond to a single 2 mg dose of ergotamine at bedtime.[26]

Ergotamine in rectal suppositories is slowly absorbed during the night and one or two used at bedtime may be effective for morning headaches. Alternatively, the administration of ergotamine by the parenteral or aerosol route at the onset of headache is usually beneficial.[26] Sublingual administration is occasionally helpful, although absorption by this route is poor.[28]

Prophylactic Therapy. In patients with closely spaced cluster headaches and in patients not responding to ergotamine, prophylactic management with methysergide (Sansert) may reduce the frequency and severity of headaches to a significant degree.[26] Amitriptyline, pizotyline, and propranolol have been advocated in the management of cluster headache,[2,26] but we are unaware of objective studies demonstrating their efficacy. Cyproheptadine (Periactin) has been shown to be effective in a few patients, but controlled studies have shown it to be of marginal value.[2,16]

DRUG MONOGRAPHS

AGENTS USED TO TREAT ACUTE ATTACKS OF MIGRAINE AND CLUSTER HEADACHE

ERGOTAMINE TARTRATE (Ergomar, Gynergen, Medihaler-Ergotamine)
ERGOTAMINE TARTRATE WITH CAFFEINE (Cafergot)

Ergotamine is the drug of choice in the symptomatic treatment of acute migraine attacks. Although gastrointestinal absorption is highly variable and usually incomplete, oral administration is the preferred route in most patients. Cafergot, a combination of ergotamine and caffeine, is more rapidly and more completely absorbed than ergotamine alone.[6,28] In patients who cannot tolerate the gastrointestinal side effects of ergotamine, rectal administration is often beneficial. Aerosol inhalation of ergotamine is effective, but nausea and vomiting are often pronounced and patients are more likely to take excessive doses by this route. In resistant or severe migraine, intramuscular or subcutaneous injection may be necessary. Selected patients should be instructed in self-administration of parenteral ergotamine. Sublingual administration of ergotamine is the least effective method of dosing;[28] patients who fail to respond to oral ergotamine will rarely benefit from sublingual administration.

Ergotamine should be given in sufficient dosage early in a migraine attack, since it is progressively less effective as the headache endures and is without effect once the headache is well established. When used properly, ergotamine provides symptomatic relief in 80 to 90% of migraineurs.[23,28]

The pharmacology of the ergot alkaloids is largely unknown. They have been shown to inhibit reuptake of serotonin by platelets, thereby preventing the precipitous fall in plasma serotonin levels that has been postulated to trigger migraine.[6] The ability of ergot alkaloids to maintain high levels of circulating norepinephrine by blocking its reuptake may also augment their vasoconstrictive action.

Contraindications—The ergot compounds are contraindicated in patients with hemiplegic migraine and in those whose prodrome involves prolonged visual impairment, paresthesias, or other neurological symptoms. Permanent hemiplegia, enduring hemianopsia, aphasia and other neurological deficits have been reported in such patients following treatment with ergot compounds. Rarely, fixed neurological deficits occur after the administration of ergotamine in the absence of contraindicating prodromata.

Because of their potent vasoconstrictive properties, the ergot compounds are contraindicated in patients with severe vascular disease (peripheral vascular disease, coronary artery disease, Raynaud's disease).[23,28–30] Their marked oxytocic activity limits their use during pregnancy.[23,28,29] The ergot compounds are relatively contraindicated in patients with active sepsis, impaired renal or hepatic function, thyrotoxicosis or significant hypertension.[23,28,29]

Adverse Reactions—Unpleasant but relatively mild side effects are commonly observed in patients receiving ergot preparations. Nausea, vomiting, polydypsia, abdominal cramps, stiffness and weakness of the legs, muscle pains in the extremities, and paresthesias of the fingers and toes are among the more commonly reported side effects. While transient paresthesias, abdominal pains, muscle pains, and cramps are common and do not contraindicate further use of ergotamine, persistent symptoms are a direct contraindication.[28,30]

Serious side effects are uncommon when ergotamine is used

properly but are nonetheless well documented.[28] They include gangrene of the extremities, angina, myocardial infarction, and profound peripheral vasospasm. It is important to note that such side effects have been observed in patients with no prior history of vascular disease.[28,30] A recent report suggests that severe ergot-induced ischemia can be reversed with sodium nitroprusside.[31]

Chronic ergotism is a particularly serious and often poorly recognized problem that may arise in patients who take excessive amounts of ergot preparations. These patients often complain of drowsiness, depression, anorexia, coldness of the extremities and, paradoxically, exacerbation of their headaches. 'Rebound' headache following withdrawal of the ergot compounds is a well known phenomenon.[16,24,28,32,33] Since rebound headaches are similar to migraine, patients often increase the dose of ergotamine. In cluster headache, patients often experience daily headaches, prompting them to take ergotamine on a daily basis for weeks at a time. Chronic ergotism can be minimized if patients are advised to limit the total dose of ergotamine to 10 mg per week,[28] and to omit one day of therapy each week.[26] In the patient who presents with signs and symptoms suggestive of chronic ergotism, all ergot preparations should be withheld and the patient should be warned of the possibility of rebound headache.[28]

Dosage in Migraine—Oral: Adults, 1 mg at onset of symptoms, repeated 30 to 60 minutes later if needed. If repeat doses were necessary, the patient should take 2 mg of ergotamine at the onset of the next attack, followed by 1 mg 30 and 60 minutes later if needed. This procedure is continued until the patient needs only one dose at the onset of the attack or until the initial dose reaches 5 mg.

Rectal: Adults, one Cafergot suppository (2 mg ergotamine tartrate and 100 mg caffeine) inserted at onset of symptoms and repeated at 45 and 90 minutes if needed. No more than 3 suppositories should be used for an attack.[2,28]

Inhalation: Adults, one application of Medihaler-Ergotamine (0.36 mg) at onset of symptoms, repeated at 5 to 10 minute intervals until the headache ceases or six applications have been given.[28]

Intramuscular, Subcutaneous: Adults, 0.5 mg at onset of attack, repeated in one hour if necessary.

Dosage in Cluster Headache—Oral: Adults, 1 or 2 mg an hour before the anticipated attack. Ergotamine is usually ineffective when taken orally at the onset of an attack.

Inhalation: Adults, one or two applications of Medihaler-Ergotamine (0.36 or 0.72 mg) at onset of symptoms.

Rectal: Adults, one or two Cafergot suppositories inserted at bedtime to prevent morning headaches.

ISOMETHEPTENE MUCATE, DICHLORALPHENAZONE, AND ACETAMINOPHEN (Midrin)

In those patients in whom ergotamine is ineffective or its side effects are intolerable, Midrin may be a useful alternative. Pharmacologically, isometheptene is an alpha and beta post-ganglionic adrenergic agonist. It appears to exert its cerebral vasoconstrictor effect without significant cardiovascular effects. Dichloralphenazone is a complex of chloral hydrate and phenazone. The efficacy of Midrin in the treatment of migraine has been shown to be due to the isometheptene.[34,35]

Although the patient response rate is less with Midrin than with ergotamine (50% versus 80–90%), Midrin has the advantage of low toxicity.[16,29,34,35] Dizziness, insomnia, nausea, vomiting, and transient 'numbness' are the most frequently reported side effects.[16,29]

Dosage in Migraine—Oral: Adults, two capsules at onset of symptoms, followed by one capsule every hour until relief is obtained. A maximum of 5 capsules should be taken in any 12 hour period.

AGENTS USED FOR PROPHYLACTIC TREATMENT OF CHRONIC MIGRAINE

AMITRIPTYLINE HYDROCHLORIDE (Elavil)
PIZOTYLINE HYDROGEN MALATE (Sandomigran)

Amitriptyline and pizotyline (pizotifen), a structurally similar compound, are as effective as methysergide as prophylactic agents.[6,16,33,36,40,44,45] In several well-designed studies, approximately 70% of patients treated with either amitriptyline or pizotyline reported a 50% decrease in the frequency, severity, and duration of migraine attacks.[33,36,44,45] Pizotyline, an investigational drug in the United States, appears to be as effective or perhaps more effective than amitriptyline in the prophylaxis of migraine. Amitriptyline is clearly more effective than the other tricyclic antidepressants currently available in the United States.

An important advantage of amitriptyline and pizotyline over

TABLE 1 Preparations and Costs of Agents Used to Treat Migraine and Cluster Headache

GENERIC NAME	TRADEMARK NAME(S)	PREPARATIONS AND 1978 COSTS
Ergotamine Tartrate	Gynergen	Tablets 1 mg—$13.50/100 Injection (solution) 0.5 mg/ml—$0.81/1-ml ampul
	Ergomar	Sublingual tablets 2 mg—$4.14/20
	Medihaler-Ergotamine	Inhalation (solution) 9 mg/ml—$6.90/2.5 ml
Ergotamine Tartrate with Caffeine	Cafergot	Tablets (ergotamine tartrate 1 mg and caffeine 100 mg)—$13.50/100 Suppository (ergotamine tartrate 2 mg and caffeine 100 mg)—$5.70/12
Isometheptene Mucate, Dichloralphenazone, and Acetaminophen	Midrin	Capsules (isometheptene mucate 65 mg, dichloralphenazone 100 mg, acetaminophen 325 mg)—$7.05/50
Methysergide Maleate	Sansert	Tablets 2 mg—$23.94/100
Amitriptyline Hydrochloride	Elavil	Tablets 10 mg—$5.27/100; 25 mg—$10.57/100; 50 mg—$18.79/100
Pizotyline Hydrogen Malate	Sandomigran	—[a]
Propranolol	Inderal	Tablets 10 mg—$4.10/100; 40 mg—$7.08/100; 80 mg—$11.32/100

[a]Not available in the United States.

methysergide is that after one or two headache-free months the drug can be discontinued and about half of the patients will not require further therapy.[33] Others will need periodic one to three month courses of therapy to maintain satisfactory control. In a few patients, almost continuous therapy is required.

Tricyclic antidepressants inhibit the reuptake of norepinephrine and serotonin centrally and peripherally.[36,40] They also possess marked antihistaminic and modest anticholinergic properties.[6,16,33,36,46] Unlike methysergide, the tricyclics do not interfere with the release of serotonin from platelets.[6] These agents are postulated to exert their prophylactic effect by repleting the deficient levels of central serotonin. It has been shown that the antimigraine properties of the tricyclic compounds are distinct from their antidepressant properties.[36,44]

Contraindications—Tricyclic antidepressants are contraindicated in patients with narrow angle glaucoma.[30]

Adverse Reactions—The most common adverse effects of amitriptyline are anticholinergic and include dry mouth, blurred vision, constipation, urinary retention, and tachycardia. Drowsiness is commonly observed during initiation of therapy but usually subsides after one to two weeks of therapy.[30,33,45] Pizotyline may stimulate appetite in some patients.[33,45] Its other adverse reactions are similar to those of amitriptyline.[16]

Drug Interactions—See Chapter 36, Antidepressants.

Dosage in Migraine—Oral: Adults, amitriptyline is initially given as 10 mg three times during the day and 20 mg at bedtime. After one to two months, if the headaches are not substantially improved, the dose may be increased to 25 mg four times a day. Despite the long half-life of amitriptyline, patients appear to have fewer adverse reactions and to have greater relief from migraine when smaller, divided doses are used rather than a single bedtime dose, as is often used in depression. Amitriptyline therapy is usually discontinued when the patient has been essentially headache-free for one to two months. It may be restarted again if migraine recurs.

Pizotyline therapy is usually initiated with 0.5 to 1 mg three times a day. The dose is increased over a period of weeks to an average maintenance dose of 1.5 to 3 mg three times a day.[16,33,45]

METHYSERGIDE MALEATE (Sansert)

Methysergide is a semisynthetic ergot derivative that is a congener of lysergic acid diethylamide (LSD). Treatment with methysergide is indicated only in patients with frequent, severe, and disabling migraine or cluster headaches; its potential for serious side effects precludes its routine use in less severe cases.[2,30,36] Methysergide is indicated for prophylactic treatment only and must be taken on a regular, daily basis. It is devoid of intrinsic vasoconstrictor properties and is of no benefit when administered intermittently or in the treatment of ongoing, acute attacks.[2,6,30] Methysergide has no place in the treatment of simple tension (muscle contraction) headache.[30] Approximately 70% of properly treated patients will have a significant decrease in the frequency and severity of migraine attacks.[6–8,36]

Methysergide appears to act as a central serotonin agonist, primarily at the brainstem raphé nuclei. Serotonergic stimulation results in an inhibition of these neurons and a correction of the 'central' hyperalgesia postulated in migraineurs.[37–39] The central serotonin agonist activity of methysergide is consistent with its similar prophylactic efficacy compared to other central serotonin agonists (eg, amitriptyline, pizotyline, 5-hydroxytryptophan, monoamine oxidase inhibitors).[6,32,33,37,38,40]

In contrast to its central effects methysergide is a potent peripheral antagonist of serotonin; it competitively blocks the serotonin receptors in blood vessels.[6,37] The primary result of this blockade is an inhibition of the increased vessel wall permeability characteristically induced by serotonin. This leads to a marked dimunition of the local, synergistic hyperalgesia induced by transudation of serotonin, prostaglandins, and plasma kinins into the substance of the vessel wall.[6,37] Methysergide also inhibits the release of histamine from mast cells and stabilizes platelets against spontaneous or induced release of serotonin.[6] The last phenomenon may be important as a precipitant of migraine attacks.[6,7]

Contraindications—Contraindications to methysergide therapy are similar to those for other ergot compounds. Methysergide should not be used in patients who are pregnant or patients with severe hypertension, severe coronary or peripheral vascular disease, or severe hepatic or renal impairment. Methysergide should be used with caution, if at all, in patients with a tendency toward thromboembolic disorders, active infections, or peptic ulcers.[30]

Adverse Reactions—Adverse reactions to methysergide often limit its use. Thirty to 50% of methysergide recipients experience one or more relatively minor side effects.[30,36] These include nausea, vomiting, leg cramps, abdominal discomfort, ataxia, paresthesias of the hands and feet, edema, weight gain, and, occasionally, hair loss.[2,6,30,36] Less common adverse effects include euphoria and hallucinations.[2,30] Other side effects associated with methysergide are uncommon but potentially life-threatening. These are fibrotic changes associated with long-term (greater than one year) uninterrupted therapy. Retroperitoneal fibrosis with ureteral obstruction and hydronephrosis and, less commonly, pleuropulmonary and cardiac fibrosis with dysphagia, chest pain, pleural effusions and the development of cardiac murmurs have been widely reported.[230,36,41–43] The fibrotic changes usually regress upon cessation of therapy but recur after rechallenge with methysergide.[2,30,41]

Myocardial infarction has been reported in patients on methysergide who were apparently free of prior cardiac disease.[30] Methysergide should be discontinued in patients who complain of unexplained flank pain, dysuria, angina, signs of phlebitis, venous obstruction, pleural friction rub or effusions, and in patients who exhibit an increase in erythrocyte sedimentation rate or serum creatinine.[30]

Dosage in Migraine and Cluster Headache—Oral: Adults, therapy is initiated with one tablet (2 mg) daily. One additional tablet is added every 3 to 4 days to a total of 3 to 4 tablets daily. The tablets should be taken in divided doses, preferably with meals.[1,2,5,30] Minor side effects (nausea, vomiting, ataxia, drowsiness) are commonly observed if the dose is increased too rapidly.[2] A therapeutic trial of at least 3 weeks is required before the patient's response to methysergide can be accurately assessed.[2,30]

Most authorities emphasize that methysergide should not be dosed continuously for longer than 6 months without a one month drug-free 'holiday.'[2,5,17] This approach appears to minimize the risk of irreversible fibrotic changes. Patients should have an annual intravenous pyelogram, a sensitive early indicator of retroperitoneal fibrosis.[2,30,41] When methysergide is discontinued, even temporarily, the dose should be slowly tapered over a period of 2 to 3 weeks to minimize the risk of severe, rebound headache.[30,33] In cluster headache, adequate drug-free periods are usually provided by withdrawing methysergide after each cluster.

PROPRANOLOL (Inderal)

Propranolol is more effective than placebo in preventing migraine, but more controlled studies are needed to establish its efficacy. It probably should be used only after amitriptyline or pizotyline have proven ineffective or caused intolerable adverse effects. Propranolol prevents vasodilation of cerebral arteries by its beta-adrenergic blocking activity, which probably accounts for its efficacy in migraine.[13–15]

Contraindications and Adverse Reactions—See Chapter 25, Antihypertensive Agents.

Dosage in Migraine—Oral: Adults, 10 mg daily initially, increased by 10 mg until a dose of 10 mg four times daily is reached. Further increases in dosage are unlikely to be beneficial if there is no response within two weeks of therapy with 10 mg four times daily. If the patient does respond, the dose may again be increased until maximal benefit is obtained or intolerable adverse effects occur. The highest doses used in most studies were 80 to 160 mg daily.[13,14] However, many patients were satisfactorily maintained on 10 mg four times daily.[15]

REFERENCES

1. Simard D, Paulson OB: Cerebral vasomotor paralysis during migraine attack. Arch Neurol 29:207–209, 1973.
2. Gilroy J, Meyer J: Headache, migraine, epilepsy, and syncope. In *Medical Neurology,* 2nd edition. New York, Macmillan, 1975, pp 302–311.
3. Hartwig H: Varieties of hemiplegic migraine. Headache 12:135–142, 1973.
4. Lundberg PO: Abdominal migraine—diagnosis and therapy. Headache 15:122–124, 1975.
5. Adams RD, Griffith JF: Migraine. In *Harrison's Principles of Internal Medicine,* 7th edition. Edited by MM Wintrobe, GW Thorn, RD Adams, et al. New York, McGraw-Hill, 1974, pp 1863–1870.
6. Fanchamps A: Pharmacodynamic principles of antimigraine therapy. Headache 15:79–90, 1975.
7. Anthony M, Lance JW: Monoamine oxidase inhibition in the treatment of migraine. Arch Neurol 21:263–268, 1969.
8. Skinhoj E: Hemodynamic studies within the brain during migraine. Arch Neurol 29:95–98, 1973.
9. Adams RD: Headache. In *Harrison's Principles of Internal Medicine,* 8th edition. Edited by GW Thorn, RD Adams, E Braunwald, et al. New York, McGraw-Hill, 1977, pp 22–25.
10. Anthony M, Lance JW: Histamine and serotonin in cluster headache. Arch Neurol 25:225–231, 1971.
11. Vardi Y, Rabey IM, Streifler M, et al: Migraine attacks. Alleviation by an inhibitor of prostaglandin synthesis and action. Neurology 26:447–450, 1976.
12. Bruyn GW: The biochemical basis of migraine: a critique. In *Clinical Neuropharmacology.* Edited by HL Klawans. New York, Raven Press, 1976, pp 185–213.
13. Diamond S, Medina JL: Double blind study of propranolol for migraine prophylaxis. Headache 16:24–27, 1976.
14. Wideroe TE, Vigander T: Propranolol in treatment of migraine. Br Med J 2:699–701, 1974.
15. Hedges TR: Isolated ophthalmic migraine: its frequency, mechanisms, and differential diagnosis. In *Neuro-Ophthalmology,* volume 6. Edited by JL Smith. St. Louis, C. V. Mosby Co., 1972, pp 140–150.
16. Diamond S, Baltes BJ, Levine HW: A review of the pharmacology of drugs used in the therapy of migraine. Headache 12:37–43, 1972.
17. Ryan RE, Diamond S, Ryan RE Jr: Double blind study of clonidine and placebo for the prophylactic treatment of migraine. Headache 15:202–206, 1975.
18. Hockaday JM, Peet KMS, Hockaday TDR: Bromocriptine in migraine. Headache 16:109–114, 1976.
19. Nattero G, Lisino F, Brandi G, et al: Reserpine for migraine prophylaxis. Headache 15:279–281, 1976.
20. Fog-Moller F, Bryndum B, Dalsgaard-Nielsen T, et al: Therapeutic effect of reserpine on migraine syndrome: relationship to blood amine levels. Headache 15:272–278, 1976.
21. Matts SGF: Metoclopramide in the treatment of migraine. Practitioner 212:887–890, 1974.
22. Pinder RM, Brogden RN, Sawyer PR, et al: Metoclopramide: a review of its pharmacological properties and clinical use. Drugs 12:81–131, 1976.

23. Brazeau P: Oxytocics. In *The Pharmacological Basis of Therapeutics,* 5th edition. Edited by LS Goodman, A Gilman. New York, Macmillan, 1975, pp 872–878.
24. Friedman AP: Migraine headache. JAMA 222:1399–1402, 1972.
25. Graham JR: Cluster headache. Headache 11:175–185, 1972.
26. Duvoisin RC: The cluster headache. JAMA 222:1403–1404, 1972.
27. Ekbom K: Clinical aspects of cluster headache. Headache 13:176–180, 1974.
28. Bradfield JM: A new look at the use of ergotamine. Drugs 12:449–453, 1976.
29. Diamond S, Medina JL: Isometheptene-A non-ergot drug in the treatment of migraine. Headache 15:211–213, 1975.
30. *American Hospital Formulary Service.* Edited by MJ Reilly. Washington, American Society of Hospital Pharmacists, 1977.
31. Carliner NH, Denune DP, Finch CS, et al: Sodium nitroprusside treatment of ergotamine-induced peripheral ischemia. JAMA 227:308–309, 1974.
32. Sicuteri F: The ingestion of serotonin precursors (l-5-hydroxytryptophan and l-tryptophan) improves migraine headache. Headache 13:19–22, 1973.
33. Schaer J: BC-105—a new serotonin antagonist in the treatment of migraine. Headache 10:67–73, 1970.
34. Ryan RE: A study of Midrin in the symptomatic relief of migraine headache. Headache 14:33–42, 1974.
35. Diamond S: Treatment of migraine with isometheptene, acetominophen, and dichloralphenazone combination: a double-blind crossover study. Headache 15:282–286, 1976.
36. Couch JR, Ziegler DK, Hassanein R: Amitriptyline in the prophylaxis of migraine. Neurology 26:121–127, 1976.
37. Appenzeller O: Pathogenesis of vascular headache of migrainous type: the role of impaired central inhibition. Headache 15:177–179, 1975.
38. Sicuteri F: Headache biochemistry and pharmacology. Arch Neurobiol 37:27–59, 1974.
39. Sicuteri F: Migraine, a central biochemical dysnociception. Headache 16:145–159, 1976.
40. Cooper JR, Bloom FE, Roth RH: *The Biochemical Basis of Neuropharmacology,* 2nd edition. New York, Oxford University Press, 1974, pp 175–201.
41. D'Arcy PF, Griffin JP: *Iatrogenic Disease.* London, Oxford University Press, 1972.
42. Graham JR, Suby HI, LeCompte PR, et al: Fibrotic disorders associated with methysergide therapy for headache. N Engl J Med 274:359–368, 1966.
43. Kunkel RS: Fibrotic syndromes with chronic use of methysergide. Headache 11:1–5, 1971.
44. Couch JR, Ziegler DK, Hassanein RS: Evaluation of amitriptyline in migraine prophylaxis. Trans Am Neurol Assoc 99:94–98, 1974.
45. Sjaastad O, Stensrud P: Appraisal of BC-105 in migraine prophylaxis. Acta Neurol Scand 45:594–600, 1969.
46. Ekbom K: Prophylactic treatment of cluster headache with a new serotonin antagonist, BC-105. Acta Neurol Scand 45:601–610, 1969.

31. AGENTS USED IN GOUT

Stephen E. Goldfinger

Unlike most forms of chronic, destructive arthritis, gout is now so readily treatable that complete remission is achievable in a great majority of cases, even when managed by the non-rheumatologist. This is true because a few potent, safe, and affordable drugs can be employed in a manner that has sound physiological rationale. Enlightened use of them requires an awareness of the intimate relationship between hyperuricemia, tophus formation, and acute gouty arthritis. This is rooted in the fact that the 'upper limit of normal' of the serum urate concentration, 7.0 mg/dl, approximates the limit of solubility of sodium urate in plasma at the physiologic pH of 7.4.[1] Thus hyperuricemia, present in 10% of adults, connotes the occurrence of biological fluid that is super-saturated with sodium urate. The tendency for excess urate to crystallize upon minor perturbations is characteristic of this metastable state. Tophi are deposited at various cartilaginous sites (eg, pinnae, tendon sheaths, articular surfaces). Acute gouty arthritis is likely a reflection of the same process, since microcrystals of sodium urate are almost always observed when joint fluid is examined.[2] These microcrystals probably incite an outpouring of the polymorphonuclear leukocytes that engulf them; the leukocytes are later destroyed by the disruptive effect of the crystals on their phagolysosomal membranes.[3,4] It is believed that the metabolic stimulation of the leukocytes produces a local decrease in pH, thus initiating a cycle in which further crystallization induces an amplified leukocytic response. The cause of the initial seeding of urate crystals—in joint fluid or elsewhere—remains a matter of speculation. Proposed explanations include trauma, cold, minor pH changes, a deficiency of plasma urate-binding protein,[5] and increased degradation of the proteoglycans that promote urate solubility in connective tissue.[6] Whatever the initiating mechanism(s), urate deposition can be *prevented* by reducing its serum concentration. The prolonged return to a subsaturation range will result in the dissolution of tophi and curtailment of gouty attacks.

Accordingly, agents used for gout fall into two categories. The first includes anti-inflammatory drugs that are given to prevent or control arthritis. These are usually prescribed for short duration and constitute the initial form of treatment, as arthritis is usually the signal for more definitive therapeutic intervention in gout. The second group of drugs are employed to reduce the serum urate concentration below 7 mg/dl. They are administered on a long-term basis to prevent urate deposition—the event common to tophus formation and arthritis.

TREATMENT OF GOUTY ARTHRITIS

Acute gouty arthritis is generally treated with either colchicine, phenylbutazone, or indomethacin. (Reports of the effectiveness of new non-steroidal anti-inflammatory agents in gout are favorable, but too preliminary to warrant their inclusion among conventionally accepted drugs.)[7]

Colchicine has been employed for gouty arthritis for centuries. Selectively accumulated in polymorphonuclear leukocytes,[8] it is thought to act by suppressing their response to sodium urate microcrystals. Malawista[9] proposes that colchicine's known action of blocking the aggregation of soluble tubulin to microtubules deprives the leukocyte of its cytoskeletal system. The latter is presumed to be necessary for margination, chemotaxis and the internal arrangement of subcellular organelles. Malawista considers colchicine to be a *weak*, general anti-inflammatory agent, one that is potent in the early phase of gout because it prevents leukocyte-mediated amplification of inflammation.[10] This formulation helps explain why colchicine is inconsistently beneficial when begun at the *peak* of a gouty attack, why it is of no value in other forms of arthritis, and why it has so little tendency to decrease host resistance to stronger stimuli of inflammation than crystals, such as pathogenic bacteria and immune complexes. Although Wallace[7] has reasoned from the potency of trimethylcolchicinic acid that colchicine's effectiveness in gout might not be due specifically to its binding to tubulin, it remains likely that the target site of colchicine is the polymorphonuclear leukocyte. An additional action on synoviocytes, which also ingest microcrystalline urate, may also occur.[11]

Unlike colchicine, phenylbutazone and indomethacin are effective in many inflammatory musculoskeletal disorders. Both are known to inhibit the biosynthesis of prostaglandins, which may play a role in initiating or perpetuating gouty arthritis.[12]

The choice between colchicine versus phenylbutazone or indomethacin in treating acute gout is related to their relative potency in the different stages of gouty inflammation. Phenylbutazone and indomethacin are more predictably effective when the attack is full-blown and for this reason, their use in this setting has largely replaced the ritual of hourly colchicine tablets taken to the point of gastrointestinal toxicity. On the other hand, colchicine is superior to indomethacin or phenylbutazone for prophylaxis. In persons predisposed to frequent gouty attacks, one colchicine tablet twice daily will often prove extremely useful, and will have fewer adverse effects than indomethacin or phenylbutazone taken chronically. Colchicine is frequently used in this manner to suppress attacks of 'paradoxical gout' that tend to occur during the first six months of hypouricemic therapy with allopurinol. The choice of drug for an *early* attack of gout is less clear; all three drugs are apt to be effective, and the decision is based on which one is best tolerated by the patient.

The same approach, in respect to phenylbutazone versus indomethacin, obtains for the treatment of the more sustained attack. Both drugs produce gastrointestinal side effects; indomethacin may cause headache, dizziness or even confusion in some patients, and phenylbutazone promotes fluid retention. Intravenous colchicine is indicated in postoperative gout when oral therapy is precluded. Corticosteroids are rarely needed to control gout and are used only in unusual circumstances. Supplementary analgesic drugs, such as propoxyphene, meperidine, and pentazocine, may be administered for pain control at the height of a gouty attack. Salicylates should be avoided, as they cause hyperuricemia at customary dosage.[13]

HYPOURICEMIC TREATMENT

Sustained reduction of serum urate to subsaturation concentrations (ie, less than 7.0 mg/dl) will result in tophus dissolution, freedom from gouty attacks and a greater chance for preservation of remaining renal function in kidneys that have already been damaged by tophaceous deposits. The value of treating asymptomatic hyperuricemia is uncertain. The rationale of such therapy would be to avert silent renal deterioration, but there are no properly randomized, long-term clinical studies to support this approach or to indicate the degree of hyperuricemia that warrants aggressive therapy. An exception to this general statement is the importance of allopurinol (along with hydration) to prevent urate nephropathy accompanying myelo- and lymphoproliferative diseases, especially when cytocidal doses of irradiation or chemotherapy are given.

There are two major pharmacological approaches to induce normouricemia. Uricosuric drugs (eg, probenecid, sulfinpyrazone) inhibit renal tubular transport of organic acids. As such, they block tubular reabsorption of urate, thus eliminating excess urate by increasing renal excretion. Allopurinol, on the other hand, reduces urate formation by inhibiting xanthine oxidase. Although allopurinol has achieved much recent popularity, uricosuric treatment remains a sound and effective method for achieving sustained normouricemia in many patients. Those most suitable for uricosuric therapy excrete normal or only slightly increased quantitites of uric acid, for they are less likely to develop uricolithiasis when tubular reabsorption is blocked. If urinary urate excretion is less than 600 mg per day on a low purine diet, uricosuric therapy is appropriate. At the initiation of therapy the hyperuricemic patient will excrete large amounts of urate, and the risk of uricolithiasis is greatest. For this reason, uricosuric treatment is begun with doses that are 1/4 to 1/3 of maintenance levels, with gradual advancement to full dosage over a two week period. Extra fluids and alkalinization of the urine also serve to reduce this risk. Uricosuric treatment may be unsuccessful in the presence of even mild azotemia, and should not be expected to work if the blood urea nitrogen exceeds 35 mg/100 ml.

XANTHINE OXIDASE INHIBITION

Allopurinol's initial promise as a safe and uniformly effective hypouricemic agent has been largely fulfilled during a decade of extensive use. In particular, important mutational or metabolic side effects have not been reported. By inhibiting the enzyme xanthine oxidase, allopurinol and its metabolite, oxpurinol, predictably retard the conversion of hypoxanthine and xanthine to uric acid.[14–16] Because these latter oxypurines have appreciably higher renal clearances than urate,[17] their serum levels remain well within solubility range. Several factors mitigate against crystalluria: (a) total purine excretion is divided among hypoxanthine, xanthine and uric acid—each of which has an independent solubility; (b) hypoxanthine, in particular, is very soluble[1]; (c) in patients who 'overproduce' urate, a net decrease in purine synthesis occurs, since xanthine and hypoxanthine are reincorporated into the nucleotide pool and thereby heighten feedback control of purine biosynthesis.[16]

Allopurinol therapy has been associated with xanthine crystalluria rarely, and only in circumstances of extraordinarily high oxypurines —the Lesch Nyhan syndrome[18] and during tumoricidal therapy.[19] The increasing popularity of allopurinol as the initial hypouricemic agent—even in patients who excrete normal or low amounts of uric acid—can be endorsed with caution, recognizing that long-range toxicity has not been totally excluded by experience to date. Specific indications that favor allopurinol include:

(a) known urate hyperexcretion or a history of uricolithiasis;
(b) azotemia;
(c) adverse reactions to uricosuric drugs.

Allopurinol can be used concomitantly with a uricosuric drug in patients with massive tophaceous deposits.

DRUG MONOGRAPHS

COLCHICINE

Colchicine is an effective agent for preventing gouty attacks in susceptible individuals and for ameliorating acute attacks of gout. In acute gout, its benefit is most predictable when instituted during the early phase of the attack. Colchicine has no effect on urate metabolism and is believed to act by inhibiting the role of polymorphonuclear leukocytes in perpetuating the attack. It may also be of diagnostic usefulness, inasmuch as other forms of arthritis are not relieved by colchicine.

Adverse Reactions—The most common adverse reaction is gastro-intestinal toxicity, manifested by diarrhea, nausea, and vomiting. Some persons will exhibit these symptoms at relatively modest doses, whereas others will be affected only at the high therapeutic range of repeated hourly doses for control of acute gout. Intravenously-administered colchicine improves the therapeutic ratio with respect to gastrointestinal disturbances.

Acute poisoning with colchicine produces marked gastrointestinal

TABLE 1 Preparations and Costs of Agents Used in Gout

GENERIC NAME	TRADEMARK NAME(S)	PREPARATIONS AND 1978 COSTS
Allopurinol	Zyloprim	Tablets 100 mg—$6.95/100; 300 mg—$18.50/100
Colchicine	generic	Tablets 0.5 mg—$2.54/100; 0.6 mg—$1.76/100
Indomethacin	Indocin	Capsules 25 mg—$11.77/100; 50 mg—$18.83/100
Phenylbutazone	Butazolidin (Azolid)	Tablets 100 mg—$9.33/100
Probenecid	Benemid generic	Tablets 500 mg—$7.96/100 Tablets 500 mg—$5.62/100
Sulfinpyrazone	Anturane	Capsules 200 mg—$12.16/100 Tablets 100 mg—$7.52/100

symptoms, with fluid loss sufficient to cause dehydration and shock. Nephrotoxicity, ascending paralysis, and delirium may also occur. Chronic overdosage may result in marrow suppression, hair loss, myopathy, and oligospermia.

Dosage—Oral: Adults, one tablet (0.5 or 0.6 mg) administered one to three times daily is used as prophylactic therapy. Recommended treatment for acute attacks is one tablet hourly until (1) substantial improvement occurs, (2) gastrointestinal symptoms are produced, or (3) a total of ten tablets have been used. Once inflammation subsides, a maintenance dose of one tablet three times daily is employed for the next 48 hours.

Intravenous: Adults, 2 mg of parenteral colchicine is diluted with saline to 20 ml and injected slowly, with special attention to avoid extravastion. This may be repeated, if necessary, 12 hours later. Intravenous administration is generally reserved for the treatment of acute gout.

INDOMETHACIN (Indocin)

See Chapter 32 for general information. For acute gout, indomethacin is given orally, 50 mg three times daily until symptoms subside. Because it competes with probenecid for the same mechanism of renal tubular secretion, inordinately high serum levels of indomethacin may occur in patients who are receiving probenecid.[20] Accordingly, a lower dose of indomethacin should be prescribed.

PHENYLBUTAZONE (Butazolidin)

See Chapter 32 for general information. For acute gout, phenylbutazone is given orally in a dose of 200 mg three to four times daily for two days; it may be given at half this dosage for the next several days if needed. Phenylbutazone has a mild uricosuric effect, but it is not definitive treatment for hyperuricemia.

ALLOPURINOL (Zyloprim)

Allopurinol is a highly effective hypouricemic agent. While useful in all patients with gout, it is of particular benefit for those who 'overproduce' uric acid, have renal insufficiency, or cannot use uricosuric drugs because of adverse reactions.

Adverse Reactions—Allopurinol is usually well tolerated; a minority of patients experience mild side effects (eg, drowsiness, gastrointestinal upset) that rarely require cessation of therapy. Permanent withdrawal of treatment is usually necessary for hypersensitivity reactions, which occur in less than 5% of patients. Such reactions include rash (most common), eosinophilia, fever, and, rarely, marrow suppression.

Interactions—Allopurinol inhibits xanthine oxidase, the enzyme which also mediates the inactivation of mercaptopurine, azathioprine and 6-thioguanine.[14,21,22] This interaction is of clinical significance. To avoid enhanced effects (and toxicity) from these antineoplastic drugs, they should be administered at 1/4 to 1/3 of customary dosage in patients concurrently receiving allopurinol.

Dosage—Oral: Adults, allopurinol is generally effective as a dose of 300 mg daily, in either divided dosage (100 mg three times daily) or a single 300 mg tablet taken once daily. Twice this amount is recommended for patients with marked hyperuricemia and large tophi; normouricemia will not be achieved until tophus dissolution occurs. Monitoring serum urate levels to check the effectiveness of treatment is recommended for allopurinol as well as probenecid therapy.

PROBENECID (Benemid)

Probenecid is a general inhibitor of renal tubular transport of organic acids. Normally, a high percentage of filtered and secreted uric acid is reabsorbed by the tubule. At customary dosage, probenecid's action of blocking urate reabsorption is of greater physiological consequence than its suppressant effect upon urate secretion, and uricosuria ensues.

The use of probenecid and colchicine in tablet combination (ColBenemid) should be avoided in the treatment of an initial attack of gout, since acute lowering of the uric acid level may perpetuate the attack. The rationale for long-term therapy with ColBenemid is questionable. Not only does it obligate the use of colchicine, which may produce diarrhea in the therapeutic range, but sustained normouricemia should minimize the need for colchicine by preventing further episodes of acute gouty attacks.

Adverse Reactions—Probenecid is a relatively safe drug. Adverse reactions other than uricolithiasis (see introduction) are generally limited to dyspepsia and rash—neither of which tend to be frequent or severe.

Interactions—Probenecid blocks the renal excretion of the penicillins and cephalosporins,[23] sulfonamides,[24] aminosalicyclic acid,[25] indomethacin[20] and nitrofurantoin[25] resulting in higher blood levels of these drugs. Decreased excretion of nitrofurantoin may diminish its effectiveness as an antibacterial agent for urinary tract infections. Caution is warranted when probenecid is given to achieve higher serum penicillin levels, since the cause of a subsequent drug rash will be difficult to interpret. Increased dosage of penicillin is generally preferred. Concurrent low-dose salicylate administration blocks probenecid inhibition of tubular reabsorption of uric acid, with consequent impairment of uricosuria.[14]

Dosage—Therapy is begun with one-half tablet (250 mg) once or twice daily and a recommended fluid intake of three liters/day to avoid uricolithiasis. The dose is advanced during the first two weeks to the maintenance level that is required to achieve sustained normouricemia. This will usually be one tablet (500 mg) two to four times daily.

SULFINPYRAZONE (Anturane)

Sulfinpyrazone, like probenecid, inhibits renal tubular reabsorption of uric acid.

Adverse Reactions—These are similar to probenecid—dyspepsia, rash and uricolithiasis. Structurally related to phenylbutazone, sulfinpyrazone may produce symptoms in patients predisposed to dyspepsia; it has not been reported to cause blood dyscrasias.

Interactions—Similar to probenecid.

Dosage—Initially, 100 mg is administered twice daily to achieve gradual reduction of the serum urate level. Maintenance therapy is usually 400 to 500 mg/day, divided into two doses.

REFERENCES

1. Klinenberg JR, Goldfinger SE, Seegmiller JE: The effectiveness of xanthine oxidase inhibitor allopurinol in the treatment of gout. Ann Intern Med 62:639–647, 1965.
2. McCarty DJ, Hollander JL: Identification of urate crystals in gouty synovial fluid. Ann Intern Med 54:452–470, 1961.
3. Seegmiller JE, Howell RR: The old and new concepts of acute gouty arthritis. Arthritis Rheum 5:616–623, 1962.
4. Schumacher HR, Phelps P: Sequential changes in human polymorphonuclear leukocytes after urate crystal phagocytosis: electron microscopic study. Arthritis Rheum 14:513–526, 1971.
5. Alvasker JO: Uric acid in human plasma. V. Isolation and identification of plasma proteins interacting with urate. Scan J Clin Lab Invest 18:227–239, 1966.
6. Katz WA: Deposition of urate crystals in gout: altered connective tissue metabolism. Arthritis Rheum 18:751–756, 1975.
7. Wallace SL: Colchicine and new anti-inflammatory drugs for the treatment of acute gout. Arthritis Rheum 18:847–851, 1975.
8. Creasey WA, Bensch KG, Malawista SE: Colchicine, vinblastine and griseofulvin: pharmacological studies with human leukocytes. Biochem Pharmacol 20:1579–1588, 1971.
9. Malawista SE, Bensch KG: Human polymorphonuclear leukocytes: demonstration of microtubules and effect of colchicine. Science 156:521–522, 1967.
10. Malawista SE: The action of colchicine in acute gouty arthritis. Arthritis Rheum 18:835–846, 1975.
11. Aguledo CA, Schumacher HR, Phelps P: Sequence of synovial changes in urate crystal-induced arthritis in the dog. Arthritis Rheum 15:100, 1972.
12. Kellermeyer RW, Naff GB: Chemical mediators of inflammation in acute gouty arthritis. Arthritis Rheum 18:765–770, 1975.
13. Yu TF, Gutman AB: A study of the paradoxical effects of salicylate in low, intermediate and high dosage on the renal mechanisms for excretion of urate in man. J Clin Invest 38:1298–1315, 1959.
14. Rundles RW, Wyngaarden JB, Hitchings GH, et al: Effects of a xanthine oxidase inhibitor on thiopurine metabolism, hyperuricemia and gout. Trans Assoc Am Physicians 76:126–140, 1963.
15. Yu TF, Gutman AB: Effect of allopurinol (4-hydroxpyracole [3,4,-d] pyrimidine) on serum and urinary uric acid in primary gout. Am J Med 37:885–898, 1964.
16. Hitchings GH: Pharmacology of allopurinol. Arthritis Rheum 18:863–870, 1975.
17. Goldfinger S, Klinenberg JR, Seegmiller JE: The renal excretion of oxpurines. J Clin Invest 44:623–628, 1965.
18. Greene ML, Fujimoto WY, Seegmiller JE: Urinary xanthine stones—a rare complication of allopurinol therapy. N Engl J Med 280:426–427, 1969.
19. Band PR, Silverberg DS, Henderson JF, et al: Xanthine nephropathy in a patient with lymphosarcoma treated with allopurinol. N Engl J Med 283:354–357, 1970.
20. Skeith MD, Simkin PA, Healey LA: The renal excretion of indomethacin and its inhibition of probenecid. Clin Pharmacol Ther 9:89–93, 1968.
21. Elion GB, Beeber S, Hitchings GH: The fate of 6-mercaptopurine in mice. Ann NY Acad Sci 60:297–303, 1954.

22. Elion GB, Callahan S, Rundles RW, et al: Relationship between metabolic fates and antitumor activities of thiopurines. Cancer Res 23:1207–1217, 1963.
23. Kaplan K, Reisberg BE, Weinstein L: Cephaloridine: antimicrobial activity and pharmacological behavior. Am J Med Sci 253:667–674, 1967.
24. Weiner IM, Washington JA, Mudge GH: On the mechanism of action of probenecid on renal tubular secretion. Bull Johns Hopkins Hosp 106:333–346, 1960.
25. Weiner IM, Mudge GH: Renal tubular mechanism for excretion of organic acids and bases. Am J Med 36:743–762, 1964.

32. ANTIRHEUMATIC AGENTS

Ronald P. Evens

The rheumatic diseases are a group of polyarthritic disorders of unknown etiology. They include rheumatoid arthritis, juvenile rheumatoid arthritis, ankylosing spondylitis, psoriatic arthritis, and Reiter's syndrome. Gouty arthritis is generally considered separately since the immediate cause of the disease (hyperuricemia) is known and can be controlled with appropriate drug therapy (see Chapter 31, Agents Used in Gout).

GENERAL THERAPEUTIC PRINCIPLES

The basic pathophysiologic process in rheumatic diseases is chronic joint inflammation,[1–5] leading to joint damage, destruction of adjacent cartilage and bone, and eventually, joint deformities.[2,6] Prostaglandins are mediators that amplify the inflammatory process. Disease activity can be assessed by the degree of inflammation, the severity and duration of pain, appearance of nocturnal pain, and the degree of morning stiffness. Rheumatic disorders are chronic and episodic with spontaneous exacerbations and remissions and are progressive with or without therapy. Treatment with drugs and other measures should be individualized and adjusted as the disease changes. Physiotherapeutic, surgical, orthopedic, and psychiatric therapy may be of equal or greater importance than drug therapy, depending on the individual patient.

Goals of drug therapy include pain relief, reduction of inflammation, and preservation of functional capacity of joints and adjoining muscles; however, complete resolution of the pathologic process ('cure') is not a reasonable goal. Optimal disease control requires individualization of therapy based on several pharmacotherapeutic principles:[1,3,5]

1. Placebo response is of considerable importance. Over a 2-year period, oral or parenteral placebo produced a satisfactory response in more than 50% of patients in one study.[4]

2. Prior to selection of new treatments, a drug history should be taken to determine response to previous antirheumatic drug therapy.

3. Oral antirheumatic drugs should be prescribed singly at first and assessed in a serial manner in each patient until the optimal drug and dosage is found.

4. Response to antirheumatic drugs is highly variable. Some patients have the same response to different drugs, whereas others respond differently to different drugs within the same class of compounds.

5. A single drug should be continued until sufficient time has elapsed to permit a full pharmacologic response. For example, aspirin or phenylproprionic acid derivatives should be given for one to two weeks, and penicillamine should be given for four to six months.

6. If treatment failure occurs, the drug dose, frequency of administration, and patient compliance should be considered before another drug is prescribed.

7. When treatment is successful, dosage should be reduced to maintenance levels, and, if possible, the drug should be discontinued during disease remissions.

The less toxic agents should be used in the early disease stages, with the more toxic agents subsequently added as prior drug therapy becomes less effective and the disease progresses (Table 1).[1,3,5] The first step frequently involves simple analgesic therapy. Low doses of aspirin (eg, 2 to 3 g/day) or acetaminophen may be used. Alternatively, other salicylates, phenylpropionic acid derivatives (fenoprofen, ibuprofen, naproxen) or propoxyphene may be used.[2,7] Also, a proper balance of rest and exercise should maximize mobility and control joint trauma in early stages.

As the disease progresses, larger doses of aspirin (3.6 to 6.0 g/day) should be used to reduce inflammation in the few involved joints—usually phalangeal and carpal joints in the hands, wrists, feet, and ankles (Table 1). Aspirin remains the drug of choice since no other nonsteroidal anti-inflammatory agent is more effective or less expensive.[8] However, many patients cannot tolerate large doses of aspirin for long periods. Before prescribing a non-salicylate drug, other forms of salicylate should be evaluated. Enteric-coated aspirin or sodium salicylate tablets and aspirin suppositories are erratically absorbed but may be useful. Similarly, choline salicylate (Arthropan), choline magnesium trisalicylate (Trilisate), or salsalate (Disalcid) may be beneficial. Because they have less gastrointestinal toxicity than aspirin, phenylpropionic acid derviatives are being promoted as first choice agents.[5] However, they probably should be used only after salicylates have failed or proved too toxic. If either of these drug categories proves inadequate or too toxic, tolmetin or sulindac (indole drugs chemically related to indomethacin) can be tried.

When control of inflammation is not achieved with a nonsteroidal drug and arthritis is moderate to severe, parenteral therapy with a gold compound or penicillamine is usually indicated (Table 1). These drugs are usually added to a nonsteroidal agent and can slow or arrest the pathogenic process. However, up to six months of therapy are required before full beneficial effects become evident, and these drugs have major dermatologic, renal, and hematologic adverse effects in many patients.

Step four includes indomethacin or phenylbutazone and the antimalarials (Table 1). Because of their toxicity, antimalarial drugs are usually used only after indomethacin or phenylbutazone have proven inadequate. Like gold compounds and penicillamine, antimalarials slow the progression of rheumatic disease.

Step five includes corticosteroids or immunosuppressive agents (Table 1). These drugs are reserved for patients who are unsuccessfully controlled by other drugs or who have major side effects. In patients with asymmetric, single joint inflammation that has significantly compromised mobility, intraarticular steroids are given prior to systemic steroid therapy.

ASSESSMENT OF THE DISEASE PROCESS AND RESPONSE TO THERAPY

Diagnostic criteria of the American Rheumatism Association allow assessment of the degree of response to treatment.[9,10] Common subjective parameters include joint pain, tenderness, swelling, and stiffness; these are tabulated singly or together in an articular index of active joints (eg, 'Lansbury articular index'). Each symptom is evaluated with a rating scale to quantitate improvement in the disease. Other subjective measures are the duration of morning stiffness, patient or observer preference of a particular therapy, ancillary analgesic intake, and ring size (joint size). Functional capacity is quantitated by evaluating the grip strength, time required to walk 50 feet, time to onset of fatigue, time to climb a specific number of stairs, and range of joint movement with flexion and extension. Bone and

TABLE 1 Steps in the Drug Treatment of Rheumatic Disease

Step 1	Analgesia with aspirin (2–3 g/day) or acetaminophen Alternative drugs: phenylpropionic acid derivatives or propoxyphene
Step 2	Salicylates, phenylpropionic acid derivatives, tolmetin, or sulindac
Step 3	Gold compounds or penicillamine
Step 4	Indomethacin or phenylbutazone Alternative drugs: antimalarials
Step 5	Adrenal corticosteroids or immunosuppressives

joint fluid changes are assessed by x-rays, radioactive isotope uptake in joints, synovial effusions, and histologic exam of synovial specimens. Immunologic disease activity is measured by erythrocyte sedimentation rate (ESR), serum rheumatoid factors, antinuclear antibodies, and cryoglobulins.

DRUG MONOGRAPHS

SALICYLATES

ASPIRIN
SODIUM SALICYLATE
CHOLINE SALICYLATE (Arthropan)
CHOLINE MAGNESIUM TRISALICYLATE (Trilisate)
SALSALATE (Disalcid)

Aspirin has been the drug of choice for rheumatoid arthritis for over 30 years.[11–14] Pain, swelling, mobility of joints, morning stiffness, and analgesic intake are routinely improved. The mechanism of action of all nonsteroidal anti-inflammatory agents like aspirin is inhibition of prostaglandin synthesis, which interrupts amplification of the inflammatory process.[2,6] About one-half of patients with mild to moderate disease will be controlled by aspirin alone.[15] Although there is not a direct relationship between therapeutic response and blood levels, a salicylate concentration of 20 to 30 mg/100 ml is generally considered the therapeutic range for anti-inflammatory action.[14–16] Once an effective daily dose is found, the frequency of administration can range from every four to eight hours with acceptably small interdose blood level fluctuation. Steady-state serum levels are achieved within about one week with chronic dosing. When a 650 mg dose is given every four hours during waking hours with a 1.3 g bedtime dose, adequate blood levels are maintained throughout the 24 hour period.[17] The pharmacokinetic properties, formulations, and adverse effects of aspirin are discussed in Chapter 28 (Mild Analgesics) and other sources.[13–16,18–22]

Sodium salicylate is as effective as indomethacin.[23] It is more rapidly absorbed than aspirin but contains substantial amounts of sodium; a 5 g daily dose provides about 31 mEq of sodium.

Choline salicylate is marketed as a solution containing 870 mg of choline salicylate, equivalent to 500 mg of salicylate, per 5 ml. This is about the same salicylate content as 650 mg of aspirin. Absorption of choline salicylate is rapid because the drug is already in solution and tablet dissolution is not necessary. Thus, choline salicylate solution provides peak salicylate blood levels more rapidly than aspirin tablets.[24–27] Since the overall bioavailability of choline salicylate and aspirin are probably similar, these differences are unimportant during chronic therapy.

Published clinical trials of choline salicylate[27–31] are limited because of many methodologic inadequacies. Therefore, the efficacy and toxicity of choline salicylate and aspirin are only empirically equated. Since choline salicylate is marketed as a solution, gastrointestinal side effects probably occur less often, but bad taste limits its usefulness.

Choline magnesium trisalicylate contains 500 mg of salicylate per tablet in the form of choline salicylate (293 mg) and magnesium salicylate (362 mg). The salicylate content is equal to that of 650 mg of aspirin. As with aspirin, the half-life of Trilisate is dose-dependent; eg, when given in a dose of 1 g twice daily the half-life is 7.6 hours; when given as 1.5 g twice daily the half-life is 18.3 hours.[32] Similar serum levels of salicylate are produced by aspirin and Trilisate.[33] In terms of duration of morning stiffness and joint involvement, Trilisate and aspirin have been shown equally effective.[34]

The adverse effects of Trilisate are similar in scope to those of aspirin but may occur less often.[34] In one study the most common reactions to Trilisate were tinnitus (5.3%) and gastrointestinal distress, nausea and pain (6%). Headache and hearing loss were also reported. Gastrointestinal blood loss was not significant with Trilisate, 1.5 g twice daily (0.9 ml/day) but was significant with aspirin, 1 g three times a day (5.1 ml/day).[35]

Salsalate, or salicylsalicylic acid, has anti-inflammatory properties similar to those of aspirin.[36] It is hydrolyzed in vivo to salicylic acid more slowly than aspirin[37] and has a half-life of about eight hours.[38] The rate of absorption is slower than that of aspirin or sodium salicylate. Steady-state salicylate blood levels after ingestion of salsalate or aspirin are about equivalent—13.5 mg/100 ml at 3 g/day, and 12.9 mg/100 ml at 3.6 g/day, respectively.[39]

Although published clinical trials on salsalate are few, it is evident that salsalate exhibits anti-inflammatory and analgesic activity in rheumatoid and musculoskeletal disorders. In a comparison with indomethacin, salsalate provided comparable relief of joint pain and inflammation in patients with rheumatoid arthritis.[40] In another study, salsalate was slightly superior or equal to aspirin for relief of symptoms of osteoarthritis, especially pain.[39] An open trial showed 73% improvement in joint pain in 66 patients with musculoskeletal-joint disease.[41] Dosage is usually 3 g/day in three divided doses; this provides salicylate equivalent to 3.6 g of aspirin.

The adverse effects of salsalate are comparable in scope to those of other salicylates. Precise frequency rates cannot be calculated due to the very few clinical trials, but they appear to be less than or equal to aspirin.[39–41] Gastric erosion and hyperemia are unusual with salsalate ingestion, in contrast to their common occurrence with aspirin.[42] Also, blood loss, based on analysis of radioactive tagged red blood cells in feces,[43] and occult blood loss[44] were similarly insignificant for salsalate and placebo but common with aspirin.

PHENYLPROPIONIC ACID DERIVATIVES

FENOPROFEN (Nalfon)
IBUPROFEN (Motrin)
NAPROXEN (Naprosyn)

Pharmacokinetic Properties—In usual doses, fenoprofen,[5,45,46] ibuprofen,[5,47–49] and naproxen[15,50,51] are well absorbed (over 80%), rapidly achieve steady-state blood levels, and are highly protein bound (95–99%). All three drugs are biotransformed in the liver, and the metabolites are excreted in the urine. However, their half-lives differ significantly, fenoprofen—2.5–3 hours, ibuprofen—1.9–2 hours, naproxen—14 hours.

The relation between dose and blood levels for naproxen is linear

TABLE 2 Preparations and Costs of Antirheumatic Agents

Generic Name	Trademark Name(s)	Preparations and 1978 Costs
Salicylates		
Aspirin	generic	Tablets 325 mg—$0.18–$4.00/100
Sodium Salicylate	generic	Tablets 325 mg—$4.50–$17.00/1,000; 650 mg—$15.63–$18.00/1,000 Tablets (enteric-coated) 325 mg—$0.75–$1.20/100; 650 mg—$0.99–2.00/100
Choline Salicylate	Arthropan	Liquid 870 mg/5 ml—$3.78/8 oz, $6.24/pint
Magnesium Salicylate	Magan	Tablets 650 mg—$6.56/100
Choline Magnesium Trisalicylate	Trilisate	Tablets (500 mg salicylate)—$10.00/100
Salsalate	Disalcid	Tablets 500 mg—$6.60/100
Phenylpropionic Acid Derivatives		
Fenoprofen Calcium	Nalfon	Capsules 300 mg—$8.61/100
Ibuprofen	Motrin	Tablets 300 mg—$6.61/60; 400 mg—$7.93/60
Naproxen	Naprosyn	Tablets 250 mg—$20.15/100
Indole Derivatives		
Indomethacin	Indocin	Capsules 25 mg—$11.77/100; 50 mg—$18.83/100
Sulindac	Clinoril	Tablets 150 mg—$22.00/100; 200 mg—$27.90/100
Tolmetin Sodium	Tolectin	Tablets 200 mg—$11.86/100
Pyrazalone Derivatives		
Oxyphenbutazone	Tandearil (Oxalid)	Tablets 100 mg—$10.96/100
Phenylbutazone	Butazolidin (Azolid)	Tablets 100 mg—$9.33/100
Gold Compounds		
Aurothioglucose	Solganal	Injection (suspension) 50 mg/ml in sesame oil—$11.05/10 ml vial

TABLE 2 *(continued)*

Generic Name	Trademark Name(s)	Preparations and 1978 Costs
Gold Sodium Thiomalate	Myochrysine	Injection (solution) 10 mg/ml—$0.61/1 ml ampul; 25 mg/ml—$0.97/1 ml ampul; 50 mg/ml—$1.37/1 ml ampul, $12.75/10 ml vial; 100 mg/ml—$1.70/1 ml ampul
Other Drugs		
Penicillamine	Cuprimine	Capsules 250 mg—$22.88/100
Mafenamic Acid	Ponstel	Capsules 250 mg—

up to approximately 500 mg/day, where the absorption process becomes saturated. Thus, higher doses produce smaller increments in blood level.[45] Food delays the absorption of all three agents and reduces peak plasma concentration (about 30%) and total absorption (about 20%), as does coadministration of aspirin or antacids.[45–51] Concomitant use of aspirin reduces absorption of fenoprofen by 46%,[45] and of naproxen by 16%.[52]

Efficacy—In rheumatoid arthritis, equivalence to aspirin has been demonstrated for fenoprofen,[53–56] ibuprofen,[57–59] and naproxen.[60–62] Also, comparable activity in osteoarthritis has been observed for fenoprofen and phenylbutazone,[63] ibuprofen and indomethacin,[64,65] and naproxen and indomethacin.[66] Consistent differences among the three propionic acid derivatives have not been established in direct comparisons.[67–69] Corticosteroid dose requirements have been lowered by naproxen coadministration.[70]

Adverse Reactions—Studies comparing these three agents with aspirin have shown the same scope of adverse reactions, although the frequency is usually lower with the phenylpropionic acid derivatives.[55,59,62–68,71–74] The degree of gastrointestinal bleeding is reduced by at least 50% in comparison to aspirin.[71–73] Also, naproxen has been given to peptic ulcer disease patients with evidence of occult blood in stools essentially absent.[75] However, all three drugs have been associated with fatal gastrointestinal hemorrhage in rare cases.[76]

Dosage—Oral: Adults. Therapeutic dosage ranges for fenoprofen are 1.2 to 2.4 g/day in 4 divided doses; ibuprofen, 1.2 to 2.4 g/day in 4 divided doses; and naproxen, 500 to 1000 mg/day in 2 divided doses.

INDOLE DERIVATIVES

INDOMETHACIN (Indocin)
SULINDAC (Clinoril)
TOLMETIN (Tolectin)

Indomethacin is the prototype indole agent. Sulindac and tolmetin are two structural analogues that have been recently marketed. *Pharmacokinetic Properties*—Gastrointestinal absorption is about 90% or greater for each agent, with peak levels within 1–2 hours for indomethacin,[77] 20–60 minutes for tolmetin,[78] and 2 to 3 hours for sulindac.[79–81] Protein binding is extensive, being 90% or greater for each agent.[77,78,80,82] Hepatic biotransformation and renal excretion with some fecal excretion of metabolites are the means of elimination.[77,79,80,82,83] Sulindac undergoes significant enterohepatic recirculation with fecal excretion of about 25% of the dose.[79,81,82] Half-lives are about 6 hours for indomethacin,[77] 1 hour for tolmetin,[78,82] and 7 hours for sulindac.[79,83] However, an active metabolite of sulindac, the sulfide compound, has an 18 hour half-life[79,83] and is considered to account for most of sulindac's action.[80] Concomitant aspirin reduces plasma levels of tolmetin by about 20%, but the interaction probably is not clinically important.[78]

Efficacy—The clinical efficacy of indomethacin in rheumatoid disease is described as good to excellent in 62% of recipients in uncontrolled trials and 25% in controlled studies.[84] Indomethacin shows no consistent superiority over aspirin,[85] ibuprofen,[86] naproxen,[65,87,88] or phenylbutazone[89–92] for rheumatoid and/or osteoarthritis. Indomethacin has been used for ankylosing spondylitis and gout in uncontrolled clinical trials.[84,93] Tolmetin is clearly superior to placebo.[94–98] Controlled comparative trials in rheumatoid arthritis exhibit similar efficacy as aspirin,[99,100] phenylbutazone,[101] or ibuprofen.[102] Sulindac has antirheumatic activity equal to or superior to lower doses of ibuprofen, 0.6–1.2 g/day,[103] and aspirin, 3.6–4.8 g/day.[104] Clinical response to sulindac is evident within 1–2 weeks.

Adverse Reactions—Adverse reactions are most frequent and serious with indomethacin. One study reported side effects in 50% of 228 patients at 1.1 or 2.9 mg/kg/day.[105] Gastrointestinal effects are common: nausea—12%, diarrhea—10%, abdominal pain—3%, and ulcers—2%.[84] Blood loss is significant, but less so than with aspirin.[105] Central nervous system effects are also common: headache—25%, vertigo and dizziness—15%; depression, psychosis and hallucinations also occur.[84] Toxicity is dose related. Daily doses of less than 150 mg caused adverse reactions in 36% of recipients, whereas 150 to 200 mg doses produced a 60–70% frequency.[84,105] Tolmetin also commonly produces gastrointestinal reactions (25% of recipients),[100] and they range from transient mild effects, such as nausea, to serious reactions requiring cessation of therapy.[95] Tolmetin produced fewer side effects than aspirin[99,100] or phenylbutazone[97] in comparative trials. Urticaria, headache, water retention, dizziness, and hypertension have also been reported.[96,98] Adverse reactions to sulindac occur in about 25% of the patients and are generally less severe than reactions to aspirin.[80] Gastrointestinal effects again predominate (18%) and include nausea, abdominal pain and constipation.[80,104] Gastric mucosal erythema, edema, hemorrhage, and erosion with fecal blood loss are minimal with sulindac and common with aspirin.[106–108] Neurologic reactions are also common with sulindac and include dizziness, drowsiness, tiredness, and headache.[80,104] Dry mouth is also a frequent complaint.[104] Platelet aggregation is inhibited, but its persistance is short (about 24 hours), and bleeding time was not changed in one report.[109]

Dosage—Oral: Adults. The usual daily dosages are 150 mg in 2 or 3 divided doses for indomethacin, 1200 mg in four divided doses for tolmetin, and 200–400 mg in two divided doses for sulindac. Indomethacin therapy should be initiated with 25 mg doses, two or three times a day, with 25 mg weekly increments until a 150 mg daily dose is achieved; higher doses usually lead to intolerable side effects. Bedtime administration of two-thirds of the daily dose, eg, 50–100 mg, is often useful to improve sleep and reduce morning stiffness.[110,111] Tolmetin therapy is usually initiated with 600–900 mg daily doses followed by weekly 200 mg increments. Doses of up to 1600 mg are effective,[97,99,101] but a daily dose of more than 1200 mg is usually not necessary.[95]

PYRAZOLONE DERIVATIVES

OXYPHENBUTAZONE (Oxalid, Tandearil)
PHENYLBUTAZONE (Azolid, Butazolidin)

Phenylbutazone and its active metabolite, oxyphenbutazone, are pyrazolone derivatives with almost identical properties.[4,112]

Pharmacokinetic Properties—Phenylbutazone has a half-life of 37 to 76 hours.[113] Protein binding is about 98%.[4] As the dose increases, plasma levels increase, but not linearly. Plasma levels do not correlate with clinical response,[114,115] but higher doses generally provide greater therapeutic effects than lower doses.[116]

Efficacy—Phenylbutazone is not consistently more effective than indomethacin,[89–92] ibuprofen,[117] or tolmetin[118] in rheumatoid arthritis or ibuprofen[119] in osteoarthritis. Superiority over low doses of aspirin (3.9 g/day) has been observed in osteoarthritis.[120,121]

Adverse Reactions—The overall frequency of unwanted effects is lower with phenylbutazone than with indomethacin, primarily because it causes few central nervous system problems.[91,92] However, phenylbutazone and oxyphenbutazone cause significant gastrointestinal irritation, including nausea, pain, stomatitis, and ulceration,[111] at least as often as indomethacin.[122] Edema has been reported in several studies,[118,119,122] and phenylbutazone should be used cautiously in patients with heart or renal disease.

The most serious adverse reaction is bone marrow depression (eg, leukopenia, pancytopenia, agranulocytosis, aplastic anemia); it has an estimated frequency of 1 in 80,000 to 150,000 patient-months of treatment.[116] Aplastic anemia occurs primarily in older patients (over 50 years of age) after three months of therapy. Agranulocytosis occurs in younger patients, usually within the first three months of therapy. Regular blood counts are advisable during prolonged therapy, but the insidiousness and spontaneity of the blood dyscrasias limit their predictable value. Patients should be advised to stop the drug and notify their physician immediately if they develop fever, sore throat, or stomatitis.

Dosage—Oral: Adults. Phenylbutazone and oxyphenbutazone are usually given in a daily dose of 200 to 400 mg, divided into two to four doses. As with other orally administered antirheumatic drugs, dosing with meals reduces gastrointestinal side effects.

GOLD COMPOUNDS

AUROTHIOGLUCOSE (Solganal)
GOLD SODIUM THIOMALATE (Myochrysine)

Pharmacokinetic Properties—Single 60 mg doses of gold sodium thiomalate produce peak blood levels of 7 μg/ml at two to eight hours.[123–125] Steady-state gold levels of 0.75–1.25 μg/ml are maintained with 50 mg given by intramuscular (IM) injection every three to four weeks. However, a correlation between serum levels and effectiveness or toxicity is not established.[126] Gold is about 92% bound to serum albumin.[127] Sites of tissue localization include liver, skin, bone, kidney, eyes, and the reticuloendothelial system.[128] Synovial concentrations are about one-half those of serum. Excretion is very slow, proceeding with a half-life of about one week and persistence of low blood levels (0.1–0.3 μg/ml) for many months.[124,125,128,129] The routes of excretion are urine (70%) and feces (30%).

Efficacy—After the introduction of parenteral gold compounds in the 1930's, they enjoyed widespread clinical acceptance. Subsequently, a long-standing controversy over the safety and effectiveness of gold compounds developed. This was finally settled by a 30-month, double-blind, placebo-controlled trial published in 1960;[130,131] their efficacy has been further confirmed in more recent reports.[126,132–134] Gold compounds produce a favorable response in about 75% of patients, with disease remission in 20 to 25% and lesser improvement in about 55%.[135]

All gold compounds have similar antiarthritic efficacy in adult and juvenile rheumatoid arthritis, as well as similar toxicity.[135–140] Aurothioglucose is more difficult to administer accurately than gold sodium thiomalate because the former is marketed as a suspension in oil that requires warming and agitation to resuspend.

Adverse Reactions—Adverse reactions to gold compounds are often major and can be life-threatening.[141–143] They are dose-related; at 25 mg per week, 18% of recipients have an adverse reaction; this increases to 40% at 100 mg per week. Dermatitis is the most common adverse reaction (20–30% incidence). This usually begins as pruritus, then progresses to almost any type of skin lesion (eg, urticarial, maculopapular, vesicular, or purpuric rash). Concomitant stomatitis and/or eosinophilia are common. The reactions are reversible within a few weeks if the drug is discontinued. Otherwise, rash may progress to fatal exfoliative dermatitis. Thus, gold therapy should be immediately discontinued when rash occurs. Gold dermatitis may be related to the vehicle; in retrospective studies of gold compounds administered in aqueous or oily vehicles, patients who received aqueous preparations had a higher frequency of dermatitis.[144,145]

Nephrotoxicity has been observed in up to 17% of gold recipients.[141–143] Albuminuria and proteinuria are found initially, and they may progress to nephrotic syndrome and eventually membranous glomerulonephritis and acute tubular necrosis. Blood dyscrasias can result from bone marrow suppression and may involve platelets, neutrophils, and/or erythrocytes. Ocular toxicity includes corneal chrysiasis with reversible gold deposition when the total dose exceeds 1 g. More serious cataracts, corneal ulceration, and retinopathy have also occurred.[146]

Dosage—Intramuscular: Adults. An adequate trial of chrysotherapy requires four to five months because of the need for careful assessment of toxicity, as well as the slow onset of effect (8 to 12 weeks).[129,141] Therapy should begin with an IM injection of 10 mg of either gold compound as a test dose. If no toxicity occurs, 25 mg is given one week later. Weekly 50 mg doses are given until a total of 0.5 to 1.0 g has been administered. If there is no response by the time 1 g has been given, the drug should be discontinued. If the patient has improved and no toxic effects have developed, dosage can be reduced to 50 mg every two weeks. In patients who have prolonged remissions, the frequency of injections can be further reduced to every three to four weeks.

ANTIMALARIAL DRUGS

CHLOROQUINE PHOSPHATE
HYDROXYCHLOROQUINE SULFATE (Plaquenil Sulfate)

Chloroquine or hydroxychloroquine are almost always used in combination with other nonsteroidal drugs where prior therapy is inadequate or parenteral treatment is not feasible.[147,148] Onset of improvement is gradual, with initial changes after at least four weeks and maximal benefit at three to six months.

Adverse Reactions—Ocular toxicity is the major complication of antimalarial therapy. These drugs concentrate in the eyes at levels 100 times greater than those in plasma. Diplopia and loss of accommodation are reversible reactions. Reversible corneal opacities occur with chronic administration, but they are asymptomatic. Retinal toxicity is the most serious effect, since antimalarials accumulate in pigmented ocular tissues. Ocular toxicity has been variably reported from less than 1% to as many as 15% of patients. High cumulative doses, eg, 550 g over 3 to 4 years, are associated with retinal toxicity. Fundoscopic diagnosis reveals edema and pigmentary changes. Blindness may result.

Central nervous system and neurologic effects include headache, dizziness, and neuromyopathy. Gastrointestinal effects (diarrhea and nausea) and cutaneous reactions (lichenoid patches, hyperpigmentation, and exfoliative dermatitis) can also occur.

Dosage—Oral: Adults. Therapy is usually initiated with loading doses, eg, chloroquine 250 mg daily at bedtime or hydroxychloroquine, 200 mg one to three times a day. Maintenance doses are lower, eg, chloroquine 250 mg two to three times a week.

ADRENAL CORTICOSTEROIDS

Systemic corticosteroids should be one of the last therapeutic alternatives because of their many serious side effects.[1-5,149] They should be used only as palliative adjunctive treatment in patients with very resistant disease, and should be given in physiologic doses (eg, prednisone, 5 to 7.5 mg/day; 10 to 12 mg maximum). Steroids are given in single morning doses to minimize interference with the normal diurnal adrenal secretion pattern. Alternate day doses are generally unsuccessful in rheumatoid disease.

Adverse Reactions—A summary of untoward reactions attributable to corticosteroids is as follows:[150,151] (1) endocrine—adrenal suppression, hyperglycemia, Cushing's syndrome; (2) musculoskeletal—osteoporosis, myopathy; (3) cardiovascular—fluid and electrolyte imbalances; (4) hematologic—superinfection; (5) ocular—glaucoma, posterior subcapsular cataracts; (6) cutaneous—bruiseability, acne, striae; (7) neurologic—euphoria, dependence, depression, psychosis; (8) gastrointestinal—gastritis. A more complete description of adverse effects may be found in Chapter 49.

Intraarticular Administration—Intraarticular corticosteroids are employed for specific asymmetric joint inflammation that restricts mobility.[149] Response is apparent within 24 hours of injection, with reduction of swelling and pain. Long-acting steroid suspensions, such as triamcinolone hexacetonide or prednisolone tebutate, provide effects of 2 to 4 weeks duration following a single injection. The dose is dependent on the joint size, eg, knee—1 ml, ankle—0.5 ml, phalangeal—0.1 ml. Activity of the joint should be limited for about 48 hours after injection to minimize damage due to premature mobilization. The injection procedure employs an adjunctive topical anesthetic, withdrawal of excess fluid, and a flushing of the needle in situ to prevent placement of crystals in synovial membranes. If repeated at all, at least six to eight weeks should elapse between injections. Complications of intraarticular corticosteroid injections can be acute (eg, septic arthritis and crystal-induced synovitis) or delayed (eg, destructive arthropathy and cutaneous atrophy).

IMMUNOSUPPRESSIVE AGENTS

AZATHIOPRINE (Imuran)
CYCLOPHOSPHAMIDE (Cytoxan)

Cyclophosphamide and azathioprine are highly effective agents that provide partial or complete remissions in up to 75% of severely arthritic patients. However, hematologic toxicity diminishes their value.[152–155] Immunosuppressives are usually given together with corticosteroids, which permits lower steroid doses. Response follows a latent period of three to six months after initiation of therapy. Dosage of cyclophosphamide ranges from 1 to 2.5 mg/kg/day in one or two divided doses.

Adverse Reactions—Major toxicity precludes routine use of these drugs in rheumatoid arthritis. Leukopenia (2000 to 4000 per cubic mm) is routinely produced by therapeutic doses. Secondary infections, especially with herpes zoster and protozoa, is another important limitation of immunosuppressive therapy. Hemorrhagic cystitis due to a cyclophosphamide metabolite occurs frequently (up to 40%) and can range from microhematuria to overt bleeding. Bedtime dosing should be avoided to prevent retention of the metabolites overnight in the bladder. Adequate hydration and frequent bladder emptying are useful means to minimize this toxicity. Gastrointestinal reactions are also common (50% of patients) and include nausea, vomiting, oral ulcerations, abdominal pain, and diarrhea. Alopecia is observed in up to 30% of recipients. Ovarian suppression with amenorrhea can occur in women. See Chapter 19, Antineoplastic Drugs.

OTHER ANTIRHEUMATIC AGENTS

D-PENICILLAMINE (Cuprimine)

D-penicillamine has chelating activity and has been used for many years in the treatment of Wilson's disease, heavy metal poisoning, and cystinuria. More recently is has been used to treat rheumatoid arthritis, but the mechanism of its antiarthritic action is unknown.[156]

Efficacy—Clinical improvement with penicillamine occurs in more than 50% of patients,[157–163] but the duration of therapy preceding improvement varies from 1.5 to 6 months.[159,164] Penicillamine had similar efficacy to that of gold compounds in a direct comparison.[165]

Penicillamine should be considered as an alternative to gold, and should not be used before an adequate trial of more conventional modes of treatment. Downward adjustment of dosage of other anti-inflammatory drugs, especially corticosteroids, is often possible after the addition of penicillamine to the drug regimen.[159,160] Due to the severe toxicity of this drug, renal function and hematologic parameters must be closely monitored during treatment.

Adverse Reactions—Penicillamine causes adverse reactions (over 60%) more often than gold compounds, but they are less likely to require drug discontinuation.[165] Adverse effects to penicillamine include rash (26%), thrombocytopenia (17%), proteinuria, loss of taste (28%), anorexia (12%), and nausea and vomiting (22%).[157–160] Other side effects include sore lips and swollen legs. Proteinuria is common (15–20%) and can progress to the nephrotic syndrome (6%).[158,161,166] Urinary protein above two to five grams per day necessitates drug discontinuation. Agranulocytosis,[159,160] myasthenia gravis,[167] and Goodpasture's syndrome[168] are rare complications of treatment. Skin reactions are divided into early and late manifestations.[156,161,162,164,169,170] The early rash is a reversible, allergic, pruritic, morbilliform eruption, occurring within three months. The late rash occurs after five months and is a papular scaly lesion, resistant to steroids.

Dosage—Oral: Adults. The dosage range of penicillamine for adults with rheumatoid arthritis is 0.75 to 2.0 g/day.[163,164] The drug should be given after meals in divided doses, starting at low levels. A recommended regimen is 0.25 g daily for the first 14 days, followed by increases of 0.25 g daily at bimonthly intervals until an average maintenance dose of 0.75 to 1.5 g/day is achieved in 12 to 14 weeks. Clinical effects may require 6 to 8 weeks to be seen; therefore, longer intervals between dosage adjustments may be appropriate. If no improvement is seen after 6 months, the patient will probably not respond.

MEFENAMIC ACID (Ponstel)

Mefenamic acid occupies a secondary position in rheumatoid arthritis therapy.[1,4,5] At daily doses of 750 to 1000 mg/day (given in three divided doses), it is similar to aspirin in analgesic and anti-inflammatory properties. However, it has no advantage with respect to side effects. Common adverse reactions include dyspepsia (33%), diarrhea (10–15%), maculopapular rashes, headache, dizziness, and drowsiness. Gastrointestinal blood loss and hemolytic anemia are unusual effects.

REFERENCES

1. Constable TJ, Crockson RA, Crockson AP, et al: Drug treatment of rheumatoid arthritis. Lancet 1:1176–1179, 1975.
2. Smyth CJ, Bravo JF: Antirheumatic drugs: clinical pharmacology and therapeutic aspects. Drugs 10:394–425, 1975.
3. Hart FD: Which antirheumatic drug? Drugs 11:451–460, 1976.
4. Brooks PM, Buchanan WW: Current management of rheumatoid arthritis. Recent Adv Rheum 1:33–87, 1976.
5. Huskisson EC: Antiinflammatory drugs. Semin Arthritis Rheum 7:1–20, 1977.
6. Weissman G: Rheumatoid arthritis: how the non-steroidal anti-inflammatory agents work. Med Times 104:64–72, 1976.
7. Huskisson EC: Simple analgesics for arthritis. Br Med J 4:196–200, 1974.
8. Lee P, Anderson JA, Miller J, et al: Evaluation of analgesic action and efficacy of antirheumatic drugs. J Rheumatol 3:283–304, 1976.
9. Lee P, Dick WC: The assessment of disease activity and drug evaluation in rheumatoid arthritis. Recent Adv Rheum 1:1–32, 1976.
10. Ropes MW, Bennett GA, Cobb S, et al: 1958 revision of diagnostic criteria for rheumatoid arthritis. Bull Rheum Dis 9:175–176, 1958.
11. Fremont-Smith K, Bayles TB: Salicylate therapy in rheumatoid arthritis. JAMA 192:1133–1136, 1965.
12. Calabro JJ, Paulus HE: Anti-inflammatory effects of acetylsalicylic acid in rheumatoid arthritis. Clin Orthop 71:124–131, 1970.
13. Bayles TB: Salicylate therapy in rheumatoid arthritis. Med Clin North Am 52:703–706, 1968.
14. Kozin F: Aspirin therapy in the rheumatic disease. Wis Med J 75:S126–S127, 1976.
15. Smiley JD: Rheumatoid arthritis. Postgrad Med 58:17–24, 1975.
16. Rubin A, Rodda BE, Warrick P, et al: Interactions of aspirin with nonsteroidal antiinflammatory drugs in man. Arthritis Rheum 16:635–645, 1973.
17. Levy G, Giacomini KM: Rational aspirin dosage regimens. Clin Pharmacol Ther 23:247–252, 1978.
18. Canada AT, Little AH, Creighton EL: The bioavailability of enteric-coated acetylsalicylic acid: a comparison with buffered ASA in rheumatoid arthritis II. Curr Ther Res 19:554–557, 1976.
19. Canada AT, Little AH: The bioavailability of enteric-coated acetylsalicylic acid: a comparative study in rheumatoid arthritis I. Curr Ther Res 18:727–732, 1975.
20. Sutor AH, Bowie EJM, Owen CA Jr: Effect of aspirin, sodium salicylate and acetaminophen on bleeding. Mayo Clin Proc 46:178–181, 1971.
21. O'Brien JR: Effects of anti-inflammatory agents on platelets. Lancet 1:894–895, 1968.
22. Kanada SA, Kolling WM, Hindin BI: Aspirin hepatotoxicity. Am J Hosp Pharm 35:330–336, 1978.
23. Dick C, Dick PH, Nuki G, et al: Effect of antiinflammatory drug therapy on clearance of ^{133}Xe from knee joints of patients with rheumatoid arthritis. Br Med J 3:278–280, 1969.
24. Broh-Kahn RH: Choline salicylate: a new, effective and well-tolerated analgesic, anti-inflammatory and antipyretic agent. Int Rec Med Gen Pract Clin 173:217–232, 1960.
25. Wolf J, Aboody R: Choline salicylate: a new and more rapidly absorbed drug for salicylate therapy. Int Rec Med Gen Pract Clin 173:234–241, 1960.
26. Leary JF: Preliminary pharmacological comparison of choline salicylate with acetylsalicylic acid. Int Rec Med Gen Pract Clin 173:259–261, 1960.
27. Nevinny D, Gowans JDC: Observations on the usefulness of a new liquid salicylate in arthritis. Int Rec Med Gen Pract Clin 173:242–247, 1960.

28. Thomas RP: Comparative evaluation of the effectiveness of choline salicylate in treatment of arthritis and allied conditions. Int Rec Med Gen Pract Clin 173:248–254, 1960.
29. Scully FJ: Choline salicylate: an effective, well tolerated drug for treatment of rheumatic diseases. South Med J 53:12–16, 1960.
30. Brooke JW: Preliminary observations concerning the use of choline salicylate in various types of arthritis. Am Pract 11:305–308, 1960.
31. Everett AD: Choline salicylate for arthritic and rheumatic pain (letter). Lancet 2:316, 1961.
32. Cohen A, Thomas GB, Cohen EB: Serum concentration safety and tolerance of oral doses of choline magnesium trisalicylate. Curr Ther Res 23:358–364, 1978.
33. Cohen A: A comparative blood salicylate study of two salicylate tablet formulations utilizing normal volunteers. Curr Ther Res 23:772–778, 1978.
34. Lechner BJ, Blechman WJ: Double comparison—Trilisate[T.M.] tablets vs aspirin. Florida Fam Physician 28:51–58, (Winter) 1978.
35. Cohen A, Garber HE: Comparison of choline magnesium trisalicylate and acetylsalicylic acid in relation to fecal blood loss. Curr Ther Res 23:187–193, 1978.
36. Aberg G, Larsson KS: Pharmacological properties and some antirheumatic salicylates. Acta Pharmacol Toxicol 28:249–257, 1970.
37. Harthon L, Hedstrom M: Hydrolysis of salicylsalicylic acid in human blood and acetylsalicylic acid. Acta Pharmacol Toxicol 29:155–163, 1971.
38. Nordqvist P, Harthon JGL, Karlsson R: Metabolic kinetics of salicylsalicylic acid, aspirin, and sodium-salicylate in man. Nord Med 74:1074–1076, 1965.
39. Liyanage SP, Tambar PK: Comparative study of salsalate and aspirin in osteoarthrosis of the hip or knee. Curr Med Res Opin 5:450–453, 1978.
40. Deodhar SD, McLeod MM, Dick WC, et al: A short-term comparative trial of salsalate and indomethacin in rheumatoid arthritis. Curr Med Res Opin 5:185–188, 1977.
41. Regalado RG: The use of salsalate for control of long-term musculoskeletal pain: an open, non-comparative assessment. Curr Med Res Opin 5:454–460, 1978.
42. Edmar D: Effects of salicylates on the gastric mucosa as revealed by roentgen examination and the gastrocamera. Acta Radiol Diagn 11:57–64, 1971.
43. Leonards JR: Absence of gastrointestinal bleeding following administration of salicylsalicylic acid. J Lab Clin Med 74:911–914, 1969.
44. Thune S: Gastrointestinal bleeding and salicylates. Nord Med 79:352–354, 1971.
45. Rubin A, Chernish SM, Crabtree R, et al: A profile of the physiological disposition and gastrointestinal effects of fenoprofen in man. Curr Med Res Opin 2:529–544, 1974.
46. Gruber CM: Clinical pharmacology of fenoprofen: a review. J Rheumatol 3(Suppl 2):8–17, 1976.
47. Kaiser DG, Vangiessen GJ: GLC determination of ibuprofen [(I)-2-p-Isobutylphenylpropionic acid] in plasma. J Pharm Sci 63:219–221, 1974.
48. Davies EF, Avery GS: Ibuprofen: a review of its pharmacological properties and therapeutic efficacy in rheumatic disorders. Drugs 2:416–446, 1971.
49. Davis LJ: Ibuprofen. Drug Intell Clin Pharm 9:501–503, 1975.
50. Runkel R, Forchielli E, Boost G, et al: Naproxen—metabolism, excretion, and comparative pharmacokinetics. Scand J Rheumatol (Suppl 2):29–36, 1973.
51. Segre EJ: Naproxen metabolism in man. J Clin Pharmacol 15:316–323, 1975.
52. Segre E, Sevelius H, Chaplin M, et al: Interaction of naproxen and aspirin in the rotund man. Scand J Rheumatol (Suppl 2):37–42, 1973.
53. Huskisson EC, Wojtulewski JA, Berry H, et al: Treatment of rheumatoid arthritis with fenoprofen: comparison with aspirin. Br Med J 1:176–180, 1974.
54. Zuckner J, Auclair RJ: Fenoprofen calcium therapy in rheumatoid arthritis. J Rheumatol 3(Suppl 2):18–25, 1976.
55. Gum OB: Fenoprofen in rheumatoid arthritis: a controlled crossover multicenter study. J Rheumatol 3(Suppl 2):26–31, 1976.
56. Sigler JW, Ridolfo AS, Bluhm GB: Comparison of benefit to risk ratios of aspirin and fenoprofen: controlled multicenter study in rheumatoid arthritis. J Rheumatol 3(Suppl 2):49–60, 1976.
57. Dornan J, Reynolds WJ: Comparison of ibuprofen and acetylsalicylic acid in treatment of rheumatoid arthritis. Can Med Assoc J 110:1370–1372, 1974.
58. Brooks CD, Schmid FR, Biundo J, et al: Aspirin and ibuprofen in the treatment of rheumatoid arthritis. Rheumatol Physical Med 10(Suppl):9–14, 1970.
59. Blechman WJ, Schmid FR, April PA, et al: Ibuprofen or aspirin in rheumatoid arthritis therapy. JAMA 233:336–340, 1975.

60. Diamond H, Alexander S, Kuzell W, et al: A multicenter double-blind crossover comparison study of naproxen and aspirin in patients with rheumatoid arthritis. Scand J Rheumatol (Suppl 2):171–175, 1973.
61. Hill HFH, Hill AGS, Mowat AG, et al: Naproxen: a new nonhormonal anti-inflammatory agent. Ann Rheum Dis 33:12–14, 1974.
62. Alexander SJ: Clinical experience with naproxen in rheumatoid arthritis. Arch Intern Med 135:1429–1435, 1975.
63. Wojtulewski JA: Fenoprofen in the treatment of osteoarthritis. Curr Med Res Opin 2:551–555, 1974.
64. Clarke AK, Barnes CG, Goodman HV, et al: A double-blind comparison of naproxen against indomethacin in osteoarthritis. Arzneim Forsch 25:302–304, 1975.
65. Barnes CG, Goodman HV, Eade AWT, et al: A double-blind comparison of naproxen with indomethacin in osteoarthritis. J Clin Pharmacol 15:347–354, 1975.
66. Cochrane GM: A double blind comparison of naproxen with indomethacin in osteoarthritis. Scand J Rheumatol (Suppl 2):89–93, 1973.
67. Reynolds PMG, Whorwell PJ: A single blind crossover comparison of fenoprofen, ibuprofen, and naproxen in rheumatoid arthritis. Curr Med Res Opin 2:461–464, 1974.
68. Huskisson EC, Woolf DL, Balme HW, et al: Four new anti-inflammatory drugs: responses and variations. Br Med J 1:1048–1049, 1976.
69. Lewis JR: New rheumatic agents: fenoprofen calcium (Nalfon), naproxen (Naprosyn), and tolmetin sodium (Tolectin). JAMA 237:1260–1261, 1977.
70. Flores JJB, Rojas SV: Naproxen: corticosteroid-sparing effect in rheumatoid arthritis. J Clin Pharmacol 15:373–377, 1975.
71. Loebl DH, Craig RM, Culic DD, et al: Gastrointestinal blood loss: effect of aspirin, fenoprofen and acetaminophen. JAMA 237:976–981, 1977.
72. Schmid FR, Culic DD: Antiinflammatory drugs and gastrointestinal bleeding: a comparison of aspirin and ibuprofen. J Clin Pharmacol 16:418–425, 1976.
73. Arsenault A, Varady J, LeBel E, et al: Effect of naproxen on gastrointestinal microbleeding following acetylsalicylate medication. J Clin Pharmacol 15:340–346, 1975.
74. Halvorsen L, Dotevall G, Sevelius H: Comparative effects of aspirin and naproxen on gastric mucosa. Scand J Rheumatol (Suppl 2):43–47, 1973.
75. Roth SH, Boost G: An open trial of naproxen in rheumatoid arthritis patients with significant esophageal, gastric and duodenal lesions. J Clin Pharmacol 15:378–384, 1975.
76. Cuthbert MF: Adverse reactions to non-steroidal antirheumatic drugs. Curr Med Res Opin 2:600–610, 1974.
77. Hvidberg E, Lausen HH, Jansen JA: Indomethacin: plasma concentration and protein binding in man. Eur J Clin Pharmacol 4:119–124, 1972.
78. Cressman WA, Wortham GE, Plostnieks J: Pharmacokinetics of tolmetin, a new antiinflammatory agent (abstract). Clin Pharmacol Ther 15:203–204, 1974.
79. Shen T-Y, Winter CA: Chemical and biological studies on indomethacin, sulindac, and their analogs. Adv Drug Res 12:89–245, 1977.
80. Brogden RN, Heel RC, Speight TM, et al: Sulindac: a review of its pharmacological properties and therapeutic efficacy in rheumatic diseases. Drugs 16:97–114, 1978.
81. Huskisson EC: Antiinflammatory drugs. Semin Arthritis Rheum 7:1–20, 1977.
82. Selley ML, Glass J, Triggs EJ, et al: Pharmacokinetic studies of tolmetin in man. Clin Pharmacol Ther 17:599–605, 1975.
83. Duggan DE, Hare LE, Ditzler CA, et al: The disposition of sulindac. Clin Pharmacol Ther 21:326–335, 1977.
84. O'Brien WM: Indomethacin: a survey of clinical trials. Clin Pharmacol Ther 9:94–107, 1968.
85. Pinals RS, Frank S: Relative efficacy of indomethacin and acetylsalicylic acid in rheumatoid arthritis. N Engl J Med 276:512–514, 1967.
86. Royer GL Jr, Moxley TE, Hearron MS, et al: A six month double blind trial of ibuprofen and indomethacin in osteoarthritis. Curr Ther Res 17:234–248, 1975.
87. Kogstad O: A double-blind crossover study of naproxen and indomethacin in patients with rheumatoid arthritis. Scand J Rheumatol (Suppl 2):159–163, 1973.
88. Cochrane GM: A double blind comparison of naproxen with indomethacin in osteoarthritis. Scand J Rheumatol (Suppl 2):89–93, 1973.
89. Percy JS, Stephenson P, Thompson M: Indomethacin in the treatment of rheumatic diseases. Ann Rheum Dis 23:226–231, 1964.

90. Hart FD, Boardman PL: Indomethacin and phenylbutazone: a comparison. Br Med J 2:1281–1284, 1965.
91. Wright V, Walker WC, McGuire RJ: Indomethacin in the treatment of rheumatoid arthritis. A controlled trial comparing indomethacin, phenylbutazone and placebo. Ann Rheum Dis 28:157–162, 1969.
92. Hahn K-J: A comparison of phenylbutazone and indomethacin in the treatment of rheumatoid arthritis. Arzneim Forsch 23:851–854, 1973.
93. Smyth CJ, Percy JS: Comparison of indomethacin and phenylbutazone in acute gout. Ann Rheum Dis 32:351–353, 1973.
94. Berkowitz SS, Bernhard G, Bilka PJ, et al: Tolmetin versus placebo for the treatment of rheumatoid arthritis: a sequential double-blind clinical trial. Curr Ther Res 16:442–456, 1974.
95. Brooks PM, Watkins CF, Sturrock RD, et al: Clinical evaluation of tolmetin. Curr Med Res Opin 2:323–328, 1974.
96. Brown JH, Hull J, Biundo JJ: Results of a one-year trial of tolmetin in patients with rheumatoid arthritis. J Clin Pharmacol 15:455–463, 1975.
97. Cordrey LJ: Tolmetin sodium, a new anti-arthritis drug: double-blind and long term studies. J Am Geriatr Soc 24:440–446, 1976.
98. Maibach E: European experiences with tolmetin in the treatment of rheumatic diseases. Curr Ther Res 19:350–362, 1976.
99. Bain LS, El-Ghobarey AF, Collins RM, et al: Tolmetin: an evaluation of a new preparation in the treatment of rheumatoid arthritis. Br J Clin Pract 29:208–210, 1975.
100. Muller FO, Gosling JA, Erdmann GH: A comparison of tolmetin with aspirin in the treatment of osteoarthritis of the knee. S Afr Med J 51:794–796, 1977.
101. Huskisson EC, Berry H, Scott J, et al: Tolectin for rheumatoid arthritis. Rheumatol Rehabil 13:132–134, 1974.
102. McMillen JI: Tolmetin sodium vs. ibuprofen in rheumatoid arthritis patients previously untreated with either drug: a double-blind crossover study. Curr Ther Res 22:266–275, 1977.
103. Dieppe PA, Burry HC, Grahame R, et al: Sulindac in osteoarthrosis of the hip. Rheumatol Rehabil 15:112–115, 1976.
104. Huskisson EC, Scott J: Sulindac: trials of a new anti-inflammatory drug. Ann Rheum Dis 37:89–92, 1978.
105. Boardman PL, Hart FD: Side effects of indomethacin. Ann Rheum Dis 26:127–132, 1967.
106. Beirne JA, Bianchine JR, Johnson PC, et al: Gastrointestinal blood loss caused by tolmetin, aspirin and indomethacin. Clin Pharmacol Ther 16:821–825, 1974.
107. Bianchi-Porro G, Petrillo M, Caruso E, et al: Sulindac and gastric mucosa. Lancet 1:1152–1153, 1977.
108. Cohen A: Intestinal blood loss after a new anti-inflammatory drug, sulindac. Clin Pharmacol Ther 20:238–240, 1976.
109. Green D, Ts-ao C, Ross EC: Sulindac. Lancet 1:804, 1977.
110. Huskisson EC, Taylor RT, Burston D, et al: Evening indomethacin in the treatment of rheumatoid arthritis. Ann Rheum Dis 29:393–396, 1970.
111. Hobkirk D, Rhodes M, Haslock I: Night medication in rheumatoid arthritis: II. Combined therapy with indomethacin and diazepam. Rheumatol Rehabil 16:125–127, 1977.
112. Committee on the Review of Medicines: Recommendations on phenylbutazone, oxyphenbutazone, feprazone, allopurinol, colchicine, probenecid, and sulfinpyrazone. Br Med J 1:1466–1467, 1978.
113. Dick WC, Brooks PM, Buchanan WW: Phenylbutazone dose response in patients with rheumatoid arthritis. J Int Med Res 5(Suppl 2):48–51, 1977.
114. Orme M, Holt PJL, Hughes GRV, et al: Plasma concentration of phenylbutazone and its therapeutic effects—studies in patients with rheumatoid arthritis. Br J Clin Pharmacol 3:185–191, 1976.
115. Brooks PM, Walker JJ, Dick WC, et al: Phenylbutazone: a clinico-pharmacological study in rheumatoid arthritis. Br J Clin Pharmacol 2:437–442, 1975.
116. Orme MLE: Phenylbutazone: plasma concentrations and effectiveness in patients with rheumatoid arthritis. J Int Med Res 5(Suppl 2):40–47, 1977.
117. Pavelka K, Susta A, Vojtisek O, et al: Double-blind comparison of ibuprofen and phenylbutazone in a short term treatment of rheumatoid arthritis. Arzneim Forsch 23:842–846, 1973.

118. Cardoe N, Steele CE: A doubleblind crossover comparison of tolmetin sodium and phenylbutazone in the treatment of rheumatoid arthritis. Curr Med Res Opin 4:688–694, 1977.
119. Moxley TE, Royer GL, Hearron MS, et al: Ibuprofen versus buffered phenylbutazone in the treatment of osteoarthritis. J Am Geriatr Soc 23:343–348, 1975.
120. Scharff EU: A doubleblind comparison of phenylbutazone and aspirin in osteoarthritis. Curr Ther Res 16:1264–1269, 1974.
121. Rotstein J: Phenylbutazone and aspirin in osteoarthritis: a controlled study. Curr Ther Res 17:444–451, 1975.
122. Sperling IL: Adverse reactions with long-term use of phenylbutazone and oxyphenbutazone. Lancet 2:535–537, 1969.
123. Gerber RC, Paulus HE, Jennrich RI, et al: Gold kinetics following aurothiomalate therapy. J Lab Clin Med 83:778–789, 1974.
124. Gottlieb NL: Chrysotherapy. Bull Rheum Dis 27:912–917, 1977.
125. Gottlieb NL, Smith PM, Smith EM: Pharmacodynamics of Au labeled aurothiomalate in blood. Correlation with course of rheumatoid arthritis, gold toxicity, and gold excretion. Arthritis Rheum 17:171–183, 1974.
126. Anon: Gold revalued (editorial). Lancet 1:789–790, 1974.
127. Gottlieb NL, Smith PM, Smith EM: Tissue gold in a rheumatoid arthritic receiving chrysotherapy. Arthritis Rheum 15:16–32, 1972.
128. Mascarhenes BR, Grand JL, Freyberg RH: Gold metabolism in patients with rheumatoid arthritis treated with gold compounds—reinvestigated. Arthritis Rheum 15:391–402, 1972.
129. Gottlieb NL, Smith PM, Smith EM: Gold excretion correlated with clinical course during chrysotherapy in rheumatoid arthritis. Arthritis Rheum 15:582–592, 1972.
130. Empire Rheumatism Council: Gold therapy in rheumatoid arthritis. Report of a multi-center controlled trial. Ann Rheum Dis 19:95–119, 1960.
131. Freyberg RH, Block WD, Wells GS: Gold therapy for rheumatoid arthritis. Clinics 1:537–570, 1942.
132. Sigler JW, Bluhm GB, Duncan H, et al: Gold salts in the treatment of rheumatoid arthritis. Ann Intern Med 80:21–26, 1974.
133. American Rheumatism Council: A controlled trial of gold salt therapy in rheumatoid arthritis. Arthritis Rheum 16:353–358, 1973.
134. Palmer DG, Dunckley JV: Gold levels in serum during treatment of rheumatoid arthritis with gold. Aust NZ J Med 3:461–466, 1973.
135. Allegretti JE: The role of chrysotherapy in active rheumatoid arthritis. Postgrad Med 28:623–626, 1960.
136. Freyberg RH: Gold salts in the treatment of chronic arthritis: metabolic and clinical studies. Proc Staff Meet Mayo Clin 17:534–541, 1942.
137. Adams CH, Cecil RL: Gold therapy in early rheumatoid arthritis. Ann Intern Med 33:163–167, 1950.
138. Hill DF: Gold therapy for rheumatoid arthritis. Med Clin North Am 52:733–738, 1968.
139. Bland JH: Drug treatment of rheumatoid arthritis. Semin Drug Treat 1:93–118, 1971.
140. Myers AR: Chrysotherapy in rheumatoid arthritis. Mod Treat 8:761–768, 1971.
141. Bluhm GB: The treatment of rheumatoid arthritis with gold. Semin Arthritis Rheum 5:147–166, 1975.
142. Rothermich NO, Philips VK, Bergen W, et al: Chrysotherapy. A prospective study. Arthritis Rheum 19:1321–1327, 1976.
143. Anon: Gold for rheumatoid arthritis (editorial). Br Med J 1:470–472, 1971.
144. Lawrence JS: Comparative toxicity of gold preparations in treatment of rheumatoid arthritis. Ann Rheum Dis 35:171–173, 1976.
145. Lawrence JS: Factors in gold dosage and toxicity in rheumatoid arthritis. Ann Rheum Dis 12:129–135, 1953.
146. Gottlieb NL, Major JC: Ocular chrysiasis correlated with gold concentrations in the crystalline lens during chrysotherapy. Arthritis Rheum 21:704–708, 1978.
147. Popert AJ: Chloroquine: a review. Rheumatol Rehabil 15:235–238, 1976.
148. Zvaifler NJ: Antimalarials in the treatment of rheumatoid arthritis. Mod Treat 8:769–777, 1971.
149. Gifford RH: Corticosteroid therapy in rheumatoid arthritis. Med Clin North Am 57:1179–1190, 1973.

150. David DS, Grieco MH, Cushman P: Adrenal glucocorticoids after twenty years. A review of their clinically relevant consequences. J Chronic Dis 22:637–711, 1970.
151. Thompson EB, Lippman ME: Mechanism of action of glucocorticoids. Metabolism 23:159–202, 1974.
152. Urowitz MB: Immunosuppressive therapy in rheumatoid arthritis. J Rheumatol 1:364–373, 1974.
153. Andreis M: Immunosuppression in the treatment of rheumatoid arthritis. Adv Clin Pharmacol 6:81–88, 1974.
154. DeSeze S, Kahn MF: Immunosuppressive drugs in rheumatoid arthritis: clinical results. Adv Clin Pharmacol 6:89–97, 1974.
155. Currey HLF: Immunosuppressive drugs in rheumatoid arthritis—toxicity. Adv Clin Pharmacol 6:98–104, 1974.
156. Huskisson EC: Penicillamine and the rheumatologist: a review. Pharmacotherapeutics 1:24–39, 1976.
157. Multicenter Trial Group: Controlled trial of D(-)penicillamine in severe rheumatoid arthritis. Lancet 1:275–280, 1973.
158. Day AT, Golding JR, Lee PN, et al: Penicillamine in rheumatoid disease. A long term study. Br Med J 1:180–183, 1974.
159. Zuckner J, Ramsey RH, Dorner RW, et al: D-penicillamine in rheumatoid arthritis. Arthritis Rheum 13:131–138, 1970.
160. Golding JR, Wilson JV, Day AT: Observations on the treatment of rheumatoid disease with penicillamine. Postgrad Med J 46:599–605, 1970.
161. Huskisson EC, Hart DF: Penicillamine in the treatment of rheumatoid arthritis. Ann Rheum Dis 31:402–404, 1972.
162. Hill HLH: Selection of patients with rheumatoid arthritis to be treated with penicillamine and their management. Curr Med Res Opin 2:573–580, 1974.
163. Jaffe IA: The effect of penicillamine on the laboratory parameters in rheumatoid arthritis. Arthritis Rheum 8:1064–1069, 1965.
164. Jaffe IA: The treatment of rheumatoid arthritis and necrotizing vasculitis with penicillamine. Arthritis Rheum 13:436–443, 1970.
165. Huskisson EC, Gibson TJ, Balme HW, et al: Trial comparing D-penicillamine and gold in rheumatoid arthritis. Ann Rheum Dis 33:532–535, 1974.
166. Jaffe IA, Treser G, Suzuki Y, et al: Nephropathy induced by penicillamine. Ann Intern Med 69:549–556, 1968.
167. Bucknall RC, Dixon ASJ, Glick EN, et al: Myasthenia gravis associated with penicillamine treatment for rheumatoid arthritis. Br Med J 1:600–602, 1975.
168. Sternlieb I, Bennett B, Scheinberg IH: D-penicillamine induced Goodpasture's syndrome in Wilson's disease. Ann Intern Med 82:673–676, 1975.
169. Jaffe IA: Rheumatoid arthritis with arteritis. Report of a case treated with penicillamine. Ann Intern Med 61:556–560, 1964.
170. Jaffe IA, Smith RW: Rheumatoid vasculitis—report of a second case treated with penicillamine. Arthritis Rheum 11:585–592, 1968.

PSYCHOTROPIC DRUGS

33. HYPNOTICS

David J. Greenblatt and Russell R. Miller

'Insomnia' is the inability to sleep properly. Most patients with insomnia have difficulty falling asleep, do not sleep as long as they would like, or do not feel refreshed upon awakening. Hypnotic drugs provide symptomatic relief of insomnia, but they do not treat the underlying cause.

Sleep disorders can be secondary manifestations of other obvious organic pathology, such as somatic pain, skeletal muscle spasm, hypoxia, pulmonary congestion, nocturnal cough, night sweats, nocturia, or hypoglycemia. In such cases symptomatic treatment with hypnotic drugs alone may be irrational or even contraindicated. When emotional disorders such as anxiety or depression cause sleep disturbances, it is equally important that the underlying disease be treated. Therapy of depression-induced insomnia with hypnotic drugs may exacerbate a patient's depressive illness.

Most hospitalized patients have difficulty sleeping. The possibility or reality of serious organic disease, the prospect of an uncomfortable diagnostic procedure, or just the novelty of the hospital environment, can provoke enough emotional discomfort to disrupt sleep. Because medical care is a round-the-clock endeavor, hospitals are inherently unconducive to normal sleep. If the physician is certain that insomnia is not secondary to causes described above, administration of hypnotic drugs to hospitalized patients is usually justified. Their sleep disorder is temporary and reversible; moreover, the drug, the dosage, and frequency of administration are regulated entirely by professional staff.

In contrast, administration of hypnotic drugs to outpatients is much more problematic. No longer does the physician control the dosage and frequency of administration. Misuse, abuse, and overdosage are important hazards of ambulatory hypnotic drug use which do not exist in the hospital. Less serious but more common is the syndrome of hypnotic drug 'dependence,' characterized as the continued habitual use of a hypnotic drug by patients who feel they cannot sleep without medication. It is not a true physiologic addiction, but rather a compelling psychological reliance upon a drug for sleep.[1]

When ambulatory patients experience temporary insomnia because of stressful life events, hypnotic drug therapy is reasonable provided the physician prescribes a small number of pills and insures frequent follow-up. Chronic, unexplained insomnia deserves thorough medical and psychiatric evaluation. Refillable prescriptions for large numbers of pills are not justifiable.

PHARMACOLOGIC PROPERTIES

Hypnotic drugs are non-specific central nervous system (CNS) depressants. Appropriate doses induce sleep. Progressively larger doses produce deep sleep, general anesthesia, coma, and death. Most hypnotic drugs are relatively lipid-soluble at physiologic pH, and thus are rapidly and extensively distributed to body tissues, including the brain.[2–4] Furthermore, most sleep-inducing drugs are biotransformed by the liver to pharmacologically inactive metabolites. Physicians are traditionally taught that hypnotics are 'short-acting' agents, rapidly metabolized and excreted such that very little residual effect can be detected the day after a nighttime dose. This concept is both correct and incorrect, since the elimination pattern of most hypnotics has two phases: a rapid phase due mainly to drug distribution, followed by a much slower phase due to biotransformation by the liver.[5–7] Thus, the clinical effects of pentobarbital, for example, may appear to 'wear off' rapidly, but significant blood concentrations are detectable for days after a single dose.[7] Physicians should remember that elderly individuals[8–10] and those with severe liver disease[11–13] seem to have impaired drug-metabolizing capacities. This could partly explain the apparent 'sensitivity' of such patients to CNS-depressant drugs.

Hypnotics are rapidly absorbed when administered in the fasting state. When given with food, however, the absorption rate and thus the onset of clinical effects can be delayed.[7,14] Animal studies also suggest that certain antacids can impair the absorption of coadministered hypnotics.[15] Sleeping medications therefore should be given on an empty stomach whenever possible.

Numerous *short-term* controlled studies show that all commonly used prescription hypnotic drugs (Table 1) are highly effective as symptomatic treatment for occasional insomnia.[16,17] When given in adequate dosage, these drugs consistently reduce the time for onset of sleep ('sleep latency'), prolong the duration and quality of sleep, reduce the number of nocturnal awakenings, and leave the patient feeling well-rested and refreshed. Unfortunately, physicians tend to be too conservative with dosage, sometimes leading to apparent drug 'failure.' Unless specific mitigating circumstances exist, therapy should be initiated with doses in the middle or high end of the ranges listed in the individual drug monographs.

CHOICE OF A HYPNOTIC DRUG

There is no consistent evidence that any one of the available hypnotic drugs is more effective than the others for short-term therapy of less than four or five days. However, major differences in long-term efficacy, propensity to interact with other drugs, effects on dreaming, and abuse, dependence, and serious overdosage potential have been observed, and these properties strongly influence the choice of a hypnotic drug.

Abuse, Addiction, and Overdosage

Barbiturates and glutethimide are widely abused drugs. Daily ingestion of only three to four times the usual therapeutic dose can produce physiologic addiction.[18] Relatively small doses can produce deep coma and death. Methaqualone has recently become another popular drug of abuse.[19–24] Two other less commonly prescribed drugs, ethchlorvynol and methyprylon, probably also are abusable,[25,26] and can produce serious overdosage.[27] For unknown reasons, chloral derivatives are uncommonly abused and are rarely implicated in cases of intentional overdosage. Flurazepam is probably the least hazardous of hypnotic drugs with respect to the danger of abuse and overdosage.[28,29]

Drug Interactions

Enzyme Induction. Barbiturates and glutethimide stimulate the activity of hepatic microsomal drug-metabolizing enzymes.[16] The clinical activity of other drugs metabolized by this enzyme system can be diminished when barbiturates or glutethimide are coadministered.[30] The dose of an oral anticoagulant might have to be increased, for example, in a patient who is started on a barbiturate. The greatest danger, however, occurs when an anticoagulant-treated patient *stops* taking a barbiturate. Unless the anticoagulant dosage is concurrently reduced, excessive hypoprothrombinemia and serious bleeding can occur. Osteomalacia due to accelerated metabolism of vitamin D has been reported in a chronic user of glutethimide.[31]

Enzyme induction due to methaqualone and ethchlorvynol is not adequately evaluated, but has been suggested by some reports.[32–34] Chloral hydrate and flurazepam do not cause clinically important enzyme induction in man.

Protein-Binding Displacement. Chloral derivatives are metabolized first to trichloroethanol, then to trichloroacetic acid (TCA). TCA is tightly bound to plasma protein and can displace other protein-bound drugs from their binding sites. The result is an increase in the concentration of the pharmacologically active unbound fraction of the displaced drug, and a transient potentiation of its clinical effect.[35,36] Thus, transient excessive hypoprothrombinemia can occur when a chloral derivative is given to a patient receiving warfarin or bishydroxycoumarin. Other tightly protein-bound drugs such as diphenylhydantoin, phenylbutazone, or imipramine, could potentially interact with chloral derivatives in this manner, but clinically important interactions have not been adequately documented. No other hypnotic drugs cause protein-binding displacement.

Dreaming

Normal individuals spend approximately 25% of sleeping time in the rapid-eye movement (REM) or dreaming stage of sleep. Barbiturates, glutethimide, and methyprylon significantly reduce both total and percentage REM time.[16,28,29,37] Prolonged REM deprivation causes increased 'pressure' to dream. Thus, during chronic use of these drugs dreaming time can return toward normal because of 'REM breakthrough.' This often coincides with diminishing drug efficacy, and causes patients to increase the dose. If the drug is discontinued, REM time becomes supranormal. The 'REM rebound' phenomenon is frequently associated with nightmares, insomnia, and severely disordered sleep. Patients may return to drug use to suppress the unpleasant symptoms of REM rebound. Thus, dream suppression is an undesirable characteristic of barbiturates, glutethimide, and methyprylon, since it can lead to hypnotic dependence.[37] High doses of methaqualone also depress REM sleep. Ethchlorvynol is not adequately evaluated; chloral hydrate probably does not cause REM suppression. When given for several days, flurazepam produces a slight decrease in the percent of REM sleep. When given for 18 to 32 days, the percent of REM sleep is decreased considerably more, and the time that elapses between induction of sleep and the first REM episode is prolonged. However, after withdrawal of the drug, there is no rebound in REM sleep to above baseline values.[38]

Long-Term Efficacy

Although most hypnotics are effective for short-term, occasional use, nearly all fail to both induce or maintain sleep by the second week of daily administration.[37,39] In controlled studies, chronic insomniacs who had been using hypnotics other than flurazepam for months or years had as much or more difficulty sleeping as did insomniac controls who were not using medication. The only exception is flurazepam, which continues to be effective after two weeks of daily use.[38] When used for 32 days or more, a slight loss of effectiveness occurs. Since flurazepam has relatively minor effects on REM sleep compared to most other hypnotics, this could partly explain its long-term efficacy.

Other Adverse Effects

All commonly prescribed hypnotics can produce 'hangover' —unwanted residual drowsiness or heavy-headedness experienced the morning after a nighttime dose. Depending on dosage, up to 40% of hospitalized hypnotic drug takers complain of hangover. The frequency of hangover among ambulatory hypnotic users is much more difficult to determine but probably is similar. A higher percentage of subjects, many of whom are asymptomatic, have impairment of reaction time, coordination, motor function, or intellectual performance the day after taking a sleeping pill. The dangers are obvious, particularly for individuals who operate automobiles or heavy machinery.

Antihistamines

Diphenhydramine (Benadryl), hydroxyzine (Atarax, Vistaril), promethazine (Phenergan, Remsed), and other antihistamines are not included in this discussion because they are not hypnotics *per se*. Their non-specific sedative effects are actually a secondary pharmacologic property which is often exploited for sleep-inducing purposes.[40] There is no evidence that antihistamines are 'milder' or 'safer' than traditional hypnotics; like most of the drugs in Table 1, antihistamines are metabolized by the liver. Since antihistaminic agents have anticholinergic effects, they carry the additional hazard of producing atropine-like toxicity, particularly in elderly individuals.[41,42]

CONCLUSION

Flurazepam has the fewest disadvantages of currently available hypnotics and should be the hypnotic of choice in most clinical circumstances. Nitrazepam (Mogadon), a benzodiazepine hypnotic available in many other countries, has essentially the same clinical effects.[43,44] Alternatively, other benzodiazepine drugs such as diazepam (Valium), chlordiazepoxide (Librium), or chlorazepate (Tranxene) could be used. There is no evidence that they are less effective than flurazepam as hypnotics, and they probably produce no more hangover. If drug cost is of major importance, generically prescribed chloral hydrate can be substituted for flurazepam provided the patient is not taking a coumarin anticoagulant. Generically prescribed barbiturates are inexpensive, but this advantage is outweighed by their numerous hazards and disadvantages. Glutethimide is at least as hazardous as barbiturates and much more expensive; under no circumstances is it rational to prescribe this drug. Glutethimide and barbiturates are contraindicated in patients receiving oral anticoagulants. Methaqualone, methyprylon, and ethchlorvynol have no particular advantages, and thus their use can seldom be recommended.

DRUG MONOGRAPHS

CHLORAL HYDRATE C-IV

Chloral hydrate is an effective hypnotic when used on a short-term basis; by the second week of chronic use it has essentially no effect on sleep.[45] Unlike barbiturates, glutethimide (Doriden), and many other hypnotics, chloral hydrate is rarely abused or taken in overdoses.[46] Since chloral hydrate does not cause clinically important induction of hepatic microsomal enzymes, it has little effect on the metabolism of other drugs.[46] However, it does displace warfarin from its binding sites on serum proteins, and this may cause a transient potentiation of anticoagulant activity (see Interactions section). Chloral hydrate probably does not affect the dreaming or rapid-eye-movement (REM) stage of sleep.

Adverse Reactions—Symptoms of CNS depression the morning after an evening dose (hangover, disorientation, confusion, vertigo, fatigue) are the most common adverse reactions. Other adverse effects occur infrequently and are mostly minor.[47]

Interactions—In about 25% of warfarinized patients, a clearcut but transient potentiation of the hypoprothrombinemic effect of warfarin occurs when chloral hydrate is given.[48] An enhanced anticoagulant effect can appear as early as 12 hours after ingestion of 1 gm of chloral hydrate; a temporary reduction in warfarin dosage may be advisable. Because the liver metabolizes the excess free warfarin, the increased anticoagulant effect is transient. It has also been shown that chloral hydrate recipients require less warfarin during the induction phase of anticoagulation.[49] The use of other hypnotic drugs that do not interact with oral anticoagulants, such as flurazepam,[50] is preferable in warfarin recipients.

Dosage—Oral, Rectal: Adults, 0.5 to 2 gm; 1.5 and 2.0 gm doses are frequently required.[51] *Children,* 30 to 40 mg/kg/24 hours; higher doses (e.g., 100 mg/kg) are used when chloral hydrate is given to children as a sedative prior to minor suturing, etc. All orally-administered hypnotics should be given on an empty stomach.

FLURAZEPAM HYDROCHLORIDE (Dalmane) C-IV

Flurazepam has pharmacological properties similar to those of other benzodiazepines such as chlordiazepoxide (Librium) and diazepam (Valium). Numerous studies have demonstrated its efficacy as a hypnotic agent.[28] In contrast to other hypnotics, flurazepam continues to be effective during chronic therapy.[45] This may be related to its negligible interference with the dreaming or rapid-eye-movement (REM) stage of sleep.[46] When REM-suppressant drugs are withdrawn, nightmares and insomnia can occur due to 'REM rebound'; this may perpetuate drug dependence.[37] Flurazepam does not have this drawback.

Dependence and serious overdosage with flurazepam have not been reported. The drug does not cause enzyme induction; therefore, it does not interfere with oral anticoagulant therapy.[50] Chronic use of

TABLE 1 Preparations and Costs of Hypnotic Drugs

Generic Name	Trademark Name(s)	Preparations and 1978 Costs
"Short-Acting" Barbiturates		
Pentobarbital	Nembutal	Capsules 100 mg—$4.34/100
	generic	Capsules 100 mg—$1.61–$2.54/100
Secobarbital	Seconal	Capsules 100 mg—$3.51/100
	generic	Capsules 100 mg—$1.20–$2.10/100
Chloral Derivatives		
Chloral Hydrate	Noctec	Capsules 500 mg—$5.52/100
	Felsules	Capsules 500 mg—$4.20/100
	generic	Capsules 500 mg—$1.55–$3.98/100
Chloral Betaine	Beta-Chlor	Tablets 870 mg—$12.81/100
Triclofos	Triclos	Tablets 750 mg—$10.90/100
Piperidinediones		
Glutethimide	Doriden	Capsules 500 mg—$9.81/100
Methyprylon	Noludar	Tablets 200 mg—$6.43/100; 300 mg—$7.77/100
Quinazolines		
Methaqualone	Quaalude	Tablets 150 mg—$8.13/100; 300 mg—$10.73/100
	Sopor	Tablets 150 mg—$6.95/100; 300 mg—$9.58/100
Methaqualone Hydrochloride	Parest	Capsules 200 mg—$7.54/100; 400 mg—$10.75/100
Acetylinic Alcohols		
Ethchlorvynol	Placidyl	Capsules 500 mg—$9.98/100; 750 mg—$13.26/100
Benzodiazepines		
Flurazepam Hydrochloride	Dalmane	Capsules 15 mg—$7.81/100; 30 mg—$9.38/100

flurazepam results in accumulation of its active metabolite;[52] the clinical importance of this accumulation is unknown.

Adverse Reactions—Hangover or morning drowsiness is the most common side effect.[53] The frequency of hangover among hospitalized recipients of flurazepam ranged from 1.3% among those receiving less than 15 mg/day to 12.3% at doses of 30 mg/day or more in one study.[53] Hangover also occurs more often with increasing age. With flurazepam the frequency of all adverse reactions (principally hangover) increased from 1.9% among recipients under 60 to 7.1% among those 80 or over. Dose and age effects are additive. Only 2.0% of flurazepam recipients 70 or older experienced adverse reactions at doses under 15 mg/day, whereas 39.0% had adverse reactions at 30 mg/day or more.[53] Depression of respiration and circulation is minimal,[53,54] but flurazepam should always be given with caution in patients with impaired respiratory drive, in the elderly, and in those receiving other depressant drugs concurrently.

Dosage—Oral: Adults, 15 to 30 mg at bedtime. A 15 mg dose is less consistently effective than a 30 mg dose,[55,56] but the 15 mg dose should be initially prescribed for elderly patients.[53] No pediatric dosage form is available. All orally-administered hypnotics should be given on an empty stomach.

PENTOBARBITAL (Nembutal) C-II
PENTOBARBITAL SODIUM (Nembutal Sodium) C-II
SECOBARBITAL SODIUM (Seconal Sodium) C-II

Barbiturates are no longer considered hypnotic agents of choice. Therefore, they should be used only in patients who cannot tolerate flurazepam or chloral hydrate or in those who do not adequately respond to these agents. The disadvantages and hazards of barbiturate hypnotics are such that their prescribing is seldom advisable.

Barbiturates do not produce natural sleep since they inhibit the rapid-eye-movement (REM) or dreaming stage of sleep.[16] When their use is discontinued, dreaming time rebounds to supranormal levels.[38] The REM rebound phenomenon may be associated with nightmares and insomnia and can cause patients to return to the drug to suppress these unpleasant symptoms.

Barbiturates lose their hypnotic effectiveness when they are used on a chronic basis.[37] Therefore, pentobarbital and secobarbital should be given for periods of one week or less.

All barbiturate hypnotics induce increased activity of hepatic microsomal enzymes that are responsible for the biotransformation of many drugs.[30,57] Increased biotransformation can render usual doses of many drugs therapeutically ineffective. Interference by barbiturates has been a serious problem in oral anticoagulant therapy and has resulted in numerous fatalities.[30,58] In short, the use of barbiturates makes effective and safe therapy with drugs metabolized in the liver very difficult.

Barbiturates are very commonly abused, and dependence develops readily.[59,60] Physiological addiction can occur in about one month.[60] Barbiturates are the drugs most often used in attempted and successful suicides.[61–63] No specific antidote for overdoses of barbiturates is available.

Adverse Reactions—Hangover and other symptoms of CNS depression (disorientation, confusion, vertigo, ataxia) are the most common adverse effects.[47]

Interactions—As noted above, barbiturates may cause a decreased hypoprothrombinemic effect of oral anticoagulants. If the dose of anticoagulants is increased to offset this decreased effect and the barbiturate hypnotic is subsequently discontinued, then the prothrombin time may become excessively prolonged.

Barbiturates interact with adrenal corticosteroids to cause reduced serum levels and decreased systemic effects of the steroids; the probable mechanism is induction of microsomal activity.[64,65] Decreased serum levels of doxycycline (Vibramycin) have been reported when a barbiturate was given concurrently; the probable mechanism is induction of microsomal enzyme activity.[66] Decreased serum levels of griseofulvin have also been noted; the mechanism involved is unclear.[67] Chlorpromazine may be more rapidly metabolized when barbiturates are given concurrently.[68]

Dosage—Oral: Adults, 100 to 200 mg at bedtime. *Children,* proper hypnotic dose must be judged on the basis of individual age and weight. All hypnotics should be given on an empty stomach.

OTHER HYPNOTIC DRUGS

A large number of other somnifacient agents are commercially available (Table 1). None of these preparations has any advantage over the four drugs described above, and many of them have significant disadvantages.[17,37,46,69] The disadvantages include abuse and dependence, serious overdosage, suppression of rapid-eye-movement sleep, and induction of drug-metabolizing enzymes in the liver (see Introduction).

REFERENCES

1. Clift AD: Factors leading to dependence on hypnotic drugs. Br Med J 3:614–617, 1972.
2. Way WL, Trevor AJ: Sedative-hypnotics. Anesthesiology 34:170–182, 1971.
3. Parke DV: Biochemistry of barbiturates. In *Acute Barbiturate Poisoning*. Edited by H Matthew. Amsterdam, Excerpta Medica Foundation, 1971, pp 7–53.
4. Mark LC: Pharmacokinetics of barbiturates. In *Acute Barbiturate Poisoning*. Edited by H Matthew. Amsterdam, Excerpta Medica Foundation, 1971, pp 75–83.
5. Morris RN, Gunderson GA, Babcock SW, et al: Plasma levels and absorption of methaqualone after oral administration to man. Clin Pharmacol Ther 13:719–723, 1972.
6. Alvan G, Lindgren J-E, Bogentoft C, et al: Plasma kinetics of methaqualone in man after single oral doses. Eur J Clin Pharmacol 6:187–190, 1973.
7. Smith RB, Dittert LW, Griffen WO, et al: Pharmacokinetics of pentobarbital after intravenous and oral administration. J Pharmacokin Biopharm 1:5–16, 1973.
8. O'Malley K, Crooks J, Duke E, et al: Effect of age and sex on human drug metabolism. Br Med J 3:607–609, 1971.
9. Jori A, DiSalle E, Quadri A: Rate of aminopyrine disappearance from plasma in young and aged humans. Pharmacology 8:273–279, 1972.
10. Irvine RE, Grove J, Toseland PA, et al: The effect of age on the hydroxylation of amylobarbitone sodium in man. Br J Clin Pharmacol 1:41–43, 1974.
11. Branch RA, Herbert CM, Read AE: Determinants of serum antipyrine half-lives in patients with liver disease. Gut 14:569–573, 1973.
12. Mawer GE, Miller NE, Turnberg LA: Metabolism of amylobarbitone in patients with chronic liver disease. Br J Pharmacol 44:549–560, 1972.
13. Klotz U, Avant GR, Hoyumpa, P, et al: The effects of age and liver disease on the disposition and elimination of diazepam in adult man. J Clin Invest 55:347–359, 1975.
14. Johnson PC, Braun GA, Cressman WA: Non-fasting state and the absorption of a hypnotic. Arch Intern Med 131:199–201, 1973.
15. Hurwitz A, Sheehan MB: The effects of antacids on the absorption of orally administered pentobarbital in the rat. J Pharmacol Exp Ther 179:124–131, 1971.
16. Greenblatt DJ, Shader RI: The clinical choice of sedative-hypnotics. Ann Intern Med 77:91–100, 1972.
17. Miller RR, DeYoung DV, Paxinos J: Hypnotic drugs. Postgrad Med J 46:314–317, 1970.
18. Greenblatt DJ, Shader RI: Acute poisoning with psychotropic drugs. In *Psychotropic Drug Side Effects: Clinical and Theoretical Perspectives*. By RI Shader, A DiMascio, and associates. Baltimore, Williams and Wilkins, 1970, pp 214–234.
19. Brown SS, Goenechea S: Methaqualone: metabolic, kinetic, and clinical pharmacologic observations. Clin Pharmacol Ther 14:314–324, 1973.
20. Ostrenga JA: Methaqualone—a Dr. Jekyll and Mr. Hyde? Clin Toxicol 6:607–609, 1973.
21. Gerald MC, Schwirian PM: Nonmedical use of methaqualone. Arch Gen Psychiatry 28:627–631, 1973.
22. Bridge TP, Ellinwood EH: Quaalude alley: a one-way street. Am J Psychiatry 130:217–219, 1973.
23. Inaba DS, Gay GR, Newmeyer JA, et al: Methaqualone abuse: 'luding out.' JAMA 224:1505–1509, 1973.
24. Pascarelli EF: Methaqualone abuse, the quiet epidemic. JAMA 224:1512–1514, 1973.
25. Flemenbaum A, Gunby B: Ethchlorvynol (Placidyl) abuse and withdrawal. Dis Nerv Syst 32:188–192, 1971.
26. Swanson DW, Weddige RL, Morse RM: Abuse of prescription drugs. Mayo Clin Proc 48:359–367, 1973.
27. Arieff AI, Friedman EA: Coma following nonnarcotic drug overdosage: management of 208 adult patients. Am J Med Sci 266:405–426, 1973.
28. Greenblatt DJ, Shader RI, Koch-Weser J: Flurazepam hydrochloride. Clin Pharmacol Ther 17:1–14, 1975.
29. Greenblatt DJ, Shader RI: *Benzodiazepines in Clinical Practice*. New York, Raven Press, 1974.
30. Koch-Weser J, Sellers EM: Drug interactions with coumarin anticoagulants. N Engl J Med 285:487–498, 547–558, 1971.

31. Greenwood RH, Prunty FTG, Silver J: Osteomalacia after prolonged glutethimide administration. Br Med J 1:643–645, 1973.
32. Johansson S.A: Apparent resistance to oral anticoagulant therapy and influence of hypnotics on some coagulation factors. Acta Med Scand 184:297–300, 1968.
33. Cullen SI, Catalano PM: Griseofulvin-warfarin antagonism. JAMA 199:582–583, 1967.
34. Ballinger B, Browning M, O'Malley K, et al: Drug-metabolizing capacity in states of drug dependence and withdrawal. Br J Pharmacol 45:638–643, 1972.
35. Sellers EM, Koch-Weser J: Potentiation of warfarin-induced hypoprothrombinemia by chloral hydrate. N Engl J Med 283:827–831, 1970.
36. Sellers EM, Lang M, Koch-Weser J, et al: Enhancement of warfarin-induced hypoprothrombinemia by triclofos. Clin Pharmacol Ther 13:911–915, 1972.
37. Kales A, Bixler EO, Tan TL, et al: Chronic hypnotic-drug use. Ineffectiveness, drug-withdrawal insomnia, and dependence. JAMA 227:513–517, 1974.
38. Kales A, Bixler EO, Scharf M, et al: Sleep laboratory studies of flurazepam: A model for evaluating hypnotic drugs. Clin Pharmacol Ther 19:576–583, 1976.
39. Kales A, Kales JD: Sleep disorders. N Engl J Med 290:487–499, 1974.
40. Cirillo VJ, Tempero KF: The pharmacology and therapeutic use of antihistamines. Am J Hosp Pharm 33:1200–1207, 1976.
41. Greenblatt DJ, Shader RI: Drug therapy: anticholinergics. N Engl J Med 288:1215–1219, 1973.
42. Shader RI, Greenblatt DJ: Belladonna alkaloids and synthetic anticholinergics: uses and toxicity. In *Psychiatric Complications of Medical Drugs*. Edited by RI Shader. New York, Raven Press, 1972, pp 103–147.
43. James NM, Montague AF: A double blind trial of nitrazepam and flurazepam as sedatives. NZ Med J 81:246–248, 1975.
44. Lynch T, Greene VT: Double-blind crossover trial of flurazepam (Dalmane) and nitrazepam (Mogadon) in the treatment of insomnia in psychiatric patients. J Ir Coll Physicians Surg 4:87–90, 1975.
45. Kales A, Allen C, Scharf MB, et al: Hypnotic drugs and their effectiveness. All-night EEG studies of insomniac subjects. Arch Gen Psychiatry 23:226–232, 1970.
46. Greenblatt DJ, Miller RR: Rational use of psychotropic drugs. I. Hypnotics. Am J Hosp Pharm 31:990–995, 1974.
47. Greenblatt DJ, Miller RR: Hypnotics. In *Drug Effects in Hospitalized Patients*. Edited by RR Miller, DJ Greenblatt. New York, John Wiley and Sons, 1976, pp 171–191.
48. Sellers EM, Koch-Weser J: Kinetics and clinical importance of displacement of warfarin from albumin by acidic drugs. Ann NY Acad Sci 179:213–225, 1971.
49. Boston Collaborative Drug Surveillance Program: Interaction between chloral hydrate and warfarin. N Engl J Med 286:53–55, 1972.
50. Robinson DS, Amidon EL: Interaction of benzodiazepines with warfarin in man. In *The Benzodiazepines*. Edited by S Garattini, E Mussini, LO Randall. New York, Raven Press, 1973, pp 641–646.
51. Owens AH, Marshall EK: Further studies on metabolic fate of chloral hydrate and trichloroethanol. Bull Johns Hopkins Hosp 97:320–326, 1955.
52. Kaplan SA, deSilva JAF, et al: Blood level profile in man following chronic oral administration of flurazepam hydrochloride. J Pharm Sci 62:1932–1935, 1973.
53. Greenblatt DJ, Allen MD, Shader RI: Toxicity of high-dose flurazepam in the elderly. Clin Pharmacol Ther 21:355–361, 1977.
54. Finn H, Cohen R, Steen SN: Comparison of the effects of RO 5-6901, pentobarbital, and meperidine on the respiratory response to carbon dioxide. Anesth Analg (Cleve) 49:297–299, 1970.
55. Bielman P, Pinard G, Tetreault L: Flurazepam: study of its hypnotic properties in normal subjects. Int J Clin Pharmacol 6:13–17, 1972.
56. Wang RIH, Stockdale SL: The hypnotic efficacy of triazolam. J Int Med Res 1:600–607, 1973.
57. Kuntzman R: Drugs and enzyme induction. Annu Rev Pharmacol 9:21–36, 1969.
58. Robinson DS, MacDonald MG: The effect of phenobarbital administration on the control of coagulation achieved during warfarin therapy in man. J Pharmacol Exp Ther 153:250–253, 1966.
59. Swanson DW, Weddige RL, Morse RM: Abuse of prescription drugs. Mayo Clin Proc 48:359–367, 1973.

60. Wikler A: Diagnosis and treatment of drug dependence of the barbiturate type. Am J Psychiatry 125:758–765, 1968.
61. Whelton A, Snyder DS, Walker WG: Acute toxic drug ingestions at Johns Hopkins Hospital, 1963 through 1970. Johns Hopkins Med J 132:157–167, 1973.
62. Barraclough BM: Are there safer hypnotics than barbiturates? Lancet 1:57–58, 1975.
63. Matthew H: Are there safer hypnotics than barbiturates? Lancet 1:224, 1974.
64. Morselli PL, Marc V, Garattini S, et al: Metabolism of exogenous cortisol in humans. Influences of phenobarbital treatment on plasma cortisol disappearance rate. Rev Eur Etud Clin Biol 15:195–198, 1970.
65. Kuntzman R, Jacobson M, Levin W, et al: Stimulatory effect of N-phenylbarbital (phetarbital) on cortisol hydroxylation in man. Biochem Pharmacol 17:565–571, 1968.
66. Neuvonen PJ, Pentilla O: Interaction between doxycycline and barbiturates. Br Med J 1:535–536, 1974.
67. Riegelman S, Rowland M, Epstein WL: Griseofulvin-phenobarbital interaction in man. JAMA 213:426–431, 1970.
68. Forrest FM, Forrest JS, Serra MT: Modification of chlorpromazine metabolism by some other drugs frequently administered to psychiatric patients. Biol Psychiatry 2:53–58, 1970.
69. Editorial: Glutethimide—an unsafe alternative to barbiturate hypnotics. Br Med J 1:1424–1425, 1976.

34. ANTIANXIETY AGENTS

David J. Greenblatt and Richard I. Shader

When confronted with threat or danger the human organism responds in characteristic and predictable ways. The response is at least partly mediated by the sympathetic nervous system. Cardiovascular manifestations are generally prominent, and include tachycardia, increased force of cardiac contraction accompanied by the subjective sensation of palpitations, widened pulse pressure, and increased blood flow to vasculature of skeletal muscles. Accompanying signs and symptoms include tachypnea or hyperventilation, mydriasis, and tremulousness. A second category of manifestations involve the central nervous system (CNS), and includes the subjective feelings of apprehension, dread, and the need for escape, avoidance, or defense. The sensation of hyperalertness or increased response to external stimuli is also common.

This general response to perceived threat or conflict is traditionally categorized along a continuum ranging from appropriate fear to morbid or pathologic anxiety.[1–5] When the threat, danger, or impending conflict is imminent and real, we categorize the psychophysiologic response as appropriate fear, being essential to the survival of the organism. On the other hand, when perceived threat is trivial, nonexistent, or arising from internal conflict rather than external danger, the response is generally termed pathologic anxiety. The diagnosis of morbid anxiety in clinical practice is relatively straightforward when extremes are reached. In most cases, however, the distinction between anxiety and fear is not straightforward, since many individuals face very real external stresses and conflicts which reinforce and perpetuate internal conflicts. A useful approach to assessment of clinical anxiety involves an operational judgment of whether the response is adaptive or maladaptive. When the individual's response to ongoing or intermittent stress benefits his or her ability to cope with the situation, and in turn does not meaningfully interfere with interpersonal relationships and occupational function, then the response can be considered as adaptive and therefore probably not pathologic. On the other hand, when conflict and stress evoke psychophysiologic symptoms and signs which impair the person's ability to cope or which are damaging to interpersonal and occupational function, the situation is maladaptive. Generally, the patient's decision to seek medical help is a good indicator that his or her response to stress and conflict is maladaptive and may benefit from some form of intervention. However, this is not always the case—many individuals seek medical advice for trivial or transient situational stresses, while others who are essentially disabled by morbid anxiety avoid medical intervention for compelling social or ethical reasons, or even because of the disease process itself.

This operational approach to clinical anxiety is useful but clearly oversimplifies the complex nature of the syndrome. Clinical anxiety can have numerous manifestations and etiologies, which are the subject of an extensive literature.[1–5] While many anxious individuals experience both peripheral and central manifestations, this is not always the case. A large proportion of patients with anxiety do not perceive themselves as overtly anxious and in fact do not experience feelings of apprehension, dread, uneasiness, nervousness, tension, or fear. Instead, their complaints are almost entirely peripheral in nature, leading to the categorization of 'somatic' anxiety. Symptoms commonly focus upon the cardiovascular and respiratory systems, and include ill-defined chest pains, palpitations, awareness of the 'heart pounding' in the head or neck, breathlessness, hyperventilation, and fatigability. Hyperventilation can be accompanied by or lead to further weakness, dizziness, peripheral parasthesias, and tremor. Such patients generally first seek help from an internist or family physician, and often undergo extensive and expensive testing for organic disease. Objective tests generally fail to reveal organic disease, except possibly for labile systolic hypertension which is usually mild. In other patients, problems focus upon the gastrointestinal tract, and include nausea, diarrhea, vague intermittent abdominal pain, aerophagia, belching, and a feeling of bloating or 'gas'. Again, their complaints may precipitate extensive, expensive medical evaluation, including radiographic contrast studies and sometimes endoscopy. Evidence of objective organic disease is generally absent, leading to nonspecific diagnoses such as 'functional bowel disorder' or 'spastic colon'. Another category of disorders is neurologic, usually including some combination of headache, dizzy spells, visual disturbances, difficulty in concentrating, and easy distractability. Again, objective tests are normal and lead to nonspecific diagnoses such as 'tension headache'. Other manifestations of somatic anxiety in women include gynecologic disturbances such as lower abdominal pain or dyspareunia, as well as urinary frequency and urgency with no evidence of urinary tract infection or other anatomic abnormalities. Regrettably, the diagnosis of anxiety in this large group of patients with the 'somatic anxiety' syndrome usually is one of exclusion, being made only after extensive medical evaluation. Not surprisingly, non-psychiatrist physicians usually dislike dealing with such patients, since their symptoms and complaints persist despite a lack of demonstrable organic disease.

THERAPEUTIC APPROACHES TO ANXIETY

Traditional psychoanalytic theory dictates that clinical anxiety can be a manifestation of unresolved and presumably unconscious intrapsychic conflicts, derived from stressful or painful past experiences. A second source of clinical anxiety derives from ongoing or impending environmental stresses, leading to or associated with a sense of helplessness or lack of mastery. Definitive cures of anxiety derived from intrapsychic conflict require identification, clarification, and mastery of these conflicts through psychotherapeutic intervention. Anxiety resulting from external stress is directly approached by identification and removal of the stress-inducing situation. In many cases anxiety derives from a combination of internal and external stress, in which case interpersonal psychotherapy together with some manipulation of the environmental situation would constitute definitive therapy.

Unfortunately, definitive solutions through these two approaches are not feasible for many individuals. Psychotherapeutic intervention is costly, time-consuming, and may in itself be a potentially disquieting experience. Manipulation of the environment is not always possible, as in the case of persons trapped in unhappy, conflict-ridden family, marital, or occupational situations from which they cannot realistically escape.

Faced with apparently insoluble internal and external problems which can make life unpleasant if not unbearable, many such individuals seek alternative means of coping, often in the form of pharmacotherapy. Self-medication with ethanol may be the most popular and widely used pharmacologic approach to anxiety. When used judiciously and in appropriate doses, ethyl alcohol undoubtedly has some antianxiety effects. However, its concurrent adverse effects on psychomotor function, together with the well-known medical hazards of long-term ethanol ingestion, are major drawbacks of this approach. The consequent need for safer and more effective antianxiety agents has led to continuing research in this area and development of a succession of drugs used for the treatment of anxiety.

The extent of use of prescription drugs for the treatment of anxiety in clinical practice in the Western world now is staggering. From 10 to 20% of ambulatory adults in the Western world utilize prescription drugs for the treatment of anxiety and tension on a reasonably regular basis.[6,7] These findings clearly support the concept that pharmacotherapy is a widespread means of coping with anxiety. The continuing and, if anything, expanding extent of antianxiety drug use further suggests that the clinical effectiveness of these drugs is generally satisfactory, and that they do in fact provide some symptomatic relief for the majority of individuals.[8] On the other hand, there are worrisome aspects of this widespread degree of pharmacotherapy. Inasmuch as millions of Americans appear to be candidates for anxiolytic drugs, this huge pharmaceutical market has stimulated the development of an intensely competitive antianxiety drug industry whose promotional efforts may stimulate unnecessary drug use.[9–11] Although most of these drugs appear to be relatively innocuous and reasonably effective, the disquieting possibility of hitherto unidentified long-term adverse effects is always present. Finally, it is pointed out that drug therapy of anxiety may sometimes be maladaptive rather than adaptive, since drugs provide only symptomatic relief and may be used as another means of avoidance.

Clinicians who prescribe anxiolytic drugs should be aware of these potentially conflicting outcomes of treatment. Antianxiety agents by themselves do not 'cure' anxiety any more than insulin cures diabetes or nitroglycerin cures angina pectoris. Nor are anxiolytic drugs uniformly and dramatically effective for all individuals that take them. On the other hand, anxiolytic drug therapy is not necessarily counterproductive just because it is not curative. Well supervised and monitored pharmacotherapy can often be of considerable benefit, particularly when the choice of drug and dosage schedule are tailored to the needs of the individual patient.

USES OF ANXIOLYTIC DRUGS

Clinical anxiety can take many forms, and the appropriate therapeutic use of anxiolytic agents depends in large part upon the particular nature of the clinical syndrome.[1]

Intermittent Anxiety or Acute Situational Stress

Anxiety commonly takes the form of a cyclic disorder, with periodic remissions or exacerbations. The fluctuation in the severity of clinical symptomatology can be either spontaneous or associated with periodic episodes of situational stress. Many such individuals respond well to antianxiety drug therapy, particularly when treatment is focused upon the periods of exacerbation. During remission, dosage can be lowered or the drug discontinued altogether. Patients with insight into their illness sometimes can tailor their own dosage regimen to fit the fluctuating pattern of symptoms.

Chronic Anxiety

Another category of clinical anxiety appears as a more or less continuous syndrome of tension, worry, concern, and apprehension. In some cases this is a response to continuous environmental stress. In others, it represents a personality trait sometimes termed 'chronic characterological anxiety'. Superimposed upon the continuous background level of symptomatic anxiety may be further periods of remission and exacerbation, during which symptoms become relatively worse or relatively better. Such individuals appear to be candidates for long-term antianxiety drug therapy, with dosage raised or lowered if necessary to coincide with episodes of exacerbation if they occur. The effectiveness of anxiolytic drugs in this category of anxiety seems to be somewhat less than in those who are relatively symptom-free except for periods of acute exacerbation. The reasons for this are not established but may be explained either by the diminishing effectiveness of the drugs as they are given over time or by the intrinsically less drug-responsive nature of the underlying disorder.

Acute, Severe Anxiety or Agitation

Episodes of acute anxiety, fear, panic, or terror can appear in the two categories of anxious patients as described above. They also can occur in patients who are otherwise completely asymptomatic. Again, a precipitant may be evident, or the attack may be purely spontaneous. A common precipitant is the use or abuse of other drugs, as in the case of 'bad trips' due to hallucinogens.[12]

Individuals with acute panic or terror should be carefully evaluated for the possibility of a drug-induced disorder or for the occurrence of an acute psychotic state. In these two cases, more specific drug therapy may be appropriate. If clinical evaluation suggests that symptomatic therapy with a (nonspecific) sedative or antianxiety agent is indicated, treatment is usually short-term, in relatively high doses, and by the parenteral route. Although intramuscular injection of sedatives and anxiolytics is common clinical practice in such situations, absorption of the drug from the injection site may be slow and erratic. Accordingly, if parenteral therapy is thought to be indicated, slow and careful intravenous infusion is generally preferable to intramuscular injection.

Withdrawal from Ethanol and Other Addicting Drugs

Severe agitation, fearfulness, and disorientation can accompany the syndrome of withdrawal from ethanol and similar agents with addictive properties.[13] If untreated, symptoms may progress to the more serious, life-threatening syndrome of delirium tremens. Early intervention with sedative or hypnotic agents is indicated in such cases. Again, high doses are generally administered by the parenteral route. Clinical considerations in the treatment of withdrawal syndromes are described in detail elsewhere.[13]

Sleep Disorders

Since many antianxiety agents have nonspecific sedative properties, they can serve equally well as hypnotic agents if doses are increased above the usual anxiolytic level, and given all at once at bedtime.[14] In fact, many individuals with insomnia accompanied by anxiety can benefit from once-daily anxiolytic therapy, in which an appropriate dose of a drug having a long duration of action is given all at once at bedtime.[15,16] The role of benzodiazepines and other sedative-hypnotic agents in the treatment of sleep disorders is discussed in Chapter 33.

Other Uses

Anxiolytic drugs of the sedative-hypnotic category also possess muscle relaxant and anticonvulsant effects and therefore are commonly used to treat certain seizure disorders and spastic musculoskeletal disorders.[15] Drug therapy of such diseases are discussed in detail in Chapters 37 and 39. The adjunctive role of antianxiety agents in numerous other psychiatric and medical disorders will not be discussed in detail.

CATEGORIES OF ANTIANXIETY AGENTS

Many drugs have been or are in current use for the treatment of anxiety and related disorders. Most of these fall in the category of sedative-hypnotic agents, having relatively nonspecific CNS depressant properties.[17] Other categories of anxiolytic agents (such as antihistamines or major tranquilizers) may have different primary pharmacologic properties but also have secondary sedative and anxiolytic effects. One class of drugs, the beta-adrenergic receptor blocking drugs, have different pharmacologic actions, acting via blockade of peripheral (and possibly central) beta-adrenergic receptor sites rather than exerting central depressant effects.

Barbiturates

Derivatives of barbituric acid have long been used to treat clinical anxiety. The anxiolytic effects of these drugs are very nonspecific, occurring as part of generalized CNS depression.[18] Many barbiturates are relatively inexpensive and time-tested anxiolytics. However, their clinical efficacy is dubious, inasmuch as most individuals do not experience relief of anxiety without coincident nonspecific sedation which can interfere with intellectual and motor functioning.[16,19,20] Furthermore, barbiturates carry a considerable potential for abuse and addiction. Barbiturates present an additional hazard associated with overdosage, since serious and sometimes fatal intoxication can result from ingestion of doses that do not greatly exceed the usual therapeutic range.[21] Because of these drawbacks, barbiturates are generally relegated to a secondary position as anxiolytic agents.

Meprobamate and Related Propanediols

Meprobamate and tybamate also are anxiolytic drugs of the sedative-hypnotic category. They also have intraneuronal blocking properties and muscle relaxant effects,[22,23] but these appear to be of little or no clinical importance. Early pharmaceutical claims suggested that meprobamate had more specific antianxiety effects than did barbiturates. Numerous controlled studies, however, suggest that meprobamate is no more specific or effective than barbiturates and has similar hazards.[24,25] For this reason meprobamate also holds a secondary position as an anxiolytic agent.

Benzodiazepines

Numerous benzodiazepine derivatives are available for the treatment of anxiety. This class of drugs, and in particular diazepam, is clearly the most widely used category of anxiolytic agents despite their relatively high cost.[15,16] The reasons for their immense popularity are not established. Benzodiazepines do appear to be more effective, and certainly considerably safer, than barbiturates or meprobamate. Another major determinant of their popularity probably is skillful and timely pharmaceutical marketing.

Like barbiturates and meprobamate, benzodiazepines are sedative-hypnotic agents. Although they are by no means specific for anxiety, the difference between anxiolytic and nonspecific sedating doses tends to be considerably greater for benzodiazepines than for barbiturates and meprobamate. Accordingly, many individuals experience satisfactory anxiolytic effects in doses that do not produce clinically important sedation or impairment of psychomotor function. Furthermore, it appears that continued exposure to benzodiazepines results in adaptation to its central depressant effects, although not necessarily to the anxiolytic effects. Therefore, many individuals who experience sedation early in the course of therapy find that sedative effects wane despite continuation of therapy at the same dosage.

Antihistamines

Certain antihistaminic agents having secondary sedative effects are promoted for the treatment of anxiety. The most popular of these is hydroxyzine (Vistaril, Atarax).[26] As in the case of barbiturates and meprobamate, the CNS depressant effects of these drugs are very nonspecific, and it is not established that they have any particular value in the treatment of the majority of individuals with symptomatic anxiety. They may, however, be of some benefit for individuals in whom combination anxiolytic-antihistaminic therapy is indicated. This may include patients suffering from pruritic allergic dermatoses of unknown etiology in which anxiety is thought to play a contributory or precipitating role.

Major Tranquilizers (Antipsychotic Agents)

Major tranquilizers (neuroleptic or antipsychotic agents) are extensively promoted for the treatment of anxiety in ambulatory nonpsychotic individuals. The primary pharmacologic property of this class of drugs is dopaminergic receptor blockade, which appears to account for their antipsychotic properties.[27] Nonspecific sedation produced by this class of agents varies from drug to drug and is a secondary pharmacologic property. Major tranquilizers do appear to have antianxiety effects in anxious nonpsychotic individuals. The mechanism of anxiolytic effect is not well established and may not be attributable to nonspecific CNS depression.

Although appropriate doses of major tranquilizers appear to have anxiolytic effects comparable to those of benzodiazepines,[28–31] neuroleptic agents are seldom if ever the drugs of first choice in the treatment of anxiety unassociated with psychosis or other schizophrenic thought disorder. These drugs have a variety of other effects on the autonomic nervous system and other major organ systems, leading to numerous possible adverse reactions associated with usual therapeutic dosage.[27] The frequency of adverse reactions associated with the use of these drugs in nonpsychotic patients generally is unacceptably high and usually greatly exceeds those attributable to benzodiazepines, both in nature and severity. Furthermore, it is increasingly evident that long-term use of major tranquilizers carries the hazard of tardive dyskinesia, a disfiguring and sometimes irreversible disorder of involuntary movement. These important drawbacks should be considered by all clinicians who contemplate use of major tranquilizers as anxiolytics.

Antidepressants

Tricyclic antidepressants and monoamine oxidase inhibitors are sometimes prescribed for the treatment of anxiety. This approach has justification in some cases since anxious individuals can also experience concurrent manifestations of depression. As in the case of major tranquilizers, the anxiolytic effect of antidepressant agents probably is no greater than that of benzodiazepines. Furthermore, most individuals experience unwanted autonomic side effects during treatment with therapeutic doses of tricyclic antidepressants. For this reason, the general use of antidepressants in anxious patients cannot be recommended. It should be emphasized, however, that patients whose primary disorder is endogenous depression, but who also have a component of anxiety, may experience relief of both types of symptoms when tricyclic antidepressants are appropriately administered.

Beta-Adrenergic Blocking Agents

Benzodiazepines and other sedative-hypnotic agents influence the clinical manifestations of anxiety presumably due to their effects on the CNS. The use of beta blockers as anxiolytics constitutes a different approach to drug therapy, inasmuch as these agents interfere with beta-adrenergic transmission outside the central nervous system. The use of beta blockers as anxiolytics has substantial theoretical rationale, since many of the somatic manifestations of anxiety are mediated by the beta-adrenergic sympathetic system.[32] However, the clinical use of beta blockers in antianxiety therapy has not been consistently satisfactory.[16] Even for those individuals whose primary manifestations of anxiety are precisely those that are beta-adrenergically mediated (such as tachycardia, palpitations, tremor, etc.), beta blockers are not predictably effective and are certainly no more effective than benzodiazepines.[16] There does appear to be some value in short-term treatment with beta-adrenergic blockers in acutely stressful situations in which manifestations of beta-adrenergic hyperactivity interfere with performance and reinforce a self-perpetuating cycle of acute symptomatic anxiety. Examples include public speaking, job interviews, oral examinations, or athletic events.[33,34] In such cases beta blockers generally produce considerable symptomatic improvement, probably due to their ability to interrupt the cycle of beta-adrenergic hyperactivity and anxiety. The use of beta blockers as anxiolytics in these and other situations requires further evaluation.

DRUG MONOGRAPHS

BARBITURATES

AMOBARBITAL (Amytal) C-II
AMOBARBITAL SODIUM (Amytal Sodium) C-II
BUTABARBITAL SODIUM (Butisol Sodium) C-III
PHENOBARBITAL C-IV

'Intermediate-acting' and 'long-acting' barbiturates are used in the treatment of anxiety.[19,20,35,36] The distinction between intermediate and long action is mythological, since all three of these drugs have a long effective duration of action.[37]

The clinical value of barbiturates as anxiolytic agents is limited by the very narrow range between their antianxiety effects and their nonspecific depressant properties. Many individuals experience relief of anxiety only at doses that produce oversedation and impairment of psychomotor function. The advantage of barbiturates is their relatively low cost, particularly if they are prescribed (and dispensed) as generic drugs.

During long-term treatment of anxiety with barbiturates, development of adaptation or tolerance is common. That is, the drugs may lose their effectiveness despite continuation of the same dose, or even with increasing doses. This effect is partly explained by the stimulatory effect of barbiturates on hepatic microsomal enzymes,[38,39] causing steady-state blood concentrations to fall over time as the drugs stimulate their own metabolism. Furthermore, adaptation or tolerance to drug effects may also develop at their sites of action in the central nervous system.

For these and other reasons, effective doses of barbiturates vary widely between individuals. Therapy should be initiated with a relatively low dose, then gradually increased upward (with dose changes no more often than twice weekly) until clinical effectiveness is achieved or side effects limit therapy. Some degree of tolerance to nonspecific CNS depressant effects generally develops over time, without necessarily a loss of anxiolytic effect. Due to the long duration of action of barbiturates mentioned above, it is feasible and usually desirable to give the entire dose at bedtime. Some persons may require supplemental doses during the day, particularly when they face intermittent, acutely stressful situations.

See Chapters 33 and 37 for further discussion on use of barbiturates as hypnotic agents and as anticonvulsants.

Adverse Reactions—The most common unwanted effects are attributable to nonspecific CNS depression: somnolence, drowsiness, ataxia, diplopia, dysarthria, and impairment of intellectual function. Due to the enzyme inducing properties of barbiturates, some patients on long-term barbiturate therapy develop hypocalcemia and occasionally hypocalcemic bone disease.[40,41] This is attributable to the stimulatory effect of barbiturates on the catabolism of vitamin D.

Because barbiturate clearance is reduced in the elderly[42] and in those with liver disease,[43–45] lower doses should be administered to such patients.

Drug Interactions—Barbiturate treatment results in stimulation of hepatic microsomal enzymes responsible for the biotransformation of a number of drugs. Although this interaction is only rarely of clinical significance, it is always important in patients concurrently taking coumarin anticoagulants.[38,39] In coumarin-treated patients, concurrent barbiturate therapy should be avoided if at all possible; if barbiturates must be coadministered, the prothrombin time should be carefully monitored. Conversely, close monitoring of anticoagulant dosage and prothrombin times is essential after barbiturate therapy is discontinued, since 'rebound' prothrombin time prolongation may occur.

The CNS depressant effects of barbiturates are additive with those of any other drug that depresses the CNS. Of particular importance is ethanol. Persons taking barbiturates should be cautioned about the potential hazards of ethanol coingestion.

The hazards of barbiturate overdosage are substantial.[21] Serious and even fatal intoxication can occur with ingested doses exceeding the usual therapeutic dose by only 10 to 20 times. Accordingly, only small numbers of tablets should be prescribed at any given time, and the number of refills should be limited.

Dosage—Adults, 45 to 200 mg daily. Most or all of the daily dose can be given at bedtime.

PROPANEDIOLS

MEPROBAMATE (Equanil, Miltown) C-IV
TYBAMATE (Tybatran)

Despite initial enthusiasm for meprobamate as a relatively specific antianxiety agent, controlled studies performed since its release in 1955 indicate that meprobamate has no clearly documented benefits over barbiturates.[24,25] Furthermore, the spectrum of adverse reactions to meprobamate is similar to that of barbiturates. Experience with tybamate is limited, although early studies suggested that its addicting potential may be somewhat less than that of meprobamate.[46] A potential benefit of meprobamate is its low cost when prescribed as a generic compound. Tybamate, however, is an expensive drug.

Adverse Reactions—Unwanted effects of meprobamate resemble those of barbiturates. The most common is dose-related CNS depression, including drowsiness, sedation, ataxia, dysarthria, and impaired psychomotor function. Doses slightly exceeding the usual therapeutic range can produce dependence and addiction. Meprobamate overdosage is a potential medical hazard,[47] making it essential that only small number of pills be provided with any given prescription. As with most drugs, rare cases of hematologic toxicity have been reported.

Drug Interactions—Additive CNS depression occurs when propanediols are combined with other central depressant drugs. Enzyme inducing effects of meprobamate are reported in animal studies but have not been substantiated in human investigations.[38]

Dosage—Since there is little information on the relation of dose or plasma concentration of meprobamate to clinical effects, most patients are arbitrarily prescribed the same dosage, with little room for flexibility. The usual starting dose is 800 to 1600 mg a day in four divided doses. Since the elimination half-life of meprobamate is approximately 12 hours,[48] it is possible to administer the drug in doses of 600 mg twice daily. The usual dose of tybamate is 750 to 2000 mg daily in divided doses.

BENZODIAZEPINES

Benzodiazepine derivatives are by far the most common anxiolytic agents. Their advantage over barbiturates and meprobamate in terms

TABLE 1 Preparations and Costs of Antianxiety Agents

Generic Name	Trademark Name(s)	Preparations and 1978 Costs
Barbiturates		
Amobarbital	Amytal	Tablets 15 mg—$1.29/100; 30 mg—$1.72/100; 50 mg—$1.91/100; 100 mg—$3.19/100 Elixir 44 mg/5 ml—$6.18/pint
Amobarbital Sodium	Amytal Sodium	Capsules 65 mg—$2.55/100; 200 mg—$5.85/100 Injection (powder) 125 mg—$0.88/ampul; 250 mg—$1.12/ampul; 500 mg—$1.65/ampul
Butabarbital Sodium	Buticaps	Capsules 15 mg—$2.80/100; 30 mg—$3.50/100; 50 mg—$4.45/100; 100 mg—$5.10/100
	Butisol Sodium	Tablets 15 mg—$2.03/100; 30 mg—$2.68/100; 50 mg—$3.50/100; 100 mg—$4.15/100 Elixir 30 mg/5ml—$3.80/pint
Phenobarbital	generic	Tablets 15 mg—$0.50–$1.00/100; 30 mg—$0.55–$1.50/100; 60 mg—$0.70–$0.75/100; 100 mg—$0.68–$1.25/100
Propanediols		
Meprobamate	Equanil	Capsules 400 mg—$6.17/50 Tablets 200 mg—$5.64/100; 400 mg—$17.06/100
	Miltown	Tablets 200 mg—$5.20/100; 400 mg—$6.50/100; 600 mg—$10.08/100
	generic	Tablets 200 mg—$0.75–$4.85/100; 400 mg—$0.98–$2.76/100
Tybamate	Tybatran	Capsules 250 mg—$8.60/100; 350 mg—$11.20/100
Benzodiazepines		
Chlordiazepoxide	Libritabs	Tablets 5 mg—$5.84/100; 10 mg—$8.34/100; 25 mg—$12.53/100

TABLE 1 *(continued)*

Generic Name	Trademark Name(s)	Preparations and 1978 Costs
Chlordiazepoxide Hydrochloride	Librium (A-poxide) (Chlordiazachel) (SK-Lygen)	Capsules 5 mg—$5.79/100; 10 mg—$8.14/100; 25 mg—$12.49/100 Injection (powder) 100mg—$0.77/ampul
Diazepam	Valium	Tablets 2 mg—$7.46/100; 5 mg—$9.50/100; 10 mg—$14.10/100 Injection (solution) 5 mg/ml—$0.87/2-ml ampul, $3.93/10-ml vial
Clorazepate Dipotassium	Tranxene	Capsules 3.75 mg—$7.95/100; 7.5 mg—$10.19/100; 15 mg—$16.03/100
	Tranxene SD	Tablets (timed-release) 11.25 mg—$22.30/100; 22.5 mg—$26.81/100
Prazepam	Verstran	Tablets 10 mg—$9.70/100
Oxazepam	Serax	Capsules 10 mg—$7.62/100; 15 mg—$9.71/100; 30 mg—$14.32/100 Tablets 15 mg—$9.71/100
Lorazepam	Ativan	Tablets 1 mg—$10.88/100; 2 mg—$16.46/100
Antihistamines		
Hydroxyzine Hydrochloride	Atarax	Tablets 10 mg—$8.05/100; 25 mg—$11.82/100; 50 mg—$14.42/100; 100 mg—$17.71/100
	Vistaril IM	Injection (solution) 25 mg/ml—$5.56/10-ml vial; 50 mg/ml—$8.90/10-ml vial; 100 mg/ml—$1.78/2-ml vial
Hydroxyzine Pamoate	Vistaril	Capsules 25 mg—$11.82/100; 50 mg—$14.42/100; 100 mg—$17.71/100 Suspension 25 mg/5ml—$18.03/pint
Beta-Adrenergic Antagonists		
Propranolol	Inderal	Tablets 10 mg—$4.10/100; 40 mg—$7.08/100; 80 mg—$11.32/100

of safety and efficacy is reasonably well-established. However, benzodiazepines are relatively expensive.

Six benzodiazepines are available as anxiolytics, and there is no consistent evidence that any one is superior to the rest.[15,16] There are differences among drugs in pharmacokinetic characteristics, which may influence the choice of dosage schedule.[49,50]

CHLORDIAZEPOXIDE (Libritabs) C-IV
CHLORDIAZEPOXIDE HYDROCHLORIDE (A-poxide, Chlordiazachel, Librium, SK-Lygen) C-IV
DIAZEPAM (Valium) C-IV
CLORAZEPATE DIPOTASSIUM (Tranxene) C-IV
CLORAZEPATE MONOPOTASSIUM (Azene) C-IV
PRAZEPAM (Verstran) C-IV

These benzodiazepine derivatives are characterized by a long effective duration of clinical action, and accumulation during multiple-dose therapy. After initiation of therapy with one of these compounds, drug accumulation to the steady-state condition is usually complete within five to fourteen days of therapy. Pharmacologic activity may be due either to the parent compound, active metabolic products, or a combination of the two. In the case of clorazepate and prazepam, the two compounds are biotransformed to desmethyldiazepam prior to reaching the systemic circulation. Desmethyldiazepam is also a major metabolite of diazepam, and a minor metabolite of chlordiazepoxide.

Owing to extensive drug accumulation, therapy with these compounds usually can be initiated or maintained with a single daily dose at bedtime.[51–54] Alternatively, if divided doses are indicated, two-thirds of the daily dose can be given at bedtime. An example of this type of schedule would be: diazepam, 10 to 15 mg as a single dose at bedtime; or diazepam, 10 mg at bedtime and 5 mg at noon. As with all anxiolytics, there is considerable individual variation in clinical response, making careful titration of dosage and monitoring of clinical response essential. Despite drug accumulation during multiple-dose therapy, cumulative clinical sedation is usually not encountered owing to adaptation of the CNS to the effects of the drugs.

OXAZEPAM (Serax) C-IV
LORAZEPAM (Ativan) C-IV

These two benzodiazepines already have a 3-hydroxy substitution, rendering them immediately susceptible to glucuronidation in the liver, followed by excretion in the urine of the water-soluble glucuronide metabolite.[49,55] Since the elimination half-life of these two compounds is considerably shorter than those of the other benzodiazepines, they should be given on a multiple daily dose basis. In the case of oxazepam, three to four daily doses are necessary; for lorazepam, two to three doses per day is appropriate. Again, titration of dose and clinical response is essential. Attainment of steady-state is generally rapid with these two compounds, owing to their short elimination half-life.

Adverse Reactions—Dose-dependent CNS depression is the most common adverse effect. However, most patients can achieve an adequate antianxiety response without evidence of overt clinical sedation or impairment of psychomotor function. Due to CNS adaptation, drowsiness experienced early in the course of therapy may remit spontaneously despite continuation of the same dosage. Numerous other adverse effects of benzodiazepines are described,[15] but most of these are exceedingly rare and are generally not of realistic clinical concern in the great majority of patients. As with other CNS depressant drugs, patients should be cautioned about the possibility of additive effects if the drugs are combined with alcohol. However, there is no evidence of a specific synergistic or super-additive effect attributable to the combination of benzodiazepines and ethanol.[56]

The effects of age and liver disease on benzodiazepine clearance are not clearly established. It may be that these conditions do not have the same effect on the clearance of all benzodiazepines.[45,57,58] In any case, the drugs should be administered with caution to the elderly and to those with hepatic dysfunction.[59,60]

Drug Interactions—Very few, if any, clinically important drug interactions have been attributed to benzodiazepine therapy. There is no evidence that these drugs cause enzyme induction in humans. Some studies suggest an impairment of absorption of desmethyldiazepam from clorazepate when the latter is coadministered with antacids.[61] Accordingly, another benzodiazepine should probably be utilized in patients taking antacids.

Dosage—Oral: Adults, chlordiazepoxide: 15 to 100 mg a day in single or divided doses; diazepam, 40 to 60 mg a day in single or divided doses; clorazepate, 11.25 to 60 mg a day in single or divided doses; prazepam, 10 to 60 mg a day in single or divided doses; oxazepam, 30 to 120 mg a day in three or four divided doses; lorazepam, 1.5 to 6 mg a day in two or three divided doses. *Parenteral: Adults,* only chlordiazepoxide and diazepam are currently available for parenteral administration. Since they are slowly absorbed following intramuscular injection,[62–64] they should be given by slow intravenous infusion rather than an intramuscular injection whenever parenteral administration is indicated. The usual single parenteral dose is 50 to 100 mg of chlordiazepoxide or 5 to 10 mg of diazepam. Cardiovascular and respiratory depression during parenteral administration of benzodiazepines is exceedingly unusual except in individuals with serious underlying disease. Nonetheless, as with parenteral administration of any CNS depressant compound, intravenous infusion should be slow and accompanied by careful clinical monitoring. Rapid bolus injections of chlordiazepoxide and diazepam are hazardous, probably due to the irritating nature of the oily solvent vehicle.

ANTIHISTAMINES

HYDROXYZINE HYDROCHLORIDE (Atarax, Vistaril IM)
HYDROXYZINE PAMOATE (Vistaril)

The nonspecific sedative effects of hydroxyzine, an antihistaminic compound, have led to its utilization as an anxiolytic agent. Although reasonably effective as a preoperative medication, the efficacy of hydroxyzine as an oral anxiolytic agent in ambulatory individuals is not adequately established.[26] Furthermore, there is little pharmacokinetic data on the disposition of hydroxyzine in humans.

Adverse Reactions—CNS depression is the major unwanted effect. Because hydroxyzine, like other antihistamines, has anticholinergic properties, central and peripheral anticholinergic toxicity is possible. Such effects include confusion, disorientation, or delirium, as well as the usual peripheral manifestations of mydriasis, cycloplegia, dry mouth and mucous membranes, tachycardia, and impaired motility of bowel and bladder.[65] It is likely that elderly individuals are more susceptible to anticholinergic toxicity.

Drug Interactions—Hydroxyzine may be expected to have additive effects with other drugs that have anticholinergic properties. These include certain classes of phenothiazines, tricyclic antidepressants, antiparkinsonism agents, and belladonna alkaloids or other synthetic anticholinergics used to treat gastrointestinal disorders.

Dosage—Oral: Adults, 30 to 200 mg per day in divided doses. *Parenteral: Adults,* although usually given by intramuscular injection, the rate and completion of absorption of hydroxyzine when given by this route is not established. The usual dose is 25 to 100 mg.

BETA-ADRENERGIC BLOCKING AGENTS

PROPRANOLOL (Inderal)

The use of beta blocking agents in anxiolytic therapy represents a conceptual departure from therapy with other agents (listed above) that act primarily on the CNS. By virtue of their ability to block beta-adrenergic receptors, propranolol in theory could interrupt those peripheral manifestations of anxiety mediated by the beta sympathetic nervous system. Such effects include tachycardia, palpitations, feeling of the heart pounding, tremulousness, and diaphoresis. Despite the sound rationale of this approach, propranolol and other beta blockers appear to be no more effective than benzodiazepines in the treatment of anxiety, even when manifestations are mainly somatic in nature.[16]

Beta blockade may have potential value in the treatment of anxiety associated with short-term acute situational stress. At the present time, propranolol is not indicated for the treatment of anxiety by the Food and Drug Administration.

Adverse Reactions—Unwanted effects of propranolol are outlined in detail in Chapter 21. The drug should be used with great caution, if at all, in patients with cardiovascular disease whose cardiac compensation is maintained by sympathetic stimulation.[66,67] Propranolol can also precipitate bronchospasm and should be avoided in patients with a history of this disorder. It should also be used with caution in patients with diabetes, particularly those who are insulin-dependent. In healthy individuals with normal cardiovascular function, the hazards of propranolol are minimal.

Drug Interactions—Numerous drug interactions have been described for propranolol, but most of these are anecdotal in nature and have uncertain clinical significance.[68] See Chapter 21 for further discussion.

Dosage—Oral: Adults, single-dose therapy for acute anxiety, 10 to 40 mg by mouth approximately one hour prior to the anticipated stressful event. For chronic therapy, 30 to 160 mg per day in two to four divided doses. *Parenteral: Adults,* 1 to 5 mg by slow intravenous infusion with careful monitoring.

REFERENCES

1. Shader RI, Greenblatt DJ: The psychopharmacologic treatment of anxiety states. In *Manual of Psychiatric Therapeutics.* Edited by RI Shader. Boston, Little, Brown and Company, 1975, pp. 27–38.
2. Johnson G: The recognition and management of anxiety states. Med J Aust 2:643–645, 1975.
3. Lader M: The nature of anxiety. Br J Psychiatry 121:481–491, 1972.
4. Marks I, Lader M: Anxiety states (anxiety neurosis): a review. J Nerv Ment Dis 156:3–18, 1973
5. Woodruff RA Jr, Guze SB, Clayton PJ: Anxiety neurosis among psychiatric outpatients. Compr Psychiatry 13:165–170, 1972.
6. Greenblatt DJ, Shader RI, Koch-Weser J: Psychotropic drug use in the Boston area: a report from the Boston Collaborative Drug Surveillance Program. Arch Gen Psychiatry 32:518–521, 1975.
7. Parry HJ, Balter MB, Mellinger GD, et al: National patterns of psychotherapeutic drug use. Arch Gen Psychiatry 28:769–783, 1973.
8. Gardner EA: Implications of psychoactive drug therapy. N Engl J Med 290:800–802, 1974.
9. Miller RR: Prescribing habits of physicians: a review of studies on prescribing of drugs. Drug Intel Clin Pharm 7:492–500; 557–564, 1973; 8:81–91, 1974.
10. Lennard HL, Epstein LJ, Bernstein A, et al: Hazards implicit in prescribing psychoactive drugs. Science 169:438–441, 1970.
11. Muller C: The overmedicated society: forces in the marketplace for medical care. Science 176:488–492, 1972.
12. Greenblatt DJ, Shader RI: Bad trips. In *Manual of Psychiatric Therapeutics.* Edited by RI Shader. Boston, Little, Brown and Company, 1975, pp. 185–193.
13. Greenblatt DJ, Shader RI: Treatment of the alcohol withdrawal syndrome. In *Manual of Psychiatric Therapeutics.* Edited by RI Shader. Boston, Little, Brown and Company, 1975, pp. 211–235.
14. Perkins R, Hinton J: Sedative or tranquillizer? A comparison of the hypnotic effects of chlordiazepoxide and amylobarbitone sodium. Br J Psychiatry 124:435–439, 1974.
15. Greenblatt DJ, Shader RI: *Benzodiazepines in Clinical Practice.* New York, Raven Press, 1974.
16. Greenblatt DJ, Shader RI: Pharmacotherapy of anxiety with benzodiazepines and β-adrenergic blockers. In *Psychopharmacology: A Generation of Progress.* Edited by MA Lipton, A DiMascio, KF Killam. New York, Raven Press, 1978, pp. 1381–1389.
17. Greenblatt DJ, Shader RI: Psychotropic drugs in the general hospital. In *Manual of Psychiatric Therapeutics.* Edited by RI Shader. Boston, Little, Brown and Company, 1975, pp. 1–26.
18. Meares R: The place of barbiturates in psychiatric treatment. Med J Aust 1:1207–1209, 1970.

19. Lader MH, Bond AJ, James DC: Clinical comparison of anxiolytic drug therapy. Psychol Med 4:381–387, 1974.
20. Cohen J, Gomez E, Hoell NL, et al: Diazepam and phenobarbital in the treatment of anxiety: a controlled multicenter study using physician and patient rating scales. Curr Ther Res 20:184–193, 1976.
22. Berger FM: The similarities and differences between meprobamate and barbiturates. Clin Pharmacol Ther 4:209–231, 1963.
23. Ludwig BJ, Potterfield JR: The pharmacology of propanediol carbamates. Adv Pharmacol Chemother 1:173–240, 1971.
24. Laties VG, Weiss B: A critical review of the efficacy of meprobamate (Miltown, Equanil) in the treatment of anxiety. J Chronic Dis 7:500–519, 1958.
25. Greenblatt DJ, Shader RI: Meprobamate: a study of irrational drug use. Am J Psychiatry 127:1297–1303, 1971.
26. Barranco SF, Bridger W: Treatment of anxiety with oral hydroxyzine: an overview. Curr Ther Res 22:217–227, 1977.
27. Shader RI, Jackson AH: Approaches to schizophrenia. In *Manual of Psychiatric Therapeutics*. Edited by RI Shader. Boston, Little, Brown and Company, 1975, pp. 63–100.
28. Sarteschi P, Cassano GB, Castrogiovanni P, et al: Major and minor tranquilizers in the treatment of anxiety states. Arzneim Forsch 22:93–97, 1972.
29. Stevenson J, Burrows GD, Chiu E: Comparison of low doses of haloperidol and diazepam in anxiety states. Med J Aust 1:451–452, 1976.
30. Rickels K, Weise CC, Whalen EM, et al: Haloperidol in anxiety. J Clin Pharmacol 11:440–449, 1971.
31. Yamamoto J, Kline FM, Burgoyne RW: The treatment of severe anxiety in outpatients: a controlled study comparing chlordiazepoxide and chlorpromazine. Psychosomatics 14:46–51, 1973.
32. Jefferson JW: Beta-adrenergic receptor blocking drugs in psychiatry. Arch Gen Psychiatry 31:681–691, 1974.
33. Krishnan G: Oxprenolol in the treatment of examination stress. Curr Med Res Opin 4:241–243, 1976.
34. James IM, Griffith DNW, Pearson RM, et al: Effect of oxprenolol on stage-fright in musicians. Lancet 2:952–954, 1977.
35. Stotsky BA: Sodium butabarbital for emotional disorders and insomnia. Dis Nerv Syst 33:798–802, 1972.
36. General Practitioner Research Group: Phenobarbitone compared with an inactive placebo in anxiety states. Practitioner 192:147–151, 1964.
37. Parke DV: Biochemistry of the barbiturates. In *Acute Barbiturate Poisoning*. Edited by H Matthew. Amsterdam, Excerpta Medica, 1971, pp. 7–53.
38. Greenblatt DJ, Shader RI: The clinical choice of sedative-hypnotics. Ann Intern Med 77:91–100, 1972.
39. Greenblatt DJ, Shader RI, Lofgren S: Rational psychopharmacology for patients with medical diseases. Annu Rev Med 27:407–420, 1976.
40. Richens A: The clinical consequences of chronic hepatic enzyme induction by anticonvulsant drugs. Br J Clin Pharmacol 1:185–187, 1974.
41. Hahn TJ, Hendin BA, Scharp CR, et al: Serum 25-hydroxycalciferol levels and bone mass in children on chronic anticonvulsant therapy. N Engl J Med 292:550–554, 1975.
42. Richey DP, Bender AD: Pharmacokinetic consequences of aging. Annu Rev Pharmacol Toxicol 17:49–65, 1977.
43. Mawer GE, Miller NE, Turnberg LA: Metabolism of amylobarbitone in patients with chronic liver disease. Br J Pharmacol 44:549–560, 1972.
44. Alvin J, McHorse T, Hoyumpa A, et al: The effect of liver disease in man on the disposition of phenobarbital. J Pharmacol Exp Ther 192:224–235, 1975.
45. Schenker S, Hoyumpa AM Jr, Wilkinson GR: The effect of parenchymal liver disease on the disposition and elimination of sedatives and analgesics. Med Clin North Am 59:887–896, 1975.
46. Feldman HS, Mulinos MG: Lack of addiction from high doses of tybamate. J New Drugs 6:354–360, 1966.

47. Allen MD, Greenblatt DJ, Noel BJ: Meprobamate overdosage: a continuing problem. Clin Toxicol 11:501–516, 1977.
48. Hollister LE, Levy G: Kinetics of meprobamate elimination in humans. Chemotherapia 9:20–24, 1964.
49. Greenblatt DJ, Shader RI, Koch-Weser J: Pharmacokinetics in clinical medicine: oxazepam versus other benzodiazepines. Dis Nerv Syst 36(No.5,Sect.2):6–13, (May) 1975.
50. Greenblatt DJ, Shader RI: Pharmacokinetic understanding of antianxiety drug therapy. South Med J 71(Supp 2):2–9, 1978.
51. Burrows GD, Dumovic P, Smith JA, et al: A controlled comparative trial of clorazepate (Tranxene) and diazepam (Valium) for anxiety. Med J Aust 2:525–528, 1977.
52. Magnus RV, Dean BC, Curry SH: Clorazepate: double blind crossover comparison of a single nightly dose with diazepam thrice daily in anxiety. Dis Nerv Syst 38:819–821, 1977.
53. General Practitioner Research Group: A single-dose anti-anxiety drug. Practitioner 215:98–101, 1975.
54. Magnus RV: Once-a-day potassium clorazepate in anxiety. Br J Clin Pract 27:449–452, 1973.
55. Greenblatt DJ, Schillings RT, Kyriakopoulos AA, et al: Clinical pharmacokinetics of lorazepam. I. Absorption and disposition of ^{14}C-lorazepam. Clin Pharmacol Ther 20:329–341, 1976.
56. Greenblatt DJ, Shader RI, Weinberger DR, et al: Effect of a cocktail on diazepam absorption. Psychopharmacology 57:199–203, 1978.
57. Shull HJ Jr, Wilkinson GR, Johnson R, et al: Normal disposition of oxazepam in acute viral hepatitis and cirrhosis. Ann Intern Med 84:420–425, 1976.
58. Klotz U, Avant GR, Hoyumpa A, et al: The effects of age and liver disease on the disposition and elimination of diazepam in adult man. J Clin Invest 55:347–359, 1975.
59. Boston Collaborative Drug Surveillance Program: Clinical depression of the central nervous system due to diazepam and chlordiazepoxide in relation to cigarette smoking and age. N Engl J Med 288:277–280, 1973.
60. Greenblatt DJ, Allen MD, Shader RI: Toxicity of high-dose flurazepam in the elderly. Clin Pharmacol Ther 21:355–361, 1977.
61. Shader RI, Georgotas A, Greenblatt DJ, et al: Impaired absorption of desmethyldiazepam from clorazepate by coadministration of antacid. Clin Pharmacol Ther 23:129, 1978.
62. Greenblatt DJ, Shader RI, Koch-Weser J, et al: Slow absorption of intramuscular chlordiazepoxide. N Engl J Med 291:1116–1118, 1974.
63. Greenblatt DJ, Shader RI, MacLeod SM, et al: Absorption of oral and intramuscular chlordiazepoxide. Eur J Clin Pharmacol 13:267–274, 1978.
64. Hillestad L, Hansen T, Melsom H, et al: Diazepam metabolism in normal man. I. Serum concentrations and clinical effects after intravenous, intramuscular, and oral administration. Clin Pharmacol Ther 16:479–489, 1974.
65. Greenblatt DJ, Shader RI: Drug therapy: anticholinergics. N Engl J Med 288:1215–1219, 1973.
66. Greenblatt DJ, Koch-Weser J: Adverse reactions to propranolol in hospitalized medical patients: a report from the Boston Collaborative Drug Surveillance Program. Am Heart J 86:478–484, 1973.
67. Greenblatt DJ, Koch-Weser J: Adverse reactions to beta-adrenergic receptor blocking drugs: a report from the Boston Collaborative Drug Surveillance Program. Drugs 7:118–129, 1974.
68. Greenblatt DJ, Koch-Weser J: Clinical toxicity of propranolol and practolol: a report from the Boston Collaborative Drug Surveillance Program. In *Cardiovascular Drugs, Vol. 2: β-Adrenoceptor Blocking Drugs*.ugs. Edited by GS Avery. New York, ADIS Press Australasia Pty Ltd, 1977, pp. 179–195.

35. ANTIPSYCHOTIC AGENTS

David J. Greenblatt and Richard I. Shader

The availability of pharmacologic agents that are effective in mitigating the disordered behavior and thought processes of psychotic patients has revolutionized the approach to treatment of major mental illness.[1] Prior to 1950, therapeutic modalities generally focused upon custodial care, together with a variety of inconsistently effective somatic therapies (such as insulin coma) and nonspecific central depressant medications (such as barbiturates). Modern antipsychotic agents, of which chlorpromazine is the prototype, allow relatively specific pharmacotherapy of the syndrome of schizophrenia.[2] In many cases, these drugs appear to induce essentially complete remission, allowing patients to return to healthy and productive lives. Many antipsychotic agents are now available for clinical use.[2-4] They vary considerably in their spectrum of side effects and secondary pharmacologic properties, yet none has improved upon or substantially altered the general range of clinical efficacy of older drugs such as chlorpromazine.[5,6]

CLASSIFICATION OF ANTIPSYCHOTIC AGENTS

Nearly twenty antipsychotic drugs are currently available in the United States. All have similar antischizophrenic properties, yet they differ considerably in milligram potency and in secondary pharmacologic properties. The majority are phenothiazine derivatives, which can be subdivided into three major categories, depending upon the structure of a critical side-chain substituent (Table 1). *Aliphatic* phenothiazines have a dimethylaminopropyl side chain. Chlorpromazine is the prototype of this class; triflupromazine is less commonly used. Promazine also is an aliphatic phenothiazine; this drug has most of the secondary pharmacologic properties of chlorpromazine and triflupromazine, yet is very weakly antipsychotic. *Piperidine*

TABLE 1 Preparations and Costs of Antipsychotic Agents

GENERIC NAME	TRADEMARK NAME(S)	PREPARATIONS AND 1978 COSTS
PHENOTHIAZINES		
Aliphatic Compounds		
Chlorpromazine Hydrochloride	Thorazine (Chlor-Pz)	Tablets 10 mg—$3.20/100; 25 mg—$3.80/100; 50 mg—$4.40/100; 100 mg—$5.40/100; 200 mg—$6.50/100 Capsules (timed-release) 30 mg—$4.20/50; 75 mg—$5.00/50; 150 mg—$5.90/50; 200 mg—$6.30/50; 300 mg—$7.00/50 Liquid (concentrate) 30 mg/ml—$2.05/4 oz; 100 mg/ml—$11.00/8 oz Syrup 10 mg/5ml—$1.35/4 oz Injection (solution) 25 mg/ml—$0.46/1-ml ampul, $0.64/2-ml ampul, $2.95/10-ml vial Suppositories 25 mg—$2.20/12; 100 mg—$2.75/12
Triflupromazine Hydrochloride	Vesprin	Tablets 10 mg—$6.26/50; 25 mg—$9.33/50; 50 mg—$12.50/50 Suspension 50 mg/5 ml—$6.40/4 oz Injection (solution) 10 mg/ml—$1.75/1-ml ampul, $5.68/10-ml vial; 20 mg/ml—$1.54/1-ml ampul
Piperidine Compounds		
Thioridazine Hydrochloride	Mellaril	Tablets 10 mg—$7.62/100; 15 mg—$9.00/100; 25 mg—$10.38/100; 50 mg—$11.28/100; 100 mg—$13.32/100; 150 mg—$17.46/100; 200 mg—$19.98/100 Liquid (concentrate) 30 mg/ml—$5.70/4 oz; 100 mg/ml—$15.24/4 oz
Mesoridazine Besylate	Serentil	Tablets 10 mg—$7.65/100; 25 mg—$10.23/100; 50 mg—$11.56/100; 100 mg—$14.14/100 Liquid (concentrate) 25 mg/ml—$6.72/4 oz Injection (solution) 25 mg/ml—$0.64/1-ml ampul

TABLE 1 *(continued)*

Generic Name	Trademark Name(s)	Preparations and 1978 Costs
Piperacetazine	Quide	Tablets 10 mg—$11.28/100; 25 mg—$16.59/100
Piperazine Compounds		
Trifluperazine Hydrochloride	Stelazine	Tablets 1 mg—$7.85/100; 2 mg—$10.05/100; 5 mg—$11.25/100; 10 mg—$14.10/100 Injection (solution) 2 mg/ml—$4.80/10-ml vial
Acetophenazine Maleate	Tindal	Tablets 20 mg—$5.73/100
Butaperazine Maleate	Repoise Maleate	Tablets 5 mg—$8.40/100; 10 mg—$10.70/100; 25 mg—$13.60/100
Carphenazine Maleate	Proketazine	Tablets 12.5 mg—$4.20/50; 25 mg—$4.96/50; 50 mg—$6.12/50 Liquid (concentrate) 50 mg/ml—$12.24/4 oz
Fluphenazine Decanoate	Prolixin Decanoate	Injection (solution in oil) 25 mg/ml—$2.87/1-ml ampul, $13.30/5-ml vial
Fluphenazine Enanthate	Prolixin Enanthate	Injection (solution in oil) 25 mg/ml—$2.96/1-ml ampul, $13.63/5-ml vial
Fluphenazine Hydrochloride	Prolixin (Permitil)	Tablets 1 mg—$5.55/50; 2.5 mg—$7.86/50; 5 mg—$10.18/50; 10 mg—$13.22/50 Injection (solution) 2.5 mg/ml—$7.15/10-ml vial
Perphenazine	Trilafon	Tablets 2 mg—$3.25/50; 4 mg—$4.46/50; 8 mg—$5.41/50; 16 mg—$7.28/50 Tablets (timed-release) 8 mg—$18.33/100 Liquid (concentrate) 16 mg/5 ml—$4.24/4 oz Injection (solution) 5 mg/ml—$0.60/1-ml ampul

TABLE 1 *(continued)*

Generic Name	Trademark Name(s)	Preparations and 1978 Costs
Prochlorperazine	Compazine	Suppositories 2.5 mg—$3.10/12; 5 mg—$3.50/12; 25 mg—$4.35/12
Prochlorperazine Edisylate	Compazine	Liquid (concentrate) 10 mg/ml—$6.75/4 oz Syrup 5 mg/5 ml—$2.45/4 oz Injection (solution) 5 mg/ml—$1.02/2-ml ampul, $4.60/10-ml vial
Proclorperazine Maleate	Compazine	Tablets 5 mg—$8.35/100; 10 mg—$10.85/100; 25 mg—$12.70/100 Capsules (timed-release) 10 mg—$7.90/50; 15 mg—$10.25/50; 30 mg—$11.55/30; 75 mg—$13.75/50
THIOXANTHENES		
Chlorprothixene	Taractan	Tablets 10 mg—$6.90/100; 25 mg—$9.52/100; 50 mg—$11.33/100; 100 mg—$14.19/100 Liquid (concentrate) 100 mg/5 ml—$11.99/pint Injection (solution) 12.5 mg/ml—$0.84/2-ml ampul
Thiothixene	Navane	Capsules 1 mg—$8.43/100; 2 mg—$10.91/100; 5 mg—$16.01/100; 10 mg—$21.43/100; 20 mg—$29.82/100
Thiothixene Hydrochloride	Navane	Liquid (concentrate) 5 mg/ml—$17.11/4 oz Injection (solution) 2 mg/ml—$0.67/2-ml ampul
BUTYROPHENONE		
Haloperidol	Haldol	Tablets 0.5 mg—$7.06/100; 1 mg—$10.10/100; 2 mg—$15.16/100; 5 mg—$21.25/100; 10 mg—$27.35/100 Liquid (concentrate) 2 mg/ml—$4.14/½ oz Injection (solution) 5 mg/ml—$0.99/1-ml ampul

TABLE 1 *(continued)*

GENERIC NAME	TRADEMARK NAME(S)	PREPARATIONS AND 1978 COSTS
MISCELLANEOUS		
Loxapine Succinate	Loxitane	Capsules 10 mg—\$12.96/100; 25 mg—\$19.54/100; 50 mg—\$25.76/100
Molindone Hydrochloride	Moban (Lidone)	Tablets 5 mg—\$7.95/100; 10 mg—\$10.30/100; 25 mg—\$15.30/100

substituted phenothiazines include thioridazine, mezoridazine, and piperacetazine. Finally, the *piperazine* subgroup of phenothiazines includes prochlorperazine, trifluoperazine, perphenazine, fluphenazine, carphenazine, butaperazine, and acetophenazine. This last subgroup has the highest milligram potency.

A second class of antipsychotic agents are the *thioxanthenes* which are only a minor molecular modification of the phenothiazines. Two derivatives are currently available. Chlorprothixene, having an aliphatic side chain, has pharmacologic properties similar or identical to those of chlorpromazine. Thiothixene, having a piperazine substitution, closely resembles the piperazine subgroup of phenothiazines. Subsequent discussion of aliphatic and piperazine phenothiazines implicitly apply to the corresponding types of thioxanthenes.

The *butyrophenone* antipsychotic agents bear no structural similarity to phenothiazines, but have pharmacologic properties resembling the piperazine phenothiazines. Haloperidol is the only butyrophenone specifically marketed in the United States as an antipsychotic. Droperidol has similar properties, but is used almost exclusively in anesthesia.

Two newer antipsychotic agents marketed in recent years include molindone, having a *dihydroindolone* structure, and loxapine, a *dibenzoxazepine*. Despite promotional claims that these two drugs have unique advantages over older antipsychotic agents, consistent scientific evidence for these claims is lacking.[7]

PHARMACOLOGIC PROPERTIES OF ANTIPSYCHOTIC DRUGS

Antipsychotic agents have a variety of pharmacologic effects, and in clinical practice can influence the function of almost every organ system. The ability to reverse the schizophrenic thought process is only one property—most of their other pharmacologic effects are considered to be secondary. In some cases these secondary properties can be exploited for clinical indications other than schizophrenia.

Dopamine Blockade

The primary pharmacologic effect of antipsychotic agents appears to involve postsynaptic blockade of dopamine receptors in the central nervous system.[8–10] Dopaminergic hyperactivity has been implicated in the genesis of schizophrenia. Antipsychotic agents have a high affinity for dopamine receptors, and their antipsychotic potency generally parallels their affinity for these receptors.[11,12] Unwanted extrapyramidal movements induced by antipsychotic drugs probably are also explained by their dopamine blocking properties. However, the nature of the interaction with dopamine receptors still is incompletely understood, since clinical antipsychotic effects can often be achieved without the production of movement disorders.

Alpha-Adrenergic Blockade

The major consequence of this property of antipsychotic agents is postural hypotension—clearly an unwanted effect.[2–4] Male sexual dysfunction is another possible consequence.[13] Aliphatic and piperidine phenothiazines are the most potent alpha-adrenergic antagonists. Piperazine phenothiazines and butyrophenones are the weakest.

Cholinergic Blockade

Cholinergic blocking properties of antipsychotic drugs approximately parallel their adrenergic blocking effects. Aliphatic and piperidine phenothiazines are the strongest cholinergic blockers, while piperazine phenothiazines and butyrophenones are the weakest. Cholinergic antagonism may offer some 'protection' against the development of extrapyramidal movement disorders, inasmuch as the strongest cholinergic antagonists are the least likely to produce early movement disorders.[14,15] In any case, anticholinergic effects of these drugs generally lead to typical atropine-like manifestations, and are usually categorized as unwanted side effects.

Nonspecific Sedation

Aliphatic and piperidine phenothiazines, and the newer drug loxapine, have strong nonspecific sedative properties, apparently unrelated to their antipsychotic effects. Considerable sedation results from administration of chlorpromazine, chlorprothixene, thioridazine or loxapine to normal nonpsychotic persons. On the other hand, piperazine phenothiazines and butyrophenones have relatively little sedating effects and, if anything, can produce stimulation in some individuals. Any antipsychotic drug, regardless of its nonspecific sedating properties, can appear to have a calming influence on agitated, psychotic individuals whose state of agitation and hyperactivity is attributable to the underlying disease. Theoretical arguments exist for utilizing 'sedating' antipsychotic drugs for patients with psychosis accompanied by agitation or combativeness, and 'activating' compounds in those with psychoses having aspects of retardation or social withdrawal. Controlled studies have not consistently supported this theoretical distinction.[16,17]

Antiemetic Effects

Butyrophenones and piperazine phenothiazines have strong antiemetic properties, apparently mediated via the central nervous system. The drugs are highly effective in the clinical treatment of nausea and vomiting due to a variety of causes, with the interesting exception of emesis induced by labyrinthine disorders or motion sickness. Aliphatic phenothiazines are less potent antiemetics than the above two classes, and piperidine phenothiazines have little or no antiemetic activity (see Chapter 66, Antiemetic Agents).

Impairment of Temperature Regulation

Essentially all antipsychotic drugs can produce thermoregulatory impairment. Animals receiving these agents lose their ability to defend themselves against changes in environmental temperature. They become hyper- or hypothermic depending upon the temperature of their surroundings.

Thermoregulatory impairment associated with antipsychotic drugs has been exploited for therapeutic purposes, to facilitate symptomatic normalization of body temperature in patients experiencing hypo- or hyperthermia from a number of causes. This property also can constitute a potential hazard of therapy, particularly in individuals who are exposed to very high or low environmental temperatures.[18]

CLINICAL USES OF ANTIPSYCHOTIC AGENTS

Schizophrenia and Schizophreniform Thought Disorders

The syndrome or symptom complex termed psychosis or schizophrenia is complicated and varied. It can represent an idiopathic, primary mental disorder, or can be a secondary manifestation of a large number of other medical diseases, metabolic derangements, or drug-induced states. As with any other syndrome or symptom complex, possible underlying causes should be considered in the differential diagnosis. Treatment of such underlying disorders, when present, constitutes the most rational approach to therapy.

According to the formulation of Shader and Jackson,[2] disordered thought is the primary manifestation of schizophrenia. The disease typically occurs in the setting of clear consciousness, with no abnormalities of orientation or memory. Common manifestations of schizophrenic thought include: muteness or reduced initiation of verbal communication; blocking, possibly including the subjective feeling of loss of control of one's own thoughts; personalized and concrete rather than abstract thought processes, together with the use of personalized language and logic; senseless repetition of words and phrases; diffuseness of conceptual boundaries and overinclusive thinking; and difficulties in recognizing and excluding irrelevant concepts and external stimuli from those that are relevant. Other manifestations commonly associated with schizophrenia include, visual and auditory hallucinations, paranoid ideation, inappropriate affect, social withdrawal, self-neglect, or extremes of psychomotor activity (overactivity or underactivity).

Assuming that treatable underlying causes are ruled out, administration of antipsychotic agents constitutes the therapeutic approach of choice in the majority of patients for whom a somatic therapy is indicated. Despite promotional claims by drug manufacturers that specific compounds are more or less effective in some subtypes of the clinical syndrome of schizophrenia, controlled studies have failed to demonstrate consistent differences among drugs.[5-7,16,17] Any antipsychotic agent, when properly administered in appropriate dosage, has approximately the same potential to induce remission. The clinical response to antipsychotic agents can vary greatly, depending on characteristics of the patient, the disease, and the social and genetic setting. When symptoms are of relatively acute onset and associated with clear precipitating factors, when a family history of schizophrenia is absent, and when the patient's premorbid history of interpersonal, social, and occupational function is good, the likelihood for a favorable response to therapy increases. Conversely, chronic symptoms or those of insidious onset, lack of overt situational precipitants, a family history of schizophrenia, and lack of constructive interpersonal relationships are associated with an unfavorable therapeutic response. Nonetheless, in the great majority of patients, the likelihood that pharmacotherapy will lead to some degree of clinical improvement is sufficient to warrant a therapeutic trial.

Antipsychotic drug therapy of schizophrenia generally can be divided into three stages. The initial or *loading* phase usually begins in the hospital setting. The specific indications for hospitalization are controversial, and the need for hospitalization of every patient is not clearly established. Yet it is common for acute schizophrenia to be associated with management problems best dealt with in the hospital. These include: the potential for the patient to injure himself or others, inappropriate or socially unacceptable behavior, or simply the inability of the patient to care for himself. Furthermore, the loading phase of pharmacotherapy usually involves relatively high doses of potentially hazardous drugs, and is best carried out under close supervision.

Loading therapy involves administration of relatively high doses at frequent intervals until symptoms are controlled and/or clinical improvement occurs.[19] Almost every antipsychotic drug has been used for this purpose, and the superiority of one specific drug over another is not established. The duration of the loading phase can range from several hours to several days, depending on the urgency of the situation. Likewise, the route of administration depends on specific clinical needs. Parenteral (usually intramuscular) administration may be indicated in patients who are violent, or who are unable or unwilling to take oral medications. Not surprisingly, the potential for rapid onset of relatively serious side effects increases as loading therapy becomes more intensive.

A typical approach to loading is administration of 1 to 10 mg of haloperidol by intramuscular injection every 30 minutes to 4 hours, to a maximum daily dose of approximately 50 mg. At present, recommendations for a specific drug or dosage schedule must be based more upon the treating physician's clinical experience and understanding rather than specific scientifically-established guidelines.

The *early maintenance* therapeutic phase follows after control of symptoms and initial clinical improvement is achieved during the loading phase. Early maintenance usually lasts from 5 to 15 days, generally is undertaken with the patient still hospitalized, and is concurrent with interpersonal therapy aimed at beginning to help the patient clarify and understand the nature and origins of his troubled state. Transition from the loading to early maintenance phases occurs as the daily dosage is gradually lowered such that side effects are reduced in intensity, but therapeutic efficacy is not sacrificed. This generally involves a carefully monitored downward titration of dosage, with reduction of the size and/or frequency of dosing. The patient learns to adapt to the subjective sensations associated with the medication, the inevitable side effects, and the need for compliance.

The *late maintenance* phase generally coincides with discharge from the hospital. Many schizophrenic patients—particularly those with long-standing disease—require some sort of maintenance drug therapy to prevent early relapse.[20–23] However, the precise dosage and duration of therapy are not well-established, and are determined by continued clinical monitoring and follow-up. Further downward titration of dosage on an outpatient basis may be possible for patients in prolonged remission. Unfortunately, the likelihood of noncompliance increases as the duration of remission increases, and it is likely that many relapses result from failure to take medication. Problems with compliance can be reduced by a once-daily (at bedtime) dosage schedule, thereby eliminating the need for remembering multiple daily doses, and possibly also reducing the intensity of unwanted effects. The availability of long-acting parenteral antipsychotic agents (such as fluphenazine decanoate) reduces compliance problems and thereby reduces the likelihood of relapse.[24–26] Fluphenazine decanoate is given as a single 12.5- to 50-mg intramuscular injection every 10 days to 4 weeks.

Drug-Induced Agitation and Delirium

Agitation, confusion, combativeness, delirium, and unmanageable excitement or panic can be induced by a number of drugs. It can accompany withdrawal from addicting drugs such as ethanol, barbiturates, or opiates. It can also be a feature of overdosage or poisoning with certain sympathomimetic agents (such as amphetamines or methylphenidate) or with anticholinergic drugs. The value of antipsychotic drugs in the treatment of these conditions depends on the nature of the syndrome and the specific drug involved.

Ethanol Withdrawal. Although antipsychotic agents are widely used to treat agitation and delirium (delirium tremens) associated with withdrawal from ethanol, extensive evidence, including some from double-blind controlled clinical trials, strongly suggests that hazards associated with their use (such as hypotension, cardiac arrhythmias, and impaired temperature regulation) outweigh the potential benefits.[27,28] High doses of sedative-hypnotic or antianxiety agents (particularly benzodiazepine derivatives) (see Chapters 33 and 34) are as effective as antipsychotic drugs and considerably less hazardous.

Similar considerations apply to the use of antipsychotics during withdrawal from barbiturates or opiates. Less hazardous and more specific agents are available for this purpose.

Sympathomimetic Poisoning. Excessive use of certain sympathomimetic agents, such as amphetamine derivatives and methylphenidate, can lead to severe agitation and panic.[29] This syndrome is sometimes termed 'amphetamine psychosis,' but differs in some important respects from idiopathic schizophrenia described above. Conservative therapy is usually sufficient for the treatment of amphetamine-induced agitation, and includes placement of the patient in quiet surroundings with frequent reassurance that the frightening subjective symptoms are drug-induced and will terminate shortly. Sympathomimetic-induced states generally are of short duration, due to rapid clearance of the offending agent.

Occasionally, agitation and panic become unmanageably severe, or medical complications (such as hypertension and/or hyperpyrexia) supervene. In such cases, antipsychotic drugs constitute highly specific therapy, probably due to their adrenergic and/or dopaminergic blocking capacity.[29,30] A single parenteral dose is often sufficient to produce rapid reversal of subjective and objective signs. Typical doses are chlorpromazine, 25 to 100 mg intramuscularly, or haloperidol, 0.5 to 5 mg intramuscularly. The dose may be repeated in four hours if necessary.

Anticholinergic Poisoning. 'Atropine psychosis,' a state of agitated delirium, can accompany poisoning by any of a number of anticholinergic agents, including over-the-counter sleep preparations, antihistamines, antiparkinsonian agents, and tricyclic antidepressants.[29,31,32] Because most antipsychotic agents have clinically important anticholinergic properties in themselves, they should not be used to treat this syndrome. Specific therapy in the form of physostigmine, a cholinesterase inhibitor, is available for treatment of this syndrome.

Nausea and Vomiting

Symptomatic treatment of nausea and vomiting is extremely common in clinical practice. The symptoms generally appear to cause the patient great distress, eliciting prompt administration of an antiemetic by well-meaning health care professionals. However, intervention with antiemetic drugs usually is undertaken too swiftly, without due consideration of the disadvantages and hazards of pharmacotherapy. Vomiting is a relatively dramatic physiologic event, but probably causes less actual subjective distress than it appears to. Furthermore, in most cases vomiting is self-limited, and will subside without specific therapy. Since emesis is a symptom or syndrome rather than a disease in itself, and may be a secondary manifestation of more serious underlying disorders, evaluation of the underlying pathology may be complicated by administration of symptomatic therapy.[33,34] Antiemetic agents are discussed in more detail in Chapter 66.

Fever

Elevated body temperature usually indicates the presence of infection or neoplastic disease, and will remit when and if the underlying disease process is controlled. Sometimes fever by itself can be life-threatening, in particular when body temperatures greater than 104°F are reached. This can occur in severe infection, disseminated neoplastic disease, following exposure to high environmental temperatures ('heat stroke'), or after general anesthesia. Salicylates and direct body cooling are the basis of symptomatic treatment of fever. The ability of antipsychotic agents to impair temperature regulation can be exploited for adjunctive therapeutic purposes.[33,34] A typical dosage is 25 to 100 mg of parenteral chlorpromazine, used together with other symptomatic measures. Care must be taken to avoid 'overshoot,' leading to potentially dangerous hypothermia.

Anxiety

Low doses of some antipsychotic agents are promoted for the treatment of anxiety in ambulatory nonpsychotic individuals. The efficacy of antipsychotic agents in this setting probably is equivalent to that of most commonly used antianxiety agents (see Chapter 34). However, the potential hazards of antipsychotic drugs almost always outweigh the benefits. Accordingly, antipsychotic agents should seldom if ever be the first choice of pharmacotherapy for anxious nonpsychotic individuals.

Other Uses of Antipsychotic Drugs

A number of uses for antipsychotic agents are under investigation. These include: the treatment of circulatory shock accompanied by intense vasoconstriction, tetanus, choreiform movement disorders, acromegaly, and accelerated hypertension.[33,34] Considerable further evaluation is needed of the potential value of antipsychotic agents in these disorders.

ADVERSE EFFECTS

The diverse pharmacologic actions of major tranquilizers can lead to a variety of adverse reactions influencing almost every major organ system. Adverse reactions of some type almost always accompany therapeutic dosage. In fact, the choice of a particular drug in clinical practice often reflects consideration of which side effects can be accepted with the least discomfort and potential for permanent harm.

Although the qualitative nature of most adverse effects are reasonably well understood, reliable data on their incidence and severity in various treatment settings are largely lacking. Side effects appear to vary widely in incidence, depending upon the treatment setting, dosage, duration of therapy, characteristics of the patient population, coadministration of other drugs, and in particular the specific epidemiologic approach used to assess the problem. The following discussion of side effects therefore necessarily reflects, at least in part, our personal experience and interpretation of the literature.[35]

Sedation

Drowsiness, somnolence, and other manifestations of excessive nonspecific central nervous system depression are commonly associated with aliphatic and piperidine phenothiazines, and with loxapine. Epidemiologic studies of adverse reactions to chlorpromazine in both medical and psychiatric patients suggest that drowsiness is one of the most common adverse reactions.[36,37] It appears to be dose-dependent, and typically remits or subsides when dosage is lowered. In some susceptible individuals, intolerable drowsiness is associated with any dose of chlorpromazine, and use of another antipsychotic agent becomes necessary. The nonspecific sedative effects of chlorpromazine provide further rationale for its use in a single daily bedtime dose, or in two daily doses with the larger administered at bedtime.

Movement Disorders

Blockade of dopamine receptors in the basal ganglia probably accounts for a spectrum of disorders involving involuntary movement.[38–40] The frequency and severity of extrapyramidal symptoms (EPS) associated with a particular drug appear to correlate directly with its dopamine blocking potential, and inversely with its anticholinergic properties.[14,15] Two general types of EPS have been identified.

Acute, Reversible EPS. One class of involuntary movement disorders develops a few hours to a few months after initiation of therapy, and remits when the dosage is lowered, the drug is discontinued, or an antiparkinsonian agent is coadministered. In many cases, acutely-occurring EPS will subside spontaneously despite continuation of the same antipsychotic drug dosage.

Acute dystonic reactions are most commonly associated with piperazine phenothiazines, butyrophenones, and molindone, and typically afflict young individuals shortly after the initiation of therapy.[41] These reactions can be dramatic and frightening, and often involve intractable muscle spasms of eyes, face, tongue, neck, and back. They are equally dramatically reversible upon parenteral administration of an antiparkinsonian agent (such as benztropine or diphenhydramine).

Akathisia and parkinsonism tend to occur later in the course of antipsychotic drug therapy, are more insidious in onset, and arise more commonly in the elderly. It is common for akathisia (motor restlessness) to be misdiagnosed, unrecognized, or even attributed to exacerbation of the underlying disease.

Conventional antiparkinsonian agents having anticholinergic properties are highly effective in the treatment of both types of acute reversible EPS. Parenteral dosage is usually indicated for acute dystonic reactions, but oral administration is generally appropriate for the more insidious and less serious symptom complexes. Prophylactic antiparkinsonian medication is not appropriate for every patient in whom antipsychotic drug therapy is initiated, nor is it established that antiparkinsonian drugs need be continued indefinitely while the patient remains under antipsychotic drug therapy.

Tardive Dyskinesia. Unlike the acute, reversible EPS, tardive dyskinesia generally develops during long-term antipsychotic drug therapy lasting more than a year.[40,42] It appears that elderly individuals with organic brain disease are more susceptible. Grotesque involuntary movements of the face and tongue characterize the syndrome of tardive dyskinesia, which can be extremely disquieting and upsetting to the patient and family.

A most troublesome aspect of this syndrome is its potential to become irreversible, and/or its worsening upon discontinuation of the antipsychotic agent or administration of a conventional antiparkinsonian drug. Dopamine receptor hypersensitivity, consequent to long-term drug-induced dopamine blockade, is the postulated mechanism.[43,44] A number of pharmacologic treatments for tardive dyskinesia are under investigation, but none is yet generally available.

This potentially irreversible, disabling consequence of antipsychotic therapy should always be considered prior to the institution of treatment, and emphasizes the need for conservatism when antipsychotic therapy is contemplated.[45,46]

Postural Hypotension

Aliphatic and piperidine phenothiazines can cause postural hypotension by virtue of their alpha-adrenergic blocking properties. Life-threatening hypotension is a rare consequence,[47] but some degree of postural blood pressure change probably occurs in most individuals treated with these types of antipsychotic agents. Symptomatic postural hypotension generally indicates that a dosage ceiling has been achieved.

Because individual sensitivities to the hypotensive effects of antipsychotic drugs differ unpredictably, we recommend that initiation of therapy with this subclass of drugs (chlorpromazine, thioridazine, mesoridazine, chlorprothixene) start with a 'test dose' of 25 to 100 mg administered under medical observation. Supine and standing blood pressure is checked frequently during the first 4 to 6 hours after the dose, and the patient cautioned about potential problems associated with rapid changes in posture. For patients with cardiac or cerebrovascular disease in whom unwanted hypotension many lead to cardiac or cerebral ischemia, it is recommended that a different class of antipsychotic agent be considered.

Sexual Dysfunction

Male sexual dysfunction can be associated with the same antipsychotic drugs that cause postural hypotension, again due to alpha-adrenergic blockade.

Cardiac Toxicity

Cardiotoxic effects of antipsychotic agents are controversial. It is possible that the drugs predispose to the occurrence of potentially life-threatening cardiac arrhythmias in otherwise healthy individuals.[33–36] This could partly explain sporadic reports of sudden death among otherwise healthy persons receiving antipsychotic agents. However, reliable scientific documentation of a cause-and-effect relationship to the drugs is not yet available.

A number of reports have focused on thioridazine as having a particularly high potential to induce cardiac arrhythmias.[33–36,48,49] Although most of these reports are anecdotal, this drug should probably be avoided in patients with cardiac disease known to be predisposed to cardiac arrhythmias. Minor electrocardiographic (ECG) changes, in particular ST-segment depression and T-wave flattening, are noted in a large number of phenothiazine-treated individuals, particularly those receiving high doses. The changes resemble those associated with hypokalemia, and appear to be reversible with fasting or upon administration of supplemental potassium. It is not known whether thioridazine-induced ECG changes such as these portend more serious cardiac arrhythmias.

Cholinergic Blockade

Aliphatic and piperidine phenothiazines have strong anticholinergic effects. The major manifestations are peripheral, and consist of familiar atropine-like effects of tachycardia, dry mouth, blurring of vision, and reduced motility of bowel and bladder. In otherwise healthy individuals, these are troublesome but seldom serious. However, cholinergic blockade can be a potential hazard for patients with prostatic hypertrophy, ischemic heart disease, or gastrointestinal disorders associated with the potential for bowel obstruction.[50,51] In patients with open-angle glaucoma adequately controlled by topical therapy, the anticholinergic effects of this subclass of antipsychotic agents probably presents no significant hazard.[52] The potential additive anticholinergic effects of these antipsychotic agents when coadministered with other compounds having similar properties (antiparkinson agents, tricyclic antidepressants, antihistaminics, etc.) should always be considered.

Hepatotoxicity

Hepatotoxic effects occur in a small percentage of patients treated with antipsychotic drugs. The most extensive data are available for chlorpromazine, since this has been the most widely used antipsychotic drug. A cholestatic type of hepatotoxicity, associated with jaundice and elevations in serum alkaline phosphatase concentrations, appears to afflict less than 1% of chlorpromazine-treated patients.[53,54] The syndrome generally occurs within the first month of therapy, and in the vast majority of cases is reversible upon drug discontinuation. The disorder appears to be one of hypersensitivity, and there is no evidence that individuals with pre-existing liver disease are more susceptible. Chlorpromazine-induced jaundice is an indication for changing to another antipsychotic agent. Irreversible hepatic failure has been associated with chlorpromazine and other phenothiazines in very rare instances.

Hematologic Toxicity

Mild, reversible bone marrow depression, manifested mainly as mild leukopenia, can be associated with antipsychotic drug therapy. Asymptomatic, mild leukopenia warrants further monitoring, but does not necessarily require drug discontinuation. Very rare cases of aplastic anemia are reportedly associated with antipsychotic drug therapy, but a cause-and-effect relationship is very difficult to establish.

Ophthalmologic Toxicity

Lenticular opacities have been associated with antipsychotic drug therapy, but the incidence is not established. Pigmentary retinopathy appears to be a unique consequence of high-dose thioridazine therapy. It is usually reversible on drug discontinuation, but in some cases has progressed to irreversible impairment of visual acuity. For this reason, the daily dosage of thioridazine should not exceed 800 mg.

Other Adverse Effects

Numerous other relatively uncommon adverse reactions have been attributed to antipsychotic drugs. These are reviewed in detail elsewhere.[35]

DRUG MONOGRAPHS

General and class-specific pharmacologic properties, adverse reactions, and approaches to clinical use of antipsychotic agents are described in detail above. The following section will elaborate only on drug-specific properties when such information is available. Only initial doses are suggested, inasmuch as dosage schedules vary widely depending upon the clinical indication and the needs of the individual patient.

PHENOTHIAZINES—ALIPHATIC (DIMETHYLAMINOPROPYL) SUBSTITUTION

CHLORPROMAZINE HYDROCHLORIDE (Thorazine, Chlor-PZ)
TRIFLUPROMAZINE HYDROCHLORIDE (Vesprin)

Chlorpromazine was the first antipsychotic agent to be used in clinical practice, and is still among the most widely used drugs. Chlorpromazine has a complex pharmacokinetic profile since it is biotransformed into numerous metabolic products.[55] The major metabolite, chlorpromazine sulfoxide,[56] appears to be pharmacologically inactive, but several other metabolites have pharmacologic activity, and probably contribute to therapeutic and/or toxic effects of the parent compound in humans.[55,57] No reliable estimate is yet available of the elimination half-life of chlorpromazine. However, the drug does appear to have a long duration of action, making it suitable for once-daily therapy. Because the total metabolic clearance of chlorpromazine is high, a substantial fraction of an oral dose is cleared during the first pass through the liver.[55,58] Biotransformation in the wall of the small intestine may contribute to this high extraction ratio. In any case, the clinical effects of a parenteral dose are greater than those of an equivalent oral dose. Coadministration of anticholinergic or antiparkinson agents appears to enhance first-pass biotransformation, leading to lower chlorpromazine blood levels and possibly reduced clinical efficacy. The relation of plasma concentrations to clinical effects of this drug is under active investigation.[55,59,60]

The pharmacokinetic properties of triflupromazine are not well-established. No specific advantage of this compound is established. Promazine (Sparine) is an aliphatic phenothiazine derivative lacking a critical halogen substitution. This drug has greatly reduced antipsychotic efficacy in comparison to chlorpromazine, yet has most of the unwanted side effects.

Initial Dosage—Chlorpromazine: *Oral: Adults,* 25 to 100 mg. *Intramuscular: Adults,* 12.5 to 50 mg. Triflupromazine: *Oral: Adults,* 10 to 50 mg.

PHENOTHIAZINES—PIPERIDINE SUBSTITUTION

THIORIDAZINE HYDROCHLORIDE (Mellaril)
MESORIDAZINE BESYLATE (Serentil)
PIPERACETAZINE (Quide)

Thioridazine and mesoridazine also appear to have complex pharmacokinetic properties, with a number of metabolites identified.[55] The pharmacologic activity of these metabolic products is not established. The retinopathic and possible cardiotoxic effects of thioridazine are discussed above.

Initial Dosage—Thioridazine: *Oral: Adults,* 25 to 100 mg. Mesoridazine: *Oral: Adults,* 25 to 100 mg. *Intramuscular: Adults,* 12.5 to 50 mg. Piperacetazine: *Oral: Adults,* 10 to 50 mg. *Intramuscular: Adults,* 0.5 to 2 mg.

PHENOTHIAZINES—PIPERAZINE SUBSTITUTION

PROCHLORPERAZINE (Compazine)
PROCHLORPERAZINE EDISYLATE (Compazine)
PROCHLORPERAZINE MALEATE (Compazine)
TRIFLUOPERAZINE HYDROCHLORIDE (Stelazine)
BUTAPERAZINE MALEATE (Repoise Maleate)
PERPHENAZINE (Trilafon)
FLUPHENAZINE HYDROCHLORIDE (Prolixin, Permitil)
FLUPHENAZINE DECANOATE (Prolixin Decanoate)
FLUPHENAZINE ENANTHATE (Prolixin Enanthate)
ACETOPHENAZINE MALEATE (Tindal)
CARPHENAZINE MALEATE (Proketazine)

Little data are available on the kinetic properties of these compounds. There appears to be little to distinguish among them. Although prochlorperazine is commonly used as an antiemetic, specific antiemetic properties different from other piperazine phenothiazines are not established. Fluphenazine is available as sustained-release enanthate or decanoate esters administered as 'depot' intramuscular injections.

Initial Dosage—Prochlorperazine: *Intramuscular or rectal: Adults,* 2.5 to 10 mg. *Oral: Adults,* 5 to 25 mg. Trifluoperazine: *Oral: Adults,* 2 to 4 mg. *Intramuscular: Adults,* 1.5 to 2 mg. Butaperazine: *Oral: Adults,* 10 to 20 mg. Perphenazine: *Oral: Adults,* 2 to 10 mg. *Parenteral: Adults,* 2.5 to 5 mg. Fluphenazine hydrochloride: *Oral: Adults,* 0.25 to 5 mg. *Parenteral: Adults,* 1.25 to 2.5 mg. Fluphenazine enanthate or decanoate: *Intramuscular: Adults,* 12.5 to 50 mg. Acetophenazine: *Oral: Adults,* 20 to 40 mg. Carphenazine: *Oral: Adults,* 25 to 50 mg.

BUTYROPHENONE

HALOPERIDOL (Haldol)

Haloperidol has become widely used in clinical practice. Its properties are similar to those of the piperazine phenothiazines. Potential advantages include a relative lack of sedative, adrenergic-blocking, and cholinergic-blocking effects. Disadvantages include a high incidence of extrapyramidal reactions, particularly acute dystonias. Like most other antipsychotic agents, haloperidol has a high hepatic clearance,[61,62] making parenteral dosage more effective than administration of an equivalent oral dose. Haloperidol has a number of metabolites, but their pharmacologic activity is not established. For reasons that are not clear, commercially available tablet and parenteral preparations of haloperidol do not appropriately reflect the oral-parenteral dosage inequivalency.

Initial Dosage—Oral: Adults, 1 to 5 mg. *Parenteral: Adults,* 1.25 to 5 mg.

THIOXANTHENES—ALIPHATIC (DIMETHYLAMINOPROPYL) SUBSTITUTION

CHLORPROTHIXENE (Taractan)

The clinical properties of this compound closely resemble those of chlorpromazine.

Initial Dosage—Oral: Adults, 25 to 100 mg. *Intramuscular: Adults,* 12.5 to 50 mg.

THIOXANTHENES—PIPERAZINE SUBSTITUTION

THIOTHIXENE (Navane)
THIOTHIXENE HYDROCHLORIDE (Navane)

This compound resembles piperazine phenothiazines in clinical properties.

Initial Dosage—Oral: Adults, 2 to 4 mg. *Intramuscular: Adults,* 1 to 2 mg.

DIHYDROINDOLONES

MOLINDONE HYDROCHLORIDE (Moban, Lidone)

This drug appears to resemble piperazine phenothiazines in its clinical action. The place of molindone in clinical antipsychotic therapy is not yet established.[7]

Initial Dosage—Oral: Adults, 5 to 10 mg.

DIBENZOXAZEPINES

LOXAPINE SUCCINATE (Loxitane)

Loxapine is similar to aliphatic and piperadine phenothiazines. Its superiority over existing drugs is not established.[7]

Initial Dosage—Oral: Adults, 10 to 20 mg.

REFERENCES

1. Swazey JP: *Chlorpromazine in Psychiatry: A Study of Therapeutic Innovation.* Cambridge, Massachusetts, MIT Press, 1974.
2. Shader RI, Jackson AH: Approaches to schizophrenia. In *Manual of Psychiatric Therapeutics.* Edited by RI Shader. Boston, Little, Brown and Company, 1975, pp 63–100.
3. Greenblatt DJ, Shader RI: Psychotropic drugs in the general hospital. In *Manual of Psychiatric Therapeutics.* Edited by RI Shader. Boston, Little, Brown and Company, 1975, pp 1–26.
4. Greenblatt DJ, Shader RI: Rational use of psychotropic drugs. III. Major tranquilizers. Am J Hosp Pharm 31:1226–1231, 1974.
5. Davis JM: Efficacy of tranquilizing and antidepressant drugs. Arch Gen Psychiatry 13:552–572, 1965.
6. Davis JM: Comparative doses and costs of antipsychotic medication. Arch Gen Psychiatry 33:858–861, 1976.
7. Davis JM: Recent developments in the drug treatment of schizophrenia. Am J Psychiatry 133:208–214, 1976.
8. Snyder SH, Banerjee SP, Yamamura HI, et al: Drugs, neurotransmitters, and schizophrenia. Science 184:1243–1253, 1974.
9. Snyder SH: The dopamine hypothesis of schizophrenia: focus on the dopamine receptor. Am J Psychiatry 133:197–202, 1976.
10. Carlsson A: Antipsychotic drugs, neurotransmitters, and schizophrenia. Am J Psychiatry 135:164–173, 1978.
11. Seeman P, Lee T: Antipsychotic drugs: direct correlation between clinical potency and presynaptic action on dopamine neurons. Science 188:1217–1219, 1975.
12. Creese I, Burt DR, Snyder SH: Dopamine receptor binding predicts clinical and pharmacological potencies of antischizophrenic drugs. Science 192:481–483, 1976.
13. Kotin J, Wilbert DE, Verburg D, et al: Thioridazine and sexual dysfunction. Am J Psychiatry 133:82–85, 1976.
14. Snyder S, Greenberg D, Yamamura HI: Antischizophrenic drugs and brain cholinergic receptors. Arch Gen Psychiatry 31:58–61, 1974.
15. Pearl J, Spilker BA, Woodward WA, et al: Anticholinergic activity of antipsychotic drugs in relation to their extrapyramidal effects. J Pharm Pharmacol 28:302–304, 1976.
16. Hollister LE, Overall JE, Kimbell I Jr, et al: Specific indications for different classes of phenothiazines. Arch Gen Psychiatry 30:94–99, 1974.
17. Clark ML, Huber W, Charalampous KD, et al: Drug treatment in newly admitted schizophrenic patients. Arch Gen Psychiatry 25:404–409, 1971.
18. Greenblatt DJ, Greenblatt GR: Chlorpromazine and hyperpyrexia. Clin Pediatr 12:504–505, 1973.
19. Anderson WH, Kuehnle JC, Catanzano DM: Rapid treatment of acute psychosis. Am J Psychiatry 133:1076–1078, 1976.
20. Davis JM: Overview: maintenance therapy in psychiatry: I. schizophrenia. Am J Psychiatry 132:1237–1245, 1975.
21. Leff JP, Wing JK: Trial of maintenance therapy in schizophrenia. Br Med J 3:599–604, 1971.
22. Prien RF, Cole JO, Belkin NF: Relapse in chronic schizophrenics following abrupt withdrawal of tranquilizing medication. Br J Psychiatry 115:679–686, 1968.
23. Andrews P, Hall JN, Snaith RP: A controlled trial of phenothiazine withdrawal in chronic schizophrenic patients. Br J Psychiatry 128:451–455, 1976.
24. Hirsch SR, Gaind R, Pohde PD, et al: Outpatient maintenance of chronic schizophrenic patients with long-acting fluphenazine: double-blind placebo trial. Br Med J 1:633–637, 1973.
25. Groves JE, Mandel MR: The long-acting phenothiazines. Arch Gen Psychiatry 32:893–900, 1975.
26. Ayd FJ Jr: The depot fluphenazines: a reappraisal after 10 years' clinical experience. Am J Psychiatry 132:491–500, 1975.
27. Greenblatt DJ, Greenblatt M: Which drug for alcohol withdrawal? J Clin Pharmacol 12:429–431, 1972.

28. Greenblatt DJ, Shader RI: Treatment of the alcohol withdrawal syndrome. In *Manual of Psychiatric Therapeutics.* Edited by RI Shader. Boston, Little, Brown and Company, 1975, pp 211–235.
29. Greenblatt DJ, Shader RI: Bad trips. In *Manual of Psychiatric Therapeutics.* Edited by RI Shader. Boston, Little, Brown and Company, 1975, pp 185–193.
30. Angrist B, Lee HK, Gershon S: The antagonism of amphetamine-induced symptomatology by a neuroleptic. Am J Psychiatry 131:817–819, 1974.
31. Greenblatt DJ, Shader RI: Anticholinergics. N Engl J Med 288:1215–1219, 1973.
32. Greenblatt DJ, Shader RI: Psychotropic drug overdosage. In *Manual of Psychiatric Therapeutics.* Edited by RI Shader. Boston, Little, Brown and Company, 1975, pp 237–267.
33. Greenblatt DJ, Shader RI: Psychotropic drugs, medical disease, and other medical therapies. In *Seminars in Psychiatry: Drugs in Combination with Other Therapies.* Edited by M Greenblatt. New York, Grune and Stratton, 1975, pp 83–99.
34. Greenblatt DJ, Shader RI, Lofgren S: Rational psychopharmacology for patients with medical diseases. Annu Rev Med 27:407–420, 1976.
35. Shader RI, DiMascio A and associates: *Psychotropic Drug Side Effects: Clinical and Theoretical Perspectives.* Baltimore, Williams and Wilkins, 1970.
36. Swett C Jr: Adverse reactions to chlorpromazine in medical patients: a report from the Boston Collaborative Drug Surveillance Program. Curr Ther Res 18:199–206, 1975.
37. Swett C Jr: Adverse reactions to chlorpromazine in psychiatric patients. Dis Nerv Syst 35:509–511, 1974.
38. Lader MH: Drug-induced extrapyramidal syndromes. J R Coll Physicians Lond 5:87–98, 1970.
39. Donlon PT, Stenson RL: Neuroleptic induced extrapyramidal symptoms. Dis Nerv Syst 37:629–635, 1976.
40. Freedman DX: Neurological syndromes associated with antipsychotic drug use: a special report. Arch Gen Psychiatry 28:463–467, 1973.
41. Swett C Jr: Drug-induced dystonia. Am J Psychiatry 132:532–534, 1975.
42. Kobayashi RM: Orofacial dyskinesia: clinical features, mechanisms and drug therapy. West J Med 125:277–288, 1976.
43. Klawans HL Jr: The pharmacology of tardive dyskinesias. Am J Psychiatry 130:82–86, 1973.
44. Gerlach J, Reisby N, Randrup A: Dopaminergic hypersensitivity and cholinergic hypofunction in the pathophysiology of tardive dyskinesia. Psychopharmacologia 34:21–35, 1974.
45. Paulson GW, Rizvi CA, Crane GE: Tardive dyskinesia as a possible sequel to long-term therapy with phenothiazines. Clin Pediatr 14:953–955, 1975.
46. Klawans HL, Bergen D, Bruyn GW, et al: Neuroleptic-induced tardive dyskinesias in nonpsychotic patients. Arch Neurol 30:338–339, 1974.
47. Gold MI: Profound hypotension associated with preoperative use of phenothiazines. Anesth Analg 53:844–848, 1974.
48. Fowler NO, McCall D, Chou T-C, et al: Electrocardiographic changes and cardiac arrhythmias in patients receiving psychotropic drugs. Am J Cardiol 37:223–230, 1976.
49. Tri TB, Combs DT: Phenothiazine induced ventricular tachycardia. West J Med 123:412–416, 1975.
50. Davis JT, Nusbaum M: Chlorpromazine therapy and functional large bowel obstruction. Am J Gastroenterol 60:635–639, 1973.
51. Kott I, Urca I: Small bowel complications probably due to Largactil therapy. Am J Surg 121:346–348, 1971.
52. Reid WH, Blouin P, Schermer M: A review of psychotropic medications and the glaucomas. Int Pharmacopsychiatry 11:163–174, 1976.
53. Clarke AE, Maritz VM, Denborough MA: Phenothiazines and jaundice. Aust NZ J Med 4:376–382, 1972.
54. Ishak RG, Irey NS: Hepatic injury associated with the phenothiazines: clinicopathologic and follow-up study of 36 patients. Arch Pathol 93:283–304, 1972.
55. Cooper TB: Plasma level monitoring of antipsychotic drugs. Clin Pharmacokinet 3:14–38, 1978.
56. Kaul PN, Whitfield LR, Clark ML: Chlorpromazine metabolism VIII: blood levels of chlorpromazine and its sulfoxide in schizophrenic patients. J Pharm Sci 65:694–697, 1976.

57. Sakalis G, Chan TL, Gershon S, et al: The possible role of metabolites in therapeutic response to chlorpromazine treatment. Psychopharmacologia 32:279–284, 1973.
58. Dahl SG, Strandjord RE: Pharmacokinetics of chlorpromazine after single and chronic dosage. Clin Pharmacol Ther 21:437–448, 1977.
59. Sakalis G, Curry SH, Mould GP, et al: Physiologic and clinical effects of chlorpromazine and their relationship to plasma level. Clin Pharmacol Ther 13:931–946, 1972.
60. Rivera-Calimlim L, Nasrallah H, Strauss J, et al: Clinical response and plasma levels: effect of dose, dosage schedules, and drug interactions on plasma chlorpromazine levels. Am J Psychiatry 133:646–652, 1976.
61. Cressman WA, Bianchine JR, Slotnick VB, et al: Plasma level profile of haloperidol in man following intramuscular administration. Eur J Clin Pharmacol 7:99–103, 1974.
62. Forsman A, Öhman R: Applied pharmacokinetics of haloperidol in man. Curr Ther Res 21:396–411, 1977.

36. ANTIDEPRESSANTS

David J. Greenblatt and Richard I. Shader

Grief and depression belong to a continuum of mood and affect disorders analogous to fear and anxiety.[1–5] Grief is a normal human response to loss or departure of an object (whether real or abstract) with which the individual's sense of well-being is intertwined. Examples of such losses include: the death or departure of spouse, loved one, parent, or offspring; loss of an aspect of bodily function due to illness or injury (ie, severe heart disease, stroke, paralysis, amputation, blindness, etc.); or professional failure or nonrecognition (ie, lack of promotion, termination of employment, loss of a public election, etc.). Repeated frustration or lack of recognition can lead to a sense of defeat or demoralization.

Acute loss triggers first a stunned shock, followed by disbelief and sometimes anger. Once the reality of the loss is recognized and acknowledged, the bereaved person usually begins a period of 'grief work,' in which some of their investment in the lost object is gradually withdrawn and redirected towards other aspects of their lives from which they can derive pleasure and satisfaction. The normal grieving process usually lasts from several months to a year. When grief work is completed, the bereaved person may still feel a sense of loss, but the feeling can generally be tolerated without the extremely dysphoric emotional and bodily sensations of heaviness and emptiness.

Appropriate grief following object loss constitutes one end of the continuum of affective disorders, and is a form of situational or reactive depression developing in an otherwise healthy individual. Pharmacotherapy of grief or situational depression beyond the occasional and short-term use of sedative-hypnotics is seldom indicated unless grief is excessively prolonged and/or severe. In such cases, coexistence of another category of depressive disorder should be considered. Demoralization likewise does not require drug intervention. The therapeutic objective rather should be the achievement or re-establishment of some sense of mastery, which sometimes can be promoted by the 'get-away-from-it-all' vacation permitting respite from the sense of oppression or defeat.

Several systems have been used to characterize depressive disorders. None is completely satisfactory, and clinical practice always reveals patients whose disorder falls into no clear-cut category. Nonetheless, a useful and widely accepted classification scheme involves separation of the more serious depressions into *unipolar* and *bipolar* disease.[1–5] A third category includes those patients with primary schizophreniform disease with coexisting or secondary depressive manifestations. Diagnosis and treatment of this latter category is problematic—it is not established whether pharmacotherapy should be directed primarily at the psychotic or the depressive aspects of the disease. Sometimes, combination therapy is appropriate.

Unipolar depression usually describes recurrent depressive states that are cyclic or episodic in character, but generally do not involve episodes of elation or mania. Although appropriate grief or situational depression, as well as depression associated with neurotic anxiety can be viewed as forms of unipolar disease, antidepressant pharmacotherapy is generally not appropriate.[6,7] In addition to demoralized persons, another category of patients generally unresponsive or poorly responsive to somatic therapy include those with chronic characterological depression. Such patients have a lifelong pattern of poor social, interpersonal, and occupational functioning, coupled with ongoing feelings of inadequacy, unhappiness, and pessimism. Exacerbation of symptoms can follow relatively minor and ordinary stresses and disappointments of day-to-day existence. Prognosis for complete recovery is often poor, but they generally respond better to interpersonal therapy and emergence of favorable life events than to specific somatic treatment.

The subcategory of unipolar depressions most responsive to pharmacologic interventions are the 'endogenous' or 'autonomous' depressions.[8] Physicians should make every effort to identify the specific characteristics of this disease before proceeding with drug treatment. In particular, symptomatology attributable to endogenous depression should be differentiated from that accompanying reactive depression or grief. In cases of reactive depression, a clear precipitant is usually evident, and prompt remission accompanies a favorable turn of life events or simply the passage of time. Patients with reactive depression generally feel worse in the evening, and have difficulty getting to sleep. Marked weight loss is uncommon. Reactive depression can develop in any individual who has experienced a loss or narcissistic injury, and shows little or no tendency to be familial. In the case of endogenous depression, a clear precipitant, or an event serious enough to trigger severe depressive symptoms, is often absent, although it is not uncommon for reactive depression to shift into autonomous depression. Even when a precipitant can be identified and ameliorated symptomatology has become 'autonomous,' and a favorable environmental change does not lead to remission. Endogenously depressed persons generally feel worse in the morning, and suffer from early morning awakening rather than difficulty falling asleep. They experience feelings of hopelessness, worthlessness, and guilt, and their ability to experience pleasure is greatly reduced. Patients' energy and interest in outside activities also are greatly reduced, and they may suffer considerable loss of bodily weight due to anorexia. Some patients show psychomotor retardation, in which their overall level of physical activity is reduced and their posture and speech seem altered. Others are 'agitated', and engage in excessive ruminative activity and in agitated behaviors such as hand-wringing and pacing. Untreated endogenous depression is usually a recurrent disorder, with depressive episodes lasting a few weeks to a few months, then gradually evolving into periods of remission during which mood is relatively normal. The suicidal risk of endogenously depressed persons is considerable, particularly at the onset or during the 'upswing' or recovery phase when they may generate just enough energy or ambition to act upon their self-destructive feelings.

Bipolar depressive disorders also are cyclic in nature, but the disease is characterized by episodes of elation or mania.[5] True mania can be spellbinding in intensity. Patients have a greatly increased sense of energy, vitality, and well-being, leading to incessant talk and activity. Their mind races with grandiose ideas and thoughts, leading to delusional 'schemes' and 'plans', increased activity (motor, social, and sexual), easy distractability and poor judgement, and a reduced need for sleep. Patients with manic-depressive disease tend to be afflicted relatively early in life, and to have a family history of similar disorders. The depressive phase of the illness is often characterized by psychomotor retardation and hypersomnia. Successful suicide again is relatively common. Self-harm during the manic phase also is common, usually from irresponsible and ill-judged acts such as reckless automobile driving, jumping from heights, inappropriately provocative or aggressive interpersonal relations, etc. As such, untreated manic-depressive disease has a relatively poor prognosis.

TREATMENT OF DEPRESSIVE DISORDERS

This section focuses on somatic (pharmacologic or otherwise) therapies of depressive disorders.[1–5,8,9] Identification of a depressive subtype having a reasonable chance of responding to somatic treatment is essential prior to initiation of such treatment. Furthermore, somatic therapy must be instituted in the setting of a physician-patient interaction conducive to management of serious mental disease.

Electroconvulsive Therapy (ECT)

ECT continues to be the most consistently effective therapy of unipolar depressions of the endogenous or autonomous type.[10,11] Disease characteristics associated with favorable response include: intense feelings of low self-esteem, worthlessness, and pessimism; constitutional manifestations such as anorexia, weight loss, constipation (vegetative symptoms); sleep disturbance characterized by early morning awakening; and suicidal ideation or action. Patients with other forms of depressive disease, including bipolar depression, sometimes respond less favorably to ECT. The mechanism by which ECT ameliorates the depression is unknown.

Despite its effectiveness, ECT seldom should constitute the therapy of first choice. Properly administered ECT is relatively safe, but the risks generally exceed those associated with pharmacologic therapies. Furthermore, ECT may not be indicated for patients having medical diseases (such as ischemic heart disease, increased intracranial pressure, etc.) for which the risks of general anesthesia and/or systemic muscle relaxant use are substantial. Irresponsible, sensationalistic and exaggerated claims of 'brain damage' attributable to ECT, alleged by the popular media and by a few pseudo-scientists, have unfortunately frightened many patients away from what might have been a reasonable and effective choice of treatment.

Tricyclic Antidepressants

Although less consistently effective than ECT, tricyclic antidepressant derivatives usually constitute the somatic therapy of first choice for endogenously depressed individuals when such treatment is indicated.[8] Six tricyclics are currently available for clinical use. They include two dibenzazepine compounds (imipramine and desipramine), three dibenzocycloheptene compounds (amitriptyline, nortriptyline, and protriptyline), and one dibenzoxepin derivative (doxepin). Many theoretical and biochemical theories are available to support the use of one or another of these compounds in certain subclasses of patients having particular symptom complexes. In clinical terms, however, there appears to be little basis for choosing one antidepressant over another, although for unknown reasons some persons may respond better to one drug than another. The dibenzoxepin derivative doxepin is claimed to have special attributes such as fewer side effects and antianxiety as well as antidepressant properties; these claims are largely unfounded. In fact, doxepin appears to have no specific antianxiety action,[12] and it may be a relatively weak antidepressant agent at the recommended doses.[13] The clinical similarity of the various tricyclics is not surprising, when one considers, for example, that desipramine is an endogenous metabolite of imipramine, and that nortriptyline is a metabolite of amitriptyline. Fixed-combination preparations containing amitriptyline as one component (ie, amitriptyline plus perphenazine; amitriptyline plus chlordiazepoxide) are widely used in clinical practice. Although coadministration of an antidepressant with an antianxiety or antipsychotic agent may be beneficial in some individuals (see below), the routine use of such fixed combinations is not rational.

Dosage and Onset of Action. Clinical failure of tricyclic antidepressant therapy is often explained either by use of inadequate dosage or by failure to continue therapy long enough for clinical improvement to become manifest.

Clinical studies indicate that relatively high doses of tricyclic antidepressants are necessary for reasonably consistent and predictable clinical response. The usual minimum dosage level is considered to be 150 mg per day of imipramine or its equivalent.[14] Many physicians are reluctant to utilize the necessary dosage, inasmuch as an increment in side effects inevitably results. Unfortunately, use of lower doses to minimize unwanted effects also reduces the probability of clinical improvement.

The likelihood of patient acceptance of necessary therapeutic doses can be enhanced by initiation of therapy at a lower dose (ie, 75 mg per day of imipramine), then gradually increasing over a period of 1 to 2 weeks to the desired level. Administration of the entire daily dose at bedtime appears to be equally effective as a multiple daily dose schedule, and patients often experience less toxicity.[15–18]

The use of plasma tricyclic antidepressant levels to guide dosage titration is currently under active investigation. Numerous studies have suggested a possible relation between plasma concentrations and therapeutic (and/or toxic) effects.[19–29] Unfortunately, there remains some inconsistency from study to study. Furthermore, analysis of plasma concentrations is methodologically complicated, and beyond the capability of most clinical laboratories.

Although unwanted side effects of antidepressants are of rapid onset, therapeutic effects are not. A 'lag period' of from 5 days to 3 weeks generally elapses between the initiation of therapy and the onset of desired antidepressant effects.[30] Despite claims that the time of therapeutic onset may differ slightly among drugs in this class, there is no consistent evidence to this effect. Unfortunately, the rapid onset of side effects as opposed to the slow onset of therapeutic effects often leads physicians and patients to discard the therapy prematurely, with the complaint that the drug was ineffective and only made the patient miserable. Physicians should provide guidance and support of patients during this difficult phase of initiation of therapy. Therapeutic failure cannot be assumed unless the patient has received at least four weeks of full therapeutic dosage with no evidence of clinical benefit.

Common Side Effects. Several secondary pharmacologic properties of tricyclic antidepressants are commonly encountered in clinical practice.[31] In fact, therapeutic benefit usually is not achieved without the patient experiencing some combination of the following side effects, at least early in the course of therapy.

Anticholinergic-like manifestations are exceedingly common. The usual complaints are dry mouth, blurring of vision, constipation, palpitations due to tachycardia, and urinary hesitancy. Patients should be warned that such effects are likely to be encountered, particularly at the start of treatment. Not all tricyclic antidepressants, however, are equally anticholinergic.[32] Amitriptyline appears to be the most potent, desmethylimipramine the least, and imipramine in between.

Anticholinergic side effects of tricyclics are potentially hazardous for patients with prostatic hypertrophy, ischemic heart disease, or untreated glaucoma. In most patients, however, atropine-like effects pose no serious hazard but are subjectively troublesome and must be endured. They may lessen as the duration of treatment grows longer, particularly when the much more important therapeutic benefits develop. Use of the beta-adrenergic blocking agent propranolol may be of value in antagonizing tachycardia and palpitations. Recently, the cholinomimetic agent bethanechol has been suggested as a possible 'antidote' to atropine-like effects of tricyclic antidepressants.[33]

The ability of tricyclics to produce nonspecific drowsiness approximately parallels their anticholinergic potency. Amitriptyline and doxepin produce the greatest amount of sedation, protriptyline and desipramine the least, with imipramine and nortriptyline falling somewhere in between. The sedative properties of amitriptyline make it particularly suitable for once-daily bedtime therapy, especially for patients in whom sleep disturbances are a major problem.[17] The theoretical benefit of amitriptyline in cases of agitated depression, as opposed to protriptyline or desipramine in retarded depression, is not clinically established.[34]

Another common side effect of tricyclic antidepressants is a subjective feeling of agitation and restlessness, sometimes accompanied by a fine tremor. These effects, thought to be due to release of catecholamines, tend to occur early in the course of therapy and can be quite troublesome. The beta-adrenergic blocking agent propranolol is highly effective in reversing these manifestations. Low doses of a benzodiazepine antianxiety agent such as diazepam also can provide symptomatic benefit. Prophylactic mitigation of restlessness and tremor inherent in the fixed combination of amitriptyline and chlordiazepoxide (Limbitrol) may explain its alleged superiority over amitriptyline alone in some clinical studies. However, routine use of this fixed combination preparation is not recommended.

Less Common Side Effects. Cardiovascular complications of tricyclic antidepressant therapy are being increasingly recognized.[35] Postural hypotension does occur, but the incidence and significance are not established. Hypotension appears to be more common in patients with underlying cardiovascular disease. Of more concern is the potential cardiotoxic effect of tricyclics. Identified manifestations include a variety of conduction disturbances and tachyarrhythmias.[35–42] Such effects are common manifestations of overdosage with tricyclic antidepressants.[35,43–45] Patients suspected of ingesting excessive amounts of these drugs should be monitored for the possible occurrence of cardiac complications. However, the incidence and clinical significance of tricyclic antidepressant cardiotoxicity following therapeutic doses are not established. Most studies present only anecdotal evidence, and it is not known whether electrocardiographic changes in asymptomatic individuals portend more serious arrhythmias. Adequately controlled epidemiologic studies have yielded conflicting evidence.[46,47] Until the issue is settled, tricyclic antidepressants probably should be utilized with caution in patients with a history of cardiac disease, particularly those known to be predisposed to arrhythmias. The cardiotoxic effects of doxepin may be less than those of other tricyclic antidepressants.[36] However, the possibility of an increased margin of safety with recommended doses of this agent must be weighed against its probable reduced efficacy.[13]

Drug Interactions. With the possible exception of doxepin, tricyclic antidepressants interfere with the clinical action of the antihypertensive drugs guanethidine and clonidine.[48,49] For this reason, other antihypertensive agents should be used in tricyclic-treated depressed patients needing pharmacologic reduction of elevated blood pressure.

Synergistic anticholinergic effects may be expected in patients taking tricyclics together with other drugs having similar properties, such as antiparkinson agents, antihistamines, belladonna-containing preparations used to treat gastrointestinal disorders, and anticholinergic antipsychotic agents such as chlorpromazine and thioridazine. Tricyclic antidepressants may reduce the rate of gastric emptying and therefore reduce the rate of absorption of other concurrently administered drugs.[50]

The efficacy of tricyclic antidepressants may be enhanced by coadministration of thyroid hormone even in euthyroid patients.[51,52] Clinical guidelines for the use of this combination are not established.

Monoamine Oxidase (MAO) Inhibitors

The antidepressant efficacy of MAO inhibitors appears to be less than that of either ECT or of tricyclic antidepressants. However, there may be some individuals who are unresponsive to tricyclics and/or who are not candidates for ECT, in which case a therapeutic trial with an MAO inhibitor may be warranted.[53] Hazards of MAO inhibitor therapy described in most reference sources probably are exaggerated—judicious use of these drugs appears to be relatively safe. Likewise, although combination therapy with tricyclics and MAO inhibitors is traditionally thought to be very hazardous, carefully monitored combination therapy may be relatively safe and provide added therapeutic benefits in some selected individuals.[54–56]

Postural hypotension is a common complication of therapy with MAO inhibitors. Symptomatic postural hypotension generally means that the dosage ceiling has been reached. In rare cases, cardiovascular collapse has occurred. MAO inhibitors impair the ability to detoxify certain exogenous catecholamines. Cold preparations containing sympathomimetic agents should be used with caution in patients receiving these antidepressants.[57] Likewise, patients should be cautioned to avoid the ingestion of tyramine-containing foods, in particular certain types of wine and cheese. Ingestion of such foods has in rare instances caused hypertensive crisis and death.

Lithium

Lithium salts are widely used in the treatment of bipolar (manic-depressive) depressive disorders.[58–63] Lithium is not entirely specific for this disease, inasmuch as it is also effective in the treatment of unipolar depressive disease. Conversely, tricyclic antidepressants have some efficacy in bipolar disease.

Although lithium salts probably are the best of available pharmacologic therapies for manic-depressive disease, they are by no means ideal. During an acute episode of mania or hypomania when prompt management of aggressive and/or antisocial behavior is necessary, other pharmacologic agents may have to be used during the induction phase of lithium treatment. Antipsychotic agents (see Chapter 35) often are necessary for management of acute mania, during which time lithium treatment is simultaneously being initiated. The major benefits of lithium salts appear to be in the prophylaxis of both phases of the bipolar illness. However, the relapse rate may approach 50% even with well-monitored lithium prophylaxis.

A major drawback of lithium treatment is its very narrow therapeutic range. Doses slightly above those effective in disease prophylaxis may cause troublesome and sometimes serious toxicity.[58–65] For this reason, use of plasma or serum lithium concentrations is essential for therapeutic monitoring during treatment of bipolar disease. Dosage should be adjusted to maintain serum lithium concentrations in the range of 0.7 to 1.5 mEq/liter. Concentrations slightly higher than this may lead to toxic manifestations such as tremor, anorexia, nausea, increased thirst, and difficulty in concentrating.[66] More serious toxicity may develop at higher levels. Recent studies suggest that erythrocyte, rather than plasma, lithium concentrations may be the most reliable 'window' of therapeutic and/or potentially toxic effects.[67,68]

In addition to reasonably predictable, concentration-dependent toxicity, lithium can produce a variety of other side effects. Lithium impairs thyroid function, and sometimes leads to chemical signs of thyroid insufficiency.[69–78] Occasionally, clinical hypothyroidism becomes manifest. The antithyroid effects of lithium have in fact been utilized as a potential therapy for thyrotoxicosis.[79–81] Lithium also appears to antagonize either the release or the end-organ action of antidiuretic hormone (ADH),[82] leading to reports of a diabetes insipidus-like syndrome.[83] Again, this effect has been utilized therapeutically for treatment of the inappropriate-ADH syndrome.[84] Prolonged lithium therapy also may directly impair renal tubular function, leading to concentration defects and possibly overt pathological changes.[85,86] Finally, enhanced seizure activity has been reported in association with lithium treatment, although some authors claim that lithium may actually have an anticonvulsant effect.[87]

Elimination of lithium by the human body is similar to that of sodium. The ion is excreted essentially unchanged by the kidney.[88–90] Renal clearance of lithium is reduced in patients with renal insufficiency, and doses should be appropriately adjusted downward. Renal clearance of lithium is also reduced in patients receiving diuretics and in those on salt-restricted diets.[91] These latter two conditions commonly precipitate clinical lithium toxicity.

DRUG MONOGRAPHS

The previous section considered general concepts in antidepressant pharmacotherapy. Class- and drug-specific characteristics are described below.

TRICYCLIC ANTIDEPRESSANTS—DIBENZOCYCLOHEPTENES

AMITRIPTYLINE HYDROCHLORIDE (Elavil, Endep)
NORTRIPTYLINE HYDROCHLORIDE (Aventyl)
PROTRIPTYLINE HYDROCHLORIDE (Vivactil)
AMITRIPTYLINE AND CHLORDIAZEPOXIDE (Limbitrol)
AMITRIPTYLINE AND PERPHENAZINE (Triavil, Etrafon)

Except for differences in anticholinergic effects and nonspecific sedative properties, the three drugs in this class have similar clinical effects. Triavil and Etrafon, the combination preparations containing amitriptyline and perphenazine, are extensively used in clinical practice, at least in part due to a grandiose promotional scheme advocating these preparations for the treatment of patients having combinations of depression with anxiety and agitation. Controlled studies supporting these claims are unavailable. Limbitrol, the combination of amitriptyline and chlordiazepoxide, allegedly provides more rapid onset of antidepressant action in some individuals. This is probably explained by antagonism of some of the early stimulative effects of amitriptyline treatment by chlordiazepoxide (see above). Although combination therapy with an antidepressant and an antianxiety agent may be useful in some individuals, this is by no means the rule. When combination therapy is indicated, it is recommended that the components be administered and titrated as separate entities rather than as a fixed preparation.

Amitriptyline is biotransformed in the liver to nortriptyline, a pharmacologically active substance also marketed as an antidepressant drug.[92] During multiple-dose therapy with amitriptyline, both the parent compound and its metabolite are present in similar concentrations,[93,94] and it is likely that both contribute to pharmacologic activity. The possible clinical significance of other amitriptyline metabolites (primarily hydroxylated derivatives) is under investigation. Amitriptyline is extensively distributed to body tissues, such that only a small fraction of a dose is present in plasma.[95]

Although hepatic clearance of amitriptyline is high, its rate of elimination is slow because of a very large volume of distribution.[95] This property, together with the presence of at least one active metabolite, makes it quite suitable for once-daily bedtime dosage.

Biotransformation of nortriptyline and protriptyline appears to proceed via hydroxylation in the liver.[92,96,97] However, the pharmacologic activity of metabolites is not yet established. Otherwise, the kinetics of these two derivatives resemble those of amitriptyline.[96–98]

Due to high hepatic clearance and a substantial first-pass metabolic effect, systemic availability of oral preparations of these three drugs is considerably less than 100%.[97,99,100]

Dosage—Oral: Adults. Amitriptyline, initial, 50 to 75 mg per day (single or divided); usual maintenance, 150 to 200 mg per day (single or divided). *Nortriptyline,* initial, 40 to 75 mg per day (single or

TABLE 1 Preparations and Costs of Antidepressants

Generic Name	Trademark Name(s)	Preparations and 1978 Costs
Tricyclic Compounds—Dibenzocycloheptenes		
Amitriptyline Hydrochloride	Elavil (Endep)	Tablets 10 mg—$5.27/100; 25 mg—$10.57/100; 50 mg—$18.79/100; 75 mg—$26.84/100; 100 mg—$33.93/100
Nortriptyline Hydrochloride	Aventyl Hydrochloride	Capsules 10 mg—$5.29/100; 25 mg—$10.58/100 Liquid 10 mg/5 ml—$6.08/16 oz
Protriptyline Hydrochloride	Vivactil	Tablets 5 mg—$8.73/100; 10 mg—$12.67/100
Amitriptyline Hydrochloride 10 mg and Perphenazine 2 mg	Triavil 2-10 (Etrafon 2-10)	Tablets—$11.53/100
Amitriptyline Hydrochloride 25 mg and Perphenazine 2 mg	Triavil 2-25 (Etrafon)	Tablets—$14.64/100
Amitriptyline Hydrochloride 10 mg and Perphenazine 4 mg	Triavil 4-10 (Etrafon A)	Tablets—$12.87/100
Amitriptyline Hydrochloride 25 mg and Perphenazine 4 mg	Triavil 4-25 (Etrafon Forte)	Tablets—$15.97/100
Tricyclic Compounds—Dibenzazepines		
Imipramine Hydrochloride	Tofranil (Imavate) (Janimine) (Presamine) (SK-Pramine)	Tablets 10 mg—$6.22/100; 25 mg—$9.72/100; 50 mg—$19.33/100 Injection (solution) 12.5 mg/ml—$5.98/10-ml vial
Imipramine Pamoate	Tofranil-PM	Capsules (equivalent of imipramine hydrochloride) 75 mg—$28.86/100; 100 mg—$38.28/100; 125 mg—$47.72/100; 150 mg—$57.14/100
Desipramine Hydrochloride	Norpramin (Pertofrane)	Tablets 25 mg—$9.60/100; 50 mg—$18.00/100

TABLE 1 *(continued)*

Generic Name	Trademark Name(s)	Preparations and 1978 Costs
Tricyclic Compounds—Dibenzoxepin		
Doxepin Hydrochloride	Sinequan (Adapin)	Capsules 10 mg—$11.82/100; 25 mg—$15.17/100; 50 mg—$21.35/100; 100 mg—$38.63/100 Solution (concentrate) 10 mg/ml—$8.20/120 ml
Monoamine Oxidase Inhibitors—Hydrazine Derivatives		
Isocarboxazid	Marplan	Tablets 10 mg—$7.93/100
Phenelzine Sulfate	Nardil	Tablets 15 mg—$7.15/100
Monoamine Oxidase Inhibitors—Nonhydrazine Derivative		
Tranylcypromine Sulfate		Tablets 10 mg—$7.70/100
Lithium Salt		
Lithium Carbonate	Eskalith (Lithane) (Lithonate)	Capsules 300 mg—$3.00/100

divided); usual maintenance, 100 to 150 mg per day (single or divided). *Protriptyline,* initial, 10 to 15 mg per day (single or divided); usual maintenance, 30 to 45 mg per day (single or divided).

TRICYCLIC ANTIDEPRESSANTS—DIBENZAZEPINES

IMIPRAMINE HYDROCHLORIDE (Tofranil, Presamine)
IMIPRAMINE PAMOATE (Tofranil PM)
DESIPRAMINE HYDROCHLORIDE (Norpramin, Pertofrane)

Like amitriptyline, imipramine is biotransformed to a pharmacologically active substance, desipramine.[101–106] Both are present in similar concentrations during multiple-dose therapy, and both contribute to clinical effects. Desipramine is marketed as a separate-entity antidepressant drug.

Despite its high hepatic clearance, elimination of imipramine is slow due to its very large volume of distribution. As such, it is also suitable for once-daily antidepressant therapy. The kinetic characteristics of imipramine render the availability of a 'sustained-release' preparation (Tofranil PM) entirely unnecessary.

Dosage—Oral: Adults. Imipramine, initial, 50 to 75 mg per day (single or divided); usual maintenance, 150 to 200 mg per day (single or divided). *Desipramine,* initial, 50 to 75 mg per day (single or divided); usual maintenance, 150 to 200 mg per day (single or divided).

TRICYCLIC ANTIDEPRESSANTS—DIBENZOXEPINS

DOXEPIN HYDROCHLORIDE (Sinequan, Adapin)

Doxepin is less anticholinergic and is claimed to have fewer cardiotoxic effects than other tricyclic antidepressants. In addition, it also appears to be a less potent guanethidine antagonist. These potential benefits are offset by the seemingly reduced antidepressant efficacy of doxepin. It seems likely that when doxepin dosage is appropriately titrated upward, therapeutic and toxic effects probably will resemble those of other tricyclic antidepressants.[13] Promotional claims that doxepin has special antidepressant and antianxiety properties are not established in controlled clinical trials.

Like other tricyclic antidepressants, elimination of doxepin is slow, giving it cumulative properties and making it suitable for once-daily therapy. The major metabolite of doxepin is desmethyldoxepin, which is eliminated more slowly than the parent compound.[107] The pharmacologic activity of this metabolite is not established.

Dosage—Oral: Adults, initial, 50 to 75 mg per day (single or divided); usual maintenance, 150 to 200 mg per day (single or divided).

MONOAMINE OXIDASE INHIBITORS

ISOCARBOXAZID (Marplan)
PHENELZINE SULFATE (Nardil)
TRANYLCYPROMINE SULFATE (Parnate)

Differences among the MAO inhibitors in clinical efficacy and toxicity are not well-documented. MAO inhibitors appear to be less consistently effective than either ECT or tricyclic antidepressants. However, MAO inibitors may be useful in selected patients who fail to respond to the above two treatments, or in some individuals with atypical depressive disorders.

Hazards and precautions to the use of MAO inhibitors are described above.

Dosage—Oral: Adults. Isocarboxazid, 30 to 40 mg per day in divided doses. *Phenelzine,* 45 to 90 mg per day in divided doses. *Tranylcypromine,* 20 to 30 mg per day in divided doses.

LITHIUM SALTS

LITHIUM CARBONATE (Eskalith, Lithane, Lithonate)

Use of lithium carbonate in the treatment of manic-depressive disease requires caution and careful monitoring. A recent study suggests that a single serum lithium determination 24 hours after a single oral dose can be used to predict requirements at steady-state.[108] For practical purposes, however, dosage adjustment must be made using repeated serum lithium concentration determinations and careful clinical observation.

In patients with normal renal function, the usual starting dose is 300 mg 2 to 3 times daily. After three days of this schedule, a serum lithium level is determined in a sample drawn prior to the first dose of the day. A subtherapeutic level and/or a lack of clinical manifestations of toxicity, indicates that a dosage increase is indicated. The suggested increase is 300 mg per day. After three days of the new dosage schedule, another serum lithium determination is made. Using this approach, the dosage is gradually titrated upward until the 'therapeutic' antimanic range of 0.7 to 1.5 mEq/liter is reached. After attainment of therapeutic concentrations, lithium determinations can be done at less frequent intervals.

The need for dosage adjustment should be anticipated if patients experience an intercurrent illness, particularly one which could lead to volume depletion or dehydration. Downward dosage adjustments should also be anticipated if diuretic therapy is initiated or if a salt-restricted diet is undertaken.

Because of potential effects of lithium upon thyroid and renal function, appropriate indices of these functions should be measured prior to the start of treatment, then monitored periodically as therapy proceeds.

Dosage—Oral: Adults, initial, 600 to 900 mg per day in divided doses. Upward titration using the scheme described above.

REFERENCES

1. Schildkraut JJ, Klein DF: The classification and treatment of depressive disorders. In *Manual of Psychiatric Therapeutics.* Edited by RI Shader. Boston, Little, Brown and Company, 1975, pp 39–61.

2. Zung WWK: From art to science: the diagnosis and treatment of depression. Arch Gen Psychiatry 29:328–337, 1973.
3. Akiskal HS, McKinney WT Jr: Depressive disorders: toward a unified hypothesis. Science 182:20–29, 1973.
4. Hollister LE: Treatment of depression with drugs. Ann Intern Med 89:78–84, 1978.
5. Gershon S: The treatment of manic-depressive states. In *Manual of Psychiatric Therapeutics*. Edited by RI Shader. Boston, Little, Brown and Company, 1975, pp 101–114.
6. LaPolla A, Jones H: Placebo-control evaluation of desipramine in depression. Am J Psychiatry 127:335–338, 1970.
7. Paykel ES: Depressive typologies and response to amitriptyline. Br J Psychiatry 120:147–156, 1972.
8. Morris JB, Beck AT: The efficacy of antidepressant drugs: a review of research (1958 to 1972). Arch Gen Psychiatry 30:667–674, 1974.
9. Klerman GL: Drug therapy of clinical depressions—current status and implications for research on neuropharmacology of the affective disorders. J Psychiatr Res 9:253–270, 1972.
10. Salzman C: Electroconvulsive therapy. In *Manual of Psychiatric Therapeutics*. Edited by RI Shader. Boston, Little, Brown and Company, 1975, pp 115–124.
11. Hurwitz TD: Electroconvulsive therapy: a review. Compr Psychiatry 15:303–314, 1974.
12. Haskell DS, Gambill JD, Gardos G, et al: Doxepin or diazepam for anxious and anxious-depressed outpatients? J Clin Psychiatry 39:135–139, 1978.
13. Hollister LE: Doxepin hydrochloride. Ann Intern Med 81:360–363, 1974.
14. Blashki TG, Mowbray R, Davies B: Controlled trial of amitriptyline in general practice. Br Med J 1:133–138, 1971.
15. Mendels J, Schless A: A controlled comparison of doxepin h.s. and doxepin q.i.d. J Clin Pharmacol 15:534–539, 1975.
16. Mendels J, DiGiacomo J: The treatment of depression with a single daily dose of imipramine pamoate. Am J Psychiatry 130:1022–1024, 1973.
17. Snowdon JA: Double-blind comparison of 3-times daily and single night dosage of amitriptyline, with special reference to side-effects. Curr Med Res Opin 4:381–387, 1976.
18. Schorer CE: Single dose vs divided dose imipramine. Psychopharmacologia 28:115–119, 1973.
19. Ziegler VE, Co BT, Taylor JR, et al: Amitriptyline plasma levels and therapeutic response. Clin Pharmacol Ther 19:795–801, 1976.
20. Kragh-Sørensen P, Åsberg M, Eggert-Hansen C: Plasma-nortriptyline levels in endogenous depression. Lancet 1:113–115, 1973.
21. Braithwaite RA, Goulding R, Theano G, et al: Plasma concentration of amitriptyline and clinical response. Lancet 1:1297–1300, 1972.
22. Kragh-Sørensen P, Hansen CE, Åsberg M: Plasma levels of nortriptyline in the treatment of endogenous depression. Acta Psychiatr Scand 49:444–456, 1973.
23. Asberg M, Cronholm B, Sjöqvist F, et al: Relationship between plasma level and therapeutic effect of nortriptyline. Br Med J 3:331–334, 1971.
24. Kragh-Sørensen P, Hansen CE, Baastrup PC, et al: Self-inhibiting action of nortriptylin's antidepressive effect at high plasma levels. Psychopharmacologia 45:305–312, 1976.
25. Coppen A, Ghose K, Montgomery S, et al: Amitriptyline plasma-concentration and clinical effect. Lancet 1:63–66, 1978.
26. Kragh-Sørensen P, Hansen CE, Larsen N-E, et al: Long-term treatment of endogenous depression with nortriptyline with control of plasma levels. Psychol Med 4:174–180, 1974.
27. Gram LF, Reisby N, Ibsen I, et al: Plasma levels and antidepressive effect of imipramine. Clin Pharmacol Ther 19:318–324, 1976.
28. Åsberg M: Plasma nortriptyline levels—relationship to clinical effects. Clin Pharmacol Ther 16:215–229, 1974.
29. Luchins D, Ananth J: Therapeutic implications of tricyclic antidepressant plasma levels. J Nerv Ment Dis 162:430–436, 1976.
30. Oswald I, Brezinova V, Dunleavy DLF: On the slowness of action of tricyclic antidepressant drugs. Br J Psychiatry 120:673–677, 1972.
31. DiMascio A, Klerman GL, Prusoff B: Relative safety of amitriptyline in maintenance treatment of depression. J Nerv Ment Dis 160:34–41, 1975.
32. Vaillant GE: Clinical significance of anticholinergic effects of imipramine-like drugs. Am J Psychiatry 125:1600–1602, 1969.

33. Everett HC: The use of bethanechol chloride with tricyclic antidepressants. Am J Psychiatry 132:1202–1204, 1975.
34. Goldberg HL, Finnerty RJ: Which tricyclic for depressed outpatients, imipramine pamoate or amitriptyline? Dis Nerv Syst 38:785–789, 1977.
35. Jefferson JW: A review of the cardiovascular effects and toxicity of tricyclic antidepressants. Psychosom Med 37:160–179, 1975.
36. Burrows GD, Vohra J, Hunt D, et al: Cardiac effects of different tricyclic antidepressant drugs. Br J Psychiatry 129:335–341, 1976.
37. Biamino G, Fenner H, Schüren K-P, et al: Cardiovascular side effects of tricyclic antidepressants—a risk in the use of these drugs. Int J Clin Pharmacol 11:253–261, 1975.
38. Alexander CS, Niño A: Cardiovascular complications in young patients taking psychotropic drugs. Am Heart J 78:757–769, 1969.
39. Vohra J, Burrows GD, Sloman G: Assessment of cardiovascular side effects of therapeutic doses of tricyclic anti-depressant drugs. Aust NZ J Med 5:7–11, 1975.
40. Winsberg BG, Goldstein S, Yepes LE, et al: Imipramine and electrocardiographic abnormalities in hyperactive children. Am J Psychiatry 132:542–545, 1975.
41. Saraf KR, Klein DF, Gittelman-Klein R, et al: EKG effects of imipramine treatment in children. J Am Acad Child Psychiatry 17:60–69, 1978.
42. Kantor SJ, Bigger JT Jr, Glassman AH, et al: Imipramine-induced heart block: a longitudinal case study. JAMA 231:1364–1366, 1975.
43. Thorstrand C: Cardiovascular effects of poisoning with tricyclic antidepressants. Acta Med Scand 195:505–514, 1974.
44. Serafimovski N, Thorball N, Asmussen I, et al: Tricyclic antidepressant poisoning with special reference to cardiac complications. Acta Anaesth Scand Suppl 57:55–63, 1975.
45. Aquilonius S-M, Hedstrand U: The use of physostigmine as an antidote in tricyclic anti-depressant intoxication. Acta Anaesth Scand 22:40–45, 1978.
46. Boston Collaborative Drug Surveillance Program: Adverse reactions to the tricyclic-antidepressant drugs. Lancet 1:529–531, 1972.
47. Moir DC, Crooks J, Cornwell WB, et al: Cardiotoxicity of amitriptyline. Lancet 2:561–564, 1972.
48. Meyer JF, McAllister CK, Goldberg LI: Insidious and prolonged antagonism of guanethidine by amitriptyline. JAMA 213:1487–1488, 1970.
49. Mitchell JR, Cavanaugh JH, Arias L, et al: Guanethidine and related agents. II. Antagonism by drugs which inhibit the norepinephrine pump in man. J Clin Invest 49:1596–1604, 1970.
50. Greenblatt DJ, Shader RI, Lofgren S: Rational psychopharmacology for patients with medical diseases. Annu Rev Med 27:407–420, 1976.
51. Wheatley D: Potentiation of amitriptyline by thyroid hormone. Arch Gen Psychiatry 26:229–233, 1972.
52. Coppen A, Whybrow PC, Noguera R, et al: The comparative antidepressant value of L-tryptophan and imipramine with and without attempted potentiation by liothyronine. Arch Gen Psychiatry 26:234–241, 1972.
53. Robinson DS, Nies A, Ravaris CL, et al: Clinical pharmacology of phenelzine. Arch Gen Psychiatry 35:629–635, 1978.
54. Schuckit M, Robins E, Feighner J: Tricyclic antidepressants and monoamine oxidase inhibitors. Arch Gen Psychiatry 24:509–514, 1971.
55. Sethna ER: A study of refractory cases of depressive illnesses and their response to combined antidepressant treatment. Br J Psychiatry 124:265–272, 1974.
56. Ponto LB, Perry PJ, Liskow BI, et al: Tricyclic antidepressants and monoamine oxidase inhibitor combination therapy. Am J Hosp Pharm 34:954–961, 1977.
57. Cuthbert MF, Greenberg MP, Morley SW: Cough and cold remedies: a potential danger to patients on monoamine oxidase inhibitors. Br Med J 1:404–406, 1969.
58. Gershon S, Shopsin B (eds): *Lithium: Its Role in Psychiatric Research and Treatment.* New York, Plenum Press, 1973.
59. Gershon S: Lithium in mania. Clin Pharmacol Ther 11:168–187, 1970.
60. Schou M: Lithium in psychiatric therapy and prophylaxis. J Psychiatr Res 6:67–95, 1968.
61. Prien RF, Caffey EM Jr, Klett CJ: Lithium carbonate: a survey of the history and current status of lithium in treating mood disorders. Dis Nerv Syst 32:521–531, 1971.
62. Baldessarini RJ, Lipinski JF: Lithium salts: 1970–1975. Ann Intern Med 83:527–533, 1975.

63. Prien RF, Caffey EM Jr: The current status of lithium prophylaxis. Dis Nerv Syst 35:470–471, 1974.
64. Mendels J, Secunda SK, Dyson WL: A controlled study of the antidepressant effects of lithium carbonate. Arch Gen Psychiatry 26:154–157, 1972.
65. Saran BM, Gaind R: Lithium. Clin Toxicol 6:257–269, 1973.
66. Prien RF, Caffey EM Jr, Klett CJ: Relationship between serum lithium level and clinical response in acute mania treated with lithium. Br J Psychiatry 120:409–414, 1972.
67. Lyttkens L, Söderberg U, Wetterberg L: Relation between erythrocyte and plasma lithium concentrations as an index in psychiatric disease. Ups J Med Sci 81:123–128, 1976.
68. Marini JL: On the significance of the erythrocyte lithium to plasma lithium ratio. Br J Psychiatry 130:139–143, 1977.
69. Villeneuve A, Gautier J, Jus A, et al: The effect of lithium on thyroid in man. Int J Clin Pharmacol 9:75–80, 1974.
70. Luby ED, Schwartz D, Rosenbaum H: Lithium-carbonate-induced myxedema. JAMA 218:1298–1299, 1971.
71. Rogers MP, Whybrow PC: Clinical hypothyroidism occurring during lithium treatment: two case histories and a review of thyroid function in 19 patients. Am J Psychiatry 128:158–163, 1971.
72. Rifkin A, Quitkin F, Blumberg AG, et al: The effect of lithium on thyroid functioning: a controlled study. J Psychiatr Res 10:115–120, 1974.
73. Lindstedt G, Lundberg P-A, Tofft M, et al: Serum thyrotropin and hypothyroidism during lithium therapy. Clin Chim Acta 48:127–133, 1973.
74. Edhag O, Swahn A, Wester PO: Hypothyroidism following lithium treatment. Acta Med Scand 193:553–555, 1973.
75. Spaulding SW, Burrow GN, Bermudez F, et al: The inhibitory effect of lithium on thyroid hormone release in both euthyroid and thyrotoxic patients. J Clin Endocrinol Metab 35:905–911, 1972.
76. Carlson HE, Temple R, Robbins J: Effect of lithium on thyroxine disappearance in man. J Clin Endocrinol Metab 36:1251–1254, 1973.
77. Shopsin B, Shenkman L, Blum M, et al: Iodine and lithium-induced hypothyroidism. Am J Med 55:695–699, 1973.
78. Crowe MJ, Lloyd GG, Bloch S, et al: Hypothyroidism in patients treated with lithium: a review and two case reports. Psychol Med 3:337–342, 1973.
79. Lazarus JH, Richards AR, Addison GM, et al: Treatment of thyrotoxicosis with lithium carbonate. Lancet 2:1160–1162, 1974.
80. Temple R, Berman M, Carlson HE, et al: The use of lithium in Graves' disease. Mayo Clin Proc 47:872–878, 1972.
81. Temple R, Berman M, Robbins J, et al: The use of lithium in the treatment of thyrotoxicosis. J Clin Invest 51:2746–2756, 1972.
82. MacNeil S, Jennings G, Eastwood PR, et al: Lithium and the antidiuretic hormone. Br J Clin Pharmacol 3:305–313, 1976.
83. Martinez-Maldonado M, Terrell J: Lithium carbonate-induced nephrogenic diabetes insipidus and glucose intolerance. Arch Intern Med 132:881–884, 1973.
84. White MG, Fetner CD: Treatment of the syndrome of inappropriate secretion of antidiuretic hormone with lithium carbonate. N Engl J Med 292:390–392, 1975.
85. Ramsey TA, Mendels J, Stokes JW, et al: Lithium carbonate and kidney function: a failure in renal concentrating ability. JAMA 219:1446–1449, 1972.
86. Viol GW, Grof P, Daigle L: Renal tubular function in patients on long-term lithium therapy. Am J Psychiatry 132:68–70, 1975.
87. Erwin CW, Gerber CJ, Morrison SD, et al: Lithium carbonate and convulsive disorders. Arch Gen Psychiatry 28:646–648, 1973.
88. Steele TH, Manuel MA, Newton M, et al: Renal lithium reabsorption in man: physiologic and pharmacologic determinants. Am J Med Sci 269:349–363, 1975.
89. Fryö B, Petterson U, Sedvall G: Pharmacokinetics of lithium in manic-depressive patients. Acta Psychiatr Scand 49:237–247, 1973.
90. Thomsen K, Schou M: Renal lithium excretion in man. Am J Physiol 215:823–827, 1968.
91. Petersen V, Hvidt S, Thomsen K, et al: Effect of prolonged thiazide treatment on renal lithium clearance. Br Med J 3:143–145, 1974.
92. Gram LF: Metabolism of tricyclic antidepressants. Dan Med Bull 21:218–231, 1964.

93. Ziegler VE, Clayton PJ, Biggs JT: A comparison study of amitriptyline and nortriptyline with plasma levels. Arch Gen Psychiatry 34:607–612, 1977.
94. Ziegler VE, Wylie LT, Biggs JT: Intrapatient variability of serial steady-state plasma tricyclic antidepressant concentrations. J Pharm Sci 67:554–555, 1978.
95. Jørgensen A, Hansen V: Pharmacokinetics of amitriptyline infused intravenously in man. Eur J Clin Pharmacol 10:337–341, 1976.
96. Ziegler VE, Biggs JT, Wylie LT, et al: Protriptyline kinetics. Clin Pharmacol Ther 23:580–584, 1978.
97. Alván G, Borgå O, Lind M, et al: First pass hydroxylation of nortriptyline: concentrations of parent drug and major metabolites in plasma. Eur J Clin Pharmacol 11:219–224, 1977.
98. Overø KF, Gram LF, Hansen V: Kinetics of nortriptyline in man according to a two compartment model. Eur J Clin Pharmacol 8:343–347, 1975.
99. Gram LF, Overø KF: First-pass metabolism of nortriptyline in man. Clin Pharmacol Ther 18:305–314, 1975.
100. Alexanderson B, Borgå O, Alván G: The availability of orally administered nortriptyline. Eur J Clin Pharmacol 5:181–185, 1973.
101. Gram LF, Christiansen J: First-pass metabolism of imipramine in man. Clin Pharmacol Ther 17:555–563, 1975.
102. Gram LF, Søndergaard I, Christiansen J, et al: Steady-state kinetics of imipramine in patients. Psychopharmacology 54:255–261, 1977.
103. Reisby N, Gram LF, Bech P, et al: Imipramine: clinical effects and pharmacokinetic variability. Psychopharmacology 54:263–272, 1977.
104. Nagy A, Johansson R: Plasma levels of imipramine and desipramine in man after different routes of administration. Naunyn-Schmiedeberg's Arch Pharmacol 290:145–160, 1975.
105. Dencker H, Dencker SJ, Green A, et al: Intestinal absorption, demethylation, and enterohepatic circulation of imipramine. Clin Pharmacol Ther 19:584–586, 1976.
106. Gram LF, Andreasen PB, Overø KF, et al: Comparison of single dose kinetics of imipramine, nortriptyline and antipyrine in man. Psychopharmacology 50:21–27, 1976.
107. Ziegler VE, Biggs JT, Wylie LT, et al: Doxepin kinetics. Clin Pharmacol Ther 23:573–579, 1978.
108. Cooper TB, Bergner P-EE, Simpson GM: The 24-hour serum lithium level as a prognosticator of dosage requirements. Am J Psychiatry 130:601–603, 1973.

OTHER DRUGS AFFECTING THE CENTRAL NERVOUS SYSTEM

37. ANTICONVULSANT DRUGS

H. Harris Funkenstein

Since the late nineteenth century, epilepsy has been recognized as a disorder of the central nervous system (CNS) that is manifested by recurrent, transient episodes of altered CNS function. The development of the electroencephalogram (EEG) as a clinical tool and subsequent experimental studies have clearly established the relationship of seizure disorders to dysfunction of the cerebral cortex and the reticular formation.

Most classifications of seizures are based on the International Classification of Epilepsy described in 1970 by Gastaut.[1] This classification includes the three main categories:

(1) Generalized seizures that are symmetrical and without focal onset. These include absence (petit mal), grand mal (tonic-clonic), tonic, atonic, infantile spasms, and generalized myoclonus.

(2) Partial seizures with focal onset. One subcategory consists of partial seizures with elementary symptomatology that can be motor (including Jacksonian seizures), sensory, autonomic, or affective. Complex forms combine more than one of these symptoms. The second subcategory includes those partial seizures with complex symptomatology such as temporal lobe or psychomotor seizures.

(3) Partial seizures that are secondarily generalized.

Accurate characterization of the type of seizure is essential for successful management, including diagnostic evaluation and choice of drug therapy. In seizures characterized by alterations of consciousness (generalized or psychomotor seizures), descriptions from observers may be more important than the patient's own report in establishing the type of convulsive activity. In general, the EEG does not establish the type of seizure, except in the case of petit mal where bilaterally synchronous 3-per-second spike-and-wave activity during the absence is essential for the diagnosis.[2]

The EEG is most useful in assessing the possibility of a focal lesion and in distinguishing true from hysterical seizures. Frequent routine EEG recordings are not indicated in seizure patients with good control.

Microelectrode recording from human and animal epileptic foci show recurrent high-frequency rhythmic bursts in single cells coincident with membrane depolarization.[3–5] These discharges are not associated with clinical symptomatology unless they spread to adjacent or distant cortical sites. Drugs may reduce clinical seizures either by suppressing epileptic foci or by impairing transmission to other cortical areas.

The electrophysiological basis of primary generalized seizures is less clear. The term 'centrencephalic' has been coined by Penfield[6] to denote the deep, midline, possibly diencephalic origin of the symmetric spike-and-wave activity of petit mal; whether other generalized seizure disorders arise from a similar deep locus which acts on both hemispheres simultaneously is unclear.[7] In experimental animals, generalized tonic-clonic seizures can be produced from cortical lesions involving the inferior surface of the frontal lobes and other regions.

The etiology of epilepsy may be genetic, congenital or acquired; it may reflect either systemic disease or a localized CNS disease. In a particular patient the likely causes depend upon both the age of onset and the character of the seizure. In infancy, the causes include congenital lesions, perinatal encephalopathy, pyridoxine deficiency, and metabolic abnormalities (hypocalcemia, hypoglycemia). In childhood the usual causes are perinatal trauma or anoxia, or fever. Seizures in adulthood can be caused by alcohol or drug withdrawal, tumors, or trauma. Finally, seizures in the elderly usually result from cerebrovascular disease, tumors, trauma, or degenerative changes. In a large percentage of cases a specific etiology cannot be established.

Evaluation should first focus on the possibility of a treatable medical or neurologic disorder, and then on the choice of anticonvulsant. Careful history (both of the seizures themselves and of past infection, trauma or perinatal injury), complete neurological examination, EEG, and certain blood tests (complete blood count, serology, electrolytes, blood urea nitrogen, blood sugar, calcium) are required in all patients presenting with new onset of a seizure disorder. Computerized axial tomography scanning is highly desirable, especially in those with a focal component to the seizures, or focal abnormalities on EEG or neurological examination. Lumbar puncture should be performed in any patient where acute or chronic infection is possible, and in most patients with recent onset of seizures.

The decision to institute drug therapy depends on the frequency of seizures, their possible serious consequences, and their probable cause. A single seizure in an otherwise healthy individual with a normal EEG may not require medication, but this is controversial and such patients are uncommon. Seizures provoked by a metabolic abnormality, such as hyponatremia, hypo- or hyperglycemia, hypocalcemia, hypoxia or uremia, or such conditions as eclampsia, hypertensive encephalopathy or iatrogenic respiratory alkalosis, require only short-term or no therapy with anticonvulsants. Attention should be directed toward the correction of the medical condition. Withdrawal seizures require no treatment unless recurrence is due to persistent drug or alcohol abuse.[8]

The choice of anticonvulsants depends on the type of seizure. Petit mal absence attacks are treated with ethosuximide;[9] the oxazolidinediones are second choices. Benzodiazepines may be useful in selected cases, especially in pregnant women.[10] Sodium valproate may eventually become the drug of first choice. Most absence attacks persisting into adulthood, however, are not petit mal but rather atypical temporal lobe seizures. In grand mal or focal seizures, a major anticonvulsant (ie, phenytoin, phenobarbital or carbamazepine) should be started. A second drug, such as phenobarbital, carbamazepine or primidone, should be added if high therapeutic levels of the first fail to control seizures. Addition of acetazolamide around menstrual periods may aid control in women with seizures related to the menses. Myoclonic seizures are best treated with clonazepam.

Status epilepticus (recurrent or continuous seizures without regaining consciousness) is treated with intubation and adequate oxygenation, hypertonic glucose, and either diazepam or a barbiturate intravenously.[11–13] Phenytoin is usually added early to establish therapeutic levels (one gram given intravenously at a rate of 25 to 50 mg/minute) or bolster inadequate levels.[14] Failure to control status with these drugs should lead to consideration of paraldehyde or general anesthesia. In many cases, failure to correct a metabolic imbalance perpetuates 'refractory' seizures.

Epilepsy partialis continua (persistent or repeated focal seizures without loss of consciousness) calls for a more conservative combined approach of adequate phenytoin doses together with gradually increasing doses of oral or intramuscular phenobarbital up to about 60 mg four times a day. Since most focal seizures will stop spontaneously within 72 to 96 hours, observation without further drug therapy may be preferable to the administration of large doses of sedative drugs.

Several principles guide the choice and use of anticonvulsant medication. Drugs should be gradually increased to the point of tolerance or therapeutic levels before other drugs are added. Discontinuation of a drug or substitution of another should be done gradually; status epilepticus is most frequently a complication of sudden withdrawal of medication. Drug levels may be useful in determining which of several drugs can be increased to achieve better control, which drug may be responsible for side effects, and whether the patient is compliant.[15] Most anticonvulsants can be given one or two times per day; such a schedule generally ensures better adherence to a therapeutic regimen.

The emergence of increased numbers of seizures after a period of good control should prompt a search for a remediable cause —inadequate blood levels of anticonvulsant medication (secondary to poor compliance or improved metabolism) and a new intercurrent illness are two of the most frequent reasons.

DRUG MONOGRAPHS

PHENYTOIN (Dilantin)
PHENYTOIN SODIUM (Dilantin Sodium)

Phenytoin has anticonvulsant properties against all types of seizures except petit mal absences and myoclonic seizures. It acts primarily by blocking the spread of activity from epileptic foci and possibly by interference with post-tetanic potentiation. Since its introduction by Merritt and Putnam in 1938, phenytoin has become one of the two first-choice drugs for the management of grand mal, focal, and temporal lobe seizures regardless of cause.

Phenytoin is almost completely absorbed from the gastrointestinal tract, although rare cases of malabsorption have been described.[16] Intramuscular administration is not recommended because of slow and frequently erratic absorption. The plasma elimination half-life averages 24 hours, but there is considerable individual variation.

TABLE 1 Preparations and Costs of Anticonvulsants

GENERIC NAME	TRADEMARK NAME(S)	PREPARATIONS AND 1978 COSTS
Hydantoins		
Phenytoin	Dilantin	Suspension 30 mg/5 ml—$3.03/8 oz; 125 mg/5 ml—$3.98/8 oz Tablets (chewable) 50 mg—$2.73/100
Phenytoin Sodium	Dilantin Sodium	Capsules 30 mg—$2.61/100; 100 mg—$3.68/100 Injection (powder) 50 mg/ml (when diluted with special solvent provided)—$2.92
Ethotoin	Peganone	Tablets 250 mg—$4.76/100; 500 mg—$8.92/100
Mephenytoin	Mesantoin	Tablets 100 mg—$3.18/100
Barbiturates		
Phenobarbital	generic	Tablets 15 mg—$0.50–$1.00/100; 30 mg—$0.55–$1.50/100; 60 mg—$0.70–$0.75/100; 100 mg—$0.68–$1.25/100 Elixir 20 mg/5 ml—$1.45–$2.75/pint
Phenobarbital Sodium	generic	Injection (solution) 24 mg/ml—$0.31/5 ml; 30 mg/ml—$0.36/10 ml; 60 mg/ml—$0.23/2 ml; 120 mg/ml—$0.22/1 ml; 150 mg/ml—$0.23/2 ml
Mephobarbital	Mebaral	Tablets 32 mg—$4.82/250; 50 mg—$7.21/250; 100 mg—$9.68/250; 200 mg—$16.37/250
Primidone	Mysoline	Tablets 20 mg—$1.70/100; 250 mg—$5.98/100 Suspension 250 mg/5 ml—$3.50/8 oz
Succinimides		
Ethosuximide	Zarontin	Capsules 250 mg—$9.92/100 Syrup 250 mg/5 ml—$10.45/pint
Methsuximide	Celontin	Capsules 150 mg—$6.18/100; 300 mg—$9.74/100

TABLE 1 *(continued)*

Generic Name	Trademark Name(s)	Preparations and 1978 Costs
Phensuximide	Milontin	Capsules 250 mg—$6.65/100; 500 mg—$9.50/100 Suspension 300 mg/5 ml—$7.84/pint
Oxazolidinediones		
Trimethadione	Tridione	Capsules 300 mg—$4.95/100 Tablets (chewable) 150 mg—$4.38/100 Solution 200 mg/5 ml—$3.26/pint
Paramethadione	Paradione	Capsules 150 mg—$5.00/100; 300 mg—$8.28/100 Solution 300 mg/ml—$4.16/50 ml
Benzodiazepines		
Diazepam	Valium	Tablets 2 mg—$7.46/100; 5 mg—$9.50/100; 10 mg—$14.10/100 Injection (solution) 5 mg/ml—$0.86/ 2 ml, $3.93/10 ml
Clonazepam	Clonopin	Tablets 0.5 mg—$5.18/100; 1 mg—$6.44/100; 2 mg—$8.97/100
Miscellaneous		
Carbamazepine	Tegretol	Tablets 200 mg—$10.82/100
Valproic acid	Depakene	Capsules 250 mg—$14.60/100 Syrup 250 mg/5 ml—$14.60/pint

Intravenous administration, either as the undiluted material or following dilution in 200 to 500 ml of normal saline, provides effective levels and is recommended in emergencies or where oral administration is impractical. Infusion rates should not exceed 25 to 50 mg/min due to the potential of adverse cardiovascular effects.

Excretion occurs via the urine—5% unchanged, 75% oxidized and conjugated by the liver. At therapeutic levels, the enzyme systems involved are usually saturated; thus, small increments in dosage may result in major changes in plasma levels.[17]

Therapeutic efficacy correlates well with plasma levels of the drug. The usual therapeutic range is 7 to 22 μg/ml. Side effects are usually minimal (confined to slight fatigue or nystagmus) or nonexistent at these levels. Addition of a second drug or discontinuation of phenytoin should only follow failure to control seizures with high therapeutic levels. Maintenance of appropriate plasma concentrations may require from 200 to 600 mg of phenytoin per day, given as 1 to 3 doses. Establishment of therapeutic levels in an average adult not previously taking the drug requires a loading dose of approximately 1 g over 24 hours.

Adverse Reactions—Nystagmus, ataxia, diplopia, dysarthria and drowsiness in most patients occur when levels exceed 20 to 30 μg/ml. Choreiform movements often accompany intoxication in children. Persistent cerebellar deficits have been reported in some cases of chronic toxicity.[18]

Upper gastrointestinal discomfort such as anorexia, nausea, and occasionally vomiting may follow oral administration. These effects usually subside if the drug is continued or antacids given. Intravenous administration rarely produces vomiting, but precautions against aspiration should be taken.

A rash, usually morbilliform and nonpruritic, may begin 10 to 14 days after initiation of therapy. Medication should be discontinued although some authorities recommend a second trial. Very rarely, exfoliative dermatitis or erythema multiforme may result. Hirsutism has also been observed.

Gingival hypertrophy is more common in children and usually most severe where dental hygiene is poor.

Chronic administration of phenytoin has been associated with reduced serum calcium, elevated alkaline phosphatase, and rarely osteomalacia.[19] The condition appears to reflect either increased hepatic metabolism of vitamin D, reduced absorption of calcium, or both. Children receiving chronic anticonvulsants and adults with marginal diets or reduced sun exposure should probably receive supplemental vitamin D.

Although the mechanism is not fully understood, a megaloblastic anemia with low serum folate levels has been reported in phenytoin recipients.[20] The anemia is corrected by high doses of folic acid. Phenytoin therapy may be associated in the first month or two with a syndrome of generalized painless lymphadenopathy, often with skin rashes and systemic reaction. Biopsy of lymph nodes reveals reticulum cell hyperplasia, plasma cell infiltration, and focal necroses but no Reed-Sternberg cells. The condition resolves within several weeks after cessation of the drug.[21] Recently an increased incidence of phenytoin exposure was reported in a group of patients with true malignant lymphoma.[22] This observation should be further substantiated before it can be accepted. Bone marrow depression with leukopenia is common; however, serious marrow depression is rare.

An increased incidence of malformations—especially congenital heart disease, cleft lip, cleft palate and microcephaly—have been found in infants of women taking anticonvulsants during pregnancy. Although phenytoin and not epilepsy appears to play a role, the relative importance of different anticonvulsants in producing this syndrome has not been established.

Hepatitis has rarely been reported. It is more commonly related to the use of contaminated needles in drug abusers who may also have seizures.

Dosage—Oral: Adults, initial rapid loading dose, 10 to 13 mg/kg over 4 to 12 hours in single or divided doses. *Initial slow loading dose,* 400 mg daily in one or two doses for 4 to 5 days. *Maintenance,* 200 to 600 mg daily, depending on therapeutic effect and serum concentrations. Older adults often require lower doses to produce comparable serum concentrations. *Children,* 4 to 7 mg/kg daily in single or divided doses.

Intravenous: For status epilepticus, *adults,* 14 mg/kg initially followed by 100 mg orally or intravenously every 6 to 8 hours. *Children,* 15 to 20 mg/kg.

MEPHENYTOIN (Mesantoin)

Mephenytoin is a structural analog of phenytoin and has similar uses. A few patients may respond better to mephenytoin than to phenytoin.

Adverse Reactions—Mephenytoin carries an increased risk of skin rashes and of serious bone marrow depression, including aplastic anemia.[23] It reportedly causes less cerebellar disturbance, gum hypertrophy, and hirsutism. Otherwise, side effects are similar to those with phenytoin.

Dosage—Oral: 7 to 12 mg/kg daily in single or divided doses.

METHETOIN (Deltoin)
ETHOTOIN (Peganone)
ALBUTOIN (Co-Ord)

Since these hydantoins have no advantages over phenytoin and may have some disadvantages, their use is not recommended.

PHENOBARBITAL C-IV
PHENOBARBITAL SODIUM C-IV

Except for bromides, phenobarbital was the first anticonvulsant used extensively. It is effective against most forms of epilepsy including major motor seizures and both simple and complex (psychomotor) focal seizures although less preferable than phenytoin or carbamazepine for the latter. Phenobarbital is frequently used as an adjunct to phenytoin in the treatment of these seizure types. Phenobarbital may be used in children for the treatment of petit mal epilepsy and is the drug of choice in treating or preventing febrile convulsions. The major advantage of phenobarbital is its relative freedom from long-term side effects. On the other hand, phenobarbital has substantial sedative effects, accounting for its use mainly as an adjunct. Furthermore, it occasionally produces paradoxical hyperexcitability in children and the elderly.

Phenobarbital may be administered orally, intramuscularly or intravenously. It is slowly but almost completely absorbed from the gastrointestinal tract, reaching peak levels in 4 to 7 hours. About 50% of the total drug present in plasma is bound to plasma proteins. Phenobarbital is oxidized and conjugated in the liver, with both free and conjugated forms excreted via the kidneys.

Therapeutic plasma concentrations of phenobarbital range from 20 to 30 μg/ml.[24] There is considerable individual variation in response, necessitating careful monitoring and clinical judgement based on efficacy and the presence of toxic manifestations. Because of its long elimination half-life of 4 to 7 days, once-daily administration is usually sufficient to maintain stable levels. In status epilepticus, intravenous or intramuscular administration is preferred.

The mechanism of phenobarbital's action is not established. In the experimental animal, it raises seizure threshold to both electrical and chemical convulsants. Phenobarbital may also delay transmission through synaptic chains and potentiate presynaptic inhibition.[25]

Adverse Reactions—Drowsiness is common when therapy is initiated but usually remits spontaneously in 1 to 2 weeks (despite rising blood levels), or responds to changes in the time of administration. Toxic levels produce drowsiness, slurred speech, ataxia, and confusion. Children may become more irritable and hyperactive. Subtle deficits in intellectual function are frequent complaints in patients taking high therapeutic doses.

Agranulocytosis and aplastic anemia are very rare, although an early depression of the white count is not uncommon. Folate deficiency is less common than with phenytoin. Anticonvulsants may be associated with coagulation defects and even bleeding in the neonate, which is prevented by prophylactic vitamin K.[26]

Hepatitis and severe rash are rare; however, fine punctate erythema or morbilliform eruptions may occur occasionally.

Dosage—Oral: Adults, sole drug, 60 to 240 mg daily depending on therapeutic response and side effects. Once daily administration is quite feasible; when given in divided doses, the largest is given at supper or bedtime. *Adjunct drug,* 30 to 180 mg daily. *Children,* 15 to 50 mg two or three times daily.

Intramuscular, Intravenous (slow): For status epilepticus, *adults,* 200 to 400 mg. Dividing the dose between intravenous and intramuscular administration is often useful. The amount and frequency of repeated doses should depend on clinical response. Extreme caution should be exercised when other drugs have been used and when control of respiration is not assured. *Children* (intramuscular), 3 to 5 mg/kg.

MEPHOBARBITAL (Mebaral) C-IV

This N-methyl derivative of phenobarbital has a similar range of action. It is absorbed less well than phenobarbital and hence is given in higher doses. Virtually all of the drug is biotransformed *in vivo* to phenobarbital with subsequent fate as described for phenobarbital. In some patients, slower metabolism to phenobarbital may result in relatively high mephobarbital levels such that side effects (drowsiness, ataxia) are not accurately reflected by the phenobarbital level.[27] At present, there is no generally available method of measuring mephobarbital plasma levels directly. Because of its erratic absorption, this drug is not recommended.

Adverse Reactions—The adverse reactions of mephobarbital are similar to those of phenobarbital.

Dosage—Oral: Adults, 400 to 600 mg daily in divided doses. *Children:* 2.5 to 10 mg/kg.

PRIMIDONE (Mysoline)

Primidone has been used since 1952 to treat grand mal, simple focal and psychomotor epilepsy. It is frequently given together with other drugs, especially phenytoin, and as a substitute for phenobarbital. The superiority of primidone in the treatment of temporal lobe epilepsy has not been substantiated.[28] No evidence yet exists that primidone provides better seizure control than phenobarbital when both drugs are given in therapeutic amounts, although individual patients may fare better.

Primidone is rapidly absorbed from the gastrointestinal tract, but the completeness of absorption is not known. Primidone is metabolized in the liver to phenobarbital and phenylethylmalonamide. During chronic administration phenobarbital accounts for more than half of the ingested primidone. Once-daily administration will probably maintain reasonably constant therapeutic levels, but transient drowsiness may result. Therapeutic plasma concentrations of primidone range from 7 to 15 μg/ml, but phenobarbital concentrations should be measured simultaneously due to its important role in the anticonvulsant effect of primidone.

Adverse Reactions—Drowsiness, ataxia, nystagmus, and dysarthria may result from high concentrations of primidone or phenobarbital. Initial doses of primidone often lead to excessive drowsiness that probably represents high initial primidone levels; this may be managed by initiating therapy with smaller more frequent doses. Other CNS reactions that are attributed to phenobarbital may occur with primidone.

Gastrointestinal disturbances are not uncommon and may require a slow approach to final dosage over 10 to 20 days.

Megaloblastic anemia, secondary to folic acid deficiency, and skin rashes, usually maculo-papular, also may occur.

Dosage—Oral: Adults, 500 to 1500 daily. It is wise to start with low dosage, eg, 125 mg twice a day, then increase gradually. *Children,* 10 to 25 mg/kg.

CARBAMAZEPINE (Tegretol)

This compound is structurally related to the tricyclic antidepressants. It has been used for seizures since the early 1960's and also is given to treat trigeminal neuralgia and diabetes insipidus. Carbamazepine is effective by itself or adjunctively against both grand mal and focal seizure disorders, including temporal lobe epilepsy. There is some evidence that carbamazepine is the most effective drug for partial seizures with complex symptomatology. It is not recommended for petit mal. Although side effects may be serious, they are fortunately rare.

Oral carbamazepine is rapidly but incompletely absorbed and is widely distributed to body tissues. The elimination half-life is about 14 hours. More than 75% of the drug in plasma is bound to plasma proteins. Plasma levels of 6 to 8 μg/ml (measured by gas chromatography) represent a reasonable therapeutic range, although more experience is needed. Patients differ in their absorption (and possibly metabolism) of oral doses but most will obtain therapeutic levels on 600 to 1000 mg per day.

While still under active investigation, carbamazepine appears to act by reducing after-discharge and depressing synaptic transmission in selected areas of brain related to the genesis or propagation of epileptic discharges.[29]

Adverse Reactions—Nystagmus, fatiguability, drowsiness, ataxia, and dizziness are dose-related CNS effects.

Blood dyscrasias such as aplastic anemia, leucopenia, and thrombocytopenia have been reported.[30] Routine blood counts are advisable at frequent intervals after starting therapy, but hematologic complications are rare.

Mild allergic dermatitides have been seen, as well as more serious eruptions, including purpura, erythema multiforme exudativum (Stevens-Johnson syndrome) and exfoliative reactions.[31] A reversible lupus-like disorder has been observed.

Gastrointestinal disturbances (nausea, vomiting, and anorexia) and jaundice are reported.

Dosage—Oral: Adults, 600 to 1000 mg daily, given twice a day. Patients should be started at levels no higher than 200 mg twice a day, then increased gradually, 100 mg each day. *Children under 6 years of age,* 100 mg daily; *6 to 12 years,* 100 mg twice daily.

ETHOSUXIMIDE (Zarontin)

This drug is the first choice for typical petit mal absence seizures; it is preferred to the older oxazolidinediones (trimethadione and paramethadione) because of its relatively greater safety. In atypical absence seizures with frontal spike-and-wave or rhythmical slow wave activity, ethosuximide may be useful.

Oral doses are rapidly and virtually completely absorbed from the gastrointestinal tract. The drug is minimally protein-bound. Ethosuximide is largely oxidized to a ketone and an alcohol before excretion; 20% is eliminated unchanged in the urine.

Following initiation of therapy, plasma levels rise over 4 to 6 days, the half-life in adults being 50 to 60 hours, and in children 30 to 40 hours. Therapeutic plasma concentrations of 40 to 100 μg/ml are recommended although occasionally higher levels are required.[32]

Adverse Reactions—Fatigue, drowsiness, headache, and dizziness are dose-related CNS effects. Local gastrointestinal irritation can occur, particularly if the drug is given once daily.

Leucopenia and pancytopenia are rare and usually not serious. Cutaneous eruptions have been observed, although rarely Stevens-Johnson syndrome, and several investigators have reported a systemic lupus-like disorder.

Dosage—Oral: Adults and older children, 750 to 1250 mg daily in divided doses.

METHSUXIMIDE (Celontin)
PHENSUXIMIDE (Milontin)

These drugs have no advantage over ethosuximide and have the disadvantage of considerably shorter half-lives, requiring more frequent administration. They may be used in the treatment of petit mal epilepsy where ethosuximide cannot be tolerated.

Dosage—Oral: Adults and children, methsuximide, 10 to 20 mg/kg per day; phensuximide, 1 to 3 g/day in 2 to 3 doses.

TRIMETHADIONE (Tridione)
PARAMETHADIONE (Paradione)

These drugs, originally introduced by Lennox in 1945, were the major agents for the treatment of petit mal epilepsy and atypical spike-and-wave absence attacks before the introduction of ethosuximide. Though effective, their side effects make them drugs of second choice. They may occasionally precipitate grand mal attacks.

Trimethadione is absorbed rapidly from the gastrointestinal tract and is not significantly bound to plasma proteins. Both drugs are almost totally dealkylated in the liver. Trimethadione, with a plasma half-life of 14 to 16 hours, is metabolized to dimethadione, which possesses considerable anticonvulsant activity and has a much longer biological half-life.

In patients taking trimethadione on a chronic basis, dimethadione accounts for most of the anticonvulsant activity. Plasma levels of dimethadione of 600 μg/ml or higher, or trimethadione levels of 20 to 40 μg/ml, are considered therapeutic for petit mal epilepsy; levels for paramethadione are not known.

Adverse Reactions—Sedation may occur with high doses. Uncomfortable visual alterations, particularly an unpleasant glare when emerging into sunlight or a well-lit room, are common in patients taking these drugs.[33]

Edema and severe protein-losing nephropathy may occur, although the condition generally remits after drug withdrawal.[34]

Neutropenia occurs in about 20% of recipients, and occasionally pancytopenia and fatal aplastic anemia have been reported.

Other adverse effects include hepatitis, skin reactions (generalized erythema, maculopapular eruptions and exfoliative dermatitis) and, rarely, mild gastrointestinal disturbances. Congenital malformations may be more frequent in women taking these drugs; however, use of these medications in the child-bearing age group is now rare.

Dosage—Oral: Adults and children, trimethadione, 10 to 25 mg/kg in 2 to 3 doses, and therapy should be initiated slowly; paramethadione, 10 to 25 mg/kg in 2 to 3 doses.

DIAZEPAM (Valium) C-IV

Parenteral diazepam is one of the drugs of choice in the treatment of status epilepticus,[35] regardless of its etiology. It is less effective, because of its transient effect, in the treatment of focal epilepsy partialis continua. Diazepam is not generally used for the ambulatory treatment of other seizure disorders, such as myoclonus, petit mal or grand mal, because of the strong sedative action which accompanies levels sufficiently high to prevent seizures.

The drug is absorbed rapidly and nearly completely (90%) from the gastrointestinal tract. About 96% or more of diazepam is protein-bound. The elimination of diazepam after oral or intravenous administration is biphasic. The initial rapid decay during the first few hours is due to distribution. Thereafter, elimination proceeds slowly with a half-life of 20 to 50 hours, and is mirrored by appearance of desmethyldiazepam, the major metabolite of diazepam. Desmethyldiazepam is biologically active and has a very long half-life of 48 hours or more. Other hydroxylated metabolites of diazepam are conjugated to glucuronic acid and rapidly excreted in the urine. Oxazepam glucuronide is the major urinary metabolite.

Periods of several weeks may be required to reach stable plasma levels in patients taking a fixed daily dose. Optimal plasma concentrations for the prevention of epileptic seizures are not presently known.

There is some evidence that benzodiazepines act in part by augmenting presynaptic inhibition.

Adverse Reactions—CNS effects such as drowsiness, ataxia, and dysarthria are common and have limited the usefulness of this drug as the primary treatment for ambulatory seizure disorders.[10] Patients taking this drug should be warned about the possible serious consequences of concurrent alcohol ingestion.

Parenteral diazepam, especially in doses of 10 mg or more and particularly if given rapidly, may induce serious systemic hypotension and/or respiratory depression in susceptible individuals.

Skin reactions have also been observed.

Dosage—Intravenous: For status epilepticus, 5 to 10 mg given as a slow infusion over several minutes. This may be repeated once or twice, but further doses are unlikely to produce a greater effect. Caution must be exercised if other drugs, such as phenobarbital, are employed concurrently, as their depressant effects may be potentiated. *Oral:* Dosage is varied according to response, generally 15 to 30 mg per day in divided doses, or lesser amounts if other drugs are used concurrently. At present, the role of oral diazepam in seizure control is not established.

CLONAZEPAM (Clonopin) C-IV

This compound, structurally related to diazepam, is still under active investigation. Clonazepam appears useful against many seizure disorders, including typical and atypical petit mal, myoclonus, akinetic seizures, and, in parenteral form, status epilepticus. Its strong sedative action confines its use to adjunctive rather than to primary therapy.

Approximately 90% is absorbed after oral administration with peak levels reached at 3 hours. Clonazepam has an elimination half-life of about 12 hours. The major metabolic pathway involves nitroreduction to yield a pharmacologically inactive amino derivative. Early data suggest that plasma levels should exceed 15 μg/ml for myoclonus and 30 μg/ml for other types of seizures.[36] Plasma clonazepam levels should probably not exceed 50 μg/ml, a level obtained by daily doses of 10 mg. Clonazepam may depress phenytoin levels significantly in patients taking both drugs.

Adverse Reactions—Adverse reactions are generally similar to diazepam and other benzodiazepines. However, paradoxical excicment and aggressiveness appear to be quite common in children taking clonazepam.

Dosage—Oral: Adults, 2 to 8 mg in divided doses. Therapy should be started with doses no larger than 0.5 mg three times a day. *Children,* 0.1 to 0.3 mg/kg/day. The total daily dose may be increased by increments of 0.25 to 0.5 mg every third day until a maintenance dose of 0.1 to 0.2 mg/kg/day has been reached.

NITRAZEPAM (Mogadon)

This benzodiazepine derivative is particularly useful in the treatment of myoclonic seizures. It is also useful in controlling brief, irregular muscle jerks that may occur in generalized seizure disorders, during withdrawal states, as a manifestation of metabolic derangements such as hypoxic encephalopathy, and in some less common neurological disorders. Nitrazepam is not available in the United States.

About 80% of an oral dose is absorbed from the gastrointestinal tract. In the blood 85% is bound to plasma proteins. Like clonazepam, nitrazepam is biotransformed mainly by nitroreduction to form an inactive amino derivative. The elimination half-life is about 24 hours.[37] Therapeutic levels are not established.

Adverse Reactions—These are similar to those of diazepam and clonazepam. In addition, nitrazepam appears to cause increased salivary and bronchial secretions.

Dosage—Oral: Adults, 5 to 10 mg per day.

VALPROIC ACID (Depakene)

The anticonvulsant properties of sodium dipropylacetate were discovered accidentally by Meunier and colleagues in 1963 during testing of other compounds solubilized in dipropylacetic acid. Its structure, as a result, differs considerably from those of other anticonvulsants.[38]

Valproic acid possesses a wide spectrum of usefulness in the treatment of seizure disorders.[39] In petit mal attacks it equals ethosuximide in potency and may be safer. Valproic acid alone, or preferably in combination with other agents, successfully controls partial seizures with both simple and complex sympatomatology. Both generalized myoclonus and generalized tonic-clonic seizures are more easily managed when valproic acid is added to other drugs. Its usefulness in infantile spasms or hypsarrhythmia and in atypical petit mal is not fully determined. Valproic acid produces very little sedation or other serious side effects and may actually increase alertness because of the beneficial effects of concurrent reduction in doses of other anticonvulsants.

The mechanism of valproic acid's anticonvulsant action is under investigation. Cortical and cerebellar levels of gamma aminobutyric acid (GABA) are increased, possibly by an inhibition of GABA transaminase,[40] but whether this occurs at therapeutic levels and whether this change affects the small neurotransmitter fraction of the total GABA pool is uncertain. The drug reduces or blocks spread from most experimentally-induced seizure foci, and protects against a variety of epileptogenic agents.[39]

Valproic acid is rapidly absorbed from the gastrointestinal tract. Most of the circulating drug (80 to 90%) is bound to plasma proteins. Blood levels at a given daily dose vary widely between individuals. Steady-state levels are reached in 24 to 36 hours with administration three or four times per day, but interdose fluctuation can range from 40 to 140%. The elimination half-life is approximately 7 to 10 hours when valproic acid is given alone and may be reduced when given in conjunction with other drugs. Therapeutic blood levels appear to range from 50 to 100 μg/ml, which represents an average daily adult intake of 1200 to 1500 mg per day.[41]

Excretion occurs via the urine after metabolism to propylhydroxypentanoic acid and thence to propylglutamic acid. Small quantities are excreted via the biliary tract into the feces and via the lungs after degradation to carbon dioxide.

When given in conjunction with other drugs, valproic acid frequently produces significant increases in the concentrations of these other agents, especially phenobarbital and primidone.[42] This usually requires adjustment downward of the daily intake of these other drugs.

Adverse Reactions—CNS effects, transient drowsiness and sedation, are usually due to elevation in blood levels of concurrently administered drugs.

Platelet aggregation may be inhibited[43] and prolonged bleeding times and thrombocytopenia[44] have been reported rarely. Introduction of other antihemostatic drugs should be undertaken with caution; surgery may also be complicated by a bleeding diathesis.

Gastrointestinal disorders, including nausea, vomiting, diarrhea, and abdominal cramps, occur in 9 to 16% of adults and 22% of children but are usually transient. Alterations in appetite may result with either weight gain or loss. Reversible alopecia has been observed. Teratogenicity is described in experimental animals, with about the same incidence as equivalent doses of phenytoin.

Dosage—Oral: Adults, initially 250 mg three times per day, may be increased by increments of 250 mg at three-day intervals to a range of 1000 to 1500 mg per day, given three or four times. If control is unsatisfactory, doses may be further increased to 2500 mg daily or rarely even higher. *Children,* 30 to 40 mg/kg/day, starting at 400 mg per day. *Infants and young children,* 20 mg/kg/day is usually sufficient, although doses up to 50 mg/kg/day have been used. The liquid form is preferred for adjusting doses in children.

REFERENCES

1. Gastaut H: Clinical and electroencephalographic classification of epileptic seizures. Epilepsia 11:102–113, 1970.
2. Livingston S: *Comprehensive Management of Epilepsy in Infancy, Childhood and Adolescence.* Springfield, C.C. Thomas, 1972.
3. Ward AA Jr: The epileptic neurone. Epilepsia 2:70–80, 1961.
4. Matsumoto H, Ajmone-Marsan C: Cortical cellular phenomena in experimental epilepsy. Exp Neurol 9:286–326, 1964.
5. Ward AA Jr: The epileptic neuron: chronic foci in animals and man. In *Basic Mechanisms of the Epilepsies.* Edited by HH Jasper, AA Ward Jr., A Pope. Boston, Little, Brown, 1969, pp 263–288.
6. Penfield W: Epileptic automatism and the centrencephalic integrating system. Assoc Res Nerv Mental Dis 30:513–528, 1952.
7. Williams D: The propagation of epileptic events. In *Modern Trends in Neurology 5.* Edited by D Williams. London, Butterworths, 1970, pp 287–295.
8. Sampliner R, Iber FL: Diphenylhydantoin control of alcohol withdrawal seizures. Results of a controlled study. JAMA 230:1430–1432, 1974.
9. Carter S, Gold A: Current concepts. Convulsions in children. N Engl J Med 278:315–317, 1968.
10. Browne TR, Penry JK: Benzodiazepines in the treatment of epilepsy. A review. Epilepsia 14:277–310, 1973.
11. Oxbury JM, Whitty CWM: Causes and consequences of status epilepticus in adults. A study of 86 cases. Brain 94:733–744, 1971.
12. Lombroso C: Treatment of status epilepticus with diazepam. Neurology 16:629–634, 1966.
13. Prensky AI, Raff MC, Moore MJ, et al: Intravenous diazepam in the treatment of prolonged seizure activity. N Engl J Med 276:779–784, 1967.
14. Wallis W, Kutt H, McDowell F: Intravenous diphenylhydantoin in treatment of acute repetitive seizures. Neurology 18:513–525, 1968.
15. Kutt H, Penry JK: Usefulness of blood levels of antiepileptic drugs. Arch Neurol 31:283–288, 1974.
16. Kutt H, Haynes J, McDowell F: Some causes of ineffectiveness of diphenylhydantoin. Arch Neurol 14:489–492, 1966.
17. Gerber N, Lynn R, Bush M, et al: Relationship of plasma level of diphenylhydantoin (DPH) to the rate of excretion of urinary HPPH (abstract). Clin Pharmacol Ther 13:139, 1972.
18. Kokenge R, Kutt H, McDowell F: Neurological sequelae following Dilantin overdose in a patient and in experimental animals. Neurology 15:823–829, 1965.
19. Richens A, Rowe DJF: Disturbance of calcium metabolism by anticonvulsant drugs. Br Med J 4:73–76, 1970.
20. Davis RE, Woodliff HJ: Folic acid deficiency in patients receiving anticonvulsant drugs. Med J Aust 2:1070–1072, 1971.
21. Saltzstein SL, Ackerman LV: Lymphadenopathy induced by anticonvulsant drugs and mimicking clinically and pathologically malignant lymphomas. Cancer 12:164–182, 1959.

22. Hyman GA, Sommers SC: The development of Hodgkins disease and lymphoma during anticonvulsant therapy. Blood 28:416–427, 1966.
23. Robins MM, Aplastic anemia secondary to anticonvulsants. Am J Dis Child 104:614–624, 1962.
24. Buchthal F, Sversmark O, Simonsen H: Relation of EEG and seizures to phenobarbital in serum. Arch Neurol 19:567–572, 1968.
25. Woodbury DM, Kemp JW: Some possible mechanisms of action of antiepileptic drugs. Pharmakopsychiatr Neuro-psychopharmakol 3:201–226, 1974.
26. Mountain KR, Hirsch J, Gallus AS: Neonatal coagulation defect due to anticonvulsant drug treatment in pregnancy. Lancet 1:265–268, 1970.
27. Eadie MJ, Tyrer JH: Unpublished data cited in *Anticonvulsant Therapy*. Edited by MJ Eadie, JH Tyrer. Edinburgh, Churchill-Livingstone, 1974, p 92.
28. Olesen OV, Dam M: The metabolic conversion of primidone (Mysoline) to phenobarbitone in patients under long-term treatment. Acta Neurol Scand 43:348–356, 1967.
29. Kobayashi K, Inata Y, Mukawa J: Preferential action of Tegretol (G-32883) to limbic seizures. Clinical and experimental analysis. Brain Nerve (Japan) 19:999–1005, 1967.
30. Harman RRM: Carbamazepine (Tegretol) drug eruptions. Br J Derm 79:500–501, 1967.
31. Menardi H: Other antiepileptic drugs. Carbamazepine. In *Antiepileptic Drugs*. Edited by DM Woodbury, JK Penry, RP Schmidt. New York, Raven Press, 1972, pp 487–496.
32. Sherwin AL, Robb JP: Ethosuximide. Relation of plasma levels to clinical control. In *Antiepileptic Drugs*. Edited by DM Woodbury, JK Penry, RP Schmidt. New York, Raven Press, 1972, pp 443–448.
33. Sloan LL, Gilger AP: Visual effects of Tridione. Am J Ophthalmol 30:1387–1405, 1947.
34. Heymann W: Nephrotic syndrome after use of trimethadione and paradione in petit mal. JAMA 202:893–894, 1967.
35. Parsonage MJ, Harris JW: Use of diazepam in treatment of severe convulsive status epilepticus. Br Med J 3:85–88, 1967.
36. Huang CY, McLeod JG: Clonazepam in the treatment of epilepsy. Proc Aust Assoc Neurol 10:67–74, 1978.
37. Rieder J, Wendt G: Pharmacokinetics and metabolism of the hypnotic nitrazepam. Symposium on benzodiazepines. Cited in *Anticonvulsant Therapy*. Edited by MJ Eadie, JH Tyrer. London, Churchill-Livingstone, 1974, p 131.
38. Pinder RM, Brogden RM, Sperght TM, et al: Sodium valproate: a review of its pharmacological properties and therapeutic efficacy in epilepsy. Drugs 13:81–123, 1977.
39. Simon D, Penry JK: Sodium di-n-propylacetate (DPA) in the treatment of epilepsy. A review. Epilepsia 16:549–573, 1975.
40. Sawaya MCB, Horton RW, Meldrum BS: Effects of anticonvulsant drugs on the cerebral enzymes metabolizing GABA. Epilepsia 16:649–655, 1975.
41. Richens A, Ahmad S: Controlled trial of sodium valproate in severe epilepsy. Br Med J 4:225–226, 1975.
42. Windorfer A, Sauer W, Gadeke R: Elevation of diphenylhydantoin and primidone serum concentration by addition of dipropylacetate, a new anticonvulsant drug. Acta Paediatr Scand 64:771–772, 1975.
43. Richardson SGN, Fletcher DJ, Jeavons PM, et al: Sodium valproate and platelet function. Br Med J 1:221–222, 1976.
44. Winfield DA, Benton P, Espir MLE, et al: Sodium valproate and thrombocytopenia. Br Med J 2:981, 1976.

38. ANOREXIANTS

Denis Craddock

Obesity is so common in the Western World that it has come to be regarded as normal. Nevertheless, because obesity contributes to maturity-onset diabetes, coronary artery disease, and other diseases its treatment and prevention are very important. Treatment of established obesity is unrewarding, but fortunately those individuals most at risk, namely young and middle-aged men, respond best.

It is extremely difficult for some individuals to reduce caloric intake below that needed to sustain their body weight and therefore to a level necessary to lose weight. Many obese patients have an inherited tendency to gain weight easily and lose it with difficulty.[1] Due to the metabolic changes of long-standing obesity, the longer obese patients have been overweight the harder it is for them to lose weight. In some individuals when caloric intake is decreased basal metabolic rate falls by about 15%, which is enough to make losing weight difficult without becoming clinically hypothyroid.[2] In extreme cases, overweight individuals can maintain their body weight on a daily dietary intake of merely 1500 calories.[3] Maintaining intake appreciably below this level over a long period of time requires a great deal of will-power, since the obese person is being asked to forego a major part of the pleasures of eating for periods of months or even years.

Accordingly, anorectic drugs are useful for some obese patients at a certain stage in their weight-loss regimen. However, patients should attempt to alter their eating habits before resorting to these drugs.

Many obesity-promoting foods would not normally be eaten in large quantities by humans in their 'natural state'. These fall into three main categories:

(1) *Sugar and items made from it.* No one is likely to eat 2½ lbs of sugar beets daily, which is the amount necessary to produce the average daily sugar consumption in the Western World.[4] Even sugar cane is difficult to consume in sufficient quantities to produce this amount of raw sugar.

(2) *Items made from refined carbohydrate.* Natural cereal products require more chewing than refined products. They also provide indigestible fiber so that less of the total bulk of the food is absorbed. Whole meal bread, cereals made from whole grain (such as Weetabix and Shredded Wheat), and bran products are less likely to be eaten in excess than white bread, polished rice, cakes, and cookies made from white flour.

(3) *Items containing large amounts of saturated fats.* The fat of free-running animals is made up mainly of polyunsaturated fatty acids. It is only the animals reared in captivity that develop large stores of saturated fats.

Any diet which restricts the intake of the above foods is likely to be suitable for long-term use in patients who wish to control their weight. Anorectic drugs are justifiable for any patient who has lost weight on a diet and has then come to a plateau for a period of four to six weeks. Flattening of the weight curve commonly occurs with conscientious dieters when they are about halfway between their starting weight and their ideal weight. In most cases anorectic drugs enable them to lose more weight. A few individuals need drugs to help them at an earlier stage than this, and it is occasionally justifiable to start a patient on a drug at the same time as a diet. Individuals in this latter category include those who have to eat frequently because of peptic ulcer disease and those who are moderately depressed.

Anorectic drugs should only be prescribed for as long as weight continues to be lost, and the patient should invariably be seen and weighed by the physician before a further prescription is given. The one exception is in women in whom premenstrual fluid retention masks a loss of fat. Providing that prescriptions are only renewed when weight has been lost, there is no reason why anorectic drugs should not be continued for as long as weight loss continues.

LONG-TERM EFFICACY

Anorectic drugs usually become ineffective after 8 to 12 weeks, but it is uncertain whether this is due to loss of drug efficacy or to loss of patient motivation. Some treated patients continue to lose weight for as long as six months or more.[1,5,6] After losing weight with the aid of drugs, many patients regain it again slowly and require further short courses at intervals of 6 to 12 months. The increasing use of behavioral methods of treatment[7] may allow more obese patients to achieve a permanent change in their eating habits.

PHARMACOLOGIC PROPERTIES

The action of anorectic drugs is principally mediated through centers in the hypothalamus. The metabolic effects of the anorectic drugs are almost entirely due to weight loss which in itself can reverse the metabolic consequences of long-standing obesity.[8] These drugs may also increase weight loss by producing a small increase in energy expenditure.

All anorectic drugs will cause a weight loss of about 1 lb per week for eight to twelve weeks, after which they appear to lose effectiveness in most patients. The choice of drug is therefore based on consideration of the type and frequency of adverse effects, the abuse and dependence potential, and the possible effects from overdosage.

ABUSE, ADDICTION AND OVERDOSAGE

Abuse and addiction are not uncommon with the amphetamines and phenmetrazine (Preludin), and these drugs are accordingly classified under Schedule II of the Controlled Substances Act. One observer alone reported six female cases of amphetamine dependence among patients who received the drugs for obesity.[9] It is seldom justifiable to prescribe these drugs for obesity, except on rare occasions for patients who have taken them previously without adverse effects. The risk of abuse or addiction is minimal with other anorectic drugs in common usage, providing that increased energy or euphoria are regarded as warning signs.

THE RISK OF OVERDOSAGE

Overdosage of anorectic drugs classified under Schedule III or IV (all of the drugs discussed in the individual monographs below) is most commonly accidental and occurs most often in children, although occasionally an overdose is taken with suicidal intent by adults. The risk is greatest with fenfluramine, but it is present with all the others and is a further reason for strict prescribing control. Ideally, prescriptions should not be issued for more than two weeks at a time.

DRUG INTERACTIONS

The monoamine oxidase (MAO) inhibitors can cause potentially serious interaction with the amphetamines and fenfluramine, and none of the anorectic drugs should be taken within two weeks of the cessation of MAO inhibitors. Alcohol and tricyclic antidepressants can cause potentially serious interactions when taken with fenfluramine (Pondimin). This provides an additional reason why fenfluramine should not be given to depressed patients.

ADVERSE REACTIONS

Side effects severe enough to cause patients to cease taking an anorectic drug are uncommon in drug trials, but in normal clinical practice patients are under no obligation to continue treatment if it is disruptive. At least 10% of patients stop taking the drugs because of adverse reactions.

Central nervous system (CNS) stimulation resulting in nervousness, restlessness, irritability, euphoria, increased energy, and wakefulness, is common with the amphetamines and phenmetrazine, occurs occasionally with benzphetamine (Didrex), phendimetrazine (Plegine), and phentermine (Fastin, Ionamin, Wilpo), and less often with diethylpropion (Tenuate, Tepanil) and mazindol (Sanorex). It occurs occasionally with fenfluramine (Pondimin) in normal dosage, and dreaming is relatively common with this drug. Symptoms of CNS stimulation are invariably present in overdosage.

Sympathomimetic effects occur occasionally with all the anorectics, although they are much less common with fenfluramine. These include: dry mouth, blurred vision, lightheadedness, dizziness, tachycardia, palpitations, and sweating.

Gastrointestinal side effects, such as nausea, vomiting, constipation, and diarrhea, occur almost as commonly with placebos as with active drugs in controlled trials. Therefore most of them are coincidental or psychogenic in origin, with the exception of the occasional colicky abdominal pain or severe diarrhea due to fenfluramine.

INTERMITTENT USE

Providing that weight loss is continuing and there are no adverse effects, it is not of much import whether the continuing effect is directly attributable to the drug. The intermittent use of drugs has been successful in hospital trials but is not suitable for normal clinical practice; it is potentially dangerous with fenfluramine, as depression may be precipitated by sudden withdrawal of the drug.

USE IN HYPERTENSIVE PATIENTS

Although all anorectic drugs could theoretically have a slight hypertensive effect this is usually far outweighed by the hypotensive effect of weight loss. Accordingly, they can safely be used in hypertensive patients, provided blood pressure is carefully monitored. In a few hypertensive individuals the blood pressure may rise with anorectic treatment.

CONCLUSIONS

Diethylpropion (Tenuate, Tepanil) appears to be the drug of choice for most individuals, since it is at least as effective as the other agents, has fewer adverse effects and is cheaper than all except phentermine (Fastin, Ionamin, Wilpo). Mazindol (Sanorex) is a good alternative, although evaluation is still in progress. Fenfluramine (Pondimin) is preferable for patients who are especially tense without being depressed and for diabetic patients, but it should not be used for any patient with previous or current depressive symptoms. Phentermine is also relatively free of adverse effects, but the incidence of insomnia is high enough to limit its usefulness. The amphetamines and phenmetrazine (Preludin) should not be used because of the dangers of dependence and psychosis. Benzphetamine (Didrex) and phendimetrazine (Plegine) have too many adverse effects to be drugs of choice, and chlorphentermine (Pre-Sate) is potentially dangerous in long-term use.[10]

DRUG MONOGRAPHS

DIETHYLPROPION HYDROCHLORIDE (Tenuate, Tepanil) C-IV

Diethylpropion is an effective anorectic, and in its long-acting dosage form it can be taken as a single morning dose. The drug has rarely been abused or taken in overdose since its introduction in 1959.

Adverse Reactions—Untoward effects cause less than 10% of patients in clinical practice to stop taking the drug, although the incidence in clinical trials is usually less. CNS stimulation occurs in a few individuals, but these effects are rarely sufficient to discontinue the drug. In fact, patients who have suffered from CNS side effects with other drugs have been transferred to diethylpropion without a

TABLE 1 Preparations and Costs of Recommended Anorexiants

Generic Name	Trademark Name(s)	Preparations and 1978 Costs
Diethylpropion Hydrochloride	Tenuate (Tepanil)	Tablets 25 mg—$7.75/100 Tablets (timed-release) 75mg—$20.20/100
Fenfluramine Hydrochloride	Pondimin	Tablets 20 mg—$7.50/100
Mazindol	Sanorex	Tablets 1 mg—$16.50/100; 2 mg—$19.80/100
Phentermine Hydrochloride	Fastin (Wilpo)	Capsules 30 mg—$14.25/100
Phentermine Resin	Ionamin	Capsules 15 mg—$13.88/100; 30 mg—$15.32/100

continuation of the effects.[11] Insomnia is uncommon provided the long-acting form is taken before midday, or the short-acting form no later than 4 PM. Dry mouth is the most common sympathomimetic effect, and gastrointestinal adverse reactions are uncommon.

Dosage—Oral: Adults, 25 mg three times daily, not later than 4 PM, or 75 mg once daily before noon. In refractory cases or in patients over 300 lbs, the dose can be cautiously increased to twice the above level. *Children 8 years and older* can safely be given half the adult dose.

MAZINDOL (Sanorex) C-III

Mazindol is a tricyclic compound that probably acts by inhibiting the reuptake of norepinephrine by the afferent neuron and prolonging its action. It increases muscle glucose uptake by a mechanism similar to that of fenfluramine. It has a long plasma half-life, and once-daily dosage is adequate. Clinical evaluation of this drug began in 1973; thus, its relative value is still uncertain.

Adverse Reactions—Adverse effects, usually related to CNS stimulation, cause about 15% of patients to cease taking the drug in normal clinical practice. Sympathomimetic effects also occur, and constipation is fairly common. Dependence potential is probably low.

Dosage—Oral: Adults, 1 mg or 2 mg before noon. Mazindol is probably safe to use in older children but cannot yet be recommended.

PHENTERMINE HYDROCHLORIDE (Fastin, Wilpo) C-IV
PHENTERMINE RESIN (Ionamin) C-IV

Phentermine is an effective anorectic and as the ion-exchange resin it can be given in one morning dose.

Adverse Reactions—The incidence of minor CNS stimulation is similar to that of the amphetamines, and in one large trial 20% of patients complained of insomnia as compared with 6% of those on placebo.[6] Dryness of the mouth is also common. This drug is less suitable as an anorectic of first choice than either diethylpropion or mazindol.

Dosage—Oral: Adults, 15 to 30 mg in the morning. Phentermine is not recommended for children.

FENFLURAMINE HYDROCHLORIDE (Pondimin) C-IV

The central effects of fenfluramine are mediated by 5-hydroxytryptamine (5-HT) in the brainstem; a rapid reduction of 5-HT in the brain can lead to depression. Fenfluramine was widely used for a few years in Europe, mainly because of its widely-advertised metabolic effects. These are almost entirely a consequence of weight loss,[8,12] although fenfluramine increases glucose uptake by muscle,[13] thus reversing the tendency towards diabetes in patients with long-standing obesity. Fenfluramine is not as effective an anorectic as its competitors.

Adverse Reactions—Unwanted effects cause between 10% and 20% of patients to cease taking the drug in normal clinical practice. Nervousness, restlessness, and irritability are not common, but dreaming often occurs; in one series dreams assumed frightening proportions in 5 out of 20 patients.[14] The most common adverse effect is drowsiness. Although fenfluramine is not an amphetamine derivative it has a very similar structural formula, and in overdosage typical amphetamine-like effects occur.

Depression can be provoked by fenfluramine, especially in those patients with a previous history of depression and in any patient who is suddenly withdrawn from the drug. Gastrointestinal side effects are more common than with other anorectic drugs; colicky abdominal pain and severe diarrhea are not uncommon. Fenfluramine may prove to be the most suitable anorectic for obese diabetics and for patients who are especially tense without being depressed. The drug cannot be recommended for children since it may retard growth.[15]

Dependence Potential—Dependence is unlikely, but fenfluramine has been abused by young men already dependent on other drugs.[16]

Dosage—Oral: Adults, 20 to 60 mg twice daily. It is wise to start with 20 mg twice daily, as this dose causes drowsiness in some patients. The dose can be increased to 120 mg twice daily in refractory cases, or in patients weighing over 300 lbs.

REFERENCES

1. Craddock D: The aetiology of obesity. In *Obesity and its Management,* 3rd edition. London, Churchill Livingstone, 1978, pp 13–20.
2. Bray GA: The myth of diet in the management of obesity. Am J Clin Nutr 23:1141–1148, 1970.
3. Miller DS, Parsonage S: Resistance to slimming: adaptation or illusion? Lancet 1:773–775, 1975.
4. Cleave TL: *The Saccharine Disease.* Bristol, Wright, 1974.
5. McKay RHG: Long-term use of diethylpropion in obesity. Curr Med Res Opin 1:489–493, 1973.
6. Steel JM, Munro JF, Duncan LJP: A comparative trial of different regimens of fenfluramine and phentermine in obesity. Practitioner 211:232–236, 1973.
7. Stuart RB, Davis B: *Slim Chance in a Fat World: Behavioral Control of Obesity.* Champagne, Illinois, Research Press, 1972.
8. Garrow JS, Belton EA, Daniels A: A controlled investigation of the 'glycolyptic' action of fenfluramine. Lancet 2:559–561, 1972.
9. Jones HS: Fenfluramine used as a substitute for methylamphetamines and dexamphetamines in the treatment of dependence on these drugs. S Afr Med J 45(Suppl) July 31, 1971.
10. Lullman-Rauch R, Reil G-H: Chlorphentermine-induced lipisosislike ultrastructural alterations in lungs and adrenal glands of several species. Toxicol Appl Pharmacol 30:408–421, 1974.
11. Welsh AL: *Side Effects of Anti-Obesity Drugs.* Springfield, Illinois, Charles Thomas, 1962.
12. Pinder RM, Brogden RM, Sawyer PR, et al: Fenfluramine: a review of its pharmacological properties and therapeutic efficacy in obesity. Drugs 10:241–323, 1975.
13. Turtle JR, Burgess JA: Hypoglycemic action of fenfluramine in diabetes mellitus. Diabetes 22:858–867, 1973.
14. Mullen A, Wilson CWM, Wilson BPM: Dreaming, fenfluramine, and vitamin C. Br Med J 1:70–72, 1977.
15. Rayner PHW, Court JM: The effect of dietary restriction and anorectic drugs on linear growth velocity in childhood obesity. Postgrad Med J 51(Suppl 1):120–125, 1975.
16. Levin A: Abuse of fenfluramine. Br Med J 2:49, 1973.

39. SKELETAL MUSCLE RELAXANTS

Everett M. Delabarre

Centrally-acting skeletal muscle relaxants are widely prescribed for muscle spasm associated with musculoskeletal disorders and spasticity due to primary neurological disease. Drugs useful in the management of spasticity are generally not indicated in the management of muscle spasm, and drugs used to treat muscle spasm are of infrequent benefit in spasticity.

PRIMARY NEUROLOGICAL DISEASE

Centrally-acting skeletal muscle relaxants are frequently prescribed for spasticity consequent to disease or injury to the cortico-reticulo-spinal pathways. Spasticity results from increased excitability of the muscle stretch reflex and is manifested by increased myotatic reflexes, clonus, increased muscle resistance to passive stretch, and sometimes the appearance of spontaneous flexor or extensor spasms.[1,2] In general, the responsible lesions are either relatively stable and permanent or part of a progressive disease process. The need for treatment should be carefully defined in terms of patient function. Quadriceps femoris spasticity may stabilize the knee and facilitate walking in a stroke patient, and lower extremity extensor spasm in the paraplegic may aid in standing pivot transfers from bed to chair. When spasticity interferes with ambulation, self-care, or nursing management, the use of a muscle relaxant could be considered with the objective of improving function. In order to diminish unwanted muscular tension, the patient may have to endure some degree of somnolence, fatigue, or weakness, as a consequence of the medication. These reactions, as well as the clinical effectiveness of the drugs, are usually dose-related.

MUSCULOSKELETAL DISORDERS

Muscle relaxant drugs are widely used to reduce muscle spasm that is postulated to occur in musculoskeletal disorders resulting from trauma, some mechanical derangement, or an inflammatory process. This spasm is a submaximal, involuntary contraction of a muscle or group of muscles resulting from a painful musculoskeletal lesion. This muscle reaction is not associated with increased stretch reflexes, may serve to limit movement of the affected area, and may contribute to the pain if sustained. Some of the conditions leading to muscle spasm are chronic but more often they are self-limiting and of short duration. The apparent clinical response to medication may be difficult to evaluate if spontaneous improvement is occurring, rest and analgesic drugs are also employed, and placebo effect is encountered.

NON-DRUG METHODS OF CONTROLLING SPASTICITY AND MUSCLE SPASM

Ice or low temperatures may alleviate spasticity in the patient with multiple sclerosis. Treating a urinary tract infection, decubitus, or fecal impaction may decrease spasticity in the patient with spinal cord injury or multiple sclerosis. When spasticity is limited to certain muscle groups, nerve blocks, intramuscular neurolysis, or even neurectomy or rhizotomy may be effective. This direct approach is indicated if the spasticity is most severe in a single muscle group and if it could lead to contractures.

In patients with pain and muscular spasm associated with musculoskeletal disorders there are several modalities other than medication that provide symptomatic relief. These include heat application, cold application (including ethyl chloride and fluoromethane spray), rest, selective exercise, transcutaneous nerve stimulation, and various orthotic devices. Medication is frequently substituted because these modalities are more costly, unavailable, more time-consuming, or the physician is uncertain how they should be employed.

THE IDEAL MUSCLE RELAXANT

A muscle relaxant useful in neurological and musculoskeletal problems associated with muscular hypertonus ideally should have a wide separation between the spasticity-reducing dose and that producing sedation or weakness. The drug should decrease skeletal-muscular tension with no or minimal effects on voluntary movement or breathing. It should be intermediate to long-acting and suitable for oral or intravenous administration. By these criteria no centrally-acting agent now available is entirely satisfactory.[3]

No single drug is effective in all situations. Development of effective drugs has been hampered by a limited understanding of the pathophysiological mechanisms of abnormal muscle tone. An evaluation of the clinical efficacy of such agents is difficult, and animal screening procedures for evaluation may not be adequate.[4–6] Agents effective when given parenterally may be only marginally effective when given in much larger doses by mouth.

SKELETAL MUSCLE RELAXANTS: THE CLINICAL SPECTRUM

The search for 'interneuronal' depressants acting on the spinal cord was stimulated by early reports on the propanediol derivative mephenesin in 1946.[7] To be effective this agent had to be given intravenously; in addition, its half-life was short, and it could cause hemolysis. Analogs of mephenesin have often proven too weak, at least when given orally, to be of much clinical value.[3] The classes of compounds that have been or are now in use include: mephenesin and related propanediol derivatives, benzazole derivatives, benzodiazepines, a tricyclic amine, a gamma aminobutyric acid derivative, dantrolene, and several miscellaneous agents.

Unlike all of the other drugs, dantrolene acts not centrally but at the level of the sarcoplasmic reticulum; it is the only drug of its class.

Clinically the most useful muscle relaxant drugs in patients with lesions of the central nervous system and resulting spasticity are dantrolene, diazepam, and baclofen. The latter has been extensively used in Europe and the United Kingdom but only recently has been approved for use in the United States.

Evidence for the value of agents promoted for the relief of painful muscle spasm associated with various musculoskeletal disorders is more controversial. It is not sufficient to recommend their routine use as a substitute for appropriate physiotherapeutic measures.[3,8] Several of these drugs are available in combination with analgesics. If symptomatic relief is obtained, it would be difficult in a given instance to determine to what extent this was due to the muscle relaxant component rather than the analgesic.

DRUG MONOGRAPHS

BACLOFEN (Lioresal)

Baclofen is a derivative of gamma aminobutyric acid, a naturally occurring inhibitory neurotransmitter in the spinal cord. It may act by blocking impulse conduction in preterminal axons or by hyperpolarization of afferent terminals at the spinal level;[9,10] actions at supraspinal sites may also occur. Baclofen seems to be of particular value in reducing the frequency and severity of flexor or extensor spasms and in decreasing resistance to passive movement in patients with spinal cord injury or disease. There is no consistent effect on myotatic reflexes, clonus, or muscle strength. In ambulatory patients gait may not be improved.[11-17] Spasticity resulting from cerebral damage responds less often than spasticity consequent to spinal cord injury or disease.[18] Baclofen is not indicated in patients with stroke. Side effects or increased weakness may limit its usefulness in some patients with multiple sclerosis.[14]

Adverse Reactions—Adverse effects include drowsiness (usually transient), dizziness, weakness and fatigue, confusion, hypotension, and nausea. Increases in SGOT, alkaline phosphatase, and blood sugar have been reported. Baclofen should be used with caution in patients with impaired renal function. There are no data on its use in pregnant women.

Drug Interactions—The effects of baclofen are additive to those of alcohol and other central depressants.

Dosage—Oral: Adults, 5 mg three times daily initially. Increase by 5 mg each dose every three days. Daily dose should not exceed 80 mg (20 mg four times daily). Hallucinations may occur if the drug is discontinued abruptly.

CARISOPRODOL (Rela, Soma)
CARISOPRODOL WITH PHENACETIN AND CAFFEINE (Soma Compound)
CARISOPRODOL WITH PHENACETIN, CAFFEINE, AND CODEINE (Soma Compound with Codeine)

Carisoprodol, a propanediol, is a weak muscle relaxant acting by interneuronal blockade in the spinal cord and in the descending reticular formation of the brainstem.[19] Convincing objective evidence of significant relief of muscular spasm in painful musculoskeletal

TABLE 1 Preparations and Costs of Skeletal-Muscle Relaxants

GENERIC NAME	TRADEMARK NAME(S)	PREPARATIONS AND 1978 COSTS
Carisoprodol	Rela (Soma)	Tablets 350 mg—$12.76/100
	Soma Compound	Tablets (carisoprodol 200 mg, phenacetin 160 mg, and caffeine 32 mg)—$10.80/100
	Soma Compound with Codeine	Tablets (carisoprodol 200 mg, phenacetin 160 mg, caffeine 32 mg and codeine phosphate 16 mg)—$16.08/100
Chlordiazepoxide	Libritabs	Tablets 5 mg—$5.84/100; 10 mg—$8.34/100; 25 mg—$12.53/100
Chlordiazepoxide Hydrochloride	Librium	Capsules 5 mg—$5.79/100; 10 mg—$8.14/100; 25 mg—$12.49/100
Chlorzoxazone	Paraflex	Tablets 250 mg—$7.49/100
	Parafon Forte	Tablets (chlorzoxazone 250 mg and acetaminophen 300 mg)—$9.94/100
Dantrolene Sodium	Dantrium	Capsules 25 mg—$10.62/100; 50 mg—$13.80/100; 75 mg—$16.80/100; 100 mg—$18.48/100
Diazepam	Valium	Tablets 2 mg—$7.46/100; 5 mg—$9.50/100; 10 mg—$14.10/100 Injection (solution) 5 mg/ml—$.86/2-ml ampul, $3.93/10-ml vial
Meprobamate	Equanil (Miltown)	Tablets 200 mg—$5.64/100; 400 mg—$7.06/100
	generic	Tablets 200 mg—$0.75–$4.85; 400 mg—$0.95–$2.76
Methocarbamol	Robaxin	Tablets 500 mg—$7.85/100; 750 mg—$11.75/100 Injection (solution) 100 mg/ml—$1.20/10-ml ampul
	Robaxisal	Tablets (methocarbamol 400 mg and aspirin 325 mg)—$6.80/100

TABLE 1 *(continued)*

Generic Name	Trademark Name(s)	Preparations and 1978 Costs
Orphenadrine Citrate	Norflex	Tablets 100 mg—$21.90/100 Injection (solution) 30 mg/ml—$1.46/2-ml ampul
	Norgesic	Tablets (orphenadrine citrate 25 mg, aspirin 225 mg, phenacetin 160 mg, and caffeine 30 mg)—$10.56/100
	Norgesic Forte	Tablets (orphenadrine citrate 50 mg, aspirin 450 mg, phenacetin 320 mg, and caffeine 60 mg)—$19.20/100

conditions is lacking.[8,20–22] Its effects on spasticity in a variety of central nervous system lesions manifested by athetosis, dystonia, and spasticity are described as 'marginal.'[6] Carisoprodol may have some beneficial relaxant effects in selected patients with cerebral palsy.[23] If carisoprodol is used and an analgesic effect is desired, aspirin may be administered separately. Combination preparations are not recommended.

Adverse Reactions—The most common adverse reactions are sedation, drowsiness, vertigo, dizziness, and ataxia. Various allergic and idiosyncratic reactions with cutaneous manifestations, asthma, and marked central nervous system depression have been reported.

Drug Interactions—Carisoprodol is additive with alcohol and other CNS depressants or psychotropic drugs. Cross sensitization may exist with meprobamate. Enhanced metabolism of carisoprodol may result from enzyme induction in patients already receiving barbiturates and in chronic alcoholics.[24–27]

Dosage—Oral: Adults, 350 mg of carisoprodol three to four times daily.

CHLORDIAZEPOXIDE (Libritabs)
CHLORDIAZEPOXIDE HYDROCHLORIDE (Librium)

Chlordiazepoxide, a benzodiazepine derivative, is not commonly used as a muscle relaxant. It is reported to be about as effective as diazepam in neurological disorders manifesting spasticity.[27] There is no apparent reason to prefer this agent over diazepam.

Adverse Reactions and Drug Interactions—Adverse reactions and interactions are similar to those described for diazepam.

Dosage—Oral: Adults, 5 to 25 mg three to four times daily. *Children over six,* 5 mg two to four times daily; may be increased to 10 mg two to three times daily.

CHLORZOXAZONE (Paraflex)
CHLORZOXAZONE WITH ACETAMINOPHEN (Parafon Forte)

Chlorzoxazone, a benzazole compound, is too weak to be clinically effective.[3] It is usually administered in combination with acetaminophen for painful muscular spasms associated with musculoskeletal conditions. Chlorzoxazone is reported to be of occasional benefit for children with cerebral palsy, but there is no evidence that it is superior to diazepam.[28,29]

Adverse Reactions—Adverse reactions are rare and include sedation, gastrointestinal upset, and possible liver damage.

Dosage—Oral: Adults, 250 to 750 mg taken three to four times daily; chlorzoxazone with acetaminophen, two tablets taken three to four times daily.

CYCLOBENZAPRINE HYDROCHLORIDE (Flexeril)

Cyclobenzaprine, a tricyclic amine related to amitriptyline and other tricyclic antidepressants, owes its muscle relaxant activity to a reduction in descending tonic discharges on gamma and alpha motoneurons coming from supraspinal levels. It may also have some direct effect on spinal motoneurons.[30,31] Published reports documenting its value in muscle spasm associated with musculoskeletal disease are few. It has been compared with benztropine methanesulfonate in reducing rigidity in Parkinson's disease and was judged equally effective.[32] In a study on its use in patients with spasticity of spinal or cerebral origin its value was judged equal to a placebo.[33] It is not indicated in cerebral or spinal cord disease.

Adverse Reactions—The most frequent are drowsiness, dry mouth, and dizziness. Reactions reported for the related tricyclic antidepressants are possible. It has been shown to stimulate the spontaneous rate of atrial muscle and, in higher doses, to depress both chronotropic and inotropic activity, as do other tricyclic compounds.[34] It should be used with caution, if at all, in patients with known myocardial disease.

Drug Interactions—Similar to those described for amitriptyline (see Chapter 36).

Dosage—Oral: Adults, 10 mg two to four times daily. Dosage should not exceed 60 mg a day. Its use for periods longer than two to three weeks is not recommended. Its safety and efficacy in children under age 15 have not been established.

DANTROLENE SODIUM (Dantrium)

Dantrolene differs from the centrally-acting muscle relaxants in that its site of action is beyond the surface membrane of striated muscle. It dissociates excitation-contraction coupling in skeletal muscle, interfering with calcium release from the sarcoplasmic reticulum.[35–37]

The greatest value of dantrolene is for the reduction of clonus and involuntary muscular spasms.[38] It cannot effectively reduce painful muscular contractions found in various rheumatic states or musculoskeletal trauma.[39] Dantrolene should be used only when clinical manifestations of spasticity are disabling, and its administration results in improved motor function or lessened requirements for nursing care. In some instances better control of spasticity may not be demonstrable in terms of motor performance, yet the patient reports benefit in terms of improved relaxation, reduced tension, less involuntary motion, and an increased sleep span.[40]

Dantrolene will effectively reduce spasticity in patients with disease or injury of the spinal cord.[41] With continued administration beneficial effects may persist for one or more years, or they may fade, possibly because the underlying disease becomes worse. Weakness or reduced trunk stability might necessitate discontinuation of the drug.

Dantrolene may have limited value in patients with multiple sclerosis.[42–44] Because side effects are common, the benefits appear to warrant continued treatment in only a minority of patients.

Patients with hemiplegia and spasticity may show less improvement with dantrolene than those with spinal cord damage.[45–47] Clonus is reduced or abolished and motor function and gait improved, but positive effects can disappear with time. Often spasticity does not increase after the medication is discontinued.

The value of dantrolene in patients with cerebral palsy is difficult to assess.[45,49,50] It is probably useful in less than 50% of patients showing spasticity.

Dantrolene is not recommended in neurological diseases with

muscle weakness or when the control of localized spasticity can be accomplished by nerve blocks or motor point injections without loss of significant voluntary motor function. Because of induced weakness the drug is not well-tolerated by patients with amyotrophic lateral sclerosis and related disorders.[51] It is also ineffective in myotonic dystrophy.[52]

Adverse Reactions—The most common adverse reactions, seen in up to 75% of patients, are weakness, fatigue, drowsiness, and light-headedness or dizziness.[38,40,42] They usually last only a few days and are less troublesome if the starting dose is small. Patients with seizure disorders may show an increased frequency of seizures. The appearance of seizures in a patient without prior history and with a normal electroencephalogram has been reported.[50] Auditory and visual hallucinations have occurred.[53] Nausea, vomiting, diarrhea, constipation and flatulence are also common complaints but tend not to persist.[40] The most serious possible adverse effect is hepatitis, which in some instances is fatal.[38,54,55] Up to 10% of patients receiving dantrolene will develop minor and usually transient liver function abnormalities. Dantrolene's long-term safety, especially in patients with cardiac disease, remains to be established.

Dosage—Oral: Adults, initially 25 mg two or three times daily. In some instances much smaller doses than this are recommended.[49] The drug may be increased by 25 to 50 mg daily at weekly intervals. Most investigators do not recommend exceeding 600 mg daily in four divided doses. Dantrolene has been given concurrently with diazepam 2 to 10 mg three times daily, although the value of this combination is not established.

DIAZEPAM (Valium)

The benzodiazepine derivative diazepam and dantrolene are the two drugs most commonly used to manage spasticity resulting from disease or injury to the brain or spinal cord,[56,57] and may provide limited relief to sufferers of cerebral palsy.[57,58] Although diazepam is reportedly more effective than carisoprodol and methocarbamol, some studies fail to clearly demonstrate its superiority over aspirin or a placebo.[59] Diazepam and chlordiazepoxide may have some benefit in patients with reversible musculoskeletal disorders. When joint pain alone is a primary manifestation, as in rheumatoid arthritis, beneficial effects are less obvious.[60] There are reports of benefit in the rare 'stiff man' syndrome and spasmodic torticollis.[61,62] Diazepam is now the muscle relaxant of choice in the treatment of tetanus, but its value in neo-natal tetanus has been disputed.[59,63,64]

In general, diazepam is relatively safe and can be recommended for a therapeutic trial in patients with muscular hypertonus associated with neurological disorders causing significant functional impairment. Diazepam administration should not be prolonged unless the evidence of improved function with respect to ambulation, activities of daily living, or ease of nursing management is unmistakable.

Adverse Reactions—Unwanted effects of diazepam and other benzodiazepines are similar to barbiturates. Those most commonly encountered are drowsiness, fatigue, headache, and ataxia.[65] Paradoxical reactions with stimulation of portions of the central nervous system may occur but these are rare. Rapid intravenous bolus injections of diazepam may cause unexpected apnea.[66,67] Minimal effective doses should be used in the elderly and debilitated.

Drug Interactions—Diazepam and other benzodiazepines may potentiate the sedative action of various central depressant drugs including alcohol.[24,25] In combination with the latter, additive or synergistic effects detrimental to driving skills occur.[68] The hypotensive effects of various antihypertensive drugs may be potentiated. Patients treated for parkinsonism with levodopa may deteriorate on addition of diazepam.[69] Non-depolarizing muscle relaxants used in anesthesia may be potentiated.[70]

Dosage—Oral: Adults, 2 to 10 mg three to four times daily. *Children over 6 months of age,* 1 to 2 mg three to four times daily. *Intravenous:* 5 to 10 mg every two to four hours; larger doses may be required in tetanus.

MEPROBAMATE (Equanil, Miltown)

The sedative action of meprobamate (another propanediol derivative) may be more marked than carisoprodol,[6] but there is no evidence that its muscle relaxant effects differ significantly from carisoprodol.

Adverse Reactions—Adverse effects are similar to those of carisoprodol.

Dosage—Oral: Adults, 1,200 to 1,600 mg per day in four divided doses. *Children 6 to 12 years,* 100 to 200 mg taken two to three times daily.

METHOCARBAMOL (Robaxin)
METHOCARBAMOL WITH ASPIRIN (Robaxisal)

Methocarbamol is a weak skeletal muscle relaxant related to mephenesin. It has no direct effect on the innervation or contractile mechanism of the skeletal muscle fiber. Like mephenesin, methocarbamol may depress polysynaptic reflexes within the central nervous system.[3,71] If given alone, evidence indicates that methocarbamol's effectiveness is much greater when given intravenously than when administered orally,[72] but circumstances warranting intravenous administration are infrequent. Its usefulness is limited to painful musculoskeletal conditions, frequently traumatic, accompanied by local muscular spasm. Methocarbamol is not recommended for use in spasticity due to neurological disease. Symptomatic relief is likely to be greater when aspirin is administered concomitantly.[8] Whether its efficacy exceeds that of adequate doses of aspirin administered alone is not established.

Adverse Reactions—Sedation, lightheadedness, dizziness, and nausea are the most common adverse reactions and occasionally necessitate discontinuation of the drug.[73]

Drug Interactions—Methocarbamol may impair the therapeutic effect of pyridostigmine bromide in myasthenia gravis.[74]

Dosage—Oral: Adults, 1.5 g four times daily for 48 hours, then 1 g four times daily; methocarbamol with aspirin, two to three tablets four times daily.

ORPHENADRINE CITRATE (Norflex)
ORPHENADRINE CITRATE WITH ASPIRIN, PHENACETIN, AND CAFFEINE (Norgesic)
ORPHENADRINE CITRATE WITH ACETAMINOPHEN (X-Otag Plus)

Orphenadrine citrate, originally introduced for treatment of parkinsonism, is now used primarily for treatment of muscular spasms associated with painful musculoskeletal conditions. There is no convincing evidence that its efficacy is superior to that of a placebo.[3,8,75] The combination with aspirin, phenacetin, and caffeine (APC) is no more effective than APC alone, nor is combination with acetaminophen superior to orphenadrine citrate given separately with 325 mg of aspirin. Orphenadrine is not recommended for spasticity associated with neurological disease.

Adverse Reactions—Adverse reactions include tachycardia, anxiety, mental confusion, dry mouth, pupillary dilation, urinary retention, increased intra-ocular tension and reactions associated with anticholinergic agents in general, plus those of the ingredients in combinations.

Drug Interactions—Orphenadrine exhibits additive effects with anticholinergic drugs. A report of anxiety and tremors when given with propoxyphene has not been substantiated.[76] Enhanced hypoglycemic effect with tolbutamide has been reported, and severe hypoglycemia was seen when given with chlorpromazine.[77]

Dosage—Oral: Adults, 100 mg of orphenadrine citrate twice daily. The combination products are given in a dosage of one or two tablets two to four times daily. *Intramuscular, Intravenous: Adults,* 60 mg every 12 hours.

REFERENCES

1. Landau WM: Spasticity: the fable of a neurological demon and the emporor's new therapy. Arch Neurol 31:217–219, 1974.
2. Lenman JAR: Spasticity. Proc R Soc Med 63:935–937, 1970.
3. Domino EF: Centrally acting skeletal muscle relaxants. Arch Phys Med Rehabil 55:369–373, 1974.
4. Domino EF: Muscle relaxants of the mephenesin type. Ann NY Acad Sci 64:705–729, 1956.
5. Pedersen E: Clinical assessment and pharmacological therapy of spasticity. Arch Phys Med Rehabil 55:344–354, 1974.
6. Schlesinger E: The rationale of treatment of motor disorders with muscle relaxants. Ann NY Acad Sci 86:238–241, 1960.
7. Berger FM, Bradley W: Pharmacological properties of α:β-dihydroxy-γ-(2-methylphenoxy)-propane (myanesin). Br J Pharmacol 1:265–272, (Dec) 1946.
8. Schwab RS: Muscle relaxants. Practitioner 192:104–108, 1964.
9. Davidoff RA, Sears ES: The effects of Lioresal on synaptic activity in the isolated spinal cord. Neurology 24:957–963, 1974.
10. Saito K, Konishi S, Otsuka M: Antagonism between Lioresal and substance P in rat spinal cord. Brain Res 97:177–180, 1975.
11. Jones RF, Burke D, Marosszeky JE, et al: A new agent for control of spasticity. J Neurol Neurosurg Psychiatry 33:464–468, 1970.
12. Paeslack V: Lioresal in the treatment of spasticity. Postgrad Med J 48(Oct Suppl):30–32, 1972.
13. Shahani BT, Young RR: Management of flexor spasms with Lioresal. Arch Phys Med Rehabil 55:465–467, 1974.
14. Hedley DW, Maroun JA, Espir LE: Evaluation of baclofen (Lioresal) for spasticity in multiple sclerosis. Postgrad Med J 51:615–618, 1975.
15. Roussan MS, Abramson AS, Levine S, et al: Pharmacological rebound: a tool in the evaluation of antispasticity drugs. Arch Phys Med Rehabil 57:504–507, 1976.
16. Duncan GW, Bhagwan TS, Young RR: An evaluation of baclofen treatment for certain symptoms in patients with spinal cord lesions. Neurology 26:441–446, 1976.
17. McLellan DL: Co-contraction and stretch reflexes in spasticity during treatment with baclofen. J Neurol Neurosurg Psychiatry 40:30–38, 1977.
18. Pinto O de S, Poliker M, DeBono G: Results of international clinical trials with Lioresal. Postgrad Med J 48(Oct Suppl):18–23, 1972.

19. Maxwell DR, Read MA: The effects of some drugs on the rigidity of the cat due to ischemic or intercollicular decerebration. Neuropharmacology 11:849–855, 1972.
20. Hindle TH III: Comparison of carisoprodol, butabarbital, and placebo in the treatment of the low back syndrome. Calif Med 117:7–11, 1972.
21. Jones AC: The role of carisoprodol in physical medicine. Ann NY Acad Sci 86:226–230, 1960.
22. Miller AR: A comparative study of Parafon Forte tablets and Soma compound in the treatment of painful skeletal muscle conditions. Curr Ther Res 19:444–450, 1976.
23. Argy WP: Clinical evaluation of carisoprodol in cerebral palsy. Ann NY Acad Sci 86:231–232, 1960.
24. Hansten PD: *Drug Interactions.* Philadelphia, Lea and Febiger, 1975.
25. Martin EW: *Hazards of Medication.* Philadelphia, J.B. Lippincott, 1971.
26. *Evaluation of Drug Interactions,* 2nd edition. Washington, D.C., American Pharmaceutical Association, 1976.
27. Fischer FJ, Houtz SJ: Clinical and electromyographic evaluation of chlordiazepoxide, diazepam, and meprobamate in patients with cerebral palsy. Western Med 4(Supp 1):26–33, 1963.
28. Darienzo C: Muscle relaxant analgesic therapy. Dis Nerv Syst 27:189–192, 1966.
29. Berman HA, Noe O, Goodfield F: Relief of severe spasticity with chlorzoxazone. Dis Nerv Syst 25:430–433, 1964.
30. Share NN, McFarlane CS: Cyclobenzaprine: a novel centrally acting skeletal muscle relaxant. Neuropharmacology 14:675–684, 1975.
31. Barnes CD: Effects of cyclobenzaprine on brainstem motor systems. Neuropharmacology 15:643–652, 1976.
32. Potrin AR, Tourtellotte WW, Costanza A, et al: Cyclobenzaprine and benztropine methanesulfonate in Parkinson's disease: a randomized double-blind cross-over study (abstract). Clin Pharmacol Ther 21:144, 1977.
33. Ashby P, Burke D, Rao S, et al: The assessment of cyclobenzaprine in the treatment of spasticity. J Neurol Neurosurg Psychiatry 35:599–605, 1972.
34. Lemons SF, Barnes CD, Hughes MJ: The effects of cyclobenzaprine on atrial muscle (abstract). Fed Proc 36:1042, 1977.
35. Constantin LL: Contractile activation in skeletal muscle. Prog Biophys Mol Biol 29:199–224, 1975.
36. Ellis KO, Carpenter JF: Mechanism of control of skeletal muscle contraction by dantrolene sodium. Arch Phys Med Rehabil 55:362–369, 1974.
37. Putney JW Jr, Bianchi CP: Effect of dantrolene on E-C coupling in skeletal muscle. Fed Proc 32:772, 1973.
38. Joynt RL: Dantrolene sodium: long term effects in patients with muscle spasticity. Arch Phys Med Rehabil 57:212–217, 1976.
39. Nelson JR: Dantrolene sodium (Dantrium - Eaton) for relief of spasticity. West J Med 123:131, 1975.
40. Chyatte SB, Basmajian JV: Dantrolene sodium: long term effects in severe spasticity. Arch Phys Med Rehabil 54:311–315, 1973.
41. Jonsson B, Ladd H, Dahllöf AG: Effect of dantrolene on spasticity in spinal cord injuries. Scand J Rehabil Med 7:61–64, 1975.
42. Gelenberg AJ, Poskanzer DC: The effect of dantrolene sodium on spasticity in multiple sclerosis. Neurology 23:1313–1315, 1973.
43. Ladd H, Öist C, Jonsson B: The effect of dantrium on spasticity in multiple sclerosis. Acta Neurol Scand 50:397–408, 1974.
44. Tolosa ES, Soll RW, Loewenson RB: Treatment of spasticity in multiple sclerosis with dantrolene. JAMA 233:1046, 1975.
45. Steinberg FU, Ferguson KL: Effect of dantrolene sodium on spasticity associated with hemiplegia. J Am Geriatr Soc 23:70–73, 1975.
46. Jonsson B, Ladd H, Afzelius-Frick I, et al: The effect of dantrolene on spasticity in hemiplegic patients. Acta Neurol Scand 51:385–392, 1975.
47. Chipman M, Kaul S: Efficacy of dantrolene sodium in the treatment of spasticity. Neurology 22:401, 1972.
48. Chyatte SB, Birdsong JH, Robertson DL: Dantrolene sodium in athetoid cerebral palsy. Arch Phys Med Rehabil 54:365–368, 1973.

49. Haslam RA, Walcher JR, Lietman DS, et al: Dantrolene sodium in children with spasticity. Arch Phys Med Rehabil 55:384–388, 1974.
50. Denhoff E, Feldman S, Smith MG, et al: Treatment of spastic cerebral palsied children with sodium dantrolene. Dev Med Child Neurol 17:736–763, 1975.
51. Rivera VM, Breitbach WB, Swanke L: Dantrolene in amyotrophic lateral sclerosis. JAMA 233:863–864, 1975.
52. Dunne PB, Singer PA: Dantrolene ineffective in myotonic dystrophy. Lancet 1:1034, 1975.
53. Andrews LG, Muzumdar AS, Pinkerton AC: Hallucinations associated with dantrolene sodium therapy. Can Med Assoc J 112:148, 1975.
54. Schneider R, Mitchell D: Dantrolene hepatitis. JAMA 235:1590–1591, 1976.
55. Ogburn RM, Myers RL, Burdick GE: Hepatitis associated with dantrolene sodium. Ann Intern Med 84:53–54, 1976.
56. Anon: Diazepam in spasticity. Lancet 1:1161–1162, 1970.
57. Griffiths APW, Sylvester PE: Clinical trial of diazepam in adult cerebral palsy. Ann Phys Med 7(Suppl):25–29, 1964.
58. Bayliss SG, Gilbertson MP: Controlled trial of chlordiazepoxide in spastic children. Dev Med Chil Neurol 4:597–601, 1962.
59. Greenblatt DJ, Shader RI: *Benzodiazepines in Clinical Practice*. New York, Raven Press, 1974, pp 121–139.
60. Vince JD, Kremmer D: Double blind trial of diazepam in rheumatoid arthritis. Practitioner 210:264–267, 1973.
61. Gordon EE, Januszko DM, Kaufman L: A critical survey of the stiff-man syndrome. Am J Med 42:582–599, 1967.
62. Bianchine JR, Bianchine JW: Treatment of spasmodic torticollis with diazepam. South Med J 64:893–894, 1971.
63. Tempero KF: The use of diazepam in the treatment of tetanus. Am J Med Sci 266:4–12, 1973.
64. Hendrickse RG, Sherman PM: Tetanus in childhood: report of a therapeutic trial of diazepam. Br Med J 2:860–862, 1966.
65. Schmidt RT, Lee RH, Spehlman R: Treatment of spasticity in multiple sclerosis: comparison of dantrolene sodium and diazepam. Trans Am Neurol Assoc 100:235–237, 1975.
66. Steen SN, Kepes ER, Arkins RE, et al: Unexpected responses following diazepam. NY State J Med 71:578–580, 1971.
67. Doughty A: Unexpected danger of diazepam. Br Med J 2:239, 1970.
68. Linnoila M, Häkkinen S: Effects of diazepam and codeine, alone and in combination with alcohol, on simulated driving. Clin Pharmacol Ther 15:368–373, 1974.
69. Wodak J, Gilligan BS, Veale JL, et al: Review of 12 months treatment with L-dopa in Parkinson's disease with remarks on unusual side effects. Med J Aust 2:1277–1282, 1972.
70. Feldman SA, Crawley BE: Diazepam and muscle relaxants. Br Med J 1:691, 1970.
71. Crankshaw DP, Raper C: Some studies on the peripheral actions of mephenesin, methocarbamol, and diazepam. Br J Pharmacol 34:579–590, 1968.
72. Poppen JL, Flanagan ME: The use of methocarbamol for muscle spasm after lumbar and cervical laminectomies. JAMA 171:298–299, 1959.
73. Valtonen EJ: A double blind trial of methocarbamol versus placebo in painful muscle spasm. Curr Med Res Opin 3:382–385, 1975.
74. Podrizki A: Methocarbamol and myasthenia gravis. JAMA 205:938, 1968.
75. Valtonen EJ: A controlled trial of chlormezanone, orphenadrine, orphenadrine and paracetamol, and placebo in treatment of painful skeletal muscle spasms. Ann Clin Res 7:85–88, 1975.
76. Pearson RE, Salter FJ: Drug interactions?—orphenadrine with propoxyphene. N Engl J Med 282:1215, 1970.
77. Buckle RM, Guillebaud J: Hypoglycemic coma, occurring during treatment with chlorpromazine and orphenadrine. Br Med J 4:599–600, 1967.

AGENTS AFFECTING BLOOD

40. AGENTS USED TO TREAT DEFICIENCY ANEMIAS

Zareh Demirjian

Anemia, a reduction in the concentration of hemoglobin, is a common and important problem in medical practice. It is best diagnosed by measuring the volume of packed red cells (hematocrit), a simple and reliable test. The normal value depends upon age, sex, and altitude of residence.

Anemia can either be a primary illness or a secondary manifestation of a more serious condition. The wide range of possible etiologies requires that the cause of anemia be determined before therapy is initiated and that therapy be as specific as possible. Thus, the use of 'shotgun' therapy for the treatment of anemia should be avoided.

IRON DEFICIENCY ANEMIA

The three most common causes of primary anemia are iron deficiency, vitamin B_{12} deficiency, and folic acid (folate) deficiency. Iron deficiency is by far the most common cause. Hallberg, et al[1] reported an incidence of 20 to 30% in premenopausal women and 1% in men in a survey of the general population in Sweden. Studies in the United States have shown an incidence of approximately 9% in the general population. Subclinical iron deficiency is particularly common in premenopausal women.

Total body iron in a normal adult is 2 to 3.5 grams, of which two-thirds is in red blood cell hemoglobin, approximately 5% is in myoglobin and iron-containing enzymes, and the remainder stored in bone marrow, liver, and spleen.[2] Very minimal amounts of iron are lost under normal circumstances—1 mg or so per day from the shedding of cells and occult gastrointestinal blood loss. Menstruating women probably lose an additional 150 to 250 mg of iron per year.

The ordinary American diet provides about 15 mg of iron per day,[3] of which about one-tenth is absorbed. In iron deficiency anemia, iron absorption is enhanced, but the increment is insufficient to correct the deficiency. Normal daily requirements for an adult male are 0.5 to 1.0 mg; for females of reproductive age, they are 1 to 2 mg.[3] Iron is absorbed mainly from the duodenum and proximal jejunum as ferrous ions. The increased alkalinity in the small intestine causes oxidation of the ferrous ions into the nonabsorbable ferric form.

The diagnosis of iron deficiency depends on the severity of the condition. Severe iron deficiency anemia is characterized by microcytic and hypochromic red cells, with variation in their shape. The plasma iron level is low and the total iron binding capacity is high, with absent stainable iron in the bone marrow.

The body absorbs inorganic iron (eg, ferrous sulfate) better than organic iron (eg, hemoglobin). Iron tablets are the principal form of therapy for iron deficiency. Despite a variety of available preparations, there is little evidence that one product is superior to another. Sustained release preparations should be avoided because the iron is released beyond the duodenum and jejunum and, consequently, is poorly absorbed.

All iron compounds are best absorbed when taken on an empty stomach.[4] Iron absorption is impaired if tablets are taken at the same time as antacid preparations. About 10% of patients taking oral iron preparations complain of nausea, cramps, diarrhea, or constipation. Iron can be taken with meals to diminish absorption and thereby reduce side effects. Some preparations are reportedly better tolerated than ferrous sulfate. However, differences in the frequency of adverse reactions are probably due to lower iron content rather than some special property of the preparation itself. The more expensive preparations containing ascorbic acid, etc., have no proven advantage. Tolerance to iron tablets may occasionally be improved by starting with only a single tablet per day and increasing to 3 to 4 tablets per day over 1 to 2 weeks.

The inability to absorb an oral dose of iron is rare. However, occasionally one has to resort to parenteral iron in patients with excessive gastrointestinal intolerance to oral preparations and in those who cannot be relied upon to take their medication. There are many different methods for calculating the total dose of parenteral iron. A practical rule is to give 250 mg of elemental iron for each gram of hemoglobin below normal.

MEGALOBLASTIC ANEMIAS

Vitamin B_{12} and folic acid deficiency produce megaloblastic anemias. The term megaloblast was first used by Ehrlich in 1880 to describe a morphologically abnormal red cell precursor in the bone marrow. The megaloblastic anemias are a group of disorders where DNA synthesis is defective, but they are responsive to the replacement of deficient vitamin B_{12} and/or folic acid.

Vitamin B_{12}

Until the demonstration by Minot and Murphy in 1926 that feeding of liver reversed the changes of pernicious anemia, a specific type of vitamin B_{12}-responsive megaloblastic anemia, the condition was almost invariably fatal.[5] However, it was not until 1948 that vitamin B_{12} was isolated from liver extracts. Vitamin B_{12} is synthesized by microorganisms and the most intensive synthesis is by bacteria in the gastrointestinal tract.[6] The dietary sources of vitamin B_{12} (milk, eggs, meats, and seafood) are mainly of animal origin. The daily requirement is 2 to 5 μg, and the total body stores are 2000 to 5000 μg. The average western diet contains 5 to 30 μg of vitamin B_{12}; two-fifths of this is absorbed in the terminal ileum and the remaining three-fifths is excreted. Absorption takes place only if the vitamin B_{12} is bound by intrinsic factor, a glycoprotein found in human gastric juice, and secreted by the parietal cells. The large stores of vitamin B_{12} in the liver permit maintenance of vitamin B_{12} levels for 3 to 5 years even if intake or absorption are negligible.

Vitamin B_{12} is an important element in several biochemical processes. The most important of these are DNA synthesis and the maintenance of the integrity of myelin. The two most common manifestations of vitamin B_{12} deficiency are megaloblastic anemia and neurologic degeneration. The two may occur together or separately. Approximately one-third of patients with pernicious anemia have neurologic abnormalities. The disease usually develops late in life, with 90% of patients over the age of 40.[7] The highest frequency is found among people of northern European ancestry.

The two major forms of vitamin B_{12} are cyanocobalamin and hydroxocobalamin.

Folic Acid

Folic acid is mandatory for the synthesis of purine and pyrimidine, and its deficiency is associated with metabolic disorders leading to megaloblastic anemia.[8] Dietary folate consists mainly of polyglutamic forms of folic acid, and intestinal deconjugation is necessary for the hydrolysis and absorption of these polyglutamates.

Folic acid absorption occurs mainly in the duodenum and jejunum. The sources of folic acid are numerous, the richest being green leaves. Yeasts, grain, milk, and meat are other dietary sources. Excessive cooking removes a great deal of the folate from these foods. The normal western daily diet contains up to 300 μg.[9] The total body stores are estimated at 6 to 10 μg. In the absence of proper intake, body stores can last 3 to 4 months, considerably less than those of vitamin B_{12}. When requirements for folic acid are increased, as in hemolytic anemias and pregnancy, stores are more rapidly depleted and megaloblastosis with pancytopenia may occur in one week. In some postsurgical patients, acute folate deficiency has developed during parenteral nutrition without supplemental folic acid.[10] Folate deficiency also occurs in malabsorption states, in some women taking oral contraceptives, in patients taking phenytoin (diphenylhydantoin), Crohn's disease involving the jejunum, sprue, and surgical resection of the jejunum. The most common setting of folic acid deficiency is poor diet, often associated with alcoholism.

Folic acid is normally well-absorbed, with 65% of an orally administered dose recoverable in plasma, and only a small percentage excreted in urine.

DRUG MONOGRAPHS

ORAL IRON PREPARATIONS

FERROUS SULFATE (Feosol, Fer-In-Sol)
FERROUS FUMARATE (Feostat, Ircon, Toleron)
FERROUS GLUCONATE (Fergon)
FERROCHOLINATE (Chel-Iron, Ferrolip)

Ferrous sulfate has for many years been the mainstay in therapy of iron deficiency anemia. It is available as either the hydrated or dried form; the hydrated form contains 20% elemental iron whereas the dried form contains 33% iron. Thus, Feosol (dried ferrous sulfate), 200 mg tablets, provide 65 mg of elemental iron, and generic ferrous sulfate, 300 mg tablets, provide 60 mg.

Ferrous gluconate contains 11.6% elemental iron. Thus, Fergon, 320 mg tablets, contains 37 mg of iron. Due to its lower iron content, claims of improved tolerance have been made[11] but not substantiated[12] in therapeutic trials.

Ferrocholinate is a chelate of ferric hydroxide and choline dihydrogen citrate. It contains 12% elemental iron. Thus, Chel-Iron or Ferrolip, 333 mg tablets, contain 40 mg of iron.

Ferrous fumarate is a stable organic iron compound that probably tastes worse than other iron compounds.[13] It contains 33% elemental iron. Thus, Ircon or Toleron, 200 mg tablets, contain 66 mg of iron.

Adverse Reactions—Nausea, cramps, diarrhea, or constipation occur in about 10% of iron recipients.

Dosage—Oral: Adults, three to four tablets daily; dosage may be divided for better tolerance.

PARENTERAL IRON PREPARATIONS

IRON DEXTRAN INJECTION (Imferon)

Iron dextran is a colloidal solution of ferric hydroxide with dextran. It has a molecular weight of 55,000 and contains 50 mg of elemental iron per ml.

Intramuscular injection, usually 2 ml, is performed according to the 'Z track' technique. If larger doses are needed local discomfort and discoloration may occur. Iron dextran is very slowly absorbed from intramuscular injection sites; the half-life of radioactive iron in plasma is 2.5 to 3 days with a peak value of 10 days.[14] Grimes and Hult[15] found that one-third of an injected dose stays at the injection site for almost a month. Iron dextran can also be given intravenously. It is diluted in 5% dextrose in water or normal saline to a volume of 250 to 1000 ml. It is advisable to give a small intravenous test dose (0.1 ml of undiluted solution or several drops of a diluted preparation) initially to detect sensitivity. Following the test dose, the initial infusion should be slow (10 to 15 drops/minute) and then speeded up to 60 drops/minute if no side effects are observed.

Adverse Reactions—The incidence of side effects with parenteral iron is reported to be 1 to 2%, with no difference between the intravenous and intramuscular routes.[16] Most of the reactions are immediate and include: flushing, headache, bronchospasm, and rare instances of hypotension or shock. In addition, there have been

TABLE 1 Preparations and Costs of Agents Used to Treat Deficiency Anemias

Generic Name	Trademark Name(s)	Preparations and 1978 Costs
Iron Preparations		
Ferrous Sulfate	Feosol	Tablets 200 mg (65 mg iron)—$1.55/100 Elixir 220 mg/5 ml (44 mg/5 ml iron)—$1.75/12 oz
	Fer-In-Sol	Capsules 190 mg (60 mg iron)—$2.27/100 Syrup 150 mg/5 ml (30 mg/5 ml iron)—$3.43/pint Drops 75 mg/0.6 ml (15 mg/0.6 ml iron)—$1.10/15 ml, $2.25/30 ml
	generic	Tablets 300—325 mg (60–65 mg iron)—$0.50–1.67/100
Ferrous Fumarate	Ircon (Feostat) (Toleron)	Tablets 200 mg (65.7 mg iron)—$1.96/100
Ferrous Gluconate	Fergon	Capsules 435 mg (50 mg iron)—$1.98/30 Tablets 320 mg (40 mg iron)—$1.50/100 Elixir 300 mg (37.5 mg iron)—$3.30/pint
Ferrocholinate	Chel-Iron (Ferrolip)	Tablets 333 mg (40 mg iron)—$36.00/100 Liquid 417 mg/5 ml (50 mg/5 ml) iron)—$30.00/60 ml Drops 208 mg/ml (25 mg/ml) iron)—$42.00/8 oz
Iron Dextran Injection	Imferon	Injection (solution) 50 mg iron/ml—$2.10/2-ml ampul, $4.20/5-ml ampul, $8.43/10-ml vial
Vitamin B_{12} Preparations		
Cyanocobalamin	Betalin 12 Crystalline (Redisol) (Rubramin PC) (Ruvite) (Sytobex)	Injection (solution) 100 μg/ml—$0.69/10-ml vial; 1000 μg/ml—$1.45/5-ml vial; $2.28/10-ml vial
Hydroxocobalamin	alphaRedisol	Injection (solution) 1000 μg/ml—$3.18/10-ml vial

TABLE 1 *(continued)*

Generic Name	Trademark Name(s)	Preparations and 1978 Costs
Folates		
Folic Acid	Folvite	Tablets 0.25 mg—$4.17/100; 1 mg—$4.93/100
Folate Sodium	Folvite Sodium	Injection (solution) 5 mg/ml—$3.02/10-ml vial

reports of arthralgias (particularly in patients with rheumatoid arthritis) and local phlebitis, the latter being more frequent when undiluted iron is administered intravenously. In some animals, iron dextran reportedly caused carcinogenesis at the site of injection.

Dosage—Intramuscular, Intravenous: Adults, a practical rule is to give 250 mg of elemental iron for each gram of hemoglobin below normal.

VITAMIN B_{12} PREPARATIONS

CYANOCOBALAMIN

Cyanocobalamin is a water-soluble vitamin with a molecular weight of 1355.[17] It may be administered by either subcutaneous or intramuscular routes. The dosages for confirmed deficiency states are variable. One approach involves daily intramuscular injection of 100 μg for approximately one week, followed by the same dose once per month for life. Larger doses are not harmful and may assure adequate replacement. After an injection of 1000 μg, peak plasma levels are reached in approximately 24 hours and fall to less than 200 μg in a mean of 3.2 weeks. The response to therapy is rapid. Within 48 hours a sense of well-being occurs. Reticulocytosis occurs within 3 to 4 days and peaks in 5 to 7 days.

Adverse Reactions—Side effects are very rare but anaphylactic reactions have been reported in isolated instances[18] and chronic urticaria has been observed.[19]

Dosage—Intramuscular, Subcutaneous: Adults, 100 μg monthly.

HYDROXOCOBALAMIN (alphaRedisol)

Hydroxocobalamin has an hydroxyl substitution replacing the

cyano group of cyanocobalamin. It is sometimes called vitamin B_{12a}. The peak plasma levels obtained with this preparation are higher and are maintained for longer periods (mean: 7.2 weeks) than those obtained with cyanocobalamin. Whether this makes any therapeutic difference is not known.

Adverse Reactions—Same as cyanocobalamin.

Dosage—Same as cyanocobalamin.

FOLATES

FOLIC ACID (Folvite)
FOLATE SODIUM (Folvite Sodium)

These agents are indicated for the correction of folic acid deficiency, but should not be used to treat pernicious anemia or other vitamin B_{12} deficiency states. When they are used indiscriminately in patients with pernicious anemia, diagnosis becomes difficult and irreversible neurologic damage may occur if the anemia is untreated.

Adverse Reactions—Even in large doses, folic acid is free of side effects, except for occasional allergic urticaria.

Dosage—Intramuscular, Intravenous, Oral: Adults and children, up to 1 mg per day. When clinical symptoms have subsided and blood tests have returned to normal, a maintenance dose of 0.1 to 0.25 mg daily should be given.

REFERENCES

1. Hallberg L, Hallgren J, Hollander A, et al: Occurrence of iron deficiency anemia in Sweden. In *Symposia of the Swedish Nutrition Foundation,* sixth edition. Edited by J Blix. Uppsala, Almqvist and Wiksells, 1968, pp 19–27.
2. *Laboratory Medicine,* fourth edition. Edited by JB Miale. St. Louis, C.V. Mosby Company, 1972, pp 494–530.
3. Crosby WH: Iron and anemia. Disease-a-Month, Jan 1966, pp 1–72.
4. Callender ST: Oral iron therapy. Br J Haematol 18:123–125, 1970.
5. Castle WB: The contributions of George Richard Minot to experimental medicine. N Engl J Med 247:585–592, 1952.
6. Perlman D: Microbial synthesis cobamides. Adv Appl Microbiol 1:87–122, 1959.
7. Chanarin I: Pernicious anemia and other vitamin B_{12} deficiency states. Abstracts of World Medicine 44:73–85, 1970.
8. Bernstein HL, Gutstein S, Weiner S, et al: The absorption and malabsorption of folic acid and its polyglutamates. Am J Med 48:570–579, 1970.
9. Herbert V: Minimal daily adult folate requirements. Arch Intern Med 110:649–652, 1962.
10. Wardrop CAJ, Tennant GB, Heatley RV, et al: Acute folate deficiency in surgical patients on amino acid ethanol intravenous nutrition. Lancet 2:640–642, 1975.
11. Reznikoff P, Goebel WF: Ferrous gluconate. J Clin Invest 16:547–554, 1937.
12. O'Sullivan DJ, Higgins PG, Wilkinson JF: Oral iron compounds. Lancet 2:482–485, 1958.
13. Swan HT, Jowett GH: Treatment of iron deficiency with ferrous fumarate. Br Med J 2:782–787, 1959.

14. Wallerstein RO: Intravenous iron dextran complex. Blood 32:450–454, 1968.
15. Grimes HJ, Hult MSR: Metabolism of Fe^{59} dextran complex in human subjects. Br Med J 2:1074–1077, 1957.
16. Marchasin S, Wallerstein RO: Treatment of iron deficiency anemia with intravenous iron dextran. Blood 23:354–358, 1964.
17. Corcine JJ, Waxman S, Herbert V, et al: Absorption and malabsorption of vitamin B_{12}. Am J Med 48:562–569, 1970.
18. Houding G: Anaphylactic reaction after injection of vitamin B_{12}. Br Med J 3:102, 1968.
19. James J, Warin RP: Sensitivity to cyanocobalamin. Br Med J 1:262, 1971.

41. ANTICOAGULANT, ANTIPLATELET, AND FIBRINOLYTIC AGENTS

Gordon D. O. Lowe, William W. McCloskey, and David H. Lawson

The significance of thromboembolic disease cannot be underestimated. *Arterial* thromboembolism is a major contributor to myocardial infarction, stroke and renal disease—three leading causes of death in the United States.[1] *Venous* thromboembolism is responsible for the hospitalization of approximately 300,000 Americans annually, of whom over 500,000 die.[1] Consequently, various pharmacologic agents are employed in attempts to prevent the formation of thrombi or limit their extension.

Several factors contribute to the development of thrombi in large vessels. These include abnormalities in blood flow, the vessel wall, platelet adhesion and aggregation, and blood coagulation. Platelets and coagulation proteins participate in the generation of all thrombi, the relative role of each depending upon whether the thrombus is arterial or venous. A white or arterial thrombus is initiated by vascular injury and exposure to subendothelial collagen. The primary pathological event is a platelet-tissue reaction, with the coagulation cascade playing a secondary role. A red or venous thrombus is triggered by the activation of coagulation proteins, and the role of platelets appears to be of lesser importance.

ANTICOAGULANTS

Anticoagulant drugs interfere with the formation or function of those plasma proteins which interact to form fibrin, a complex protein which is a major constituent of all thrombi. These drugs may be given to prevent the development of thrombi in susceptible individuals, or to prevent their extension and subsequent embolization in situations where thrombi have already formed. The anticoagulants available for use are heparin, a natural anticoagulant which must be administered parenterally, and the coumarins and indanediones, synthetic drugs which are usually administered orally. The coumarin most commonly employed is warfarin sodium because it has an intermediate half-life. Phenindione derivatives are not recommended because of a high incidence of serious non-hemorrhagic complications such as agranulocytosis, hepatitis, nephropathy, and exfoliative dermatitis.[2]

Although anticoagulants are widely used in the management of thrombosis, objective evidence of their efficacy is often lacking. Their value in some forms of venous thromboembolism is reasonably well established, but their efficacy in arterial thromboembolism other than that arising from fibrillating atria in rheumatic heart disease or prosthetic heart valves is unclear.[3]

Indications

Since venous thromboembolism with pulmonary embolism is a leading cause of death in the general hospital population, preventive therapy is indicated in high risk patients.[3] This group includes patients over 40 with prolonged immobilization, those suffering from trauma, patients with certain neoplastic diseases, and those who have undergone major orthopedic procedures, especially hip surgery.[3] Low-dose subcutaneous heparin has replaced oral agents in the prophylaxis of postoperative thromboembolic complications except in hip surgery.[4] No control tests are required, a standard dose is used, and the risk of hemorrhage appears less than with oral anticoagulants.

Anticoagulation probably benefits patients with established venous thromboembolism. Prompt treatment of patients with acute pulmonary embolism appears to reduce the risk of recurrent embolism and lowers the mortality from 18–32% to 1–9%.[5] Although there are no controlled trials of anticoagulants in established deep vein thrombosis, indirect evidence suggests that they prevent extension and embolization of the thrombus. First, prophylactic anticoagulants in patients at risk reduce the incidence and extent of deep vein thrombosis and pulmonary embolism.[6,7] Further, untreated deep vein thrombosis is associated with pulmonary embolism, especially when proximal to the calf.[8] In contrast, when deep vein thrombosis is treated with anticoagulants, pulmonary embolism is rare; when it does occur, it is associated with poor anticoagulant response.[9,10]

The duration of therapy in patients with venous thromboembolism is controversial. Up to six months of anticoagulation has been recommended for the treatment of pulmonary embolism,[11] and as long as three months suggested for the treatment of deep venous thrombosis.[11] However, a prospective controlled trial has demonstrated that six weeks of therapy is just as effective as six months for the treatment of recurrent venous thromboembolism, unless there is a previous history of the disorder or a continuing predisposing cause.[12]

Heart valve disease has been an indication for anticoagulation, although controlled trials are lacking. The rheumatic heart with mitral stenosis is a frequent source of systemic emboli,[3] and clinical experience has shown that long-term anticoagulation decreases the occurrence of systemic thromboembolism. Similarly, the incidence of thromboembolism is high in patients with prosthetic heart valves who are not anticoagulated.[13] More recently developed valves appear less likely to cause emboli, which may reduce the need for anticoagulation.

The value of anticoagulant therapy in acute myocardial infarction is not established. Early studies describing the benefits of short-term anticoagulant therapy were poorly designed. Subsequent studies do not demonstrate a reduction in mortality with short-term anticoagulation, although some trials suggest a reduction in thromboembolic events.[14,15] An International Review Group concluded that long-term anticoagulant therapy (1–2 years) probably results in a slight reduction in mortality in males under 55 with either previous angina or infarction.[16] The risk of hemorrhage and of other complications must be weighed against the benefit to a minority of treated patients.

Oral anticoagulants are commonly given for weeks to months after coronary artery bypass surgery to prevent graft thrombosis, but controlled trials demonstrating their efficacy are lacking. Also, there is no evidence that anticoagulation is effective in patients with angina or peripheral arterial disease.

The value of anticoagulation in patients with cerebral artery disease remains unresolved. While most trials of reasonable design suggest that oral anticoagulants reduce the incidence of transient cerebral ischemic attacks for at least a year, long-term benefit and effect on mortality is unproven. There is no definite proof that anticoagulants are of value in the acute phase of stroke or when given long-term after a completed stroke.

ANTIPLATELET DRUGS

Because of the role that platelets play in the formation of thrombi, particularly in arterial and other high flow systems, drugs that inhibit platelet function are used to prevent some thrombotic diseases. The list of agents used includes aspirin, clofibrate, dipyridamole, hydroxychloroquine, sulfinpyrazone, and dextrans (Table 1). Since the efficacy of these drugs in thrombotic disease is not fully established and they have other primary uses that are covered in other chapters, the antiplatelet drugs are only briefly discussed here.

Platelet survival time is shortened in patients with prosthetic heart valves, a condition that correlates with the incidence of thromboembolism.[17] Dipyridamole[18] and sulfinpyrazone[19] prolong platelet survival to normal in these patients and possibly reduce thromboembolism. Sullivan, Harken and Gorlin[20] report that dipyridamole in combination with warfarin is more effective in reducing the number of thromboembolic complications in patients with prosthetic heart valves than warfarin alone.

Blakely and Gent[21] have shown a significant reduction in death from cerebrovascular causes in a group of institutionalized elderly males who were given 600 mg of sulfinpyrazone compared to placebo-treated controls. More recently the Anturane Reinfarction Trial Research Group reported that sulfinpyrazone prevented cardiac death in patients who had recently suffered a myocardial infarction.[22] This multicenter trial was a randomized, double-blind study comparing sulfinpyrazone (200 mg four times a day) with placebo in over 1400 patients with a recently documented infarction. There was a 57.2% reduction in the annual sudden-cardiac-death rate ($p = 0.015$) in the sulfinpyrazone-treated group, indicating that the drug may be effective in reducing cardiac deaths during the first year after a myocardial infarction.

The Boston Collaborative Drug Surveillance Program found a highly significant negative association between regular aspirin intake and nonfatal myocardial infarction in three case-control studies.[23,24] A prospective study in Wales demonstrated that individuals with recent myocardial infarction who received 300 mg of aspirin a day had a reduction in total mortality as compared to those who received placebo, although the results were statistically inconclusive.[25]

The Newcastle[26] and Scottish Physicians[27] studies conclude that

TABLE 1 Clinical Effects of Antiplatelet Drugs[a]

	Aspirin		Dipyridamole		Sulfinpyrazone		Other Drugs
	Yes	No	Yes	No	Yes	No	Yes
Transient Ischemic Attacks	31–33	34*	34*	31, 35	36		
Acute Myocardial Infarction	23, 25, 37						Clofibrate 26–28
Prosthetic Devices							
1. Shunts, membranes	38	39	34, 40		41		
2. Heart valves		18*	18,* 21, 42		19		
Renal Disease and Graft Rejection		43	44–46				
Microangiography	47–51		48–51				Dextran 52
Venous Thrombosis	53, 54 55,** 56**	57,** 58,** 59**	56,** 60	34,** 53, 59,** 61	62		Chloroquine 63**
Longevity		64			21, 22		

[a]Drug was either effective (yes) or ineffective (no) in reducing the number of clinical events, prolonging platelet survival (*), or preventing the uptake of ^{125}I fibrinogen in the legs (**). (Adapted from reference 29 with permission).

clofibrate protects patients with ischemic heart disease against fatal and nonfatal sequelae. Krasno and Kidera[28] similarly report a favorable effect of clofibrate. In none of these studies was a relation between clofibrate's antilipidemic effect and protective effect demonstrated, thus the drug's antiplatelet properties may be responsible for its beneficial effect.[29]

Other studies with aspirin, dipyridamole and clofibrate fail to show a significant difference in favor of antiplatelet therapy.[30]

Antiplatelet drugs have been advocated for the treatment of peripheral vascular disease, but good evidence for clinical efficacy is lacking.[30]

Although platelets are believed to play a more important role in the formation of arterial thrombosis, antiplatelet drugs have been employed for the prevention of postoperative deep vein thrombosis. In orthopedic surgery, dextran 70 is the most effective of these agents.[30] However, low-dose heparin is still the only drug that prevents fatal pulmonary embolism in patients following general surgery.[30]

A summary of the clinical effects of antiplatelet drugs in various disorders, including some not discussed here, is presented in Table 1.

FIBRINOLYTIC AGENTS

Anticoagulant and antiplatelet drugs may be of benefit in preventing thrombus formation, but they are of little value in the treatment of established clots.[65] Consequently, fibrinolytic (thrombolytic) agents have been developed to lyse clots that have already formed. By converting plasminogen to the active proteolytic enzyme plasmin, fibrinolytic drugs produce a local thrombolysis.

The two fibrinolytic agents most commonly employed are urokinase and streptokinase. The most promising indication for streptokinase and urokinase appears to be venous thrombosis.[66] Studies by Briggs[67] and Kakkar et al[68] demonstrate successful clot lysis in patients with venous thrombosis treated with streptokinase. Experience with urokinase is more limited; Silver et al[69] report clinical improvement in four of nine patients treated with this plasminogen activator.

Successful fibrinolytic therapy is more likely when treating fresh clots, although thrombi older than ten days have been lysed.[65] Plasminogen activators are no more effective than anticoagulants in preventing pulmonary embolism.[65] Because rethrombosis may occur after termination of therapy, conventional anticoagulation should follow urokinase or streptokinase treatment.[65]

Although the use of fibrinolytic agents in the therapy of pulmonary embolism has been well studied, their value is not established.[66] The two Urokinase Pulmonary Embolism Trials failed to demonstrate a decrease in mortality or morbidity among patients with pulmonary embolism treated with urokinase and streptokinase as compared to those treated with heparin.[70,71]

Both urokinase and streptokinase have major disadvantages. Severe bleeding complications can occur. Both drugs are expensive, especially urokinase. Streptokinase is antigenic, thus allergic reactions may occur.[65] Urokinase is pyrogenic, although the greater purity of newer preparations has somewhat reduced this problem.[65]

Thus, although fibrinolytic therapy has considerable potential, more studies must be done before its value in thromboembolic disease can be established more clearly.

DRUG MONOGRAPHS

HEPARIN SODIUM

Heparin sodium is a naturally occurring sulfated mucopolysaccharide with powerful anticoagulant activity when given parenterally in doses of 20,000 to 60,000 units per day. Its anticoagulant effect is primarily due to its potentiation of antithrombin which inhibits the conversion of fibrinogen to fibrin. In addition, heparin inhibits the action of several other activated coagulation factors (factors IX, X, XI, and XII).[72] The action of heparin begins shortly after an intravenous injection and lasts for several hours. To prevent fluctuations in the anticoagulant effect, heparin may be given in a continuous infusion of 1,000 to 2,000 units hourly rather than in the more usual dosage of 5,000 to 10,000 units every four to six hours.

Due to the risks of hemorrhage and wide individual variation in dosage required, heparin therapy should be controlled by regular estimations of plasma clotting time. Tests such as the whole blood clotting time, partial thromboplastin time, and thrombin clotting time are useful. Whole blood clotting time should be prolonged by a factor of 1.5 to 2.5 times control.

Heparin is usually prescribed for patients requiring immediate anticoagulation. These include patients with venous thrombosis in whom embolism is a potentially fatal complication, patients with severe pulmonary or systemic embolization, and patients undergoing cardiac bypass surgery, arterial surgery, or hemodialysis. Heparin may also be instilled into cannulae to prevent local clotting—in which case the patient remains free of a general anticoagulant effect. It can also be given subcutaneously in lower doses of 5,000 units two or three times daily for prophylaxis against venous thrombosis in patients at high risk (eg, patients over 40 years undergoing major general surgery).[73]

Adverse Reactions—Hemorrhage, the major adverse reaction, appears to occur most frequently in elderly females.[74] Other adverse effects include hypersensitivity,[75] alopecia,[76] and osteoporosis[77] (after long-term use), although all of these are uncommon. Thrombocytopenia can also occur, and it is probably wise to monitor the platelet count in all patients receiving heparin.[78] Protamine sulfate can be used to instantly neutralize heparin activity.

WARFARIN SODIUM (Coumadin)

Warfarin is an intermediate-acting coumarin anticoagulant that is usually given orally. It reduces the hepatic synthesis of four vitamin K dependent coagulation factors—prothrombin, VII, IX and X, and the plasma concentrations of these factors decline at varying rates over the ongoing 72 to 90 hours. These effects can be reversed by vitamin K administration. Dosage of warfarin should be controlled by regular measurement of the prothrombin time (or an equivalent test). When patients are also receiving heparin therapy, measurement of prothrombin time should not be done within five hours of an intravenous bolus of heparin. Controlled infusion of heparin, however, does not significantly affect the results of this test.[79]

Drug Interactions—Since warfarin is highly protein-bound (97% or more), small changes in the degree of binding may lead to large, although transient, changes in the amount of circulating free warfarin and hence in its anticoagulant activity. Many drugs can displace warfarin from its binding sites, eg, salicylates, phenylbutazone, clofibrate, sulfonamides, nalidixic acid, ethacrynic acid, tolbutamide, phenytoin. If given to patients on long-term warfarin therapy, these drugs could lead to an increased anticoagulant effect and thereby increase the likelihood of hemorrhage. Unfortunately, the frequency and severity of clinically important interactions of this type is not adequately established.

TABLE 2 Preparations and Costs of Antithrombotic Agents

Generic Name	Trademark Name(s)	Preparations and 1978 Costs
Anticoagulants		
Heparin Sodium	Liquaemin Sodium (Panheprin)	Injection (solution) 1000 units/ml—$2.60/10-ml vial; 5000 units/ml—$7.15/10-ml vial; 10,000 units/ml—$6.20/4-ml vial; 20,000 units/ml—$14.25/5-ml vial; 40,000 units/ml—$22.50/5-ml vial
Warfarin Sodium	Coumadin (Panwarfin)	Tablets 2 mg—$5.05/100; 2.5 mg—$5.05/100; 5 mg—$5.60/100; 7.5 mg—$6.80/100; 10 mg—$8.10/100; 25 mg—$13.50/100
Antiplatelet Drugs		
Aspirin	generic	Tablets 325 mg—$0.18–$4.00/100
Dipyridamole	Persantine	Tablets 25 mg—$10.06/100
Sulfinpyrazone	Anturane	Capsules 200 mg—$12.16/100 Tablets 100 mg—$7.52/100
Fibrinolytic Agents		
Streptokinase	Streptase	Injection (powder) 100,000 units—$12.19/vial; 250,000 units—$23.84/vial; 750,000 units—$57.89/vial
Urokinase	Abbokinase	Injection (powder) 250,000 units—$175.00/vial

Since warfarin is a competitive inhibitor of vitamin K, drugs which interfere with the synthesis (broad spectrum antibiotics) or absorption (mineral oil, cholestyramine) of vitamin K may lead to an increased anticoagulant effect in patients receiving warfarin.

Since warfarin is metabolized in the liver, drugs that alter liver microsomal enzyme activity may have a profound effect on anticoagulant activity. Drugs that reduce microsomal enzyme activity, such as disulfiram, metronidazole, clofibrate, allopurinol, chloramphenicol, chlorpromazine and reserpine, may enhance anticoagulant activity. Drugs that enhance the microsomal enzymes, such as barbiturates, phenytoin, rifampin, dichloralphenazone, and spironolactone, may reduce anticoagulant activity. Drug interactions with warfarin are extensively reviewed elsewhere.[80–82]

Adverse Reactions—The major adverse effect of warfarin is hemorrhage. It occurs in some 5 to 7% of patients during short-term therapy. The most common sites of hemorrhage are the gastrointestinal tract, skin, and urinary tract.[75] Allergic reactions to warfarin are exceedingly rare. Hemorrhagic gangrene[83] and purple toes[84] have been reported but are rare phenomena.

In patients receiving long-term therapy with warfarin, spontaneous hemorrhage occurring at a time of satisfactory anticoagulant control should suggest the presence of an underlying lesion.

In pregnant mothers, fetal deaths may occur during warfarin treatment.[85] Although few complications have been reported in breast-fed children whose mothers are taking warfarin,[86] care should be exercised since warfarin is excreted in breast milk.

Dosage—Warfarin therapy is often started with a loading dose of 20 mg, followed in 24 to 48 hours by a maintenance dose that is determined by the results of control tests. Anticoagulation may, however, be instituted without a loading dose.[87] Optimum therapeutic prothrombin times have not been definitely established, but the generally accepted range is 1.5 to 2.5 times the control prothrombin time.[79] The customary maintenance dose of warfarin can be determined only by titration of the individual patient, and usually lies in the range of 3 to 10 mg daily. Care should be exercised in initiating anticoagulant therapy particularly in the elderly, or those with low protein levels in whom the ratio of free:bound warfarin may be higher than in normal subjects.[88]

STREPTOKINASE (Streptase)
UROKINASE (Abbokinase)

Streptokinase and urokinase are plasminogen activators that are used therapeutically to lyse thrombi. They differ in mode of action and dosage, but the clinical results of treatment are similar. Therapy with streptokinase may be complicated by immunoresistance in isolated cases and require more frequent laboratory monitoring than urokinase therapy. Treatment with urokinase, however, is more expensive.

Streptokinase and urokinase should be used only by physicians who have wide experience in the management of thromboembolic disease and under conditions that allow for appropriate clinical and laboratory monitoring. Bleeding complications occur more frequently than during oral anticoagulant therapy and are more severe and more difficult to manage.

Chemistry and Pharmacokinetics.—Streptokinase is an enzymatic protein produced by group C β-hemolytic streptococci. Like other streptococcal proteins, it is antigenic to man. Immune antibodies to streptokinase are present to a variable extent in all individuals, probably as a result of previous streptococcal infection. They react immediately with streptokinase to render it biologically inert. Studies with radioactive streptokinase have demonstrated two disappearance rates after intravenous administration—a short half-life of approximately 18 minutes due to antibody neutralization and a long half-life of about 83 minutes that occurs in the absence of antibodies.[89]

Urokinase is a protein isolated from tissue cultures of human kidney cells. It is not antigenic to man; therefore its use is not complicated by the presence of neutralizing antibodies.[90] After infusion, urokinase is cleared from the circulation with a plasma half-life of 10 to 15 minutes.[91]

Both streptokinase and urokinase are not absorbed from the gastrointestinal tract and must be given intravenously.

Clinical Pharmacology.—Streptokinase activates human plasminogen indirectly by first combining with plasminogen in equimolecular proportions to form an 'activator complex,' which then activates the remaining non-complexed plasminogen to plasmin.[92] The amount of plasmin generated depends on the relative amounts of streptokinase and plasminogen present. When the ratio of streptokinase to plasminogen is low, only small amounts of activator are formed and most of the plasminogen remains available for conversion into plasmin. When the ratio of streptokinase to plasminogen is high, most available plasminogen is complexed as activator and little is available to form plasmin. With currently recommended infusion schedules, which aim at high activator and low plasmin levels, the initial phase of plasmin generation and the resulting plasma proteolytic state are transient. Plasmin generated during the initial stages of streptokinase infusion produces a coagulation defect, which is due partly to digestion of fibrinogen, fibrin, and factors V and VIII[93] and partly to the presence of large amounts of fibrinogen or fibrin degradation products, which act as circulating anticoagulants. The sustained high level of plasminogen activator during the recommended maintenance infusion results in digestion of the fibrin structure of hemostatic plugs as well as thrombi and so produces bleeding from recent wounds, even when the plasma coagulation defect is slight.[94] The effect on coagulation after intravenous administration may persist for up to 12 hours after discontinuation.[93] Effective blood levels and disappearance rate are dependent upon availability of substrates and are only relative indices of pharmacologic effects of the drug.[95]

Urokinase enzymatically activates the endogenous fibrinolytic system by directly converting plasminogen to plasmin.[96] Its infusion, like streptokinase, produces a plasma coagulation defect due to the action of plasmin on fibrinogen, fibrin, and factors V and VIII. However, in comparison with streptokinase, the coagulation defect can be more predictably controlled by altering the infusion rate of urokinase. As with streptokinase, the infusion of urokinase is followed promptly by increased fibrinolytic activity which may persist for up to 12 hours after discontinuation.[97]

Indications—Venous thrombosis. Streptokinase has been shown to accelerate lysis of recent, radiographically documented, venous thrombi in random and non-random controlled cooperative studies.[68,98–102] Experience with urokinase is considerably more limited,[69] and it is not approved for this indication in the United States. The benefits of treating deep vein thrombosis with a fibrinolytic agent must be weighed against the risk of causing serious hemorrhage. The greatest potential benefits are in patients with major thromboses likely to cause lifelong venous insufficiency or other severe sequelae. Whether fibrinolytic therapy of deep venous thromboses will decrease the frequency of pulmonary embolization has not been established.

Pulmonary embolism. Two studies organized by the United States National Heart and Lung Institute compared the effects of urokinase infused for 12 or 24 hours, streptokinase infused for 24 hours, and heparin on the rate of resolution of recent submassive or massive pulmonary emboli.[70,71] All three fibrinolytic regimens produced greater resolution of emboli at 24 hours than heparin, and 24 hours of treatment with urokinase or streptokinase had no advantage over 12-hour treatment with urokinase. However, after the first week, lung scan improvement in heparin-treated patients was similar to that in urokinase-treated patients. A third, smaller study showed greater resolution of emboli after 72 hours of streptokinase therapy than after heparin.[103]

Arterial occlusion. Uncontrolled studies indicate that streptokinase treatment produces partial or complete lysis of 50 to 75% of limb artery occlusions less than three days old.[104,105] Since rapid removal of obstruction is often necessary to preserve limb viability, and fibrinolytic therapy acts slowly, it is indicated only when surgery is contraindicated.[104]

Myocardial infarction. A number of randomized trials have evaluated the effects of fibrinolytic treatment after myocardial infarction. Some well-designed studies have shown no effect of fibrinolytic therapy, while others have shown variable evidence of benefit.[95,106,107]

Arteriovenous cannula occlusion. Streptokinase can be used for clearing of totally or partially occluded arteriovenous cannulae as an alternative to surgical revision when acceptable flow cannot otherwise be achieved. According to the manufacturer, approximately 50% of totally occluded cannulae and 80% of partially occluded cannulae can be cleared sufficiently to resume dialysis by treatment with streptokinase.

Other indications. Chronic arteriosclerotic peripheral artery disease,[108,109] retinal vascular occlusion,[104] and the hemolytic uremic syndrome[110] are conditions that have been treated with plasminogen activators. All of the studies on these uses are uncontrolled, often with small numbers of treated patients.

Adverse Reactions—Hemorrhagic complications occur with equal frequency with both drugs; blood vessel punctures and skin incisions are the most common sites. One or more units of blood were needed in 13 to 18% of individuals in the National Heart and Lung Institute pulmonary embolism study. The antifibrinolytic drug aminocaproic acid (Amicar) can be given. Mild temperature elevation of more than 0.8°C occurred in 24% of 54 patients treated with streptokinase; only one patient had a temperature above 40°C during treatment; in contrast mild temperature elevation occurred in 16% of 113 urokinase recipients. Allergic reactions were seen in 3 of 54 streptokinase recipients and 1 of 113 urokinase recipients.[71]

Contraindications—Predisposition to bleeding, allergy, or systemic infection and recent cerebral embolism, thrombosis or hemorrhage are contraindications. Concurrent use of anticoagulants and fibrinolytic agents is not recommended. Since fibrinolytic agents may alter platelet function, the concurrent use of antiplatelet drugs should be avoided.

Dosage and Cost Comparison—For complete details of dosage, see the manufacturer's literature. Because of antibodies to streptokinase in most individuals, a loading dose is necessary. Heparin therapy is recommended after fibrin therapy to prevent further thrombosis, but it should not be initiated until the thrombin clotting time has decreased to less than twice control values.

In a patient with a massive pulmonary embolism a 24-hour course of streptokinase (3 million units) will cost about $300; a 72-hour course (7.5 million units) will cost about $700. A 12-hour course of urokinase (4 million units) will cost $2,800. However, since laboratory monitoring and pretesting requirements are higher with streptokinase the difference in cost may not be so dramatic.

REFERENCES

1. Wessler S: Anticoagulant therapy. JAMA 228:757–761, 1974.
2. Gallus AS, Hirsh J: Antithrombotic drugs. Drugs 12:41–68, 1976.
3. Naussbaum M, Moschos C: Anticoagulants and anticoagulation. Med Clin North Am 60:855–869, 1976.
4. Wessler S, Yin ET: Theory and practice of mini-dose heparin in surgical patients. Circulation 47:671–676, 1973.
5. Thomas DP: Heparin and pulmonary embolism. In *Heparin—Chemistry and Clinical Usage.* Edited by VV Kakkar, DP Thomas. New York, Academic Press, 1976, pp 189–199.
6. Sevitt S, Gallagher NG: Prevention of venous thrombosis and pulmonary embolism in injured patients. Lancet 2:981–989, 1959.
7. Morris GK, Mitchell JRA: Warfarin sodium in prevention of deep venous thrombosis and pulmonary embolism in patients with fractured neck of femur. Lancet 2:869–872, 1976.
8. Kakkar VV, Howe CT, Flanc C, et al: Natural history of postoperative deep vein thrombosis. Lancet 2:230–232, 1969.
9. O'Sullivan EF, Hirsh J, McCarthy RA, et al: Heparin in the treatment of venous thromboembolic disease; administration, control and results. Med J Aust 2:153–159, 1968.
10. Basu D, Gallus AS, Hirsh J, et al: A prospective study of the value of monitoring heparin therapy with the activated partial thromboplastin time. N Engl J Med 287:324–327, 1972.
11. Aggeler PM, Kosmin M: Anticoagulant prophylaxis and treatment of venous thromboembolic disease. In *Thrombosis.* Edited by S Sherry, KM Brinkhous, E Genton, et al. Washington, National Academy of Sciences, 1969, pp 639–689.
12. O'Sullivan EF: Duration of anticoagulant therapy in venous thromboembolism. Med J Aust 2:1104–1107, 1972.
13. Pluth J, McGoo DL: Current status of heart valve replacement. Mod Concepts Cardiovas Dis 48:65–70, 1974.
14. Hilden T, Iversen K, Raaschow F, et al: Anticoagulants in acute myocardial infarction. Lancet 2:327–331, 1961.
15. Medical Research Council Working Party: Assessment of short term anticoagulant administration after cardiac infarction. Br Med J 1:335–342, 1969.
16. An International Anticoagulant Review Group: Collaborative analysis of long term anticoagulant administration after acute myocardial infarction. Lancet 1:203–209, 1970.
17. Weily HS, Steele PP, Davis H, et al: Platelet survival in patients with substitute heart valves. N Engl J Med 290:534–537, 1974.
18. Harker LA, Slichter SJ: Studies of platelet and fibrinogen kinetics in patients with prosthetic heart valves. N Engl J Med 283:1302–1305, 1970.

19. Weily HS, Genton E: Altered platelet function in patients with prosthetic mitral valves: effects of sulfinpyrazone therapy. Circulation 42:967–972, 1970.
20. Sullivan JM, Harken DE, Gorlin R: Pharmacologic control of thromboembolic complications of cardiac valve replacement. N Engl J Med 284:1391–1394, 1971.
21. Blakely JA, Gent M: Platelets, drugs and longevity in a geriatric population. In *Platelets, Drugs and Thrombosis*. Edited by J Hirsh, JF Cade, AS Gallus, et al. Basel, S Karger, 1975, pp 284–291.
22. Anturane Reinfarction Trial Research Group: Sulfinpyrazone in the prevention of cardiac death after myocardial infarction. N Engl J Med 298:289–295, 1978.
23. Boston Collaborative Drug Surveillance Program: Regular aspirin intake and acute myocardial infarction. Br Med J 1:440–443, 1972.
24. Jick H, Miettinen OS: Regular aspirin intake and acute myocardial infarction. Br Med J 1:1057, 1976.
25. Elwood PC, Cochrane AL, Burr ML, et al: A randomized controlled trial of acetylsalicylic acid in the secondary prevention of mortality from myocardial infarction. Br Med J 1:436–440, 1974.
26. Five-year study by a group of physicians of the Newcastle upon Tyne region: Trial of clofibrate in the treatment of ischemic heart disease. Br Med J 4:767–775, 1971.
27. Report by a research committee of the Scottish Society of Physicians: Ischemic heart disease. A secondary prevention trial using clofibrate. Br Med J 4:775–784, 1971.
28. Krasno LR, Kidera GJ: Clofibrate in coronary heart disease. Effect on morbidity and mortality. JAMA 219:845–851, 1972.
29. Weiss HJ: Antiplatelet drugs—a new pharmacologic approach to the prevention of thrombosis. Am Heart J 92:86–102, 1976.
30. Verstraete M: Are agents affecting platelet functions clinically useful? Am J Med 61:897–914, 1976.
31. Harrison MJG, Marshall J, Meadows JC, et al: Effect of aspirin on amaurosis fugax. Lancet 2:743–744, 1971.
32. Mundall J, Quintero P, von Kaulla KN, et al: Transient monocular blindness and increased platelet aggregability treated with aspirin. Neurology 22:280–285, 1972.
33. Dyken ML, Kolar OJ, Jones FH: Differences in the occurrence of carotid transient ischemic attacks associated with antiplatelet aggregation therapy. Stroke 4:732–736, 1973.
34. Harker LA, Slichter SJ: Platelet and fibrinogen consumption in man. N Engl J Med 287:999–1005, 1972.
35. Acheson J, Danta G, Hutchinson EC: Controlled trial of dipyridamole in cerebral vascular disease. Br Med J 1:614–615, 1969.
36. Evans GE: Effects of drugs that suppress platelet surface interaction on incidence of amaurosis fugax and transient cerebral ischemia. Surg Forum 23:239–241, 1972.
37. Craven LL: Experiences with aspirin in the nonspecific prophylaxis of coronary thrombosis. Miss Valley J 75:38–40, 1953.
38. Lindsay RM, Prentice CRM, Ferguson D, et al: Reduction of thrombus formation on dialyser membranes by aspirin and RA 233. Lancet 2:1287–1290, 1972.
39. Andrassy K, Ritz E, Bornefeld M: Hypercoaguability and thrombotic AV cimino fistula complication and their prevention with acetyl salicylic acid (abstract). In *Proceedings of Third Meeting of International Society of Thrombosis and Hemostasis*. Washington, 1972, p 412.
40. Rittenhouse EA, Hessel EA, Ito CS, et al: Effect of dipyridamole on microaggregate formation in the pump oxygenator. Ann Surg 175:1–9, 1972.
41. Kaeggi A, Pineo GF, Schimizu A, et al: Arteriovenous-shunt thrombosis. Prevention by sulfinpyrazone. N Engl J Med 290:304–306, 1974.
42. Sullivan JM, Harken DE, Gorlin R: Pharmacologic control of thromboembolic complications of cardiac valve replacement. A preliminary report. N Engl J Med 279:576–580, 1968.
43. Trygstad CW, Bang NU, Heidenreich RO: A controlled trial of aspirin in childhood glomerular disorders. Thromb Diath Haemorrh 30:12–17, 1973.
44. Kincaid-Smith P: Modification of the vascular lesions of rejection in cadaveric renal allografts by dipyridamole and anticoagulants. Lancet 2:920–922, 1969.
45. Mathew TH, Clyne DH, Nanra RS, et al: A controlled trial of oral anticoagulants and dipyridamole in cadaveric renal allografts. Lancet 1:1307–1310, 1974.

46. Griepp RB, Dong E, Stanson EB, et al: Advances in human heart transplantation. Transplant Proc 5:835–839, 1973.
47. Jobin F, Delage JM: Aspirin and prednisone in microangiopathic hemolytic anemia. Lancet 2:208–210, 1970.
48. Giromini M, Bouvier CA, Dami R, et al: Effect of dipyridamole and aspirin in thrombotic microangiopathy. Br Med J 1:545–546, 1972.
49. Ross EC, Redondo D, Borges WH: Thrombotic thrombocytopenic purpura, survival following treatment with aspirin, dipyridamole and prednisone. JAMA 228:1141–1143, 1974.
50. Amir J, Krauss S: Treatment of thrombotic thrombocytopenic purpura with antiplatelet drugs. Blood 42:27–33, 1973.
51. Facharki LR, Walworth C, McIntyre OR: Antiplatelet therapy for thrombotic thrombocytopenic purpura. N Engl J Med 285:408–409, 1971.
52. Cuttner J: Splenectomy, steroids and dextran 70 in thrombotic thrombocytopenic purpura. JAMA 227:397–402, 1974.
53. Salzman EW, Harris WH, DeSanctis RW: Reduction in venous thromboembolism by agents affecting platelet function. N Engl J Med 284:1287–1292, 1971.
54. Zekert F, Kohn P, Vormittag E: Prophylaxis of thromboembolic diseases in traumatologic patients. A randomized double blind study with acetylsalicylic acid (abstract). In *Proceedings of Fourth Meeting of International Society of Thrombosis and Hemostasis.* Vienna, 1973, p 246.
55. Hey DM, Burckhardt D, Heinrich D, et al: Antithrombotic treatment by means of ASA in patients with major hip joint operation (abstract). In *Proceedings of Third Meeting of International Society of Thrombosis and Hemostasis.* Washington, 1972, p 426.
56. O'Sullivan EF, Renney JTG: Antiplatelet drugs in the prevention of postoperative deep vein thrombosis (abstract). In *Proceedings of Third Meeting of International Society of Thrombosis and Hemostasis.* Washington, 1972, p 438.
57. Butterfield WJH, British Medical Research Council: Effect of aspirin on postoperative venous thrombosis. Lancet 2:441–444, 1972.
58. O'Brien JR, Tulevski V, Etherington M: Two in vivo studies comparing high and low aspirin dosage. Lancet 1:338–400, 1971.
59. Wood EH, Prentice CRM, McGrouther DA, et al: Trial of aspirin and RA 233 in prevention of postoperative deep vein thrombosis. Thromb Diath Haemorrh 30:18–24, 1973.
60. Quick AJ, Clesceri L: Influence of acetylsalicylic acid and salicylamide on the coagulation of blood. J Pharmacol Exp Ther 128:95–98, 1960.
61. Browse NL, Hall JH: Effect of dipyridamole on the incidence of clinically detectable deep-vein thrombosis. Lancet 2:718–721, 1969.
62. Steele P, Weily HS, Genton E: Platelet survival and adhesiveness in recurrent venous thrombosis. N Engl J Med 288:1145–1152, 1973.
63. Carter AE, Eban R: Prevention of postoperative deep vein thrombosis in legs by orally administered hydroxychloroquine sulfate. Br Med J 3:94–95, 1974.
64. Heikinheimo R, Jarvinen K: Acetylsalicylic acid and arteriosclerotic-thromboembolic diseases in the aged. J Am Geriatr Soc 19:403–405, 1971.
65. Ockene IS, Dalen JE: The role of fibrinolytic agents in the treatment of thromboembolism. In *Thrombosis, Platelets, Anticoagulation and Acetylsalicylic Acid.* Edited by E Donoso, JI Haft. New York, Stratton Intercontinental Medical Book Corporation, 1976, pp 44–59.
66. Streptokinase (editorial). Br Med J 1:927–928, 1977.
67. Briggs JC: Thrombolytic therapy in arterial and venous thrombosis. Aust Ann Med 19(Suppl I):19–24, 1970.
68. Kakkar VV, Flanc C, Howe CT, et al: Treatment of deep vein thrombosis; a trial of heparin, streptokinase and arvin. Br Med J 1:806–810, 1969.
69. Silver D: Urokinase in the management of acute arterial and venous thrombosis. Arch Surg 97:910–916, 1968.
70. Urokinase-pulmonary embolism trial. Phase I results. JAMA 214:2163–6172, 1970.
71. Urokinase-streptokinase pulmonary embolism trial. Phase II results. JAMA 229:1606–1613, 1974.
72. *Human Blood Coagulation, Haemostasis and Thrombosis,* 2nd Edition. Edited by R Biggs. Oxford, Blackwell Scientific Publications, 1976.

73. International Multicentre Trial: Prevention of fatal post-operative pulmonary embolism by low doses of heparin. Lancet 2:45–51, 1975.
74. Jick H, Slone D, Borda IT, et al: Efficacy and toxicity of heparin in relation to age and sex. N Engl J Med 279:284–286, 1968.
75. Levine WG: Anticoagulants: heparin and oral anticoagulants. In *The Pharmacological Basis of Therapeutics,* 4th Edition. Edited by LS Goodman, A Gilman. New York, Macmillan, 1976, pp 1445–1463.
76. Zinn WJ: Side reactions of heparin in clinical practice. Am J Cardiol 14:36–38, 1964.
77. Gilfillan GC, Nichols G, Asher JD: Heparin osteoporosis. Ann Intern Med 63:921–922, 1965.
78. Deykin D: Heparin therapy: regimens and management. Drugs 13:46–51, 1977.
79. Salzman EW, Deykin D, Shapiro RM, et al: Management of heparin therapy: controlled prospective trial. N Engl J Med 292:1046–1050, 1975.
80. Sigell LT, Flessa HC: Drug interactions with anticoagulants. JAMA 214:2035–2038, 1970.
81. Deykin D: Warfarin therapy. N Engl J Med 283:691–694, 801–803, 1970.
82. Koch-Weser J, Sellers EM: Drug interactions with coumarin anticoagulants. N Engl J Med 285:487–498, 547–558, 1971.
83. Verhagen H: Local haemorrhage and necrosis of the skin and underlying tissues during anticoagulant therapy with dicumarol or dicumafyl. Acta Med Scand 148:453–462, 1954.
84. Feder W, Auerbach R: 'Purple toes': an uncommon sequela of oral coumarin drug therapy. Ann Intern Med 55:911–917, 1961.
85. Gordon RR, Dean T: Foetal deaths from antenatal anticoagulant therapy. Br Med J 2:719–721, 1955.
86. Eckstein HB, Jack B: Breast feeding and anticoagulant therapy. Lancet 1:672–673, 1970.
87. O'Reilly RA, Aggeler PM: Studies on coumarin anticoagulant drugs: initiation of warfarin therapy without a loading dose. Circulation 38:169–177, 1968.
88. Hayes MJ, Langman MJS, Short AH: Changes in drug metabolism with increasing age: I. Warfarin binding and plasma proteins. Br J Clin Pharmacol 2:69–73, 1975.
89. Fletcher AP, Alkjaersig N, Sherry S: The clearance of heterologous proteins from the circulation of normal and immunized man. J Clin Invest 37:1306–1315, 1958.
90. Genton E, Claman HN: Urokinase: antigenic studies in patients following thrombolytic therapy. J Lab Clin Med 75:619–621, 1970.
91. Fletcher AP, Alkjaersig N, Sherry S, et al: The development of urokinase as a thrombolytic agent. Maintenance of a sustained thrombolytic state in man by its intravenous infusion. J Lab Clin Med 65:713–731, 1965.
92. Trobisch H: Streptokinase and fibrinolysis. Postgrad Med J 49(Suppl 5):17–20, 1973.
93. Fletcher AP, Alkjaersig N, Sherry S: The maintenance of a sustained thrombolytic state in man. I. Introduction and effects. J Clin Invest 38:1096–1110, 1959.
94. Cade JF, Basu D, Muckle TJ, et al: Effects of thrombolytic therapy on hemorrhage from postoperative wounds. Thromb Diath Haemorrh 32:592–599, 1974.
95. Brogden RN, Speight TM, Avery GS: Streptokinase: a review of its clinical pharmacology, mechanism of action and therapeutic uses. Drugs 5:357–445, 1973.
96. Kjeldgaard NO, Ploug J: Urokinase. An activator of plasminogen from human urine. II. Mechanism of plasminogen activation. Biochim Biophys Acta 24:283–289, 1957.
97. Bell WR: Thrombolytic therapy: a comparison between urokinase and streptokinase. Semin Thromb Hemostas 2:1–13, 1975.
98. Gormsen J, Laursen B: Treatment of acute phlebothrombosis with streptase. Acta Med Scand 181:373–383, 1967.
99. Browse NL, Thomas ML, Pim HP: Streptokinase and deep vein thrombosis. Br Med J 3:717–720, 1968.
100. Robertson BR, Nilsson IM, Nylander G: Thrombolytic effect of streptokinase as evaluated by phlebography of deep venous thrombi of the leg. Acta Chir Scand 136:173–180, 1970.
101. Tsapogas MJ, Peabody RA, Wu KT, et al: Controlled study of thrombolytic therapy in deep vein thrombosis. Surgery 74:973–984, 1973.
102. Duckert F, Müller G, Nyman D, et al: Treatment of deep vein thrombosis with streptokinase. Br Med J 1479–481, 1975.
103. Tibbut DA, Davies JA, Anderson JA, et al: Comparison by controlled clinical trial of streptokinase and heparin in treatment of life-threatening pulmonary embolism. Br Med J 1:343–347, 1974.

104. Schmutzler R, Koller F: Thrombolytic therapy. In *Recent Advances in Blood Coagulation.* Edited by L Poller. London, JA Churchill, 1969, pp 229–235.
105. Dotter CT, Rösch J, Seaman AJ: Selective clot lysis with low-dose streptokinase. Radiology 111:31–37, 1974.
106. Simon TL, Ware JH, Stengle JM: Clinical trials of thrombolytic agents in myocardial infarction. Ann Intern Med 79:712–719, 1973.
107. Anon: Controlled trial of urokinase in myocardial infarction. A European Collaborative Study. Lancet 2:624–626, 1975.
108. Verstraete M, Vermylen J, Donati MB: The effect of streptokinase infusion on chronic arterial occlusions and stenoses. Ann Intern Med 74:377–382, 1971.
109. Persson AV, Thompson JE, Patman RD: Streptokinase as an adjunct to arterial surgery. Arch Surg 107:779–784, 1973.
110. Stuart J, Winterborn MH, White RHR, et al: Thrombolytic therapy in haemolytic-uraemic syndrome. Br Med J 3:217–221, 1974.

42. HEMOSTATIC AGENTS

Gordon D. O. Lowe and David H. Lawson

Hemostatic drugs can be classified as either local or systemic preparations. Local hemostatic agents are applied topically to promote clot formation in areas of capillary oozing on body surfaces and internally during surgery. They are eventually absorbed. Such agents include thrombin, gelatin sponge, oxidized cellulose, and collagen fibrils. Systemic hemostatic agents are given to correct specific generalized hemostatic deficiencies seen in a wide variety of clinical situations and include vitamin K preparations, aminocaproic acid and tranexamic acid, antihemophilic factor, fibrinogen, and other blood derivatives.

NORMAL AND ABNORMAL HEMOSTASIS AND FIBRINOLYSIS

Coagulation

The sequence of events promoting hemostasis when a blood vessel is damaged may be summarized as follows: (1) The vessel contracts, affording transient hemostasis. (2) Blood platelets adhere to the edges of the damaged vessel wall and to each other; this platelet aggregate forms an initial, loose hemostatic plug. (3) At the same time the coagulation system is activated, resulting in the formation of fibrin strands which reinforce the platelet plug; this platelet-fibrin meshwork firmly and finally seals the vessel defect. (4) The fibrinolytic system is activated, breaking down fibrin; under normal circumstances this proceeds slowly over a period of days, in parallel with tissue repair processes.

The coagulation and fibrinolytic systems are shown in greater detail in Figure 1. Fibrin is formed from circulating fibrinogen (factor I) by the enzyme thrombin. Thrombin is itself formed from a circulating plasma precursor, prothrombin (factor II) as a result of the interaction of other plasma protein coagulation factors. All coagulation factors are identified by Roman numerals in a standard international classification, and all are synthesized in the liver except factor VIII whose site of synthesis is uncertain. Prothrombin is converted to thrombin by the interaction of factor V, factor X, phospholipid (from damaged tissues or platelets) and calcium (formerly known as factor IV). This 'final common pathway' of thrombin formation, and hence fibrin formation, can be activated by either of two systems—the extrinsic or intrinsic systems.

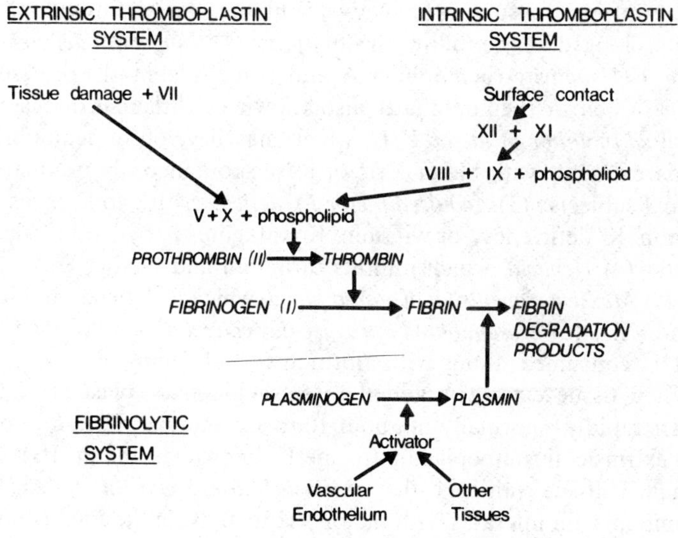

FIGURE 1. Coagulation and fibrinolytic systems.

When blood is taken by clean venipuncture, placed in a glass tube, and incubated at 37°C, clotting normally occurs within 5 to 10 minutes (whole blood clotting time). All factors required for coagulation are present in the blood, hence this coagulation pathway is termed the *intrinsic system*. Surface contact with glass initiates interaction of factors XII and XI. Activated factor XI then activates factor IX, which interacts with factor VIII, phospholipid, and calcium to activate the final common pathway of thrombin and fibrin formation discussed above. This pathway is an amplification system;

increasing amounts of activated coagulation factors are formed at each stage of the process.

The function of this intrinsic system is crudely tested by the whole blood clotting time. More reproducible tests are the partial thromboplastin time (re-calcification of citrated plasma) and activated partial thromboplastin time (prior activation with kaolin surface and cephalin phospholipid). However, these screening tests may be insensitive to moderate defects of factor VIII or factor IX, and if hemophilia is suspected, then specific assays of factor VIII and factor IX should be performed.

The intrinsic system is defective, and the partial thromboplastin time prolonged, in the following situations: (1) *Congenital deficiency of factor VIII activity* (hemophilia A and von Willebrand's disease) or *factor IX activity* (hemophilia B, also known as Christmas disease). (2) *Acquired inhibitor of factor VIII,* which may develop in hemophiliacs after treatments with factor VIII or arise spontaneously in otherwise normal subjects. (3) *Acquired factor IX deficiency* due to liver disease, vitamin K deficiency, or vitamin K antagonism by oral anticoagulants. (4) *Heparin,* which inhibits thrombin and factors IX, X, and XI. (5) *Massive transfusion of stored blood,* which is deficient in factors V and VIII. (6) *Disseminated intravascular coagulation,* in which factor VIII is consumed along with fibrinogen and factor V.

When tissue extract is added to fresh blood or plasma, clotting occurs rapidly—normally in about 10 to 15 seconds. The addition of this extrinsic thromboplastin (formerly known as factor III) from damaged tissue initiates the *extrinsic thromboplastin system;* the thromboplastin interacts with factor VII to activate the final common pathway of thrombin and fibrin formation. The function of this extrinsic system is tested by the prothrombin time; a standard tissue thromboplastin is added to citrated plasma which is then re-calcified.

The extrinsic system is defective and the prothrombin time prolonged in the following disorders and therapies: (1) *Acquired deficiency of factors II (prothrombin), VII, and X* due to liver disease, vitamin K deficiency, or vitamin K antagonism by oral anticoagulants. These three factors, along with factor IX discussed above, are synthesized in adequate amounts only when liver function is reasonably intact and adequate supplies of vitamin K are available. Concentrates of factors II, VII, IX and X (prothrombin complex concentrates or factor IX concentrates) are available for the correction of such combined defects. (2) *Heparin therapy,* which inhibits factor X and thrombin. (3) *Massive transfusion of stored blood,* which is deficient in labile factor V. (4) *Disseminated intravascular coagulation,* in which various coagulation factors are consumed.

Fibrinolysis

The mechanisms of the fibrinolytic system are not as well understood as those of the coagulation systems. Fibrin is converted into soluble breakdown products (fibrin degradation products) by the enzyme plasmin. Plasmin can also digest fibrinogen to form similar products; such products are therefore termed fibrinogen/fibrin degradation products (FDP). Plasmin is formed from a circulating plasma precursor, plasminogen, which is incorporated into clots along with fibrin during coagulation. Activators of plasminogen are present in all body tissues, especially vascular endothelium; coagulation factor XII can also initiate fibrinolysis. FDP are anticoagulants; like heparin, they inhibit the conversion of fibrinogen to fibrin by thrombin.

In many clinical situations, bleeding may occur because of a marked deficiency of plasma fibrinogen, accompanied by increased fibrinolytic activity and high levels of anticoagulant FDP. A rapid screening test for this *defibrination syndrome* is the thrombin clotting time, in which thrombin is added to citrated plasma. The thrombin clotting time is prolonged with a marked deficiency of plasma fibrinogen, and/or high levels of FDP. (Heparin, which also inhibits thrombin, will also prolong the thrombin time). Marked fibrinogen deficiency will also result in a small clot in clotting time tests.

The defibrination syndrome usually arises from *disseminated intravascular coagulation* (DIC), which may complicate a wide variety of acute illnesses and operations; a more chronic form is seen in malignant diseases, retained dead fetus, and giant hemangioma. The coagulation system is activated by release of thromboplastins from damaged tissues or by widespread damage to the endothelial lining of small blood vessels. There is secondary activation of the fibrinolytic system, which digests fibrinogen and fibrin to their degradation products. Clinical features include (1) thrombosis; (2) hemolytic anemia, due to damage to red cells by fibrin strands in the capillaries; and (3) bleeding, due to depletion of fibrinogen, platelets, factor VIII and factor V, and to the anticoagulant action of FDP.

Less commonly, defibrination arises from primary activation of the fibrinolytic system, resulting in the conversion of fibrinogen to degradation products and consequent bleeding. Such *primary pathological fibrinolysis* occurs in similar situations to DIC (postpartum, after surgery, and complicating malignant disease). Therapeutic activation of the fibrinolytic system, to lyse thromboemboli, may be effected with urokinase or streptokinase. Bleeding may then occur if there is excessive consumption of fibrinogen and production of degradation products.

GENERAL MANAGEMENT OF SYSTEMIC HEMOSTATIC DEFECTS

Diagnosis

Accurate diagnosis is essential for proper management of generalized hemostatic defects. Frequently the defect is obvious—for example, bleeding in patients on anticoagulant therapy, patients known to be thrombocytopenic, or in known hemophiliacs. Laboratory tests are usually required to provide specific diagnosis and to guide replacement therapy.

A family history of bleeding or a past history of prolonged bleeding after injury or surgery (especially after extraction of teeth, tonsillectomy, or childbirth) are commonly found in patients with congenital coagulation defects, such as the hemophilias. However, one-third of hemophiliacs give no family history, and mild hemophiliacs may appear to have normal coagulation after minor hemostatic stresses, yet may bleed profusely after major trauma or surgery. It is essential to distinguish hemophilia A (factor VIII deficiency) from the less common hemophilia B (factor IX deficiency, Christmas disease) so that the appropriate factor may be replaced. The presence of a factor VIII inhibitor will also influence therapy.

Anticoagulant and fibrinolytic therapy are usually obvious causes of defective hemostasis. Less obvious are drugs and chemicals causing thrombocytopenia, and drugs such as aspirin and dextran that produce defects in platelet function rather than reduction in number of platelets. Renal failure and paraproteinemias also cause functional abnormalities of platelets. Purpura with enlargement of liver, spleen or lymph nodes suggest the possibility of thrombocytopenia from reticulo-endothelial neoplasia. Liver disease, obstructive jaundice, or malabsorption suggest a defect of vitamin K-dependent clotting factors. Defibrination syndromes can complicate obstetric accidents (septic abortion, antepartum hemorrhage, retained dead fetus), surgery (especially prostatic, lung, and cardiac bypass), acute hemolysis (transfusion reactions, burns, snakebite), septicemias, and malignancy. Massive transfusion of stored blood, deficient in platelets and labile coagulation factors (V, VIII), may also cause bleeding.

The pattern of bleeding differs in platelet defects and coagulation factor defects. In platelet deficiency, bleeding occurs soon after injury and may be alleviated by pressure; purpura and oozing from venipuncture sites are common. In clotting factor defects, bleeding is commonly delayed for some hours after injury and is not alleviated by pressure; large spreading subcutaneous bruises and bleeding into muscles and joints are characteristic.

Blood samples for hemostatic screening should be taken by clean venipuncture at sites distant from intravenous infusions. Samples commonly taken are an E.D.T.A. sample for blood count, blood film and platelet count, a citrated sample kept on ice for coagulation tests (thrombin time, prothrombin time, activated partial thromboplastin time), and a sample for fibrinogen/fibrin degradation products (if defibrination is suspected). Initial results should be available within an hour and will indicate whether a hemostatic defect is due to thrombocytopenia, to coagulation factor deficiency, or to both. Further tests of coagulation or fibrinolysis, or further investigation of thrombocytopenia, may then be indicated. If the hemostatic defect is due to blood vessel or platelet dysfunction, the coagulation screen will be normal.

General Management of Acute Hemorrhage

Unless intravascular volume is maintained with intravenous fluids, plasma, or blood and shock prevented, small blood vessels can be damaged and DIC may occur, which will increase the coagulation defect. Treatment of the underlying disorder is especially important in the defibrination syndromes, and, as in cases of abruptio placentae, may be all that is required.

General Management of Chronic Hemostatic Defects

In congenital bleeding disorders, accurate diagnosis, screening of relatives for cases and carriers, and genetic counseling are most important. Patients should be educated on the risks of trauma, surgery, and tooth extraction, and provided with a card stating the type and severity of the disorder, blood group, and physician or reference center. A 'physician-alert' bracelet may be valuable in case of accident. Patients should be warned not to take salicylates, which impair platelet function and exacerbate bleeding. Intramuscular injections should be avoided as large, painful, crippling hematomas may occur.

Despite the benefits of modern replacement therapy, persons with severe hemophilia commonly have problems with chronic arthropathy, education, employment, personal relationships, and drug addiction. Such patients are best managed at a hemophilia center where physicians, surgeons, hematologists, physiotherapists, social workers, and dentists communicate regularly and are aware of optimal management of these special problems.

SYSTEMIC HEMOSTATIC AGENTS

Systemic hemostatics are grouped into those that are derived from blood and those that are not. The latter group includes protamine, vitamin K preparations, and fibrinolytic inhibitors. The only use of protamine sulfate is to neutralize heparin in the event of major bleeding during heparin therapy. It is discussed in Chapter 41, Anticoagulant, Antiplatelet, and Antifibrinolytic Agents.

Vitamin K Preparations

Vitamin K is required for the hepatic synthesis of coagulation factors II, VII, IX, and X. Vitamin K therapy may be needed in (1) bleeding due to vitamin K deficiency, and (2) bleeding during treatment with oral anticoagulant drugs. 'Vitamin K' is a general name for a group of napthoquinone derivatives. The commonly used vitamin K preparations are synthetic compounds. They include the fat-soluble substances phytonadione (vitamin K_1) and menadione, and the water-soluble salts of menadione—menadione sodium bisulfite (Hykinone) and menadiol sodium diphosphate (Synkayvite). Phytonadione is the preferred drug since it has a more rapid and potent effect and is less toxic to neonates.

Most dietary vitamin K comes from leafy green vegetables. Another source of the vitamin is the endogenous bacterial flora of the gut. Pure dietary deficiency is rare but may occur in patients with steatorrhea who are on low fat diets and in patients on long-term parenteral nutrition. Reduction of the normal bowel flora by prolonged antibacterial therapy may reduce bacterial synthesis of vitamin K and thereby cause deficiency. Significant vitamin K deficiency can also arise from failure of intestinal absorption. Naturally-occurring vitamin K is fat-soluble and normally is absorbed with fat; it is not absorbed when deficiencies of bile salts (as in obstructive jaundice) or pancreatic lipase (as in pancreatic insufficiency) are present. Extensive intestinal resection or disease may also produce vitamin K deficiency by reduction of jejunal fat absorption or ileal bile salt reabsorption.

Hemorrhagic disease of the newborn is due to deficiency of vitamin K dependent coagulation factors and is an exaggeration of the physiological deficiency of these factors during the first week of life. The pathogenesis of the syndrome is complex, and vitamin K deficiency is only one aspect. Deficiency may be due to lack of vitamin K-forming bacteria in the neonatal gut, maternal deficiency, or maternal ingestion of antagonist drugs (eg, oral anticoagulants, salicylates). Breast feeding is a risk factor since human milk contains only about 25% of the vitamin K present in cow's milk. In addition, the immature liver synthesizes less of the clotting factors; this is more marked in premature babies. There is also an increased risk of hemorrhagic disease in traumatic and hypoxic deliveries. Phytonadione may be given to the neonate for prevention or treatment, but small doses should be used since a rise in unbound bilirubin may occur, due to its displacement from plasma albumin or reduced hepatic conjugation with glucuronic acid. This effect is more marked with the water-soluble vitamin K analogues, which may also cause hemolysis in patients with glucose 6-phosphate dehydrogenase deficiency and kernicterus in infants. Prophylaxis is more effective when given to the neonate than when given antepartum to the mother; a single intramuscular injection of phytonadione (1.0 mg) is given on delivery to infants at risk because of prematurity, traumatic or hypoxic delivery, or maternal drug ingestion; some centers give prophylaxis to all newborns. In the treatment of hemorrhage, phytonadione (1.0 mg) is given intramuscularly or intravenously, and repeated every 8 hours if indicated.

DRUG MONOGRAPH

PHYTONADIONE (AquaMephyton, Konakion, Mephyton)

Phytonadione may be given orally, intramuscularly, and intravenously. Intravenous injections should be given slowly since adverse effects (flushing, sweating, sensation of chest constriction, cyanosis, peripheral circulatory failure) may occur. Intravenous injection is usually reserved for hemorrhage during oral anticoagulant therapy. The usual dose range is 5 to 50 mg in 24 hours. Large doses render the patient refractory to further oral anticoagulant therapy for several days.

Parenteral therapy is indicated in malabsorption states; the intramuscular route is generally used. An example is correction of hemostasis before surgery in patients with obstructive jaundice. Here, the dose of phytonadione is 10 to 20 mg daily, and the response —synthesis of vitamin K-dependent clotting factors—is assessed by the return of a prolonged prothrombin time to normal. Vitamin K will not correct the prothrombin time or the bleeding tendency in jaundiced patients if a major part of the clotting factor defect is due to hepatocellular dysfunction.

Fibrinolytic Inhibitors

These synthetic drugs competitively inhibit activators of plasminogen that convert plasminogen to plasmin. As a result, they prevent breakdown of formed fibrin clot. They are used to prevent or treat bleeding in which local or general fibrinolysis is thought to play a role. Their use carries a risk of formation of unlysable fibrin with consequent thrombotic occlusion. Two fibrinolytic inhibitors are available—aminocaproic acid and tranexamic acid. The latter drug is more potent, acts longer, and has fewer side effects, but it is not available in the United States.

In hemophilia, whether due to factor VIII deficiency or factor IX deficiency, prophylactic antifibrinolytic agents given before and after dental extraction reduce post-extraction bleeding and factor replacement requirements,[1,2] presumably by inhibition of fibrinolytic enzymes from saliva and buccal tissue. The first dose should be given orally or intravenously before extraction, and oral therapy continued for 7 to 10 days. Synovial fluid contains high levels of fibrinolytic activator that might perpetuate hemarthrosis in hemophilia, but there is insufficient evidence that antifibrinolytic prophylaxis reduces spontaneous musculoskeletal bleeding. Hematuria may respond to fibrinolytic inhibitors (presumably due to inactivation of endogenous urokinase), but in view of the risk of ureteral obstruction, this therapy should only be used as a last resort.

The prostate gland is rich in plasminogen activators which are released into urine during and after prostatectomy, and they may play a role in postoperative hematuria. Prophylactic antifibrinolytic therapy reduces blood loss after prostatic surgery;[3] this type of therapy is started intravenously during surgery and continued after the operation (intravenously or orally) until macroscopic hematuria is no longer evident.

Endometrial plasminogen activators are increased in women with idiopathic menorrhagia, and fibrinolytic inhibitors reduce menstrual bleeding in this condition[4] as well as in menorrhagia due to intrauterine contraceptive devices; treatment is given from the first day of profuse bleeding. Such therapy is less well established than estrogen/progestogen treatment, and the possibility of thrombotic side effects should be remembered.

Bleeding commonly occurs during thrombolytic therapy with plasminogen activators (urokinase, streptokinase) and is due to depletion of plasma fibrinogen and high levels of FDP. In severe hemorrhage, excessive fibrinolysis can be reversed by cessation of thrombolytic therapy and slow intravenous injection of aminocaproic acid (100 mg/kg every six hours) or tranexamic acid (15 mg/kg every eight hours). In pathological defibrination when laboratory tests suggest that the primary disorder is fibrinolysis rather than DIC, the value of fibrinolytic inhibitor therapy is not established.

Fibrinolytic inhibitors also inhibit activation of plasma enzymes that consume C1′ inhibitor (C1′ is the first component of the complement system), and they have been used successfully in the long-term prophylaxis and treatment of minor attacks of visceral edema in patients with the rare disorder of hereditary angioedema due to C1′ inhibitor deficiency.[5]

DRUG MONOGRAPHS

TRANEXAMIC ACID

Tranexamic acid, an investigational drug in the United States, is well absorbed orally with a peak effect at about two hours. A more rapid effect can be obtained by intravenous injection which should be given slowly to avoid hypotension. Elimination is largely by renal excretion; accumulation may occur in renal insufficiency and dosage adjustments are required, although their extent is not yet established.

TABLE 1 Preparations and Costs of Hemostatic Agents

GENERIC NAME	TRADEMARK NAME(S)	PREPARATIONS AND 1978 COSTS
Systemic Hemostatic Agents		
Phytonadione	Mephyton AquaMephyton (Konakion)	Tablets 5 mg—$11.55/100 Injection (solution) 2 mg/ml—$0.50/0.5-ml ampul; 10 mg/ml—$0.97/1-ml ampul, $2.55/2.5-ml vial, $5.08/5-ml vial
Tranexamic Acid[a]		Tablets 250 mg Injection (solution) 100 mg/ml—5-ml ampul
Aminocaproic Acid	Amicar	Tablets 500 mg—$12.41/100 Syrup 1.25 g/5 ml—$37.16/pint Injection (solution) 250 mg/ml—$6.33/20-ml vial
Antihemophilic Factor	Factorate (Hemofil) (Humafac)	Injection 225 AHF units (with diluent)—$45.00/vial
Factor IX Complex (Human)	Konyne (Proplex)	Injection (with diluent and administration set)—$62.90/vial
Human Fibrinogen	Parenogen	Injection (powder) 1 g (with diluent and intravenous set)—$23.22/vial
Local Hemostatic Agents		
Absorbable Gelatin Sponge	Gelfoam	Blocks 20 × 60 × 3 mm—$2.88 Powder—$2.80/1 g Many forms available
Oxidized Cellulose	Oxycel (Surgical)	Many forms available
Thrombin	generic	Powder 1,000 units—$3.51/30-ml vial
Microfibrillar Collagen Hemostat	Avitene	Powder—$33.00/g

[a]Not marketed in the United States.

Adverse Reactions—Gastrointestinal disturbances and allergic reactions occasionally occur. More serious reactions are local or general arterial or venous thrombosis, which may be due to inhibition of physiological fibrinolysis. Similarly, unlysable clot causing ureteric obstruction and permanent renal failure has been reported in hemophiliacs treated for hematuria with aminocaproic acid.[6]

Dosage—Oral or Intravenous: Adults, 10 to 15 mg/kg (0.5 to 1.0 g) every eight hours.

AMINOCAPROIC ACID (Amicar)

Aminocaproic acid is less potent, is shorter acting, and has more adverse effects than tranexamic acid. Absorption, elimination, and action are similar to tranexamic acid.

Dosage—Oral or Intravenous: Adults, 50 to 100 mg/kg (2 to 6 g) every six hours.

Blood Products

General Principles. The cost of collection, processing, storage and delivery of blood and blood products makes them expensive. Since the products are heterogeneous mixtures of proteins from other individuals, the risk of immunologic reactions and of the transmission of diseases, particularly viral hepatitis, always exists; these risks are dose-related. The proper blood product must be selected for the appropriate degree of correction of the individual patient's hemostatic defect or defects. Specific therapy is most economical. Because of the risk of circulatory overload, the less concentrated products, such as plasma, can only be administered in limited quantities. Thus, blood and blood products should be used cautiously, and the relative risks of bleeding and adverse effects should be carefully balanced. The type and degree of hemostatic defect should be determined by laboratory tests, and close collaboration with a specialist in blood disorders is desirable.

Adverse Effects. (1) *Circulatory overload.* Pulmonary edema may occur following infusion of large quantities of blood or plasma, particularly in the normovolemic, the severely anemic, the elderly, and patients with heart disease. The infusion should be stopped and appropriate treatment of pulmonary edema instituted. Preventive measures include slow infusion and the administration of a diuretic.

(2) *Allergic reactions.* Allergic reactions to gamma globulins, leukocyte antigens, or platelet antigens are more common in patients with an allergic history and in those who have received multiple infusions of blood products. The incidence of reactions may be

reduced, but not entirely eliminated, by prophylactic administration of an antihistamine or corticosteroid; this should be considered in such patients, particularly those with a history of previous reactions. These drugs should be given separately to the patient and not added to the blood product. Minor reactions (headache, malaise, nausea, urticaria, pyrexia, skin edema) may be treated by stopping or slowing the infusion and the administration of an antihistamine, such as chlorpheniramine (10 mg by slow intravenous injection, then 4 mg orally every 4 to 6 hours). Major reactions (asthma, laryngeal edema, anaphylaxis) should be treated immediately by stopping the infusion and giving subcutaneous or intramuscular epinephrine, 0.1 to 0.5 mg (0.1 to 0.5 ml of a 1:1000 solution), intravenous chlorpheniramine, 10 to 20 mg, and intravenous hydrocortisone, 100 to 200 mg. Epinephrine is by far the most effective antidote. Oxygen and cardiopulmonary support may also be necessary.

(3) *Hemolytic reactions.* These are usually complications of whole blood transfusions, but plasma and plasma fractions also contain small amounts of iso-antibodies, and repeated large infusions may cause hemolysis.

(4) *Pyrogenic reactions.* Fever may be part of an allergic or hemolytic reaction, or due to pyrogens from bacterial contamination of the blood product or transfusion apparatus. Septic shock and death may result. Careful aseptic technique and disposable apparatus have reduced such complications.

(5) *Viral hepatitis.* As with infective hepatitis, overtly jaundiced patients represent only a fraction of those with post-transfusion hepatitis, since most cases are subclinical and revealed only by screening for abnormal liver function.[7] Blood products prepared from large pools of donors, such as clotting factor concentrates, are particularly hazardous since the virus from a single donor can be distributed throughout the batch and remain infective. Patients who have not received such concentrates frequently in the past are at greatest risk.[8] Persons with a history of jaundice or drug addiction should be excluded from blood donation; the hepatitis risk is also greater in products derived from the blood of paid donors as compared to volunteer donor blood,[7] and volunteer blood is preferable. About 25% of blood donors who are carriers of viral hepatitis can be identified by screening for the surface antigen of hepatitis B (classical long-incubation serum hepatitis). The risk of transmitted hepatitis can be further reduced by screening potential

donors and blood products. More recently serologic tests have been developed for hepatitis A (classical short-incubation infectious hepatitis), which can also be transmitted parenterally. However, most cases of post-transfusion hepatitis are not due to well-characterized viruses.[9]

Principles of Replacement Therapy in Clotting Factor Deficiencies. In patients with hemorrhage due to thrombocytopenia, the level of platelets may be raised by the infusion of fresh blood, platelet-rich plasma, or platelet concentrate. In those with coagulation factor deficiencies, the deficient factor or factors as well as the degree of deficiency should both be identified if possible. General guidelines for adequate replacement therapy have been defined by observation of clinical response in large numbers of patients treated in special units and are best established for the hemophilias. However, they are only guidelines, since within- and between-patient variations in hemostatic response to replacement therapy are considerable.

Blood products used in replacement therapy are as follows.

(1) *Whole blood* and *plasma* which contain stable coagulation factors but not the labile factors V and VIII; *fresh plasma* and *fresh frozen plasma* (F.F.P.) contain these factors.

(2) *Cryoprecipitate* and *factor VIII concentrates* (antihemophilic factor) [Factorate, Hemofil, Humafac] which are rich in factor VIII and are used in the management of hemophilia A and von Willebrand's disease.

(3) *Factor IX concentrates* (prothrombin complex concentrates) [Konyne, Proplex] which are rich in factors II, VII, IX, and X and are used in the management of hemophilia B (factor IX deficiency) as well as acquired defects of these factors.

(4) *Fibrinogen concentrates* (Parenogen) which are used in defibrination syndromes.

Hemophilia A. This is the most common congenital bleeding disorder. Patients with hemophilia A are deficient in factor VIII (antihemophilic factor) activity. The severity of bleeding depends on plasma factor VIII activity.[10] When less than 5% of normal, bleeding into muscles and joints commonly occurs, either spontaneously or following minor trauma; spontaneous bleeding is particularly common in patients with a level of 1% or less. Spontaneous bleeding is uncommon in patients with levels of 5 to 25%, but can occur after minor trauma; serious bleeding may occur after major trauma or surgery. Patients with levels of 25 to 50% of normal (borderline levels for normal hemostasis) bleed excessively only after major trauma or surgery.

The plasma level of factor VIII required to treat bleeding, or to prevent bleeding after surgery, depends on the type, size, and duration of the trauma or hemorrhage.[10] Traumatic bleeds, large bleeds, and bleeds in muscles, bleeds that endanger the airway or compress arteries or nerves and bleeds not treated within a few hours of onset require higher plasma levels. For early spontaneous hemarthroses a level of 5 to 20% immediately after infusion is sufficient. Larger musculoskeletal bleeds, especially in dangerous sites, and dental extractions will require a post-infusion level of 20 to 40%. In major surgery, trauma, or hemorrhage in the central nervous system, immediate levels of 80 to 100% are desirable.

Since the half-life of infused factor VIII in the circulation is about 12 hours, the level after 24 hours will be only one-quarter of the initial level. Doses of factor VIII should be given before the plasma level falls dangerously low, and in major bleeds, trauma, or surgery infusions may have to be repeated every 8 to 12 hours. For optimal replacement therapy, the factor VIII level before and after infusion should be monitored in such patients.

The duration of treatment also depends on the type of bleeding. A single dose may be sufficient for a small hemarthrosis treated early; larger bleeds may require several daily doses and major surgery may require 10 to 14 days of treatment. The frequency of doses may be reduced from every 8 hours to every 24 hours if progress is satisfactory. Orthopedic surgery or wound complications may necessitate even more prolonged treatment. At some centers selected patients are given regular prophylactic factor VIII infusions.

The amount of material necessary to achieve a given plasma factor VIII level depends on the type, potency, and volume of the material as well as the patient's plasma volume. Approaches to dosage calculations are available elsewhere.[10]

Factor VIII levels in whole blood and plasma decline rapidly with storage and hence they are inadequate for factor VIII replacement. In the treatment of hemophilia, they should be used solely for red cell and plasma volume replacement. Fresh plasma or fresh frozen plasma may be used to treat minor bleeds, since a rise in factor VIII level of 20% may be achieved in a 70 kg man by infusion of about 1 liter. Problems of volume overload and time delays in preparation and infusion of plasma are reduced by the use of plasma fractions rich in factor VIII—cryoprecipitate or factor VIII concentrates.

DRUG MONOGRAPHS

CRYOPRECIPITATE

Cryoprecipitate is made by rapid freezing and cold-thawing of plasma, and is easily prepared in hospital blood banks. It contains 40 to 80% of the original factor VIII activity and is rich in fibrinogen.[11] An average bag of cryoprecipitate from a pint of blood contains about 60 units of factor VIII (1 unit of factor VIII activity is the amount present in 1 ml of fresh pooled citrated normal plasma) and an average dose for an early musculoskeletal bleed is 600 to 900 units (10 to 15 bags). A small dose may be drawn up and infused in large syringes; larger doses are pooled and infused via a blood product drip set. Gel formation suggests activated clotting factors and the pack should not be given. Large doses of cryoprecipitate may be given to achieve high plasma factor VIII levels (up to 100%) without hypervolemia for the treatment of serious bleeding and for hemostatic cover of major surgery; this has revolutionized the management of hemophilia in the last ten years. Cryoprecipitate has been used for home treatment but is less satisfactory than factor VIII concentrate since it must be stored frozen and then thawed. The main disadvantage of cryoprecipitate is the variation in potency of different batches. A high plasma fibrinogen level results from frequent infusions and occasionally causes hemolysis, platelet dysfunction, and transient proteinuria.

ANTIHEMOPHILIC FACTOR [Factor VIII Concentrates] (Factorate, Hemofil, Humafac)

In recent years lyophilized concentrates of factor VIII have been produced from human plasma or cryoprecipitate. These concentrates are stable for several months when stored at about 4°C and may be kept in a domestic refrigerator, allowing early treatment of minor bleeds in the home of selected patients. Treatment may be given by the patient himself, a relative, nurse, or general practitioner. Home treatment has undoubtedly improved the quality of life of patients with severe hemophilia; however careful selection, education and follow-up of patients is required.

Each batch of concentrate is assayed for Factor VIII activity and the amount per vial (usually 150 to 500 units) is stated on the label. The product is reconstituted with about 20 ml of Water for Injection with sterile precautions; this takes about 10 minutes. Gel formation suggests activated clotting factors and the vial should not be given. The concentrate is drawn up in a large syringe and infused at a rate not exceeding 10 ml per minute, otherwise vasomotor reactions may occur.

Unlike cryoprecipitate, the potency of factor VIII concentrates is known and the plasma level of factor VIII is more predictable. One problem with the concentrates is that the large pool of donors increases the risk of hepatitis; the risk is greatest in patients with mild hemophilia who have not received multiple infusions of blood products in the past, and some physicians prefer to treat minor bleeds in such patients with single donor or small pool products.[8]

Patients with Factor VIII Inhibitors. At some stage in their lives, about 10% of treated hemophiliacs develop antibodies to factor VIII that destroy its activity. The appearance of an inhibitor does not correlate with the amount, frequency, or type of factor VIII replacement therapy, and should be suspected if the clinical response or plasma factor VIII level response to replacement therapy is poor. An inhibitor assay should be done routinely prior to surgery or dental extraction. If further infusions of factor VIII are given, their activity is rapidly destroyed by the inhibitor, and, in addition, the inhibitor level often rises. Left untreated, the antibody level slowly falls over a year or two, sometimes to undetectable levels, but returns within 5 to 10 days of further factor VIII infusion. Therefore, in patients with high levels of inhibitors, only serious bleeds should be treated. Once the decision to treat has been made, treatment should be intensive with large doses of factor VIII before the antibody levels rise.[12] Removal of the antibodies by plasmaphoresis, and suppression of the antibodies by corticosteroids or azathioprine have been tried, but the results are usually disappointing. Bypassing of the factor VIII state of the coagulation cascade by prothrombin complex concentrates (see below) is more promising;[13,14] however there is a risk of thrombosis with these products and their use is still experimental.

Occasionally factor VIII inhibitors develop in non-hemophiliacs, especially the elderly, those with immune disorders, and postpartum women. The manifestations are similar to hemophilia, and treatment is the same.

Von Willebrand's Disease. The characteristics of this congenital bleeding disorder are: (1) a moderate deficiency of factor VIII activity; (2) a prolonged and progressive rise in factor VIII following infusion of plasma or serum, which presumably contain an inducer of endogenous factor VIII synthesis; (3) a prolonged skin puncture bleeding time, presumably due to various morphological and functional abnormalities of platelets, the most sensitive of which is ristocetin-induced aggregation. The interrelationship of these characteristics is unclear and the extent of defect varies between patients, suggesting that the syndrome may actually be a group of disorders. Bleeding severe enough to warrant treatment can usually be controlled by raising the plasma factor VIII to an appropriate level, as in the treatment of hemophilia A. Small daily doses of fresh frozen plasma are often sufficient since they induce endogenous factor VIII formation, although 24 to 48 hours may elapse before peak levels are reached. More rapid correction of factor VIII levels may be achieved with cryoprecipitate or factor VIII concentrates, although they may be less effective stimulants of factor VIII synthesis. These plasma fractions may also correct the prolonged bleeding time and platelet functional abnormalities.

Hemophilia B (Christmas Disease). Hemophilia A and B are clinically indistinguishable, but B hemophiliacs have congenital deficiency of factor IX activity rather than factor VIII. The levels of factor IX required for hemostasis are similar to those of factor VIII required in hemophilia A, and the principles of replacement therapy are also similar even though the products used are different.

The half-life of infused factor IX in the circulation is longer than that of factor VIII—about 24 hours—hence once daily doses are sufficient for most bleeds. Doses given every 12 hours may be required to maintain high plasma levels in major bleeds or surgery. The recovery of factor IX activity in the circulation is less complete than the recovery of infused factor VIII, possibly because the smaller molecular weight of factor IX allows extravascular distribution.[10]

Stored whole blood and plasma lose factor IX activity much more slowly than factor VIII activity, but the risk of volume overload limits their use for any but minor bleeds. Fresh plasma or fresh frozen plasma may be used to treat minor bleeds; a rise in factor IX level of 5 to 10% may be achieved in a 70 kg man by infusion of 1 to 1.5 liters of fresh plasma.

DRUG MONOGRAPH

FACTOR IX CONCENTRATES [Prothrombin complex concentrates] (Konyne, Proplex)

These preparations are used to treat major bleeds or to cover major surgery in patients with hemophilia B. Plasma levels of 50 to 100% can be achieved by infusion of relatively small volumes. Factor IX concentrates are much more convenient for treating minor bleeds than fresh frozen plasma; however as in hemophilia A some physicians prefer to treat minor bleeds with single-donor or small pool plasma since the risk of hepatitis is less.

At present, factor IX cannot be separated from factor II (prothrombin), factor X, and (not in all preparations) factor VII. Factor IX concentrates are therefore also termed prothrombin complex concentrates, and they may be used for treating bleeding in the rare congenital deficiencies of factor II, factor X, or factor VII, as well as the much more common acquired deficiencies of these factors—liver disease (see below) and oral anticoagulant therapy.

As with factor VIII concentrates, factor IX concentrates are lyophilized, stored in a refrigerator, and reconstituted with sterile water. They are suitable for home therapy. Gel formation suggests activated clotting factors (see below), and the vial should not be given. The rate of infusion should not exceed 10 ml per minute. The amount of assayed factor IX, and sometimes the level of other factors, is stated on the vial.

Factor IX concentrates are prepared from large pools of donors and have a fairly high risk of hepatitis. Thromboembolic complications, which include local thrombosis and disseminated intravascular coagulation, can be fatal.[15,16] Such complications may arise from activation of clotting factors during the manufacturing process; screen tests for thrombogenicity are now performed and some preparations contain heparin to neutralize activated factors. Some 'activated' preparations have been used in the treatment of patients with factor VIII inhibitors (see above), however relatively 'non-activated' concentrates have also been used successfully.[14]

Other Congenital Coagulation Disorders. Fibrinogen (factor I) may be given to patients with afibrinogenemia or abnormal fibrinogens (dysfibrinogenemia) as plasma, cryoprecipitate or fibrinogen concentrate (see section on defibrination below). Deficiency of factors II, VII or X can be treated with plasma or prothrombin complex concentrates as mentioned above. Deficiency of factors V or XI can be treated with fresh or fresh frozen plasma. Factor XIII, which has been omitted from Figure 1 for clarity, converts soluble fibrin polymer to insoluble fibrin polymer; congenital deficiency may be treated with fresh frozen plasma.

Acquired Deficiency of Factors II, VII, IX and X. Acquired deficiency of 'prothrombin complex' factors may be due to vitamin K deficiency, oral anticoagulant therapy, or hepatocellular dysfunction. In bleeding due to vitamin K deficiency or oral anticoagulant therapy, vitamin K may control the hemorrhage (see section on vitamin K above) but in severe bleeding replacement of coagulation factors may be indicated, using plasma or prothrombin complex concentrates (see above).

Bleeding in patients with hepatocellular disease does not usually respond to vitamin K, and factor replacement may be required in serious bleeding or prior to surgery. However, recovery of infused factors in the circulation, and clinical response, are often disappointing. Fresh plasma or fresh frozen plasma may be used, but dosage is limited by volume overload. Prothrombin complex concentrates are more potent but carry the risk of viral hepatitis and thromboembolic complications;[17] the latter may occur because the liver normally either removes activated clotting factors from the circulation or inactivates them. The relative contribution of the deficient factors to bleeding is uncertain. Similarly, the relative value of plasma, concentrates containing factor VII, and concentrates lacking factor VII is unclear. It is logical to monitor individual factor levels in addition to coagulation times and to aim for 'hemostatic' levels—factor II, 40% of normal; factor VII, 10%; factor IX, 40% and factor X, 20%. However, the efficacy, safety, and choice of blood products in liver disease requires further study. Patients with liver disease may also have low levels of platelets (consider replacement if the platelet count is under 50,000 per cmm), fibrinogen (replace with plasma or fibrinogen concentrate to 100 mg/100 ml), and factor V (replace with fresh or fresh frozen plasma to 15% of normal)—all of which may contribute to bleeding.

Defibrination Syndrome. In bleeding due to defibrination, treatment of the underlying cause and effective supportive care are essential. In the special case of bleeding during thrombolytic therapy with urokinase or streptokinase, the use of fibrinolytic inhibitors may be considered (see above). Plasma fibrinogen may be raised to a hemostatic level (100 mg/100 ml) with blood, plasma, cryoprecipitate, or fibrinogen concentrate.

In disseminated intravascular coagulation, other clotting factors are consumed, particularly the labile factor VIII and factor V. Platelets may also be consumed. Factor VIII may be replaced by fresh plasma, cryoprecipitate, or factor VIII concentrates; factor V by fresh or fresh frozen plasma; and platelets by platelet concentrates. Fresh whole blood provides volume, red cells, platelets, and all clotting factors and may be valuable in urgent situations. However, bleeding may be due largely to circulating anticoagulant fibrinogen/fibrin degradation products (FDP) rather than to deficiency of clotting factors or platelets.

The use of heparin and fibrinolytic inhibitors in defibrination syndromes is controversial. Management of defibrination syndrome is discussed in detail elsewhere.[18]

DRUG MONOGRAPH

FIBRINOGEN CONCENTRATE (Parenogen)

Fibrinogen is available as a freeze-dried powder which is stored under refrigeration and reconstituted with sterile water. The risk of hepatitis is high (up to 20%), and many physicians prefer to use cryoprecipitate if a more potent source of fibrinogen than plasma or blood is required.

Massive Transfusion of Stored Blood. When bleeding patients receive massive transfusions of stored blood, (eg, more than 8 units in 24 hours) plasma levels of platelets and the labile coagulation factors (VIII and V) may fall and thereby contribute to bleeding. Two units of fresh blood or fresh frozen plasma per 10 units of blood are usually sufficient to prevent or treat these deficiencies; additional platelet transfusions may be required if thrombocytopenia is severe. The large quantities of infused citrate lower plasma calcium levels, and this may also contribute to bleeding. To prevent calcium depletion, slow intravenous injection of 10 ml of 10% calcium gluconate per 5 units of transfused blood has been recommended.

LOCAL HEMOSTATIC AGENTS

The local hemostatic agents are applied topically to areas of capillary oozing. They promote clot formation and are eventually absorbed. They have few adverse effects but will interfere with healing if infection is present at the site of application.

DRUG MONOGRAPHS

ABSORBABLE GELATIN SPONGE (Gelfoam)

This agent is useful in highly vascular areas that are difficult to suture. It is insoluble in water and is usually moistened with sterile sodium chloride or thrombin solution.

OXIDIZED CELLULOSE (Oxycel, Surgicel)

This agent is a form of surgical gauze. When exposed to blood, it expands and forms an artificial clot; it does not participate in the normal clotting mechanism. Oxidized cellulose is useful in surgical procedures to control moderate bleeding when suturing or ligation is impractical or ineffective. It should not be used for permanent packing or implantation in fractures because it interferes with bone regeneration and will cause cyst formation. The Oxycel brand should not be used as a surface dressing except for immediate control of hemorrhage, since it inhibits epithelialization; silver nitrate or other corrosives should not be applied prior to its use. The hemostatic action of oxidized cellulose is not increased by other hemostatic agents, and thrombin is destroyed by its low pH.

THROMBIN

Thrombin is a plasma protein. The commercial product is prepared from prothrombin of bovine origin, and is used topically to control capillary oozing. It will clot whole blood, plasma, or a solution of fibrinogen without the addition of other substances. It may initiate clot formation when combined with gelatin sponge or fibrin foam. When applied to denuded tissue, thrombin is rapidly neutralized by antithrombins and its activity is reduced as a result of fibrin absorption.

MICROFIBRILLAR COLLAGEN HEMOSTAT (Avitene)

This preparation is a powder that consists of fibrils of shredded purified bovine collagen. It acts rapidly and is easily applied to most areas where hemostasis is necessary.

REFERENCES

1. Walsh PN, Rizza CR, Matthews JM, et al: Epsilon-aminocaproic acid therapy for dental extractions in hemophilia and Christmas disease: a double-blind controlled trial. Haematologica 20:463–475, 1971.
2. Forbes CD, Barr RD, Reid C, et al: Tranexamic acid in control of haemorrhage after dental extraction in haemophilia and Christmas disease. Br Med J 1:311–313, 1972.
3. McNicol GP, Fletcher AP, Alkjaersig N, et al: The use of epsilon-aminocaproic acid, a potent inhibitor of fibrinolytic activity, in the management of post-operative hematuria. J Urol 86:829–837, 1961.
4. Vermylen J, Verhaegen-Declerq ML, Verstraete M, et al: A double-blind study of the effect of tranexamic acid in essential menorrhagia. Thromb Diath Haemorrh 20:583–587, 1968.
5. Hadjiyannaki K, Lachmann PJ: Hereditary angio-oedema: a review with particular reference to pathogenesis and treatment. Clin Allergy 1:221–233, 1971.
6. Gobbi F: Use and misuse of aminocaproic acid (letter). Lancet 2:472–473, 1967.
7. Gocke DJ: A prospective study of post-transfusion hepatitis. JAMA 219:1165–1170, 1972.
8. Kasper CK, Kipnis SA: Hepatitis and clotting-factor concentrates (letter). JAMA 221:510, 1972.
9. Mosley, JW, Redeker AG, Feinstone SM, et al: Multiple hepatitis viruses in multiple attacks of acute viral hepatitis. N Engl J Med 296:75–78, 1977.
10. Rizza CR: The management of patients with coagulation factor deficiencies. In *Human Blood Coagulation, Haemostasis and Thrombosis*. Edited by R Biggs. Oxford, Blackwell Scientific, 1976, pp 365–398.
11. Pool JG, Shannon AE: Production of high potency concentrates of antihemophilic globulin in a closed bag system. N Engl J Med 273:1443–1447, 1965.
12. Rizza CR, Biggs R: The treatment of patients who have factor VIII antibodies. Br J Haematol 24:65–82, 1973.
13. Kurczynski FM, Penner JA: Activated prothrombin concentrate for patients with factor VIII inhibitors. N Engl J Med 291:164–167, 1974.
14. Lowe GDO, Harvie A, Forbes CD, et al: Successful treatment with prothrombin complex concentrate of postoperative bleeding in a haemophiliac with a factor VIII inhibitor. Br Med J 2:1110–1111, 1976.
15. Kasper, CK: Postoperative thromboses in hemophilia B (letter). N Engl J Med 289:160, 1973.
16. Blatt PM, Lundblad RL, Kingdon HS: Thrombogenic materials in prothrombin complex concentrates. Ann Intern Med 81:766–770, 1974.
17. Gazzard BA, Lewis ML, Ash G, et al: Coagulation factor concentrate in the treatment of the haemorrhagic diathesis of fulminant hepatic failure. Gut 15:993–998, 1974.
18. Merskey C: Defibrination syndrome. In *Human Blood Coagulation, Haemostasis and Thrombosis*. Edited by R Biggs. Oxford, Blackwell Scientific, 1976, pp 492–535.

43. AGENTS USED TO TREAT HYPERGLYCEMIA

Sigrid A. Hagg

Diabetes is a disease of absolute or relative insulin lack, although other hereditary or environmental factors may be involved in its pathogenesis. Insulin, a polypeptide hormone which combines with membrane receptors to allow glucose uptake, has actions on nutrients other than glucose. It enhances transport and incorporation of amino acids into protein in muscle, affects transport of ions into tissues, and inhibits the breakdown of fat. Glucagon opposes these actions. Blood glucose is maintained in the normal physiological range by minute-to-minute variations in the supply of nutrients reaching the cell under the influence of permissive quantities of insulin. If sufficient quantities of insulin are not present, uncontrolled wasting of the body occurs. Relative insulin lack appears in the presence of obesity in which peripheral tissues are resistant to the action of endogenous or exogenous insulin. If ideal body weight can be achieved, endogenous insulin is frequently adequate to maintain normal blood glucose. Glucagon is abnormally high in the diabetic state, contributing to the hyperglycemia and production of ketone bodies from fat.[1]

The institution of an appropriate diet to achieve or maintain normal body weight is the most important task in the successful treatment of diabetes. The addition of insulin or oral agents may also be necessary to relieve symptoms and prevent acute complications, such as diabetic ketoacidosis and hyperosmolar coma. The goal of long-term therapy is to avoid late complications involving the microvascular and nervous systems. Ideal long-term treatment would mimic the normal physiological control of blood glucose. Although this is not possible with the available modes of therapy, the development of glucose sensors coupled to insulin delivery systems offers promise for the future.[2] Recent studies in animals and man strongly suggest that reduction of blood glucose levels will decrease the incidence of microvascular complications of diabetes.[3]

Physicians should establish definite criteria for control. At the Joslin Clinic, control is assessed by measurement of fasting and three hour postprandial blood glucose values. Control is considered good if 70% of whole-blood glucose values are less than 110 mg/100 ml, and fair if less than 130 mg/100 ml. All others are considered to be poorly controlled. Corresponding values for serum or plasma are 15% higher. These figures are somewhat arbitrary, but provide a reference point for clinical decision-making.

Objectives of therapy differ between juvenile-onset diabetics (patients of whatever age who are lacking in endogenous insulin and ketosis-prone) and adult-onset diabetics (patients who have relative insulin insufficiency, often associated with the insulin resistance of obesity).[4] In the former group, insulin is almost always necessary except during periods of remission; in the latter group, insulin may be required only during unusual stress, and weight reduction is the primary goal. In both groups, the effect of exercise to enhance glucose uptake by muscle and to alter energy balance can be used to advantage. Many studies have shown the effectiveness of diet therapy in adult-onset diabetes; the degree of response in most instances is related to the degree of successful weight reduction. In a recent study of 118 patients with mild adult-onset diabetes, two months of dietary treatment resulted in adequate control of blood glucose in 59% and improved glucose tolerance in almost all patients.[5] Insulin or oral agents are required to control symptoms in patients who fail to respond adequately to diet, exercise, and weight reduction.

DRUG MONOGRAPHS

INSULINS

Long-term therapy of diabetics who need insulin includes regularity in timing of meals and exercise. An intermediate-acting insulin as a single dose or a combination of an intermediate- and rapid-acting insulin should be given to approximate normoglycemia. Optimal control involves education of the patient and analysis of his metabolic state and behavior over time, with appropriate adjustment of insulin dosage.

In acute decompensated diabetes, where prolonged or severe insulin lack results in ketoacidosis or hyperosmolar coma, the goals of treatment are to restore fluid and electrolyte losses as well as to provide adequate insulin to inhibit lipolysis (the breakdown of fat) and gluconeogenesis (the production of glucose from protein). Conventional treatment of these states has been to administer relatively large (50 to 100 units) doses of short-acting insulin intravenously or subcutaneously at intervals of two to four hours until blood glucose levels are normal and acidosis is corrected. Recently, the use of low-dose insulin (6 to 10 units/hr) by constant infusion techniques[6–8] has confirmed earlier reports[9] demonstrating that large doses of insulin are usually unnecessary and carry the risk of hypoglycemia later in treatment. Two cautions are necessary in employing low-dose insulin for the treatment of ketoacidosis and hyperosmolar coma. In rare instances, patients in diabetic ketoacidosis may manifest resistance to insulin, with increasing blood glucose and worsening clinical state during low-dose insulin infusions. The use of 'automatic' methods may deflect the physician's attention from the clinical state of the patient and the need for close monitoring of blood glucose, acid-base balance, and fluid and electrolyte status.

Glucose-insulin-potassium infusions have also been effective in lactic acidosis.[10]

Adverse Reactions—Hypoglycemia may occur with any preparation of insulin and may be due to excessive dosage, inappropriate timing of meals or exercise, failure to mix suspensions of intermediate-acting insulin before withdrawal from a vial, and irregular absorption from subcutaneous injection sites. Many patients require less insulin during periods of good control than early in therapy when the blood sugar is high. Patients with insulin resistance receiving large doses of insulin may experience a sudden drop in insulin requirement with consequent hypoglycemia. The duration of action of insulin is prolonged with larger doses, and the requirement for insulin must be determined individually for each patient. Replacement of fluids and insulin during treatment of diabetic ketoacidosis or hyperosmolar coma may result in magnesium deficiency[11] as well as hypokalemia and hypophosphatemia. An additional problem may be encountered during the hyperglycemic rebound which follows hypoglycemia, due to counter-regulatory hormones. If low blood sugar has not been recoginzed, the consequent hyperglycemia and ketonuria may be misinterpreted, resulting in increased insulin doses.

Drug Interactions—Drugs interfere with insulin action by opposing counter-regulatory hormones or by independent actions to raise or lower blood glucose levels (Table 1). Guanethidine,[12] propranolol,[13] and monoamine oxidase inhibitors[14] enhance or prolong the hypoglycemic response to insulin, probably by interfering with counter-regulation by catecholamines. Epinephrine produces glycogenolysis and inhibits the peripheral utilization of glucose, opposing the action of insulin. Corticosteroids increase insulin requirements, since they enhance gluconeogenesis and produce peripheral insulin resistance. Oral contraceptives appear to cause insulin resistance and decreased control of diabetes.[15] Thyroid replacement therapy may increase insulin requirements. Anabolic steroids,[16] phenylbutazone,[17] alcohol and salicylates,[18] and tetracycline[19] enhance the effect of insulin by unknown mechanisms. Thiazide diuretics may worsen glucose tolerance by producing potassium depletion which impairs insulin release.[20] Diazoxide appears to act directly to interfere with insulin release.[21] The antineoplastic agent cyclophosphamide may produce hypoglycemia in insulin-treated patients.[22]

Characteristics of Insulin Preparations—Some characteristics are described in Table 2. Treatment with insulin is usually accompanied by the production of antibodies due to contamination of the insulin preparation by minute amounts of proinsulin and other proteins. The presence of antibodies may relate to the stability of diabetic control.[23,24] With the introduction of purer insulin preparations over the years, clinical evidence of impaired insulin responsiveness because of antibodies to insulin is infrequent. Further purification of semilente insulin by gel filtration yields monocomponent insulin, which causes little or no antibody response.[25] The use of monocomponent insulin is associated with a decrease in insulin requirement, suggesting that antibodies may retard the action of insulin and delay its availability to the tissues.[26,27] Monocomponent insulin may be useful in the treatment of severe insulin resistance. It is not commercially available, but may be obtained in special instances from the manufacturer, Eli Lilly and Co.

Regular, Crystalline or Short-Acting Insulin—This form of insulin was the first to become available shortly after the discovery of insulin. It is extracted from pork or beef pancreas in the form of zinc crystals. It is the only preparation to be used for intravenous injection during treatment of diabetic ketoacidosis or hyperosmolar coma, or by any route for control of hyperglycemia by intermittent injection during such acute stress as surgery, infection or trauma. It may be mixed with intermediate-acting insulins (NPH or protamine zinc) to achieve control of late-morning hyperglycemia with a single injection. It is

TABLE 1 Drugs That May Interact with Insulin or Oral Hypoglycemic Agents

Drug	Interaction	Hypoglycemic Agent
Alcohol	Additive hypoglycemic effect; impairs gluconeogenesis; disulfiram-like reaction with sulfonylureas	Insulin Sulfonylureas Phenformin
Dicumarol Sulfonamides	Increase duration of action or serum levels; may cause hypoglycemia	Sulfonylureas
Chloramphenicol Phenylbutazone Salicylates Tetracycline	Increase duration of action or serum levels; may also have direct hypoglycemic effect	Insulin Sulfonylureas
Thiazides	Promote glucose intolerance; interfere with insulin release	Insulin Sulfonylureas
Monoamine oxidase inhibitors	Enhance or prolong hypoglycemic response	Insulin Sulfonylureas
Propranolol	Interferes with glycogenolysis, glucagon release and glucose-induced insulin release; may cause hypoglycemia or hyperglycemia	Insulin Sulfonylureas
Guanethidine	Has hypoglycemic action and may decrease insulin requirements	Insulin
Epinephrine	Increases blood glucose by inhibiting peripheral uptake and promoting glycogenolysis	Insulin Sulfonylureas
Oral contraceptives	Produce peripheral insulin resistance; may cause hyperglycemia	Insulin Sulfonylureas
Glucocorticoids	Enhance gluconeogenesis and cause peripheral insulin resistance; may cause hyperglycemia	Insulin Sulfonylureas
Thyroid hormones	May produce hypoglycemia or hyperglycemia	Insulin
Phenothiazines	Promote glucose intolerance; interfere with insulin release	Insulin Sulfonylureas

TABLE 1 *(continued)*

Drug	Interaction	Hypoglycemic Agent
Clofibrate	Increase duration of action or serum levels	Sulfonylureas
Anabolic Steroids (Methandrostenolone and Related Compounds)	Have hypoglycemic action	Sulfonylureas Phenformin

supplied as zinc crystals in an acid solution of pH 3.0 In making mixtures, the regular insulin should always be drawn into the syringe first, to avoid contamination by the protein precipitants or buffers present in the modified insulin. Semilente is essentially identical in action to crystalline insulin. It is supplied as a turbid solution in neutral acetate buffer.

Intermediate- and Long-Acting Insulins—Because of the desire for control of blood glucose by less frequent injections, insulin preparations were modified to retard absorption from subcutaneous injection sites and provide slower and more prolonged action. NPH and PZI insulins are produced by mixing insulin with protamine and zinc to form a uniform suspension in phosphate buffer; greater quantities of protamine produce a more prolonged duration of action. Protein precipitants are not used in the lente insulin series. By increasing the amount of zinc in solution of acetate buffer, the action of semilente is altered to form ultralente which has a slow and prolonged action similar to protamine zinc insulin (PZI). An intermediate-acting insulin similar to NPH (lente insulin) is produced by mixing semilente and ultralente insulins in a 30:70 ratio. The lente series has the advantage of fewer hypersensitivity reactions to the protein precipitant, although there is generally no reason to alter therapy in patients who are adequately controlled and accustomed to using NPH. Insulin mixtures may be recommended when needed in individual cases. Crystalline insulin may be mixed with NPH or PZI to provide more rapid onset of action. When added to PZI, the ratio of regular insulin to PZI must be from 2:1 to 3:1; this excess is not required when mixing regular insulin with NPH, since this contains

TABLE 2 Characteristics of Insulin Preparations

Preparation	pH	Maximum Action (hr)	Duration of Action (hr)	Added Protein	Buffer	Appearance
Rapid-Acting						
Regular	3.0	0.5–1	5–7	None	None	Clear
Semilente	7.2	1–2	12–16	None	Acetate	Turbid
Monocomponent semilente	7.2	1–2	10–15	None	Acetate	Turbid
Intermediate-Acting						
Isophane (NPH)	7.2	2–8	18–24	Protamine	Phosphate	Turbid
Lente	7.2	2–8	18–24	None	Acetate	Turbid
Long-Acting						
Protamine zinc (PZI)	7.2	8–12	24–36	Protamine	Phosphate	Turbid
Ultralente	7.2	8–14	24–36	None	Acetate	Turbid

only small amounts of protein precipitant. Similarly, the insulins of the lente series may be mixed with each other.

Complications of Insulin Treatment—The major complications of insulin treatment are lipoatrophy, insulin allergy, and insulin resistance. A decrease in subcutaneous fat may occur at the site of insulin injection, or occasionally remote from it. Lipoatrophy is most common in patients of both sexes under the age of 20, and in women over the age of 20.[28] Localized areas of hypertrophy are also common but generally are not mentioned by patients. The changes in adipose tissue occur after about six months of treatment, even with only a few injections in the same location. Atrophy may be reduced or diminished by injecting crystalline or monocomponent insulin into the margins of the atrophic region.[29]

About one-fourth to one-third of patients have mild skin reactions with burning or itching at the site of injection a few hours after the dose. This usually occurs in the first few weeks of insulin treatment and disappears after weeks or months of continued insulin. Generalized allergic reactions, angioneurotic edema, laryngeal edema, or anaphalytic shock are rare.[30] Mild reactions of this type may be treated with antihistamines. Severe reactions in patients who definitely require insulin should be treated by a desensitization procedure, in which crystalline insulin is injected subcutaneously, beginning with a 1/1000 unit dose which is then doubled at hourly intervals. If needed for treatment of ketoacidosis, large doses of insulin may have to be given with corticosteroid coverage.

Insulin resistance generally refers to patients who require greater than 200 units daily for more than two days. It is a self-limited condition rarely lasting for more than two years.[31] In some patients, thousands of units are required daily.[32] Insulin resistance may be associated with underlying conditions such as acanthosis nigricans,[33] acromegaly, hemochromatosis, Cushing's syndrome, or infection. High levels of insulin antibodies may occasionally limit the action of insulin. Treatment often requires several injections daily, and the dose must be individualized. Crystalline insulin is available as a suspension of zinc crystals containing 500 units/ml and may be administered using tuberculin syringes for patients requiring large doses. Larger doses of insulin usually have a prolonged effect, often allowing management with a single dose of regular insulin. A change from beef to pork insulin or the use of monocomponent insulin may enhance hypoglycemic effectiveness; in severe instances, corticosteroids are required.

Preparations—Insulin is available in 10 ml vials labeled as U-40, U-80, and U-100 which contain 40, 80, and 100 units per ml, respectively. U-40 and U-80 will soon be unavailable since it is felt that only one standard concentration of 100 units/ml should be available; a single standard syringe with a small bore for accurate measurement of the insulin dose will be marketed. Patients whose prescriptions do not indicate pure beef or pork insulin usually receive the less expensive preparation, a mixture of insulin extracted from both species. Insulin should be refrigerated, although the preparations are quite stable and need not be refrigerated for travel. NPH, PZI and lente insulins should be resuspended before withdrawal, otherwise the dose may be variable and unpredictable. For further details on insulin preparations see Table 3.

ORAL HYPOGLYCEMIC AGENTS

Since their introduction 20 years ago, oral hypoglycemic drugs have been widely used in the treatment of maturity-onset diabetes. The recent University Group Diabetes Program (UGDP) report of enhanced cardiovascular mortality has emphasized the lack of basic information on their mechanism of action and toxic effects and has led to a thorough reevaluation of their indications for use. Because these agents relieve the clinical symptoms related to hyperglycemia and obviate the need for daily insulin injections, they have had a high degree of patient acceptance and have been convenient for physicians. Unfortunately, this has frequently led to an inadequate emphasis on diet and weight reduction.

The UGDP Study—This prospective clinical evaluation of oral hypoglycemic agents, begun in 1957, raised serious questions about the long-term safety and effectiveness of these drugs.[34,35] Patients with recently diagnosed adult-onset diabetes, ie, those most likely to respond to oral agents, were randomly assigned to treatment groups and followed under double-blind conditions. Subjects were given one of four treatments: placebo; fixed-dose tolbutamide (1.5 g/day); fixed-dose insulin calculated for body surface area, or variable-dose insulin to approximate normoglycemia. Later, a fifth group treated with phenformin (0.1 g/day) was added. The results of the study were unexpected. Blood glucose was controlled only in the variable insulin group. In the phenformin and tolbutamide groups, there were more than twice as many cardiovascular deaths than in patients treated

TABLE 3 Preparations and Costs of Insulins

GENERIC NAME	OTHER NAME(S)	PREPARATIONS AND 1978 COSTS[a]
Rapid-Acting		
Insulin Injection	Regular Insulin Crystalline Zinc Insulin Regular Iletin	Injection (solution) 40 units/ml—$1.93/10-ml vial; 80 units/ml—$3.62/10-ml vial; 100 units/ml—$4.56/10-ml vial
Prompt Insulin Zinc Suspension	Semilente Iletin Semilente Insulin	Injection (suspension) 40 units/ml—$2.28/10-ml vial; 80 units/ml—$4.16/10-ml vial; 100 units/ml—$5.20/10-ml vial
Intermediate-Acting		
Isophane Insulin Suspension	NPH Iletin NPH Insulin	Injection (suspension) 40 units/ml—$2.28/10-ml vial; 80 units/ml—$4.16/10-ml vial; 100 units/ml—$5.20/10-ml vial
Insulin Zinc Suspension	Lente Iletin Lente Insulin	Injection (suspension) 40 units/ml—$2.28/10-ml vial; 80 units/ml—$4.16/10-ml vial; 100 units/ml—$5.20/10-ml vial
Long-Acting		
Protamine Zinc Insulin Suspension	PZI Protamine, Zinc and Iletin	Injection (suspension) 40 units/ml—$2.28/10-ml vial; 80 units/ml—$4.16/10-ml vial; 100 units/ml—$5.20/10-ml vial
Expanded Insulin Zinc Suspension	Ultralente Iletin Ultralente Insulin	Injection (suspension) 40 units/ml—$2.28/10-ml vial; 80 units/ml—$4.16/10-ml vial; 100 units/ml—$5.20/10-ml vial

[a]Costs are average prices of all manufacturers' preparations from mixed bovine–porcine sources. Single source preparations, which are available for all types of insulin, are usually more expensive.

with insulin or placebo. A significant increase in heart rate and in systolic and diastolic blood pressure was also noted in the phenformin-treated group. In addition, after eight years of follow-up, there was no evidence in this study that control of blood glucose levels was effective in delaying or preventing diabetic vascular complications. These findings stimulated debate for and against the use of oral agents.[36–38] Satisfactory answers to some of the questions raised will require further research. For example, the possibility remains that baseline variations between the groups in age, blood glucose, cardiovascular risk factors, and concurrent use of other drugs, each not statistically significant, may have had a cumulative influence on cardiovascular mortality. Nonfatal cardiovascular events were not compared, although recent review of the data demonstrated that the groups did not differ in degree of retinopathy during the study, and that 50% of patients in all groups developed hypertension. Data on risk factors such as cigarette smoking were not obtained. In addition, the fixed-dose regimen which was necessary for the double-blind design is not customarily used by practicing physicians. Despite these and other objections, the UGDP study remains the most extensive prospective trial of oral agents. In the retrospective study of 2500 patients reported from the Joslin Clinic,[39] no increase in cardiovascular mortality was noted. However, other clinical studies have substantiated the increased risk of myocardial infarction[40] and ventricular arrhythmias[41] in patients taking oral agents. After careful review of the shortcomings of the UGDP study, the Biometric Society[42] concluded that the baseline differences between the groups could not account for the increase in cardiovascular mortality observed. The importance of controlled prospective clinical trials of drugs is evident, since toxic effects occurring at low frequency may not be detectable by any other method. The study has also stimulated research into the basic mechanisms of action of the hypoglycemic compounds. The UGDP study has made a strong case for more careful selection of patients for oral therapy and increased emphasis on diet and weight reduction in the management of maturity-onset diabetes.

The UGDP results may or may not be applicable to other sulfonylureas. Rational therapy will depend on improved understanding of factors influencing toxicity as well as the onset and progression of diabetic vascular disease.

When diet and weight reduction are ineffective or impossible, the physician must choose between insulin and oral agents. Insulin is the safer and more effective way to achieve control of blood glucose. Although most authorities would withhold full approval from the oral agents, the decision to use the drugs rests with the patient and the physician. Patients should be informed of the potential risks and should participate in the decision to use these medications.

TABLE 4 Characteristics of Oral Hypoglycemic Compounds

Drug	Dose (min–max)	Duration of Action (hr)	Time of Peak Concentration After Oral Dose (hr)	Elimination Half-Life (hr)	Dose Frequency	Preparations and 1978 Costs
Sulfonylureas						
Tolbutamide (Orinase)	0.5–2.0 g	6–12	3–5	5–6	Divided	Tablets 500 mg—$5.93/50
Chlorpropamide (Diabinese)	0.1–0.5 g	24–60	4–6	35	Single	Tablets 100mg—$6.67/100; 250 mg—$14.01/100
Acetohexamide (Dymelor)	0.25–1.5 g	12–24	3	1–2	Single or Divided	Tablets 250 mg—$3.47/50; 500 mg—$6.05/50
Tolazamide (Tolinase)	0.1–1.0 g	6–18	4–6	7	Single or Divided	Tablets 100 mg—$7.04/100; 250 mg—$14.87/100
Glibenclamide[a]	2.5–3.0 g	15	4	5–7	Single	
Biguanides						
Phenformin Hydrochloride (DBI, Meltrol-25)	50–100 mg	4–6	2–4	3	Divided	Tablets 25 mg—$6.06/100
Phenformin Hydrochloride (DBI-TD, Meltrol-50)	50–150 mg	8–12	—	—	Single or Divided	Tablets (timed-release) 50 mg—$13.52/100

[a]Glibenclamide is not marketed in the United States.

Pharmacologic Properties and Mechanisms of Action—There are two classes of oral hypoglycemic drugs—the sulfonylureas and the biguanides. Clinically important properties and doses are shown in Table 4. Dosage in excess of the maximum listed is rarely more effective.

All sulfonylurea agents acutely lower blood glucose by inducing insulin release from the pancreas. Therefore, they are ineffective in patients who lack endogenous insulin. However, in patients receiving chronic therapy, the blood glucose lowering effect persists, but insulin levels are no longer increased.[43] Tolbutamide restores pancreatic responsiveness to subthreshold levels of glucose, suggesting that it enhances insulin release.[44] An alteration in the kinetics of insulin release may explain the improved glucose tolerance during chronic sulfonylurea therapy.[45] Sulfonylureas may alter glucagon levels in diabetics; such an effect might partially account for their glucose lowering action.[46]

Extrapancreatic actions of the sulfonylureas[47] have received increased attention as a result of the UGDP report. The newer and more potent agents, such as glibenclamide, may dissociate the toxic and therapeutic actions of these drugs.

After oral administration, sulfonylureas are rapidly absorbed. They are hydroxylated in the liver to active and inactive products which are almost totally excreted in the urine. Much of the activity of acetohexamide is due to its metabolic product, hydroxyhexamide, which is six times more potent that the parent compound.[47] Sulfonylureas are largely bound to plasma proteins[48] and are distributed in the extracellular space.[49] In therapeutic doses, these drugs appear to be equally effective. Thus, the choice of agents depends on the experience of the physician and the cost and convenience for the patient.

Phenformin, the only biguanide available in the United States has recently been withdrawn from unlimited distribution by the Secretary of Health, Education, and Welfare because of concern for its ability to produce lactic acidosis. It remains available, however, for selected patients. Phenformin is effective in lowering blood glucose in diabetic patients, but has no hypoglycemic effect in normal humans.[50] Basal and stimulated insulin levels are reduced by phenformin treatment, an effect thought to be secondary to its glucose-lowering action.[51] The drug probably acts at multiple sites, producing decreased hepatic gluconeogenesis, inhibition of oxidative enzymes with increased anaerobic glycolysis, and decreased glucose absorption from the small intestine.[52] Phenformin has been used to treat hypoglycemia due to rapid intestinal glucose absorption[53] and has been suggested for the obese diabetic because of its anorexogenic effect.[54]

Phenformin is absorbed after oral administration and widely distributed to body tissues. About one-third of the administered dose is inactivated in the liver by hydroxylation, and the metabolic products as well as the active drug are excreted in the urine.[55] This may account for increased toxicity in patients with impaired renal function.

Hazards and Side Effects—Side effects, as opposed to toxic effects with objective organic change, occur in less than 5% of sulfonylurea recipients.[56] Acute side effects with biguanides may occur in as many as 60%.[57] These have included metallic taste, weakness and malaise, minor skin irritation, and anorexia and nausea. Hepatic toxicity with cholestatic jaundice has occurred with sulfonylurea therapy,[56] although this should be distinguished clinically from the alterations of liver function which are associated with poorly controlled diabetes.[58] Hematologic toxicity has occurred rarely, with transient leukopenia or other blood dyscrasias.[56,59] Both chlorpropamide and tolbutamide may produce the syndrome of inappropriate antidiuretic hormone. These drugs cause dilutional hyponatremia by increasing renal tubular sensitivity to antidiuretic hormone as well as by enhancing its release from the posterior pituitary.[60,61] Sulfonylureas have a goitrogenic effect in animals and man which is rarely observed clinically.

Lactic acidosis has been associated with biguanide therapy, particularly when impaired renal function limits drug excretion.[62] Since 1959, when phenformin was first marketed, the FDA has received approximately 240 case reports of lactic acidosis associated with its use, with death resulting in 50%.[63] Review of these patients indicated that lactic acidosis occurred at low doses and without impaired renal function in some patients. Several case reports have linked the drug with acute pancreatitis.[64] Currently it is considered a drug of last resort, indicated only for symptomatic diabetics unresponsive to diet and sulfonylureas in whom insulin cannot be used. The maximum recommended dose is now 100 mg per day. Further investigation may result in its withdrawal from the market. In addition, the evidence suggests that it would be prudent to re-evaluate individual patients now taking phenformin to determine if a safer approach is possible.

The increase in cardiovascular mortality during treatment with sulfonylureas or biguanides is the major toxic effect so far reported. In therapeutic concentrations sulfonylureas, but not biguanides, activate adenyl cyclase in human cardiac muscle and have a positive inotropic effect on cardiac muscle in animals.[65] These actions may account for the apparent cardiac toxicity.

Interactions—Sulfonylureas interact by a variety of mechanisms with many commonly-used drugs (Table 1). Alcohol and salicylates, because of their direct hypoglycemic action, may precipitate hypoglycemic coma in patients receiving sulfonylureas.[17] A disulfiram-like reaction (severe nausea and vomiting) has been reported in 10% of chlorpropamide recipients, but it appears to be less common with other sulfonylureas.[66] Propranolol, by interfering with glycogenolysis and glucagon release, enhances the hypoglycemic action of the sulfonylureas.[13] Drugs which oppose the action of the sulfonylureas to facilitate insulin release include thiazide diuretics and propranolol. Chlorpromazine and related compounds cause hyperglycemia in diabetic and nondiabetic patients[67,68] by inhibiting pancreatic insulin release.[69,70] They may interfere with the action of sulfonylureas to promote insulin release. Oral contraceptives and glucocorticoids produce peripheral insulin resistance; the latter also enhance gluconeogenesis. In addition, drugs may effect the absorption, metabolism or excretion of the sulfonylureas. Dicumarol, sulfonamides or phenylbutazone are known to increase circulating unbound tolbutamide concentrations and prolong the effective half-life of the drug in man.[71] These drugs displace sulfonylureas from serum albumin,[72] although this may not be the sole mechanism for the enhanced hypoglycemic effect. They also interfere with the hydroxylation of sulfonylureas, which is rate-limiting for their metabolism in the liver.[45] Clofibrate may enhance the hypoglycemic effect of the sulfonylureas but not phenformin by two mechanisms. It competes with chlorpropamide for renal tubular secretion sites, prolonging the half-life of chlorpropamide and decreasing its excretion.[73] It also displaces chlorpropamide and other sulfonylureas from plasma protein binding sites, enhancing hypoglycemic activity.[74,75] Phenylbutazone inhibits the renal excretion of hydroxyhexamide, the active metabolite of acetohexamide.[76] Methandrostenolone and other anabolic steroids lower blood sugar in normal subjects and some diabetics and may decrease insulin requirements.[77] These drugs do not appear to enhance the hypoglycemic response to insulin directly, and the exact mechanism of action is unknown.[78] Androgen therapy prolongs the half-life of antipyrine and possibly other drugs such as sulfonylureas or phenformin which are metabolized by hepatic hydroxylating enzymes.[79]

Ethanol potentiates the effect of phenformin to decrease lactate utilization.[52]

Therapeutic Use—In patients who are unwilling or unable to use insulin, oral agents may be employed with the aim of controlling the blood glucose. These drugs are most likely to be effective in maturity-onset diabetics over 40 years of age who have had diabetes for less than 10 years and who can be controlled on less than 20 units of insulin per day. Oral agents are contraindicated in ketosis-prone patients or in insulin-dependent juvenile-onset diabetics. They should never be used in ketoacidosis or in patients during pregnancy, surgery, stress or infection. They may lead to severe toxic effects in the presence of cardiac, renal or hepatic disease.

Therapy is initiated using the minimum effective dose and increasing this at weekly intervals until the desired degree of control is reached. Patients who do not respond to maximal doses within one month are considered to have primary failure, although some may respond after weight reduction or insulin therapy. Secondary failure occurs in 10 to 25% of patients who respond initially. The majority of patients who are not controlled on sulfonylureas or phenformin alone will respond to concurrent use of both drugs. However, since indications for use of either of these drugs are now more limited, combination therapy should be considered the last and least attractive alternative.

In patients who are not eventually controlled on oral agents, insulin by daily injection is indicated. Evaluation is made difficult by the cyclic nature of diabetes. During stable periods, oral agents or insulin in doses less than 20 units/day may achieve control, while at other times oral agents may be inadequate and higher doses of insulin required. It is evident that insulin offers greater flexibility in the treatment of such patients.

Preparations and costs of oral hypoglycemic agents are included in Table 4.

REFERENCES

1. Gerich JE, Lorenzi M, Schneider V, et al: Effects of somatostatin on plasma glucose and glucagon levels in human diabetes mellitus. N Engl J Med 291:544–547, 1974.
2. Soeldner JS, Chang KW, Aisenberg S, et al: Diabetes mellitus: a bioengineering approach:

an implantable glucose sensor. In *Diabetes Mellitus*. Edited by SS Fajans. Washington, DHEW Publication No. (NIH)78–854, 1976, pp 267–277.
3. Cahill GF, Etzwiler DD, Freinkel N: 'Control' and diabetes. N Engl J Med 294:1004–1005, 1976.
4. West KW: Diet therapy of diabetes: an analysis of failure. Ann Intern Med 79:425–434, 1973.
5. Doar JWH, Wilde CE, Thompson ME, et al: Influence of treatment with diet alone on oral glucose tolerance test and plasma sugar and insulin levels in patients with maturity-onset diabetes mellitus. Lancet 1:1263–1266, 1975.
6. Page MM, Alberti KGMM, Greenwood R, et al: Treatment of severe diabetes mellitus by insulin infusion. Br Med J 2:687–690, 1974.
7. Kidson W, Casey J, Kraegen E, et al: Treatment of severe diabetes mellitus by insulin infusion. Br Med J 2:691–694, 1974.
8. Semple PF, White C, Manderson WG: Continuous intravenous infusion of small doses of insulin in treatment of diabetic ketoacidosis. Br Med J 2:694–698, 1974.
9. Shaw CE Jr, Hurwitz GE, Schmukler M, et al: A clinical and laboratory study of insulin dosage in diabetic acidosis: comparison with small and large doses. Diabetes 11:23–30, 1962.
10. Fulop M, Hoberman D: Phenformin-associated metabolic acidosis. Diabetes 25:292–296, 1976.
11. Wacker WEC, Parisi AF: Magnesium metabolism. N Engl J Med 278:712–717, 1968.
12. Gupta KK: Guanethidine and glucose tolerance in diabetics (letter). Br Med J 3:679, 1968.
13. Gerich JE, Langlois M, Noaces C, et al: Adrenergic modulation of pancreatic glucagon secretion in man. J Clin Invest 53:1441–1446, 1976.
14. Cooper AJ, Ashcroft G: Modification of insulin and sulfonylurea hypoglycemia by monoamineoxidase inhibitor drugs. Diabetes 16:272–274, 1967.
15. Reder JA, Tulgan H: Impairment of diabetic control by norethynodrel with mestranol. NY J Med 67:1073–1074, 1967.
16. Landon J: The effect of anabolic steroids on blood sugar and plasma insulin levels in man. Metabolism 12:924–925, 1963.
17. Anturane[R] product information. Geigy Pharmaceuticals, July, 1969.
18. Seltzer HS: Drug-induced hypoglycemia: a review based on 473 cases. Diabetes 21:955–966, 1972.
19. Miller JB: Hypoglycemic effect of oxytetracycline (letter). Br Med J 2:1007, 1966.
20. Conn JW: Hypertension, the potassium ion and impaired carbohydrate tolerance. N Engl J med 273:1135–1143, 1965.
21. Seltzer HS, Allen EW: Hyperglycemia and inhibition of insulin secretion during administration of diazoxide and trichlormethiadide in man. Diabetes 18:19–28, 1969.
22. Hartshorn EA: Drug interactions: antineoplastics. Drug Intelligence 3:196, 1969.
23. Dixon K, Exon PD, Hughes HR: Insulin antibodies in aetiology of labile diabetes. Lancet 1:343–347, 1972.
24. Schlichtkrull J, Brange J, Christiansen AH, et al: Clinical aspects of insulin-antigenicity. Diabetes 21(Suppl 2):649–656, 1972.
25. Vinik AI, Joffe BI, Seftel HC, et al: Clinical aspects of monocomponent insulins in the treatment of diabetes. S Afr Med J 50:587–591, 1976.
26. Logie AW, Stowers JM: Hazards of monocomponent insulins. Br Med J 1:879–880, 1976.
27. Olefsky S, Shreeve DR, Sutcliffe CH: Brittle diabetes. Q J Med 43:113–125, 1974.
28. Marble A, Reynold AE: Atrophy and hypertrophy of subcutaneous fat due to insulin. Trans Assoc Am Physicians 62:219–224, 1949.
29. Ferland L, Erlich RM: Single-peak insulin in the treatment of fat atrophy. J Pediatr 86:741–743, 1975.
30. Hanauer L, Batson JM: Anaphylactic shock following insulin injection. Case report and review of the literature. Diabetes 10:105–109, 1961.
31. Shipp JC, Cunningham RW, Russell RO, et al: Insulin resistance: clinical features, natural course and effects of adrenal steroid treatment. Medicine 44:165–186, 1965.
32. Field JB, Johnson P, Herring B: Insulin resistant diabetes associated with increased endogenous plasma insulin followed by complete remission. J Clin Invest 40:1672–1683, 1961.
33. Tucker WR, Klink D, Goetz F, et al: Insulin resistance and acanthosis nigricans. Diabetes 13:395–399, 1964.

34. University Group Diabetes Program: A study of the effects of hypoglycemic agents on vascular complications in patients with adult-onset diabetes. Diabetes 19(Suppl 2):747–830, 1970.
35. University Group Diabetes Program: A study of the effects of hypoglycemic agents on vascular complications in patients with adult-onset diabetes. Diabetes 24(Suppl 1):65–184, 1975.
36. Seltzer HS: A summary of criticisms of the findings and conclusions of the University Group Diabetes Program. Diabetes 21:976–979, 1972.
37. Roth J, Prout TE, Goldfine ID, et al: Sulfonylureas: effects *in vivo* and *in vitro*. Ann Intern Med 75:607–621, 1971.
38. Chalmers TC: Settling the UGDP controversy. JAMA 231:624–625, 1975.
39. Ferguson BD: The oral hypoglycemic compounds. Med Clin North Am 49:929–938, 1965.
40. Boyle D, Bhatia SK, Hadden DR, et al: Ischaemic heart-disease in diabetics. Lancet 1:338–339, 1972.
41. Soler NG, Bennett MA, Lamb P, et al: Coronary care for myocardial infarction in diabetes. Lancet 1:475–477, 1974.
42. Report of the Committee for the Assessment of Controlled Trials of Hypoglycemic Agents. JAMA 231:583–608, 1975.
43. Chu P, Conway MJ, Krouse HA, et al: The pattern of response of plasma insulin and glucose to meals and fasting during chlorpropamide therapy. Ann Intern Med 68:757–769, 1968.
44. Grodsky GM, Schmid FG, Manning M, et al: Comparison of the independent and interrelated effects of glucose and sulfonylureas in insulin release in the perfused pancreas. In *Pharmacology and the Future of Man,* vol. 3. Edited by GT Okita, GH Acheson. Basel, Karger, 1973, pp 230–237.
45. Karam JH, Matin SB, Forsham PH: Antidiabetic drugs after the University Group Diabetes Program (UGDP). Annu Rev Pharmacol 15:351–366, 1975.
46. Samols E, Tyler JM, Mialhe P: Suppression of pancreatic glucagon release by the hypoglycemic sulfonylureas. Lancet 1:174–176, 1969.
47. Galloway JA, McMahon RE, Culp HW, et al: Metabolism, blood levels, and rate of excretion of acetohexamide in human subjects. Diabetes 16:118–127, 1967.
48. Wichinsky H, Glasser EJ, Perkal S: Protein interactions of sulfonylurea compounds. Diabetes 11(Suppl 1):18–25, 1962.
49. Hellman B, Sehlin J, Taljedal I-B: The pancreatic β-cell recognition of insulin secretogogues. II. Site of action of tolbutamide. Biochem Biophys Res Commun 45:1384–1388, 1971.
50. Fajans SS, Moorehouse JA, Doorenbos H: Metabolic effects of phenethylbiguanides in normal subjects and in diabetic patients. Diabetes 9:194–201, 1960.
51. Stout RW, Brunzell JD, Bierman EL, et al: Effect of phenformin on glucose-insulin interrelationships. Diabetes 23:624–630, 1974.
52. Kreisberg RA, Owen WC, Siegal AM: Hyperlacticacidemia in man: ethanol-phenformin synergism. J Clin Endocrinol Metab 34:29–35, 1972.
53. Permutt MA, Kelly J, Bernstein R, et al: Alimentary hypoglycemia in the absence of gastrointestinal surgery. N Engl J Med 288:1206–1210, 1973.
54. Danowski TS: Diabetes mellitus and obesity: phenformin hydrochloride as a research tool. Metabolism 16:865–869, 1967.
55. Beckman R: The fate of biguanides in man. Ann NY Acad Sci 148:820–832, 1968.
56. O'Donovan DJ: Analysis of long-term experience with tolbutamide (Orinase) in the management of diabetes. Curr Ther Res 1:69–87, 1959.
57. Baird RW, Hall JG: Cholestatic jaundice from tolbutamide. Ann Intern Med 53:194–197, 1960.
58. Bradley RF, Sagild U, Scheilenleib F: Diabetes mellitus and liver function. N Engl J Med 253:454–458, 1955.
59. Balodimos MC, Camerini-Advalos RD, Marble A: Nine years experience with tolbutamide in the treatment of diabetes. Metabolism 15:957–970, 1966.
60. Moses AM, Numann P, Miller M: Mechanism of chlorpropamide induced antidiuresis in man: Evidence for release of ADH and enhancement of peripheral action. Metabolism 22:59–66, 1973.
61. Hagen GA, Fraley TF: Hyponatremia due to sulfonylurea compounds. J Clin Endocrinol Metab 31:570–575, 1970.

62. Colwell JA: Therapy with oral hypoglycemic agents. In *Diabetes Mellitus: Diagnosis and Treatment,* vol. 3. Edited by SS Fagans, KE Sussman. New York, American Diabetes Association, 1971, pp 153–158.
63. FDA Drug Bulletin 7:6–7, 1977.
64. Chase HS Jr, Mogan GR: Phenformin-associated pancreatitis. Ann Intern Med 87:314–315, 1977.
65. Levey GS, Lasseter KC, Palmer RF: Sulfonylureas and the heart. Annu Rev Med 25:69–74, 1974.
66. Podgarny H, Bressler R: Biochemical basis of the sulfonylurea-induced Antabuse syndrome. Diabetes 17:679–683, 1968.
67. Thonnard-Neuimann E: Phenothiazines and diabetes in hospitalized women. Am J Psychiatry 124:978–982, 1968.
68. Hiles BH: Hyperglycemia and glycosuria following chlorpromazine therapy. JAMA 162:1651–1653, 1956.
69. Proakis AG, Borowitz JL: Blockage of insulin release by certain phenothiazines. Biochem Pharmacol 23:1693–1700, 1974.
70. Ammon HP, Orci L, Steinke J: Effect of chlorpromazine (CPA) on insulin release *in vivo* and *in vitro* in the rat. J Pharmacol Exp Ther 187:423–429, 1973.
71. Cristensen LK, Hansen JM, Kristensen M: Sulphaphenazole-induced hypoglycemia attacks in tolbutamide-treated diabetes. Lancet 2:1298–1301, 1963.
72. Judis J: Binding of sulfonylureas to serum proteins. J Pharm Sci 61:89–93, 1972.
73. Petitpierre B, Perrin L, Rudhardt M, et al: Behavior of chlorpropamide in renal insufficiency and under the effect of associated drug therapy. Int J Clin Pharmacol Ther Toxicol 6:120–124, 1972.
74. Ryan JR: The metabolic spectrum of halofenate. Int J Clin Pharmacol Biopharm 12:239–243, 1975.
75. Jain AK: Potentiation of hypoglycemic effect of sulfonyureas by halofenate. N Engl J Med 293:1283–1286, 1975.
76. Field JB, Ohta M, Boyle C, et al: Potentiation of acetohexamide hypoglycemia by phenylbutazone. N Engl J Med 277:889–894, 1967.
77. Landon VW, Samols E: The effect of anabolic steroids on blood sugar and plasma insulin levels in man. Metabolism 12:924–935, 1963.
78. Tiwari NM, Namaji KJ, Joshi BK, et al: Effect of anabolic steroids on insulin induced hypoglycemia in rats. J Exp Med Sci 11:98–100, 1968.
79. Sotaniemi EA, Kontturi MJ, Larmi TK: Drug metabolism and androgen control therapy in prostatic cancer. Clin Pharmacol Ther 14:413–417, 1973.

44. AGENTS USED TO TREAT HYPERLIPIDEMIA AND ATHEROSCLEROSIS

Ann M. Lees and Robert S. Lees

Hyperlipidemia, an increased blood plasma concentration of one or more lipids (of which cholesterol and triglycerides are the two most often measured), affects at least 5% of the North American population, depending on what levels are considered abnormal. Plasma lipid concentrations associated with an above average risk of atherosclerotic cardiovascular disease are usually considered 'abnormal.' Thus, the upper limit of normal in adults for plasma cholesterol[1] is about 220 mg/100 ml and for plasma triglycerides, 140 mg/100 ml. Patients with fasting levels consistently above these limits are considered to have hyperlipidemia.

Hyperlipidemia may be a primary metabolic disorder, or it may be secondary to other diseases such as alcoholism, uncontrolled diabetes, renal failure, or myxedema. It may also be iatrogenic, as in patients on oral contraceptives. Hyperlipidemia caused by diet should be considered as primary, since not everyone on an improper diet becomes hyperlipidemic. Treatment of primary hyperlipidemia is the subject of this chapter. Secondary hyperlipidemia is best treated by treating the primary disease, with the exception of renal failure, where treatment of the accompanying hyperlipidemia may be appropriate.[2]

SCREENING FOR HYPERLIPIDEMIA

In the initial screening for hyperlipidemia, plasma cholesterol and glyceride concentrations are measured after a 12 to 16 hour overnight fast. The measurements can be made at low cost by automated methods.[3] Plasma glycerides vary widely throughout the day in relation to fat intake. Their concentration should ordinarily be measured 12 to 16 hours after the last meal, because it is most stable and reproducible at that time. The plasma cholesterol concentration, on the other hand, varies relatively little through the day, making random samples reasonably accurate. Because plasma lipids normally vary with diet and stress, accurate evaluation of patients with a personal or family history of hyperlipidemia is best achieved by obtaining three sets of lipid values at two- to four-week intervals. The means of these values serve as a baseline to determine if treatment is necessary and to judge its efficacy. For general screening of patients in whom hyperlipidemia is not suspected, one set of values every two to five years is enough if the values are normal and the patient's clinical status remains unchanged.

Lipoprotein Electrophoresis

'Plasma lipids' are not present as such but are bound chemically to specific proteins and circulate in plasma as lipoproteins whose concentrations cannot be accurately predicted by plasma lipid measurements alone. Precise quantitative measurement of individual lipoprotein classes is difficult and time consuming. However, semiquantitative measurement by lipoprotein electrophoresis is quite easily done on paper or thin-layer agarose gel.[3] The second and third blood samples drawn from patients whose first set of lipid values is abnormal should be accompanied by lipoprotein electrophoresis. The two electrophoretic patterns and the three sets of lipid values determine the phenotype of the patient's hyperlipidemia.[4,5] The phenotype of untreated patients gives information which is useful in selecting the most appropriate treatment and in predicting response.[4,5]

Phenotyping also helps to identify patients with increased platelet sensitivity to aggregating agents,[6] and patients with coagulation abnormalities who may be at increased risk for thromboembolism[7] (see Antiplatelet and Anticoagulant Therapy below). It also aids in prediction of the likelihood of such complications of hyperlipidemia as xanthomatosis and atherosclerosis even though most phenotypes are genetically heterogeneous.[8,9]

Types of Hyperlipidemia

Type I. Type I hyperlipidemia is rare,[10] but should be considered in any patient from infancy to adulthood presenting with acute or recurrent abdominal pain, eruptive xanthomas, lipemia retinalis, and extremely lipemic blood which may look like chocolate milk or cream of tomato soup. Triglyceride values will be in the thousands because of chylomicronemia. Atherosclerosis is rare in Type I patients.

Type II. Elevated plasma cholesterol resulting from increased beta lipoprotein concentrations, with or without elevated triglycerides,[10] is the hallmark of this syndrome, which occurs in 40 to 45% of hyperlipidemic patients. It should be suspected in patients with cardiovascular disease and/or xanthomas, or in completely asymptomatic patients with a family history of such disorders. The risk of developing atherosclerotic disease at an early age is high in Type II patients. The blood platelets of these patients are abnormally sensitive to aggregating agents *in vitro;* this may explain the early and severe morbidity from thrombotic complications associated with the Type II syndrome.[6]

Type III. About 5% of hyperlipidemic patients fall into the Type III category. They have a characteristic abnormal lipoprotein pattern associated with approximately equal elevations of both cholesterol and triglycerides.[10] Peripheral vascular disease and certain kinds of xanthomas are common. A striking feature of the disease is the lability of the hyperlipidemia, which is very responsive to therapy.

Type IV. Moderately elevated plasma triglycerides, because of increased pre-beta lipoproteins, with normal or near normal cholesterol levels, are characteristic of Type IV.[10] This category accounts for 40 to 45% of hyperlipidemic patients. Triglyceride levels usually do not exceed 1000 mg/100 ml. Xanthomas are seldom seen in Type IV patients, who are often not recognized until their cardiovascular disease is symptomatic. Earlier detection would be greatly facilitated if patients with a family history of cardiovascular disease were screened for elevated plasma triglycerides, as well as for elevated cholesterol.

Type V. About 5% of hyperlipidemic patients are Type V. These patients have an increase in plasma pre-beta lipoproteins and chylomicrons, often to very high levels.[10] As in Type I, abdominal pain and creamy blood are frequently seen in Type V and eruptive xanthomas may also occur. Unlike Type I, these sequelae seldom occur before early adulthood in Type V. Also unlike Type I, Type V patients are often obese, and their obesity exacerbates both the lipemia and the symptoms of the disease. Although Type V patients are at higher than average risk for atherosclerosis, it generally occurs less often and at a later age than in Types II, III and IV.

GENERAL PRINCIPLES OF THERAPY

The purpose of long-term, lipid-lowering therapy is to prevent, arrest, or cause regression of atherosclerosis and xanthomatosis. Xanthoma regression can be demonstrated in some patients, but clearly beneficial effects on the course of atherosclerosis are more difficult to document. The Coronary Drug Project findings[11] are often cited as evidence that lipid-lowering drug therapy does not alter the course of atherosclerosis. However, in that study the degree of cholesterol reduction was minimal (less than 10%); many patients were not hyperlipidemic and thus may have been inappropriate candidates for evaluating lipid-lowering therapy. Also, atherosclerosis is correlated with many other risk factors in addition to hyperlipidemia, and no attempt was made to modify any of these other factors. Third, although the drugs studied, clofibrate and nicotinic acid, did not influence overall mortality, they clearly had a beneficial effect on other important parameters, particularly non-fatal cardiovascular events. Lastly, the study dealt only with patients who had a previous myocardial infarction and therefore sheds no light on the primary prevention of atherosclerotic disease. A recent clinical study of lipid-lowering by dietary change[12] does offer reasonably convincing evidence that primary prevention or arrest of atherosclerosis is possible.

Prevention, arrest, or regression of atherosclerosis and xanthomatosis requires attention not only to hyperlipidemia but to several other risk factors as well. Although often very difficult to achieve, cessation of smoking is of utmost importance.[13–16] Treatment of hypertension is also vital, since elevated blood pressure is as important as hyperlipidemia as a risk factor for the development of atherosclerosis.[16–19] When cholesterol and triglycerides are both elevated, treatment of the hyperglyceridemia takes precedence; often plasma cholesterol will then fall to normal levels without specific therapy. If the hypercholesterolemia is treated first in patients with even only modest hypertriglyceridemia, a severe exacerbation of the latter may occur.

Dietary Therapy

The importance of dietary therapy, both quantitative and qualitative, as the primary treatment for hyperlipidemia has often been stressed.[20–23] In some patients, dietary therapy alone may be sufficient to reduce plasma lipids to acceptable levels. Except in severely atherosclerotic patients, the effect of diet therapy alone should be observed before drug therapy is started. As with smoking, changes in dietary habits can be very difficult to achieve. Many hyperlipidemic patients are overweight and the almost invariable lipid-lowering seen with weight reduction[24,25] strongly supports the concept that the synergy of gluttony and sloth makes an important contribution to the development of atherosclerosis. Details of dietary therapy have been outlined elsewhere.[26] Briefly, for weight reduction we prescribe a diet 700 calories a day below the usual intake, with low to moderate cholesterol content (200 to 500 mg/day). For weight maintenance, dietary cholesterol should be kept moderate (300 to 500 mg/day).

We see no value in diets with greatly increased polyunsaturated fat content since they are often expensive, unpalatable, and may increase the risk of gallstones[27] or have other undesirable effects.[28]

A low-cholesterol (<200 mg/day), low-saturated fat diet is appropriate for patients whose glycerides have fallen to normal with weight reduction, but whose cholesterol is still elevated. If glycerides are not normal when the patient is at stable lower body weight, a redetermination of phenotype by lipoprotein electrophoresis is appropriate. Type IV patients should be maintained on a relatively low carbohydrate diet in which calories are distributed in the following proportion: carbohydrate, 40 to 50%; protein, about 15%; and fat, 35 to 45%. Type III or V patients should be maintained on a moderately fat-restricted diet, with about 30% of calories from fat and 55% from carbohydrate. Diets very low in carbohydrate or of low simple sugar content generally are not well accepted.

Lipid-Lowering Drugs

Unless cardiovascular symptoms are present, lipid-lowering drug therapy should not be started until the maximum effect of diet has been achieved. Drug therapy of hyperlipidemia is not an emergency intervention and, in asymptomatic patients, should be instituted only as an adjunct to dietary therapy. The two major categories of lipid-lowering drugs are listed in Table 1. The poorly absorbed drugs

TABLE 1 Drugs Used in the Treatment of Hyperlipidemia

Generic Name	Trademark Name(s)	Primarily Lowers		Primary Site of Action	
		TC[a]	TG[b]	Intestinal	Systemic
Cholestyramine Resin	Questran	X		X	
Colestipol	Colestid	X		X	
Neomycin Sulfate	—	X		X	
Sitosterols	Cytellin	X		X	
Probucol	Lorelco	X		X?	X?
Clofibrate	Atromid-S	variable	X		X
Niacin (Nicotinic Acid)	—	X	X		X
Norethindrone[c] Acetate	Norlutate		X		X
Oxandrolone[d]	Anavar		X		X

[a]TC = total plasma cholesterol.

[b]TG = plasma triglycerides.

[c]May have androgenic effects in some women.

[c]Has considerable androgenic activity.

which act in the gastrointestinal tract lower plasma cholesterol by inhibiting cholesterol or bile acid absorption, thereby increasing fecal excretion. When plasma glycerides are normal, these drugs often produce a mild increase in their plasma concentrations, though seldom to abnormal levels. When glycerides are abnormally elevated, the bile-acid binding resins in particular may cause striking further glyceride elevations. Because they are so poorly absorbed, their side effects, when present, are usually limited to the gastrointestinal tract. They are especially useful in children.

The absorbable drugs, whose primary action is systemic rather than intestinal, lower triglycerides, and sometimes cholesterol, in a variety of ways. Since they are absorbable, they are seldom used in children. Fortunately, hypertriglyceridemia requiring drug therapy rarely occurs in children, and the non-absorbable drugs are available to treat childhood hypercholesterolemia.

Efficacy of Lipid-Lowering Drugs. Establishing the efficacy of a lipid-lowering drug is difficult. First, no available drug will lower lipids significantly in all patients for whom it is theoretically appropriate. Second, most of the recognized phenotypes, particularly Types II and IV (80 to 90% of hyperlipidemic patients), represent a mixture of as yet incompletely defined genotypes; for example, some patients with Type II hyperlipidemia respond to lipid-lowering drug therapy more readily than others. Third, if a particular drug is used only in patients whose hyperlipidemia is refractory to other agents, the former may appear to be less efficacious than it really is, because some forms of hyperlipidemia respond poorly to any lipid-lowering drug.

With these problems in mind, the following scheme will be used to describe the efficacy of the lipid-lowering drugs discussed in this chapter. (The percentages given are in addition to the percent lowering achieved by diet alone.)

A *highly effective* drug may be expected to lower lipids more than 20% in at least 50% of patients.

A *moderately effective* drug may be expected to lower lipids by 10% or more in at least 50% of patients.

A *slightly effective* drug may be expected to lower lipids by less than 10% in at least 50% of patients.

These designations will apply to all uses of a drug, whether as the drug of choice or as a 'second-line' drug when the drug of choice has failed. Whether or not the designated percentage decreases will bring a specific patient's lipids within normal limits depends on the pre-treatment lipid concentrations, as well as the nature of the patient's hyperlipidemia, and will not be considered as an element in the definition of efficacy.

Multiple Lipid-Lowering Drug Therapy. Some patients with elevated cholesterol do not have an adequate lipid-lowering response to any single drug. For these patients, two or even three drugs may be prescribed in combination, at moderate dose levels, rather than increasing the dose of a single drug to near toxic levels. Finding the best drug combination requires patience and persistence, since it must be found by trial and error and may take as long as a year. The correct combination, once found, may remain effective indefinitely. Hepatic toxicity most often limits the use of multiple drug therapy in doses high enough to reduce lipids effectively. Thus, the usual liver enzyme tests should be monitored frequently until an effective combination has been found. They should be rechecked periodically as long as the regimen is continued.

Monitoring Therapy. Plasma cholesterol concentrations of 200 mg/100 ml or less, and triglyceride concentrations of 100 mg/100 ml or less, are associated with a low risk of developing atherosclerosis. Thus, these are the levels towards which we aim both diet and drug therapy. Normally, three sets of fasting cholesterol and triglyceride values are obtained at two to four week intervals before any therapy is begun. The means of these values serve as a baseline against which the efficacy of subsequent therapy is measured. Additional lipid estimations are obtained at monthly intervals after starting or changing treatment, until the results are similar for two consecutive months.

After an adequate regimen has been achieved, lipid values are obtained at decreasing intervals of two, three, four and six months, then yearly, as long as the patient's clinical condition remains stable. If therapy includes a drug, or drugs, in addition to diet, the patient should be checked for drug side effects.

If a given regimen has not adequately lowered plasma lipids after three or four months, another treatment should be added or substituted.

It is also important to assess cardiovascular function with yearly resting and exercise electrocardiograms, palpation of peripheral arterial pulses at each office visit, and documentation of arterial bruits[29] when possible. Symptoms of cardiovascular disease also should be carefully graded and recorded at each office visit.

ANTITHROMBOTIC AND ANTICOAGULANT THERAPY

Hyperlipidemia and atherosclerosis appear to be associated with changes in hemostatic mechanisms which lead both to thrombosis and to intravascular coagulation.

In vitro, even in the absence of clinically apparent atherosclerosis, platelets from Type II, and to a lesser degree from Type IV, patients have increased sensitivity to aggregating agents.[6] Both Type II and Type IV patients also have increased plasma concentrations of high molecular weight fibrinogen derivatives and lower than expected concentrations of fibrin degradation products, suggesting that these patients have both accelerated intravascular coagulation and decreased fibrinolysis.[7] *In vivo,* patients with clinical signs and symptoms of atherosclerosis have increased platelet destruction as evidenced by shortened platelet half-life and accelerated intravascular coagulation as evidenced by shortened fibrinogen half-life.[30]

Although not yet complete,[31] the evidence that antithrombotic drugs effectively prevent initial or recurrent thrombotic events in atherosclerotic patients is suggestive enough to cause many physicians to use such drugs in the treatment of hypercholesterolemic patients with angina, peripheral vascular, or cerebrovascular disease. Their symptoms often abate, although it is not yet clear whether there is a decrease in the number of detectable thromboembolic events. For a more detailed discussion of antithrombotic drugs, see Chapter 41.

Anticoagulants are commonly used, especially in patients with cerebrovascular disease, as well as for the prevention of systemic embolus in patients with chronic atrial fibrillation.

DRUG MONOGRAPHS

CHOLESTYRAMINE (Questran)
COLESTIPOL (Colestid)

Cholestyramine and colestipol are high molecular weight anion-exchange resins which interrupt the enterohepatic circulation of bile acids by binding the bile acids in the intestinal lumen. Both resins are moderately to highly effective plasma cholesterol-lowering agents.[32–36] Their high molecular weight makes them virtually unabsorbable.

Cholestyramine was developed first[37,38] following the observation that oral ferric chloride, a toxic, low molecular weight, bile acid binding agent, could prevent hypercholesterolemia in cholesterol-fed fowl.[39] Cholestyramine is an insoluble powder which must be mixed with liquid before ingestion (see Adverse Reactions). Its taste and odor make it unpalatable to many patients and led to the development of colestipol, which is tasteless and odorless,[40] but still has a gritty consistency similar to that of cholestyramine. Like cholestyramine, colestipol is an insoluble powder which must be mixed with liquid before ingestion.

Both resins exchange chloride ions for bile acids in the gastrointestinal tract. The resulting decrease in bile acid reabsorption produces a compensatory increase in oxidation of cholesterol to form new bile acids, as well as increased fecal excretion of acidic steroids.[32,41–43] The net change in plasma cholesterol depends on the balance between cholesterol loss in bile acids and the compensatory increase in cholesterol synthesis,[41–43] as well as possible mobilization of cholesterol from tissue stores, including xanthomas. After a year or more of resin therapy, xanthomas have been reported to diminish in many patients.[32–34,42] The effect of the resins on dietary cholesterol absorption is variable[32,41–43] and probably does not play a significant role in lowering plasma cholesterol levels.

Triglyceride levels are sometimes increased by resin therapy.[34,36,43] Normal levels usually do not become abnormal, but some patients with already abnormal levels may develop a marked and persistent increase in plasma triglycerides (see Adverse Reactions). While resin therapy reduces low-density lipoprotein (LDL) cholesterol and may elevate very low-density lipoprotein (VLDL) triglycerides, it has no significant effect on high-density lipoprotein (HDL) cholesterol.[34,44]

In summary, resins are moderately to highly effective in lowering plasma cholesterol in patients with normal or near normal plasma glycerides. Because they are not absorbed, they are the drugs of choice in children. For severe hypercholesterolemia, a resin is often useful as one component of a multiple-drug regimen.[26,45] However, their relative lack of palatability and gastrointestinal side effects (see Adverse Reactions) limit their usefulness in long-term therapy.

Resins are also useful for relieving pruritus associated with elevated serum levels of bile acids.

Adverse Reactions—The most common adverse effect of the resins is constipation, which is frequent and occasionally intolerable; also common is a feeling of fullness or bloating.[32–34,36,40] Constipation is sometimes improved with the use of a stool softener. Constipation is not usually a problem with resin therapy in children,[35] although it may occur transiently when therapy is begun.[46,47] The taste and consistency of the resins, which are insoluble, gritty powders, may also be objectionable. Because they swell considerably in water and may form a thick mass with insufficient water, intestinal obstruction may result[48] if the resins are taken dry or packed in capsule form.

Hyperglyceridemia may occur in patients whose plasma glycerides are normal or already elevated. This effect is usually mild, but in some patients whose glycerides are high before treatment, the bile acid binding resins may provoke severe hyperglyceridemia.[36] They should be stopped in such patients and alternative agents used.

Drug Interactions—Cholestyramine and colestipol may interact with other drugs in two ways: either directly by anion exchange or adsorption; or indirectly, by decreasing the availability of bile acids and thus interfering with absorption of fat soluble substances. Cholestyramine given to hypothyroid patients simultaneously with thyroxine decreases thyroxine absorption by direct binding.[49] Thyroxine malabsorption is decreased when thyroxine is administered four to five hours after cholestyramine ingestion.[49] Intestinal absorption of digitalis glycosides is also reduced by cholestyramine through direct binding.[50] Because of the enterohepatic circulation of some digitalis compounds, this effect may be more difficult to overcome by adjusting the time of drug administration. Cardiac function and serum glycoside levels should be closely monitored in patients on digitalis who start or discontinue resin therapy, and the dosage of digitalis adjusted as necessary. Cholestyramine reportedly binds a number of other drugs, *in vitro,* particularly warfarin.[51] However, *in vivo* animal studies suggest that the effect of the interaction may be minimal.[51] In another study, a hypercholesterolemic patient was treated for one year with both cholestyramine (12 g/day) and warfarin; warfarin was taken about six hours after cholestyramine, and the patient's prothrombin time and warfarin dose remained unchanged from pre-cholestyramine treatment levels.[52] Another substance which is bound by cholestyramine is the folate anion. Children on long-term cholestyramine therapy may develop lower than normal serum and red cell folate levels, without however, becoming anemic.[35,53] While some investigators recommend supplementary folic acid therapy,[35,53] others do not.[46,47] In any case, hemoglobin and serum folic acid levels should be measured periodically in children on long-term resin therapy.

Indirect interactions between resins and fat soluble substances have been reported, but are of little clinical significance. Mean serum concentrations of vitamins A and E may decrease in children on long-term cholestyramine therapy, but the levels were either within normal limits[53] or not significantly below normal,[46] and supplementary fat-soluble vitamins were not prescribed.[46,53] Colestipol therapy produced no change in vitamin E levels of children.[47] The plasma levels of vitamins D and K, as judged indirectly by plasma calcium, alkaline phosphatase, and prothrombin time, appeared to be adequate in children.[53] In an adult patient with severe impairment of hepatic function, the prothrombin time became markedly abnormal after four months of cholestyramine therapy but was corrected with supplementary oral vitamin K, 10 mg daily.[52]

In summary, children on long-term resin therapy should have hemoglobin and plasma folic acid measurements at periodic intervals; supplementary folic acid (1 mg/day) should be prescribed if necessary. Adults simultaneously taking both digitalis and resin should have cardiac function and serum glycoside levels monitored when resin therapy is begun or discontinued. Prothrombin times of patients on coumarin anticoagulants may or may not be altered by resin therapy. Whenever possible, other drugs should be taken one hour before or five hours after the resin.

Dosage—Oral: Adults and Children, Cholestyramine, 8 to 24 grams daily in divided dose. Colestipol, 10 to 30 grams daily in divided dose. Twice daily dosage is probably equally as effective as 3 or 4 times daily dosage.[35,54] The drug is usually taken, well-mixed, in water, fruit juice, applesauce, or carbonated beverages. It may be baked in cookies for children.

NEOMYCIN SULFATE (Mycifradin Sulfate)

Neomycin, an aminoglycoside antibiotic, was first noted to lower the plasma cholesterol of a patient receiving the drug orally for a Salmonella infection of the gastrointestinal tract.[55] Subsequently, low doses of oral neomycin (0.5 to 2 g daily) were found to lower plasma cholesterol an average of 22% in 16 patients for periods ranging from one to three years.[56] Further studies have confirmed the moderate to high efficacy of neomycin as a lipid-lowering drug.[57–63]

The mechanism of the hypocholesterolemic effect of neomycin is unclear. One study[57] showed that neomycin precipitated fatty acids, cholesterol, and usually bile acids (6 out of 7 subjects) from micelles in the small intestine. In another study[58] the micellar content of fatty acids and bile acids was not decreased by neomycin.

There is also disagreement on whether or not fecal excretion of neutral and acidic steroids is increased by neomycin. If neomycin precipitates intestinal bile acids which are essential for cholesterol incorporation into micelles, then increased excretion of both acidic and neutral steroids might be expected. Some studies have shown this[59,60] but others have not. One showed an increase in bile acid excretion only,[61] whereas another found consistent increases in the excretion of neutral but not acidic steroids.[62]

An additional possibility is that neomycin acts in part by its effect on the intestinal bacterial flora. Normal bacterial conversion of cholesterol and primary bile acids is greatly altered by neomycin.[62]

TABLE 2 Preparations and Costs of Drugs Used in the Treatment of Hyperlipidemia

Generic Name	Trademark Name(s)	Preparations and 1978 Costs
Cholestyramine	Questran	Packets 4 g—$16.87/50 Can 378 g (with 4-g measuring scoop)—$12.80
Colestipol	Colestid	Packets 5 g—$8.44/30 Can 500 g (with 5-g measuring scoop)—$25.00
Neomycin Sulfate	generic	Tablets 500 mg (equivalent to 350-mg base)—$7.70–$30.72/100
	Mycifradin Sulfate	Tablets 500 mg—$28.59/100
Sitosterols	Cytellin	Suspension (3 g = 1 tablespoonful)—$5.81/pint
Probucol	Lorelco	Tablets 250 mg—$18.30/112, $18.80/120
Clofibrate	Atromid-S	Capsules 500 mg—$7.10/100
Niacin (Nicotinic Acid)	generic	Tablets 500 mg—$0.99–$3.61/100
Norethindrone Acetate	Norlutate	Tablets 5 mg—$8.19/50
Oxandrolone	Anavar	Tablets 2.5 mg—$6.25/100

The frequency and severity of nausea and diarrhea (see Adverse Reactions) associated with neomycin therapy may differ widely,[56,63] depending upon whether it is taken in the fasting or the non-fasting state. Many patients who start on 0.5 to 1.0 g of neomycin per day immediately after meals have no difficulty with nausea or diarrhea. Others may experience these symptoms transiently and find that they wear off with continued therapy. Severe symptoms, requiring discontinuation of neomycin, are uncommon (see Adverse Reactions).

Neomycin is useful for adults with mild to moderate hypercholesterolemia whose degree of risk warrants cholesterol lowering drug therapy. Because of the possibility of systemic side effects, (see Adverse Reactions), it is not ordinarily used in children.

Adverse Reactions—Nausea and/or diarrhea occur in some patients on doses as low as 0.5 to 1.0 g per day. At the Massachusetts Institute of Technology Arteriosclerosis Center, 13 of 95 patients (14%) who were started on neomycin in this dose range had to stop the drug because of nausea or diarrhea.

Large oral doses of neomycin (12 g per day), which induce steatorrhea, produce malabsorption of carotene, sodium, potassium, calcium, vitamins B_{12} and K, iron, glucose and xylose, as well as fat.[64,65] Even much lower doses of neomycin (3 g per day) may cause steatorrhea and decreased absorption of xylose.[66] However, with neomycin doses of 0.5 to 2 g daily, others have found no steatorrhea,[62,67] and at the MIT Arteriosclerosis Center, no clinical evidence of nutrient malabsorption has been seen in patients on up to 2 g of neomycin a day for as long as five years.

Deafness and impairment of renal function have *not* been associated with oral administration of 0.5–2.0 g of neomycin per day. However, since most absorbed neomycin is excreted by the kidney,[68] its use in patients with abnormal renal function should be avoided. Periodic audiograms may be done as a precautionary measure in patients on long-term neomycin therapy.

Interactions—Oral neomycin in single doses ranging from 1 to 3 g has been reported to decrease intestinal absorption of digoxin in humans.[69] Since it may decrease the absorption of any drug, neomycin should be taken as far removed in time as possible from any other drugs. In addition, the plasma level and therapeutic effects of other drugs should be monitored when neomycin therapy is begun or terminated, and appropriate changes in dosage made as needed.

Dosage—Oral: Adults, Neomycin sulfate, 0.5–2.0 g daily in divided dose. For patients with mild hypercholesterolemia, 0.5 g (1 tablet) in the morning or evening may suffice. In more severe disease 0.5 g three times daily or 1 g twice daily may be required to lower plasma cholesterol adequately. The drug should be taken with or immediately after meals.

SITOSTEROLS (Cytellin)

Sitosterols are naturally occurring plant sterols which have different aliphatic side chains than cholesterol. The present commercial preparation is obtained from pine trees (tall oil) and contains about 90% beta sitosterol and about 10% of other plant sterols, chiefly stigmasterol.[70] The first report that plant sterols could prevent hypercholesterolemia in animals came from Peterson in 1951.[71] Since that time, the sources and preparations of beta sitosterol have varied, but generally the compound is slightly to moderately effective in lowering the total plasma cholesterol and LDL cholesterol concentrations in Type II patients.[70,72–77] The advantages of beta sitosterol are a very low incidence of side effects, relative palatability, low cost, and the convenience of a single daily dose.[70] On the other hand, the drug is, at best, only moderately effective. For patients whose hypercholesterolemia is mild (between 250 and 300 mg/100 ml on dietary therapy alone) but whose risk of developing atherosclerotic disease is high, beta sitosterol could be the appropriate first drug. The efficacy of beta sitosterol varies widely from patient to patient, but when effective it decreases plasma cholesterol by 10 to 15%.[70] Beta sitosterol therapy is sometimes[70] but not always[75,77] associated with an increase in plasma triglycerides, but seldom to abnormal levels. The drug's effect on HDL levels is variable and insignificant.[75,77] For patients with moderate or severe hypercholesterolemia, beta sitosterol may be combined with other lipid-lowering drugs, such as niacin (nicotinic acid), neomycin, resins, or clofibrate.[78,79]

Beta sitosterol is poorly absorbed. It exerts its hypocholesterolemic effect in the intestine by inhibiting cholesterol absorption[76,80] via any of several possible mechanisms.[81]

In summary, beta sitosterol alone may be a useful adjunct to dietary therapy in patients with mild hypercholesterolemia. In those with more severe disease, beta sitosterol may be useful when combined with another lipid-lowering agent.

Adverse Reactions—There have been no reports of adverse reactions to beta sitosterol therapy. Although absorption of beta sitosterol by normal adults is no more than 5% of the dose,[81] there is one report that children whose diets are enriched in plant sterols (for example, infants fed commercial formula, or children fed diets high in polyunsaturated fats) have elevated plasma levels of these sterols.[82] The clinical significance of such elevations is unknown, but in one report two sisters with abnormally high beta sitosterol absorption had high plasma sitosterol levels and xanthomatosis while on a normal diet.[83] Fortunately, beta sitosterol is measured as cholesterol in all the commonly used methods for cholesterol estimation; any patient in whom the plasma cholesterol rises significantly with beta sitosterol therapy should discontinue the drug.

Dosage—Oral: Adults, although higher doses were previously thought necessary, it now appears that the maximal adult response to beta sitosterol is obtained with 3 g once a day (one tablespoon of the 20% suspension).[70] *Children,* maximal response may occur with 3 g twice daily.[70]

PROBUCOL (Lorelco)

Probucol, a substituted dithioacetal, is a new cholesterol-lowering agent. In some long-term human studies, probucol is moderately effective in lowering plasma cholesterol[84–86] and may cause diminution or disappearance of xanthelasmas.[85] Others, however, found that while individual Type II patient responses varied widely, there was no change in the mean response between placebo and probucol periods in patients already on lipid-lowering diets.[87] In one early study, the initial response of Type II patients was very good, but six to seven months after probucol therapy was begun the mean change in serum cholesterol was only questionably significant.[88] This finding was supported in a later study which showed a moderately good maximal cholesterol decrease at three months, followed by a slow rise to give only a slight net decrease (9%) by nine months.[89] Probucol was more effective in mild than severe hypercholesterolemia.[89] Probucol has a variable effect on plasma triglycerides[84–86] and is not recommended for lowering them. In one study probucol significantly lowered both LDL and HDL cholesterol but had no effect on VLDL cholesterol.[84]

Probucol appears to have two major advantages over other hypocholesterolemic agents: minimal clinical side effects (see Adverse Reactions), and no adverse effects on hepatic function, carbohydrate tolerance, or prothrombin time.[85,87–89] The mechanism of action of probucol is unknown although it may decrease hepatic and/or intestinal cholesterol synthesis.[88]

A potentially serious problem with probucol is accumulation in adipose tissue.[90] Although less than 10% of orally administered probucol is absorbed, in animal studies only about 10% of the amount absorbed was excreted after 30 hours.[90] Thus, if human metabolism of the drug is comparable, a patient taking the recommended dose of 1 g per day, absorbing 5% of the dose, and excreting 10% of that amount, could accumulate as much as 16 g of probucol in one year. Since the half-life of the drug is long, side effects, if they occurred, might be long-lasting. Six months after stopping the drug, the average plasma level of probucol in eight patients was still 20% of the peak level.[90]

During a two-year study of probucol in dogs, 12 out of 32 apparently healthy dogs died.[90] Subsequent studies showed that the myocardium of dogs is sensitized to epinephrine by probucol, leading to ventricular fibrillation; there were no premonitory electrocardiographic changes to indicate that myocardial sensitization had developed.[90,91] Sensitization did not occur in four other animal species.[90,91] Arrhythmias so far have not been associated with probucol therapy in humans.

In summary, probucol's effectiveness as a hypocholesterolemic agent is reported to vary from slight to moderate in Type II patients. The drug's effect on triglycerides is variable, and it is not recommended for the treatment of primary hypertriglyceridemia. Recognized side effects from probucol are minimal (see Adverse Reactions). However, the desirability of using probucol in place of other cholesterol-lowering agents is uncertain in view of its accumulation in adipose tissue, its slow rate of disappearance from plasma, and its association with ventricular fibrillation in dogs.

Adverse Reactions—There are no recognized serious side effects of probucol therapy.[84,86,87] Minor adverse reactions are limited to the gastrointestinal tract and include diarrhea and flatulence.[85,90] A few patients are reported to have marked plasma triglyceride elevations on probucol therapy. When this persists, the drug should be discontinued.

The significance of the drug's accumulation in adipose tissue (see above) is unknown and should be investigated more fully. The association of probucol therapy with unheralded ventricular fibrillation in dogs, suggests the need for caution in the use of the drug in patients with arrhythmias (see above).

Dosage—Oral: Adults (only), 500 mg, morning and evening with meals.

CLOFIBRATE (Atromid-S)

Clofibrate is a systemically active, branched-chain fatty acid ester, ethyl-p-chlorophenoxyisobutyrate (CPIB), whose lipid-lowering effect in patients was first noted in 1962.[92] Androsterone was previously thought to enhance the hypolipidemic effect of clofibrate, but this now appears incorrect.[93,94] The drug circulates in the plasma as the free fatty acid, bound to albumin.

The action of clofibrate is difficult to characterize. It can lower both plasma cholesterol and triglycerides to varying degrees depending on the type of hyperlipidemia. In one study of more than 60 hyperlipidemic patients followed for up to 6 years, clofibrate produced no significant effect on cholesterol or triglycerides in Type I patients, but caused a marked lowering of triglycerides in Type III (-44%), IV (-44%), and V (-59%) patients, with similar effects on cholesterol in Type III (-39%) and V (-23%) patients.[95] In Type II patients, the drug produced only moderate lowering of both cholesterol (-15%) and triglycerides (-16%); it lowered cholesterol only slightly in Type IV patients (-8%).[95] These results are consistent with other studies.[93,94] Many investigators find that clofibrate lowers plasma triglycerides more effectively than cholesterol and recommend its use primarily for Types III, IV, and V.[21,22,26,96] A minority opinion holds that in Type IIa patients, with normal triglycerides, as opposed to Type IIb patients, whose triglycerides are elevated, clofibrate is a very effective cholesterol-lowering agent.[97] Prolonged clofibrate therapy in Type II patients selected for study because of their good response to the drug may result in gradual disappearance of xanthomas.[98]

Clofibrate's mechanism of action is incompletely understood. Its effects on several hepatic enzymes in animals are summarized elsewhere.[99] In human studies clofibrate lowers plasma free fatty acid levels,[100] which could decrease the acyl groups available for triglyceride synthesis. It also increases biliary and fecal cholesterol output, while decreasing fecal bile acid excretion.[101] In hypercholesterolemic patients who respond to clofibrate, both VLDL and LDL levels are decreased.[98] In hyperglyceridemic patients whose glycerides are lowered by clofibrate, complex reciprocal lipoprotein changes occur. In general, LDL and HDL concentrations increase, while VLDL decrease in concentration.[25] The net result may be an increase in total plasma cholesterol levels even as glyceride levels are decreased. In such cases, one should either add a second, cholesterol-lowering drug such as neomycin, niacin, or resin, or substitute another glyceride-lowering drug.[26]

Two large scale secondary prevention trials have demonstrated that clofibrate significantly reduces morbidity and mortality in patients who already have ischemic heart disease.[102,103] A third study, the Coronary Drug Project,[11] showed no beneficial effect of clofibrate in men who had had a myocardial infarction. In the latter study, many of the patients were not hyperlipidemic and clofibrate produced no significant cholesterol-lowering in the group as a whole, although triglycerides were lowered by 22%. A primary prevention study has shown that the drug may lower the risk of developing ischemic heart disease in asymptomatic patients,[104] regardless of whether the patients were hyperlipidemic or whether clofibrate influenced their hyperlipidemia.

The beneficial effect of clofibrate in ischemic heart disease may be the result of direct effects on platelets and on intravascular coagulation. In platelets of hypercholesterolemic patients, clofibrate may reduce stickiness,[105,106] may prolong survival time and may decrease turnover,[106] as well as reverse hypersensitivity to aggregating agents.[107] The decreased platelet sensitivity to aggregating agents in Type II patients is associated with decreased intravascular coagulation and increased fibrinolysis.[108] When a maximal antithrombotic effect is sought, for example, in patients with transient cerebral ischemic attacks, clofibrate can be used in combination with aspirin or dipyridamole (see Antithrombotic Drugs below).

In summary, clofibrate is most often the drug of choice for lowering plasma triglycerides in patients with primary hypertriglyceridemia who do not respond adequately to dietary therapy alone. It may also be effective in some patients with increased plasma cholesterol levels, but other drugs are likely to lower cholesterol more effectively in Type II patients. Independent of its hypolipidemic action, clofibrate may be a useful antithrombotic agent in patients with or without elevated blood lipids.

Adverse Reactions—Gastrointestinal discomfort, particularly nausea, is the most common side effect of clofibrate therapy[11,102,104] and occurs in 5 to 10% of patients. General malaise, particularly myalgia, is also common. Since malaise and myalgia are common and nonspecific symptoms, their association with clofibrate therapy may be considerably underestimated. In some patients serum creatine phosphokinase (CPK) levels rise[11] and very rarely a severe reversible myopathy, with myalgia, muscle swelling, stiffness, and weakness, accompanied by elevations in CPK and aldolase, occurs.[109]

Decreased libido and/or breast tenderness occur in some men.[11,104] Liver enlargement may also occur;[11] hepatic transaminase levels are sometimes elevated,[11,92,94] but the changes are reversible and clinical signs of hepatotoxicity are unusual. A small but significant increase in the incidence of cholelithiasis in men taking clofibrate has been reported.[11,110] Slight to moderate weight gain also occurs in some patients.[11,111] Uncommonly, exteme weight gain may necessitate discontinuation of the drug. The cause of the increased weight is not clear but the drug does have an antidiuretic effect[112] and can cause an increase in appetite.[11] Several other isolated effects, such as hair loss and skin rash have also been reported.[11,102,104]

Drug Interactions—Clofibrate enhances the effects of coumarin anticoagulants;[113] the dosage of anticoagulant should be reduced by one-third to one-half in patients started on clofibrate, and the anticoagulant effects should be carefully monitored.

Hepatotoxicity may also be increased if clofibrate is given with another systemically active lipid-lowering drug.

Dosage—Oral: Adults, 1.5 to 2 g daily in divided dose. In adults of body weight over 50 kg (110 lbs), 1 g twice daily is usually the optimal dose. The drug is not generally used in children.

NIACIN [NICOTINIC ACID]

Niacin, a B vitamin which prevents pellagra, is the only lipid-lowering drug which is highly effective in lowering both plasma cholesterol and triglycerides. It was first found to lower cholesterol levels in humans by Altschul and co-workers in 1955.[114] The effect is independent of the compound's action as a vitamin and requires much greater doses than are necessary for pellagra prevention. Following Altschul's investigations, several long-term clinical trials,[115–118] using doses ranging from 1.5 to 7 g daily, showed that nicotinic acid is a highly effective cholesterol-lowering agent. These early reports focused on the drug's effect on plasma cholesterol. However, nicotinic acid lowers plasma triglycerides equally as well as cholesterol.[21,22,26] In assessing the benefit of niacin therapy, the Coronary Drug Project found a significant decrease in the five-year incidence of 'definite, non-fatal myocardial infarction,' which occurred in 8.9% of nicotinic acid-treated patients in contrast to 12.2% of placebo-treated patients.[11] A similar significant decrease occurred in the five year incidence of 'definite or suspected fatal or non-fatal stroke' (7.7% vs 9.7%). In patients with xanthomas and xanthelasmas, marked diminution of the lesions sometimes occurs with niacin therapy; less frequently, the lesions disappear.[117]

Niacin lowers the plasma free fatty acid (FFA) concentration within thirty minutes after oral administration, apparently by inhibiting fatty acid mobilization from adipose tissue.[119] This effect is followed within hours by lower plasma triglycerides.[120] Presumably the decreased availability of FFA leads to decreased hepatic production of triglycerides and VLDL. Plasma cholesterol levels do not fall until several days after niacin therapy is begun.[120] Niacin increases fecal endogenous neutral steroid excretion in humans[121] consistent with a direct effect on cholesterol metabolism. Animal studies indicate that niacin may inhibit hepatic cholesterol synthesis[122] at a step between acetate and mevalonate formation.[123] Altschul's original hypothesis[114] that niacin acts by increasing *in vivo* oxidation of cholesterol appears unlikely, although the drug does enhance hepatic mitochondrial oxidation of cholesterol in rats.[124] Interestingly, the closely related compound, niacinamide, does not lower plasma cholesterol.[114,116]

In summary, niacin is the drug of choice when maximal lowering of cholesterol and/or triglycerides is sought in patients at risk for the development of atherosclerotic disease or who already have such disease. Those in the latter group sometimes experience improvement in their clinical status while on niacin therapy. However, the drug should be used with caution in patients with a history of prior liver disease or peptic ulcer; its use is contraindicated in those whose liver function tests are abnormal before treatment is begun, or who have active ulcer disease.

Adverse Reactions—The most prominent immediate side effect of niacin therapy is cutaneous flushing, often accompanied by pruritus and occasionally by urticaria.[11,115–118,125] Flushing occurs shortly after ingestion of the drug in almost all patients but usually subsides within a week or two with continuing therapy.[115–118,125] It is seldom necessary to discontinue the drug or to decrease the dosage because of flushing. Starting with small doses (100 to 150 mg) and working up gradually does not seem to lessen the incidence or severity of this symptom. Similarly, modified forms of niacin such as buffered or sustained release preparations, or the alcohol form, nicotinyl alcohol, have no special advantage. Sustained release preparations can even exacerbate several of the side effects of the drug.[126,127] Taking niacin with meals can help to decrease the severity of flushing. Dryness of the skin, hyperpigmentation (especially in the axilla and groin) and acanthosis nigricans are uncommon but do occur.[11,115–118] They disappear when the drug is discontinued.

Gastrointestinal irritation occurs quite commonly in patients taking niacin; symptoms include anorexia, nausea, vomiting, diarrhea, and abdominal pain.[11,117,118,125] Taking the drug immediately after meals or at bedtime may alleviate such symptoms, but occasionally the drug must be discontinued. Activation of peptic ulcer has been associated with niacin therapy in a few patients.[125,128] Patients with known active ulcer disease should not be started on niacin.

The drug also may impair glucose metabolism in some patients. Some non-diabetic patients develop carbohydrate intolerance[129] and some diabetic patients become more difficult to regulate.[115,125,130] In the Coronary Drug Project, the fasting plasma glucose was 106 mg/100 ml in patients on placebo (n=1613 patients) and 109.3 mg/100 ml in those on niacin (n=588 patients), while the one-hour post-challenge plasma glucose values were 174.8 mg/100 ml and 184.9 mg/100 ml in placebo-treated (n=1577) and niacin treated (n=578) patients respectively.[11] Because of the large numbers of patients studied, these changes do have statistical significance.[11] Niacin should be used with caution in patients with diabetes. It is often well tolerated by patients with chemical and mild adult-onset diabetes whose disease is controlled by diet alone. Blood glucose should be measured frequently in such patients, and niacin stopped if clinically important deterioration in glucose tolerance occurs. Juvenile, brittle, or insulin-requiring diabetics should not ordinarily be treated with niacin.

A potentially more serious consequence of niacin therapy is impaired hepatic function. The drug should not be started in patients with abnormal control liver function tests. Scattered reports of jaundice, particularly with sustained-release preparations of niacin, have appeared.[126,127,131,132] One study of hepatic biopsies from patients with normal liver function tests who were taking plain niacin revealed histologically normal hepatic tissue, although electron microscopic studies did show some changes in the endoplasmic reticulum and mitochondria.[133] The Coronary Drug Project did not report jaundice in any patient on niacin, nor did liver function tests become abnormal.[11] Most studies have found one or more abnormal liver function tests in some patients during the course of niacin therapy.[115,117,118,133,134] The changes were usually mild and transitory even though therapy was continued.[117,118,134] Abnormalities of liver function return to normal soon after cessation of nicotinic acid therapy.[117,118] Liver function should be monitored routinely and the drug discontinued if persistent, serious abnormalities develop. Monitoring is especially important when combination lipid-lowering therapy is employed.

Hyperuricemia also occurs in many patients treated with niacin.[117,118,126] It is usually transient and disappears while the patients remain on the drug, but may persist in a few patients as long as the drug is continued.[117,118,126] Uric acid levels should be measured at regular intervals during niacin therapy; if levels rise above 10 mg/100 ml in an asymptomatic patient, coadministration of allopurinol should be considered. Rarely, acute gouty arthritis is precipitated by niacin.[117,118,126] Temporarily discontinuing niacin, treating the gout, and then restarting niacin in combination with allopurinol usually prevents a recurrence of gout. Pre-existing gout is not necessarily a contraindication to the use of niacin.

The Coronary Drug Project reported an increased incidence of cardiac arrhythmias, particularly atrial fibrillation, in patients on niacin.[11]

Although some side effects are common with niacin therapy, many are transitory and do not usually necessitate withdrawal of the drug. At the MIT Arteriosclerosis Center, 23 of 144 patients (16%) discontinued niacin therapy because of side effects, which were all cutaneous or gastrointestinal. None of the patients had cardiac arrhythmias.

Drug Interactions—Niacin may act synergistically with thiazide diuretics to increase plasma uric acid. If the uric acid level in an asymptomatic patient exceeds 10 mg/100 ml, it should be lowered by concurrent administration of allopurinol in order to prevent gout. Niacin may also potentiate the effects of antihypertensive drugs, including both ganglionic blocking agents and direct vasodilators. Niacin should be started with caution in such patients, and the dose of the antihypertensive drugs adjusted as necessary.

Dosage—The drug is usually begun at a dose of 0.5 g three times daily after meals. If flushing or itching is troublesome, a single 0.5 g dose may be given after dinner or at bedtime for a few days to a few weeks until the annoying side effects disappear. The dose may then be increased to 1 g three or four times daily. Doses higher than 4 g daily are rarely needed and increase the risk of serious side effects.

Reassurance by the physician that the annoying initial side effects will eventually disappear, while the therapeutic effect continues, usually convinces the patient to remain on the drug during the critical first few weeks of therapy.

NORETHINDRONE ACETATE (Norlutate)
OXANDROLONE (Anavar)

Norethindrone acetate is a synthetic progestational steroid derived from nortestosterone. Oxandrolone, which is structurally similar to norethindrone, is an anabolic, weakly androgenic synthetic steroid also derived from nortestosterone. Norethindrone alcohol (Norlutin) is also available but is less potent than the acetate.

Oxandrolone was noted in 1968 to lower the plasma triglycerides of patients with Type III and Type V hyperlipoproteinemia.[135] A year later, norethindrone acetate was reported to be moderately effective in lowering plasma triglycerides in patients with Type V hyperlipoproteinemia.[136] Both drugs are moderately effective in lowering triglycerides in hyperglyceridemic patients, but are usually not used unless dietary therapy and therapy with clofibrate or niacin have failed. When necessary, either drug may be used in combination with clofibrate or nicotinic acid. Norethindrone acetate and oxandrolone may also lower triglycerides in Type III and Type IV patients,[135–137] but are most frequently used in Type V patients, who are more likely to be refractory to other drugs. Triglyceride levels may start to decline within three days after starting therapy but may not reach their lowest levels for four weeks or longer.[135–138] Use of these drugs is associated with decreases in the plasma concentrations of chylomicrons and VLDL.[135–137] While a decrease in plasma triglycerides is the rule, plasma cholesterol is only variably decreased. Type V patients, whose severe hyperlipidemia is associated with recurrent acute abdominal attacks and pancreatitis, often experience relief with norethindrone acetate or oxandrolone therapy, even when their triglycerides do not fall to normal. Therapy is associated with an increase in plasma postheparin lipolytic activity.[136–138] Recent studies with oxandrolone[139] suggest that the drug increases the activity of a hepatic lipase. The increase in this lipase may explain the action of both drugs.

Adverse Reactions—Since norethindrone is a progestational steroid, it is more commonly prescribed for women than men, but can also be used in men with Type V hyperlipoproteinemia who are unresponsive to other drugs (including oxandrolone). Norethindrone should not be used in patients with benign or malignant changes in tissues which respond to sex hormones.

Norethindrone, which is also used in oral contraceptives, may produce changes in the reproductive cycle in women.

Oxandrolone has weak androgenic activity and may produce masculinization in women. It is ordinarily prescribed only for male Type V patients, although it may be used in women with Type V whose hypertriglyceridemia is refractory to other drugs (including norethindrone acetate).

At the MIT Arteriosclerosis Center, two patients on long-term oxandrolone therapy developed mild to moderate hypertension. Fluid retention and edema have often been reported with this drug. Other side effects are not significant, but the drug should not be used in patients with carcinoma of the breast or prostate.[22] Oxandrolone apparently has no adverse effects on hepatic function[135,137] or carbohydrate metabolism.[137]

Dosage—Oral: Adults, Norethindrone acetate, 5 mg once daily; Oxandrolone, 2.5 mg three times daily. Neither drug has been used in children.

ANTITHROMBOTIC DRUGS

ASPIRIN
CLOFIBRATE (Atromid-S)
DIPYRIDAMOLE (Persantine)
SULFINPYRAZONE (Anturane)

The most feared consequences of hyperlipidemia are atherosclerosis and its sequelae—heart attack, stroke and peripheral vascular occlusion. These complications are often, but not always, thrombotic or thromboembolic in nature. For this reason, many physicians treat patients having clinically evident atherosclerosis with drugs which have been shown to inhibit platelet aggregation *in vitro,* in the expectation that *in vivo* thrombogenesis will also be inhibited or prevented.[26,31,140] Patients at high risk for atherosclerosis, eg, those with a familial form of Type II hyperlipoproteinemia, may also be treated prophylactically with antithrombotic drugs. Finally, in some patients whose arterial disease has traditionally been treated with anticoagulants (those with transient cerebral ischemic attacks or coronary artery bypass grafts), antithrombotic drugs have been used in clinical trials as alternative therapy.

The rationale for the use of these drugs is as follows. Patients with atherosclerotic arterial thrombosis or embolus have increased platelet turnover, as do those with prosthetic arterial grafts.[3] In these patients, platelet kinetics are returned toward normal by antithrombotic drugs. The platelets of patients with hypercholesterolemia are hypersensitive *in vitro* to standardized aggregation stimuli,[6] and experimental animals with dietary hypercholesterolemia have increased platelet turnover as well as evidence of arterial endothelial damage.[141] Antithrombotic drugs prevent platelet thrombi from occluding experimentally narrowed coronary arteries[142] and silastic arterio-venous shunts in man[143]; they also prevent the *in vitro* platelet hypersensitivity of hypercholesterolemia.[107]

Despite encouraging *in vitro* studies[107,108,144,145] as well as *in vivo* studies of platelet and fibrinogen turnover with and without antithrombotic drug therapy,[31,146] the routine use of these drugs in the prevention and treatment of atherosclerotic complications cannot be recommended until the potential risks and benefits are more clearly established.

Clinical trials of antithrombotic drugs are reviewed in detail elsewhere.[31,147] The results are generally encouraging but inconclusive because most studies either are not randomized or utilize small sample sizes. Nevertheless, ongoing studies in patients with both coronary and cerebral vascular disease should allow definitive evaluation of aspirin, clofibrate, sulfinpyrazone, and dipyridamole as well as certain combinations of these drugs.[31,104,147] Until these data are available, the drugs may be used empirically in patients at risk or with symptomatic atherosclerosis. At the MIT Arteriosclerosis Center, patients with angina pectoris, transient cerebral ischemia, or peripheral vascular insufficiency are tried on these agents. Where clearcut clinical improvement occurs, they are continued on a long-term basis. A brief description of each of the antithrombotic drugs in general use follows. For a more detailed discussion, see Chapter 41.

Aspirin has profound effects on platelet behavior *in vitro*. While initial platelet adhesion and *in vitro* aggregation are not affected, usual doses of aspirin prevent platelet nucleotide release and prevent the normal conversion of platelet arachidonic acid to prostaglandins and thromboxanes.[144,148] *In vivo*, aspirin may decrease the occurrence of both arterial and venous thromboembolism[31] although it does not seem to affect platelet kinetics[30]—a dissociation between laboratory and clinical findings which is common with antithrombotic drugs. Aspirin is frequently used to complement or potentiate the effects of other antithrombotic drugs.[30] The side effects and drug interactions of aspirin are discussed in Chapter 27.

Clofibrate (Atromid-S), given to hypercholesterolemic patients, prevents the *in vitro* platelet hypersensitivity otherwise seen in hypercholesterolemia[107] and reduces active intravascular coagulation also found in these patients.[108] *In vivo,* clofibrate has been reported to decrease the incidence of myocardial infarction and death in previously asymptomatic patients[104] as well as in those with symptomatic coronary artery disease.[102,103] In another study, clofibrate had no apparent effect on cardiovascular mortality.[11] It has been reported to prevent transient cerebral ischemia in several individual case reports and to reduce accelerated platelet turnover in patients with coronary disease.[146] The side effects associated with clofibrate therapy and its many interactions with other drugs are discussed above.

Dipyridamole (Persantine) is a pyrimidine derivative originally used as a coronary vasodilator, although it dilates peripheral vascular smooth muscle as well. However, it was soon discovered to inhibit platelet aggregation[149] and has been used in many clinical and laboratory studies of thrombosis and its prevention,[30,31,147,149] including one convincing study on the prevention of thromboembolism from prosthetic heart valves.[150] Like clofibrate, its efficacy may be enhanced by concomitant administration of aspirin.[30] Side effects include flushing, tachycardia, and postural hypotension, probably attributable to its peripheral vasodilating effects. These do not usually occur in the dosage used to prevent thrombosis (100 to 150 mg per day) when the drug is used in conjunction with aspirin.[30] Nausea and vomiting, diarrhea, and epigastric pain may also occur, presumably from direct gastric irritation. As with all antithrombotic drugs, pathological bleeding may occur, particularly in hypertensive patients and these drugs should not ordinarily be given until hypertension is reasonably well controlled.

Sulfinpyrazone (Anturane, see Chapters 31 and 41), a drug closely related to phenylbutazone (Butazolidine, see Chapter 32) but which lacks its anti-inflammatory properties, was originally used as a uricosuric agent. However, it shares with other anti-arthritic drugs a potent antiplatelet activity.[31,145] Its ability to inhibit platelet activity *in vitro* is well established;[145] it increased platelet survival in patients with prosthetic heart valves,[151] and prevented thrombosis of extracorporeal silastic arteriovenous shunts in one clinical trial.[143] However, sulfinpyrazone did not reduce the incidence of strokes or stroke death in a large well-controlled multicenter trial,[152,153] nor did it potentiate the effect of aspirin.[153] Gastric irritation, epigastric pain, nausea and vomiting, bleeding and dermatitis are the major side effects of sulfinpyrazone therapy.[140]

To summarize, the use of antiplatelet or antithrombotic drugs may be prophylactic or therapeutic in patients with hyperlipidemia and atherosclerosis. However, clinical verification of their efficacy is incomplete. In patients at high risk or with atherosclerotic symptoms, the use of antithrombotic drugs may be warranted on an empirical basis. Justification for long-term use in an individual patient is greatest when the drugs appear to control clinical signs and symptoms.

Dosage—Oral: Adults, Aspirin 0.6 g twice daily; Clofibrate 1 g twice daily in patients over 50 kg body weight, 0.5 g three times daily in patients under 50 kg body weight; Dipyridamole 50 mg two to three times daily; Sulfinpyrazone 200 mg three to four times daily.

REFERENCES

1. Kannel WB, Castelli WP, Gordon T, et al: Serum cholesterol, lipoproteins, and the risk of coronary heart disease. Ann Intern Med 74:1–12, 1971.
2. Lees RS, Wilson DE, Schonfeld G, et al: The familial dyslipoproteinemias. Prog Med Genet 9:237–290, 1973.
3. Hatch FT, Lees, RS: Practical methods for plasma lipoprotein analysis. Adv Lipid Res 6:1–68, 1968.
4. Lees RS, Fredrickson DS: The differentiation of exogenous and endogenous hyperlipidemia by paper electrophoresis. J Clin Invest 44:1968–1977, 1965.
5. Fredrickson DS, Lees RS: A system for phenotyping hyperlipoproteinemia. Circulation 31:321–327, 1965.
6. Carvalho AC, Colman RW, Lees RS: Platelet function in hyperlipoproteinemia. N Engl J Med 290:434–438, 1974.
7. Carvalho AC, Lees RS, Vaillancourt RA, et al: Intravascular coagulation in hyperlipidemia. Thromb Res 8:843–857, 1976.
8. Goldstein JL, Schrott HG, Hazzard WR, et al: Hyperlipidemia in coronary heart disease. II. Genetic analysis of lipid levels in 176 families and delineation of a new inherited disorder, combined hyperlipidemia. J Clin Invest 52:1544–1568, 1973.
9. Lees RS: A progress report on lipoprotein phenotyping. J Lab Clin Med 82:529–533, 1973.
10. Fredrickson DS, Levy RI, Lees RS: Fat transport in lipoproteins—an integrated approach to mechanisms and disorders. N Engl J Med 276:32–44, 94–103, 148–156, 215–226, 273–281, 1967.
11. Coronary Drug Project: Clofibrate and niacin in coronary heart disease. JAMA 231:360–381, 1975.
12. Miettinen M, Turpeinen O, Karvonen MJ, et al: Effect of cholesterol-lowering diet on mortality from coronary heart disease and other causes. Lancet 2:835–838, 1972.
13. Smoking and Health: Report of the Advisory Committee to the Surgeon General of the Public Health Service, U.S. Department of Health, Education, and Welfare, Public Health Service Publication No. 1103. Washington, Government Printing Office, 1964.
14. Doyle JT, Dawber TR, Kannel WB, et al: The relationship of cigarette smoking to coronary heart disease. JAMA 190:886–890, 1964.

15. Heyden S, Cassel JC, Bartel A, et al: Body weight and cigarette smoking as risk factors. Arch Intern Med 128:915–919, 1971.
16. Duncan GW, Lees RS, Ojemann RG, et al: Concomitants of atherosclerotic carotid artery stenosis. Stroke 8:665–669, 1977.
17. Kannel WB, Dawber TR, Kagan A, et al: Factors of risk in the development of coronary heart disease—six-year follow-up experience: The Framingham Study. Ann Intern Med 55:33–50, 1961.
18. Freis ED: Hypertension and atherosclerosis. Am J Med 46:735–740, 1969.
19. Tyroler HA, Heyden S, Bartel A, et al: Blood pressure and cholesterol as coronary heart disease risk factors. Arch Intern Med 128:907–914, 1971.
20. Lees RS, Wilson DE: The treatment of hyperlipidemia. N Engl J Med 284:186–195, 1971.
21. Levy RI, Morganroth J, Rifkind BM: Treatment of hyperlipidemia. N Engl J Med 290:1295–1301, 1974.
22. Yeshurun D, Gotto AM, Jr.: Drug treatment of hyperlipidemia. Am J Med 60:379–396, 1976.
23. Lewis B: *The Hyperlipidaemias.* London, Blackwell Scientific Publications, 1976, pp 341–380.
24. Olefsky J, Reaven GM, Farquhar JW: Effects of weight reduction on obesity. Studies of lipid and carbohydrate metabolism in normal and hyperlipoproteinemic subjects. J Clin Invest 53:64–76, 1974.
25. Wilson DE, Lees, RS: Metabolic relationships among the plasma lipoproteins. J Clin Invest 51:1051–1057, 1972.
26. Lees RS, Lees AM: Therapy of the hyperlipidemias. Postgrad Med 60:99–107, (Sep) 1976.
27. Sturdevant RAL, Pearce ML, Dayton S: Increased prevalence of cholelithiasis in men ingesting a serum-cholesterol-lowering diet. N Engl J Med 288:24–27, 1973.
28. Dayton S, Pearce ML, Hashimoto S, et al: A controlled clinical trial of a diet high in unsaturated fat in preventing complications of atherosclerosis. Circulation 40 (Suppl II):1–63, 1969.
29. Duncan GW, Gruber JO, Dewey CF, Jr, et al: Evaluation of carotid stenosis by phonoangiography. N Engl J Med 293:1124–1128, 1975.
30. Harker LA, Slichter SJ: Platelet and fibrinogen consumption in man. N Engl J Med 287:999–1005, 1972.
31. Genton E, Gent M, Hirsch J, et al: Platelet-inhibiting drugs in thrombotic disease. N Engl J Med 293:1174–1178, 1236–1240, 1296–1300, 1975.
32. Hashim SA, VanItallie TB: Cholestyramine resin therapy for hypercholesterolemia. JAMA 192:289–293, 1965.
33. Fallon HJ, Woods JW: Response of hyperlipoproteinemia to cholestyramine resin. JAMA 204:1161–1164, 1968.
34. Glueck CJ, Ford S Jr, Scheel D, et al: Colestipol and cholestyramine resin: comparative effects in familial Type II hyperlipoproteinemia. JAMA 222:676–681, 1972.
35. West RJ, Lloyd JK: Use of cholestyramine in treatment of children with familial hypercholesterolemia. Arch Dis Child 48:370–374, 1973.
36. Lees AM, McCluskey MA, Lees, RS: Results of colestipol therapy in Type II hyperlipoproteinemia. Atherosclerosis 24:129–140, 1976.
37. Tennent DM, Siegal H, Zanetti ME, et al: Plasma cholesterol lowering action of bile acid binding polymers in experimental animals. J Lipid Res 1:469–473, 1960.
38. Bergen SS Jr, VanItallie TB, Tennent DM, et al: Effect of an anion exchange resin on serum cholesterol in man. Proc Soc Exp Biol Med 102:676–679, 1959.
39. Siperstein MD, Nichols CW Jr, Chaikoff IL: Effects of ferric chloride and bile on plasma cholesterol and atherosclerosis in the cholesterol-fed bird. Science 117:386–389, 1953.
40. Parkinson TM, Gundersen K, Nelson NA: Effects of colestipol (U-26,597A), a new bile acid sequestrant, on serum lipids in experimental animals and man. Atherosclerosis 11:531–537, 1970.
41. Moore RB, Crane CA, Frantz ID Jr: Effect of cholestyramine on the fecal excretion of intravenously administered cholesterol-4-14C and its degradation products in a hypercholesterolemic patient. J Clin Invest 47:1664–1671, 1968.
42. Moutafis CD, Myant NB: The metabolism of cholesterol in two hypercholesterolaemic patients treated with cholestyramine. Clin Sci 37:443–454, 1969.
43. Miller NE, Clifton-Bligh P, Nestel PJ: Effects of colestipol, a new bile-acid-sequestering resin, on cholesterol metabolism in man. J Lab Clin Med 82:876–890, 1973.

44. Witztum JL, Schonfeld G, Weidman SW: The effects of colestipol on the metabolism of very-low-density lipoproteins in man. J Lab Clin Med 88:1008–1018, 1976.
45. Goodman DS, Noble RP, Dell RB: The effects of colestipol resin and of colestipol plus clofibrate on the turnover of plasma cholesterol in man. J Clin Invest 52:2646–2655, 1973.
46. Glueck CJ, Fallat RW, Tsang RC: Pediatric familial Type II hyperlipoproteinemia: therapy with diet and cholestyramine resin. Pediatrics 52:669–679, 1973.
47. Glueck CJ, Fallat RW, Mellies M, et al: Pediatric familial Type II hyperlipoproteinemia: therapy with diet and colestipol resin. Pediatrics 57:68–74, 1976.
48. Cohen MI, Winslow PR, Boley SJ: Intestinal obstruction associated with cholestyramine therapy. N Engl J Med 280:1285–1286, 1969.
49. Northcutt RC, Stiel JN, Hollifield JW, et al: The influence of cholestyramine on thyroxine absorption. JAMA 208:1857–1861, 1969.
50. Caldwell JH, Bush CA, Greenberger NJ: Interruption of the enterohepatic circulation of digitoxin by cholestyramine. J Clin Invest 50:2638–2644, 1971.
51. Gallo DG, Bailey KR, Sheffner AL: The interaction between cholestyramine and drugs. Proc Soc Exp Biol Med 120:60–65, 1965.
52. Bressler R, Nowlin J, Bogdonoff MD: Treatment of hypercholesterolemia and hypertriglyceridemia by anion exchange resin. South Med J 59:1097–1103, 1966.
53. West RJ, Lloyd JK: The effect of cholestyramine on intestinal absorption. Gut 16:93–98, 1975.
54. Gundersen K, Cooper EE, Ruoff G, et al: Cholesterol-lowering effect of colestipol hydrochloride given twice daily in hypercholesterolemic patients. Atherosclerosis 25:303–310, 1976.
55. Samuel P, Steiner A: Effect of neomycin on serum cholesterol level in man. Proc Soc Exp Biol Med 100:193–195, 1959.
56. Samuel P, Holtzman CM, Goldstein J: Long-term reduction of serum cholesterol levels of patients with atherosclerosis by small doses of neomycin. Circulation 35:938–945, 1967.
57. Thompson GR, Barrowman J, Gutierrez L, et al: Action of neomycin on the intraluminal phase of lipid absorption. J Clin Invest 50:319–323, 1971.
58. Hardison WGM, Rosenberg IH: The effect of neomycin on bile salt metabolism and fat digestion in man. J Lab Clin Med 74:564–573, 1969.
59. Powell RC, Nunes WT, Harding RS, et al: The influence of nonabsorbable antibiotics on serum lipids and the excretion of neutral sterols and bile acids. Am J Clin Nutr 11:156–168, 1962.
60. Faloon WW, Rubulis A, Rubert M: Cholesterol lowering and fecal bile acid and neutral sterol alteration during oral neomycin. Clin Res 17:158, 1969.
61. Goldsmith GA, Hamilton JG, Miller ON: Lowering of serum lipid concentrations. Mechanisms used by unsaturated fats, nicotinic acid and neomycin: excretion of sterols and bile acids. Arch Intern Med 105:512–517, 1960.
62. Sedaghat A, Samuel P, Crouse JR, et al: Effects of neomycin on absorption, synthesis and/or flux of cholesterol in man. J Clin Invest 55:12–21, 1975.
63. Faergeman O: Effects and side effects of treatment of hypercholesterolemia with cholestyramine and neomycin. Acta Med Scand 194:165–167, 1973.
64. Jacobson ED, Chodos, RB, Faloon WW: An experimental malabsorption syndrome induced by neomycin. Am J Med 28:524–533, 1960.
65. Gordon SJ, Haro EN, Paes IC, et al: Studies of malabsorption and calcium excretion induced by neomycin sulfate. JAMA 204:127–134, 1968.
66. Hvidt S, Kjeldsen K: Malabsorption induced by small doses of neomycin sulfate. Acta Med Scand 173:699–705, 1963.
67. Samuel P, Meilman E, Siil TE: Dietary lipids and reduction of serum cholesterol levels by neomycin in man. J Lab Clin Med 70:471–479, 1967.
68. Hawkins JE: Pharmacology of neomycin. In *Neomycin: Its Nature and Practical Application.* Edited by SA Waksman. Baltimore, Williams and Wilkins, 1958, pp 130–146.
69. Lindenbaum J, Maulitz RM, Butler VP: Inhibition of digoxin absorption by neomycin. Gastroenterology 71:399–404, 1976.
70. Lees AM, Mok HYI, Lees RS, et al: Plant sterols as cholesterol-lowering agents: clinical trials in patients with hypercholesterolemia and studies of sterol balance. Atherosclerosis 28:325–338, 1977.

71. Peterson DW: Effect of soybean sterols in the diet on plasma and liver cholesterol in chicks. Proc Soc Exp Biol Med 78:143–147, 1951.
72. Best MM, Duncan CH, VanLoon EJ, et al: The effects of sitosterol on serum lipids. Am J Med 19:61–70, 1955.
73. Farquhar JW, Smith RE, Dempsey ME: The effect of beta-sitosterol on the serum lipids of young men with arteriosclerotic heart disease. Circulation 14:77–82, 1956.
74 Riley FD, Steiner A: Effect of sitosterol on the concentration of serum lipids in patients with coronary atherosclerosis. Circulation 16:723–729, 1957.
75. Farquhar JW, Sokolow M: Response of serum lipids and lipoproteins of man to beta-sitosterol and safflower oil—a long-term study. Circulation 17:890–899, 1958.
76. Kudchodkar BJ, Horlick L, Sodhi HS: Effects of plant sterols on cholesterol metabolism in man. Atherosclerosis 23:239–248, 1976.
77. Oster P, Schlierf G, Heuck C, et al: Sitosterol in type II hyperlipoproteinemia. In *Lipoprotein Metabolism*. Edited by H Greten. Berlin, Springer-Verlag, 1976, pp 125–130.
78. Berge KG, Achor RWP, Barker NW, et al: Nicotinic acid, sitosterol, and safflower oil. Am Heart J 58:849–853, 1959.
79. Grundy SM, Mok HYI: Colestipol, clofibrate, and phytosterols in combined therapy of hyperlipidemia. J Lab Clin Med 89:354–366, 1977.
80. Grundy SM, Ahrens EH, Davignon J: The interaction of cholesterol absorption and cholesterol synthesis in man. J Lipid Res 10:304–315, 1969.
81. Salen G, Ahrens EH Jr, Grundy SM: Metabolism of beta-sitosterol in man. J Clin Invest 49:952–967, 1970.
82. Mellies M, Glueck CJ, Sweeney C, et al: Plasma and dietary sterols in children. Pediatrics 57:60–67, 1976.
83. Bhattacharyya AK, Connor WE: Beta sitosterolemia and xanthomatosis. A newly described lipid storage disease in two sisters. J Clin Invest 53:1033–1043, 1974.
84. LeLorier J, DuBreuil-Quidoz S, Lussier-Cacan S, et al: Diet and probucol in lowering cholesterol concentrations. Arch Intern Med 137:1429–1434, 1977.
85. Harris RS, Gilmore HR III, Bricker LA, et al: Long-term oral administration of probucol in the management of hypercholesterolemia. J Am Geriatr Soc 22:167–175, 1974.
86. Nash DT: Probucol: a new cholesterol lowering agent. J Med 6:305–315, 1975.
87. Brown HB, deWolfe VG: The additive effect of probucol on diet in hyperlipidemia. Clin Pharmacol Ther 16:44–50, 1974.
88. Miettinen TA: Mode of action of a new hypocholesterolemic drug (DH-581) in familial hypercholesterolemia. Atherosclerosis 15:163–176, 1972.
89. Miettinen TA, Toivonen I: Treatment of severe and mild hypercholesterolaemia with probucol and neomycin. Postgrad Med J 51 (Suppl 8):71–75, 1975.
90. Probucol Product Literature. Indianapolis, Dow Chemical Company, 1977.
91. Marshall FN, Lewis JE: Sensitization to epinephrine-induced ventricular fibrillation produced by probucol in dogs. Toxicol Appl Pharmacol 24:594–602, 1973.
92. Oliver MF: Reduction of serum-lipid and uric-acid levels by an orally active androsterone. Lancet 1:1321–1323, 1962.
93. Oliver MF: Further observations on the effects of atromid and of ethyl chlorophenoxyisobutyrate on serum lipid levels. J Atherosclerosis Res 3:427–444, 1963.
94. Hellman L, Zumoff B, Kessler G, et al: Reduction of serum cholesterol and lipids by ethyl chlorophenoxyisobutyrate. J Atherosclerosis Res 3:454–466, 1963.
95. Lees RS, Ahrens EH Jr: Unpublished observations, 1969.
96. Hunninghake DB, Tucker DR, Azarnoff DL: Long-term effects of clofibrate (Atromid-S) on serum lipids in man. Circulation 39:675–683, 1969.
97. Pichardo R, Boulet L, Davignon J: Pharmacokinetics of clofibrate in familial hypercholesterolemia. Atherosclerosis 26:573–582, 1977.
98. Scott PJ, Hurley PJ: Effect of clofibrate on low-density lipoprotein turnover in essential hypercholesterolemia. J Atherosclerosis Res 9:25–34, 1969.
99. Sirtori CR, Torreggiani D, Fumagalli R: Mechanism of action of hypolipidemic drugs. Adv Exp Med Biol 63:123–133, 1974.
100. Rifkind BM: Effect of CPIB ester on plasma free fatty acid levels in man. Metabolism 15:673–675, 1966.
101. Grundy SM, Ahrens EH Jr, Salen G, et al: Mechanisms of action of clofibrate on cholesterol metabolism in patients with hyperlipidemia. J Lipid Res 13:531–551, 1972.

102. Trial of clofibrate in the treatment of ischaemic heart disease. Five-year study by a group of physicians of the Newcastle upon Tyne region. Br Med J 4:767–775, 1971.
103. Ischaemic heart disease: a secondary prevention trial using clofibrate. Report by a research committee of the Scottish Society of Physicians. Br Med J 4:775–784, 1971.
104. Krasno LR, Kidera GJ: Clofibrate in coronary heart disease. JAMA 219:845–851, 1972.
105. Carson P, McDonald L, Pickard S, et al: Effect of clofibrate with androsterone (Atromid) and without (Atromid-S) on blood platelets and lipids in ischemic heart disease. Br Heart J 28:400–403, 1966.
106. Glynn MF, Murphy EA, Mustard JF: Effect of clofibrate on platelet economy in man. Lancet 2:447–448, 1967.
107. Carvalho AC, Colman RW, Lees RS: Clofibrate reversal of platelet hypersensitivity in hyperbetalipoproteinemia. Circulation 50:570–574, 1974.
108. Carvalho AC, Lees RS, Vaillancourt RA, et al: Effect of clofibrate on intravascular coagulation in hyperlipoproteinemia. Circulation 56:114–118, 1977.
109. Langer T, Levy RI: Acute muscular syndrome associated with administration of clofibrate. N Engl J Med 279:856–858, 1968.
110. Coronary Drug Project: Gallbladder disease as a side effect of drugs influencing lipid metabolism. N Engl J Med 296:1185–1190, 1977.
111. MacMillan DC, Oliver MF, Simpson JD, et al: Effect of ethylchlorophenoxyisobutyrate on weight, plasma volume, total body-water, and free fatty acids. Lancet 2:924–926, 1965.
112. Moses AM, Howanitz J, vanGemert M, et al: Clofibrate-induced antidiuresis. J Clin Invest 52:535–542, 1973.
113. Oliver MF, Roberts SD, Hayes D, et al: Effect of Atromid and ethyl chlorophenoxyisobutyrate on anticoagulant requirements. Lancet 1:143–144, 1963.
114. Altschul R, Hoffer A, Stephen JD: Influence of nicotinic acid on serum cholesterol in man. Arch Biochem Biophy 54:558–559, 1955.
115. Mahl M, Lange K: A long-term study of the effect of nicotinic acid medication on hypercholesterolemia. Am J Med Sci 246:673–677, 1963.
116. Parsons WB Jr, Flinn JH: Reduction in elevated blood cholesterol levels by large doses of nicotinic acid: preliminary report. JAMA 165:234–238, 1957.
117. Berge KG, Achor RWP, Christensen NA, et al: Hypercholesterolemia and nicotinic acid. Am J Med 31:24–36, 1961.
118. Christensen NA, Achor RWP, Berge KG, et al: Hypercholesterolemia: effects of treatment with nicotinic acid for three to seven years. Dis Chest 46:411–416, 1964.
119. Carlson LA, Oro L: The effect of nicotinic acid on the plasma free fatty acids. Demonstration of a metabolic type of sympathicolysis. Acta Med Scand 172:641–645, 1962.
120. Carlson LA, Oro L, Ostman J: Effect of nicotinic acid on plasma lipids in patients with hyperlipoproteinemia during the first week of treatment. J Atherosclerosis Res 8:667–677, 1968.
121. Miettinen TA: Effect of nicotinic acid on catabolism and synthesis of cholesterol in man. Clin Chim Acta 20:43–51, 1968.
122. Schade H, Saltman P: Influence of nicotinic acid on hepatic cholesterol synthesis in rabbits. Proc Soc Exp Biol Med 102:265–267, 1959.
123. Gamble W, Wright LD: Effect of nicotinic acid and related compounds on incorporation of mevalonic acid into cholesterol. Proc Soc Exp Biol Med 107:160–162, 1961.
124. Kritchevsky D, Whitehouse MW, Staple E: Oxidation of cholesterol-26-C_{14} by rat liver mitochondria: effect of nicotinic acid. J Lipid Res 1:154–158, 1960.
125. Belle M, Halpern MM: Oral nicotinic acid for hyperlipidemia with emphasis on side effects. Am J Cardiol 2:449–452, 1958.
126. Christensen NA, Achor RWP, Berge KG, et al: Nicotinic acid treatment of hypercholesterolemia: comparison of plain and sustained-action preparations and report of two cases of jaundice. JAMA 177:546–550, 1961.
127. Kohn RM, Montes M: Hepatic fibrosis following long acting nicotinic acid therapy: a case report. Am J Med Sci 258:94–99, 1969.
128. Parsons WB Jr: Activation of peptic ulcer by nicotinic acid. JAMA 173:1466–1470, 1960.
129. Gurian H, Adlersberg D: The effect of large doses of nicotinic acid on circulating lipids and carbohydrate tolerance. Am J Med Sci 237:12–22, 1959.

130. Molnar GD, Berge KG, Rosevear JW, et al: The effect of nicotinic acid in diabetes mellitus. Metabolism 13:181–190, 1964.
131. Rivin AU: Jaundice occurring during nicotinic acid therapy for hypercholesterolemia. JAMA 170:2088–2089, 1959.
132. Pardue WO: Severe liver dysfunction during nicotinic acid therapy. JAMA 175:137–138, 1961.
133. Baggenstoss AH, Christensen NA, Berge KG, et al: Fine structural changes in the liver in hypercholesterolemic patients receiving long-term nicotinic acid therapy. Mayo Clin Proc 42:385–399, 1967.
134. Parsons WB Jr: Studies of nicotinic acid use in hypercholesterolemia. Arch Intern Med 107:653–667, 1961.
135. Sachs BA, Wolfman L: Effect of oxandrolone on plasma lipids and lipoproteins of patients with disorders of lipid metabolism. Metabolism 17:400–410, 1968.
136. Glueck CJ, Brown WV, Levy RI, et al: Amelioration of hypertriglyceridaemia by progestational drugs in familial Type V hyperlipoproteinaemia. Lancet 1:1290–1291, 1969.
137. Glueck CJ: Effects of oxandrolone on plasma triglycerides and postheparin lipolytic activity in patients with Types III, IV, and V familial hyperlipoproteinemia. Metabolism 20:691–702, 1971.
138. Glueck CJ, Levy RI, Fredrickson DS: Norethindrone acetate, postheparin lipolytic activity, and plasma triglycerides in familial Types I, III, IV and V hyperlipoproteinemia. Ann Intern Med 75:345–352, 1971.
139. Ehnholm C, Huttunen JK, Kinnunen PJ, et al: Effect of oxandrolone treatment on the activity of lipoprotein lipase, hepatic lipase and phospholipase A1 of human postheparin plasma. N Engl J Med 292:1314–1317, 1975.
140. Blakely JA, Gent M: Platelets, drugs and longevity in a geriatric population. In *Platelets, Drugs and Thrombosis*. Edited by J Hirsh. Basel, Karger, 1975, pp 284–291.
141. Ross R, Harker L: Hyperlipidemia and atherosclerosis. Science 193:1094–1100, 1976.
142. Folts JD, Crowell EB, Rowe GG: Platelet aggregation in partially obstructed vessels and its elimination with aspirin. Circulation 54:365–370, 1976.
143. Kaegi A, Pineo GF, Shimizu A, et al: Arteriovenous-shunt thrombosis: prevention by sulfinpyrazone. N Engl J Med 290:304–306, 1974.
144. Smith JB, Willis AL: Aspirin selectively inhibits prostaglandin production in human platelets. Nature New Biol 231:235–237, 1971.
145. Mustard JF, Packham MA: Factors influencing platelet function: adhesion, release, and aggregation. Pharmacol Rev 22:97–187, 1970.
146. Steele P, Rainwater J, Ellis JE Jr, et al: Effect of platelet suppressant drugs on shortened platelet survival time in patients with coronary artery disease. Circulation 54 (Supp II):124, 1976.
147. Klimt CR, Doub N: Clinical trials in thrombosis: secondary prevention of myocardial infarction. Thromb Haemostas 35:49–56, 1976.
148. Hamberg M, Samuelsson B: Prostaglandin endoperoxides. Novel transformations of arachidonic acid in human platelets. Proc Nat Acad Sci (USA) 71:3400–3404, 1974.
149. Emmons PR, Harrison MJG, Honour AJ, et al: Effect of dipyridamole on human platelet behavior. Lancet 2:603–606, 1965.
150. Sullivan JM, Harken DE, Gorlin R: Pharmacologic control of thromboembolic complications of cardiac-valve replacement. N Engl J Med 284:1391–1394, 1971.
151. Weily HS, Genton E: Altered platelet function in patients with prosthetic mitral valves: effects of sulfinpyrazone therapy. Circulation 42:967–972, 1970.
152. Gent M: Canadian cooperative study of recent recurrent presumed cerebral emboli (RRPCE). In *Platelets, Drugs and Thrombosis*. Edited by J Hirsh. Basel, Karger, 1975, pp 253–257.
153. The Canadian Cooperative Study Group: A randomized trial of aspirin and sulfinpyrazone in threatened stroke. N Engl J Med 299:53–59, 1978.

45. VITAMINS

Bruce Weiner

DRUG MONOGRAPHS

LIPID-SOLUBLE VITAMINS

VITAMIN A

The major source of natural vitamin A is fish liver oils; it is also found in lesser quantities in eggs, dairy products, and meats. Vitamin A precursors, which the body converts to active vitamin A, are found in green parts of plants, carrots, apricots, peaches and yellow corn.

Deficiency—Xerophthalmia is the eye disease that occurs after long-term vitamin A deficiency.[1–4] Vitamin A deficiency may initially be manifested as decreased acuity in dim light, referred to as nyctalopia or night blindness.[5–7] Dark adaptation depends on the accumulation of visual purple, and vitamin A is essential for its regeneration.[8] Xerosis conjunctivae may occur later and is characterized by thickening and drying of the conjunctival epithelium and destruction of the mucous glands. As the deficiency state continues, keratomalacia may develop; the cornea becomes cloudy and Bitot's spots, small foam-like plaques, form on the conjunctiva.[9] Finally, corneal ulceration, perforation and infection, may cause loss of vision.

In vitamin A deficiency, epithelial tissue degeneration occurs in the mucous membranes of the digestive and respiratory tracts and in the lacrimal and salivary glands.[10] The eye manifests the greatest degree of degeneration, resulting from reduced lacrimal gland secretion. Hyperkeratotic changes occur in the skin, causing dryness and scaliness, accompanied by loss of elasticity, wrinkles, diminished sweat and oil secretion, and increased pigmentation.[11]

Abnormal keratinization occurs in the respiratory and digestive tract mucous membranes as a result of hypovitaminosis A.[12] Clinical sequelae can include pulmonary infection and diarrhea.

Vitamin A regulates the activities of osteoclasts and osteoblasts. In deficiency, all epiphyseal-cartilage development ceases. Cells stop dividing; nearly mature cells undergo no further change.[13] Induced deficiency in dogs leads to slight overgrowth of periosteal bone,[14] but skeletal changes secondary to vitamin A deficiency in humans are not clearly identified.[15]

Indications—Vitamin A, except for its usage in deficiency states, has few proven clinical indications. Although rare in the United States, hypovitaminosis A is prevalent in underdeveloped countries[16,17] —especially in the Orient. In India, for example, once yearly prophylactic administration of 300,000 IU of vitamin A to children reduces the incidence of ocular signs of vitamin A deficiency.[18]

Hypovitaminosis A usually occurs when dietary intake is inadequate[19] and in those with malabsorption syndromes.[20] Supplementation is useful in diseases that impair vitamin A absorption, eg, tropical sprue, cystic fibrosis, infantile or adult celiac disease, biliary obstruction, or total gastrectomy.

Use of vitamin A for skin diseases is controversial. The drug has been used to treat lesions associated with deficiency of the vitamin, including ichthyosis, Darier's disease, and pityriasis rubra pilaris. Even in these instances the efficacy of vitamin A is questionable.[21] Topical Vitamin A may be helpful in reversing corticosteroid-induced impairment of wound healing.[22] Vitamin A acid (retinoic acid) has been used topically in the treatment of oral lichen planus,[23] palmoplantar keratoderma,[24] and acne vulgaris.[25] In the latter condition, an eight-week, twice daily topical application of vitamin A acid is recommended.[26]

Overdosage—The American Arctic explorer, Kane, first described hypervitaminosis A in 1857 after he ingested polar bear liver.[27] This acute toxicity due to ingestion of a single large dose is self-limited. Symptoms include nausea and vomiting, headache, and vertigo.[28] Acute hypervitaminosis A is often seen in infants after accidental ingestion of large doses,[29] and is characterized by vomiting, drowsiness, and fontanelle bulging. Recovery is usually rapid and complete following lumbar puncture and vitamin A abstinence.[30,31]

The chronic form of hypervitaminosis A occurs after daily ingestion of moderately large quantities over a considerable period of time.[32,33] The minimum toxic dose in adults is 41,000 IU daily for 8 years.[34] Manifestations include hepatic, cutaneous, and neurological changes.[35] In two cases of daily ingestion of 100,000 to 1,250,000 IU for five to eight years, liver changes were evidenced by spider angiomas, palmar erythema, hepatocellular dysfunction, fibrosis, portal hypertension, and ascites.[36]

In one case a 51 year-old female ingested 600,000 IU per day for more than three years; neurological changes included headache, nystagmus, diplopia, depression, and schizophrenic manifestations.[37] A 15 year-old male who was given 300,000 IU daily for a similar length of time developed papilledema and simulated acute encephalitis.[38]

Skin changes occur in all instances of vitamin A overdose. Early manifestations include pruritus and a fine cutaneous desquamation over the trunk and extremities. Later, there is soreness and fissuring at the corners of the mouth and nasal apertures, dry rough skin, alopecia, and abnormal pigmentation.[39]

In children, prolonged administration of large quantities of vitamin A result in such bony changes as periosteal swelling, hyperostoses, and premature closure of the epiphyses.[40]

VITAMIN D

Compounds collectively termed vitamin D include the natural vitamin (D_3, cholecalciferol) as well as the prepared vitamin (D_2, ergocalciferol). D_3 is acquired from animal sources in the diet and synthesized in the skin upon exposure to sunlight.[41,42] Cholecalciferol is then hydroxylated in the liver to 25-hydroxycholecalciferol (25-HCC)[43–45] the major circulating form.[46,47] Although relatively inactive, 25-HCC is converted in the kidney to 1,25-dihydroxycholecalciferol[48] (1,25-DHCC), the most active hormone form, or to 24,25-dihydroxycholecalciferol (24,25-DHCC),[49] which is less active.[50] Ergocalciferol is found in fish and oils and fortified foods such as milk and margarine, and undergoes biotransformation similar to that of cholecalciferol. The two compounds are equally potent in man.

Normal daily requirements for vitamin D are 100 IU (2.5 μg) for adults and 400 IU (10 μg) for children less than 5 years of age. Such dosage will prevent nutritional osteomalacia and rickets.[51]

Vitamin D facilitates normal calcium and phosphorus metabolism, stimulates intestinal calcium absorption, and allows normal bone development.

Deficiency—Deficiency of vitamin D causes rickets in children and osteomalacia in adults. In children, demineralization occurs in the epiphyses, resulting in deformities. In adults, deficiency develops slowly, causing more extensive weakening of the skeleton.

Although rare in the United States, nutritional vitamin D deficiency occurs in those countries that do not fortify foodstuffs, in malnourished populations, and in people who have no exposure to sunshine. The latter includes mainly the institutionalized elderly.[52] Patients with seizure disorders receiving long-term anticonvulsant therapy can develop hypocalcemia and osteomalacia due to stimulation of vitamin D catabolism by anticonvulsant drugs[53,54] (see below). Deficiency is also common among Asians living in England, especially those who are vegetarians.[55]

Patients with malabsorption syndromes, whether inherited or secondary to gastrectomy, may also develop simple deficiency osteomalacia.[56,57] Chronic obstructive jaundice and primary biliary cirrhosis can be associated with malabsorption of vitamin D and osteomalacia.[58,59] Fanconi syndrome following bowel surgery and hepatitis have also been attributed to a deficiency of vitamin D.[60,61] In premature infants neonatal hypocalcemia may result from vitamin D deficiency.[62]

Indications—Vitamin D reportedly reduces the number of seizures in epileptics,[63,64] and has been found useful in reverting or preventing osteodystrophy secondary to long-term hemodialysis.[65,66] Metabolic or vitamin D-resistant rickets, although unresponsive to microgram dosages of vitmain D, is correctable with large doses of the drug.[67] The use of vitamin D metabolites instead of the parent compound greatly improves the chance of success while minimizing toxicity.[68] Vitamin D dependency (pseudodeficiency rickets), an autosomal recessive disorder, is also responsive to 1α-hydroxycholecalciferol,[69] a synthetic form of vitamin D_3. This synthetic derivative is also useful in children with chronic renal failure and hypoparathyroidism.[70]

Drug Interactions—Vitamin D and anticonvulsant drugs can interact significantly.[71–79] Osteomalacia has resulted from chronic therapy with anticonvulsants.[74,76,77] Barbiturate and hydantoin anticonvulsants may stimulate microsomal enzymes in the liver that inactivate vitamin D.[72,74] The exact mechanism of this drug-induced osteomalacia is unclear.[78] However, phenobarbital markedly decreases vitamin D plasma half-life and increases formation of biologically inactive vitamin D metabolites.[79] Anticonvulsants reported to interact with vitamin D include phenobarbital, phenytoin, phenaturide, and primidone.[75] Patients receiving such drugs require supplemental doses of vitamin D to maintain positive calcium balance and insure proper bone growth.[71]

Overdosage—Consumption of high doses of vitamin D results in several adverse effects,[80,81] including hypercalcemia[82–87] and metastatic calcification of soft tissue, kidneys, bronchi, arteries, and periauricular tissue.[84] Pancreatitis,[85] hypertension,[86] and renal failure secondary to nephrocalcinosis[84,87] also can follow excessively rapid increases in vitamin D dosage. Symptoms of overdosage include nausea, vomiting, constipation, abdominal pain, dehydration, polyuria, muscle weakness, anorexia, and headache.[88] Long-term consumption of high doses of vitamin D might increase the likelihood of myocardial infarction.[89]

VITAMIN E

Vitamin E, a fat-soluble vitamin, functions as an antioxidant. Of the eight known tocopherols, the alpha form, designated vitamin E, is the most powerful antioxidant. The vitamin is present in large quantities in vegetable oils, leafy vegetables, certain nuts, and whole cereal grains.

Deficiency—Vitamin E deficiency can occur in adults with intestinal malabsorption, in malnourished infants, and in preterm or other low weight neonates. Physical manifestations include edema of the legs, labia, scrotum, and eyelids; tachypnea; restlessness; and a watery nasal discharge.[90] Hemolytic anemia[90–92] is present, presumably due to oxidative damage to the erythrocyte membrane.

Vitamin E deficiency has been demonstrated in patients with long-standing obstructive jaundice, probably due to impaired absorption. Deficiency contributes to the decreased erythrocyte survival associated with the disease.[93]

Vitamin E deficiency may be an important feature of thalassemia.[94]

Indications—Besides its use in rare deficiency states, vitamin E has few indications. It has been advocated for use in several types of heart disease, including angina pectoris,[95] ischemic heart disease, and congestive heart failure. In a randomized double-blind trial, vitamin E was ineffective in the treatment of angina.[96] Long-term therapy with vitamin E may improve intermittent claudication.[97]

Infants with a birth weight below 2000 g should be given oral doses of alpha-tocopherol acetate, 5 to 25 IU per day, to reduce the risk of deficiency.[98] However, gastrointestinal absorption of currently available preparations is unpredictable and intramuscular administration may be preferable.[99]

Vitamin E, presently being sold in enormous amounts to the consuming public, has been claimed to be useful in curing skin problems, alleviating pain of arthritis, preventing ulcers, and improving sex drive. Despite an extensive examination of the medical literature the Food and Drug Administration has found no scientific evidence that vitamin E will do any of the dramatic things that it has been claimed to do.

Overdosage—There is little evidence that excessive amounts of vitamin E are harmful. However, impairment of wound healing in animals suggests caution during use of large doses.[100] In an uncontrolled study, weakness and fatigue accompanied supplementary vitamin E ingestion.[101]

Drug Interactions—In an anecdotal report, addition of vitamin E to the therapeutic regimen of a patient taking warfarin and clofibrate reduced levels of vitamin K-dependent coagulation factors leading to bleeding.[102]

Concurrent administration of iron (ferrous sulfate) and vitamin E during the first few months of life results in slightly impaired absorption of the vitamin.[103] In preterm infants requiring supplemental vitamin E, iron probably should be withheld until 3 months of age.[98]

WATER-SOLUBLE VITAMINS

THIAMINE HYDROCHLORIDE (Vitamin B_1)

Thiamine is present in practically all plant and animal tissues, particularly in rice and yeast. Breakfast foods, including bread and cereals, are enriched with thiamine.

Deficiency—Deficiency, referred to as beriberi, may take several forms. Dry beriberi consists of neuropathic changes, including paresthesias, muscle weakness and wasting, partial anesthesia, and wrist and foot drop.[104] Wet beriberi, also termed the cardiac edematous form, is a syndrome of edema and congestive heart failure. Impaired cortical function can also occur, resulting in Wernicke's and Korsakoff's syndromes. The most striking signs of these syndromes are forgetfulness, impaired intellectual function, nystagmus, and ataxia. Although thiamine administration may cure Wernicke's encephalopathy, Korsakoff's psychosis is often irreversible. Other symptoms of deficiency include anorexia, constipation, nausea and vomiting.[105]

Deficiency occurs in those areas of the world where a large portion of the diet consists of polished rice. Thiamine deficiency during pregnancy develops early and remains constant until delivery due to the ability of the fetus to sequester thiamine.[106] Chronic alcohol intake interferes with the absorption, intake, or utilization of thiamine, and alcoholics often have chronic thiamine deficiency.

Indications—In addition to overt deficiency, thiamine is indicated as general prophylaxis in pregnancy and chronic alcoholism.[107] In chronic alcoholics a daily dose of 5 to 10 mg is advised. In the acute alcoholic, 100 mg may be given intramuscularly or intravenously to potentially reverse neuropathies or central nervous system disturbances.

RIBOFLAVIN (Vitamin B_2)

Riboflavin is widely distributed in all leafy vegetables, in the flesh of warm blooded animals, and in fish. Deficiency results in both oral and ocular lesions. Oral lesions include glossitis, angular stomatitis, and cheilosis. Ocular changes are more serious, including photophobia, visual fatigue, burning of the eyes, and corneal vascularization. Deficiency is seen in chronic alcoholism and pregnancy. In a study of 651 pregnant women, 40% were significantly riboflavin-depleted.[108]

PYRIDOXINE HYDROCHLORIDE (Vitamin B_6)

Pyridoxine is present in low concentrations in all animal and plant tissues.

Deficiency—Deficiency is characterized by skin, central nervous system, and hematologic abnormalities. Seborrhea-like lesions are seen about the eyes, nose, and mouth, and glossitis and cheilosis may be present. Peripheral neuritis and, rarely, seizures may occur with drug-induced pyridoxine deficiency. Such chemical antagonists include desoxypyridoxine, isoniazid, hydralazine, and penicillamine. Hypochromic anemia and lymphopenia may also accompany pyridoxine deficiency.

Indications—Pyridoxine, 50 to 100 mg daily, is administered concurrently with isoniazid in the treatment of tuberculosis for prophylaxis against peripheral neuritis. Several inborn metabolic errors, including pyridoxine-dependent convulsions, benefit from large-dose therapy.[109] Pregnant women and women taking oral contraceptives require substantially larger amounts of vitamin B_6 to maintain adequate serum levels.[110,111] In pregnancy a daily intake of 2.5 mg is recommended, an increase of 0.5 mg over usual requirements.[112] Recently, pyridoxine reportedly reduced the severity of bronchial asthma in many, but not all, asthmatic children.[113]

Drug Interactions—Pyridoxine enhances peripheral metabolism of levodopa, thereby reducing the amount of levodopa available for transport into the brain.[114] A low pyridoxine plasma concentration was reported in a patient with parkinsonism who developed a burning sensation of his feet during levodopa therapy.[115] Patients on levodopa therapy are advised to avoid taking multivitamin preparations containing more than the recommended dietary allowance of pyridoxine.[116]

NIACIN (Nicotinic Acid)
NIACINAMIDE (Nicotinamide)

Niacin and niacinamide are found in various foodstuffs and in rich supply in meat, fish, and wheat.

Deficiency—Endemic in maize-eating areas, niacin deficiency (pellagra) is relatively rare in the United States. Clinical manifestations ('the three D's of pellagra') include: (1) Diarrhea, and other gastrointestinal disorders. (2) Dementia, including depression, memory loss, and confusion. (3) Dermatitis, which is the most striking. Pellagrous dermatitis is usually confined to light-exposed areas.

Indications—Niacin, but not nicotinamide, has been used as a so-called peripheral vasodilator, and to enhance cerebral blood flow in senile dementia.[117] Niacin has also been used in schizophrenia,[118,119] and as a hypocholesterolemic agent (see Chapter 44).[117] Adverse reactions limit its usefulness.

Adverse Reactions—In usual doses niacin causes pruritus and flushing, burning or tingling of the ears, face, and hands. Jaundice has also been reported following moderate doses.[120]

ASCORBIC ACID (Vitamin C)

Unlike most animal species, humans are unable to synthesize vitamin C and therefore must acquire it from dietary sources. The vitamin is found in oranges and other citrus fruits, melons, tomatoes, broccoli, asparagus, cabbage, berries, brussel sprouts, and cauliflower.[121,122]

The recommended dietary allowance of vitamin C for infants and children is 35 to 40 mg daily. In adults, 45 mg per day will maintain an adequate body supply,[123] while in pregnancy a higher dose (60 mg) is recommended.[124] With an adequate diet, supplemental sources are unnecessary.

Deficiency—Long-term deficiency of vitamin C results in scurvy. Characteristics of scurvy include excessive capillary bleeding, defective wound healing, disturbances of bone growth, loosening of the teeth secondary to gum changes, muscle weakness, hyperkeratosis, petechiae, ecchymoses, and arthralgias.[125,126]

Reduced levels of ascorbic acid have been found in women taking contraceptive pills,[125,127] chronic alcoholics,[128] and in patients with peptic ulcer disease, regional enteritis,[129] malabsorption syndromes, and primary biliary cirrhosis.[130] Coronary atherosclerosis could be caused by a long-term deficiency of ascorbic acid.[131–133]

Indications—Except for scurvy, which can be prevented by the administration of 10 mg daily,[134] vitamin C has few clinically proven indications. Since vitamin C is essential for proper wound healing,[135] extensively burned patients may benefit from its usage. Postsurgical patients[136] and those with decubitus ulcers[137] may similarly benefit. A recent report suggests a possible therapeutic effect of vitamin C in the treatment of lepromatous leprosy.[138]

Pauling has advocated daily ingestion of 1 to 3 g of vitamin C as protection against the common cold,[139] but the studies cited by Pauling to support his claims have defects in design or reporting that rendered their results uninterpretable.[140–142] Some investigations demonstrate no efficacy of vitamin C against the common cold,[143–147] while others have shown that vitamin C does not prevent the appearance of the common cold but may reduce cold symptoms.[148,149] An attempt at replication of one such study failed to confirm the initial findings.[147] Thus, usage of ascorbic acid in any dosage for the treatment and/or prophylaxis of the common cold appears unjustified.

Vitamin C has been used to acidify the urine in patients susceptible to urinary tract infections and those taking prophylactic urinary tract antiseptics such as methenamine mandelate (Mandelamine).

Adverse Reactions—Very large doses of ascorbic acid may be harmful,[150–152] leading to hyperoxaluria by degradation to its metabolite oxalate.[153,154] Theoretically, attacks of gouty arthritis or renal calculi could be potentiated in predisposed persons,[155] but this has not been reported even with doses of 3 to 30 g per day.[156,157] A common side effect of large doses is diarrhea.[157]

Drug Interactions—Vitamin C, 1 g daily, reportedly inactivates substantial amounts of vitamin B_{12} when ingested with food;[158] others refute this claim.[159] The vitamin may increase iron absorption.[160] Anecdotal reports suggest a possible interaction with warfarin. One patient's prothrombin time was shortened following concurrent administration of ascorbic acid and the anticoagulant.[161] A similar report found no such interference.[162] Unusual resistance to warfarin in a patient consuming large amounts of vitamin C has been observed.[163]

Laboratory Test Interactions—Vitamin C causes false negative results when testing for urinary glucose with glucose oxidase enzyme strips (Bili Labstix). The vitamin also causes false positive results of the copper reduction test (Clinitest) for determining urine glucose.[164]

MULTIVITAMINS

Although oral multiple-vitamin preparations are widely advertised and accepted by the public as useful, clinical proof of their value is lacking. The primary therapeutic use of individual vitamins is to correct specific deficiency states. Deficiency may be due to genetic factors, insufficient dietary intake, or malabsorption. Deficiency states requiring replacement with both fat-soluble and water-soluble vitamins, as found in many popular multiple-vitamin preparations are not identified.

Fat-soluble vitamins are stored in the liver, and, under conditions of dietary deprivation, are utilized. Deficiencies are exceedingly rare, and, since urinary excretion is minimal, toxicity may occur when they are taken to excess.[165,166] Water-soluble vitamins, on the other hand, are readily excreted in the urine, and blood levels may fall following reduced intake or under stressful conditions.

Multiple-vitamin supplements are widely used to prevent vitamin deficiency during pregnancy[167] and lactation, in chronic alcoholics, during weight reduction,[168] in the elderly, in a variety of intercurrent illnesses (both brief and prolonged) and with oral contraceptive use.[169] However, there is no evidence that vitamin preparations are needed in these situations. Examples of widely used multivitamin preparations

TABLE 1 Preparations and Costs of Vitamins

Generic Name	Trademark Name(s)	Preparations and 1978 Costs
Lipid-Soluble		
Vitamin A	generic	Capsules 10,000 units—$0.95–$2.98/100; 25,000 units—$2.98/100; 50,000 units—$1.50–$3.60/100
	Aquasol-A	Drops 5,000 units/ml—$6.55/30 ml
		Injection (solution) 50,000 units/ml—$4.22/5-ml vial
	generic	Cream 100,000 units/oz—$0.46/½ oz; $1.25/2 oz; $5.25/1 lb; $21.00/5 lb
		Lotion 100,000 units/oz—$1.00/4 oz
Ergocalciferol (Vitamin D_2)	Deltalin Drisdol Calciferol	Capsules 50,000 units—$3.74/100
		Liquid 8,000 units/ml—$5.89/60 ml
		Injection (oil) 500,000 units—$5.50/10 ml
Vitamin E (Alpha-tocopherol)	Aquasol E (E-Ferol) (Eprolin)	Capsules 30 units—$3.66/100; 100 units—$8.52/100; 400 units—$4.68/100
		Drops 50 units/ml—$2.16 ea
		Elixir 33.3 units/5 ml—$3.18/ 8 oz
	E-Ferol	Injection (solution) 200 mg/ml—$2.88/10-ml vial
Water-Soluble		
Thiamine Hydrochloride (Vitamin B_1)	generic (Betalin S) (Bewon)	Tablets 10 mg—$0.30–$0.85/100; 25 mg—$0.35–$0.98/100; 50 mg—$0.55–$1.35/100; 100 mg—$0.80–$1.60/100; 250 mg—$1.50–$3.60/100
		Injection (solution) 100 mg/ml—$0.27–$0.47/1-ml ampul; $0.80–$1.21/10 ml vial; $1.88–$2.19/20 ml vial; $0.80–$2.48/30-ml vial; 200 mg/ml—$0.90–$0.93/30-ml vial
Riboflavin (Vitamin B_2)	generic	Tablets 5 mg—$0.50–$1.35/100; 10 mg—$0.45–$1.86/100; 25 mg—$0.70–$1.95/100

TABLE 1 *(continued)*

Generic Name	Trademark Name(s)	Preparations and 1978 Costs
Pyridoxine Hydrochloride (Vitamin B_6)	generic (Hexa-Betalin) (Hexavibex)	Tablets 10 mg—\$0.48–\$1.13/100; 25 mg—\$0.70–\$1.35/100; 50 mg—\$0.82–\$2.10/100; 100 mg—\$1.35–\$3.35/100 Injection (solution) 50 mg/ml—\$0.83/10-ml vial; 100 mg/ml—\$0.75–\$3.30/10-ml vial; \$2.50–\$3.10/30 ml vial
Niacin	generic	Tablets 25 mg—\$0.30–\$0.71/100; 50 mg—\$0.40–\$1.25/100; 100 mg—\$0.59–\$2.10/100; 500 mg—\$1.33–\$2.28/100 Injection (solution, sodium salt) 10 mg/ml—\$0.72/10-ml vial
Niacinamide	generic	Tablets 25 mg—\$0.30–\$0.63/100; 50 mg—\$0.40–\$1.25/100; 100 mg—\$0.50–\$1.06/100; 500 mg—\$1.00–\$2.42/100 Injection (solution) 100 mg/ml—\$1.02/5-ml vial
Ascorbic Acid (Vitamin C)	generic	Tablets 50 mg—\$0.772/100; 100 mg—\$0.52–\$1.18/100; 250 mg—\$0.70–\$1.77/100; 500 mg—\$1.00–\$2.90/100
	Cevalon	Injection 50 mg/ml—\$0.57/10-ml vial; 500 mg/ml—\$0.34/1-ml ampul

containing the water-soluble vitamins include: Allbee with C, Becotin with C, Berocca C, and Stresscaps.

Obstetricians commonly prescribe vitamin and mineral supplements during pregnancy to insure adequate levels of nutrients to both mother and fetus. Again, there is no evidence that such supplements are needed. Although vitamin deficiency has been recognized during pregnancy in poorly nourished women,[170] the vitamins in the standard diet of the average American are more than sufficient for normal fetal development. Supplementation may in fact increase the likelihood of

TABLE 2 Recommended Daily Dietary Allowances[a]

	Weight (kg)	Height (cm)	A (IU)	D (IU)	E (IU)	Ascorbic Acid (mg)	Thiamine B_1 (mg)	Riboflavin B_2 (mg)	Pyroxidine B_6 (mg)	Niacin (mg)
Infants (0–1 yr)	6–9	60–71	2000	400	4–5	35	0.3–0.5	0.4–0.6	0.3–0.4	5–8
Children (1–10 yr)	13–30	86–135	2000–3800	400	7–10	40	0.7–1.2	0.8–1.2	0.6–1.2	9–16
Males										
11–50 yr	44–67	158–172	5000	400	12–15	45	1.4–1.5	1.5–1.8	1.6–2.0	18–20
51+ yr	70	172	5000	—	15	45	1.2	1.5	2.0	16
Females										
11–50 yr	44–58	155–162	4000	400	12	45	1.0–1.2	1.2–1.4	1.6–2.0	13–16
51+ yr	58	162	4000	—	12	45	1.0	1.1	2.0	12
Lactating			6000	400	15	80	1.3–1.5	0.5	2.5	4
Pregnant			5000	500	15	60	1.3–1.5	0.3	2.5	2

[a] Adapted from Food and Nutrition Board, Academy of Sciences—National Research Council *Recommended Daily Dietary Allowances,* revised 1974.

hypervitaminosis.[171,172] When a proper maternal diet cannot be achieved, the direct relationship between the rapid equilibration of vitamins between maternal and fetal circulations suggests that supplementation may be enhanced.[173,174] Oral or parenteral supplementation following birth of a premature infant may also be appropriate.[167]

Because some elderly persons have erratic dietary habits, a multivitamin supplement with iron may be the safest and least expensive way to prevent nutritional deficiency and anemia.[175] Malabsorption syndromes, being more common in the geriatric population, can necessitate multivitamin supplementation.[177] However, the majority of elderly persons consuming a well-balanced diet have no greater need for vitamins than do other adults. Deficiency states of fat-soluble vitamins (A, D and E), are exceedingly rare and toxicity may occur with continued supplementation. Water-soluble vitamins (B vitamins and C), in contrast, are eliminated in the urine relatively rapidly, but excessive supplementation of these vitamins in the elderly can also lead to toxicity because of the reduction of renal function associated with aging.

Surgeons often administer intravenous supplements of water-soluble vitamins postoperatively, with the rationale that many patients are already deficient in some essential nutrients and that their postoperative nutrition may be inadequate for some days. This practice has questionable justification.[178]

Because women taking oral contraceptives often have reduced body levels of thiamine, riboflavin, pyridoxine, folic acid and ascorbic acid, daily supplementation with these vitamins might theoretically be beneficial.[179–182] Berocca Tablets (Roche) is one such combination product containing these vitamins. In contrast, body levels of the lipid-soluble vitamins A and E are significantly higher in oral contraceptive users than in non-users.[183,184]

Multivitamin preparations are often used indiscriminately and unjustifiably, are a waste of money, and may constitute an obstacle to nutrition education. Many people would prefer to rely on an all-inclusive dose of a supplement than to make sure that they eat a well-balanced diet.[185]

REFERENCES

1. DeLuca HF: Functions of the fat-soluble vitamins. Am J Clin Nutr 28:339–345, 1975.
2. Oomen HA: Clinical epidemiology of xerophthalmia in man. Am J Clin Nutr 22:1098–2005, 1969.

3. McLaren DS, Oomen HA, Escapini H: Ocular manifestations of vitamin A deficiency in man. Bull WHO 34:357–361, 1966.
4. Patwardhan VN: Hypovitaminosis A and epidemiology of xerophthalmia. Am J Clin Nutr 22:1106–1118, 1969.
5. Hecht S: Rods, cones, and chemical basis of vision. Physiol Rev 17:239–290, 1937.
6. McDonald R, Adler FH: Effect of anoxemia on the dark adaptation of normal and of the vitamin A deficient subject. Arch Opthalmol 22:980, 1939.
7. Noell WK, Albrecht R: Vitamin A deficiency effect on retina: dependence on light. Science 172:72–80, 1971.
8. Lyle TK, Cross AG, Cook CAG: *May and Worth's Manual of Diseases of the Eye,* 13th Edition. Philadelphia, F.A. Davis Company, 1968, pp 177, 202, 704.
9. Grayson M, Keats RH: *Manual of Diseases of the Cornea.Boston, Little Brown, 1969, p. 189.*
10. DeLuca L, Maestri N, Bonanni F, et al: Maintenance of epithelial cell differentiation: the mode of action of vitamin A. Cancer 30:1326–1331, 1972.
11. Korting GW: *The Skin and Eye.* Philadelphia, W.B. Saunders, 1973, pp 133–134.
12. Anon: Vitamin A and the skin. Br J Dermatol 82:197–199, 1970.
13. Wolbach SB: Vitamin A deficiency and excess in relation to skeletal growth. J Bone Joint Surg 45:171–192, 1947.
14. Mellanby E: *A Story of Nutritional Research.* Baltimore, Williams & Wilkins, 1950.
15. Bourne GH: *The Biochemistry and Physiology of Bone,* 2nd Edition. New York, Academic Press, 1972, pp 203–204.
16. Gopalan C, Venkatchalam PS, Bhavani B: Studies of vitamin A deficiency in children. Am J Clin Nutr 8:833–840, 1960.
17. Roels OA, Trout ME, Dvjaquier R: Carotene balances on boys in Ruanda where vitamin A deficiency is prevalent. J Nutr 65:115–127, 1958.
18. Swaminathan MC, Susheela TP, Thimmayamma BVS: Field prophylactic trial with a single annual oral massive dose of vitamin A. Am J Clin Nutr 23:119–122, 1970.
19. Sharman IM: An unusual case of self-imposed vitamin A deficiency. Am J Clin Nutr 22:1134, 1969.
20. Ames SR: Factors affecting absorption, transport and storage of vitamin A. Am J Clin Nutr 22:934–935, 1969.
21. Mali JWH, Mier PD: Vitamin A preparations in dermatological practice. Int J Dermatol 14:198–200, 1975.
22. Ehrlich HP, Hunt HK: The effects of cortisone and anabolic steroids on the tensile strength of healing wounds. Ann Surg 170:203–206, 1969.
23. Gunther SH: Vitamin A acid in treatment of oral lichen planus. Arch Dermatol 107:277, 1973.
24. Gunther SH: Vitamin A acid in the treatment of palmoplantar keratoderma. Arch Dermatol 106:854–857, 1972.
25. Bradford LG, Montes LF: Topical application of vitamin A acid in acne vulgaris. South Med J 67:683–687, 1974.
26. Christiansen JV, Gadborg E, Ludvigsen K, et al: Topical vitamin A acid and systemic oxytetracycline in the treatment of acne vulgaris—a controlled clinical trial. Dermatologica 149:121–128, 1974.
27. Kane EK: *Arctic Explorations in the Years 1853, 1854, 1855, Volume I.* Philadelphia, Childs & Peterson, 1856, p. 392.
28. Knudson AG, Rothman PE: Hypervitaminosis A: a review with a discussion of vitamin A. Am J Dis Child 85:316–334, 1953.
29. Persson BR, Tunell E, Kengren K: Chronic vitamin A intoxication during the first half year of life. Acta Pediatr Scand 54:49–60, 1965.
30. Marie J, See G: Acute hypervitaminosis A of the infants: its clinical manifestations with benign acute hydrocephalus and pronounced bulge of the fontanelle—a clinical and biological study. Am J Dis Child 87:731–736, 1954.
31. Gerber A, Raab AP, Subel AE: Vitamin A poisoning in adults. Am J Med 16:729–745, 1954.
32. Joseph HW: Hypervitaminosis A and carotenemia. Am J Dis Child 67:33–43, 1944.
33. Sulzberger MD, Lazar MP: Hypervitaminosis A: report of a case in an adult. JAMA 146:788–793, 1951.
34. Bergen SS, Roels OA: Hypervitaminosis A: report of a case. Am J Clin Nutr 16:265–269, 1965.

35. Morrice G Jr, Havener WH, Kapetansky F: Vitamin A intoxication as a cause of pseudotumor cerebri. JAMA 173:1802–1805, 1960.
36. Russell RM, Boyer JL, Bagheri SA, et al: Hepatic injury from chronic hypervitaminosis A resulting in portal hypertension and ascites. N Engl J Med 291:435–440, 1974.
37. Dibenedetto RJ: Chronic hypervitaminosis A in an adult. JAMA 201:130–132, 1967.
38. Mikkelsen B, Ehlers N, Thomsen HG: Vitamin A intoxication causing papilledema and simulating acute encephalitis. Acta Neurol Scand 50:642–650, 1974.
39. Muenter MD, Perry HO, Ludwig J: Chronic vitamin A intoxication in adults. Am J Med 50:129–136, 1971.
40. Stimson WH: Vitamin A intoxication in adults: report of a case with a summary of the literature. N Engl J Med 265:369–373, 1961.
41. McLaughlin M, Fairney A, Lester E, et al: Seasonal variations in serum 25-hydroxycholecalciferol in healthy people. Lancet 1:536–538, 1974.
42. Gupta MM, Round JM, Stamp TCB: Spontaneous cure of vitamin D deficiency in Asians during summer in Britain. Lancet 1:586–589, 1974.
43. Ponchon G, Kennan AL, DeLuca HF: Activation of vitamin D by the liver. J Clin Invest 48:2032–2037, 1969.
44. Olson EB Jr, Knutson JC, Bhattacharyya MH, et al: The effect of hepatectomy on the synthesis of 25-hydroxyvitamin D_3. J Clin Invest 57:1213–1220, 1976.
45. DeLuca HF: 25-Hydroxycholecalciferol. Arch Intern Med 124:442–450, 1969.
46. Blunt JW, DeLuca HF, Schnoes HK: 25-Hydroxycholecalciferol. A biologically active metabolite of vitamin D_3. Biochemistry 7:3317–3322, 1968.
47. Ponchon G, DeLuca HF: The role of the liver in the metabolism of vitamin D. J Clin Invest 48:1273–1279, 1969.
48. DeLuca HF: The kidney as an endocrine organ involved in the function of vitamin D. Am J Med 58:39–47, 1975.
49. DeLuca HF: Vitamin D endocrinology. Ann Intern Med 85:367–377, 1976.
50. Ponchon G, DeLuca HF: Metabolities of vitamin D_3 and their biologic activity. J Nutr 99:157–167, 1969.
51. Committee on Nutrition, American Academy of Pediatrics: The proplylactic requirement and the toxicity of vitamin D. Pediatrics 31:512–525, 1963.
52. Stamp TCB, Exton-Smith AN, Richens A: Classical rickets and osteomalacia in Britain. Lancet 2:308, 1976.
53. Richens A, Rowe DJF: Disturbance of calcium metabolism by anticonvulsant drugs. Br Med J 4:73–76, 1970.
54. Richens A, Rowe DJF: Anticonvulsant osteomalacia. Br Med J 4:684–685, 1971.
55. Goel KM, Logan RW, Arneil GC, et al: Florid and subclinical rickets among immigrant children in Glascow. Lancet 1:1141–1145, 1976.
56. Morgan DB, Paterson CR, Pulvertaft CN, et al: Osteomalacia after gastrectomy. Lancet 2:1089–1091, 1965.
57. Wortsman J, Pack CYC, Bartter FC, et al: Pathogenesis of osteomalacia in secondary hyperparathyroidism after gastrectomy. Am J Med 52:556–564, 1972.
58. Atkinson M, Nordin BEC, Sherlock S: Malabsorption and bone disease in prolonged obstructive jaundice. Q J Med 25:299–312, 1956.
59. Kehayoglou AK, Agnew JE, Holdsworth CD, et al: Bone disease and calcium absorption in primary biliary cirrhosis. Lancet 1:715–719, 1968.
60. Guignard JP, Torrado A: Proximal renal tubular acidosis in vitamin D deficient rickets. Acta Pediatr Scand 62:543–546, 1973.
61. Chesney RW, Harrison HE: Fanconi syndrome following bowel surgery and hepatitis reversed by 25-hydroxycholecalciferol. J Pediatr 86:857–861, 1975.
62. Rosen JF, Roginsky M, Nathenson G, et al: 25-Hydroxyvitamin D plasma levels in mothers and their premature infants with neonatal hypocalcemia. Am J Dis Child 127:220–223, 1974.
63. Christiansen C, Rodbro P, Sjo O: 'Anticonvulsant action' of vitamin D in epileptic patients? A controlled pilot study. Br Med J 2:258–259, 1974.
64. Christiansen C, Rodbro P: Effect of vitamin D_2 on serum phenytoin. A controlled therapeutic trial. Acta Neurol Scand 50:661–664, 1974.
65. Teitelbaum SL, Bone JM, Stein PM, et al: Calcifediol in chronic renal insufficiency. JAMA 235:164–167, 1976.

66. Avioli LV, Birge SJ, Slatopolsky E: The nature of vitamin D resistance of patients with chronic renal disease. Arch Intern Med 124:451–454, 1969.
67. Brickman AS, Coburn JW, Kurokawa K, et al: Actions of 1,25-dihydroxycholecalciferol in patients with hypophosphatemic, vitamin-D-resistant rickets. N Engl J Med 289:495–498, 1973.
68. DeLuca HF: Vitamin D today. Disease-A-Month, 28–33, March, 1975.
69. Reade TM, Scriver CR, Glorieux FH, et al: Response to crystalline 1α-hydroxyvitamin D_3 in vitamin D dependency. Pediatr Res 9:593–599, 1975.
70. Balsan S, Garabedian M, Sorgniard R, et al: 1,25-Dihydroxyvitamin D_3 and 1α-hydroxyvitamin D_3 in children: biologic and therapeutic effects in nutritional rickets and different types of vitamin D resistance. Pediatr Res 9:586–593, 1975.
71. Peterson P, Gray P, Tolman KG: Calcium balance in drug-induced osteomalacia: response to vitamin D. Clin Pharmacol Ther 19:63–67, 1976.
72. Hunter J, Maxwell JD, Stewart DA, et al: Altered calcium metabolism in epileptic children on anticonvulsants. Br Med J 4:202–204, 1971.
73. Hahn TJ, Hendin BA, Scharp CR, et al: Effect of chronic anticonvulsant therapy on serum 25-hydroxycholecalciferol levels in adults. N Engl J Med 287:900–904, 1972.
74. Dent CE, Richens A, Rowe DJF, et al: Osteomalacia with long-term anticonvulsant therapy in epilepsy. Br Med J 4:69–72, 1970.
75. Richens A, Rowe DJF: Disturbance of calcium metabolism by anticonvulsant drugs. Br Med J 4:73–76, 1970.
76. Tolman KG, Jubiz W, Sannella JJ, et al: Osteomalacia associated with anticonvulsant drug therapy in mentally retarded children. Pediatrics 56:45–51, 1975.
77. Hahn TJ, Hendin BA, Scharp CR, et al: Serum 25-hydroxycalciferol levels and bone mass in children on chronic anticonvulsant therapy. N Engl J Med 292:550–554, 1975.
78. Burt R, Freston JW, Tolman KG: The influence of phenobarbital on biotransformation of 25-hydroxycholecalciferol. J Clin Pharmacol 16:393–398, 1976.
79. Hahn TJ: Anticonvulsant therapy and vitamin D. Ann Intern Med 78:308–309, 1973.
80. Food and Nutrition Board, National Research Council: Hazards of overuse of vitamin D. Am J Clin Nutr 28:512–513, 1975.
81. Committee on Nutrition: The prophylactic requirement and the toxicity of vitamin D. Pediatrics 31:512–525, 1963.
82. Shetty KR, Ajlouni K, Rosenfeld PS, et al: Protracted vitamin D intoxication. Arch Intern Med 135:986–988, 1975.
83. Counts SJ, Baylink DJ, Shen FH, et al: Vitamin D intoxication in an anephric child. Ann Intern Med 82:196–200, 1975.
84. Irnell L: Metastatic calcification of soft tissue on overdosage of vitamin D. Acta Med Scand 185:147–152, 1969.
85. Leeson PM, Fourman P: Acute pancreatitis from vitamin D poisoning in a patient with parathyroid deficiency. Lancet 1:1185–1186, 1966.
86. Blum M, Kirsten M, Worth MH: Reversible hypertension. JAMA 237:262–263, 1977.
87. Leeson PM, Fourman P: Increased sensitivity to vitamin D after vitamin D poisoning. Lancet 1:1182–1185, 1966.
88. Palmisano PA: Vitamin D: a reawakening. JAMA 224:1526–1527, 1973.
89. Linden V: Vitamin D and myocardial infarction. Br Med J 3:647–650, 1974.
90. Ritchie JH, Fish MG, McMaster V, et al: Edema and hemolytic anemia in premature infants, a vitamin E deficiency syndrome. N Engl J Med 279:1185–1190, 1968.
91. Melhorn DK, Gross S, Childres G: Vitamin E dependent anemia in the premature infant. I. Effects of large doses of medicinal iron. J Pediatr 79:569–580, 1971.
92. Hassan H, Hashim SA, VanItallie TB, et al: Syndrome in premature infants associated with low plasma vitamin E levels and high polyunsaturated fat diet. Am J Clin Nutr 19:147–157, 1966.
93. Powell LW: Vitamin E deficiency in human liver disease and its relation to haemolysis. Aust NZ J Med 3:355–360, 1973.
94. Zannos-Mariolea L, Tzortzatov F, Dendaki-Svalaki K, et al: Serum vitamin E levels with beta-thallasemia major: preliminary report. Br J Haematol 26:193–199, 1974.
95. Toone WM: Effects of vitamin E: good and bad (letter). N Engl J Med 289:979–980, 1973.
96. Anderson TW: Vitamin E in angina pectoris. Can Med Assoc J 110:401–406, 1974.
97. Haeger K: Long-time treatment of intermittent claudication with vitamin E. Am J Clin Nutr 27:1179–1181, 1974.

98. Dallman PR: Iron, vitamin E, and folate in the preterm infant. J Pediatr 85:742–752, 1974.
99. Graeber JE, Williams ML, Oski FA: The use of intramuscular vitamin E in the premature infant. J Pediatr 90:282–284, 1977.
100. Ehrlich HP, Tarver H, Hunt TK: Inhibitory effects of vitamin E on collagen synthesis and wound repair. Ann Surg 175:235–240, 1972.
101. Cohen HM: Effects of vitamin E: good and bad (letter). N Engl J Med 289:980, 1973.
102. Corrigan JJ, Marcus FI: Coagulopathy associated with vitamin E ingestion. JAMA 230:1300–1301, 1974.
103. Melhorn DK, Gross S, Childers G: Vitamin E-dependent anemia in the premature infant. II. Relationships between gestational age and absorption of vitamin E. J Pediatr 79:581–588, 1971.
104. vonMuralt H: The role of thiamine in neurophysiology. Ann NY Acad Sci 98:499–507, 1962.
105. Sebrell WH Jr: A clinical evaluation of thiamine deficiency. Ann NY Acad Sci 98:563–567, 1962.
106. Heller S, Sakeld RM, Korner WF: Vitamin B_1 status in pregnancy. Am J Clin Nutr 27:1221–1224, 1974.
107. Zbinden G: Therapeutic use of vitamin B_1 in diseases other than beriberi. Ann NY Acad Sci 98:550–561, 1962.
108. Heller S, Salkeld RM, Korner WF: Riboflavin status in pregnancy. Am J Clin Nutr 27:1225–1230, 1974.
109. Hunt AD Jr, Stokes J, McGrory WW, et al: Pyridoxine dependency: report of a case of intractable convulsions in an infant controlled by pyridoxine. Pediatrics 13:140–145, 1945.
110. Anon: Requirements of vitamin B during pregnancy. Nutr Rev 34:15–16, 1976.
111. Driskell JA, Geders JM, Urban MC: Vitamin B_6 status of young men, women, and women using oral contraceptives. J Lab Clin Med 87:813–821, 1976.
112. National Academy of Sciences, National Research Council, Food and Nutrition Board: Recommended Dietary Allowances, Ed. 8, NAS ISBN 0–309–02216–9, pp 1–20, 25–48, 74–77, 1974.
113. Collipp PJ, Goldzier S, Weiss N, et al: Pyridoxine treatment of childhood bronchial asthma. Ann Allergy 35:93–97, 1975.
114. Van Woert MH: Low pyridoxine diet in parkinsonism (letter). JAMA 219:1211, 1972.
115. Golden RL, Mortati FS, Schroeter GA: Levodopa, pyridoxine, and the burning feet syndrome (letter). JAMA 213:628, 1970.
116. Duvoisin RC, Yahr MD, Cote LD: Pyridoxine reversal of L-dopa effects on parkinsonism. Trans Am Neurol Assoc 94:81–84, 1969.
117. Darby WJ, McNutt KW, Todhunter EN: Niacin. Nutr Rev 33:289–297, 1975.
118. Wittenborn JR, Weber ESP, Brown M: Niacin in the long-term treatment of schizophrenia. Arch Gen Psychiatry 28:308–315, 1973.
119. Wittenborn JR: A search for responders to niacin supplementation. Arch Gen Psychiatry 31:547–552, 1974.
120. Sugerman AA, Clark CG: Jaundice following the administration of niacin. JAMA 228:202, 1974.
121. Dillon HL: Recommended daily allowances of vitamins C and D for infants and children. JAMA 235:859, 1976.
122. Horowitz I, Fabry EM, Gerson CD: Bioavailability of ascorbic acid in orange juice. JAMA 235:2624–2625, 1976.
123. Harper AE: The recommended dietary allowances for ascorbic acid. Ann NY Acad Sci 58:491–497, 1975.
124. Rivers JM, Devine MM: Relationships of ascorbic acid to pregnancy, and oral contraceptive steroids. Ann NY Acad Sci 58:465–482, 1975.
125. Barnes MJ: Function of ascorbic acid in collagen metabolism. Ann NY Acad Sci 58:264–277, 1975.
126. Hodges RE, Hood J, Canham JE, et al: Clinical manifestations of ascorbic acid deficiency in man. Am J Clin Nutr 24:432–443, 1971.
127. Horwitt MK, Harvey CC, Dahm CH: Relationship between levels of blood lipids, vitamins C, A, and E, serum copper compounds and urinary excretions of tryptophan metabolites in women taking oral contraceptive therapy. Am J Clin Nutr 28:403–412, 1975.

128. O'Keane M, Russell RI, Goldberg A: Ascorbic acid status of alcoholics. J Alcoholism, 7:6–11, 1972.
129. Gerson CD: Ascorbic acid deficiency in clinical disease including regional enteritis. Ann NY Acad Sci 258:483–490, 1975.
130. Beattie AD, Sherlock S: Ascorbic acid deficiency in liver disease. Gut 17:571–575, 1976.
131. Sokoloff B, Hori M, Saelhof CC, et al: Aging, atherosclerosis and ascorbic acid metabolism. J Am Geriatr Soc 14:1239–1260, 1966.
132. Shaffer CF: Ascorbic acid and atherosclerosis. Am J Clin Nutr 23:27–30, 1970.
133. Spittle CR: Atherosclerosis and vitamin C. Lancet 2:1280–1281, 1971.
134. Goldsmith GA: Human requirements for vitamin C and its use in clinical medicine. Ann NY Acad Sci 92:230–245, 1961.
135. Schwartz PL: Ascorbic acid in wound healing—a review. J Am Diet Assoc 56:477–503, 1970.
136. Cranden JH, Lennihan R, Mikal S, et al: Ascorbic acid economy in surgical patients. Ann NY Acad Sci 92:246–267, 1961.
137. Taylor TV, Rimmer S, Day B, et al: Ascorbic acid supplementation in the treatment of pressure-sores. Lancet 2:544–546, 1974.
138. Skinshes OK: Vitamin C for patients with leprosy. JAMA 233:188, 1975.
139. Pauling L: *Vitamin C and the Common Cold.* San Francisco, W.H. Freeman, 1970, pp 26–38.
140. Anon: Vitamin C and the common cold. Med Lett Drugs Ther 12:105–106, 1970.
141. Anon: Vitamin C—were the trials well controlled and are large doses safe? Med Lett Drugs Ther 13:46–48, 1971.
142. Beaton GH, Whalen S: Vitamin C and the common cold. Can Med Assoc J 105:355–357, 363, 1971.
143. Dykes MHM, Meier P: Ascorbic acid and the common cold. JAMA 231:1073–1079, 1975.
144. Karlowski TR, Chalmers TC, Frenkel LD, et al: Ascorbic acid for the common cold. JAMA 231:1038–1042, 1975.
145. Chalmers TC: Effects of ascorbic acid on the common cold. Am J Med 58:532–536, 1975.
146. Schwartz AR, Togo Y, Harnsky RB, et al: Evaluation of the efficacy of ascorbic acid in prophylaxis of induced rhinovirus 44 infection in man. J Infect Dis 128:500–505, 1973.
147. Coulehan JL, Eberhard S, Kapner L, et al: Vitamin C and acute illness in Navajo schoolchildren. N Engl J Med 295:973–977, 1976.
148. Anderson TW, Reid DBW, Beaton GH: Vitamin C and the common cold: a double blind trial. Can Med Assoc J 107:503–508, 1972.
149. Coulehan JL, Reisinger KS, Rogers KD, et al: Vitamin C prophylaxis in a boarding school. N Engl J Med 290:6–10, 1974.
150. Lamden MP: Dangers of massive vitamin C intake. N Engl J Med 284:336–337, 1971.
151. Brown RG: Possible problems of large intakes of ascorbic acid. JAMA 224:1529–1530, 1973.
152. Rhead WJ, Schrauzer GN: Risks of long-term ascorbic acid overdosage. Nutr Rev 29:262–263, 1971.
153. Smith LH, Fromm H, Hofmann AF: Acquired hyperoxaluria, nephrolithiasis, and intestinal disease. N Engl J Med 286:1371–1375, 1972.
154. Baker EM, Saari JC, Tolbert BM: Ascorbic acid metabolism in man. Am J Clin Nutr 19:371–378, 1966.
155. Stein HB, Hasan A, Fox IH: Ascorbic acid-induced uricosuria. Ann Intern Med 84:385–388, 1976.
156. Poser E: Large ascorbic acid intake (letter). N Engl J Med 287:412, 1972.
157. Hoffer A: Ascorbic acid and toxicity. N Engl J Med 285:635–636, 1971.
158. Herbert V, Jacob E: Destruction of vitamin B_{12} by ascorbic acid. JAMA 230:241–242, 1974.
159. Newmark HL, Scheiner J, Marcus M, et al: Stability of vitamin B_{12} in the presence of ascorbic acid. Am J Clin Nutr 29:645–649, 1976.
160. Cook JD, Monsen ER: Vitamin C, the common cold, and iron absorption. Am J Clin Nutr 30:235–241, 1977.
161. Rosenthal G: Interaction of ascorbic acid and warfarin (letter). JAMA 215:1671, 1971.
162. Hume R. Johnstone JMS, Weyers E: Interaction of ascorbic acid and warfarin (letter). JAMA 219:1479, 1972.
163. Smith EC, Skalski RJ, Johnson GC, et al: Interaction of ascorbic acid and warfarin (letter). JAMA 221:1166, 1972.

164. Mayson JS, Schumaker O, Nakamura RM: False negative tests for urinary glucose in the presence of ascorbic acid. Am J Clin Pathol 58:297–299, 1972.
165. Pitkin RM: Vitamins and minerals in pregnancy. Clin Perinatol 2:221–232, 1975.
166. Kopple JD, Swendseid ME: Vitamin nutrition in patients undergoing maintenance hemodialysis. Kidney Int 7(Suppl 2):79–84, 1975.
167. Malone JI: Vitamin passage across the placenta. Clin Perinatol 2:295–307, 1975.
168. Griboff SI, Berman R: A double blind clinical evaluation of a phenylpropanolamine-caffeine-vitamin combination and a placebo in the treatment of exogenous obesity. Curr Ther Res 17:535–543, 1975.
169. Larsson-Cohn U: Some effects of oral contraceptives on vitamins and on carbohydrate and lipid metabolism. Acta Obstet Gynecol Scand 54(Suppl):5–12, 1976.
170. Kaminetzky HA, Langer A, Baker H, et al: The effect of nutrition in teen-age gravidas on pregnancy and the status of the neonate. Am J Obstet Gynecol 115:639–646, 1973.
171. Thompson MF, Morse EH, Merrow SB: Nutrient intake of pregnant women receiving vitamin-mineral supplements. J Am Diet Assoc 64:382–385, 1974.
172. Averback P: Anencephaly associated with megavitamin therapy (letter). Can Med Assoc J 114:995, 1976.
173. Baker H, Frank O, Thomson AD, et al: Vitamin profile of 174 mothers and newborns at parturition. Am J Clin Nutr 28:59–65, 1975.
174. Kaminetzky HA, Baker H, Frank O, et al: The effect of intravenously administered water-soluble vitamins during labor in normovitaminemic and hypovitaminemic gravidas on maternal and neonatal blood vitamin levels at delivery. Am J Obstet Gynecol 120:697–703, 1974.
175. Jukes TH, Borsook H: Nutritional management of the anemic geriatric patient. Geriatrics 29:147–152, (May) 1974.
176. Marton, RA: Vitamins in western diets. Proc Nutr Soc 35:23–29, 1976.
177. Balack JA, Dobbins WO III: Maldigestion and malabsorption: making up for lost nutrients. Geriatrics 29:157–166, (May) 1974.
178. Taylor KB: Uses and abuses of vitamin therapy. Ration Drug Ther 9:1–6, (Oct) 1975.
179. Briggs M, Briggs MH: Changes in biochemical indices of vitamin nutrition in women using oral contraceptives during treatment with Surbex 500. Curr Med Res Opin 2:626–630, 1974–1975.
180. Shojania AM, Hornady GJ, Barnes PH: The effect of oral contraceptives on folate metabolism. Am J Obstet Gynecol 111:782–791, 1971.
181. Editorial: Vitamins and the pill. Can Med Assoc J 111:211, 1974.
182. Larsson-Cohn U: Oral contraceptives and vitamins—a review. Am J Obstet Gynecol 121:84–90, 1975.
183. Smith JL, Goldsmith GA, Lawrence JD: Effects of oral contraceptive steroids on vitamin and lipid levels in serum. Am J Clin Nutr 28:371–376, 1975.
184. Ahmed F, Bamji MS, Iyengar L: Effect of oral contraceptive agents on vitamin nutrition status. Am J Clin Nutr 28:606–615, 1975.
185. Gascon-Barre M, Mongeau E, Dubue MB: Use of vitamin and mineral supplements by urban school children: prevalence and justification. Can J Publ Health 64:537–547, 1973.

46. LIQUID NUTRITIONAL FORMULAS

Ronni Chernoff, Maurice E. Shils, and Abby S. Bloch

Liquid nutritional formulas, given orally or by tube, are designed to replace or supplement intake of food. They may be prepared individually from appropriate ingredients, or a commercially prepared product may be used. Hospital formulas of the past were largely based on whole milk, skim milk, and cream. However, it is now appreciated that many adults (especially Blacks and Chinese) have insufficient lactase concentrations in the intestinal brush border to digest large amounts of milk.[1] Milk intolerance also may occur in patients with gastric or intestinal resection, intestinal radiation damage, and diseases that adversely affect normal intestinal function.[2] Thus, the composition of standard hospital formulas has been modified to ensure adequate nutrition without excessive lactose.

Commercially prepared liquid formulas vary greatly in composition and method of preparation. Some are simply blenderized natural foods, while others are made with nutrients derived in purified form from natural or synthetic foods. The latter products are often called 'chemically defined,' 'elemental,' or 'defined formula' diets. They contain highly absorbable nutrients with little nondigestible residue, and are primarily useful in patients with malabsorption.[2]

Since the nutritional requirements of patients who are unable to digest and/or absorb nutrients properly are largely unknown, the rationale for selecting a liquid nutritional product, whether prepared in the hospital kitchen or commercially, is empirical. Comparative studies of the effectiveness of the various preparations have not been done in such patients.

INDICATIONS

While many patients require liquid feedings, most do not need defined formula diets, since there is no malabsorption or other predisposing state. Thus, for patients with dysphagia or inadequate intake of regular foods, the need is for food dispersed in water. They will tolerate blended or semi-purified foods orally or by tube. Too often, such patients are given 'empty-calorie' fluids, such as clear soups, tea, or soft drinks, rather than appropriate nutritional supplementation in liquid form.[4]

Defined formula liquid nutrients may be indicated in patients with some metabolic and gastrointestinal diseases (Table 1). They are also useful in renal failure, in hypermetabolic states, and for certain other indications. Physicians, dietitians, and nutritionists must evaluate the nutritional and clinical status of each patient in order to use defined formula diets effectively.

TABLE 1 Clinical Problems for Which Defined Formula Diets May Be Appropriate[a]

Inborn errors of metabolism	Hypermetabolic states
	Severe trauma
Gastrointestinal disease	Major burns
Ulcerative colitis	
Granulomatous bowel disease	Incidental uses
Chronic partial obstruction	Preoperative bowel preparation
Malabsorption syndromes	Nonallergic food source
Short bowel syndrome	Food supplement
Infantile diarrhea	Toilet management problems
Fistulas	Protection of bowel mucosa against damaging agents
Pancreatitis	Feeding of premature infants
Renal failure	Feeding of anorectic patients

[a]Reproduced from reference 2.

SELECTION OF A LIQUID NUTRITIONAL FORMULA

Selection of the specific formula should be based upon a knowledge of the principle constituents—protein sources, carbohydrates, fat, minerals and vitamins.

Protein Sources

Protein is derived either from: (1) intact protein in the form of puréed meat, eggs, or milk; (2) protein isolates from milk (casein), soybeans, or egg white; (3) hydrolyzed protein (casein) with added amino acids to make a complete amino acid mix; or (4) as crystalline amino acids. The digestibility of proteins in various gastrointestinal states is largely unknown. When there is severe pancreatic insufficiency or malabsorption secondary to a short or damaged small bowel, amino acids may be better absorbed as either hydrolyzed protein, di- and tripeptides, or free amino acids than from intact protein. Absorption of certain di- and tripeptides may also be more efficient than that of individual free amino acids, but comparative data on the use of these peptides in nonmalabsorptive states is lacking. Patients differ in the degree of their intestinal dysfunction; in some, a slow drip of a formula with intact protein may be just as well digested and absorbed as the amino acids from the hydrolysates or free amino acids.[2] When digestion or absorption is normal, or is only slightly impaired, there is no reason to use a preparation containing free amino acids, since they are expensive and tend to be low in fat.

Carbohydrates

Carbohydrate is the major source of calories in liquid nutritional formulas. The nature of the carbohydrate is of importance. Glucose or sucrose were used in the early formulations which were also low in fat; the large quantities required created a very high osmolality with associated problems of abdominal discomfort and diarrhea. These have been overcome by the use of starches, dextrins, and glucose oligosaccharides. Oligosaccharides are soluble polymers of glucose containing 5 or more glucose molecules; these are hydrolyzed by enzymes in the intestinal mucosa without the need for pancreatic amylase. The low osmolality formulas are useful when diarrhea or the 'dumping syndrome' is of concern. Since oligosaccharides and longer chain carbohydrates are not sweet, they can be included in relatively large amounts and be mixed with sucrose or glucose to meet individual patient taste preferences. In the commerical defined-formula diets, the percentage of calories derived from carbohydrates ranges from approximately 40 to 90%.[2]

Fat

Fat may contribute from 1% or less to as much as 47% of calories in commercial formulas, depending on the product. Most of the commercial formulas contain long-chain fats such as corn oil, soy oil, or safflower oil. Only a few products contain medium-chain triglycerides; of those that do, most combine it in varying amounts with a long-chain triglyceride such as soy or corn oil. MCT is a bland medium-chain oil derived from coconut oil. The fatty acids vary from 6 to 10 carbons in length and have the unique biochemical property of being able to pass through the intestinal epithelium directly into the portal system as free fatty acids and monoglycerides. One gram of MCT yields 8 kilocalories, and long-chain fat contributes 9 kilocalories per gram. Fat does not increase the osmolality of the formula; its presence in a formula often improves palatability.

When significant maldigestion or malabsorption is present, a diet which is low in fat or which contains MCT oil may be useful. Fat can then be progressively added as tolerance is demonstrated. MCT is absorbed better than long-chain fat when: (1) there is damage to the endothelium of the intestinal mucosa which inhibits the required resynthesis of long-chain fats; (2) the transport of fat from the epithelial cell into the lymphatic system is impaired by obstruction of the lymphatic flow; or (3) there are decreased amounts of conjugated bile salts or pancreatic enzymes in the upper small bowel.

Ingestion and absorption of large amounts of MCT may be associated with ketosis and acidosis. MCT should be used with caution in patients with hepatic cirrhosis or portacaval shunts who are predisposed to hepatic encephalopathy.[2]

Minerals and Vitamins

The commercial defined-formula diets contain all the essential minerals, including trace elements, as well as vitamins in amounts which meet or exceed the National Academy of Science—National Research Council's Recommended Dietary Allowances.[2]

In selecting a specific formula, route of administration and flow rate should be considered. For example, the composition of the specific formulation in terms of osmolality and the type and amounts of carbohydrates, amino acids, and fats may be critical when the formula is fed rapidly to certain patients such as those with high subtotal gastrectomy or those on jejunostomy feedings. These same factors may pose little or no problem in the same patient when a formulation is fed by slow drip over many hours.

Many patients may require liquid feedings because of dysphagia or for supplementation of an inadequate intake of regular foods, even though they do not have maldigestion or malabsorption. Such individuals do not require defined-formula diets with hydrolysates or purified amino acids; their need is for food dispersed in water. Too often such patients are given relatively large amounts of 'empty calorie' fluids instead of optimal nutritional supplementation in liquid form. Patients with maldigestion and malabsorption may need special formulas that are more readily absorbed than the usual hospital liquid formulas.

Palatability and acceptability become key factors when a formula is to be taken by mouth for many days, weeks or months. When milk intolerance is not present, varied formulations of the milk products, eggs and fruits are useful. When there is milk intolerance, defined formula diets low in lactose and with intact protein are useful. Palatability is appreciably greater with preparations containing intact protein than with those containing protein hydrolysates or free amino acids. Furthermore, those with free amino acids are more expensive than those with intact protein. Cost may be reduced for the patient at home by developing a diet which can be prepared by the patient or family and for which materials can be purchased in bulk.[3] Many commercial defined-formula diets with intact proteins are now cheaper and have greater palatability than commercial liquid diets made of natural foods such as meat, eggs and fruit juices.

COMMERCIAL PRODUCTS

A large number of commercially prepared liquid formulas are marketed. These vary greatly in composition and cost. The composition of some of these products, according to manufacturer's analyses, is summarized in Tables 2 and 3; the amount of individual components in the volume needed to give 1000 kilocalories is given. The products can be divided into categories on the basis of:

Completeness of Nutritional Content

Products listed in Table 2 are adequate as the sole source of nutrition, while those described in Table 3 are designed to supplement dietary intake or to meet special metabolic needs.

Presence of Fiber or Residue

Some of the products in Table 2-A contain moderate residue (see footnote c); all other products in Table 2 are low-residue.

TABLE 2 Commercially Prepared Liquid Nutrients Designed to Provide Complete Nutrition

Product (Manufacturer) Volume A[b] Volume B[c]	Protein Content (g) Source(s)	Fat Content (g) Source(s)	Carbohydrate Content (g) Source(s)	Carbohydrate Lactose (g)	mOsm/kg
A. Intact Protein Containing Milk[d]					
Compleat B (Doyle) A = 1,000 ml B = 1,600 ml	40.0 Beef Nonfat milk	40.0 Corn oil	120.0 Sucrose 23.0 Maltodextrin, Vegetables, Fruits, Orange juice } 73.4	24.4	490
Formula 2 (Cutter) A = 1,000 ml B = 2,000 ml	37.5 Nonfat milk Beef	40.0 Corn oil Egg yolks	122.5 Sucrose Vegetables Orange juice Farina Dextrose	37.5	435–510
Meatbase Formula 142 (Hosp. Diet Prod.) A = 667 ml B = 1,000 ml	33.0 Beef Soy protein isolate Nonfat dry milk	48.2 Corn oil	107.6 Dextrose Fruit Vegetables		725
C.I.B.[e,f] (Carnation) A = 880 ml B = 1,373 ml	55.2 Nonfat milk Soy protein Na caseinate	27.6 Milk fat	124.1 Sucrose Corn syrup solids Lactose	84.0	
Meritene Liquid[e] (Doyle) A = 1,000 ml B = 1,200 ml	60.0 Concentrated skim milk Na caseinate	33.3 Vegetable oil Monodiglycerides	115.0 Corn syrup solids Sucrose	56.7	700–750
Meritene + Milk[e,f] (Doyle) A = 995 ml B = 1,095 ml	65.1 Nonfat milk Whole milk	32.5 Milk fat	112.0 Corn syrup solids	97.5	690
Nutri-1,000[e] (Syntex) A = 960 ml B = 1,920	38.0 Skim milk	52.0 Corn oil	95.6 Sucrose 30.7 Corn syrup solids 14.8	50.1	500
Sustacal Liquid[e] (Mead Johnson) A = 1,000 ml B = 1,080 ml	60.3 Concentrated skim milk Na + Ca caseinate Soy protein	23.0 Soy oil	137.8 Sucrose 97.2 Corn syrup solids 25.4	16.7	625
Sustacal + Milk[e,f] (Mead Johnson)	60.3 Nonfat milk Whole milk	24.4 Milk fat	134.4 Sucrose 36.2 Corn syrup solids 11.8	85.8	756
Sustagen + Water[e] (Mead Johnson) A = 600 ml B = 1,050 ml	60.0 Nonfat milk Whole milk Ca caseinate	8.6 Milk fat	171.4 Corn syrup solids 104.7 Glucose 9.3	57.3	1,334
B. Intact Protein, Protein Isolates—Low Lactose, Low Residue					
Ensure[e] (Ross) A = 960 ml B = 1,920 ml	35.0 Na + Ca caseinate 30.6 Soy protein 4.4	35.0 Corn oil	136.7 Corn syrup solids 98.3 Sucrose 38.4	0	450
Ensure Plus[e] (Ross) A = 676 ml B = 1,920 ml	36.6 Na + Ca caseinate Soy protein	35.5 Corn oil	133.2 Corn syrup solids Sucrose	0	600
Isocal (Mead Johnson) A = 960 ml B = 1,920 ml	32.5 Na caseinate Soy protein	42.0 Soy oil 33.6 MCT 8.4	125.0 Corn syrup solids	0	350
Isomil[g] (Ross)	30.0 Soy protein isolate L-methionine	54.0 Soy oil Coconut oil Corn oil	102.0 Corn syrup Sucrose	0	

Minerals[a]										
Ca (mg)	P (mg)	Mg (mg)	Fe (mg)	I (μg)	Cu (mg)	Mn (mg)	Zn (mg)	Na (mEq)	K (mEq)	Cl (mEq)
625.0	1,687.5	250.0	11.3	93.8	1.3	2.5	9.4	67.9	33.7	22.9
720.0	560.0	100.0	12.6	75.0	1.0	0.2	7.5	26.1	45.1	53.5
646.8	710.2	264.0	11.9	100.0	1.7		9.9	31.5	27.1	
1,206.9	972.4	403.5	15.9	129.3	2.0		13.7	37.0	63.3	
1,250.0	1,250.0	333.3	15.0	125.0	1.7	3.3	12.5	39.8	42.7	47.0
2,168.6	1,807.2	361.4	16.3	136.1	1.8	3.6	13.5	39.3	71.1	64.6
1,150.0	900.0	200.0	9.0	75.0	1.0	1.3	7.5	21.7	35.9	31.0
1,000.0	916.7	375.0	16.7	138.9	1.9	2.8	13.9	40.2	52.7	(43.8)
1,611.2	1,333.4	375.0	16.7	138.9	1.9	2.8	13.9	40.2	64.8	37.6
1,828.6	1,371.4	228.6	10.3	85.7	1.1	2.9	11.4	29.8	51.3	
500.0	500.0	200.0	9.0	75.0	1.0	2.0	15.0	30.4	30.8	28.2
422.5	422.5	211.3	9.5	70.4	1.1	1.4	15.9	30.6	32.5	30.2
600.0	500.0	200.0	9.0	75.0	1.0	2.5	10.0	21.7	32.1	28.2
1,050.0	750.0	75.0	18.0	225.0	0.8		7.5	19.6	27.3	22.4

TABLE 2 *(continued)*

Product (Manufacturer) Volume A[b] Volume B[c]	Protein Content (g) Source(s)	Fat Content (g) Source(s)	Carbohydrate Content (g) Source(s)	Lactose (g)	mOsm/kg
Lolactene (Doyle) A = 1,250 ml B = 1,150 ml	66.2 Nonfat dry milk Na caseinate	23.5 Vegetable oil Monodiglycerides	132.4 Corn syrup solids 27.3 Sucrose 10.4 Glucose 46.7 Galactose 46.7	<4.0	670
Mull-Soy[g] (Syntex) A = 1,500 ml	48.0 Soy flour	55.5 Soy oil	79.5 Sucrose Invert sucrose	0	252
Neo Mull-Soy[g] (Syntex) A = 1,500 ml	27.0 Soy protein isolate L-Methionine	52.5 Soy oil	96.0 Sucrose	0	275
Osmolite (Ross) A = 960 ml B = 1,820 ml	36.7 Na + Ca caseinate Soy protein isolate	37.9 MCT Corn oil Soy oil	142.9 Corn syrup solids	0	300
Precision HN (Doyle) A = 950 ml B = 2,950 ml	41.7 Egg white solids	0.5 Vegetable oil Monodiglycerides	206.7 Malto-dextrin 193.9 Sugar 12.8	0	557
Precision Isotonic (Doyle) A = 1,042 ml B = 1,560 ml	30.0 Egg white solids	31.3 Vegetable oil Monodiglycerides	150.0 Maltodextrin Sugar	0	300
Precision LR (Doyle) A = 900 ml B = 1,710 ml	23.7 Egg white solids	0.7 Vegetable oil Monodiglycerides	224.7 Malto-dextrin 209.4 Sugar 15.3	0	500-545
Portagen (Mead Johnson) A = 1,000 ml B = 960 ml	35.0 Na caseinate	47.7 MCT 41.0 Corn oil 5.5 Lecithin 1.3	115.0 Malto-dextrin 83.5 Sucrose 28.8 Other 2.5	<0.3	357
ProSobee[g] (Mead Johnson) A = 1,500 ml	37.5 Soy protein isolate L-Methionine	50.0 Soy oil	100.0 Sucrose 62.0 Corn syrup solids 38.0	0	258
C. Hydrolyzed Protein, Amino Acids—Low Lactose, Low Residue					
Flexical (Mead Johnson) A = 1,000 ml B = 2,000 ml	22.4 Hydrolyzed casein Amino acids	34.0 Soy oil 27.4 MCT 6.6	154.0 Sugar 100.9 Dextrin 48.4 Citrate 4.7	0	550
Nutramigen[g] (Mead Johnson) A = 1,500 ml	32.5 Hydrolyzed casein	39.0 Corn oil	130.0 Sucrose 93.6 Tapioca starch 36.4	0	443
Pregestimil[g] (Mead Johnson) A = 1,500 ml	32.5 Hydrolyzed casein	41.0 MCT 36.6 Corn oil 5.2	130.0 Glucose 91.0 Tapioca starch 39.0	0	590
Vital (Ross) A = 1,000 ml B = 1,500 ml	4.17 Hydrolyzed whey Soy Meat amino acids	10.4 Sunflower oil	185.0 Glucose oligosaccharides Polysaccharides	1.7 Sucrose Hydrolyzed corn starch	450
Vivonex (Eaton) A = 1,000 ml B = 1,800 ml	20.4 Crystalline amino acids	1.4 Safflower oil	226.3 Glucose oligosaccharides	0	500

Minerals[a]										
Ca (mg)	P (mg)	Mg (mg)	Fe (mg)	I (μg)	Cu (mg)	Mn (mg)	Zn (mg)	Na (mEq)	K (mEq)	Cl (mEq)
2,353.0	2,058.8	441.2	19.9	166.2	2.2	4.4	16.5	47.9	79.0	57.2
1,875.0	1,250.0	117.2	15.6	234.4	1.6	2.2	12.5	28.1	66.1	
1.250.0	950.0	120.0	15.6	234.4	0.6	4.0	4.8	26.2	41.2	14.1
500.0	500.0	200.0	9.0	75.0	1.0	2.0	15.0	21.7	21.8	21.1
333.3	333.3	133.3	6.0	50.0	0.7	1.3	5.0	40.6	22.2	32.0
667.0	667.0	266.0	12.0	100.0	1.3	2.7	10.0	34.8	25.6	30.1
526.3	526.3	210.5	9.5	78.9	1.1	2.1	7.9	27.5	20.2	28.2
937.8	604.4	208.4	18.8	72.9	1.6	3.1	9.4	20.4	32.1	24.2
1,185.0	795.0	111.0	18.8	72.0	0.9	1.7	8.0	27.0	28.5	18.0
600.0	500.0	200.0	9.0	75.0	1.0	2.5	10.0	15.2	32.0	35.2
945.0	705.0	111.0	18.8	72.0	0.9	1.7	6.3	21.0	25.5	19.5
945.0	705.0	111.0	18.8	72.0	0.9	1.7	6.3	21.0	25.5	19.5
666.7	666.7	266.6	12.0	100.0	1.3	1.3	10.0	17.0	30.0	19.0
443.3	443.3	194.3	5.6	80.0	1.1	1.6	6.9	37.4	30.0	50.8

TABLE 2 *(continued)*

PRODUCT (MANUFACTURER) VOLUME A[b] VOLUME B[c]	PROTEIN CONTENT (G) SOURCE(S)	FAT CONTENT (G) SOURCE(S)	CARBOHYDRATE CONTENT (G) SOURCE(S)	CARBOHYDRATE LACTOSE (G)	MOSM/KG
Vivonex HN (Eaton) A = 1,000 ml B = 3,000 ml	45.6 Crystalline amino acids	0.9 Safflower oil	202.4 Glucose oligosaccharides	0	850

[a]Ca = calcium; P = phosphorous; Mg = magnesium; Fe = iron; I = iodine; Cu = copper; Mn = manganese; Zn = zinc; Na = sodium; K = potassium; Cl = chloride.

[b]Volume to give 1,000 kcal. Protein, fat, carbohydrate, and mineral contents given in this table are base upon this volume.

[c]Volume needed to meet 100% of Recommended Daily Dietary Allowances, including vitamins.

[d]Compleat B, Formula 2, and Meatbase Formula 142 contain moderate residue; all others are low residue.

[e]Vanilla flavor used.

[f]Whole milk added.

[g]Infant formula.

Lactose Content

Products listed in Table 2-A have moderate to high lactose levels; those in sections B and C have little or no lactose.

Amino Acid Sources

Table 2-A includes products with intact protein derived from meat, milk products and/or eggs. Table 2-B includes products with intact protein as semipurified isolates from milk, soybean or eggs. Table 2-C includes products with casein hydrolysate supplemented with amino acids and products with amino acids only.

DRAWBACKS WITH COMMERCIAL FORMULATIONS

Being intrinsically complete, commercial defined-formula diets are both an advantage and a problem to the physician and dietitian. They are easy to order, store, and administer. However, problems may arise because of their fixed composition. Patients with metabolic disorders may be unable to tolerate the amounts of one or more nutrients in the formula given in the volumes necessary to meet overall nutritional requirements.[3] Such a formulation may actually be hazardous for such patients. This is true, for example, in patients with renal disease who cannot tolerate the levels of protein, sodium, potassium, phosphate or magnesium present in a given formulation, in patients on corticosteroids who are accumulating salt and water and cannot tolerate the amount of sodium present, or in those with hypercalcemia who should not be ingesting the amount of calcium present. The physician must be wary in each instance of specific composition and possible contraindications. In these situations the

Minerals[a]										
Ca (mg)	P (mg)	Mg (mg)	Fe (mg)	I (μg)	Cu (mg)	Mn (mg)	Zn (mg)	Na (mEq)	K (mEq)	Cl (mEq)
266.6	266.6	116.7	3.3	48.0	0.6	0.9	3.7	33.5	18.0	52.4

dietitian must modify the formula either by adding the desired ingredients while diluting out those that are undesirable or, alternatively, by preparing a completely different preparation from specific nutrients.

Individual ingredients are available and can be combined with the proper medical prescription and the services of a trained dietitian. Three examples of formulations which can be prepared in the hospital are given in Table 4. The latter two should not be used without the direct orders and close monitoring of a physician. The first is a general tube feeding formula, the second is a palatable defined-formula for oral or tube feeding, and the third is designed for tube feeding in patients with pancreatic insufficiency, severe malabsorption, or related problems. Modifications of major nutrients and electrolytes are easily accomplished.[2]

Manufacturers could overcome the limitation of fixed formulations by preparing formula diets in modular form, with certain critical items such as fat or sodium and potassium salts made available in separate containers to be added or modified as needed.

TUBE FEEDING

The preferred method of feeding patients is by the oral route, when the gastrointestinal tract is functioning normally. However, tube feedings using nasopharyngeal, esophagostomy, gastrostomy, or jejunostomy tubes may be essential in patients who have mechanical difficulties in chewing or swallowing, who are comatose, or who have impaired digestive function because of surgical excisions, partial obstruction, fistulas, or radiation damage. In theory, such feedings should work well. In practice, however, numerous problems may arise. Many patients who have had prior experience with nasogastric tubes are strongly opposed to further encounters with them. A medium- or fine-bore silastic tube is tolerated much better than is the

TABLE 3 Commercially Prepared Liquid Nutrients Designed to Supplement Food Intake[a]

Product (Manufacturer)	Amount Needed to Give 1,000 C	Protein (G)	Fat (G)	Carbohydrate (G)	Sodium (mEq)	Potassium (mEq)	Type
Amin-Aid (McGaw)	213 g dry weight or 489 ml standard dilution	9.4	31.7	168.6	2.88	2.88	Formula for renal failure therapy
Cal-Power (General Mills)	550 g liquid	0.6	0	272.0	2.39	0.70	Carbohydrate source
Cho-Free (Syntex)	1,304 ml undiluted	46.9	91.3	0.5	41.34	59.21	Low carbohydrate formula
Citrotein Doyle	263.4 g dry weight	60.5	2.6	184.2	45.80	26.80	Calorie supplement
Controlyte (Doyle)	198.0 g dry weight	Trace	48.0	143.0	1.30	0.20	Low protein, low electrolyte calorie source
dp High p.e.r. Protein (General Mills)	258 g dry weight	206.0	10.0	21.0	22.40	9.90	Protein supplement and low electrolytes
EMF (Control Drugs)	500 ml liquid	250.0	0	0	53.00	5.10	Protein source
Gevral (Lederle)	284.8 g dry weight	170.9	5.7	66.8	18.57	3.65	Protein-calorie supplement
Hy-Cal (Beecham-Massengill)	407 ml liquid	0.1	0.1	244.1	2.41	0.07	Carbohydrate source

Lipomul-Oral (Upjohn)	166.7 ml liquid	0.1	111.1	1.1	2.90	0.09	Fat source
Liprotein (Upjohn)	183.7 g dry weight	82.7	64.3	22.1	8.00	42.46	Calorie source
Lofenalac (Mead Johnson)	1,500 ml standard dilution	32.5	39.0	130.0	21.00	25.50	Low phenylalanine formula
Lonalac (Mead Johnson)	1,500 ml standard dilution or 196 g dry weight	53.0	54.7	74.2	1.70	48.08	Low sodium-high protein source
Lytren (Mead Johnson)	268 g dry weight or 3,333 ml standard dilution	0	0	253.0	100.00	83.30	Calorie and electrolyte source
MCT Oil (Mead Johnson)	120.5 g liquid	0	120.5	0	0	0	Medium-chain triglycerides
Pedialyte (Ross)	5,000 ml liquid	0	0	250.0	150.0	100.00	Calorie and electrolyte source
Polycose (Ross)	250.0 g dry weight	0	0	235.0	12.0	0.30	Oligosaccharides
Probana (Mead Johnson)	1,500 ml standard dilution	60.0	32.0	118.0	40.50	46.50	High protein banana powder formula for celiac condition and diarrhea
Sumacal (Hospital Diet Products)	360 ml liquid	0	0	250.0	10.40	1.15	Concentrated carbohydrate source and low electrolytes

[a]Reproduced from reference 2.

TABLE 4 Examples of Formulas Prepared in Hospital (for 1,000 Kcal)[a]

Memorial Sloan-Kettering Cancer Center
Blenderized Tube Feeding

A general formula for patients with normal absorption. Sodium restriction to varying degrees is achieved by omission of salt and use of low salt vegetables. Potassium restriction is achieved by modification of orange juice.

Carrots, canned	45 g
Chopped beef	105 g
Corn oil	30 g
Dark Karo syrup	90 g
Egg, cooked	68 g
Farina, cooked	114 g
Nonfat milk powder	20 g
Orange juice	180 ml
Salt	1.5 g
Water or vegetable juice	450 g
Wax beans, canned	30 g
Poly-Vi-Sol vitamins with iron	1 tablet/day

DeR Oral or Tube Feeding

A palatable low residue-defined formula as supplement. When used as only source of nutrition, magnesium oxide or chloride and trace elements are added. Modifications are easily made as needed.

Calcium caseinate	31 g
Chocolate syrup	36 g
Cornstarch, cooked	40 g
Dextrose, anhydrous or oligosaccharides	80 g
Egg, cooked	45 g
Gevral protein	4.5 g
Oil (corn or MCT)	27 g
Potassium chloride	2.0 g
Water	600 ml
Poly-Vi-Sol vitamins with iron	1 tablet/day

T-#23 Tube Formula

A formula with casein hydrolysate for use in patients with serious malabsorption, pancreatic insufficiency, inflammatory bowel disease, or intestinal fistulae. Modifications are easily made.

Alcolec[b]	1.0 g
Calcium lactate	0.9 g
Calcium phosphate	0.9 g
DL-methionine	0.23 g

TABLE 4 Examples of Formulas Prepared in Hospital (for 1,000 Kcal)[a]

DL-tryptophan	0.23 g
Egg, cooked	45 g
Hy-Case, SF[c]	34 g
Magnesium chloride	(as needed)
Oil (corn or MCT) [initially low]	23 g
Oligosaccharides (Polycose)	169 g
Potassium gluconate and/or chloride	(as needed)
Sodium chloride and/or bicarbonate	(as needed)
Trace elements	2 ml
Water	690 ml
Poly-Vi-Sol vitamins with iron	1 tablet/day

[a]Reproduced from reference 2.

[b]Lecithin (emulsifying agent) if oil is used.

[c]Hydrolyzed casein.

usual rubber feeding tube. Once patients can be induced to permit insertion of such tubes, they are usually willing to keep them in place. A fine-bore tube does, however, require a finely dispersed formula to prevent plugging of the tube. Blenderized formulas of regular food usually do not flow well, whereas the highly dispersed defined formula diets of low viscosity flow easily.[2]

The potential hazard of formulas being aspirated must always be considered. This can be minimized by slow feeding of the formula to prevent accumulation in the stomach and by having the patient's head and chest kept at a 30° angle or higher while being fed. As a general policy, tube feedings should be avoided when the potential for aspiration is significant.

The need for a surgical procedure to insert esophagostomy, gastrostomy or jejunostomy feeding tubes all too often discourages physicians from using tube feedings. With jejunostomy feedings the formula should be given slowly, particularly if it contains significant amounts of soluble sugars, until it has been demonstrated that the patient can tolerate the formula and the rate without developing the dumping syndrome. Lower osmolality formulas may be infused more rapidly.[2]

CONCLUSIONS

The large number of commercial preparations listed in Tables 2 and 3 offers a complex array from which choices must be made. It is suggested that physicians and dietitians who prescribe such formulations perform their own taste test, review the composition, select a limited number of different types, and carefully observe patient reaction to them. By using this approach, a specific selection of liquid formulas can be stocked to meet individual patient nutritional needs.

REFERENCES

1. Gray GM: Carbohydrate digestion and absorption. N Engl J Med 292:1225–1230, 1975.
2. Shils ME, Bloch AS, Chernoff R: Liquid formulas for oral and tube feeding. Clinical Bulletin Memorial Sloan-Kettering Cancer Center 6(4):151, 1976.
3. Chernoff R, Bloch AS: Liquid feedings: considerations and alternatives. J Am Diet Assoc 70:389–391, 1977.
4. O'Hara JG, Kennedy S, Lizewski W: Effects of long-term elemental nasogastric feeding on elderly debilitated patients. Can Med Assoc J 108:977–980, 1973.

SUGGESTED READINGS

1. Kaminski MV: Enteral hyperalimentation. Surg Gynecol Obstet 143:12–16, 1976.
2. Young EA, Heuler N, Russell P, et al: Comparative nutritional analysis of chemically defined diets. Gastroenterology 69:1338–1345, 1975.

47. TOTAL PARENTERAL NUTRITION

Joseph M. Sceppa

Total parenteral nutrition (TPN) is a form of intravenous therapy designed to maintain or advance nutritional status. It involves infusing amino acids, an adequate source of calories, and small amounts of other essential substances.[1–5] Prior to the development of TPN in the late 1960's, intravenous solutions containing protein hydrolysates and low concentrations of dextrose (eg, 5%) were given in unsuccessful attempts to maintain nutritional status.[6–9] Although the amount of protein in these solutions was adequate to maintain tissues and prevent catabolism, the supply of calories was not. As a result, the protein hydrolysate was consumed as a source of calories. In 1959, Moore[10] suggested specific non-protein calorie-to-nitrogen ratios of 150–200 to 1 for optimal utilization of infused amino acids or protein.[10] Dudrick, working initially with beagle dogs, increased the concentration of dextrose to 20%.[1] Because of the irritating nature of such concentrated dextrose solutions, he infused the TPN (then known as hyperalimentation) solution into large diameter vessels, such as the superior vena cava. This technique effectively maintained homeostasis in many patients who were unable to ingest sufficient nutrients, and it dramatically improved their prognosis. More recently, a fat emulsion that can be infused in peripheral veins as a source of calories has come into use, and it has simplified TPN therapy for many patients. This concentrated caloric source increases total fluid volumes and approximately doubles TPN fluid costs. It has been employed in a large number of pediatric and adult patients who could not tolerate placement of a central venous catheter.

NUTRITIONAL DEMANDS

Post-surgical energy requirements for a 70 kg adult male vary from approximately 1800 to 2100 kcal (25 to 30 kcal/kg) for uncomplicated convalescence.[11] Additional factors encountered in hospitalized patients add to caloric needs. Severe trauma or widespread sepsis can double the requirement.[12] Fever increases the caloric requirement approximately 13% for each degree Centigrade rise in body temperature.[13]

The recommended daily allowance of protein established by the National Academy of Sciences is 0.8 g per kg per 24 hours. This totals 56 g for a 70 kg male, and is equivalent to 9 g of nitrogen, which is well below the requirements advocated by others in the field.[14] When abnormal tissue turnover exists, such as the 30 g of nitrogen necessary in burn patients, it must be replaced along with proportional increases in calories.[10]

High calorie-to-nitrogen ratios of from 150 to 200 kcal/g of nitrogen were originally advocated for parenteral nutrition.[10,11,15,16] It now seems that minimal physical activity requires a calorie-to-nitrogen ratio of approximately 150.[15,17]

Indications for total parenteral nutrition include enterocutaneous fistulae, short gut syndrome, radiation sickness, inflammatory bowel disease, extensive burns, intractable diarrhea, renal failure, and reversible liver failure.

CENTRALLY ADMINISTERED TOTAL PARENTERAL NUTRITION

In central TPN therapy, a solution containing a nitrogen source and concentrated dextrose (20–25%) is administered into a large central vein, such as the superior vena cava, through an indwelling catheter. The cathether allows maximal dilution and thereby minimizes thrombosis and phlebitis.[1-4] Methods for catheter placement have been described elsewhere.[4,5,18,19] The infusion is initiated at a slow rate (50 ml/hr) and is increased over two to three days to 100 to 125 ml/hr as tolerated. An alternative method consists of starting a half-strength solution and infusing it at 100–125 ml/hr. The concentration is increased to full-strength over 2 to 3 days. This second method may increase the risk of contamination since greater manipulation of the solution is involved; electrolyte concentrations would also have to be adjusted.

Formulation

TPN solutions should be freshly prepared in a laminar airflow hood using aseptic technique. Intravenous fluid manufacturers cannot

TABLE 1 Basic Formulation for Adult Central TPN Solution[a]

Component	From 500 ml of Travasol 8.5% with Electrolytes	Additions	Concentration per 1000 ml of Final Solution
Amino Acids	42.5 g	—	42.5 g
Dextrose	—	250 g[b]	250 g
Sodium	35 mEq	—	35 mEq
Potassium	30 mEq	—	30 mEq
Calcium	—	5 mEq[c]	5 mEq
Magnesium	5 mEq	3 mEq[d]	8 mEq
Chloride	35 mEq	—	35 mEq
Phosphate	30 mEq	—	30 mEq
Acetate	65 mEq	—	65 mEq

[a]This solution provides 1020 kcal—850 kcal from the dextrose and 170 kcal from the Travasol.

[b]Provided by 500 ml of 50% dextrose solution.

[c]Provided by 5.5 ml of 10% calcium gluceptate solution.

[d]Provided by 0.75 ml of 50% magnesium sulfate solution.

prepare amino acid solutions with concentrated dextrose. These solutions when autoclaved produce a Maillard or browning reaction as the amino groups form condensation products with aldehydes and impart a brown color to the fluid. The basic formulation for an adult central TPN solution is prepared by mixing 500 ml of a protein hydrolysate or amino acid solution with 500 ml of a concentrated source of dextrose. Table 1 describes an adult TPN solution obtained by mixing 500 ml of 8.5% Travasol with Electrolytes (crystalline amino acids with electrolytes), 500 ml of 50% dextrose solution, and small amounts of some additional electrolytes. Other preparations of crystalline amino acids (Table 2) or protein hydrolysates (Table 3) may be used. However, the use of only one or two nitrogen sources is preferable because of differences in electrolyte and amino acid content.

Electrolytes. Many different suggestions for the electrolyte composition of TPN solutions have been published.[20–22] One approach is to prepare each TPN solution individually according to each

TABLE 2 Comparison of Crystalline Amino Acid Solutions

Trademark (Manufacturer)	Aminosyn (Abbott)			Freamine II (McGaw)	Travasol (Travenol)			Veinamine (Cutter)
	3.5%	5%	7%	8.5%	3.5%	5.5%	8.5%	8%
Amino Acids (g/100 ml)								
Essential								
L-Isoleucine	0.252	0.360	0.510	0.590	0.167	0.263	0.406	0.493
L-Leucine	0.329	0.470	0.660	0.770	0.216	0.340	0.526	0.347
L-Lysine	0.252[a]	0.360[a]	0.510[a]	0.870[a]	0.202[b]	0.318[b]	0.492[b]	0.667[b]
L-Methionine	0.140	0.200	0.280	0.450[c]	0.202	0.318	0.492	0.427
L-Phenylalanine	0.154	0.220	0.310	0.480	0.216	0.340	0.526	0.400
L-Threonine	0.182	0.260	0.370	0.340	0.146	0.230	0.356	0.160
L-Tryptophan	0.056	0.080	0.120	0.130	0.063	0.099	0.152	0.080
L-Valine	0.280	0.400	0.560	0.560	0.160	0.252	0.390	0.253
Total Grams (%)	1.645	2.350	3.320	4.190	1.372	2.160	3.340	2.827
Total Grams/Container	15.270/ 1000 ml	11.230/ 500 ml	15.865/ 500 ml	19.700/ 500 ml	6.860/ 500 ml	10.800/ 500 ml	16.700/ 500 ml	14.135/ 500 ml

Nonessential								
L-Histidine	0.105	0.105	0.210	0.240	0.153	0.241	0.372	0.237
L-Arginine	0.343	0.490	0.690	0.310	0.363	0.570	0.880	0.749
L-Glutamic acid	—	—	—	—	—	—	—	0.426
L-Aspartic acid	—	—	—	—	—	—	–	0.400
Glycine	0.448	0.640	0.900	1.700	0.725	1.140	0.760	3.387
L-Proline	0.300	0.430	0.610	0.950	0.146	0.230	0.356	0.107
L-Alanine	0.448	0.640	0.900	0.600	0.725	1.140	1.760	—
L-Serine	0.147	0.210	0.300	0.500	—	—	—	00
L-Cysteine	—	—	—	0.020	—	—	—	—
L-Tyrosine	0.031	0.044	0.066	—	0.014	0.022	0.034	—
Total Grams (%)	1.822	2.604	3.676	4.320	2.126	3.343	5.171	5.306
Total Grams/Container	18.220	13.020	18.380	21.600	10.630	16.715	25.855	26.530
% Essential amino acids	47.4	47.4	47.4	49.2	39.2	39.2	39.2	47.7

[a] As the acetate.

[b] As the hydrochloride.

[c] As DL methionine.

TABLE 3 Protein Hydrolysate Solutions[a]

TRADEMARK NAME(S)	MANUFACTURER	PROTEIN	VOLUMES AVAILABLE
Amigen 5%	Travenol	Casein	500 and 1000 ml
Amigen 5% and Dextrose 5%	Travenol	Casein	500 and 1000 ml
Amigen 10%	Travenol	Casein	500 ml in 1000-ml fill

[a]Other protein hydrolysate solutions (Aminosol, C.P.H., and Hyprotigen) were available until recently but were withdrawn by order of the Food and Drug Administration.

recipient's serum electrolyte concentrations. However, since many electrolytes are largely intracellular, serum concentrations do not necessarily reflect total body content, especially for potassium, phosphate, and calcium. Another method is to prepare a standard formulation that is tolerated by the majority of adult patients. At our hospital, adults with adequate renal function are given such a standard solution (Table 1), and they show positive nitrogen balance without important electrolyte imbalances. Standardization allows optimal pharmacy work patterns and culturing of the solution before administration. When one department, such as the pharmacy, prepares all solutions and gathers patient data, the basic formulation can be modified as the increasing pool of patient data dictates. When a standard formulation is used, the capability to prepare individualized TPN solutions for patients with renal impairment or specific electrolyte abnormalities should be retained.

When preparing any TPN solution, the electrolytes present in the hydrolysate solution or amino acids must be considered.

Potassium requirements should include 3 mEq for every gram of nitrogen retained as well as enough to replace urinary losses.[20,22] Concentrations of 30 to 40 mEq per liter are adequate to initiate therapy; however, subsequent electrolyte determinations are necessary.[23]

Sodium concentrations of 30 to 40 mEq per liter of TPN satisfy the majority of adult patients.[4,21,24,25]

Calcium in the range of 4 to 5 mEq per liter is acceptable.[20,22,23,26] Calcium and phosphate should be added separately and the solution shaken to minimize the risk of precipitation of calcium phosphate.[27]

For every gram of nitrogen retained, 0.5 to 0.6 mEq of *magnesium* is utilized.[20,23] Concentrations of 5 to 8 mEq of magnesium per liter meet these and other requirements.[28]

Phosphate exists simultaneously in a monovalent ($H_2PO_4^-$) and divalent ($HPO_4^{=}$) form in the extracellular fluid.[29] The ratio of the two forms is dependent on the pH. At a physiological pH of 7.4 the ratio of ($HPO_4^{=}$):($H_2PO_4^-$) is 4:1. Thus, the average valence of phosphate in blood is 1.8. Since the pH of hydrolysate or amino acid solutions vary, their phosphate content varies accordingly. Thus, a description of phosphate availability in TPN ideally should specify mM of phosphate or mg of phosphorus. Phosphate should be added to TPN solutions with caution. Each commercially available potassium phosphate solution is a different strength, and some of the products have been incorrectly labeled (Table 4).

TABLE 4 Commercial Potassium Phosphate Solutions

	Concentration	
Manufacturer	Phosphate (mM/mL)	Potassium (mEq/mL)
Abbott	3	4.4
Invenex	3	4.4

We continue to use the term 'mEq' for phosphate on our TPN label because some commercially available solutions are labelled as such. Phosphate concentrations of 5 to 20 mEq per liter should prevent hypophosphatemia,[23] which has been reported in TPN recipients.[30-32] Periodic phosphate blood levels should be obtained.

Chloride is supplied in approximately the same ratio as sodium.[20,22,23] If hyperchloremic acidosis presents, bicarbonate precursors such as acetate or gluconate are indicated. Hyperchloremic metabolic acidosis was associated with FreAmine, a solution containing amino acids as chloride salts.[33-35] This product was replaced by FreAmine II in 1975; it utilizes acetate salts of the individual amino acids. Other companies that market crystalline amino acid solutions also use acetate salts.

Several manufacturers have recently marketed electrolyte concentrates (eg, Hyperlyte) that will speed preparation of standard TPN solutions.

Iron salts should not be added to standard formulations as precipitation may occur.

Vitamins. Vitamins should be added to parenteral nutrition solutions. There is no commercially available parenteral multivitamin preparation which meets the National Academy of Sciences National Research Council's 'Recommended Dietary Allowances' (RDA) for all essential vitamins. However, M.V.I. (USV Pharmaceutical Corporation) provides sufficient quantities of A, C, D, and E as well as all of the B-complex vitamins except folic acid and vitamin B_{12}; it does not provide vitamin K (Table 5). If 2.0 ml of M.V.I. concentrate are infused daily, most vitamin requirements are met. Another method is to administer this product once weekly and give only water-soluble vitamins on remaining days.[36] Larger portions of certain vitamins may be excreted by the kidneys when they are given intravenously as opposed to oral administration.[37] The availability of vitamin A from TPN solutions has recently been questioned.[38] Folic acid, vitamin B_{12}, and vitamin K_1 (phytonadione) should also be provided if total parenteral nutrition is to continue for long periods of time. Recent work by Shils indicates changes in parenteral RDA figures.[39]

Trace Elements. Theoretically, deficiencies of every trace element found in man can exist.[40–44] Contaminants of intravenous solutions supply at least some zinc and copper,[45,46] but reports of clinical deficiencies of these two trace elements exist.[47–50] Chromium deficiency has also been confirmed recently.[51] Formulations are available for trace element concentrates.[25,52–54] Since 1973 we have used trace element formulations (Tables 6 and 7) based on the works of Shils (Table 8).[25,55] It should be noted that these formulae are suggested rather than well-established requirements.[56] Since parenteral administration bypasses the protective intestinal mucosal barrier which prevents absorption of excessive amounts of these elements,[56] trace elements should be given cautiously. Suggestions that trace elements be supplied by plasma infusions have been abandoned due to the danger of hepatitis and lack of uniform concentrations of trace elements in plasma.

Complications

Serious hazards associated with the use of centrally-administered TPN solutions can be divided into three distinct groups[57]: (a)

TABLE 5 Daily Vitamin Requirements

	Recommended Dietary Allowances[a]		2 ml of M.V.I. Concentrate	Proposed Parenteral Requirements[b]	
Vitamin	Adult	Children (1–10 yr)		Adult	Children
Fat Soluble					
Vitamin A (IU)	4000–5000	2000–3000	4000	3300	2300
Vitamin D_2 (IU)	400	400	400	200	400
Vitamin E (IU)	12–15	4–10	2	10	7
Vitamin K_1 (μg)	2	7–10	—	—	0.2
Water Soluble					
Ascorbic Acid (mg)	45	40	200	100	80
Folic Acid (μg)	400	100–300	—	400	140
Niacinamide (mg)	12–20	9–16	40	40	17
Riboflavin (mg)	1.1–1.8	0.8–1.2	4	3.6	1.4
Thiamine (mg)	1.0–1.5	0.7–1.2	20	3.0	1.2
Pyridoxine (mg)	1.6–2.0	0.6–1.2	6	4.0	1.0
Vitamin B_{12} (μg)	3	1.0–2.0	—	5.0	1.0

[a]Established by the Food and Nutrition Board of the National Academy of Sciences—National Research Council.

[b]Adapted from ME Shils: Parenteral multivitamins: times for changes. Bull Parenteral Drug Assoc 30:226–233, 1976.

TABLE 6 Pediatric Trace Element Formulation

TRACE ELEMENT	MG/ML	MG OF SALT[a]
Zinc	240	500 $ZnCl_2$ 1200 $ZnSO_4 \cdot 5H_20$
Copper	80	200 $CuSO_4$
Manganese	80	200 $MnSO_4 \cdot H_2O$
Fluoride	320	711 NaF
Iodide	40	47 NaI

[a]See footnote to Table 7 for method of preparation.

technical mishaps associated with the placement of the catheter; (b) metabolic disorders related to the composition of the fluid; (c) infection.

Technical Mishaps. Placement of the catheter may be associated with the following complications:

1. puncture or laceration of the subclavian artery
2. air embolus from aspiration of air while the catheter is being inserted
3. pneumothorax from puncture of the pleura
4. hydrothorax from infusion into the pleural space
5. brachial plexus injury
6. mediastinal hematoma from laceration of innominate vein
7. injury to thoracic duct
8. pericardial tamponade from atrial puncture.

Later complications include accidental dislodgement of the catheter, leakage of fluid out of the vein and into the subcutaneous tissue or out of the wound, and breakage of the catheter at the point where it is tied into the vein. Careful attention to details of placement and fixation of the catheter will minimize these complications.

Secondary complications related to the catheter include thrombosis of the superior vena cava, intrahepatic abscess (from accidental placement of the catheter in an intrahepatic vein), and pulmonary embolus, secondary either to vena cava thrombosis or candida endocarditis.

TABLE 7 Adult Trace Element Formulation[a]

Trace Element	mg/ml	mg of Salt
Zinc	1	2.05 $ZnCl_2$ 5.00 $ZnSO_4 \cdot 5\ H_2O$
Copper	0.3	0.75 $CuSO_4$
Manganese	0.3	1.00 $MnSO_4 \cdot H_2O$
Fluoride	0.3	0.66 NaF
Iodide	0.33	0.039 NaI

[a]100 ml of adult trace element concentrate are prepared by dissolving 100 times each of the salt amounts listed above except sodium iodide (eg, 205 mg of zinc chloride) in enough sterile water to produce 100 ml. Small doses of iodide may be obtained by diluting the commercially available parenteral solution. This solution is passed through a 0.22-μm filter into a sterile vial and autoclaved. One milliliter of this concentration is added to each 1000 ml of adult TPN solution.

Complications of central venous catheterization and techniques for prevention are discussed in detail elsewhere.[26,58]

Metabolic Derangements. Table 9 summarizes the major metabolic problems associated with total parenteral nutrition. Patients on central TPN often require exogenous insulin. We titrate the patient with regular insulin subcutaneously. Once titrated at a uniform dose over 24 hours, that dose of insulin is added to the TPN solution. In this manner changes in fluid rate also cause proportional changes in

TABLE 8 Suggested Approximate Daily Intravenous Requirements for Trace Elements [52]

Trace Element	Infants and Young Children	Adults
Zinc	20–40 μg/kg[a]	2–4 mg[a]
Copper	10–20 μg/kg[a]	0.5–1.0 mg
Fluorine	1 μg/ml (1 ppm)	1–2 mg[a]
Iodine	3–5 μg/kg[a]	1–2 μg/kg
Manganese	10–20 μg/kg[b]	1–2 μg

[a]Inadequate data—range very uncertain.

[b]Probably human requirement but not definite—range very uncertain.

TABLE 9 Metabolic Problems Associated with Parenteral Hyperalimination [51]

PROBLEMS	POSSIBLE ETIOLOGIES
I. Glucose Metabolism	
A. Hyperglycemia	Excessive total dose or rate of infusion of glucose; inadequate endogenous insulin
1. Glycosuria	
2. Osmotic diuresis	
3. Hyperosmolar nonketotic dehydration	
4. Coma	
B. Ketocidosis in diabetes mellitus	Inadequate endogenous insulin response; inadequate exogenous insulin therapy
C. Postinfusion hypoglycemia	Persistence of endogenous insulin production secondary to prolonged stimulation of islet cells by high carbohydrate infusion
II. Amino Acid Metabolism	
A. Hyperchloremic metabolic acidosis	Excessive chloride and monohydrochloride content of crystalline amino acid solutions
B. Serum amino acid imbalances	Unphysiologic amino acid profile of the nutrient solution
C. Hyperammonemia	Excessive ammonia in protein hydrolysate solutions; arginine, ornithine, aspartic acid and/or glutamic acid deficiency in amino acid solutions; primary hepatic disorder
D. Prerenal azotemia	Excessive protein hydrolysate or amino acid infusion
III. Essential Fatty Acid Metabolism	
A. Scrum deficiencies of phospholipid linoleic and/or arachidonic acids; serum elevations of 5, 8, 11-eicosatrienoic acid	Inadequate essential fatty acid administration; inadequate vitamin E administration
IV. Calcium and Phosphorous Metabolism	
A. Hypophosphatemia	Inadequate phosphorous administration, redistribution of serum phosphorous into cell and/or bone
1. Decreased erythrocyte 2,3-diphosphoglycerate	
2. Increased affinity of hemoglobin for oxygen	
3. Aberrations of erythrocyte intermediary metabolites	

TABLE 9 *(continued)*

PROBLEMS	POSSIBLE ETIOLOGIES
B. Hypocalcemia	Inadequate calcium administration; reciprocal response to phosphorus repletion without simultaneous calcium infusion
C. Hypercalcemia	Excessive calcium administration with or without high doses of albumin
D. Vitamin D deficiency; Hypervitaminosis D	Inadequate or excessive vitamin D administration
V. Miscellaneous	
A. Hypokalemia	Inadequate potassium intake relative to increased requirements for protein anabolism
B. Hyperkalemia	Excessive potassium administration especially in metabolic acidosis
C. Hypomagnesemia	Inadequate magnesium administration relative to increased requirements for protein anabolism
D. Anemia	Iron deficiency; folic acid deficiency; vitamin B_{12} deficiency; copper deficiency
E. Bleeding	Vitamin K deficiency
F. Hypervitaminosis A	Excessive vitamin A administration
G. Elevations in SGOT, SGPT, and serum alkaline phosphatase	Enzyme induction secondary to accelerated glucose metabolism, possible hepatotoxicity secondary to amino acid imbalance; excessive glycogen and/or fat deposition in the liver

exogenous insulin infused. Published reports indicate that significant amounts of insulin are lost due to adsorption on glass and polyvinyl chloride administration sets.[59–63] Enough insulin is received intravenously to maintain the blood glucose levels within acceptable limits.

Sepsis. Indwelling catheters are inevitably associated with a risk of infection.[64–67] Total parenteral nutrition solutions support the growth of both bacteria and fungi.[68–70] Production of a 'fibrin sleeve' from indwelling central venous catheters may serve as a locus for an infection.[71] The combined incidence of bacterial and fungal infections ranges from 0 to 27%.[72–85] The higher incidences of infection were associated with the addition of dextrose, vitamins, etc. by personnel at the nursing station.[75] Central venous pressure monitoring and medication administration through the TPN line were often the cause of infection. Reductions in septic complications have been accomplished through rigid adherence to a protocol and the use of a TPN team.[58,78–87] Infections can be minimized by observing the following guidelines.[79]

1. TPN is initiated when the patient's clinical requirements outweigh the significant risks involved.
2. TPN therapy should be the responsibility of a team of individuals including at least a nurse, a physician, and a pharmacist.
3. TPN solutions should be prepared, catheters placed, delivery systems maintained, and fluid administered according to a detailed protocol incorporating adequate infection control measures.
4. All TPN components and additives should be mixed by a trained member of the hospital staff using aseptic technique.
5. The insertion of a TPN catheter should be considered a surgical procedure. Persons involved should wash, gown, glove, and mask.
6. The site of catheter placement should be shaved, draped, and thoroughly disinfected.
7. After the intravenous administration route is established, the catheter should be securely anchored to prevent irritating to-and-fro motion and to avoid potential transport of cutaneous bacteria into the puncture wound.
8. With aseptic technique the catheter site should be inspected and disinfected periodically.
9. Administration of fluid at a site should be discontinued immediately if signs of inflammation, purulence, thrombosis, or extravasation of fluid are observed.
10. Although the rationale is unsupported and undocumented, some investigators remove catheters and initiate therapy at another site every 30 days even if there have been no complications.[88]
11. The TPN system should not be used to measure the central venous pressure, administer blood products or 'piggyback' medications, or obtain blood samples.
12. Although not clearly justified, micropore filters (0.45 and 0.22

micrometer) theoretically reduce the hazard of infection from intrinsically contaminated solutions.

13. TPN solutions and sets should be changed at least every 24 hours.

14. TPN should be considered immediately in the differential diagnosis of fever. TPN fluid should be aseptically cultured along with the catheter tip. Fungal septicemia and bacteremia may spontaneously resolve when the offending infusion system is removed.

Unless fungal infections have been a problem when the 'team' concept and a protocol are in use, the use of an 'amphotericin flush' is not indicated.[89]

Protocol

Once a protocol has been instituted and approved by the medical staff, strict adherence must be enforced. The protocol should include information on fluid composition and instructions for slowly initiating TPN and tapering discontinued infusions.[86] A 'minimum standard' for metabolic monitoring which includes specific tests with optimum frequency should be provided. A procedure for regular line care, approved by the nursing department, should be included.[88] Ideally, patient data are collected and reviewed to ascertain adherence to the protocol and act as a utilization review mechanism.

Pharmacist Role

As more emphasis is placed on variations in parenteral nutrition regimens as well as changes within any one regimen, the responsibility placed on the department of pharmacy has grown. A survey by Kaminski and Stolar revealed significant discrepancies between actual and recommended practices and a high incidence of complications.[90] The use of a team approach of physicians, pharmacists, nurses and other health professionals is needed to develop protocols, standard formulas, and optimal guidelines for the safe and rational use of TPN.[91,92] Many patients cared for at home on TPN require even more detailed instructions for preparation and administration of these complex preparations.[93,94]

Pediatric Use

Protein requirements in premature and full-term infants have been adequately reviewed.[95] Weight gains of 15 g per kg have been reported.[87] Two grams of casein per kilogram of body weight is more than adequate for full-term infants.

The concentration of pediatric TPN solutions differs from adult solutions. The dextrose concentration is commonly 20% and the concentration of protein or amino acids is 2 to 3.3%.[87,96–99] Synthetic amino acids are more completely utilized, thus a 2% concentration is probably adequate. Gradually increasing administration rates to 125 ml/kg/24 hours supplies fluid, dextrose (25 g/kg), and protein (2.5–4 g/kg) requirements.[87] Infusion rates for older children parallel their fluid requirements.

Electrolyte requirements significantly exceed adult needs on a weight basis.[52] Sodium requirements range from 3 to 5 mEq/kg/day, while potassium needs vary from 2 to 5 mEq/kg/day.[52,87] Calcium varies from 0.5 to 2 mEq/kg/day, and magnesium ranges between 0.25 mEq and 0.5 mEq/kg/day. Ions such as calcium and potassium, for which the serum concentration is not an adequate indicator of total body amounts, must be carefully considered; if total body requirements are not met in the daily formulation, deficits will occur.

For infants weighing less than 5 kg, catheters are inserted through an external or internal jugular vein cut-down. This is safer than the subclavian puncture since the subclavian vein in children of this weight range is quite small. The proximal catheter end is then tunnelled subcutaneously through a small exit wound in the scalp.[96,97,99–103] This procedure allows easier catheter care and decreases the chance of infection. Before the dressing is applied to the exit site, the catheter is coiled to prevent accidental dislodgement. After X-ray confirmation of the catheter tip placement, the infusion is begun.

The pediatric formula that has been used at New England Medical Center Hospital since 1973 is given in Table 10. The original casein hydrolysate nitrogen source was changed to synthetic amino acids because of manufacturers' production difficulties with protein hydrolysates. The TPN solution is prepared in 2 liter evacuated containers without vitamins. Daily fluid quotas for each patient are filtered into smaller evacuated containers through 0.22-micrometer membrane filters in the pharmacy. Vitamins are added to each daily quota prior to dispensing. This insures that each child receives vitamins based on a daily requirement rather than on a fluid basis. Solutions are delivered to patients by an infusion pump through a 0.22- to 0.45-micrometer filter in-line. Filtration limits bacterial and particulate contamination and prevents accidental infusion of air into patients if infusion bottles run dry.

TABLE 10 Pediatric Central TPN Solution

Component	Each 125 ml Contains	Each 1000 ml Contains
Amino Acids	3.75 g	30 g
Dextrose	25 g	200 g
Sodium	3.8 mEq	30 mEq
Potassium	3.8 mEq	30 mEq
Calcium	3.13 mEq	25 mEq
Magnesium	2.0 mEq	16 mEq
Chloride	3.13 mEq	25 mEq
Phosphate	2.5 mEq	20 mEq
Trace Elements		
Zinc	30 μg	240 μg
Copper	10 μg	80 μg
Manganese	10 μg	80 μg
Fluoride	40 μg	320 μg
Iodide	5 μg	40 μg

Each 24-hour supply contains:

M.V.I. Concentrate 3 ml
Vitamin B_{12} 10 μg
Vitamin K_1 1 mg
Folic Acid 1 mg

TPN In Renal Failure

For patients with renal failure, Nephramine (McGaw), a modified preparation containing only essential amino acids, is available (Table 11). It is a 5.1% solution supplied in 250 ml bottles. When 250 ml of Nephramine is diluted with 500 ml of 70% dextrose, the resulting TPN solution contains 1.7% essential amino acids and 47% dextrose. Administration of 750 ml supplies Rose's recommended daily allowances of essential amino acids.[104] This TPN solution is titrated by frequent blood sugar determinations and is given at the rate of 60 to 100 ml/hr.[105–107] Elevated blood urea nitrogen serves as a source for synthesis of non-essential amino acids.[108–110]

TABLE 11 Composition of Essential Amino Acid Injection (Nephramine)[a]

Amino Acids	g/100 ml	g/250ml 12.8
L-Isoleucine	0.56	1.40
L-Leucine	0.88	2.20
L-Lysine	0.64	1.60
(L-Lysine Acetate)	0.90	
L-Methionine	0.88	2.20
L-Phenylalanine	0.88	2.20
L-Threonine	0.40	1.00
L-Tryptophan	0.20	0.50
L-Valine	0.65	1.62
Total Amino Acids	5.1	12.8
Total Nitrogen	0.58	1.46

[a]Addition of 500 ml of dextrose 70% to 250 ml of Nephramine 5.1% produces a solution of 750 ml with 1190 nonprotein calories (350 g dextrose x 3.4 cal/g) and 1.46 g nitrogen. The nonprotein calorie to nitrogen ratio is 815:1.

Histidine and arginine are not present in Nephramine and this may preclude its use in infants.

Intracellular electrolytes such as potassium, magnesium, and phosphate are closely titrated while sodium is administered to balance losses. Nursing personnel must have particular concern for aseptic technique due to the high susceptibility of uremic patients to infection.

Reports of administration of alpha keto precursors of essential amino acids to chronic renal failure patients are of interest.[111] The majority of these keto acids are converted in the liver or other organs to essential amino acids. This substitution of the ketone group by an amino group reportedly lowers the serum urea nitrogen, slows the disease progression, and defers the need for dialysis.

TPN In Hepatic Failure

Some cirrhotic patients with hepatic encephalopathy have abnormal plasma amino acid concentrations.[112,113] In these patients, the aromatic amino acids (phenylalanine, tryptophan, and tyrosine) are significantly elevated while levels of branched-chain amino acids (leucine, isoleucine and valine) are depressed. Hepatic coma may result in part from the inability of the liver to remove aromatic amino acids from the portal blood.[112–114] Aromatic amino acids with the branched-chain amino acids compete for active transport across the blood brain barrier. The higher levels of the serotonin precursor tryptophan favors increased synthesis of serotonin which is associated with sleep. An investigational solution, 'FO80' (McGaw) has a higher than normal ratio of branched-chain to aromatic amino acids (Table 12). Hepatic coma has been reversed with this solution.[112–114]

PERIPHERALLY ADMINISTERED TOTAL PARENTERAL NUTRITION

With the recent marketing of Intralipid, a parenteral fat emulsion, an alternative to central TPN is available. Administration of this product through a peripheral vein eliminates complications related to a central catheter and hypertonic glucose. Since Intralipid is a soybean oil emulsion, it is different from the cottonseed oil emulsion (Lipomul) used in the 1950's.[115,116] Fever, jaundice, and coagulation were linked to a toxic non-extractable substance in the cottonseed oil, and the emulsifying agent caused red blood cell aggregation.[117,118] Intralipid, 10% and 20%, has been used safely in Europe since the 1960's and in Canada for over 5 years. Availability in the United States has been limited. The emulsion, currently produced in Sweden, is inspected by the Food and Drug Administration for sterility and pyrogens prior to domestic release; only the 10% emulsion is currently FDA-approved for use in the U.S.

Fat provides 9 kcal/g, whereas carbohydrates and proteins provide approximately 4 kcal/g.[119] Glycerol has been added to the soybean oil to raise the osmolarity to 280 mOs/L and increase the caloric content to 1.1 kcal per ml; the emulsifying agent is egg yolk phosphatide. Since the fat particles in Intralipid are greater than 0.5 micrometer in diameter, they cannot pass through a micropore filter. Further,

TABLE 12 Comparison of Amino Acid Composition

Amino Acid	Freamine II g/1000 ml	FO 80[b] g/100 ml
Essential		
L-Isoleucine[a]	2.95	4.50
L-Leucine[a]	3.85	5.50
L-Lysine HCL	3.85	3.80
L-Methionine	2.25	0.50
L-Phenylalanine	2.40	0.50
L-Threonine	1.70	2.25
L-Tryptophan	0.65	0.38
L-Valine[a]	2.80	4.20
Nonessential		
L-Alanine	3.00	3.75
L-Arginine	1.55	3.00
L-Histidine	1.20	1.20
L-Proline	4.75	4.00
L-Serine	2.50	2.50
Glycine	9.00	4.50
L-Cysteine HCL	0.02	0.20
Total Amino Acids	42.47	40.78

[a]Branched-chain amino acids.
[b]For investigational use (McGaw Labs).

because Intralipid is an emulsion, the amino acids must be given as a second infusion. The two fluids are administered simultaneously through a 'Y' set at the needle (Figure 1). The amino acids solution may contain dextrose 5% along with standard electrolytes and vitamins. Administration of both fluids continuously appears to protect the vein from the effects of the hypertonic amino acid-dextrose-electrolyte solution.[116,117]

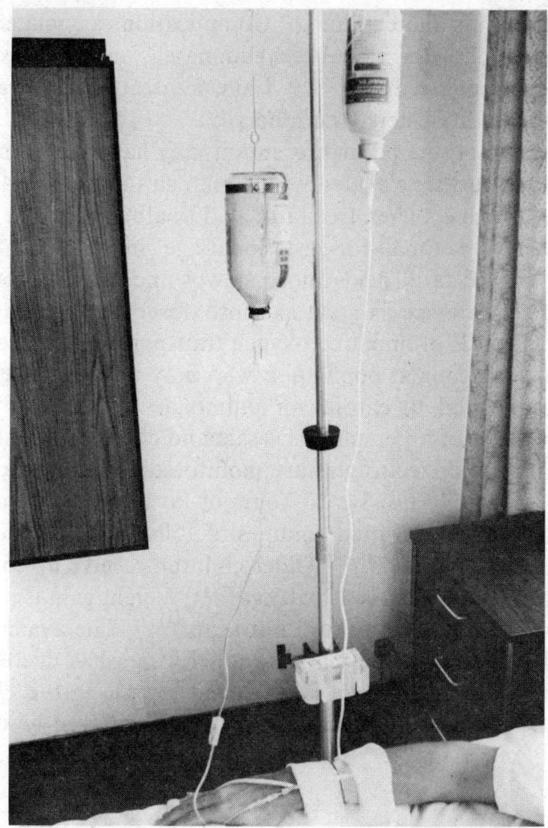

FIGURE 1. Peripheral administration of soybean oil emulsion and amino acid solution.

In adults the daily dose of Intralipid should not exceed 2.5 g (25 ml) per kg per day and it should account for a maximum of 60% of total calories. This could be approximated by administering 1500 ml (1650 kcal) of the fat emulsion along with 2000 ml of the amino acid 4.25%, dextrose 5% solution (700 kcal). Fluid volumes in the peripheral system are, therefore, higher than those of the central TPN system. Recent reports attest to the safety and efficacy of this fat emulsion when used in combination with an amino acid-dilute dextrose solution.[120–124] There appears to be a need for some carbohydrate, whether as glycerol or dextrose, to allow protein to be spared.[125,126]

Intralipid has drastically altered the concept of total parenteral nutrition in infants and children.[127] Complications associated with the central venous catheter have been eliminated, and the frequency of infections has been reduced.[128,129] Fungal infections are rarely seen when TPN is administered peripherally.

The neonate and the premature infant may have the normally high bilirubin levels further elevated with administration of Intralipid.[130,131] Bilirubin is displaced when free fatty acid to albumin molar ratios are greater than 6.[131] Small-for-gestational-age infants hydrolyze triglycerides to free fatty acids more slowly and have free fatty acid values more than twice as great as those observed in gestational age infants.[130] Hazards of impaired oxygen transport are a more common concern in this neonatal population who may already have impaired oxygenation related to cardiac or pulmonary diseases.[132]

The overall use of fat emulsions is safe and efficacious when plasma lipid clearance and electrolytes are monitored.[133] Infants commonly receive up to 4 g (40 ml)/kg/24 hours of fat added to their nitrogen source and receive total fluid volumes of 150 ml/kg/24 hours and 60 to 100 kcal/kg/24 hours.[127–129] Older children receive up to 3 g/kg of Intralipid, 100 ml/kg, and 60 kcal/kg.[127,128] Weight gain is not as great with this regimen as with central nutrition.[134,135] The availability of a 20% Intralipid emulsion in Canada and Europe has decreased total fluids.[136,137] If such a product is approved for use in the USA, more total calories would be available than with presently used fluid volumes.

Peripheral TPN Without Fat Emulsions

In infants who cannot tolerate fats, limited growth may occur with a peripherally administered amino acid-dextrose solution, given at a rate of 200 to 250 ml/kg/24 hours.[128,138] When 1% amino acids and 10% dextrose are given at this high rate, approximately 100 kcal/kg are provided. Patients with renal or cardiovascular impairment would obviously not be candidates for such large solute loads.

For premature newborns who experience episodes of apnea when fed orally, we have used a 2% amino acid and 10% dextrose solution given peripherally with or without a fat emulsion. When fat emulsions are not administered, we administer 120 to 150 ml/kg/24 hours; these volumes provide 50 to 63 kcal/kg. This is used more for short-term maintenance than for long-term weight gain.

PROTEIN SPARING

The concept of replacing the traditional postsurgical 5% dextrose and electrolyte solution with an 'isotonic' 3% amino acid and electrolyte solution was advanced in the early 1970's by Blackburn, et al.[139,140] When compared to the starvation state, dextrose infusions produce elevated insulin levels in order to utilize the carbohydrate.[140] The antilipolytic effect of the insulin curtails fat mobilization and ketosis and mandates further protein breakdown for calories. Nitrogen balance is less negative when a 3% amino acid solution (infused at the rate of 1 g/kg/24 hours) is given in place of 5% glucose.[141–144] Increasing infusion concentrations of amino acids results in hypertonic solutions, but this allows administration of as much as 1.7 g/kg with normal fluid volumes.[142,143]

It is unclear whether the incorporation of 5% dextrose into the infusion increases the protein sparing effect of 'isotonic' amino acids and electrolytes alone.[145–148] More definitive evaluation of the 'nitrogen balance' concept as it relates to 3% amino acid solutions as the sole caloric source for short-term needs must be completed. Turnover of 3-methylhistidine, found excreted in the urine, is related to muscle protein breakdown.[149] The finding that amino acid infusions reduce excretion of 3-methylhistidine indicates that the decrease in negative nitrogen balance is related to preservation of muscle tissue.[149]

REFERENCES

1. Dudrick SJ, Wilmore DW, Vars HM: Long-term total parenteral nutrition with growth in puppies and positive nitrogen balance in patients. Surg Forum 18:356–357, 1967.
2. Dudrick SJ, Wilmore DW, Vars HM, et al: Long-term parenteral nutrition with growth, development, and positive nitrogen balance. Surgery 64:134–142, 1968.
3. Wilmore DW, Dudrick SJ: Growth and development of an infant receiving all nutrients exclusively by vein. JAMA 203:860–864, 1968.
4. Dudrick SJ, Wilmore DW, Vars HM, et al: Can intravenous feeding as the sole means of nutrition support growth in the child and restore weight loss in the adult? An affirmative answer. Ann Surg 169:974–984, 1969.
5. Das JB, Filler RM, Rubin VG, et al: Intravenous dextrose-amino acid feeding: the metabolic response in the surgical neonate. J Pediatr Surg 5:127–135, 1970.
6. Elman R, Weiner DO: Intravenous alimentation: with special reference to protein (amino acid) metabolism. JAMA 112:796–802, 1939.
7. Martin GJ, Thompson MR: Intravenous alimentation with amino acids: a review. Medicine 22:73–86, 1943.
8. Geyer RP: Parenteral nutrition. Physiol Rev 40:150–186, 1960.
9. Rhoads JE: Diuretics as an adjuvant in disposing of extra water employed as a vehicle in parenteral hyperalimentation. Fed Proc 21:389, 1962.
10. Moore FD: *Metabolic Care of the Surgical Patient*. Philadelphia, W.B. Saunders Co., 1959, pp 459–468.

11. Van Way CW III, Meng HC, Sandstead HH: Nitrogen balance in postoperative patients receiving parenteral nutrition. Arch Surg 110:272–276, 1975.
12. Clowes GHA Jr, O'Donnell TF, Blackburn GL, et al: Energy metabolism and proteolysis in traumatized and septic man. Surg Clin North Am 56:1169–1184, 1976.
13. Kinney JM, Roe CF: Caloric equivalents of fever: I. Patterns of postoperative response. Ann Surg 156:610–622, 1962.
14. Myers RN, Smink RD, Goldstein F: Parenteral hyperalimentation—five years' clinical experience. Am J Gastroenterol 62:313–324, 1974.
15. Kinney JM: Calories: Nitrogen: Disease and injury relationship. In, *Total Parenteral Nutrition.* Edited by PL White, ME Nagy. Acton, Publishing Sciences Group, Inc., 1974, pp 81–91.
16. Beal JM, Cornell GN, Gilder H: Factors influencing nitrogen metabolism in surgical patients. Surgery 36:468–484, 1954.
17. Long CL, Crosby F, Geiger JW, et al: Parenteral nutrition in the septic patient: nitrogen balance, limiting plasma amino acids, and calorie to nitrogen ratios. Am J Clin Nutr 29:380–391, 1976.
18. Wilmore DW, Dudrick SJ: Safe long-term venous catheterization. Arch Surg 98:256–258, 1969.
19. Dudrick SJ: Total intravenous feeding: when nutrition seems impossible. Drug Therapy 1:11–20, (Feb) 1976.
20. Hull RL: Physiochemical considerations in intravenous hyperalimentation. Am J Hosp Pharm 31:236–243, 1974.
21. Madan PL, Madan KD, Palumbo JF: Total parenteral nutrition. Drug Intel Clin Pharm 10:684–696, 1976.
22. Shils ME: Minerals. In, *Total Parenteral Nutrition.* Edited by PL White, ME Nagy. Acton, Publishing Sciences Group, Inc., 1974, pp 257–275.
23. Dick W, Seeling W: Water and electrolyte requirements during parenteral nutrition. In, *Parenteral Nutrition.* Edited by FW Ahnefeld, C Burri, W Dick, M Halmagyi. Heidelberg, Springer-Verlag, 1974, pp 99–112.
24. Randall HT: Fluid, electrolyte, and acid-base balance. Surg Clin North Am 56:1019–1058, 1976.
25. Shils ME, Wright WL, Turnbull A, et al: Long-term parenteral nutrition through an external arteriovenous shunt. N Engl J Med 283:341–344, 1970.
26. Ryan JA Jr: Complications of total parenteral nutrition. In, *Total Parenteral Nutrition.* Edited by JE Fischer. Boston, Little, Brown and Company, 1976, pp 55–100.
27. Kaminski MV Jr, Harris DF, Colin CF, et al: Electrolyte compatibility in a synthetic amino acid hyperalimentation solution. Am J Hosp Pharm 31:244–246, 1974.
28. Electrolyte requirements in total parenteral nutrition. McGaw Medical Information Bulletin. March, 1972.
29. Turco SJ, Burke WA: Methods of ordering and use of intravenous phosphate (mEq vs mM). Hosp Pharm 10:320–326, 1975.
30. Travis SF, Sugerman HJ, Ruberg RL, et al: Alteration of red cell glycolytic intermediates and oxygen transport as a consequence of hypophosphatemia in patients receiving intravenous hyperalimentation. N Engl J Med 285:763–768, 1971.
31. Silvis SE, Paragas PD, Jr: Paresthesias, weakness, seizures and hypophosphatemia in patients receiving hyperalimentation. Gastroenterology 62:513–520, 1972.
32. Craddock PR, Yawata Y, Van Santen L, et al: Acquired phagocyte dysfunction: a complication of the hypophosphatemia of parenteral hyperalimentation. N Engl J Med 290:1403–1407, 1974.
33. Chan JCM: The influence of synthetic amino acid and casein hydrolysate on the endogenous production and urinary excretion of acid in total intravenous alimentation. Pediatr Res 6:789–796, 1972.
34. Chan JCM, Asch MJ, Lin S, et al: Hyperalimentation with amino acid and casein hydrolysate solutions: mechanism of acidosis. JAMA 220:1700–1705, 1972.
35. Heird WC, Dell RB, Driscoll JM, et al: Metabolic acidosis resulting from intravenous alimentation mixtures containing synthetic amino acids. N Engl J Med 287:943–948, 1972.
36. Giovanoni R: The manufacturing pharmacy solutions and incompatibilities. In, *Total Parenteral Nutrition.* Edited by JE Fischer. Boston, Little, Brown and Company, 1976, pp 27–53.

37. Greene HL: Vitamins in total parenteral nutrition. Drug Intel Clin Pharm 6:355–360, 1972.
38. Hartline JV, Zachman RD: Vitamin A delivery in total parenteral nutrition solution. Pediatrics 58:448–451, 1976.
39. Shils ME: Parenteral multivitamins: time for changes. Bull Parenteral Drug Assoc 30:226–233, 1976.
40. Hankins DA, Riella MC, Scribner BH, et al: Whole blood trace element concentrations during total parenteral nutrition. Surgery 79:674–677, 1976.
41. Fleming CR, Hodges RE, Hurley LS: A prospective study of serum copper and zinc levels in patients receiving total parenteral nutrition. Am J Clin Nutr 29:70–77, 1976.
42. Solomons NW, Layden TJ, Rosenberg IH, et al: Plasma trace metals during total parenteral alimentation. Gastroenterology 70:1022–1025, 1976.
43. Hull RL, Cassidy D: Trace element deficiencies during total parenteral nutrition. Drug Intel Clin Pharm 11:536–541, 1977.
44. Jacobson S, Wester PO: Balance study of twenty trace elements during total parenteral nutrition in man. Br J Nutr 37:107–126, 1977.
45. Hoffmann RP, Ashby DM: Trace element concentrations in commercially available solutions. Drug Intel Clin Pharm 10:74–76, 1976.
46. Bozian RC, Shearer C: Copper, zinc, and manganese content of four amino acid and protein hydrolysate preparations. Am J Clin Nutr 29:1331–1332, 1976.
47. Vilter RW, Bozian RC, Hess EV, et al: Manifestations of copper deficiency in a patient with systemic sclerosis on intravenous hyperalimentation. N Engl J Med 291:188–191, 1974.
48. Palmisano DJ: Nutrient deficiencies after intensive parenteral alimentation (letter). N Engl J Med 29:799, 1974.
49. Tucker SB, Schroeter AL, Brown PW, et al: Acquired zinc deficiency cutaneous manifestations typical of acrodermatitis enteropathica. JAMA 235:2399–2402, 1976.
50. Okada A, Takagi Y, Itakura T, et al: Skin lesions during intravenous hyperalimentation: zinc deficiency. Surgery 80:629–635, 1976.
51. Jeejeebhoy KN, Chu RC, Marliss EB, et al: Chromium deficiency, glucose intolerance, and neuropathy reversed by chromium supplementation, in a patient receiving long-term total parenteral nutrition. Am J Clin Nutr 30:531–538, 1977.
52. Shils ME: Guidelines for total parenteral nutrition. JAMA 220:1721–1729, 1972.
53. Dudrick SJ, Rhoades JE: New horizons for intravenous feeding. JAMA 215:939–949, 1971.
54. Hull RL: Use of trace elements in intravenous hyperalimentation solutions. Am J Hosp Pharm 31:759–761, 1974.
55. Shils ME: Minerals in total parenteral nutrition. Drug Intel Clin Pharm 6:385–393, 1972.
56. Shils ME: More on trace elements in total parenteral nutrition solutions (letter). Am J Hosp Pharm 32:141–142, 1975.
57. Dudrick SJ, MacFayden BV Jr, Van Buren CT, et al: Parenteral hyperalimentation: metabolic problems and solutions. Ann Surg 176:259–264, 1972.
58. Ryan JA Jr, Abel RM, Abbott WM, et al: Catheter complications in total parenteral nutrition: a prospective study of 200 consecutive patients. N Engl J Med 290:757–761, 1974.
59. Hill JB: The adsorption of 131-I insulin to glass. Endocrinology 65:515–517, 1959.
60. Wiseman R Jr, Baltz BE: Prevention of insulin 131-I adsorption to glass. Endocrinology 68:354–356, 1961.
61. Weisenfeld S, Podolsky S, Goldsmith L, et al: Adsorption of insulin to infusion bottles and tubing. Diabetes 17:766–771, 1968.
62. Petty C, Cunningham NL: Insulin adsorption by glass infusion bottles, polyvinyl chloride infusion containers, and intravenous tubing. Anesthesiology 40:400–404, 1974.
63. Weber SS, Wood WA, Jackson EA: Availability of insulin from parenteral nutrient solutions. Am J Hosp Pharm 34:353–357, 1977.
64. Collins RN, Braun PA, Zinner SH, et al: Risk of local and systemic infection with polyethylene intravenous catheters: a prospective study of 213 catheterizations. N Engl J Med 279:340–343, 1968.
65. Banks DC, Yates DB, Cawdrey HM, et al: Infection from intravenous catheters. Lancet 1:443–445, 1970.
66. Peter G, Lloyd-Still JD, Lovejoy FH: Local infection and bacteremia from scalp vein needles and polyethylene catheters in children. J Pediatr 80:78–83, 1972.
67. Glover JL, O'Brien SA, Jolly L: Infusion catheter sepsis: an increasing threat. Ann Surg 173:148–151, 1971.

68. Goldman DA, Martin WT, Worthington JW: Growth of bacteria and fungi in total parenteral nutrition solutions. Am J Surg 126:314–318, 1973.
69. Rowlands DA, Wilkinson WR, Yoshimura N: Storage stability of mixed hyperalimentation solutions. Am J Hosp Pharm 30:436–438, 1973.
70. Deeb EN, Natsios GA: Contamination of intravenous fluids by bacteria and fungi during preparation and administration. Am J Hosp Pharm 28:764–767, 1971.
71. Hoshal VL Jr, Ause RG, Haskins PA: Fibrin sleeve formation on indwelling subclavian central venous catheters. Arch Surg 102:353–358, 1971.
72. Groff DB: Complications of intravenous hyperalimentation in newborns and infants. J Pediatr Surg 4:460–464, 1969.
73. Boeckman CR, Krill CE: Bacterial and fungal infections complicating parenteral alimentation in infants and children. J Pediatr Surg 5:117–126, 1970.
74. Maki DG, Goldman DA, Rhame FS: Infection control in intravenous therapy. Ann Intern Med 79:867–887, 1973.
75. Curry CR, Quie PG: Fungal septicemia in patients receiving parenteral hyperalimentation. N Engl J Med 285:1221–1224, 1971.
76. Ashcraft KW, Leape LL: Candida sepsis complicating parenteral feeding. JAMA 212:454–456, 1970.
77. Beatley DW, Lepper MH: Septicemia related to indwelling venous catheter. JAMA 206:1749–1752, 1968.
78. Dillon JD Jr, Schaffner W, Van Way CW III, et al: Septicemia and total parenteral nutrition distinguishing catheter-related from other septic episodes. JAMA 223:1341–1344, 1973.
79. Goldman DA, Maki DG: Infection control in total parenteral nutrition. JAMA 223:1360–1364, 1973.
80. Nelson R: Minimizing systemic infection during complete parenteral alimentation of small infants. Arch Dis Child 49:16–20, 1974.
81. Saunders RA, Sheldon GF: Septic complications of total parenteral nutrition: a five-year experience. Am J Surg 132:214–220, 1976.
82. Copeland EM III, MacFadyen BV, Dudrick SJ: Prevention of microbial catheter contamination in patients receiving parenteral hyperalimentation. South Med J 67:303–306, 1974.
83. Skoutakis VA, Martinez DR, Miller WA, et al: Team approach to total parenteral nutrition. Am J Hosp Pharm 32:693–697, 1975.
84. Powell JR, Cupit GC: Developing the pharmacist's role in monitoring total parenteral nutrition. Drug Intel Clin Pharm 8:576–580, 1974.
85. Sanderson I, Deitel M: Intravenous hyperalimentation without sepsis. Surg Gynecol Obstet 136:577–585, 1973.
86. Leape L, Sceppa J, Barza M, et al: Guidelines for total parenteral nutrition. J Maine Med Assoc 65:320–324, 1974.
87. Heird WC, Winters RW: Total parenteral nutrition. J Pediatr 86:2–16, 1975.
88. Phillips KJ: Nursing care in parenteral nutrition. In, *Total Parenteral Nutrition.* Edited by JE Fischer. Boston, Little, Brown and Company, 1976, pp 101–110.
89. Brennan MF, Goldman MH, O'Connell RC, et al: Prolonged parenteral alimentation: candida growth and the prevention of candidemia by amphotericin instillation. Ann Surg 176:265–272, 1972.
90. Kaminski MV Jr, Stolar MH: Parenteral hyperalimentation—a quality of care survey and review. Am J Hosp Pharm 31:228–235, 1974.
91. Swenson JP, Edwards D, Chamberlain M, et al: A total parenteral nutrition protocol. Drug Intel Clin Pharm 11:714–720, 1977.
92. Conrad WF, Gassett RH, Goupil DA: A service-integrated approach to clinical pharmacy practice through a hyperalimentation program. Am J Hosp Pharm 30:695–697, 1973.
93. Tsallas G, Baun DC: Home care total parenteral alimentation. Am J Hosp Pharm 29:840–846, 1972.
94. Ivey M, Riella M, Mueller W, et al: Long-term parenteral nutrition in the home. Am J Hosp Pharm 32:1032–1036, 1975.
95. Waisman HA, Kerr GR: Amino acid and protein metabolism in the developing fetus and the newborn infant. Pediatr Clin North Am 12:551–572, 1965.
96. Filler RM, Eraklis AJ: Care of the critically ill child: intravenous alimentation. Pediatrics 46:456–461, 1970.

97. Filler RM, Eraklis AJ, Rubin VG, et al: Long-term total parenteral nutrition in infants. N Engl J Med 281:589–594, 1969.
98. Stegink LD, Baker GL: Infusion of protein hydrolysates in the newborn infant: plasma amino acid concentrations. J Pediatr 78:595–602, 1971.
99. Lloyd-Still JD, Shwachman H, Filler RM: Intravenous hyperalimentation in pediatrics. Am J Dig Dis 17:1043–1051, 1972.
100. Driscoll JM, Heird WC, Schullinger JN, et al: Total intravenous alimentation in low-birthweight infants: a preliminary report. J Pediatr 81:145–153, 1972.
101. Heird WC, MacMillan RW, Winters RW: Total parenteral nutrition in the pediatric patient. In, *Total Parenteral Nutrition.* Edited by JE Fischer. Boston, Little, Brown and Company, 1976, pp 253–284.
102. Feliciano DV, Telando RL: Total parenteral nutrition in infants and children. Mayo Clin Proc 51:647–654, 1976.
103. Wilmore DW, Groff DB, Bishop HC, et al: Total parenteral nutrition in infants with catastrophic gastrointestinal anomalies. J Pediatr Surg 4:181–189, 1969.
104. Rose WC, Wixom RD: The amino acid requirements of man. XVI. The role of nitrogen intake. J Biol Chem 217:997–1004, 1955.
105. Abel RM, Abbott WM, Fischer JE: Acute renal failure. Treatment without dialysis by total parenteral nutrition. Arch Surg 103:503–515, 1971.
106. Abel RM, Abbott WM, Back CH, et al: Essential L-amino acids for hyperalimentation in patients with disordered nitrogen metabolism. Am J Surg 128:317–323, 1974.
107. Dudrick SJ, Steiger E, Long JM: Renal failure in surgical patients. Treatment with intravenous essential amino acids and hypertonic dextrose. Surgery 68:180–186, 1970.
108. Rose WC, Dekker EE: Urea as a source of nitrogen for the biosynthesis of amino acids. J Biol Chem 223:107–121, 1956.
109. Giordano C: Use of exogenous and endogenous urea for protein synthesis in normal and uremic subjects. J Lab Clin Med 62:231–246, 1963.
110. Giovannetti S, Maggiore Q: A low-nitrogen diet with protein of high biologic value for severe chronic ureamia. Lancet 1:1000–1004, 1964.
111. Walser M: Treatment of renal failure with keto acids. Hosp Practice 10:59–66, (Jun) 1975.
112. Fischer JE, Funovics JM, Aquirre A, et al: The role of plasma amino acids in hepatic encephalopathy. Surgery 78:276–290, 1975.
113. Fischer JE, Rosen HM, Ebeid AM, et al: The effect of normalization of plasma amino acids on hepatic encephalopathy in man. Surgery 80:77–91, 1976.
114. Munro HN, Fernstrom JD, and Wurtman RJ: Insulin, plasma amino acid imbalance and hepatic coma. Lancet 1:722–724, 1975.
115. Jeejeebhoy KN, Anderson GH, Sanderson I, et al: Total parenteral nutrition: nutrient needs and technical tips, part I. Mod Med Canada 29:832–841, 1974.
116. Meng HC: Use of fat emulsions in parenteral nutrition. Drug Intel Clin Pharm 6:321–330, 1972.
117. Wilmore DW, Moylan JA, Helmkamp GM, et al: Clinical evaluation of a 10% intravenous fat emulsion for parenteral nutrition in thermally injured patients. Ann Surg 178:503–513, 1973.
118. Dietel M, Kaminsky V: Total nutrition by peripheral vein—the lipid system. Can Med Assoc J 111:152–154, 1974.
119. Eckart J: Requirement and utilization of fats. In, *Parenteral Nutrition.* Edited by FW Ahnefeld, C Burri, W Dick, M Halmagyi. Heidelberg, Springer-Verlag, 1974, pp 80–98.
120. Zohrab WJ, McHattie JD, Jeejeebhoy KN: Total parenteral alimentation, with lipid. Gastroenterology 64:583–592, 1973.
121. Yeo MT, Gazzaniga AB, Bartlett RH, et al: Total intravenous nutrition experience with fat emulsions and hypertonic glucose. Arch Surg 106:792–796, 1973.
122. Hansen LM, Hardie WR, Holdago J: Fat emulsion for intravenous administration: clinical experience with intralipid 10%. Ann Surg 184:80–88, 1976.
123. Silberman H, Freehauf M, Fong G, et al: Parenteral nutrition with lipids. JAMA 283:1380–1382, 1977.
124. Gazzaniga AB, Bartlett RH, Shobe JB: Nitrogen balance in patients receiving either fat or carbohydrate for total intravenous nutrition. Ann Surg 182:163–168, 1975.
125. Brennan MF, Fitzpatrick GF, Cohen KH, et al: Glycerol: major contributor to the short-term protein sparing effect of fat emulsions in normal man. Ann Surg 182:386–394, 1975.

126. Long TM, Wilmore DW, Mason AD, et al: Effect of carbohydrate and fat intake on nitrogen excretion during total intravenous feeding. Ann Surg 185:417–422, 1977.
127. Coran AG: Total intravenous feeding of infants and children without the use of a central venous catheter. Ann Surg 179:445–449, 1974.
128. Filler RM, Coran AG: Total parenteral nutrition in infants and children: central and peripheral approaches. Surg Clin North Am 56:395–412, 1976.
129. Puri P, Guiney EJ, O'Donnell B: Total parenteral feeding in infants using peripheral veins. Arch Dis Child 50:133–136, 1975.
130. Andrew G, Chan G, Schiff D: Lipid metabolism in the neonate. I. The effects of intralipid infusion on plasma triglyceride and free fatty acid concentrations in the neonate. J Pediatr 88:273–278, 1976.
131. Andrew G, Chan G, Schiff D: Lipid metabolism in the neonate. II. The effect of intralipid on bilirubin binding in vitro and in vivo. J Pediatr 88:279–284, 1976.
132. Bryan H, Shennan A, Griffin E, et al: Intralipid—its rational use in parenteral nutrition of the newborn. Pediatrics 58:787–790, 1976.
133. Asch MJ, Sperling M, Fiser R, et al: Metabolic and hormonal studies comparing three parenteral nutrition regimens in infants. Ann Surg 182:62–65, 1975.
134. Gunn T, Brown RS, Pencharz P, et al: Total parenteral nutrition in malnourished infants with intractable diarrhea. Can Med Assoc J 117:357–360, 1977.
135. O'Neill JA, Meng HC, Caldwell M, et al: Variations in intravenous nutrition in the management of catabolic states in infants and children. J Pediatr Surg 9:889–897, 1974.
136. Harries JT: Intravenous feeding in infants. Arch Dis Child 46:855–862, 1971.
137. Wei P, Hamilton JR, LeBlanc AE: A clinical and metabolic study of an intravenous feeding technique using peripheral veins as the initial infusion site. Can Med Assoc J 106:969–974, 1972.
138. Fox HA, Krasna IH: Total intravenous nutrition by peripheral vein in neonatal surgical patients. Pediatrics 52:14–20, 1973.
139. Blackburn GL, Flatt JP, Clowes GHA: Peripheral intravenous feeding with isotonic amino acid solutions. Am J Surg 125:447–454, 1973.
140. Blackburn GL, Flatt JP, Clowes GHA, et al: Protein sparing therapy during periods of starvation with sepsis or trauma. Ann Surg 177:588–594, 1973.
141. Freeman JB, Stegink LD, Fry LK: Evaluation of amino acid infusions as protein sparing agents in normal adult subjects. Am J Clin Nutr 28:477–481, 1975.
142. Freeman JB, Stegink LD, Meyer PD: Metabolic effects of amino acid vs dextrose infusion in surgical patients. Arch Surg 110:916–925, 1975.
143. Schulte WJ, Condon RE, Kraus MA: Positive nitrogen balance using isotonic crystalline amino acid solution. Arch Surg 110:914–915, 1975.
144. Hoover HC, Grant JP, Gorschboth C, et al: Nitrogen-sparing intravenous fluids in postoperative patients. N Engl J Med 293:172–175, 1975.
145. Moore FD, Brennan MR: Intravenous amino acids (editorial). N Engl J Med 293:194–195, 1975.
146. Editorial: Postoperative feeding and metabolism. Lancet 2:263–264, 1975.
147. Greenberg GR, Marliss EB, Anderson GH, et al: Protein-sparing therapy in postoperative patients. Effects of added hypocaloric glucose or lipid. N Engl J Med 294:1411–1416, 1976.
148. Freeman JB, Stegink LD, Wittine MF, et al: The current status of protein sparing. Surg Gynecol Obstet 144:843–849, 1977.
149. Kaminski MV, Dunn NP, Wannemacher RW Jr, et al: Specific muscle protein-sparing postoperative dextrose-free amino acid infusions. J Parenteral Enteral Nutr 1:147–151, 1977.

48. INTRAVENOUS FLUIDS

David A. Henry and David H. Lawson

Intravenous fluids are among the most commonly prescribed drugs in hospitalized patients in the United States.[1] In 1974 an estimated 100 million large volume parenteral solutions were administered in the United States.[2] Up to 54% of medical inpatients in one U.S. hospital participating in the Boston Collaborative Drug Surveillance Program received intravenous fluids, as compared with 7% in an Israeli hospital.[3] Moreover, when a comparison was made between two Scottish hospitals that participated in this study, considerable differences in the frequency of intravenous fluid use were apparent, even in comparable groups of patients.[3] Thus, major differences exist in the use of this type of therapy—both between and within countries.

INDICATIONS FOR INTRAVENOUS THERAPY

Parenteral fluids are indicated primarily to replace fluids previously lost from the body or to maintain homeostasis in those who are unable to do so unaided.

Replacement Therapy

Sudden major loss of body fluids requires rapid replacement which can be achieved only by the intravenous route. The choice of fluid is guided by the clinical problem. Whole blood is the appropriate treatment for hemorrhage and is occasionally used in the emergency management of massive fluid loss from burns. When blood is not available, other colloid solutions such as reconstituted plasma, plasma protein fractions or dextran solutions can be used, although the latter may interfere with subsequent blood grouping and may have a detrimental effect on blood coagulation.[4] Normal saline is now the frequent first choice in acute blood loss when blood is not available.

Normal saline is frequently used to replace fluids lost during prolonged vomiting, diarrhea, intestinal obstruction, ileus, and the recovery phase of acute renal failure. In these disorders the addition of potassium is essential. The clinical use of potassium supplements is reviewed elsewhere.[5,6]

Dextrose 5% in water is indicated to replace depleted extracellular water, as in diabetes insipidus, following excessive sweating, or during prolonged coma. This solution may, however, be inappropriate under certain circumstances, such as nonketotic diabetic coma, when hypotonic saline is the fluid of choice.[7]

Maintenance Therapy

In a number of clinical situations, oral fluid intake is precluded for a limited period; examples are peritonitis after abdominal surgery, or during severe systemic infection or prolonged coma. Under these circumstances, maintenance intravenous therapy must supply the entire fluid and electrolyte requirements of the patient. Assuming that any deficiencies have already been corrected, the fluid requirement of the average adult is around 25 to 40 ml/kg body weight per day. The average requirement for sodium is approximately 135 to 170 mEq per day, and for potassium, approximately 80 to 100 mEq per day. In practice, the average adult is given two liters of fluid in 24 hours, using 5% dextrose and normal saline with added potassium supplements. The normal kidney effectively conserves sodium under conditions of restricted intake, thus relieving the physician of the need for obsessional attempts at providing the exact physiological requirements for each patient. Unfortunately, such mechanisms are less effective in conserving potassium homeostasis, so greater care is required with this ion than with either sodium or water intake.

Emergency Venous Access

Establishment of an intravenous line is often considered essential in the management of many clinical situations, even when disordered fluid balance is not a prominent feature. This attitude undoubtedly results from a fear that access to a vein to inject essential drugs will otherwise prove difficult in the event of a sudden deterioration in the patient's condition. The need for establishing an infusion when a patient experiences serious arrhythmias following myocardial infarction is evident, but the provision of parenteral fluids for every individual admitted with a dubious history of chest pain or a questionable gastrointestinal bleed is unjustified. The potential benefits of routine intravenous therapy should be balanced against the potential hazards. Where doubt remains, the use of an indwelling cannula containing a heparin solution ('heparin lock') should be sufficient for most needs.

HAZARDS OF INTRAVENOUS THERAPY

Thrombophlebitis

Thrombophlebitis is primarily a physicochemical phenomenon and is uncommon within 24 hours of catheterization of a peripheral vein.[8] After this period, the incidence increases in relation to the length of time the catheter is left *in situ*.[9] This complication occurs more frequently with dextrose infusions, possibly due to their extremely low pH.[10–12] Attempts to reduce the incidence of thrombophlebitis by using buffered dextrose solutions or by adding heparin or hydrocortisone to the infusion fluids have been only partially successful.[8,13–15] Despite the high prevalence of post-catheterization thrombophlebitis, pulmonary embolization appears to be uncommon unless the thrombus extends to involve the deep venous system—a rare complication usually arising from catheterization of peripheral veins in the lower limb.

Infection

Infusion-associated sepsis is potentially serious, since the organisms have direct access to the circulation. Many potential sources of infection arise during the manufacture and administration of parenteral fluids. Recent incidents in the United States and Great Britain involving large-scale contamination of parenteral fluids during manufacture resulted in patients developing nosocomial septicemia—a potentially fatal condition.[16,17]

The subject of infection control in intravenous therapy has been extensively reviewed by Maki and coworkers.[9] They highlighted four major areas in which sepsis could complicate the use of parenteral fluids.

(1) *Catheter insertion.* Skin flora are frequent contaminants of intravenous catheters, and adequate sterilization of the skin of both operator and patient prior to venipuncture is an essential although

frequently neglected procedure.[11] Solutions containing chlorhexidine, alcohol, and iodine are effective antiseptics[18–21] although the latter may produce allergic reactions or cutaneous burns, particularly when used in high concentrations.[22] Shaving of hair from venipuncture sites is not essential and may increase the risk of introducing organisms by alterations of skin flora.[23]

(2) *Type of catheter.* The relation of long-life plastic catheters to infusion-related sepsis is controversial. The frequency with which organisms can be isolated from catheters varies widely, from 4 to 45% in different series.[11,24] Sepsis is particularly common with infusions sited in the lower extremities,[25] where long-life catheters are frequently used. Moreover, the proportion of positive cultures from catheters increases with time in all sites.[24] Although no clear-cut relationship has been demonstrated between bacterial isolation from catheters and infusion-related septicemia, both these complications are much more common when the catheter is left in place for more than 48 hours.[9] The higher prevalence of bacterial isolation from plastic as opposed to steel catheters has led to the belief that plastic catheters are associated with greater risk of infection.[9] One possible explanation for this finding is the smaller bore of metal cannulae, which results in less trauma to the venous endothelium.[26] However, it is more likely that fluid extravasation from the vessel occurs at an earlier stage with the metal device, thereby necessitating a more frequent change of cannula.[9] This also explains the current popularity of plastic catheters.

(3) *Thrombophlebitis.* Although most investigators agree that physical trauma or chemical irritation are the prime causes of phlebitis, prospective studies have shown a possible association between the occurrence of thrombophlebitis and infusion-related septicemia. In particular, during the much publicized 'Abbott incident,' a higher rate of thrombophlebitis was found among infected patients than among those who did not develop sepsis.[9]

(4) *Contaminated infusion fluids.* Bacterial contamination of infusion fluids can occur during manufacture or as a result of any medical or nursing procedure which disturbs the integrity of the container or administration set. Failure of commercial sterilization techniques is probably rare, but when it occurs the results can be devastating.[27] A study conducted by the Center for Disease Control in Atlanta revealed 378 cases of septicemia in 25 hospitals after the nationwide use of a batch of infected infusion fluid.[16] The organisms isolated in this and other similar outbreaks were of the *Enterobacter*

group. These bacteria are rare pathogens in man that have an unusual ability to survive the normally bacteriocidal environment of strongly acidic dextrose solutions.[28,29] Their isolation in blood cultures indicates the possibility of a contaminated infusion.[27]

Infection of infusion fluids can also occur following trauma to the container; tiny cracks in glass bottles or micropunctures of the newer plastic bags provide portals of entry for invading organisms.[9] Contamination can result from injection of drugs into the infusion fluid or administration set, and airborne invasion may result from the use of airways for ventilation of the older rigid containers.[30]

Discovery of contamination usually occurs after the recognition of an adverse event in a patient, since visible changes in appearance of solutions occurs only with very heavy contamination.[27] When contamination is suspected, the infusion should be discontinued immediately with removal of both administration set and catheter.

Volume Overload

When excessive volumes of isotonic intravenous fluids are administered to a healthy individual, the increase in venous return to the heart stimulates cardiac output and can increase urine volume to a maximum of approximately 16 ml/min. With an increased solute load after infusion of hypertonic saline, mannitol, or urea, an osmotic diuresis may occur with even higher urine flow rates. If an increase in cardiac output or glomerular filtration cannot be sustained because of cardiac or renal disease, a rise in pulmonary and, later, systemic venous pressure will ensue with accumulation of fluid in these areas. Since defective handling of sodium accompanies most cardiac and many renal diseases, serious volume overload occurs most frequently when such patients receive infusions of saline and, in particular, hypertonic solutions. Early signs of fluid retention should be watched for whenever a patient with known cardiac or renal disease receives intravenous fluids.

Air Embolism

Venous air embolism is usually considered the most dramatic complication of parenteral fluid therapy. In fact, it is probably necessary to inject air at a rate of 70 to 100 ml/sec to a total of over 200 ml to produce sudden death as the result of acute cor pulmonale.[31]

Infusing fluid into a peripheral vein in a dependent limb using a nonpressurized system, it is highly unlikely that such a large volume of air could be introduced, and the risk is lessened even further by the use of flexible nonventilated containers. The safety of modern infusion techniques is illustrated by a review of over 116,000 blood transfusions in which no recorded cases of fatal air embolism occurred.[32]

Central venous catheters, however, are more hazardous. Air embolism has been reported as a fatal hazard of percutaneous puncture of the subclavian vein.[33,34] The risks are greater when the patient is hypovolemic and the catheter is inserted in the sitting or semi-recumbent position.[31] The resulting negative pressure in a large vessel can introduce a substantial volume of air quickly, either during the catheterization procedure or if the infusion set subsequently becomes detached from the hub of the catheter by accident.[33,35] Insertion of central venous catheters by the internal jugular or subclavian route should only be carried out with the patient tilted in a head-down position.

Particulate Matter

The possible circulatory effects of the injection of particulate matter are seldom considered and generally receive much less attention than some of the more obvious hazards of parenteral fluid therapy. To be visible to the naked eye, particles in suspension must be greater than 50 microns in diameter.[36] Thus, visible clarity of the solution will not guarantee its safety, since invisible particles as small as 12 microns in diameter will not pass through the smallest capillaries and will be trapped in the pulmonary vascular bed.[37] The particulate content of commercial infusion fluids is fairly high, although improved manufacturing techniques have reduced this form of contamination.[38] The most common foreign substance is rubber, in the form of fragments dislodged from bungs during autoclaving.[39] The increasing use of disposable plastic containers should reduce this source of contamination. However, many other different types of particles have been found in intravenous solutions, varying from metal fragments to fibers, molds, and even insects. The opening of large numbers of glass ampuls in the preparation of an injection carries the hazard of introducing glass fragments into the body.[40–42]

Little is known about the effects of particulate matter on the body. It is likely the lungs bear the main burden of any injury. Cellulose fibers are particularly irritating, stimulating the formation of granulomata.[40] Pulmonary hypertension and respiratory failure have been noted among recipients of long-term intravenous therapy, and it is possible that pulmonary edema may sometimes be due to particulate damage in the lungs rather than volume overload.[43]

Chemical Contamination

The advent of disposable nonvented flexible fluid containers has undoubtedly reduced the risk of contamination of intravenous solutions by bacteria and particulate matter. The long-term effects of this change, however, are not known. Interest has recently centered around the possible toxicity of chemicals used in the plasticizing of polyvinyl chloride (PVC). These substances, in particular di-2-ethylhexylphthalate (DEHP), can leech out of the walls of the container and accumulate in the tissues of patients receiving blood transfusions or treatment with parenteral fluids.[44] Although the significance of this finding remains to be established, the possible toxic effects of the plasticizers and stabilizers utilized in the production of PVC will require further investigation, particularly in patients receiving long-term parenteral fluid therapy or multiple blood transfusions.

CHOICE OF PARENTERAL FLUIDS

More than 70 different basic large volume solutions are marketed in the United States. This is surprising, since the great majority of clinical situations can be managed with 5% dextrose and normal saline solutions, with the addition of potassium chloride as required. The use of mixed solutions, particularly those claiming to contain balanced quantities of electrolytes, should be discouraged since they may foster a false sense of security in the clinician who is often unaware both of the exact components contained in the solution and of the needs of the particular patient.

DRUG MONOGRAPHS

SALINE SOLUTIONS

NORMAL SALINE

Sodium chloride 0.9% solution (normal saline) contains 154 mEq of sodium and of chloride per liter. It has, therefore, a slightly higher osmolarity and sodium content than normal plasma. This is not a major disadvantage as its main use is the replacement of deficiencies of extracellular fluid volume. The use of normal saline should be avoided when the patient has a high serum sodium concentration—a situation that requires the use of solutions which replace extracellular water alone. Although hypernatremia and hyperchloremia can be induced by overtreatment with normal saline, volume overload with resulting pulmonary edema is a more common result.

HALF-STRENGTH SALINE

Sodium chloride 0.45% solution contains 77 mEq of sodium and of chloride per liter. It is hypo-osmolar with respect to plasma and can be used to replace deficiencies of extracellular water. It is most commonly used in the treatment of hyperosmolar diabetes mellitus where the use of dextrose is inadvisable and there is a need to provide large amounts of fluid without an excess of sodium ions.

HYPERTONIC SALINE

Solutions of sodium chloride with strengths ranging from 1.8 to 5.0% are available for the treatment of severe sodium depletion, but they should be used with the greatest caution. Hyponatremia frequently indicates water overload with resulting hemodilution, and the total body sodium is often normal or even high.[45] The use of hypertonic saline solutions in this situation may induce or aggravate pre-existing cardiac failure with fatal consequences. If genuine sodium deficiency appears to be present and the serum sodium concentration is dangerously low (less than 120 mEq/ml), hypertonic saline may be infused slowly; if necessary, a short-acting diuretic may be used to prevent fluid overload. This situation arises infrequently.

CARBOHYDRATE SOLUTIONS

DEXTROSE 5%

Water can be infused most conveniently in the form of 5% dextrose. This is a safe solution whose osmolarity (277 mOsm/l) is slightly less than that of plasma. The glucose content is quickly metabolized in normal individuals, although the nutrient value is slight (190 calories per liter). Dextrose solutions are acidic and tend to induce thrombophlebitis.[10] The low pH (3.5 to 5.0) should also be considered when large volumes have to be infused quickly, especially in patients with pre-existing acid-base disturbances.

HIGHER STRENGTH DEXTROSE SOLUTIONS

Dextrose solutions with strengths varying from 10 to 50% are available, the more concentrated being valuable for the immediate correction of hypoglycemia. Ten to 20% solutions provide 380 to 760 calories per liter and can be used to manage conditions such as hepatic or renal failure where a high calorie intake in the form of carbohydrate is indicated. These high-concentration dextrose solutions are intensely irritating to peripheral veins and, therefore, should be infused through long catheters into the superior or inferior vena cava.

FRUCTOSE (Levulose)

Since fructose is rapidly metabolized independently of insulin, its use has been advocated as a calorie source in the treatment of conditions such as diabetes mellitus and liver failure. It has also been used successfully in the treatment of acute alcohol intoxication.[46] Unfortunately, during fructose infusion the rate of lactate formation exceeds its clearance, with the consequent accumulation of lactate in the blood. This tendency to develop lactic acidosis is particularly marked in liver failure,[47] diabetes mellitus, and in the presence of ethanol,[48] and it may preclude the use of fructose in the very conditions in which it should be of greatest value.

ALKALINE SOLUTIONS

SODIUM BICARBONATE

Sodium bicarbonate is the most convenient solution for the correction of metabolic acidosis. It is usually prepared locally in the hospital pharmacy. A 1.43% solution provides 170 mEq of sodium and bicarbonate ions per liter; it is the safest strength for routine use but is not widely available. Unfortunately, rapid correction of acidosis with this solution requires injection of a large volume of fluid; this has led to the use of an 8.4% solution in emergencies. This solution contains 100 mEq of sodium bicarbonate per 100 ml, thus simplifying the calculation of requirements. During the chaos of cardiac arrest, patients often receive larger doses than intended, with consequent sodium overload and metabolic alkalosis. This complication may seriously compromise the likelihood of successful resuscitation.[49,50] The high sodium content of bicarbonate solutions is a drawback when they are used in renal failure, and rapid correction of acidosis in this condition engenders risk of acute tetany if intravenous calcium supplements are not provided.

TROMETHAMINE (Tham)

Tromethamine is an organic buffer, usually available as a 0.3 M solution adjusted to a pH of approximately 8.6 through the addition of acetic acid. It is hypertonic but free of sodium ions. Its use has been advocated in the treatment of most types of acidosis; because of its unique ability to neutralize carbonic acid, it was originally considered valuable in the management of respiratory failure. Experience with tromethamine in this situation has revealed that correction of acidosis is associated with further respiratory depression; modern techniques of assisted ventilation have obviated the need for buffering solutions. Because it is eliminated entirely by the kidney, tromethamine is contraindicated in uremia. A further hazard is hypoglycemia, which can result from infusion of large amounts of tromethamine. There is currently no evidence to support the use of tromethamine in preference to bicarbonate solutions in the management of acidosis.[51]

SODIUM LACTATE

When lactate is infused into normal individuals, it is metabolized to bicarbonate. Unfortunately, this conversion is markedly delayed in the presence of tissue anoxia, and excessive lactate accumulation may occur with worsening acidosis.[48] A number of proprietary mixed electrolyte solutions contain lactate as a bicarbonate precursor, and they are best avoided in situations where this conversion may be impaired.

SODIUM ACETATE

The problems associated with the use of sodium lactate do not occur with sodium acetate, since it is converted to bicarbonate in the citric acid cycle even under anaerobic conditions. It offers no real advantage over bicarbonate solution except that it is cheaper and can be stored for longer periods in hot climates.[52]

AGENTS USED TO TREAT ALKALOSIS

Metabolic alkalosis is almost always accompanied by deficiency of chloride and potassium ions, correction of which using normal saline with added potassium chloride will often partly reverse the acid-base disturbance. When more rapid correction of alkalosis is necessary, administration of ammonium chloride can provide a positive balance of hydrogen ions.[53] However, its intravenous use is accompanied by the danger of ammonia accumulation with resulting encephalopathy. Because of this hazard, some workers have advocated the infusion of hydrochloric acid in the treatment of severe alkalosis.[54] Hydrochloric acid must be given through a central venous catheter, since extravasation from peripheral veins may result in severe tissue necrosis. A further hazard is hemolysis—this has occurred after the infusion of 0.3 N hydrochloric acid. The use of hydrochloric acid should be confined to solutions with a concentration of 0.15 N or less.[55]

INTRAVENOUS POTASSIUM THERAPY

Potassium chloride is available as a 15% (by weight) solution containing 2 mEq/ml. This solution must never be injected in the undiluted form as cardiac arrest will result. It is customary to add potassium chloride to infusion bottles in a concentration of 40 mEq/l, and infusion rates generally should not exceed 10 mEq per hour.[6] In clinical situations characterized by rapid changes in the plasma potassium concentration, such as the diuretic phase of renal failure or during a forced alkaline diuresis, potassium can be infused at rates exceeding 20 mEq per hour, but this should only be attempted in the presence of biochemical and electrocardiographic monitoring. Fatal hyperkalemia has occurred after the addition of potassium chloride to modern flexible containers in the upright position because of pooling of the added potassium at the bottom of the container.[56,57] Adequate mixing of these solutions must be ensured prior to the commencement of an infusion.

CALCIUM SALTS

Calcium is given intravenously only when rapid correction of hypocalcemia is necessary, or when the patient is unable to maintain normal calcium balance by the oral route. Various solutions are available for injection, but in practice a 10% solution of calcium chloride (1.3 mEq/ml) or calcium gluconate (0.45 mEq/ml) will meet most requirements.

Calcium salts are highly irritating, and necrosis with subsequent sloughing of tissue has followed extravasation of solutions containing calcium chloride.[58] In this respect calcium gluconate is safe and is preferable.[59] Injections of calcium should be given slowly as transient hypercalcemia may induce acute cardiac arrhythmias. Calcium salts are incompatible with a number of drugs in solutions,[59] and if mixed with sodium bicarbonate precipitation of insoluble calcium carbonate will result.[60]

MAGNESIUM SALTS

Magnesium is the principal intracellular divalent cation and is essential to the functional integrity of almost every organ and tissue in the body. Despite the identification of magnesium deficiency in a wide range of disease states, including diabetes mellitus, hepatic cirrhosis, intestinal malabsorption, and patients on long-term diuretic therapy,[61–64] controversy still exists as to the benefits of magnesium supplementation in these conditions.

The approximate human daily requirement for magnesium is 20 to 40 mEq, but the normal kidney effectively conserves this cation under conditions of reduced intake.

Intravenous magnesium replacement may be necessary in severe deficiency states. Magnesium sulfate as a 10% solution (0.81 mEq/ml) is preferred. The main hazard associated with its use is hypermagnesemia characterized by neuromuscular blockade and respiratory depression. Calcium and magnesium ions have mutually opposing and competitive actions on the body; thus intravenous calcium gluconate will partially reverse the effects of acute magnesium intoxication.

MIXED SOLUTIONS

A large variety of mixed electrolyte solutions are available. The number of products and the diversity of their content is both confusing and potentially hazardous.

DRUG MONOGRAPHS

PREMIXED POTASSIUM SOLUTIONS

In order to circumvent the problems associated with the addition of potassium chloride to flexible fluid containers (see section on potassium therapy), several manufacturers now provide premixed solutions of potassium chloride in dextrose or saline. These solutions are safe so long as the user is aware of the exact potassium content; this should be clearly marked on the container.

DEXTROSE/SALINE MIXTURES

A solution containing 0.45% saline and 2.5 to 3% dextrose has the theoretical advantage of providing a fluid which is approximately iso-osmolar with plasma while containing only a modest quantity of sodium and chloride ions. This solution is not widely available, and the more commonly used mixture of 0.9% saline and 5% dextrose is undesirable in view of its high osmolarity.

MULTIPLE ELECTROLYTE SOLUTIONS

A large number of products claim to contain 'balanced' mixtures of essential electrolytes. Some of these solutions represent attempts to reduce the excess of sodium and chloride ions present in normal saline by substituting cations such as potassium, calcium, and magnesium or anions such as lactate or acetate. The resulting mixtures vary widely in their constitution and bear little relationship to the actual electrolyte requirements of most patients. As stated earlier, the great majority of clinical situations can be managed with judicious use of 0.9% saline or 5% dextrose with the addition of other electrolytes as determined by the needs of the individual patient. In practice, the only cation which should be routinely considered is potassium.

REFERENCES

1. Miller RR: Drug surveillance utilizing epidemiologic methods: a report from the Boston Collaborative Drug Surveillance Program. Am J Hosp Pharm 30:584–592, 1973.
2. Report of the Comptroller General of the U.S.A.: Recalls of large volume parenterals. Liquid drugs administered intravenously or by other non-oral means. March 12, 1976, (MSD-76-67).
3. Lawson DH: Intravenous fluids in medical in-patients. Br J Clin Pharmacol 4:299–303, 1977.

4. Berliner A, Lackner H: Hemorrhagic diathesis after prolonged infusion of low molecular weight dextran. Am J Med Sci 261:397–403, 1972.
5. Lawson DH: Clinical use of potassium supplements. Am J Hosp Pharm 32:708–711, 1975.
6. Lawson DH: Potassium therapy. Br J Hosp Med 16:392–398, (Oct) 1976.
7. Lucas CP, Grant N, Dally WJ, et al: Diabetic coma without ketoacidosis. Lancet 1:75–77, 1963.
8. Daniell HW: Heparin in the prevention of infusion phlebitis—a double-blind controlled study. JAMA 226:1317–1321, 1973.
9. Maki DG, Goldman DA, Rhame FS: Infection control in intravenous therapy. Ann Intern Med 79:867–887, 1973.
10. Page BH, Raine G, Jones PF: Thrombophlebitis following intravenous infusion (letter). Lancet 2:778, 1952.
11. Banks DC, Cawdrey HM, Harries MG, et al: Infection from intravenous catheters. Lancet 1:443–445, 1970.
12. Clementson CAB, Moshfeghi MM: Strange effects of dextrose 5% in water (letter). N Engl J Med 280:332, 1969.
13. Fonkalsrud E, Pederson BM, Murphy J, et al: Reduction of infusion thrombophlebitis with buffered glucose solutions. Surgery 63:280–284, 1968.
14. Daniell HW: Heparin prevention of catheter thrombosis (letter). JAMA 216:1200, 1971.
15. Clark PB, Polak A, Hajnal J: A clinical trial of hydrocortisone in the prevention of transfusion thrombophlebitis. Postgrad Med J 36:55–56, 1960.
16. Maki DG, Rhame FS, Mackel DC, et al: Nationwide epidemic of septicemia caused by contaminated intravenous products. I. Epidemiologic and clinical features. Am J Med 60:471–485, 1976.
17. Meers PD, Calder MW, Mazhar MM, et al: Intravenous infusion of contaminated dextrose solution. The Devonport incident. Lancet 2:1189–1192, 1973.
18. Lowbury EJL, Lilly HA, Bull JP: Disinfection of the skin of operation sites. Br Med J 2:1039–1044, 1960.
19. Lilly HA, Lowbury EJL: Disinfection of the skin: an assessment of some new preparations. Br Med J 3:674–676, 1971.
20. Lowbury EJL, Lilly HA: Use of 4% chlorhexidine detergent solution (Hibiscrub) and other methods of skin disinfection. Br Med J 1:510–515, 1973.
21. Selwyn S, Ellis H: Skin bacteria and skin disinfection reconsidered. Br Med J 1:136–140, 1972.
22. White JJ, Wallace CK, Burnett LS: Drug letter—skin disinfection. Johns Hopkins Med J 126:169–176, 1970.
23. Altemeier WA: Prevention of post-operative infections: operating theatre practice. In *Infections in Hospitals.* Edited by REO Williams, RA Shooter. Oxford, Oxford University Press, 1963, p 207.
24. Fuchs PC: Indwelling intravenous polyethylene catheters—factors influencing the risk of microbial colonization and sepsis. JAMA 216:1447–1450, 1971.
25. Crane C: Venous interruption for septic thrombophlebitis. N Engl J Med 262:947–951, 1960.
26. Crossley K, Matsen JM: The scalp-vein needle. A prospective study of complication. JAMA 220:985–987, 1972.
27. Anon: Contaminated infusion fluids (editorial). Br Med J 2:546, 1976.
28. Maki DG, Martin WT: Nationwide epidemic of septicemia caused by contaminated infusion products. IV. Growth of microbial pathogens in fluids for intravenous infusion. J Infect Dis 131:267–272, 1975.
29. Guynn JB, Poretz DM, Duma RJ: Growth of various bacteria in a variety of intravenous fluids. Am J Hosp Pharm 30:325–326, 1973.
30. Hansen JS, Hepler CD: Contamination of intravenous solution by airborne microbes. Am J Hosp Pharm 30:326–331, 1973.
31. Ordway CB: Air embolus via CVP catheter without positive pressure. Ann Surg 179:479–481, 1974.
32. Baker RJ, Moinichen SL, Myhus LM: Transfusion reaction: a reappraisal of surgical incidence and significance. Ann Surg 169:684–693, 1969.
33. Flanagan PJ, Gradisar IA, Gross RJ, et al: Air embolus—a lethal complication of subclavian venipuncture. N Engl J Med 281:488–489, 1969.

34. Lucas CR, Irini F: Air embolus via subclavian catheter (letter). N Engl J Med 281:966–967, 1969.
35. Hoshal VL, Fink GH: The subclavian catheter (letter). N Engl J Med 281:1425, 1969.
36. Groves MJ: The size distribution of particles contaminating parenteral solutions. Analyst 94:992–1001, 1969.
37. Kramer W, Tanja JJ, Harrison WL: Precipitates found in admixtures of potassium chloride and dextrose 5% in water. Am J Hosp Pharm 27:548–553, 1970.
38. Turco SJ, Davis NM: Particulate matter in intravenous infusion fluids—phase 3. Am J Hosp Pharm 30:611–613, 1973.
39. Garvan JM, Gunner BW: Intravenous fluids: a solution containing particles must not be used. Med J Aust 2:140–145, 1963.
40. Anon: Particles in veins (editorial). Br Med J 1:307, 1973.
41. Dumas RJ: Thomas Latta, what have we done?—the hazards of intravenous therapy. N Engl J Med 294:1178–1180, 1976.
42. Turco S, Davis NM: Glass particles in intravenous injections. N Engl J Med 287:1204–1205, 1972.
43. Turco SJ, Davis NM: Detrimental effects of particulate matter on the pulmonary circulation. JAMA 217:81–82, 1971.
44. Anon: A further hazard of intravenous therapy (editorial). Br Med J 3:262, 1975.
45. Anon: Hyponatraemia (editorial). Lancet 1:1334–1335, 1976.
46. Patel AR, Paton AM, Rowan T, et al: Clinical studies on the effect of laevulose on the rate of metabolism of ethyl alcohol. Scott Med J 14:268–271, 1969.
47. Bergstrom J, Furst P, Gallyas F, et al: Aspects of fructose metabolism in normal man. Acta Med Scand Suppl 542:57–64, 1972.
48. Woods HF, Alberti KGMM: Dangers of intravenous fructose. Lancet 2:1354–1357, 1972.
49. Anon: Sodium bicarbonate in cardiac arrest (editorial). Lancet 1:946–947, 1976.
50. Bishop RL, Weisfeldt ML: Sodium bicarbonate administration during cardiac arrest. Effect on arterial pH, pCO_2, and osmolality. JAMA 235:506–509, 1976.
51. Bleich HL, Schwartz WB: Tris buffer (THAM). An appraisal of its physiological effects and clinical usefulness. N Engl J Med 274:782–786, 1966.
52. *Martindale: The Extra Pharmacopoeia,* 26th edition. Edited by NW Blacow. London, Pharmaceutical Press, 1972, p 1704.
53. Gamble JL, Ross SG: The factors in the dehydration following pyloric obstruction. J Clin Invest 1:403–423, 1975.
54. Harken AH, Gabel RA, Fence V: Hydrochloric acid in the correction of metabolic acidosis. Arch Surg 110:819–821, 1975.
55. Williams SE: Molar solutions and molar concentrations (letter). Br Med J 1:643, 1977.
56. Williams RHP: Potassium overdosage: a potential hazard of non-rigid parenteral fluid containers. Br Med J 1:714–715, 1973.
57. Lankton JW, Siler JN, Neigh JL: Hyperkalemia after administration of potassium from nonrigid parenteral fluid containers (letter). Anesthesiology 39:660–661, 1973.
58. Anon: Dangerous drips (editorial). Lancet 1:291, 1976.
59. *Martindale: The Extra Pharmacopoeia,* 26th edition. Edited by NW Blacow. London, Pharmaceutical Press, 1972, p 363.
60. Mizrahi A, London RD, Gribetz D: Neonatal hypocalcemia—its causes and treatment. N Engl J Med 278:1163–1165, 1968.
61. Jackson CE, Meier DW: Routine serum magnesium analysis: correlation with clinical state in 5,100 patients. Ann Intern Med 69:743–748, 1968.
62. Lim P, Jacob E: Magnesium deficiency in liver cirrhosis. Q J Med 41:291–300, 1972.
63. Muldowney FP, McKenna TJ, Kyle LH, et al: Parathormone-like effect of magnesium replenishment in steatorrhoea. N Engl J Med 282:61–68, 1970.
64. Lim P, Jacob E: Magnesium deficiency in patients on long-term diuretic therapy for heart failure. Br Med J 3:620–622, 1972.

HORMONES AND AGENTS AFFECTING HORMONAL MECHANISMS

49. ADRENAL CORTICOSTEROIDS

Lloyd Axelrod

The adrenal cortex secretes three clinically important classes of steroid hormone: glucocorticoids, mineralocorticoids and androgens. Cortisol (hydrocortisone) is the principal glucocorticoid in man; aldosterone is the principal mineralocorticoid. This chapter is concerned with the clinical use of glucocorticoids and mineralocorticoids, both natural and synthetic. These agents are indicated for replacement therapy in patients with glucocorticoid or mineralocorticoid deficiency, or both. Glucocorticoids are widely used in pharmacologic doses as anti-inflammatory and immunosuppressive agents. Mineralocorticoids are occasionally employed in patients with orthostatic hypotension due to autonomic dysfunction. The use of androgens is considered in the following chapter. The division of adrenal corticosteroids into three functional classes should not obscure the fact that many compounds have properties of more than one class.

GLUCOCORTICOIDS

Pharmacology

Glucocorticoids are 21-carbon steroid molecules with numerous metabolic and physiologic effects. Glucocorticoids influence plasma glucose concentrations, blood pressure, inflammatory and immune response, and neuropsychiatric function. Glucocorticoids can suppress the secretion of adrenocorticotropic hormone (ACTH) from the pituitary gland via a negative feedback system.

The important differences among the available glucocorticoid compounds are: duration of action, relative glucocorticoid potency, and relative mineralocorticoid potency (Table 1).[1] The slight differences in circulating half-lives of the glucocorticoids contrast

TABLE 1 Commonly Used Glucocorticoids

Duration of Action[a]	Glucocorticoid Potency[b]	Equivalent Glucocorticoid Dose (mg)	Mineralocorticoid Activity
Short-Acting			
Cortisol (Hydrocortisone)	1	20	Yes[c]
Cortisone	0.8	25	Yes[c]
Prednisone	4	5	No
Prednisolone	4	5	No
Methylprednisolone	5	4	No
Intermediate-Acting			
Triamcinolone	5	4	No
Long-Acting			
Betamethasone	25	0.60	No
Dexamethasone	30	0.75	No

[a]This classification is based on the duration of ACTH suppression following a single large dose of a glucocorticoid equivalent in anti-inflammatory activity to 50 mg of prednisone. Short-acting glucocorticoids suppress ACTH for 24 to 36 hours, intermediate-acting steroids for 48 hours, and long-acting steroids for well over 48 hours.[2]

[b]The values given for glucocorticoid potency are relative. Cortisol is arbitrarily assigned a value of one. These values are approximations derived from several sources.[1–11]

[c]Mineralocorticoid effects are dose related. At doses close to or within the basal physiologic range for glucocorticoid activity, no such effect may be detectable.

with the marked differences in potency and the duration of ACTH suppression.[1] Commonly-used glucocorticoids are categorized as short-, intermediate- and long-acting on the basis of the duration of ACTH suppression following a single dose, equivalent in anti-inflammatory activity to 50 mg of prednisone (Table 1).[1–11]

The existence of glucocorticoid activity depends on the presence of a hydroxyl group at carbon number 11 of the steroid molecule. Thus, cortisone and prednisone, which are 11-keto compounds, lack glucocorticoid activity until converted *in vivo* to cortisol and prednisolone, the corresponding 11-beta-hydroxyl compounds.[12,13] This transformation occurs predominantly in the liver.[14] All glucocorticoid preparations that are marketed for topical or local use are 11-beta-hydroxyl compounds, thus eliminating the need for biotransformation.

In normal subjects, plasma cortisol levels after oral administration of cortisone are much lower than after equal oral doses of cortisol.[15] This suggests that while oral cortisone may be adequate replacement therapy in chronic adrenal insufficiency, it is unwise to use this agent orally when pharmacologic effects are sought. In contrast, comparable plasma prednisolone levels are achieved in normal subjects following equivalent oral doses of prednisone and prednisolone.[15,16] Plasma cortisol levels after an intramuscular injection of cortisone acetate rise little or not at all, in contrast to the marked rises that follow the intramuscular injection of hydrocortisone.[17–22] Although cortisone acetate intramuscularly has long been used for perioperative management, it may not provide adequate plasma cortisol levels and offers no advantage over hydrocortisone by the same route (see section on dosage).

Plasma cortisol levels are normal in patients with liver disease.[23] Although cortisol clearance is reduced in cirrhotics, the hypothalamic-pituitary-adrenal homeostatic mechanism appears to be intact. Thus, a decreased rate of metabolism is accompanied by decreased synthesis of cortisol.[23]

Under normal physiologic conditions, cortisol, and to a lesser extent its synthetic derivatives, are primarily bound to corticosteroid-binding globulin (CBG, transcortin), an alpha-globulin, in the plasma, CBG is a vehicle for the transportation of the steroid; the bound steroid is not active. Albumin binds most of the remaining glucocorticoid (10 to 15%) not complexed with CBG, leaving only a small portion of the steroid unbound and free to exert its physiologic and pharmacologic actions.

In the presence of active liver disease, there is impairment of the conversion of prednisone to the active metabolite prednisolone, as well as reduced protein-binding of prednisolone, largely attributable to low serum albumin concentrations.[16] An increased frequency of prednisone side effects is observed at low serum albumin levels;[24] possibly both findings reflect impaired hepatic function. Thus, prednisolone may produce a more predictable effect than prednisone in patients with active liver disease. If the serum albumin level is low, doses should be reduced. There is no evidence that a reduction in dose is necessary in patients with hypoalbuminemia and normal hepatic function, as in patients with nephrotic syndrome.

Glucocorticoid therapy appears to be well-tolerated in pregnancy.[25] Although glucocorticoids cross the placenta, at present there is no convincing evidence that this produces hypothalamic-pituitary-adrenal suppression or Cushing's syndrome in the neonate.[25] Nor is there evidence that glucocorticoids increase the incidence of congenital defects in humans.[25] Due to low concentrations of prednisone and prednisolone in breast milk, the administration of these drugs to the mother of a nursing infant is unlikely to produce deleterious effects.[26,27]

Adverse Reactions

Adverse reactions to glucocorticoids include the diverse manifestations of Cushing's syndrome and hypothalamic-pituitary-adrenal suppression (Table 2).[7,28–31] Iatrogenic Cushing's syndrome differs from spontaneous Cushing's syndrome in several respects (Table 3).[32,33] These differences may be explained in part by the fact that in iatrogenic Cushing's syndrome due to exogenous glucocorticoids ACTH is suppressed, whereas in spontaneous, ACTH-dependent Cushing's syndrome elevated ACTH output results in bilateral adrenal hyperplasia. In the former circumstance the secretion of adrenocortical androgens and mineralocorticoids is not increased. When ACTH output is elevated, the secretion of adrenal androgens[34–37] and mineralocorticoids[38–40] may be increased. The augmented secretion of adrenal androgens may account for the higher incidence of virilism, acne and menstrual irregularities reported in the spontaneous form of Cushing's syndrome, and the enhanced production of mineralocorticoids may explain the higher incidence of hypertension.

Complications that are virtually unique to iatrogenic Cushing's syndrome arise following prolonged use or large doses of glucocorticoids. This is the case with benign intracranial hypertension,[41,42] posterior subcapsular cataract,[43] and aseptic necrosis of bone.[44–48]

The association of glucocorticoid therapy and peptic ulcer disease is controversial.[49–51] A review of prospective controlled studies of adrenal corticosteroid therapy indicated that the overall frequency of peptic ulcer disease was not increased, but the occurrence of peptic ulcer was related to the duration of therapy and the total dose of steroids.[50] In studies when patients were not excluded because of a prior ulcer, ulcers developed more frequently in patients who received steroids than in those who did not.[50] Thus, the magnitude of any association between glucocorticoid therapy and peptic ulcer disease is small and is related to the total dose and duration of therapy.

TABLE 2 Adverse Reactions to Glucocorticoids

Ophthalmic
- Posterior subcapsular cataracts, increased intraocular pressure, and glaucoma, exopthalmos

Cardiovascular
- Hypertension
- Congestive heart failure in predisposed patients

Gastrointestinal
- Peptic ulcer disease (see text), pancreatitis

Endocrine–Metabolic
- Truncal obesity, moon facies, supraclavicular fat deposition, posterior cervical fat deposition (buffalo hump), mediastinal widening (lipomatosis), hepatomegaly due to fatty liver (rare)
- Acne, hirsutism or virilism, impotence, menstrual irregularities
- Suppression of growth in children
- Hyperglycemia; diabetic ketoacidosis; hyperosmolar, nonketotic diabetic coma; hyperlipoproteinemia
- Negative balance of nitrogen, potassium, and calcium
- Sodium retention, hypokalemia, metabolic alkalosis
- Secondary adrenal insufficiency

Musculoskeletal
- Myopathy
- Osteoporosis, vertebral compression fractures, spontaneous fractures
- Aseptic necrosis of femoral and humoral heads and other bones

Neuropsychiatric
- Convulsions
- Benign intracranial hypertension (pseudotumor cerebri)
- Alterations in mood or personality
- Psychosis

Dermatologic
- Facial erythema, thin fragile skin, petechiae and ecchymoses, violaceous striae, impaired wound healing
- Panniculitis (following withdrawal)

Immune, Infectious
- Suppression of delayed hypersensitivity
- Neutrophilia, monocytopenia, lymphocytopenia, decreased inflammatory responses
- Susceptibility to infections

TABLE 3 Natural Versus Iatrogenic Cushing's Syndrome

More common in natural Cushing's syndrome
Hypertension
Acne
Menstrual disturbances or impotence in males
Hirsutism or virilism
Striae
Purpura
Plethora
Virtually unique to iatrogenic Cushing's syndrome
Benign intracranial hypertension
Glaucoma
Posterior subcapsular cataract
Pancreatitis
Aseptic necrosis of bone
Panniculitis
Nearly equal frequency in both syndromes
Obesity
Psychiatric symptoms
Edema[a]
Poor wound healing

Source: Adapted from Ragan [33] and Christy [32].

[a]The incidence of edema in iatogenic Cushing's syndrome may depend on the glucocorticoid employed. Ragan utilized cortisone [33].

Glucocorticoid therapy, especially daily therapy, may suppress the immune response to skin tests for tuberculosis.[52] Tuberculin skin testing is advisable prior to the initiation of glucocorticoid therapy when possible. Routine isoniazid prophylaxis for corticosteroid-treated patients, even those with positive tuberculin skin tests, is probably not indicated.[53]

Some patients respond to and develop side effects of glucocorticoids more readily than others, due at least in part to variations in the rate of metabolism of the glucocorticoids. In asthmatic patients failure to respond to glucocorticoids correlates with an increased clearance of cortisol.[54,55] No such differences in prednisolone clearance were found in patients with a variety of disorders other than asthma.[56]

In patients who develop side effects, the clearance of prednisolone is lower and the circulating half-life longer than in those who do not.[56]

Many symptoms associated with glucocorticoid withdrawal, including anorexia, myalgia, nausea, emesis, lethargy, headache, fever, desquamation, arthralgia, weight loss and postural hypotension, can occur with normal plasma levels of glucocorticoids[57] and in patients with normal responsiveness of the hypothalamic-pituitary-adrenal system.[58,59] Thus, the 'steroid withdrawal syndrome' does not depend on the absence of glucocorticoids from the circulation or the impairment of hypothalamic-pituitary-adrenal responsiveness. There is no satisfactory explanation for these observations.

Interactions

The metabolism of glucocorticoids is accelerated by compounds that induce hepatic microsomal enzyme activity, such as phenytoin,[60–62] barbiturates[62–64] and rifampin.[65,66] Administration of these compounds can increase the steroid requirement of a patient with adrenal insufficiency[65] or lead to deterioration in the condition of a patient whose underlying disorder is well-controlled by glucocorticoid therapy.[63,64,66] These substances should be avoided if possible in patients receiving steroids. Diazepam does not alter the metabolism of glucocorticoids[62] and is preferable to barbiturates. If an inducer of hepatic microsomal enzyme activity must be used in a patient on steroids, an increase in the required dosage of the steroid should be anticipated.

The concurrent administration of a glucocorticoid and a salicylate may reduce serum salicylate levels; conversely, reduction of the steroid dose during administration of a fixed dose of a salicylate may lead to higher and possibly toxic serum salicyclate levels.[67] The mechanism of this interaction is not established, but may reflect increased renal clearance of salicylates.[67]

Glucocorticoids may increase requirements for insulin or oral hypoglycemic agents, antihypertensive drugs, or glaucoma medications. They may also alter the requirement for sedative-hypnotic or antidepressant therapy. Digitalis toxicity can result from hypokalemia induced by glucocorticoids, as from hypokalemia of any cause.

Considerations Prior to the Use of Glucocorticoids as Pharmacologic Agents

Table 4 summarizes important considerations in the initiation of glucocorticoid therapy.[68] The more severe the underlying disorder, the more readily glucocorticoid therapy can be justified. Thus, steroid therapy is usually employed in patients with status asthmaticus,

TABLE 4 Considerations Prior to the Use of Glucocorticoids as Pharmacologic Agents

1. How serious is the underlying disease?
2. How long will therapy be required?
3. What is the anticipated effective steroid dose?
4. Is the patient predisposed to any of the known hazards of glucocorticoid therapy *(see* Table 49.2)?
5. Which glucocorticoid preparation should be employed?
6. Have other modes of therapy been utilized—
   to minimize the glucocorticoid dosage?
   to minimize the side effects of glucocorticoid therapy?
7. Is an alternate day regimen indicated?

Source: Modified from Thorn [68].

chronic active hepatitis, transplantation rejection, severe pemphigus, or diseases of comparable severity. Such treatment generally should not be administered to patients with rheumatoid arthritis or mild bronchial asthma. The latter patients should receive more conservative therapy first. They may experience symptomatic relief from glucocorticoids, but steroid withdrawal may prove difficult for this very reason. As a result, they may unnecessarily experience Cushing's syndrome and hypothalamic-pituitary-adrenal suppression.

The anticipated duration of glucocorticoid therapy is another critical consideration. The use of glucocorticoids for one or two weeks for a condition such as poison ivy or allergic rhinitis is unlikely to be associated with serious side effects if there is no contraindication to their use. Because so many complications are dose- and time-related, the smallest possible dose should be prescribed for the shortest possible period.[29,31,69] If hypoalbuminemia due to hepatic disease is present, the dose should be appropriately reduced.[16,24] If chronic treatment is indicated, consideration should be given to the use of an alternate day schedule.

Whenever possible a local steroid preparation should be used, since systemic effects are minimal when these substances are properly administered. Examples are topical therapy in dermatologic disorders, steroid enemas in ulcerative proctitis and steroid aerosols in bronchial asthma and allergic rhinitis. The intra-articular injection of steroids may be of value in carefully selected patients if strict aseptic technique is employed.[70] Repeated injections should be avoided.[70]

Agents that have minimal or no mineralocorticoid activity should be used when a glucocorticoid is prescribed for pharmacologic purposes. If the dose is to be tapered over a few days, a long-acting agent may be undesirable. For alternate day therapy a short-acting agent that generally does not cause sodium retention (eg, prednisone, prednisolone, or methylprednisolone) should be used. There is no indication for glucocorticoid conjugates that are designed to achieve a prolonged duration of action (several days or several weeks) following a single intramuscular injection. The dose of such agents cannot be regulated precisely, the duration of action cannot be estimated reliably, and it is not possible to taper the dose rapidly in the event of an adverse reaction such as a steroid-induced psychosis. The use of such preparations may produce hypothalamic-pituitary-adrenal suppression more often than comparable doses of the same glucocorticoid given orally.[71]

Supplementary agents to minimize the steroid dose and to minimize the side effects of systemic glucocorticoids should always be considered. In asthma, for example, disodium cromoglycate and bronchodilators should be utilized.

Hypothalamic-Pituitary-Adrenal Suppression

There are few well-documented cases of acute adrenocortical insufficiency following chronic glucocorticoid therapy and no such cases following ACTH therapy.[1] Therefore the minimal duration of glucocorticoid therapy that can produce hypothalamic-pituitary-adrenal suppression must be ascertained from studies of adrenocortical weight and adrenocortical responsiveness to provocative tests.[1,32,72] Adrenocortical atrophy is detectable five days after the onset of glucocorticoid therapy.[73] Abnormalities in responsiveness to ACTH and metyrapone are observed in some but not all patients within three days of initiation of treatment with glucocorticoids.[1,32,72] There is no evidence of clinically significant hypothalamic-pituitary-adrenal suppression in patients who have received ACTH therapy.[1] On the basis of the available evidence any patient who has received a glucocorticoid in doses equivalent to 20–30 mg of prednisone per day for more than a week should be suspected of having hypothalamic-pituitary-adrenal suppression.[1] If the doses are closer to but above the physiologic range, one month is probably the minimal interval.[1]

The stress of general anesthesia and surgery is not hazardous to patients on replacement doses (no more than 25 mg hydrocortisone, 5 mg prednisone, 4 mg triamcinolone, or 0.75 mg dexamethasone),[74] if the steroid is given early in the day.[75] If doses of this size are given late in the day suppression may occur due to inhibition of the diurnal release of ACTH.[75,76]

During recovery from hypothalamic-pituitary-adrenal suppression, hypothalamic-pituitary function returns before adrenocortical function.[77] Twelve months must elapse following withdrawal of large doses of glucocorticoids given for a prolonged period before homeostatic function, including responsiveness to stress, returns to normal.[1,77,78] Since the time course of recovery from smaller doses and shorter courses of therapy is not known, persistence of hypothalamic-pituitary-adrenal suppression should be suspected for twelve months after a course of glucocorticoid therapy at supraphysiologic doses lasting more than a few weeks. The course of recovery from suppression of the contralateral adrenal cortex by the products of an adrenocortical tumor may exceed twelve months.[78,79] Recovery from suppression induced by exogenous glucocorticoids may be more rapid in children than adults.[80]

The adrenocortical response to an ACTH test is a useful guide to the presence or absence of suppression. The maximal response of the plasma cortisol level to ACTH corresponds to the maximal plasma cortisol level observed during the induction of general anesthesia and surgery in patients who have received glucocorticoid therapy.[81–84] This is so when one uses a six-hour infusion of ACTH[83,84] or a rapid intravenous injection of synthetic ACTH with measurement of the plasma cortisol level just before and then 30 minutes[82] or 60 minutes[81] after the injection. A normal response to ACTH preoperatively is unlikely to be followed by markedly impaired secretion of cortisol during anesthesia and surgery in steroid treated patients.

Alternate Day Glucocorticoid Therapy

Alternate day glucocorticoid therapy is defined as the administration of a short-acting glucocorticoid with no significant mineralocorticoid effect (such as prednisone, prednisolone or methylprednisolone) once every 48 hours in the morning, at about 8:00 a.m. The objective is to minimize the adverse effects of glucocorticoids while retaining therapeutic effectiveness. Alternate day glucocorticoid therapy should be considered whenever glucocorticoids are indicated for a protracted period, but is not necessary when the anticipated duration of therapy is no longer than several weeks.

An alternate day regimen can prevent or ameliorate the manifestations of Cushing's syndrome,[1,85–106] including somatic and psychological manifestations, as well as quantifiable endpoints such as high blood pressure,[88,91,93,99,106] retarded linear growth rate in children,[90,104–106] decreased somatomedin levels,[102] altered leukocyte kinetics,[96,101,103] impaired responsiveness to skin testing for delayed hypersensitivity,[89,103] and elevated urinary excretion rates of nitrogen and potassium.[92]

Patients on alternate day glucocorticoid therapy may have some suppression of basal steroid levels, but they have normal or nearly normal responsiveness to provocative tests such as ACTH stimulation tests,[86,107,108] insulin-induced hypoglycemia,[90,109] and the metyrapone test.[87] They also have less suppression of hypothalamic-pituitary-adrenal function than patients on daily therapy.[86,110,111]

Alternate day glucocorticoid therapy is as effective or nearly as effective in controlling a diverse group of diseases as daily therapy in divided doses. This approach has been utilized with apparent benefit in patients with the following disorders: childhood nephrotic syndrome,[88] adult nephrotic syndrome,[97,112] renal transplantation,[91,93,98,99,104,106,113–115] mesangiocapillary glomerulonephritis,[116] lupus nephritis,[117] ulcerative colitis,[118] rheumatoid arthritis,[119] acute rheumatic fever,[120] myasthenia gravis,[121–125] Duchenne muscular dystrophy,[126] asthma,[105,108,110,127,128] sarcoidosis,[95,100] alopecia areata and other chronic dermatoses,[85] and pemphigus vulgaris.[120,129] Alternate day therapy is not as effective as daily therapy in giant cell arteritis;[130] however, there were few adverse effects of steroids and no evidence of progression of the arteritis on the alternate day regimen, so there may be a role for this approach in giant cell arteritis.[131] With two exceptions,[114,130] there are no randomized prospective trials in which the effect of alternate day therapy is compared to the effect of the same agent given in divided daily doses.

Alternate day therapy may not be necessary during the initial stages of therapy or during exacerbation of the underlying disease. Nevertheless, patients with childhood and adult nephrotic syndrome,[88,90,97,112] lupus nephritis,[117] rheumatoid arthritis,[119] myasthenia gravis,[121–124] asthma,[107,108,127] sarcoidosis,[95,100] rheumatic fever,[120] pemphigus vulgaris,[129] a variety of ocular diseases[132] and several other disorders have been treated with an alternate day regimen as initial therapy with apparent benefit. It appears to be easier to establish treatment with alternate day steroids than to convert from daily therapy in patients with rheumatoid arthritis.[119,133] Studies in recipients of renal transplants have initially used daily therapy and then converted to an alternate day schedule.[91,93,98,99,104,106,113–115] On the other hand, alternate day therapy was unsuccessful in relieving the manifestations of an acute fulminant case of ulcerative colitis[118] and a case of pemphigus vulgaris[120] when used as initial therapy. Thus, an alternate day schedule as initial therapy may be beneficial in some disorders but ineffective in others.

Alternate day therapy may be hazardous in the presence of adrenocortical insufficiency of any cause because the patient is unprotected against glucocorticoid insufficiency during the last twelve hours of the forty-eight-hour cycle.[86,91,119] In a patient who has been on glucocorticoids for more than a brief period, or who may have adrenal insufficiency on another basis, adequacy of hypothalamic-pituitary-adrenal function should be determined before the initiation of an alternate day program. It may be possible to surmount this obstacle by giving a small dose of a short-acting glucocorticoid (ie, 10 mg of hydrocortisone) in the afternoon of the second day; this approach has not been studied.

Alternate day glucocorticoid therapy may fail to prevent or ameliorate the manifestations of Cushing's syndrome or hypothalamic-pituitary-adrenal suppression if a short-acting glucocorticoid is not used, or if it is used incorrectly.[2,107,134,135] For example, the use of prednisone four times per day on alternate days may be less successful than use of the same total dose once every forty-eight hours.

An abrupt alteration from daily to alternate day therapy should be avoided because the prolonged use of daily-dose glucocorticoids may have resulted in hypothalamic-pituitary-adrenal suppression. Patients with normal function of the hypothalamic-pituitary-adrenal axis may experience withdrawal symptoms in these circumstances and have exacerbation of the underlying disease.[104]

No program of conversion from continuous therapy to alternate day therapy has been proven to be optimal. One approach is to gradually increase the dose on the first day of each two-day period and to gradually decrease the dose on the second day. Concurrently one may gradually reduce the frequency of drug administration each day, until the total dose for each day is given in the morning. It is not clear how often such changes should be made. This probably depends on the underlying disease involved, the duration of previous glucocorticoid therapy, the personality of the patient, and the physician's ability to utilize adjunctive therapy. In any event, the conversion should be made as quickly as the patient will tolerate it. If the patient develops evidence of adrenal insufficiency, of the steroid withdrawal-syndrome or of an exacerbation of the underlying disease, the previously effective regimen should be reinstituted and then tapered more gradually. Changes in the dose should be approximately 10 mg of prednisone (or equivalent) at total daily doses of more than 40 mg, 5 mg at total doses of more than 20 mg, and 2.5 mg at lower doses. At small total daily doses, an absolute change of dose represents a larger percentage change in dose than at large total daily doses. The interval between chages in dose may be as short as one day or as long as many weeks.

Also, optimal results from alternate day glucocorticoid therapy may not be achieved because of failure to utilize supplemental therapy for the underlying disorder. Conservative (non-glucocorticoid) therapy is often used until a glucocorticoid is initiated, at which time these less toxic therapeutic measures are ignored. Utilization of adjunctive therapy may facilitate the use of the lowest possible dose of glucocorticoids. On alternate day therapy, these measures should be used especially during the end of the second day, when symptoms may be prominent. The potential benefits of disodium cromoglycate and bronchodilators in asthma, of non-steroidal anti-inflammatory agents in the rheumatic diseases and of sulfasalazine in inflammatory bowel disease should not be neglected. Supplemental therapy may be especially helpful in disorders where the patient is likely to experience symptoms of the disease on the day off therapy, such as asthma and rheumatoid arthritis. In illnesses in which disabling symptoms are less likely to appear on the alternate day, such as the childhood nephrotic syndrome, less difficulty may be encountered.

Alternate day therapy may fail because of failure to inform the patient about the purposes of this regimen. Because glucocorticoids may induce euphoria, a patient may be reluctant to accept modification of a schedule of frequent doses. Careful explanation of the risks of glucocorticoid excess, attuned to the patient's intellectual and emotional ability to comprehend, will maximize the likelihood of success.

Daily Single Dose Glucocorticoid Therapy

In some situations alternate day therapy fails because the patient experiences symptoms of the underlying disease during the last few hours of the second day. In these cases single dose glucocorticoid therapy may be of value. This regimen appears to be as effective as divided daily doses in controlling such underlying diseases as rheumatoid arthritis, systemic lupus erythematosus, and polyarthritis.[136–138] In giant cell arteritis, a daily dose in the morning is nearly as effective as daily therapy in divided doses, although alternate day therapy is not.[130] Daily single dose therapy appears to reduce the likelihood that a patient will develop hypothalamic-pituitary-adrenal suppression.[138–141] On the other hand, the manifestations of Cushing's syndrome are probably not prevented or ameliorated by a daily single dose regimen.[136,137]

Withdrawal of Patients from Glucocorticoids

The decision to discontinue glucocorticoid therapy provokes apprehension among physicians. The untoward consequences of such an action include precipitation of adrenocortical insufficiency, the steroid withdrawal syndrome, or an exacerbation of the underlying disease. Rarely, the syndrome of nodular panniculitis may occur.[142–145] When there is any possibility that the underlying illness may flare up, the glucocorticoid should be withdrawn gradually, over an interval of weeks to months, with frequent reassessment of the patient.

There is no proven means of hastening a return of normal hypothalamic-pituitary-adrenal function once inhibition has resulted from glucocorticoid therapy. The use of ACTH does not appear to prevent or reverse the development of glucocorticoid-induced adrenal insufficiency.[59,146–148] Conversion to an alternate day schedule permits but does not accelerate recovery.[119,128] In children, alternate day glucocorticoid therapy may delay recovery.[111]

Recovery from steroid-induced adrenal insufficiency is time-dependent and spontaneous. During this interval small doses (10 to 20 mg) of hydrocortisone in the morning may alleviate withdrawal symptoms.

Glucocorticoids versus ACTH

Disorders that respond to glucocorticoid therapy also respond to ACTH therapy if the adrenal cortex is normal. However, there is no evidence that ACTH is superior to glucocorticoids for the treatment of any disorder when comparable doses are used.[1,7,149] In fact, hydrocortisone and ACTH, when given intravenously in pharmacologically equivalent dosage (determined by plasma cortisol levels and urinary steroid excretion rates) are equally effective in the treatment of inflammatory bowel disease.[150] Since ACTH does not appear to offer any therapeutic advantage, glucocorticoids are preferable for therapeutic purposes;[1] they can be administered orally, the dose can be regulated precisely, the effectiveness does not depend on adrenocortical responsiveness, and they produce a lower incidence of certain side effects such as acne, hypertension and increased pigmentation.[151]

Indications

Glucocorticoids have a place in the treatment of all of the disorders listed in Table 5,[7,152] but they are not indicated for all patients with these diseases. They should only be used in patients in whom the expected benefits outweigh the risks.

The use of glucocorticoids is controversial or of no proven benefit for the treatment of a variety of conditions including alcoholic hepatitis (with the possible exception of those patients with hepatic encephalopathy whose liver function has not deteriorated to the point where liver biopsy would be contraindicated),[153] chronic obstructive lung disease (unless there is objective evidence of an asthmatic component, such as eosinophilia), Bell's palsy, Guillain-Barre syndrome, Wegener's granulomatosis, and shock (except septic shock). Because of the variability in the course of these diseases it is often impossible to assess the response of an individual patient to glucocorticoid therapy.

Dosage

The optimal dosage of a glucocorticoid depends upon whether treatment is for adrenocortical insufficiency or for anti-inflammatory or immunosuppressive purposes.

Adrenocortical Insufficiency. Treatment includes chronic replacement therapy for acute adrenal insufficiency and coverage for intercurrent illness, surgery or other stress. Cortisone acetate, 15 to 50 mg daily, is the glucocorticoid commonly used for *chronic replacement therapy* in patients with primary or secondary adrenocortical insufficiency.[154] Usually, half to two-thirds of the dose is taken upon arising in the morning and the balance taken in the early afternoon. A common regimen is 25 mg on arising and 12.5 mg in the early

TABLE 5 Indications for Glucocorticoid Therapy

Adrenocortical Diseases
Primary adrenocortical insufficiency
Secondary adrenocortical insufficiency
Congenital adrenal hyperplasia
Isolated glucocorticoid deficiency

Other Endocrine and Metabolic Diseases
Vitamin D intoxication
Hypercalcemia of cancer
Antibody-mediated insulin resistance
Subacute thyroiditis (rarely)

Ophthalmic Diseases
Conjunctival inflammation (severe)
Stevens–Johnson syndrome (acute, severe)
Scleritis, episcleritis (severe)
Postoperative corneal transplantation with graft rejection
Herpes zoster ophthalmicus with intraocular involvement
Iridocyclitis (severe)
Posterior vitreous, retinal or uveal inflammation
Endophthalmitis (pyogenic, in conjunction with systemic antibiotic)
Optic neuritis (inflammatory)
Sympathetic ophthalmia
Orbital inflammation
  Pseudomotor
Endocrine exophthalmos with or without myopathy
  Superior orbital fissure inflammation
Postoperative inflammation following glaucoma, retinal or vitreous surgery
Ocular trauma with severe vitreous or retinal involvement

Cardiac Diseases
Acute idiopathic pericarditis
Postmyocardial infarction syndrome (Dresslers syndrome)
Postpericardiotomy syndrome

Pulmonary Diseases
Asthma
Aspiration pneumonia

Pulmonary Diseases (Continued)
Fat embolism
Berylliosis
Acute pulmonary insufficiency from pulmonary metastases
Allergic pneumonitis
  Pulmonary infiltrates and eosinophilia
  Allergic alveolitis
Respiratory distress syndrome of the newborn
Acute chemical pneumonitis (including smoke inhalation)

Gastrointestinal Diseases
Inflammatory bowel disease (ulcerative colitis and Crohn's disease)
Nontropical sprue

Hepatic Diseases
Chronic active hepatitis

Renal Diseases
Lipoid (minimal change) nephrosis
Idiopathic membranous nephropathy
Renal transplantation

Neurological Diseases
Cerebral edema or increased intracranial pressure
Myasthenia gravis
Multiple sclerosis
Tuberculous meningitis with actual or impending hydrocephalus (concurrently with chemotherapy for tuberculosis)

Dermatologic Diseases
Pemphigus vulgaris
Bullous pemphigoid
Dermatitis herpetiformis
Erythema multiforme (Stevens–Johnson syndrome)
Generalized exfoliative dermatitis
Mycosis fungoides
Severe contact dermatitis
Atopic dermatitis

TABLE 5 *(continued)*

Dermatologic Diseases (continued)
Vasculitis
Actinic reticuloid
Alopecia areata
Drug eruptions
Toxic epidermal necrolysis
Lichen planus

Hematologic Diseases
Congenital red cell aplasia
Acquired red cell aplasia
Autoimmune hemolytic anemia
Idiopathic thrombocytopenic purpura
Thrombotic thrombocytopenic purpura
Bone marrow transplantation

Neoplastic Diseases
(Usually in combination with other agents)
Multiple myeloma
Hodgkin's disease
Non-Hodgkin's lymphoma
Acute lymphocytic leukemia
Chronic lymphocytic leukemia
Acute myelogenous leukemia
Breast cancer

Infectious Diseases
Infectious mononucleosis
Septic shock

Granulomatous Diseases
Sarcoidosis
Granulomatous hepatitis

Collagen-Vascular and Rheumatic Diseases
Rheumatoid arthritis
Acute rheumatic fever (with carditis)
Dermatomyositis
Gouty arthritis (rarely)
Polyarteritis nodosa
Polymyalgia rheumatica—giant cell arteritis
Systemic lupus erythematosus
Mixed connective tissue disease
Reflex sympathetic dystrophy

Miscellaneous Allergic Diseases
Allergic rhinitis
Serum sickness
Drug hypersensitivity reactions
Urticarial transfusion reactions
Angioedema
Urticaria
Laryngeal edema or anaphylaxis (epinephrine is drug of choice)

Miscellaneous
Hemangioma of liver or skin

Note: Glucocorticoids are only indicated for selected patients with most of the diseases included in this table (excluding adrenocortical disorders). Glucocorticoids are indicated for those patients in whom the anticipated benefits outweigh the risks. The decision to use glucocorticoids should be made only after review of (1) the general considerations pertinent to the use of these steroids as pharmacologic agents (see previous section of this chapter) and (2) the specific indications for the disease in question.

This table is limited to indications for systemic glucocorticoid therapy. It does not consider indications for topical or local steroid therapy for ophthalmic use, for topical or intralesional dermatologic application, for inhalation therapy, for intra-articular or local orthopedic injection, or for rectal enemas.

afternoon, but there are considerable differences in requirement, depending in part on body size. The dose must be individualized; the patient's sense of well-being is the best guide to therapy. Proper timing of the doses is essential. If the morning dose is delayed, the patient may experience more than the usual difficulty in getting going in the morning; occasionally a patient will find it helpful to take the morning dose about thirty minutes before actually getting out of bed.

The optimal time for the afternoon dose varies from patient to patient. If given too early, the patient will become fatigued early in the evening. If given too late, the patient will become fatigued before the dose is given and will be unable to fall asleep at night. An occasional patient will not need an afternoon dose. There is no substitute for trial and error. The euphoria often associated with the initiation of treatment of the newly diagnosed patient with Addison's disease frequently gives way to malaise for weeks to months; this malaise is often due to an improper total dose or improper timing of one or both doses. Hydrocortisone in comparable doses is also a suitable agent, although cortisone appears to give a smoother plasma cortisol response curve.[154] The patient with primary adrenocortical insufficiency also requires mineralocorticoid therapy and liberal salt intake (see below).

Primary adrenocortical insufficiency is completely treatable and probably does not alter life expectancy if properly managed. However, an acute adrenocortical crisis can be fatal. Every precaution must be exercised to avoid such a catastrophe. The patient must always wear proper emergency identification, such as a bracelet or necklace, indicating that he or she has adrenal insufficiency and is taking cortisone. The patient must also be adequately instructed about the function of the adrenal glands and the proper response to intercurrent illnesses and other emergencies. The patient and close relatives should be aware that the dose of cortisone acetate must be increased during times of stress. As a rule of thumb the dose of cortisone acetate is doubled for one degree of fever and tripled for two degrees of fever. For higher fevers (and severe illness) the patient should contact the physician, since high fever may be a manifestation of glucocorticoid insufficiency. The patient and a close relative should be taught to administer intramuscular injections, provided with an injectable glucocorticoid such as hydrocortisone, and instructed to inject 100 mg of hydrocortisone (or equivalent) immediately in the event of a severe illness, inability to take steroids by mouth, or symptoms of adrenocortical insufficiency. This should provide interim coverage until the patient is adequately evaluated by a physician. During a severe illness, the physician may administer as much as 100 to 150 mg of hydrocortisone (or equivalent) daily in divided doses.

For an acute crisis large doses of parenteral steroids should be used to aproximate the maximal cortisol secretion rate in normal persons—approximately 200 to 300 mg per 24 hours.[155–159] A patient who is thought to have acute adrenocortical insufficiency should receive 100 mg of hydrocortisone as an intravenous bolus, and then 100 mg by continuous infusion intravenously every 8 hours for at least 24 hours, after which the dose can be tapered. This should be accompanied by large amounts of intravenous saline and glucose, depending upon the degree of volume depletion.

Perioperative management is designed to simulate the cortisol secretion rate of patients with normal hypothalamic-pituitary-adrenal function who undergo surgery. This rate approaches the maximal adrenocortical response to stimulation by ACTH in normal subjects.[22] No clinical trials have defined the minimal effective dose. For minor procedures under local anesthesia or for routine dental work, it is generally sufficient to double or triple the usual glucocorticoid dose. For general anesthesia, hydrocortisone is usually given as follows:

Day before surgery—50 mg intramuscularly at midnight

Day of surgery—100 mg intramuscularly 1 to 2 hours before induction of anesthesia, then 50 mg intramuscularly every 6 hours; 100 mg should be given intravenously during procedure

In uncomplicated cases hydrocortisone may be tapered as follows:

1st postoperative day—50 mg intramuscularly every 6 hours
2nd postoperative day—50 mg intramuscularly every 8 hours
3rd postoperative day—50 mg intramuscularly every 12 hours
4th postoperative day—25 mg intramuscularly every 8 hours
5th postoperative day—25 mg intramuscularly every 12 hours

Thereafter, the patient can return to preoperative replacement doses orally or intramuscularly, as the postoperative situation dictates.

Mild elevations of plasma steroid levels were observed before surgery in some[160–162] but not all[163] studies. Preoperative preparation the evening before surgery (such as shaving the operative area and administering an enema) evokes a major cortisol secretory response,[162] indicating the need for initiation of glucocorticoid coverage the night before surgery when possible.

The use of hydrocortisone for perioperative management of patients with primary adrenocortical insufficiency has the advantage that at high doses this agent has mineralocorticoid activity. At doses below about 100 mg per day of hydrocortisone it may be necessary to use a mineralocorticoid agent as well; fludrocortisone orally or desoxycorticosterone acetate (DOCA) intramuscularly can be used (see below). In any case, care must be taken to assure that salt intake is adequate, and that intraoperative and postoperative fluid losses are replaced. In patients with secondary adrenocortical insufficiency, mineralocorticoid replacement is generally not required. If mineralocorticoid activity is contraindicated (because of congestive heart failure, for example), then comparable parenteral doses of a glucocorticoid other than hydrocortisone can be used.

Although cortisone acetate has long been used for perioperative management, hydrocortisone is the preferred agent. Intramuscular cortisone acetate injections at high doses produce little or no rise in the plasma cortisol level, in contrast to hydrocortisone.[17–22]

Anti-Inflammatory or Immunosuppressive Therapy. The glucocorticoid dose required for anti-inflammatory or immunosuppressive therapy is quite variable and depends on the disease under treatment. Generally, the dose ranges from just above that needed for chronic replacement therapy up to about 60 mg of prednisone or its equivalent daily. Although much larger doses are sometimes recommended for diseases such as asthma, central nervous system involvement in systemic lupus erythematosus and cerebral edema, no controlled studies have established the need for such large doses. To the contrary, in acute asthma massive doses have been shown to offer no additional benefit.[164] If the patient must also receive a hepatic microsomal enzyme inducer, the metabolism of the glucocorticoid will be accelerated (see Drug Interactions, above), and larger daily doses may be needed.

Preparations and Costs

Available preparations and costs of commonly used glucocorticoids are shown in Table 6.

MINERALOCORTICOIDS

Pharmacology

Mineralocorticoids are 21-carbon steroids characterized by their effects on fluid and electrolyte balance. They promote renal sodium reabsorption and potassium excretion. Deficiency results in hyponatremia, volume depletion, hypotension, hyperkalemia, and a hyperchloremic metabolic acidosis.[165,166] Mineralocorticoid excess is associated with retention of sodium and water, hypertension, potassium depletion, hypokalemia and a metabolic alkalosis.[166]

TABLE 6 Corticosteroid Preparations and Costs

GENERIC NAME	TRADEMARK NAME(S)	PREPARATIONS AND 1978 COSTS
Glucocorticoids		
Cortisone Acetate[a]	Cortone Acetate	Tablets 5 mg—$1.58/50; 25 mg—$13.81/100 Injection (suspension) 25 mg/ml—$6.58/20-ml vial; 50 mg/ml—$6.58/10-ml vial
	generic	Tablets 25 mg—$4.40–$9.40/100
Hydrocortisone	Hydrocortone (Cortef)	Tablets 10 mg—$4.50/100; 20 mg—$8.60/100
	generic	Tablets 20 mg—$2.75–$6.84/100
Hydrocortisone Sodium Phosphate[b]	Hydrocortone Phosphate	Injection (solution) 50 mg/ml—$2.53/2-ml vial, $3.15/2-ml disposable syringe, $12.22/10-ml vial
Hydrocortisone Sodium Succinate[b]	Solu-Cortef	Injection (powder) 100 mg—$3.44/vial; 250 mg—$8.40/vial; 500 mg—$16.34/vial; 1 g—$30.90/vial
Prednisone	Meticorten (Delta-Dome) (Deltasone) (Orasone)	Tablets 1 mg—$1.61/100; 5 mg—$2.69/100
	generic	Tablets 5 mg—$1.05–$9.60/100; 10 mg—$3.04–$3.50/100; 20 mg—$4.15–$7.71/100; 50 mg—$14.50/100
Prednisolone	Sterane (Delta-Cortef)	Tablets 5 mg—$4.04/100
	generic	Tablets 5 mg—$1.20–$10.45/100
Prednisolone Sodium Phosphate[b]	Hydeltrasol	Injection (solution) 20 mg/ml—$4.03/2-ml vial, $8.81/5-ml vial
Prednisolone Sodium Succinate[b]	Meticortelone Soluble	Injection (powder) 50 mg/vial—$4.99/vial
Prednisolone Tebutate[a]	Hydeltra-T.B.A.	Injection (suspension) 20 mg/ml—$1.28/1-ml vial, $4.90/5-ml vial

TABLE 6 *(continued)*

Generic Name	Trademark Name(s)	Preparations and 1978 Costs
Methylprednisolone	Medrol	Tablets 2 mg—$3.83/30; 4 mg—$7.24/30; 16 mg—$33.39/50
Methylprednisolone Acetate[a]	Depo-Medrol	Injection (aqueous suspension) 20 mg/ml—$6.79/5-ml vial; 40 mg/ml—$4.18/1-ml vial, $13.18/5-ml vial, $23.45/10-ml vial; 80 mg/ml—$7.44/1-ml vial, $23.45/5-ml vial, $5.66/1-ml disposable syringe
Methylprednisolone Sodium Succinate[b]	Solu-Medrol	Injection (powder) 40 mg—$4.81/vial; 125 mg—$12.76/vial; 500 mg—$40.71/vial; 1 g—$69.58/vial
Triamcinolone	Aristocort (Kenacort)	Tablets 1 mg—$3.18/50; 2 mg—$3.83/30; 4 mg—$7.37/30; 8 mg—$19.43/50; 16 mg—$23.23/30
Triamcinolone Acetonide[a]	Kenalog-10 Kenalog-40	Injection (aqueous suspension) 10 mg/ml—$3.18/5-ml vial; 40 mg/ml—$2.54/1-ml vial, $10.73/5-ml vial, $20.38/10-ml vial
Betamethasone	Celestone	Tablets 0.6 mg—$18.82/100
Betamethasone Acetate and Betamethasone Sodium Phosphate[a]	Celestone Soluspan	Injection (aqueous suspension, containing betamethasone acetate 3 mg and betamethasone sodium phosphate 3 mg/ml)—$10.15/5-ml vial
Dexamethasone	Decadron (Dexameth) (Hexadrol)	Tablets 0.25 mg—$6.85/100; 0.5 mg—$12.33/100; 0.75 mg—$15.40/100; 1.5 mg—$28.56/100; 4 mg—$48.06/100
	generic	Tablets 0.75 mg—$3.50–$8.50/100
Dexamethasone Sodium Phosphate[b]	Decadron Phosphate Hexadrol Phosphate	Injection (solution) 4 mg/ml—$1.63/1-ml vial, $7.55/5-ml vial, $29.31/25-ml vial; 10 mg/ml—$26.55/10-ml vial

Mineralocorticoids		
Fludrocortisone Acetate	Florinef Acetate	Tablets 0.1 mg—$6.09/100
Desoxycorticosterone Acetate[a]	Percorten Acetate (Doca Acetate)	Solution (in sesame oil) 5 mg/ml—$10.00/10-ml vial

[a]For intramuscular use only when injected.
[b]For intramuscular or intravenous use.

Excessive secretion or administration of a mineralocorticoid causes sodium retention with consequent fluid retention and gain in weight. The patient will retain several hundred mEq of sodium and gain several kg of weight. If mineralocorticoid excess persists, 'mineralocorticoid escape' occurs; further sodium retention and weight gain do not occur. During this escape phenomenon, urinary sodium excretion will rise until the patient comes into balance, and urinary sodium excretion reflects intake. Thus, patients with mineralocorticoid excess often will not retain sufficient fluid to develop peripheral edema (although occasional patients will do so) unless there is an additional cause for edema such as hypoalbuminemia or right ventricular failure. The absence of edema therefore does not exclude the possibility of mineralocorticoid excess.

Aldosterone is the principal, but not the only, mineralocorticoid in man. Desoxycorticosterone, corticosterone and cortisol (hydrocortisone) are also secreted in amounts sufficient to cause salt retention in certain situations.[38,40] The mineralocorticoids used clinically are fludrocortisone (9-alpha-fluorohydrocortisone) and desoxycortisone acetate (DOCA) (see below). When hydrocortisone is given in large doses (eg, 100 mg daily) a mineralocorticoid effect may be anticipated.[167–169] Aldosterone is not available for use clinically although it is a potent mineralocorticoid and is essentially devoid of glucocorticoid effect. It would be of limited value because of its brief duration of action.[167,169,170]

Fludrocortisone is the preferred mineralocorticoid for oral use.[167–173] The introduction of the fluorine atom in the 9-alpha position enhances the mineralocorticoid potency and, to a lesser extent, the glucocorticoid potency of hydrocortisone.[167–169,172,174–176] At recommended doses fludrocortisone is an effective mineralocorticoid but is essentially free of glucocorticoid activity. Its duration of action is approximately twelve to twenty-four hours.[167–170]

Desoxycorticosterone acetate (DOCA) may be used intramuscularly when a patient is unable to take fludrocortisone orally. It is essentially free of glucocorticoid activity and lasts for approximately twenty-four hours.

If the patient also needs a large dose of a glucocorticoid one can use hydrocortisone. A dose of 100 mg daily will provide mineralocorticoid activity.[167–169]

Fludrocortisone, one mg per day orally, is equivalent to aldosterone, one mg per day in four divided intramuscular doses.[169,170] An oral dose of fludrocortisone, 0.1 mg daily, is comparable to an intramuscular dose of desoxycorticosterone acetate, 2.5 mg daily.

Neither desoxycorticosterone pivalate nor DOCA pellets have any current indication. Desoxycorticosterone pivalate is a repository preparation that has no advantage over fludrocortisone for the long-term management of the usual patient with mineralocorticoid deficiency. Its disadvantages include the need for intramuscular injections and the difficulty in determining the proper dose and frequency of injections. DOCA pellets for subcutaneous implantation were of great value before cortisone and fludrocortisone were available.

No mineralocorticoid will increase the sodium stores of a sodium-depleted patient. The effectiveness of a mineralocorticoid hormone depends on substrate availability; patients with mineralocorticoid deficiency need not only the hormone but also salt and water. Both hormonal therapy and proper fluid and electrolyte administration are necessary if one is to achieve an optimal clinical response.

Adverse Reactions

The adverse reactions of mineralocorticoid therapy are those of mineralocorticoid excess: fluid retention, hypertension, hypokalemia and potassium depletion and metabolic alkalosis.

Drug Interactions

Mineralocorticoid activity is antagonized by spironolactone; the latter has no effect in patients with hypoaldosteronism.

Anything that promotes salt loss, such as diuretics, will impair mineralocorticoid efficacy. For patients ordinarily needing a diuretic (for the treatment of hypertension or fluid retention, for example), the desired effect may be achieved by modification of the dose of mineralocorticoid, the intake of salt or both. Drugs that alter sweating or promote vomiting or diarrhea may alter salt balance and therefore alter the effectiveness of a mineralocorticoid.

Indications

Mineralocorticoid therapy is indicated for the conditions included in Table 7.

TABLE 7 Indications for Mineralocorticoid Therapy

Primary adrenocortical insufficiency
Isolated hypoaldosteronism
Salt-losing forms of congenital adrenal hyperplasia
Chronic orthostatic hypotension due to autonomic insufficiency
Multiple systems atrophy (Shy–Drager syndrome)
Idiopathic orthostatic hypotension
Diabetic autonomic neuropathy

Dosage

The usual dosage of fludrocortisone is 0.1 mg daily, but may range from 0.1 mg on alternate days to 0.2 mg daily. Generally the starting dose is 0.1 mg daily, with adjustments made according to clinical response. Orthostatic vital signs are of great value in assessing the adequacy of mineralocorticoid replacement therapy. A marked rise in the heart rate or a fall in blood pressure upon standing may precede other manifestations of mineralocorticoid deficiency.

Desoxycorticosterone acetate is given by daily intramuscular injection. The usual dose is 2.5 mg per day with a range of 1 to 5 mg per day.

Preparations and Costs

Recommended preparations and costs of mineralocorticoids are shown in Table 6.

REFERENCES

1. Axelrod L: Glucocorticoid therapy. Medicine 55:39–65, 1976.
2. Harter JG: Corticosteroids: their physiologic use in allergic disease. NY State J Med 66:827–840, 1966.

3. Boland EW: 16-α-methyl corticosteroids. Calif Med 88:417–422, 1958.
4. Boland EW, Liddle GW: Metabolic and antirheumatic activities of 6-methylprednisolone (Medrol). Ann Rheum Dis 16:297–306, 1957.
5. Bondy PK: The adrenal cortex. In *Duncan's Diseases of Metabolism,* seventh edition. Edited by PK Bondy, LE Rosenberg. Philadelphia, WB Saunders Company, 1974, pp 1105–1180.
6. Bunim JJ, Black RL, Lutwak L, et al: Studies on dexamethasone, a new synthetic steroid, in rheumatoid arthritis—a preliminary report. Arthritis Rheum 1:313–331, 1958.
7. Cope CL: *Adrenal Steroids and Disease,* second edition. London, Pitman Medical, 1972.
8. Kleeman CR, Koplowitz J, Maxwell MH: Metabolic effects of two newer adrenal analogs, 6-methylprednisolone (Medrol) and 6-methyl-9α-fluoro-21-desoxyprednisolone (9α-fluoro-21-desoxymedrol). Metabolism 7:425–440, 1958.
9. Liddle GW: Studies of structure-function relationships of steroids. II. The 6α-methylcorticosteroids. Metabolism 7:405–415, 1958.
10. Liddle GW: Clinical pharmacology of the anti-inflammatory agents. Clin Pharmacol Ther 2:615–635, 1961.
11. Liddle GW: The adrenal cortex. In *Textbook of Endocrinology,* fifth edition. Edited by RH Williams. Philadelphia, WB Saunders Company, 1974, pp 233–283.
12. Hollander JL, Brown EM Jr, Jessar RA, et al: Hydrocortisone and cortisone injected into arthritic joints. JAMA 147:1629–1635, 1951.
13. Robinson RCV, Robinson HM Jr: Topical treatment of dermatoses with steroids. South Med J 49:260–266, 1956.
14. Jenkins JS: The metabolism of cortisol by human extra-hepatic tissues. J Endocrinol 34:51–56, 1966.
15. Jenkins JS, Sampson PA: Conversion of cortisone to cortisol and prednisone to prednisolone. Br Med J 2:205–207, 1967.
16. Powell LW, Axelsen E: Corticosteroids in liver disease: studies on the biological conversion of prednisone to prednisolone and plasma protein binding. Gut 13:690–696, 1972.
17. Nelson DH, Sandberg AA, Palmer JG, et al: Blood levels of 17-hydroxycorticosteroids following the administration of adrenal steroids and their relation to levels of circulating leukocytes. J Clin Invest 31:843–849, 1952.
18. Gemzell CA, Franksson C: Blood levels of 17-hydroxycorticosteroids in normal and adrenalectomized men following administration of cortisone acetate. Acta Endocrinol 12:218–224, 1953.
19. Plumpton FS, Besser GM, Cole PV: Corticosteroid treatment and surgery. 2. The management of steroid cover. Anaesthesia 24:12–18, 1969.
20. Banks P: The adreno-cortical response to oral surgery. Br J Oral Surg 8:32–44, 1970.
21. Kehlet H, Nistrup Madsen S, Binder C: Cortisol and cortisone acetate in parenteral glucocorticoid therapy? Acta Med Scand 195:421–423, 1974.
22. Kehlet H: A rational approach to dosage and preparation of parenteral glucocorticoid substitution therapy during surgical procedures. A short review. Acta Anaesth Scand 19:260–264, 1975.
23. Peterson RE: Adrenocortical steroid metabolism and adrenal cortical function in liver disease. J Clin Invest 39:320–331, 1960.
24. Lewis GP, Jusko WJ, Burke CW, et al: Prednisone side-effects and serum-protein levels, a collaborative study. Lancet 2:778–781, 1971.
25. Schatz M, Patterson R, Zeitz S, et al: Corticosteroid therapy for the pregnant asthmatic patient. JAMA 233:804–807, 1975.
26. Katz FH, Duncan BR: Entry of prednisone into human milk (letter). N Engl J Med 293:1154, 1975.
27. McKenzie SA, Selley JA, Agnew JE: Secretion of prednisolone into breast milk. Arch Dis Child 50:894–896, 1975.
28. David DS, Grieco MH, Cushman P Jr: Adrenal glucocorticoids after twenty years, a review of their clinically relevant consequences. J Chronic Dis 22:637–711, 1970.
29. deLange WE, Doorenbos H: Corticotrophins and corticosteroids. In *Side Effects of Drugs,* vol. 7. Edited by L Meyler, A Herxheimer. Amsterdam, Excerpta Medica, 1972, pp 516–539.
30. Janoski AH, Shaver JC, Christy NP, et al: On the pharmacologic actions of 21-carbon hormonal steroids ('glucocorticoids') of the adrenal cortex in mammals. In *Handbuch der Experimentellen Pharmakologie,* vol. XIV, part 3 (The Adrenocortical Hormones). Edited by HW Deane, BL Rubin. Berlin, Springer-Verlag, 1968, pp 256–368.

31. Newman S: Hormone-induced diseases. In *Diseases of Medical Progress: A Study of Iatrogenic Disease*. Edited by RH Moser. Springfield, Illinois, Charles C Thomas, 1969, pp 361–417.
32. Christy NP: Iatrogenic Cushing's syndrome. In *The Human Adrenal Cortex*. Edited by NP Christy. New York, Harper and Row, 1971, pp 395–425.
33. Ragan C: Corticotropin, cortisone and related steroids in clinical medicine: practical considerations. Bull NY Acad Med 29:355–376, 1953.
34. Deller JJ Jr, Wegienka LC, Conte NF, et al: Testosterone metabolism in idiopathic hirsutism. Ann Intern Med 63:369–376, 1965.
35. Futterweit W, Freeman R, Siegel GL, et al: Clinical applications of a gas chromatographic method for the combined determination of testosterone and epitestosterone glucuronide in urine. J Clin Endocrinol Metab 25:1451–1456, 1965.
36. Jailer JW, Vande Wiele R, Christy NP, et al: Studies in Cushing's syndrome. III. Urinary 17-ketosteroids in patients with bilateral adrenal cortical hyperplasia. J Clin Invest 38:357–365, 1959.
37. James VHT: The excretion of individual 17-oxosteroids in Cushing's syndrome. J Endocrinol 23:119–127, 1961.
38. Biglieri EG, Shambelan M, Slaton PE Jr: Effect of adrenocorticotropin on desoxycorticosterone, corticosterone and aldosterone excretion. J Clin Endocrinol Metab 29:1090–1101, 1969.
39. Melby JC, Dale SL, Wilson TE: 18-hydroxy-deoxycorticosterone in human hypertension. Circ Res, Suppl II to vols 28 and 29:143–152, 1971.
40. Schambelan M, Slaton PE Jr, Biglieri EG: Mineralocorticoid production in hyperadrenocorticism. Am J Med 51:299–303, 1971.
41. Intracranial hypertension and steroids (leading article). Lancet 2:1052–1053, 1964.
42. Walker AE, Adamkiewicz JJ: Pseudotumor cerebri associated with prolonged corticosteroid therapy. JAMA 188:779–784, 1964.
43. David DS, Berkowitz JS: Ocular effects of topical and systemic corticosteroids. Lancet 2:149–151, 1969.
44. Heimann WG, Freiberger RH: Avascular necrosis of the femoral and humeral heads after high-dosage corticosteroid therapy. N Engl J Med 263:672–675, 1960.
45. Velayos EE, Leidholt JD, Smyth CJ, et al: Arthropathy associated with steroid therapy. Ann Intern Med 64:759–771, 1966.
46. Harrington KD, Murray WR, Kountz SL, et al: Avascular necrosis of bone after renal transplantation. J Bone Joint Surg 53A:203–215, 1971.
47. Fisher DE, Bickel WH: Corticosteroid-induced aseptic necrosis: a clinical study of seventy-seven patients. J Bone Joint Surg 53A:859–873, 1971.
48. Park WM: Spontaneous and drug-induced aseptic necrosis. In *Aseptic Necrosis of Bone*. Edited by JK Davidson. Amsterdam, Excerpta Medica, 1976, pp 213–269.
49. Fenster LF: The ulcerogenic potential of glucocorticoids and possible prophylactic measures. In *Steroid Therapy*. Edited by DL Azarnoff. Philadelphia, WB Saunders Company, 1975, pp 42–48.
50. Conn HO, Blitzer BL: Nonassociation of adrenocorticosteroid therapy and peptic ulcer. N Engl J Med 294:473–479, 1976.
51. Langman MJS, Cooke AR: Gastric and duodenal ulcer and their associated diseases. Lancet 1:680–683, 1976.
52. Bovornkitti S, Kangsadal P, Sathirapat P, et al: Reversion and reconversion rate of tuberculin skin reactions in correlation with the use of prednisone. Dis Chest 38:51–55, 1960.
53. Schatz M, Patterson R, Kloner R, et al: The prevalence of tuberculosis and positive tuberculin skin tests in a steroid-treated asthmatic population. Ann Intern Med 84:261–265, 1976.
54. Dwyer J, Lazarus L, Hickie JB: A study of cortisol metabolism in patients with chronic asthma. Australas Ann Med 16:297–304, 1967.
55. Schwartz HJ, Lowell FC, Melby JC: Steroid resistance in bronchial asthma. Ann Intern Med 69:493–499, 1968.
56. Kozower M, Veatch L, Kaplan MM: Decreased clearance of prednisolone, a factor in the development of corticosteroid side effects. J Clin Endocrinol Metab 38:407–412, 1974.
57. Good TA, Benton JW, Kelley VC: Symptomatology resulting from withdrawal of steroid hormone therapy. Arthritis Rheum 2:299–321, 1959.

58. Amatruda TT Jr, Hollingsworth DR, D'Esopo ND, et al: A study of the mechanism of the steroid withdrawal syndrome. Evidence for integrity of the hypothalamic-pituitary-adrenal system. J Clin Endocrinol Metab 20:339–354, 1960.
59. Amatruda TT Jr, Hurst MM, D'Esopo ND: Certain endocrine and metabolic facets of the steroid withdrawal syndrome. J Clin Endocrinol Metab 25:1207–1217, 1965.
60. Choi Y, Thrasher K, Werk EE Jr, et al: Effect of diphenylhydantoin on cortisol kinetics in humans. J Pharmacol Exp Ther 176:27–34, 1971.
61. Haque N, Thrasher K, Werk EE Jr, et al: Studies on dexamethasone metabolism in man: effect of diphenylhydantoin. J Clin Endocrinol Metab 34:44–50, 1972.
62. Stjernholm MR, Katz FH: Effects of diphenylhydantoin, phenobarbital, and diazepam on the metabolism of methylprednisolone and its sodium succinate. J Clin Endocrinol Metab 41:887–893, 1975.
63. Brooks SM, Werk EE, Ackerman SJ, et al: Adverse effects of phenobarbital on corticosteroid metabolism in patients with bronchial asthma. N Engl J Med 286:1125–1128, 1972.
64. Brooks PM, Buchanan WW, Grove M, et al: Effects of enzyme induction on metabolism of prednisolone. Clinical and laboratory study. Ann Rheum Dis 35:339–343, 1976.
65. Edwards OM, Courtenay-Evans RJ, Galley JM, et al: Changes in cortisol metabolism following rifampicin therapy. Lancet 2:549–551, 1974.
66. Buffington GA, Dominguez JH, Piering WF, et al: Interaction of rifampin and glucocorticoids. Adverse effect on renal allograft function. JAMA 236:1958–1960, 1976.
67. Klinenberg JR, Miller F: Effect of corticosteroids on blood salicylate concentration. JAMA 194:131–134, 1965.
68. Thorn GW: Clinical considerations in the use of corticosteroids. N Engl J Med 274:775–781, 1966.
69. Boston Collaborative Drug Surveillance Program: Acute adverse reactions to prednisone in relation to dosage. Clin Pharmacol Ther 13:694–698, 1972.
70. Fitzgerald RH Jr: Intrasynovial injection of steroids. Uses and abuses. Mayo Clin Proc 51:655–659, 1976.
71. Carson TE, Daane TA, Weinstein RL: Long-term intramuscular administration of triamcinolone acetonide. Effect on the hypothalamic-pituitary-adrenal axis. Arch Dermatol 111:1585–1587, 1975.
72. Paris J: Pituitary-adrenal suppression after protracted administration of adrenal cortical hormones. Proc Mayo Clin 36:305–317, 1961.
73. Salassa RM, Bennett WA, Keating FR, et al: Postoperative adrenal cortical insufficiency: occurrence in patients previously treated with cortisone. JAMA 152:1509–1515, 1953.
74. Danowski TS, Bonessi JV, Sabeh G, et al: Probabilities of pituitary-adrenal responsiveness after steroid therapy. Ann Intern Med 61:11–26, 1964.
75. Nichols T, Nugent CA, Tyler FH: Diurnal variation in suppression of adrenal function by glucocorticoids. J Clin Endocrinol Metab 25:343–349, 1965.
76. Chamberlain MA, Keenan J: The effect of low doses of prednisolone compared with placebo on function and on the hypothalamic pituitary adrenal axis in patients with rheumatoid arthritis. Rheumatol Rehab 15:17–23, 1976.
77. Graber AL, Ney RL, Nicholson WE, et al: Natural history of pituitary-adrenal recovery following long-term suppression with corticosteroids. J Clin Endocrinol Metab 25:11–16, 1965.
78. Livanou T, Ferriman D, James VHT: Recovery of hypothalamo-pituitary-adrenal function after corticosteroid therapy. Lancet 2:856–859, 1967.
79. Kyle LH, Meyer RJ, Canary JJ: Mechanism of adrenal atrophy in Cushing's syndrome due to adrenal tumor. N Engl J Med 257:57–61, 1957.
80. Morris HG, Jorgensen JR: Recovery of endogenous pituitary-adrenal function in corticosteroid-treated children. J Pediatr 79:480–488, 1971.
81. Jasani MK, Freeman PA, Boyle JA, et al: Studies of the rise in plasma 11-hydroxycorticosteroids (11-OHCS) in corticosteroid-treated patients with rheumatoid arthritis during surgery: correlations with the functional integrity of the hypothalamic-pituitary-adrenal axis. Q J Med 37:407–421, 1968.
82. Kehlet H, Binder C: Value of an ACTH test in assessing hypothalamic-pituitary-adrenocortical function in glucocorticoid-treated patients. Br Med J 2:147–149, 1973.
83. Marks LJ, Donovan MJ, Duncan FJ, et al: Adrenocortical response to surgical operations in patients treated with corticosteroids or corticotropin prior to surgery. J Clin Endocrinol Metab 19:1458–1470, 1959.

84. Sampson PA, Winstone NE, Brooke BN: Adrenal function in surgical patients after steroid therapy. Lancet 2:322–325, 1962.
85. Reichling GH, Kligman AM: Alternate-day corticosteroid therapy. Arch Dermatol 83:980–983, 1961.
86. Harter JG, Reddy WJ, Thorn GW: Studies on an intermittent corticosteroid dosage regimen. N Engl J Med 269:591–596, 1963.
87. Fleisher DS: Pituitary-adrenal responsiveness after corticosteroid therapy in children with nephrosis. J Pediatr 70:54–59, 1967.
88. Soyka LF: Treatment of the nephrotic syndrome in childhood: use of an alternate-day prednisone regimen. Am J Dis Child 113:693–701, 1967.
89. MacGregor RR, Sheagren JN, Lipsett MB, et al: Alternate-day prednisone therapy: evaluation of delayed hypersensitivity responses, control of disease and steroid side effects. N Engl J Med 280:1427–1431, 1969.
90. Sadeghi-Nejad A, Senior B: Adrenal function, growth, and insulin in patients treated with corticoids on alternate days. Pediatrics 43:277–283, 1969.
91. Reed WP, Lucas ZJ, Cohn R: Alternate-day prednisone therapy after renal transplantation. Lancet 1:747–749, 1970.
92. Walton J, Watson BS, Ney RL: Alternate-day vs shorter interval steroid administration. Arch Intern Med 126:601–607, 1970.
93. Siegel RR, Luke RG, Hellebusch AA: Reduction of toxicity of corticosteroid therapy after renal transplantation. Am J Med 53:159–169, 1972.
94. Soyka LF: Alternate-day corticosteroid therapy. Adv Pediatr 19:47–70, 1972.
95. Block AJ, Light RW: Alternate day steroid therapy in diffuse pulmonary sarcoidosis. Chest 63:495–500, 1973.
96. Chai H, Gilbert A: The effect of alternate-day prednisone on the white blood count in children with chronic asthma. J Allergy Clin Immunol 51:65–70, 1973.
97. Gulati PD, Malik GB, Vaishnava H: Alternate-day steroid therapy in adult nephrotics. J Med 4:266–275, 1973.
98. McEnery PT, Gonzalez LL, Martin LW, et al: Growth and development of children with renal transplants. Use of alternate-day steroid therapy. J Pediatr 83:806–814, 1973.
99. Sampson D, Albert DJ: Alternate day therapy with methylprednisolone after renal transplantation. J Urol 109:345–348, 1973.
100. Sheagren JN, Simon HB, Rich RR: Therapy of sarcoidosis initiated with alternate-day prednisone. J Natl Med Assoc 65:391–398, 1973.
101. Dale DC, Fauci AS, Wolff SM: Alternate-day prednisone: leukocyte kinetics and susceptibility to infections. N Engl J Med 291:1154–1158, 1974.
102. Elders MJ, Wingfield BS, McNatt ML, et al: Glucocorticoid therapy in children: effect on somatomedin secretion. Am J Dis Child 129:1393–1396, 1975.
103. Fauci AS, Dale DC: Alternate-day prednisone therapy and human lymphocyte subpopulations. J Clin Invest 55:22–32, 1975.
104. Potter DE, Holliday MA, Wilson CJ, et al: Alternate-day steroids in children after renal transplantation. Transplant Proc 7:79–82, 1975.
105. Reimer LG, Morris HG, Ellis EF: Growth of asthmatic children during treatment with alternate-day steroids. J Allergy Clin Immunol 55:224–231, 1975.
106. Diethelm AG, Sterling WA, Hartley MW, et al: Alternate-day prednisone therapy in recipients of renal allografts: risks and benefits. Arch Surg 111:867–870, 1976.
107. Easton JG, Busser RJ, Heimlich EM: Effect of alternate-day steroid administration on adrenal function in allergic children. J Allergy Clin Immunol 48:355–360, 1971.
108. Kuzemko JA, Lines JG: Adrenal cortical function in asthmatic children on alternate day steroids. Arch Dis Child 46:366–370, 1971.
109. Ackerman GL, Nolan CM: Adrenocortical responsiveness after alternate-day corticosteroid therapy. N Engl J Med 278:405–409, 1968.
110. Falliers CJ, Chai H, Molk L, et al: Pulmonary and adrenal effects of alternate-day corticosteroid therapy. J Allergy Clin Immunol 49:156–166, 1972.
111. Morris HG, Neuman I, Ellis EF: Plasma steroid concentrations during alternate-day treatment with prednisone. J Allergy Clin Immunol 54:350–358, 1974.
112. Bolton WK, Atuk NO, Sturgill BC, et al: Therapy of the idiopathic nephrotic syndrome with alternate day steroids. Am J Med 62:60–70, 1977.
113. Bell MJ, Martin LW, Gonzales LL, et al: Alternate-day single-dose prednisone therapy: a method of reducing steroid toxicity. J Pediatr Surg 7:223–229, 1972.

114. McDonald FD, Horensten ML, Schork MA, et al: A randomized, controlled, prospective study of the effect of alternate-day prednisone on renal transplant function. Proc Dialysis Transplant Forum 2:5–7, 1972.
115. Reimold EW: Intermittent prednisone therapy in children and adolescents after renal transplantation. Pediatrics 2:235–240, 1973.
116. McAdams AJ, McEnery PT, West CD: Mesangiocapillary glomerulonephritis: changes in glomerular morphology with long-term alternate-day prednisone therapy. J Pediatr 86:23–31, 1975.
117. Ackerman GL: Alternate-day steroid therapy in lupus nephritis. Ann Intern Med 72:511–519, 1970.
118. Cocco AE, Mendeloff AL: An evaluation of intermittent corticosteroid therapy in the management of ulcerative colitis. Johns Hopkins Med J 120:162–169, 1967.
119. Carter ME, James VHT: Effect of alternate-day, single-dose, corticosteroid therapy on pituitary-adrenal function. Ann Rheum Dis 31:379–383, 1972.
120. Haim S, Benderly A, Shafrir A, et al: Alternate-day corticosteroid regimen. Dermatologica 142:171–176, 1971.
121. Jenkins RB: Treatment of myasthenia gravis with prednisone. Lancet 1:765–767, 1972.
122. Engel WK, Festoff BW, Patten BM, et al: Myasthenia gravis. Ann Intern Med 81:225–246, 1974.
123. Seybold ME, Drachman DB: Gradually increasing doses of prednisone in myasthenia gravis: reducing the hazards of treatment. N Engl J Med 290:81–84, 1974.
124. Brunner NG, Berger CL, Namba T, et al: Corticotropin or corticosteroids in generalized myasthenia gravis: comparative studies and role in management. Ann NY Acad Sci 274:577–595, 1976.
125. Mann JD, Johns TR, Campa JF: Long-term administration of corticosteroids in myasthenia gravis. Neurology 26:729–740, 1976.
126. Drachman DB, Toyka KV, Myer E: Prednisone in Duchenne muscular dystrophy. Lancet 2:1409–1412, 1974.
127. Walsh SD, Grant IWB: Corticosteroids in treatment of chronic asthma. Br Med J 2:796–802, 1966.
128. Portner MM, Thayer KH, Harter JG, et al: Successful initiation of alternate-day prednisone in chronic steroid-dependent asthmatic patients. J Allergy Clin Immunol 49:16–26, 1972.
129. Rabhan NB, Kopf AW: Alternate-day prednisone therapy for pemphigus vulgaris. Arch Dermatol 103:615–622, 1971.
130. Hunder GG, Sheps SG, Allen GL, et al: Daily and alternate day corticosteroid regimens in treatment of giant cell arteritis: comparison in a prospective study. Ann Intern Med 82:613–618, 1975.
131. Abruzzo JL: Alternate-day prednisone therapy. Ann Intern Med 82:714, 1975.
132. Schutz S, Newhouse R, Dello Russo J: Alternate-day steroid regimen in the treatment of ocular disease. Br J Ophthalmol 52:461–463, 1968.
133. Ansell BM, Bywaters EGL: Alternate-day corticosteroid therapy in juvenile chronic polyarthritis. J Rheumatol 1:176–186, 1974.
134. Jasani MK, Boyle JA, Dick WC, et al: Corticosteroid-induced hypothalamo-pituitary-adrenal axis suppression: prospective study using two regimens of corticosteroid therapy. Ann Rheum Dis 27:352–359, 1968.
135. Rabhan NB: Pituitary-adrenal suppression and Cushing's syndrome after intermittent dexamethasone therapy. Ann Intern Med 69:1141–1148, 1968.
136. Dubois EL, Adler DC: Single-daily dose oral administration of corticosteroids in rheumatic disorders: an analysis of its advantages, efficacy and side effects. Curr Ther Res 5:43–56, 1963.
137. Nugent CA, Ward J, MacDiarmid WD, et al: Glucocorticoid toxicity: single contrasted with divided daily doses of prednisolone. J Chronic Dis 18:323–332, 1965.
138. Myles AB, Schiller LGF, Glass D, et al: Single daily dose corticosteroid treatment. Ann Rheum Dis 35:73–76, 1976.
139. DiRaimondo VC, Forsham PH: Pharmacophysiologic principles in the use of corticoids and adrenocorticotropin. Metabolism 7:5–24, 1958.
140. Grant SD, Forsham PH, DiRaimondo VC: Suppression of 17-hydroxycorticosteroids in plasma and urine by single and divided doses of triamcinolone. N Engl J Med 273:1115–1118, 1965.
141. Myles AB, Bacon PA, Daly JR: Single daily dose corticosteroid treatment: effect on adrenal function and therapeutic efficacy in various diseases. Ann Rheum Dis 30:149–153, 1971.

142. Smith RT, Good RA: Sequelae of prednisone treatment of acute rheumatic fever. Clin Research Proc 4:156–157, 1956.
143. Taranta A, Mark H, Haas RC, et al: Nodular panniculitis after massive prednisone therapy. Am J Med 25:52–61, 1958.
144. Vince DJ: Nodular panniculitis after massive prednisone therapy. Can Med Assoc J 79:840–841, 1958.
145. Spagnuolo M, Taranta A: Post-steroid panniculitis. Ann Intern Med 54:1181–1191, 1963.
146. Young II, DeFilippis V, Meyer FL, et al: Maintenance of adrenal cortical responsiveness during prolonged corticoid therapy. Arch Intern Med 100:1–10, 1957.
147. Fleischer N, Abe K, Liddle GW, et al: ACTH antibodies in patients receiving depot porcine ACTH to hasten recovery from pituitary-adrenal suppression. J Clin Invest 46:196–204, 1967.
148. Carter ME, James VHT: An attempt at combining corticotrophin with long-term corticosteroid therapy: with a view to preserving hypothalamic-pituitary-adrenal function. Ann Rheum Dis 29:409–414, 1970.
149. Allander E: ACTH or corticosteroids? A critical review of results and possibilities in the treatment of severe chronic disease. Acta Rheum Scand 15:277–296, 1969.
150. Kaplan HP, Portnoy B, Binder HJ, et al: A controlled evaluation of intravenous adrenocorticotropic hormone and hydrocortisone in the treatment of acute colitis. Gastroenterology 69:91–95, 1975.
151. Savage O, Copeman WSC, Chapman L, et al: Pituitary and adrenal hormones in rheumatoid arthritis. Lancet 1:232–235, 1962.
152. Azarnoff DL: *Steroid Therapy*. Philadelphia, WB Saunders Company, 1975.
153. Lesesne HR, Fallon HJ: Treatment of liver disease with corticosteroids. In *Steroid Therapy*. Edited by DL Azarnoff, Philadelphia, WB Saunders Company, 1975, pp 96–110.
154. Kehlet H, Binder C, Blichert-Toft M: Glucocorticoid maintenance therapy following adrenalectomy: assessment of dosage and preparation. Clin Endocrinol 5:37–41, 1976.
155. Cope CL, Black E: The production rate of cortisol in man. Br Med J 1:1020–1024, 1958.
156. Peterson RE: The miscible pool and turnover rate of adrenocortical steroids in man. Rec Progr Hormone Res 15:231–274, 1959.
157. Peterson RE, Nokes G, Chen PS, et al: Estrogen and adrenocortical function in man. J Clin Endocrinol Metab 20:495–514, 1960.
158. Ichikawa Y: Metabolism of cortisol-4-C^{14} in patients with infectious and collagen diseases. Metabolism 15:613–625, 1966.
159. Thomas JP, El-Shaboury AH: Aldosterone secretion in steroid-treated patients with adrenal suppression. Lancet 1:623–625, 1971.
160. Franksson C, Gemzell CA: Adrenocortical activity in the preoperative period. J Clin Endocrinol Metab 15:1069–1072, 1955.
161. Price DB, Thaler M, Mason JW: Preoperative emotional states and adrenal cortical activity. Arch Neurol Psychiat 77:646–656, 1957.
162. Czeisler CA, Mooreede MC, Regestein QR, et al: Episodic 24-hour cortisol secretory patterns in patients awaiting elective cardiac surgery. J Clin Endocrinol Metab 42:273–283, 1976.
163. Hammond WG, Vandam LD, Davis JM, et al: Studies in surgical endocrinology. IV. Anesthetic agents as stimuli to change in corticosteroids and metabolism. Ann Surg 148:199–211, 1958.
164. Britton MG, Collins JV, Brown D, et al: High-dose corticosteroids in severe acute asthma. Br Med J 2:73–74, 1976.
165. Michelis MF, Murdaugh HV: Selective hypoaldosteronism: an editorial revisited after 15 years. Am J Med 59:1–5, 1975.
166. Biglieri EG: A perspective on aldosterone abnormalities. Clin Endocrinol 5:399–410, 1976.
167. Goldfien A, Laidlaw JC, Haydar NA, et al: Fluorohydrocortisone and chlorohydrocortisone, highly potent derivatives of compound F. N Engl J Med 252:415–421, 1955.
168. Renold AE, Haydar NA, Reddy WJ, et al: Biological effects of fluorinated derivatives of hydrocortisone and progesterone in man. Ann NY Acad Sci 61:582–590, 1955.
169. Thorn GW, Renold AE, Morse WI, et al: Highly potent adrenal cortical steroids: structure and biological activity. Ann Intern Med 43:979–1000, 1955.
170. Thorn GW, Sheppard RH, Morse WI, et al: Comparative action of aldosterone and 9-alpha-fluorohydrocortisone in man. Ann NY Acad Sci 61:609–619, 1955.

171. Liddle GW, Pechet MM, Bartter FC: Enhancement of biological activities of corticosteroids by substitution of halogen atoms in 9 α position. Science 120:496–497, 1954.
172. Garrod O, Nabarro JDN, Pawan GLS, et al: Metabolic effects of 9 α-fluorohydrocortisone and of cortisone in adrenal insufficiency. Lancet 2:367–370, 1955.
173. Hart FD: Treatment of adrenocortical deficiency states. Br Med J 1:417–422, 1957.
174. Boland EW, Headley NE: Preliminary clinical trials with 9-α-fluorohydrocortisone acetate in rheumatoid arthritis. Ann Rheum Dis 14:291–296, 1954.
175. Wakai CS, Prickman LE: Effects of 9 α-fluorohydrocortisone acetate administered to patients with asthmatic bronchitis. Proc Mayo Clin 29:663–665, 1954.
176. Ward LE, Polley HF, Slocumb CH, et al: The effects of aldosterone (electrocortin) and of 9 α-fluorohydrocortisone acetate on rheumatoid arthritis: preliminary report. Proc Mayo Clin 29:649–663, 1954.

50. ANDROGENS

William F. Crowley, Jr. and Lloyd Axelrod

Treatment with androgens can be divided into two broad categories on the basis of dosage and mechanism of action. *Replacement therapy* for hypogonadal males is designed to achieve physiologic plasma levels of androgen and is mediated by high-affinity target organ receptors specific for androgens. When virilization is the principal goal of androgen therapy, testosterone congeners are the predominant class of androgens used. When *anabolic therapy* is desired, the plasma levels of androgen required are usually pharmacologic, the results are less clearly receptor-mediated, and the desired metabolic effects often require synthetic androgens in which virilization is partially dissociated from anabolic effects.

ANDROGEN PHYSIOLOGY IN NORMAL ADULT MALES

In adult males testosterone is secreted almost exclusively from the testes; the normal production rate is 7,000 μg/24 hours.[1] Gonadal secretion of testosterone is under direct control of the pituitary via secretion of luteinizing hormone (LH), which causes testosterone release by the Leydig cells of the testes. Once secreted, testosterone is transported in the plasma by a high-affinity binding globulin, testosterone-estrogen binding globulin (TEBG).[2]

TEBG preferentially binds testosterone over estrogen with high affinity, and consequently is an important determinant of the bound and free fraction of circulating androgens. Upon arrival at the target organ the free fraction of androgen enters the cell, where it has three possible metabolic fates. One involves direct binding to the high-affinity cytoplasmic receptor that exhibits strong stereospecificity for testosterone.[3] This androgen-receptor complex then enters the nucleus, binds to DNA and initiates a series of transcriptional events specific for each target tissue. A second fate for androgens is direct reduction to dihydrotestosterone (DHT). DHT has an even higher affinity for the androgen receptor than testosterone itself. Moreover, in certain target organs, such as the external genitalia of the male, an absolute requirement for this metabolic conversion is present. The remaining fate for androgens is metabolism to estrogens. This conversion appears to be very important in the expression of certain central nervous system effects of androgens, most notably gonadotropin control.[4]

The circulating level of 'testosterone' measured by radioimmunoassay is 300 to 1,000 ng/100 ml in males and 20 to 80 ng/100 ml in females. Most radioimmunoassays of testosterone do not distinguish between testosterone and DHT in establishing normal values. However, the physiologic ratio of testosterone to DHT in the peripheral circulation is 10 to 1, so these normal levels are largely a reflection of testosterone dynamics.

ANDROGEN PHYSIOLOGY IN NORMAL ADULT FEMALES

Control of androgen synthesis in the female is less clearly understood. The production rate of testosterone in normal women is 250 μg/24 hours. Only 50% of this is derived from direct secretion by the ovaries and adrenal glands; the remainder reflects peripheral (extraglandular) conversion from less potent androgens of gonadal and adrenal origin. This contrasts with the male in whom over 90% of testosterone is derived from direct secretion.[1,5] The circadian periodicity of the secretion of androstenedione (a weak androgen precursor of testosterone) with higher levels early in the morning suggests control by adrenocorticotropic hormone (ACTH); however, another pituitary hormone may specifically regulate adrenal androgen production.[6] Ovarian androgen production occurs predominantly in the theca cells and is under LH control as is Leydig cell function in the male.

PREPARATIONS AND DOSES

Androgens are defined functionally on the basis of their androgenic and/or myogenic properties in bioassays and not on the basis of their chemical structures. Seminal vesicle weight is used to define androgenic function while a variety of muscle responses such as *levator ani* weight are used to assess myogenic function. The majority of androgens available for therapy fall into one of three structural classes (Table 1).

Testosterone Esters

Single oral doses of testosterone produce only transient elevations of the plasma testosterone level and are largely metabolized by the gastrointestinal tract.[7] Thus it is necessary to conjugate testosterone to an aliphatic or aromatic side chain via an ester linkage. Conjugation retards absorption from parenteral sites of administration and prolongs the duration of biologic effect. The duration of elevation of plasma testosterone levels following a single dose of the testosterone esters varies from testosterone propionate, with a duration of one to three days, to testosterone enanthate with a duration of 14 to 21days.[8,9] Treatment with any of the testosterone esters results in a transient increase of the plasma testosterone level to supraphysiologic values, followed by a gradual decline. In order to avoid this 'peak and valley' effect, preparations containing mixtures of short- and long-acting esters are employed. However, the bioavailability of testosterone in these preparations is not well-established.[9] Chemical structures, usual dosage, preparations and costs of androgens are given in Table 1.

Testosterone Analogues

As with estrogens and glucocorticoids, modification of testosterone by the addition of a methyl group at the 17α position and fluorine at the 9α position yields compounds that are far more potent than testosterone and are stable at very low pH levels. Hence, 17α-methyltestosterone (methyltestosterone) and 9α-fluoro-17α-methyltestosterone (fluoxymesterone) can be administered by mouth. Since these compounds bind poorly to TEBG and cannot be aromatized to estrogens, they have a somewhat different spectrum of target organ effects than testosterone. For example, fluoxymesterone treatment is associated with persistent elevation of gonadotropin secretion in castrates because it is not aromatized by the central nervous system.[4] Also, the free levels of these androgen analogues in the plasma are higher than those occurring with testosterone administration. In addition, this class of compounds results in rather high portal vein androgen concentrations and a higher incidence of hepatotoxicity than other preparations.

Synthetic Androgens

Synthetic compounds contain a combination of a 17α substitution

TABLE 1 Chemical Structure, Usual Dosage, Preparations and Costs of Commonly Used Androgens

GENERIC NAME	CHEMICAL STRUCTURE
Testosterone Esters	
Testosterone Propionate	$O-COCH_2CH_3$; O
Testosterone Cypionate	$O-COCH_2CH_2-$; O
Testosterone Enanthate	$O-CO(CH_2)_5CH_3$; O
Testosterone Analogues	
Fluoxymesterone	OH; CH_3; HO; F; O
Methyltestosterone	OH; CH_3; O
Synthetic Androgens	
Methandrostenolone	OH; CH_3; O

Usual Dosage	Preparations and 1978 Costs
Adults, 50 mg IM every 3 days	Neo-Hombreol Injection (solution in sesame oil) 50 mg/ml—$3.70/10-ml vial
Adults, 200–300 mg IM every 14–21 days	Depo-Testosterone Injection (solution in cottonseed oil) 50 mg/ml—$5.94/10-ml vial; 100 mg/ml—$2.19/1-ml ampul, $11.58/10-ml vial; 200 mg/ml—$3.80/1-ml ampul, $20.79/10-ml vial T-Ionate-P.A. Injection (solution in cottonseed oil) 200 mg/ml—$9.35/10-ml vial
Adults, 200–300 mg IM every 14–21 days	Delatestryl Injection (solution in sesame oil) 200 mg/ml—$3.74/1-ml syringe, $9.94/5-ml vial
Adults, 10–20 mg orally daily	Halotestin Tablets 2 mg—$11.23/100; 5 mg—$13.90/50; 10 mg—$20.61/50
Adults, 30–50 mg orally daily	Metandren Tablets (oral) 10 mg—$11.20/100; 25 mg—$26.70/100 Tablets (buccal) 5 mg—$6.10/100; 10 mg—$11.20/100 Oreton Methyl Tablets (oral) 10 mg—$9.87/100; 25 mg—$24.38/100 Tablets (buccal) 10 mg—$9.87/100
Adults, 5 mg orally daily initially; 2.5–5 mg daily for maintenance	Dianabol Tablets 2.5 mg—$7.95/100; 5 mg—$12.00/100

TABLE 1 *(Continued)*

Generic Name	Chemical Structure
Nandrolone Decanoate	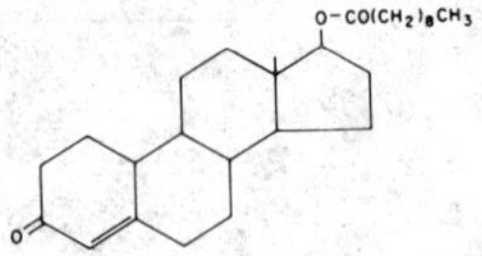 O–CO(CH$_2$)$_8$CH$_3$; O
Nandrolone Phenpropionate	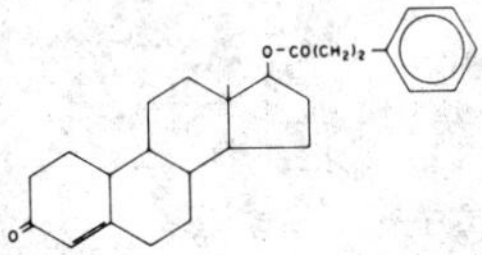 O–CO(CH$_2$)$_2$–; O
Oxandrolone	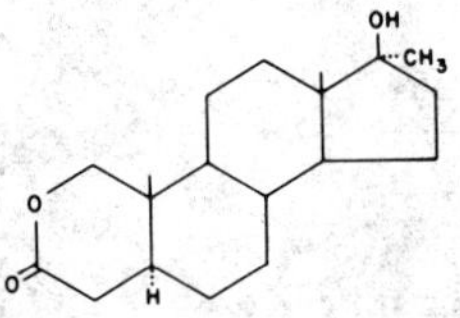 OH; CH$_3$; O; O; H
Oxymetholone	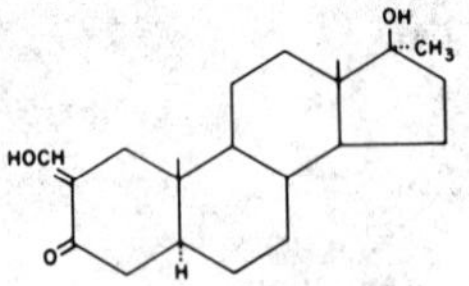 OH; CH$_3$; HOCH; O; H
Stanozolol	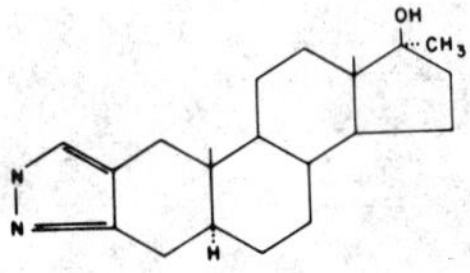 OH; CH$_3$; N; N; H

with an A ring modification, resulting in an altered spectrum of androgen activity.[10] Most of these derivatives produce anabolic effects out of proportion to virilization. This dissociation may be advantageous in certain circumstances, as in the treatment of females and prepubertal patients. However, none of these compounds is totally free of virilizing activity. The 17α substitution also provides stability via the oral route, offering increased ease of administration.

Usual Dosage	Preparations and 1978 Costs
Adults, 50–100 mg IM (deep) every 3–4 weeks Children, 2–13 years, 25–50 mg every 3–4 weeks	Deca-Durabolin Injection (solution in sesame oil) 50 mg/ml—$4.65/1-ml ampul, $8.45/2-ml vial; 100 mg/ml—$15.75/2-ml vial
Adults, 25–50 mg IM (deep) weekly Children, 2–13 years, 12.5–25 mg every 2–4 weeks	Durabolin Injection (solution in sesame oil) 25 mg/ml—$1.80/1-ml ampul, $7.60/5-ml vial; 50 mg/ml—$6.24/2-ml vial
Adults, 5–10 mg orally daily	Anavar Tablets 2.5 mg—$6.25/100
Adults, 5–10 mg orally daily Children, 1.25–5 mg daily depending on age	Adroyd Tablets 5 mg—$6.65/50; 10 mg—$24.94/100 Anadrol Tablets 50 mg—$30.00/100
Adults, 6 mg orally daily Children, 6–12 years, 2–6 mg daily; under 6 years, 2 mg daily	Winstrol Tablets 2 mg—$8.04/100

INDICATIONS

Replacement Therapy

Prior to institution of androgen therapy in hypogonadal men, the etiology of the androgen deficiency must be determined. Primary testicular failure must be distinguished from that attributable to hypothalamic or pituitary disease. Pituitary tumors or hypothalamic lesions should be recognized and treatment undertaken prior to institution of androgen therapy. Similarly, certain primary testicular deficiencies carry systemic implications. For example, the gonadal failure of myotonic dystrophy may be a presenting feature of this syndrome. Moreover, the patient's psychological and social history should be assessed to determine whether androgen replacement therapy is appropriate. Therapy is not without side effects and can often be disruptive to a patient who is well compensated in the hypogonadal state.

Hematologic Indications

Androgens stimulate erythropoiesis at multiple levels. Most androgens increase serum erythropoietin levels in animals and in humans.[11,12] Lesser elevations of erythropoiesis occur in anephric patients, implying that androgens increase both the renal and the extrarenal production of erythropoietin.[13]

Androgens also directly stimulate differentiation of cultured erythroblastic stem cells.[14] Lastly, the 5β-hydroxy metabolites of several steroids, including testosterone and progesterone, in themselves can stimulate erythropoiesis. This stimulation is stereospecific; the 5α metabolites are ineffective.[15] Androgens not only increase production of circulating hemoglobin, but also alter the functional capacity of the erythrocyte. Administration of androgens is followed by the appearance of increased levels of red cell 2,3-diphosphoglycerate.[16] Based on this evidence androgens have been employed in the treatment of several forms of bone marrow failure.

Anemia Associated with Renal Failure. Bleeding, nutritional deficiency states, hemolysis, and medications often contribute to the pathogenesis of the 'anemia of uremia'. While vigilant medical therapy and hemodialysis can ameliorate most of these problems, severe anemia generally persists and can limit the activity of uremic patients. Low serum erythropoietin levels and a hypoproliferative bone marrow picture are characteristic features of this anemia.[17]

Androgen therapy is effective in the treatment of the anemia oı renal failure (Table 2).[13,17–24] Although the increase in red cell mass is only modest, it is often masked by a larger rise of plasma volume. Therefore, the increment in red cell volume and not the rise of the hematocrit is the most reliable way to monitor response. Such mild increments in red cell mass can be quite beneficial. The anemia of uremia is usually severe and symptomatic; hence, even mild increases in oxygen-carrying capacity may produce notable clinical improve-

TABLE 2 Androgen Therapy in the Anemia of Renal Failure

Reference	Androgen[a]	Dose/Week	Duration (months)	No. of Males	No. of Females	Increase in RBC Mass	Response Rate (%)	Increase in Hematocrit (%)	Transfusion Requirements
DeGowin [18] 1970	TE	400 mg	2.5–4	2	0	—	10	5–7	↓
Richardson [19] 1970	TE	400–600 mg	1–11	15	0	353 ml (4.4 ml/kg)	87	5–6	↓
Shaldon [20] 1971	T	250 mg	3–6	20	5	—	100	4–8	↓
Shaldon [13] 1971	TE	500 mg	3	4	1	465 ml	100[c]	9	
Davies]21[1972	OM	500 mg	1.5–3	55	0	—	0	—	
Fried [22] 1973	TP	300 mg	3–4	11	0	—	100[b] 0[c]	7	
Eschbach [23] 1973	FM	70–210 mg	6	6	8	—	93	5	↓
Williams [24] 1974	NP	200 mg	3	10	8	5 ml/kg	100	4	
Hendler [17] 1974	NP	100 mg	3	22	0	227 ml	80	5	↓

[a]TE = Testosterone Enanthate; T = Testosterone; OM = Oxymetholone; TP = Testosterone Propionate; FM = Fluoxymesterone; NP = Nandrolone Proprionate.

[b]Non-nephrectomized patients.

[c]Nephrectomized patients.

ment. Also, the reduced transfusion requirements lessen the risk of hepatitis. Finally, increases in body weight and serum creatinine in the absence of a rise in BUN suggest beneficial effects upon nutrition,[17,19] and often coincide with an increase in appetite and a sense of well-being.

The beneficial effects of androgen therapy probably occur only after treatment for extended periods of time. Androgen therapy must be continued for a minimum of three months before this treatment can be adequately evaluated. Additionally, the dosage employed is pharmacologic, often exceeding physiologic replacement levels by a factor of 1.5 to 4 (Table 2). Although the proper choice of androgen is not established, several androgens seem equally effective. Oral androgens have the disadvantages of uncertainty of absorption and difficulty of administration during intercurrent vomiting; moreover, these 17α-hydroxylated substances impart a high risk of cholestatic hepatitis. Hepatotoxicity may, of course, result in jaundice, a particularly disconcerting event in a hemodialysis unit. Parenteral androgens require frequent intramuscular injections with local side effects such as bleeding and abscess formation, both of which may be lessened with proper antiseptic technique and use of a 21 gauge needle.

Aplastic Anemia. The role of androgens in the management of aplastic anemia is more controversial. Controlled studies in humans[25] and animals[26] have failed to demonstrate any effect of the synthetic androgen nandrolone phenpropionate in aplastic anemia. The human study employed a double-blind protocol, administration for three months, and a dosage that was effective in renal failure.[17,25] However, only seven patients were evaluated, two of whom were subsequently omitted from the study. Two of the remaining five patients responded to treatment in an unspecified way. Similarly, the animal study[26] employed busulfan-treated mice, a model of aplastic anemia not necessarily relevant to humans. The remaining clinical studies of androgen use in aplastic anemia have utilized historical controls, either the previous period of observation in patients under study or previous experience in allegedly similar patients within an institution. Unfortunately, historical controls are not adequate since spontaneous fluctuations in severity of the disease, remissions, changes in referral patterns, and improvement in general supportive care can occur within an institution over the periods of interest.[27]

The deficits of these studies are further compounded by the marked heterogeneity of the patient population.[27,28] Some studies have demonstrated such a high mortality rate within the first three to six months in subpopulations of patients with aplastic anemia that an adequate trial of androgen therapy is impossible.[29] Thus, patients destined to be long-term survivors may be over-represented in any large scale study of androgen therapy in aplastic anemia that lasts longer than 3 to 6 months.[27–32]

On the other hand, androgen therapy can have a beneficial effect on red cell mass in patients with aplastic anemia, especially those with congenital or prepubertal disease. This improvement disappears with the removal of the androgen only to reappear with the reinstitution of hormonal therapy. Similar effects upon white blood cells and platelets are less striking and the extremely low survival rate of these patients is not due to anemia, but rather to bleeding and infection.[27–35] Thus, while androgens may ameliorate the symptoms of anemia, there is no convincing evidence that they influence survival. Hence, androgen treatment is reserved for those patients in whom the severity of symptoms due to anemia justifies the risk of side effects. Moreover, it has been suggested that the transition of certain patients from aplastic anemia to acute leukemia occurs more frequently during androgen therapy than would be expected by chance.[36] Controlled studies will be required to establish this fact, however.

Other Hematologic Disorders. Androgens have been advocated for use in myeloid metaplasia,[37] sickle cell anemia,[38] and cyclic neutropenia.[39] However, no controlled studies exist to support their use for these indications.

Constitutional Short Stature

The characteristic feature of patients with constitutional short stature appears to be a proportional retardation of both height age (HA) and bone age (BA) when compared to chronologic age (CA). The onset of puberty, albeit delayed, ultimately results in reversal of this abnormality, thus suggesting that androgens might play a role in therapy of these patients. Treatment became possible when synthetic androgens achieving partial separation of the anabolic effects from virilization were developed. It was hoped that these compounds might accelerate height age to a greater extent than bone age and ultimately influence both the rate of change and the ultimate height.

Most studies have employed oxandrolone (Table 3). Androgens may temporarily accelerate linear growth, but long-term studies indicate that they do not significantly alter the predicted height.[40–50] In several dramatic cases, a rapid advancement of height age occurred while the patient was on androgen therapy, but the fortuitous appearance of puberty during androgen therapy may have explained this. Hence, androgens for short stature should be limited to those patients in whom there is an actual deficiency of androgens. Concomitant growth hormone deficiency will diminish the effect of androgen administration. Optimal growth rate in patients with combined growth hormone and androgen deficiency occurs only when both are corrected concurrently.[51–54]

Male Infertility

It was initially observed that morphologic improvements in the seminiferous tubules of institutionalized patients occurred after a course of testosterone suppression therapy.[55] Subsequently, these observations were applied to patients with oligospermia.[56] However, the initial observations were made by testicular biopsy and not on seminal fluid analysis; this mode of treatment represents an extrapolation from the pilot study. Nevertheless, several investigators have employed 'testosterone rebound' in patients with idiopathic oligospermia. This therapy utilizes androgens in pharmacologic doses to produce azospermia. Testosterone is then discontinued with the expectation that a rebound will occur during which the sperm count improves compared with levels observed before therapy. No controlled studies have established the efficacy of this regimen. Furthermore, the period of observation prior to the institution of therapy in most studies is inadequate. Since large spontaneous variations occur in the characteristics of seminal fluid, an abbreviated control period makes it difficult to assess the actual effects of treatment.[57]

Endometriosis

Androgen therapy of endometriosis has been variably successful.[58] Major drawbacks include the virilizing effects of most androgens, the duration of therapy required to reverse endometriosis, and unpredictable response. Synthetic progestational agents with mild anabolic properties are currently the treatment of choice (see Chapter 51).

Hereditary Angioneurotic Edema

Recurrent attacks of urticaria, abdominal pain, and life-threatening upper airway obstruction characterize this syndrome. It is caused by a deficiency in an androgen-sensitve enzyme, C′1 esterase, an inhibitor of the first component of complement. Double-blind controlled studies indicate that androgen therapy is effective in this disorder, decreasing the frequency and severity of attacks.[59–61] Derivatives of 19-nortestosterone have also been used with similar success.[62]

Carcinoma of the Breast

Androgens have been used in the therapy of metastatic breast cancer,[63] but oral estrogen and antiestrogen therapy is preferred when the tumor appears to be endocrine sensitive.[64] Androgens may act by binding to the estrogen receptor.[65]

CONTRAINDICATIONS

Since carcinoma of the prostate may be improved by castration and aggravated by testosterone, presence of this malignancy is a contraindication to androgen usage. Similarly, hepatic or breast carcinoma with possible or demonstrated androgen dependency are contraindications. Fetal virilization represents a potential hazard of androgen therapy during pregnancy. Finally, the increased plasma volume associated with androgens requires careful monitoring when androgens are used in patients with congestive heart failure, liver disease, nephrosis, and other conditions associated with fluid retention.

ADVERSE REACTIONS

The most common adverse reaction associated with androgens is hepatotoxicity. Cholestatic jaundice is associated with androgen therapy and probably occurs more often with 17α-methyl substituted androgens.[66] Less common but more serious side effects include a variety of hepatic neoplasms. Focal nodular hyperplasia and peliotic hepatitis (multiple blood-filled cysts) are the more benign of these lesions and can present with hepatic masses, tenderness or more dramatic manifestations such as rupture and peritoneal bleeding.[67] Hepatocellular carcinomas occur during androgen therapy and show

TABLE 3 Androgen Treatment for Constitutional Short Stature

Reference	No. of Patients	Androgen and Dose	Duration of Therapy	↑HA>BA[a]	Comments
Danowski [42] 1965	12	Oxandrolone 10–40 mg/day	13–17 mo	—[b]	No controls; wide variety of endocrine disorders studied;
Zangeneh [41] 1967	24	Oxandrolone 0.1 mg/kg/day	16 mo	44%	"Control" growth period before therapy; bone age tended to advance faster than height age in younger patients
Danowski [40] 1967	20	Oxandrolone 10–80 mg/day	"up to 52 mo"	—[b]	No controls; wide variety of endocrine disorders studied
Geller [43] 1968	20	Oxandrolone 0.15–0.25 mg/kg/day	11 pts—6 mo 9 pts > 12 mo	—[b]	No controls; use of correction factor for calculation of HA makes results difficult to compare
Limbeck [44] 1971	28	Oxandrolone 0.25 mg/kg/day	—[b]	14%	Historical controls; ↓HA/BA in 25%
Bettman [45] 1971	27	Oxandrolone 0.05, 0.1, 0.2 mg/kg/day	6 mo	—[b]	"Control" growth period before therapy; all doses equipotent
Jackson [46] 1973	9	Oxymetholone 0.25 mg/kg/day	2–6 mo	11%	"Control" growth period before therapy; adverse effect upon younger patients

Kaplan [47] 1973	19 (21 controls)	Methyltestosterone 10–20 mg/day	4–10 mo	—[b]	Controls retrospective; therapy had no effect upon predicted height
		Fluoxymesterone 5–10 mg/day	4–6 mo		
		Testosterone Enanthate 200 mg/mo	3–4 mo		
Marti-Henneberg [48] 1975	9 (8 contols)	Oxandrolone 1 mg/kg/day	6–33 mo	—[b]	Controlled study; no significant differences between controls and treated patients; ? decrease in testicular volume in treated patients
Ruvalcaba [49] 1976	20	Oxandrolone 0.25–0.5 mg/kg/day	6 mo–2 yr	—[b]	Controlled study; Down's syndrome patients; no significant effect upon predicted height
Moore [50] 1976	130	Oxymetholone 0.25 mg/kg/day	up to 4 yr	38%	"Control" growth period before therapy

[a]Increase in height age (HA) relative to increase in bone age (BA).
[b]Information not given.

striking amelioration after withdrawal of androgens.[68,69] These hepatic effects necessitate periodic monitoring with physical examination and laboratory determinations, but they are fortunately rare. Lastly, the occurrence of priapism mandates immediate discontinuation of androgens with reinstitution at a lower dose when this symptom has disappeared.

DRUG INTERACTIONS

Several of the androgens, including testosterone, nandrolone, methandrostenolone and oxymetholone, interact with anticoagulant compounds.[70] This interaction is poorly characterized but may decrease requirements for coumarin and indandione anticoagulants.

Several anabolic steroids have been reported to increase serum levels of oxyphenbutazone, a metabolite of phenylbutazone. However, an increased incidence of untoward effects of phenylbutazone during administration of an anabolic steroid is not established.

Androgens reduce concentrations of thyroid binding globulin, a result opposite to the effect of estrogens. Low-normal serum thyroxine levels and elevated T_3 resin uptake values may occur in euthyroid patients receiving androgens.[71]

REFERENCES

1. Odell WD, Swerdloff RS: Abnormalities of gonadal function in men. Clin Endocrinol 8:149–181, 1978.
2. Anderson DC: Sex-hormone binding globulin. Clin Endocrinol 3:69–96, 1974.
3. Griffin JE, Punyashthiti K, Wilson JD: Dihydrotestosterone binding by cultured human fibroblasts: comparison of cells from control subjects and from patients with hereditary male pseudohermaphroditism due to androgen resistance. J Clin Invest 57:1342–1351, 1976.
4. Vigersky RA, Easley RB, Loriaux DL: Effect of fluoxymesterone on the pituitary-gonadal axis: the role of testosterone estradiol-binding globulin. J Clin Endocrinol Metab 43:1-9, 1976.
5. Givens JR: Hirsutism and hyperandrogenism. Adv Intern Med 21:221–248, 1976.
6. Parker L, Odell W: Control of adrenal androgen secretion by a new pituitary factor: cortical androgen stimulating hormone (CASH). Clin Res 25:299A, 1977.
7. Johnsen SG, Bennett EP, Jensen VG: Therapeutic effectiveness of oral testosterone. Lancet 2:1473–1475, 1974.
8. Nieschlag E, Cuppers HJ, Wiegelmann W, et al: Bioavailability and LH suppressing effect of different testosterone preparations in normal and hypogonadal men. Horm Res 7:138–145, 1976.
9. Asbjorn A, Vogt JH: Plasma testosterone values in different forms of testosterone treatment. Acta Endocrinol 60:537–542, 1969.
10. Krieg M, Voigt KD: Biochemical substrate of androgenic actions at a cellular level in prostate, bulbocavernosus/levator ani and in skeletal muscle. Acta Endocrinol 85:43–89, 1977.
11. Alexanian R: Erythropoietin and erythropoiesis in anemic man following androgen. Blood 33:564–572, 1969.

12. Mirand EA, Gordon AS, Wenig J: Mechanism of testosterone action in erythropoiesis. Nature 206:270–272, 1965.
13. Shaldon S, Patyna WD, Kaltwasser D, et al: The use of testosterone in bilateral nephrectomized dialysis patients. Trans Am Soc Artif Intern Organs 17:104–107, 1971.
14. Jepson J: Mechanism of action of androgens on erythropoiesis. In *Androgens in the Anemia of Bone Marrow Failure.* Palo Alto, Syntex Laboratories, 1971, pp 3–12.
15. Levere RD, Mizoguchi H: Effect of certain 5β-H steroid metabolites on hemoglobin synthesis in cultured human marrow cells. In *Androgens in the Anemia of Bone Marrow Failure.* Palo Alto, Syntex Laboratories, 1971, pp 15–27.
16. Parker JP, Beirne GJ, DeSai JN, et al: Androgen-induced increase in red cell 2,3-diphosphoglycerate. N Engl J Med 287:381–383, 1972.
17. Hendler ED, Goffinet JA, Ross S, et al: Controlled study of androgen therapy in anemia of patients on maintenance hemodialysis. N Engl J Med 291:1046–1051, 1974.
18. DeGowin RL, Lavender AR, Farland H, et al: Erythropoiesis and erythropoietin in patients with chronic renal failure treated with hemodialysis and testosterone. Ann Intern Med 72:913–918, 1970.
19. Richardson JR, Weinstein MD: Erythropoietic response of dialyzed patients to testosterone administration. Ann Intern Med 73:403–407, 1970.
20. Shaldon S, Koch KM, Opperman F, et al: Testosterone therapy for anemia in maintenance dialysis. Br Med J 3:212–215, 1971.
21. Davies M, Muckle TJ, Cassells-Smith A, et al: Oxymetholone in the treatment of anaemia in chronic renal failure. Br J Urol 44:387–394, 1972.
22. Fried W, Jonasson O, Lang G, et al: The hematologic effect of androgen in uremic patients: study of packed cell volume and erythropoietin response. Ann Intern Med 79:823–827, 1973.
23. Eschbach JW, Adamson JW: Improvement in the anemia of chronic renal failure with fluoxymesterone. Ann Intern Med 78:527–532, 1973.
24. Williams JS, Stein JH, Ferris TF: Nandrolone decanoate therapy for patients receiving hemodialysis: a controlled study. Arch Intern Med 134:289–292, 1974.
25. Branda RF, Amsden TW, Jacob HS: Randomized study of nandrolone therapy for anemias due to bone marrow failure. Arch Intern Med 137:65–69, 1977.
26. Morley A, Remes J, Trainor K: A controlled trial of androgen therapy in experimental chronic hypoplastic marrow failure. Br J Haematol 32:533–536, 1976.
27. Li FP, Alter BP, Nathan DG: The mortality of acquired aplastic anemia in children. Blood 40:153–162, 1972.
28. Lynch RE, Williams DM, Reading JC, et al: The prognosis in aplastic anemia. Blood 45:517–528, 1975.
29. Davis S, Rubin AD: Treatment and prognosis in aplastic anemia. Lancet 1:871–873, 1972.
30. Shahidi NT, Diamond LK: Testosterone-induced remission in aplastic anemia. Am J Dis Child 98:293–302, 1959.
31. Hast R, Skarberg KO, Engstedt L, et al: Oxymetholone treatment in aregenerative anemia. II. Remission and survival—a prospective study. Scand J Haematol 16:90–100, 1976.
32. McCredie KB: Oxymetholone in refractory anaemia. Br J Haematol 17:265–273, 1969.
33. Shahidi NT: Aplastic anemia in childhood and the results of androgen therapy. In *Androgens in the Anemia of Bone Marrow Failure.* Palo Alto, Syntex Laboratories, 1971, pp 33–41.
34. Shahidi NT: Androgens and erythropoiesis. N Engl J Med 289:72–80, 1973.
35. Shahidi NT: Anabolic androgenic hormone. Am J Med 62:546–548, 1977.
36. Delamore IW, Geary CG: Aplastic anaemia, acute myeloblastic leukaemia and oxymetholone. Br Med J 2:743–745, 1971.
37. Gardner FH, Nathan DG: Androgens and erythropoiesis. III. Further evaluation of testosterone treatment of myelofibrosis. N Engl J Med 274:420–426, 1966.
38. Alexanian R, Nadell J: Oxymetholone treatment for sickle cell anemia. Blood 45:769–777, 1975.
39. Rigberg SV, Brodsky I: Potential role of androgens and the anabolic steroids in the treatment of cancer: a review. J Med 6:271–290, 1975.
40. Danowski TS, Weir TF, Girdany B, et al: Oxandrolone therapy in stunting and in ovarian dysgenesis. Clin Pharmacol Ther 8:548–553, 1967.
41. Zangeneh F, Steiner MM: Oxandrolone therapy in growth retardation of children. Am J Dis Child 113:234–241, 1967.

42. Danowski TS, Lee FA, Cohn RE, et al: Oxandrolone therapy of growth retardation. Am J Dis Child 109:526–532, 1965.
43. Geller J: Oxandrolone effect on growth and bone age in idiopathic growth failure. Acta Endocrinol 59:307–316, 1968.
44. Limbeck GA, Ruvalcaba RHA, Mahoney CP, et al: Studies on anabolic steroids. IV. The effects of oxandrolone on height and skeletal maturation in uncomplicated growth retardation. Clin Pharmacol Ther 12:798–805, 1971.
45. Bettman HK, Goldman HS, Abramowicz M, et al: Oxandrolone treatment of short stature: effect on predicted mature heights. J Pediatr 79:1018–1023, 1971.
46. Jackson ST, Rallison ML, Buntin WH, et al: Use of oxandrolone for growth stimulation in children. Am J Dis Child 126:481–484, 1974.
47. Kaplan JG, Moshang T, Bernstein R, et al: Constitutional delay of growth and development: effects of treatment with androgen. J Pediatr 82:38–44, 1973.
48. Marti-Henneberg C, Niirianen AK, Rappaport R: Oxandrolone treatment of constitutional short stature in boys during adolescence: effect on linear growth, bone age, pubic hair and testicular development. J Pediatr 86:783–788, 1975.
49. Ruvalcaba RHA, Limbeck GA, Tattoni DS, et al: Studies of anabolic steroids. VIII. Adult statures of males with Down syndrome treated with oxandrolone during childhood. J Pediatr 88:504–505, 1976.
50. Moore DC, Tattoni DS, Limbeck GA, et al: Studies of anabolic steroids. V. Effect of prolonged oxandrolone administration on growth in children and adolescents with uncomplicated short stature. Pediatrics 58:412–422, 1976.
51. Zachmann M, Prader A: Anabolic and androgenic effect of testosterone in sexually immature boys and its dependency on growth hormone. J Clin Endocrinol Metab 30:85–95, 1970.
52. MacGillivray MH, Kolotin M, Munschaver RW: Enhanced linear growth responses in hypopituitary dwarfs treated with growth hormone plus androgen versus growth hormone alone. Pediatr Res 8:103–108, 1974.
53. Aynsley-Green A, Zachmann M, Prader A: Interrelation of the therapeutic effects of growth hormone and testosterone on growth in hypopituitarism. J Pediatr 89:992–999, 1976.
54. Tanner JM, Whitehouse RH, Hughes PCR, et al: Relative importance of growth hormone and sex steroids for the growth at puberty of trunk length, limb length, and muscle width in growth hormone-deficient children. J Pediatr 89:1000–1008, 1976.
55. Heller CG, Nelson WO, Hill IB, et al: Improvement in spermatogenesis following depression of the human testis with testosterone. Fertil Steril 1:415–422, 1950.
56. Rowley MJ, Heller CG: The testosterone rebound phenomenon in the treatment of male infertility. Fertil Steril 23:498–504, 1972.
57. MacLeod J, Gold R: The male factor in infertility. J Urol 66:436–456, 1951.
58. Katayama KP, Manuel M, Jones HW, et al: Methyltestosterone treatment of infertility associated with pelvic endometriosis. Fertil Steril 27:83–86, 1976.
59. Spalding DW: Methyltestosterone therapy for hereditary episodic edema (hereditary angioneurotic edema). Ann Intern Med 53:739–745, 1960.
60. Davis PJ, Davis FB, Charache P: Long-term therapy of hereditary angioedema (HAE): preventive management with fluoxymesterone and oxymetholone in severely affected males and females. Johns Hopkins Med J 135:391–398, 1974.
61. Rosse WF, Logue GL, Silberman HR: The effect of synthetic androgens on the clinical course and C′1 esterase inhibitor (C′1 INH) levels in hereditary angioneurotic edema (HANE). Clin Res 24:482A, 1976.
62. Gelfand JA, Sherins RJ, Alling DW, et al: Treatment of hereditary angioedema with danazol. N Engl J Med 295:1444–1448, 1976.
63. American Medical Association Council on Drugs: Androgens and estrogens in the treatment of disseminated mammary carcinoma. JAMA 172:1271–1283, 1960.
64. Legha SS, David HL, Maggia FM: Hormonal therapy of breast cancer: new approaches and concepts. Ann Intern Med 88:69–77, 1978.
65. Zava DT, McGuire WL: Pharmacologic effects of androgens in human breast cancer cells are mediated by estrogen receptor (Abstract 247). Chicago, 59th Annual Meeting Endocrine Society, 1977.
66. Foss GL, Simpson SL: Oral methyltestosterone and jaundice. Br Med J 1:259–263, 1959.

67. Bagheri SA, Boyer JL: Peliosis hepatis associated with androgen-anabolic steroid therapy. Ann Intern Med 81:610–618, 1974.
68. Bernstein MS, Hunter RL, Yachnin S: Hepatoma and peliosis hepatis developing in a patient with Fanconi's anemia. N Engl J Med 284:1135–1136, 1971.
69. Farrell GC, Uren RF, Perkins KW, et al: Androgen-induced hepatoma. Lancet 1:430–431, 1975.
70. *Evaluation of Drug Interactions,* second edition. Washington, American Pharmaceutical Association, 1976, pp 289–291.
71. Barbosa J, Seak AS, Doe RP: Effects of anabolic steroids on haptoglobin, plasminogen, fibrinogen, transferrin, ceruloplasmin, antitrypsin, β-glucuronidase, and total serum proteins. J Clin Endocrinol Metab 33:388–398, 1971.

51. ESTROGENS, PROGESTINS, AND OVULATORY AGENTS

Charles Y. Kawada and Martin Farber

ESTROGENS

Estrogens vary in chemical structure and milligram potency but are similar in biologic effect. Many estrogenic preparations are steroids similar to the natural hormones—17-beta estradiol, estrone, and estriol. Conjugation or slight alterations of the estrane nucleus protects them from degradation in the gastrointestinal tract and renders them active when given by mouth. A second group of estrogens, including diethylstilbestrol, chlorotrianisene, and dienestrol, are non-steroidal, synthetic substances.

Estrogens influence the female reproductive system as well as other organ systems. They cause endometrial proliferation, an increase in myometrial tone, an increase in the quantity of cervical mucous to render it more penetrable to sperm, and cornification of the vaginal mucosa. Estrogens regulate pituitary gonadotropin secretion by a feedback mechanism. Stimulation of epithelial growth of breast tissue is estrogen-mediated. Other effects include acceleration of epiphyseal closure, sodium retention, impaired carbohydrate metabolism, and a positive calcium balance.

Therapeutic Uses

Estrogens are most extensively used in combination with progestins in oral contraceptives (see Chapter 57). They are commonly administered alone for the amelioration of menopausal vasomotor symptoms (hot flashes, etc.); six million women-years of estrogens are prescribed annually in the United States.[1] Atrophic vaginitis may be treated with systemic estrogens although the topical application of an estrogen cream suffices in most cases.

Estrogens have been advocated for the treatment of several other menopausal phenomena. Their usefulness for the prevention of osteoporosis is still very controversial, although recent data have added credence to the value of estrogens in this context.[2,3] Current data suggest that estrogens should not be administered for prevention of atherosclerotic heart disease.[4] In fact, estrogens may actually increase the risk of atherosclerotic heart disease, but this point is still controversial.[5,6] There is little evidence that estrogens are useful for menopausal depression or decreased libido.

Estrogens are also indicated for women with primary amenorrhea and gonadal dysgenesis (Turner's syndrome). Estrogen therapy will cause normal development of secondary sexual characteristics and menses in patients with otherwise complete lack of ovarian function.

Estrogens may be used to symptomatically treat dysfunctional uterine bleeding, although progestins are preferred in most cases. Intravenous estrogens may control acute uterine hemorrhage faster than progestins when no anatomic uterine pathology exists. In the treatment of endometriosis, estrogens are frequently used in combination with progestins because estrogens help to maintain the endometrial lining for long periods of time. Estrogens are also effective in the treatment of dysmenorrhea, presumably by suppressing ovulation. However, estrogen-progestin combinations in the form of oral contraceptives are usually used for this purpose. Postpartum breast engorgement and lactation can sometimes be suppressed by estrogens.

Diethylstilbestrol has been approved as a postcoital contraceptive.[7] Other estrogens are indicated in the treatment of disseminated prostatic carcinoma (see Chapter 19).

Adverse Effects

Potential adverse side effects include deep venous thrombophlebitis, pulmonary embolus, cerebral thrombosis,[8] myocardial infarction,[5] adenomatous hyperplasia of the endometrium, and endometrial adenocarcinoma.[9,10] Vaginal adenocarcinoma in female offsprings is strongly associated with the maternal ingestion of diethylstilbestrol in the first trimester of pregnancy.[11] The association of estrogens and breast cancer is controversial.

The most frequent initial side effects of estrogen ingestion are nausea and vomiting; they disappear with continued treatment. Other gastrointestinal effects include abdominal pain, diarrhea, and anorexia. Headaches, breast enlargement and tenderness, breakthrough bleeding, and fluid retention are relatively common. Hypertension, impaired carbohydrate metabolism, impaired liver function, and premature epiphyseal closure are potentially more serious. A definite correlation has been shown between estrogen therapy and gallbladder disease.[12] In addition, benign liver adenomas have been correlated with estrogen-progestin use.[13] Congenital abnormalities including cardiovascular defects and limb-reduction defects have been reported in offsprings of those mothers who ingested estrogen-progestin combination drugs during the first trimester of pregnancy.[14,15]

Drug Interactions

Most reports of interactions are based on observations of combination oral contraceptives, making it difficult to determine which component is responsible for the effect. Estrogens increase thyroid-binding globulin, thereby increasing protein-bound iodine, decreasing free thyroxine, and decreasing triiodothyronine uptake. Theoretically, patients with no endogenous thyroid hormone production may require an increase in exogenous thyroid when taking estrogens.[16,17]

Estrogens appear to inhibit oral anticoagulant activity, possibly due to an increase in serum levels of vitamin K-dependent clotting factors.[18] Other interactions include potentiation of tricyclic antidepressant activity[19] and reduction of both pyridoxine and folic acid levels.[20,21] Phenobarbital increases the metabolism of estrogens and thereby may increase estrogen requirements for therapeutic effectiveness.

DRUG MONOGRAPHS

CONJUGATED ESTROGENS AND OTHER ESTRONES

CONJUGATED ESTROGENS (Premarin)
ESTERIFIED ESTROGENS (Menest)
ESTRONE PIPERAZINE SULFATE (Ogen)

Conjugated estrogens are principally a mixture of sodium estrone sulfate and sodium equilin sulfate obtained from the urine of pregnant mares. The vaginal cream is used as local therapy for atrophic vaginitis. The parenteral form has been used to stop dysfunctional uterine bleeding when rapid onset of effects is desired. Esterified estrogens are a combination of sodium salts of estrone and are also obtained from the urine of pregnant mares.

Estrone piperazine sulfate is estrone conjugated with sulfate and stabilized with piperazine for oral use. This form of estrogen has no advantage over conjugated or esterified estrogens, except that it is tasteless and has no urine odor.

Adverse Reactions—The association between estrogens and the development of endometrial carcinoma has implicated primarily conjugated estrogens.[9] Patients with endometrial carcinoma have increased levels of circulating estrone, suggesting (but not proving) a causal relationship.[22] For other adverse reactions and interactions, see the introductory section on estrogens.

Dosage for Estrogen Deficiency States—Oral: Conjugated estrogens: 0.625 to 2.5 mg daily 3 weeks of the month. Esterified estrogens: 0.3 to 1.25 mg daily for 3 weeks of the month. Estrone piperazine sulfate: 0.625 to 2.5 mg daily for 3 weeks of the month.

Dosage for Atrophic Vaginitis—Topical: Conjugated estrogen cream: one application of vaginal cream daily for the first week, then twice weekly thereafter.

Dosage for Dysfunctional Uterine Bleeding—Intravenous: When rapid cessation of bleeding is necessary, conjugated estrogens (25 mg) are administered and repeated every 6 to 12 hours until the bleeding stops.

ESTRADIOL

ETHINYL ESTRADIOL (Estinyl, Feminone)
MICRONIZED ESTRADIOL (Estrace)
ESTRADIOL CYPIONATE (Depo-Estradiol)
ESTRADIOL VALERATE (Delestrogen)

17-beta estradiol is the most potent of the naturally-occurring estrogens. The ethinyl component of ethinyl estradiol makes it about twenty times more active than the naturally-occurring compound. A micronized form of estradiol is also available for oral administration. These orally active preparations are used mainly for estrogen deficiency states. There is no specific advantage of these oral medications over conjugated estrogens except that parenteral prep-

TABLE 1 Preparations and Costs of Estrogens, Progestins, and Ovulatory Agents

GENERIC NAME	TRADEMARK NAME(S)	PREPARATIONS AND 1978 COSTS
Estrogens		
Conjugated Estrogens	Premarin	Tablets 0.3 mg—$3.30/100; 0.625 mg—$4.78/100; 1.25 mg—$7.46/100; 2.5 mg—$13.55/100 Injection (powder) 25 mg—$4.04/vial with 5-ml diluent Vaginal cream 0.625 mg/g—$4.00/42.5-g tube
Esterified Estrogens	Menest (Amnestrogen) (Evex) (SK-Estrogen)	Tablets 0.3 mg—$2.65/100; 0.625 mg—$4.23/100; 1.25 mg—$7.19/100; 2.5 mg—$6.63/50
Estrone Piperazine Sulfate	Ogen	Tablets 0.75 mg—$4.65/100; 1.5 mg—$7.33/100; 3 mg—$9.95/100/ 6 mg—$16.15/100
Ethinyl Estradiol	Estinyl (Feminone)	Tablets 0.02 mg—$3.16/100; 0.05 mg—$5.34/100; 0.5 mg—$10.82/100
Estradiol, micronized	Estrace	Tablets 1 mg—$4.39/100; 2 mg—$7.26/100
Estradiol Cypionate	Depo-Estradiol Cypionate (E-Ionate P.A.)	Injection (solution in cotton-seed oil) 1 mg/ml—$3.79/10-ml vial; 5 mg/ml—$5.93/5-ml vial
Estradiol Valerate	Delestrogen (Duratrad) (Estra-L)	Injection (solution in sesame oil) 10 mg/ml—$5.44/5-ml vial; (solution in castor oil) 20 mg/ml—$2.87/1-ml ampul, $7.78/5-ml vial; 40 mg/ml—$13.67/5-ml vial
Estradiol Valerate and Testosterone Enanthate	Deladumone OB	Injection (solution in sesame oil) estradiol valerate 8 mg and testosterone enanthate 180 mg/ml—$5.17/2-ml vial
Diethylstilbestrol	generic	Tablets 0.25 mg—$1.05/100; 0.5 mg—$0.60–$1.60/100; 1 mg—$0.50–$3.19/100; 5 mg—$0.53—3.63/100

Dienestrol	DV	Vaginal cream 0.01%—$4.20/ 3 oz tube
Chlorotrianisene	TACE	Capsules 12 mg—$9.10/100; 25 mg—$10.50/60; 72 mg—$31.20/48
Progestins		
Progesterone	Proluton (Lipo-Lutin) generic	Injection (solution in castor oil) 50 mg/ml—$9.04/10-ml vial Injection (solution in oil) 50 mg/ ml—$1.00–$9.71/10-ml vial
Hydroxyprogesterone Caproate	Delalutin	Injection (solution in castor oil) 125 mg/ml—$3.90/2-ml ampul, $12.92/10-ml vial; 250 mg/ml—$11.74/5-ml vial
Medroxyprogesterone Acetate	Provera	Tablets 2.5 mg—$3.58/25; 10 mg—$6.03/25
	Depo-Provera	Injection (aqueous suspension) 100 mg/ml—$15.06/5-ml vial; 400 mg/ml—$11.84/1-ml ampul, $26.00/2.5-ml vial, $98.71/10-ml vial
Danazol	Danocrine	Capsules 200 mg—$96.00/100
Norethindrone	Norlutin	Tablets 5 mg—$7.45/50
Norethindrone Acetate	Norlutate	Tablets 5 mg—$8.19/30
Norethynodrel and Mestranol	Enovid 5 mg	Tablets (norethynodrel 5 mg and mestranol 0.075 mg)—$16.60/100
Ovulatory Agents		
Clomiphene Citrate	Clomid	Tablets 50 mg—$41.25/30
Human Menopausal Gonadotropin (Menotropins)	Pergonal	Injection (powder containing 75 IU of FSH activity and 75 IU of LH activity)—$12.00/vial
Human Chorionic Gonadotropin	Antuitrin-S (A.P.L.) (Follutein)	Injection (powder) 5,000 USP units—$10.65/vial

arations of estradiol derivatives are longer-acting than conjugated estrogens. However, the frequent irregular vaginal bleeding subsequent to their use makes the parenteral preparations difficult to administer successfully. Estradiol valerate with testosterone is commonly used for the prevention of postpartum breast engorgement. This is given as a single parenteral injection at the time of delivery.

Adverse Reactions—Because of the association of estrone with endometrial carcinoma, the use of non-estrone estrogens has been advocated. However, estradiol is largely converted to estrone in vivo.[23]

See the general statement on estrogens for other adverse reactions and interactions.

Dosage for Estrogen Deficiency States—Oral: Ethinyl estradiol: 0.02 to 0.05 mg daily for 3 weeks of the month. Micronized estradiol: 1 to 2 mg daily for 3 weeks of the month.

Intravenous: Estradiol cypionate: 1 to 5 mg weekly. Estradiol valerate: 5 to 40 mg every 2 to 4 weeks.

DIETHYLSTILBESTROL

Diethylstilbestrol (DES) is a non-steroidal stilbene derivative with estrogenic activity similar to steroidal estrogens. It is available for oral or parenteral administration but generally is not used parenterally because other longer-acting parenteral injections are available. DES is used for the treatment of estrogen deficiency states and is much less expensive than conjugated estrogens. It is also used for postcoital contraception and is efficacious if therapy is commenced within 72 hours of unprotected intercourse. Another use is in the treatment of postpartum breast engorgement.

Adverse Reactions—Maternal ingestion of DES during pregnancy is associated with the development of vaginal or cervical adenosis or adenocarcinoma in female offsprings.[24] Therefore, if DES is used as a postcoital contraceptive and pregnancy ensues, termination of the pregnancy must be contemplated.

In doses used for replacement therapy, minimal gastrointestinal symptoms occur, but in the high doses used for postcoital contraception nausea and vomiting are frequent.

For further information about adverse effects and interactions, see the general statement on estrogens.

Dosage for Estrogen Deficiency States—Oral: 0.1 to 0.5 mg daily for 3 weeks of the month.

Dosage for Postcoital Contraception—Oral: 25 mg two times a day for 5 days. Therapy must begin within 72 hours of unprotected intercourse.

Dosage for Postpartum Breast Engorgement—Oral: 5 mg twice a day for three days.

DIENESTROL (DV)

Dienestrol, like stilbestrol, is a non-steroidal estrogen derived from stilbene. It may be administered orally or applied topically. Its use orally has no advantages over other oral estrogens, and no oral preparations are marketed. Dienestrol is primarily used as an intravaginal cream for atrophic vaginitis or prepubertal vulvovaginitis.

Adverse Reactions—Significant absorption of dienestrol from the vaginal mucosa occurs; therefore systemic side effects are possible. The same precautions and contraindications exist as for systemic therapy. For further information on adverse effects and interactions, see the general statement on estrogens.

Dosage—Topical: Apply once daily for 1 or 2 weeks, then once or twice weekly.

CHLOROTRIANISENE (Tace)

Chlorotrianisene is a non-steroidal estrogen derived from diethylstilbestrol. Its main use is for the prevention of postpartum breast engorgement. It is most effective when given immediately after delivery, but even then it is not uniformly effective.

Adverse Reactions—See the general statement on estrogens.

Dosage—Oral: 72 mg twice a day for 2 days. The first dose should be given as close to delivery as possible.

PROGESTINS

Progestins simulate the effects of progesterone. Most were developed because of the need for an orally-active progesterone derivative. They fall into two general categories—those derived from progesterone and those derived from 19-nortestosterone. In addition to progestational effects, many of the 19-nortestosterone derivatives have androgenic and estrogenic activity.

Progestins induce a secretory endometrium, diminish cornification of the vaginal epithelium, relax uterine smooth muscle, and decrease the volume of cervical mucous. Some of their extragenital effects include stimulation of alveolar tissue growth in the breast and the induction of a hypothalamically-mediated rise in the basal body temperature. Thus, progestins can counteract the effects of estrogens.

Clinical Use

Progestins are most widely used in oral contraceptives in combination with estrogens. Occasionally, they are given alone for contraception (see Chapter 52). The injectable form of medroxyprogesterone acetate is an effective contraceptive, although it has not received Food and Drug Administration approval for this use.[25]

Progestins also are widely used to treat dysfunctional uterine bleeding when no anatomic uterine lesion exists. Estrogens and progestins, alone or in combination, are effective.

Progestins are also used to treat endometriosis. Because of breakthrough bleeding when progestins are used alone for long-term therapy, estrogen-progestin combinations are often preferred. Danazol, a derivative of the progestin ethisterone, has recently become available for treatment of endometriosis.

Progestins can be used to test for adequate levels of endogenous estrogens. In patients with amenorrhea, an indication of endogenous estrogen production, presumably of ovarian origin, is obtained by eliciting uterine withdrawal bleeding subsequent to progestin administration. If no withdrawal bleeding occurs, this suggests inadequate ovarian function. The progestin withdrawal test can be used to test for pregnancy. Because of the possible androgenic and teratogenic effects of progestins, this test is not recommended.[14,15,26]

Decreased spontaneous and threatened abortion rates have been reported with the use of progestins, although these indications are still very controversial. Progestins also may be useful in the prevention of premature labor.[27]

Other possible uses for progestins include the treatment of premenstrual tension, dysmenorrhea, and mastodynia, but these uses have not been well substantiated. High doses of injectable progestins are used for palliation of metastatic endometrial and breast carcinoma (see Chapter 19). Furthermore, adenomatous hyperplasia of the endometrium, a premalignant lesion, may be successfully treated with long-term progestins when surgery is not advised.[28]

Adverse Reactions

Therapeutic doses of progestins generally produce minimal side effects. Nausea, edema, and irregular vaginal bleeding are the most common. With prolonged use of high doses, weight gain, decreased libido, depression, jaundice, and congestive heart failure have been reported. Certain androgenic progestins may produce masculinization of the female fetus if used during pregnancy.[26]

Most serious side effects of oral contraceptives have been attributed to the estrogenic component, but there are some progestin-related effects. Progestins may affect clotting parameters, although the estrogenic component appears to be more closely implicated. There is also evidence that progestins are diabetogenic.[29] Congenital abnormalities have been reported with estrogen-progestin use in the first trimester of pregnancy.[30,31]

Interactions

No drug interactions have been conclusively attributed to progestins alone.

DRUG MONOGRAPHS

COMPOUNDS DERIVED FROM PROGESTERONE

PROGESTERONE (Lipo-Lutin, Proluton)
HYDROXYPROGESTERONE CAPROATE (Delalutin)
MEDROXYPROGESTERONE ACETATE (Depo-Provera, Provera)
DANAZOL (Danocrine)

These compounds all are either natural progesterone or derived from progesterone, and have only progestational effects. They differ in duration of action.

Progesterone itself can be given only parenterally since it is degraded within the gastrointestinal tract. It is relatively short-acting and requires repeated doses, ie, at least every other day. Progesterone is used mainly to control dysfunctional uterine bleeding and as a test for ovarian function.

Hydroxyprogesterone caproate is an esterified derivative of progesterone and can be administered only parenterally. Its main advantage is a long duration of action (about two weeks). This compound is used mainly to control dysfunctional uterine bleeding, and also for threatened and habitual abortions and premature labor. The use of a progestin for habitual abortions and premature labor is still very controversial.

Medroxyprogesterone acetate is a synthetic derivative of progesterone which can be given either orally or intramuscularly. The oral form is most commonly used as therapy for dysfunctional uterine bleeding and also as a test for ovarian function. The parenteral form of medroxyprogesterone acetate has a duration of action of about one week for every 50 mg given. It has been successfully used for the treatment of endometriosis and of adenomatous hyperplasia of the endometrium. Its use as an injectable contraceptive is not yet Food and Drug Administration approved.[25]

Danazol, a derivative of ethisterone, the first orally active progestin, is classified as a progestin because of its use in the treatment of endometriosis. Danazol is a potent inhibitor of gonadotropin secretion and has mainly androgenic side effects with very little progestational activity. It is indicated for those who do not respond to or cannot tolerate other medications specific for endometriosis.

Adverse Reactions—The most common effects are nausea, edema, and irregular vaginal bleeding. Other reported effects include weight gain, decreased libido, depression, jaundice, and congestive heart failure. With progesterone derivatives, no estrogenic or androgenic effects have been noted. Danazol is the sole exception; its androgenic effects include acne, hirsutism, weight gain, and decreased breast size.

Dosage for Amenorrhea and Dysfunctional Uterine Bleeding—Intramuscular: Progesterone: 100 mg with withdrawal bleeding 2 to 6 days later. Hydroxyprogesterone caproate: 125 to 250 mg with withdrawal bleeding about 2 weeks later.

Oral: Medroxyprogesterone acetate: 10 mg daily for five days with withdrawal bleeding 2 to 7 days later.

Dosage for Endometriosis—Intramuscular: Medroxyprogesterone acetate: 100 mg every 2 weeks for four doses, then 100 mg every 4 weeks for up to 6 months.

Oral: Danazol: 400 mg two times a day for 3 to 6 months.

Dosage for Adenomatous Hyperplasia—Intramuscular: Medroxyprogesterone acetate: 100 mg for 4 doses then 400 mg every 4 weeks for six months.

Dosage for Threatened or Habitual Abortions (not of proven efficacy)—Intramuscular: Progesterone: 25 to 50 mg daily for threatened abortions; 5 to 20 mg for habitual abortions. Hydroxyprogesterone caproate: 250 mg daily.

Oral: Medroxyprogesterone acetate: 50 mg daily if bleeding present, then 50 mg weekly for threatened abortions. For habitual abortions, 50 mg weekly.

19-NORTESTOSTERONE DERIVATIVES

NORETHINDRONE (Norlutin)
NORETHINDRONE ACETATE (Norlutate)
NORETHYNODREL WITH MESTRANOL (Enovid)

The 19-nortestosterone derivatives are available only in oral form and are the principal progestins used for contraception because of their more consistent ability to suppress gonadotropin secretion, relative to other progestins. Some of these derivatives (such as norgestrel and ethynodiol) are used exclusively for contraception (see Chapter 52). Other indications include dysfunctional uterine bleeding and endometriosis. Norethynodrel, although not a true 19-nortestosterone derivative, is available with mestranol for contraception and for the treatment of endometriosis.

Adverse Reactions—Many of the adverse reactions are similar to progesterone-derived progestins. Nausea, edema, and irregular vaginal bleeding are most commonly encountered. Other symptoms include weight gain, decreased libido, depression, and jaundice. Androgenic effects with some estrogenic symptoms, due to the metabolites of 19-nortestosterone derivatives, are occasionally encountered. Androgenic effects include hirsutism, alopecia, acne, hypomenorrhea, and occasionally complete amenorrhea. Masculinization of the female fetus has been reported when 19-nortestosterone derivatives have been used in the first trimester of pregnancy.[26]

Dosage for Dysfunctional Uterine Bleeding—Oral: Norethindrone: 5 mg daily for 20 days. Norethindrone acetate: 2.5 mg daily for 20 days. Enovid: 5 mg daily for 20 days.

This regimen may be continued for up to six months if total amenorrhea is desired.

Dosage for Endometriosis—Oral: Norethindrone: 10 mg daily for 2 weeks, then increase dose 5 mg every 2 weeks until the dose is 30 mg daily. This is continued for up to six months. Same regimen is followed for norethindrone acetate at one-half the dose. Enovid: 5 mg daily for 2 weeks, then increasing every 2 weeks up to 20 mg daily for up to six months.

OVULATORY AGENTS

In 15% of infertile couples, anovulation is the etiologic factor. Anovulatory women may be divided into two categories. The first includes those with normal plasma gonadotropin and estrogen levels who do not ovulate. The second includes those who have deficient gonadotropin levels and ovarian function so that ovulation cannot occur. Specific therapy for each category of anovulation is currently available by the administration of clomiphene citrate for the former and human menopausal gonadotropin (HMG) for the latter. In general, only specialists trained in ovulation induction should administer these drugs because of the potentially complex treatment course and the potential for major complications.

Since clomiphene citrate and HMG have different indications, they will be discussed separately. Human chorionic gonadotropin (HCG) is ineffective by itself and is used for ovulation induction only in conjunction with clomiphene citrate or HMG.

Clomiphene Citrate

Clomiphene citrate is an orally active non-steroidal estrogen antagonist structurally related to chlorotrianisene (TACE). Its mechanism of action is not clearly understood, but it appears to promote the secretion of gonadotropins by the pituitary gland. Clomiphene citrate may also have a direct effect on ovarian steroidogenesis.[32]

Clinical Use. Clomiphene citrate is used to induce ovulation in anovulatory or oligoovulatory women who desire pregnancy. Success rates are highest in those women who have adequate endogenous estrogen production, as demonstrated by withdrawal bleeding after progestin administration.[33,34]

Approach to Therapy. Treatment is generally begun on the fifth day following an induced or spontaneous menses, starting with 50 mg daily for five days. The patient is instructed to record her basal body temperature daily. A temperature rise of 0.2 to 0.6 degrees sustained for 12 to 16 days is excellent evidence for ovulation. This regimen is continued for two cycles and if ovulation is not achieved the dose may then be increased to 100 mg. Some investigators have advocated dosages as high as 200 mg daily for five days.[35] Ovulation occurs in about 70% of patients, although the conception rate is only about 30% of those who do ovulate.[36]

The use of HCG in conjunction with clomiphene has been advocated to augment a midcycle surge of luteinizing hormone in those who do not ovulate with clomiphene citrate alone.[34] 5,000 to 10,000 IU of HCG is given in one intramuscular dose on the seventh to ninth day following the last clomiphene pill when there are indications that follicular maturation is at a peak.

Human menopausal gonadotropin may be used in those women refractory to clomiphene citrate and HCG administration.

Adverse Reactions. Ovarian cyst formation is reported in as many as 20% of recipients. Usually the cysts are small, but occasionally massive enlargement with the development of ascites occurs.[37] Therefore, pelvic examinations before and during therapy should be performed and the medication discontinued if a cyst develops.

Hot flashes have been reported in about 10% of recipients, possibly due to the anti-estrogenic effect of clomiphene citrate. Other side effects include visual disturbances, abdominal discomfort, nausea, and breast discomfort. Multiple pregnancies must also be considered an adverse effect since this increases fetal wastage. The rate of multiple pregnancies with clomiphene therapy is about 8%, as compared to 1% with spontaneous ovulation.

Human Menopausal Gonadotropin

Human menopausal gonadotropin (HMG) is a purified preparation of follicle stimulating hormone (FSH) and luteinizing hormone (LH) from the urine of postmenopausal females. It is indicated for anovulatory patients with hypogonadotropic hypogonadism. Ovulation induction is not as successful in these patients compared to those who respond to clomiphene.[38] Induction of ovulation with clomiphene alone and then with clomiphene plus HCG, should first be tried even in this category of patients, since some of them will respond to clomiphene.

Clinical Use. Because of potential hazards of HMG (see below), it should be reserved for anovulatory women with adequate ovarian function. Very high levels of serum gonadotropins, especially FSH, suggest ovarian failure, excluding these women from HMG therapy.

Approach to Therapy. HMG is administered intramuscularly in increasing doses, starting with one ampul, until a satisfactory ovarian response is achieved. The estrogen response is monitored by urinary or plasma estrogen levels. The drug is continued for 9 to 12 days, and then followed by 5,000 to 10,000 IU of HCG to trigger ovulation.

Ovulation is induced in about 75% of cases, while pregnancy occurs in about 25% of those who ovulate. A 25% spontaneous abortion rate in induced cycles is no higher than that in the general population.[39]

Adverse Reactions. Most serious complications of HMG are due to ovarian hyperstimulation, leading to ovarian enlargement, abdominal distention, and weight gain. With severe hyperstimulation, the above changes plus abdominal pain, nausea and vomiting, ascites, hydrothorax, hypovolemia, hypotension, and oliguria occur secondary to accumulation of fluid in the peritoneal cavity.[40] Treatment is supportive, and removal of the stimulus is usually followed by resolution of the syndrome. Once the syndrome is diagnosed, repeated pelvic examinations are hazardous because they might cause ovarian rupture with intraperitoneal hemorrhage. HMG therapy should be monitored by repeated measurement of urinary or plasma estrogen levels,[41] and by pelvic examinations to detect ovarian enlargement prior to administration of HCG.

The incidence of multiple pregnancies following HMG induction of ovulation is 20 to 25%[39,42] and three-quarters of these are twins. The multiple pregnancy rate is directly related to the dose of HMG. Since prematurity is increased in multiple gestations and the fetal death rate increases with the rate of prematurity, the fetal death rate is increased in HMG-induced pregnancies.[43]

Other reported side effects of HMG include nausea, vomiting, diarrhea, and fever. As with clomiphene citrate, congenital malformations are not increased in frequency.

DRUG MONOGRAPHS

CLOMIPHENE CITRATE (Clomid)

Clomiphene citrate is indicated for ovulation induction in women who do not ovulate regularly but who show evidence for adequate gonadotropin secretion and ovarian estrogen production. Occasionally even those without adequate gonadotropins and estrogens will respond to clomiphene citrate solely, or with the addition of HCG.

Adverse Reactions—Ovarian cyst formation is the side effect of greatest concern, although the risk is decreased with lower doses of clomiphene. Other adverse effects include abdominal discomfort, hot flashes, nausea, and breast discomfort. The increase in multiple pregnancies can be considered an adverse effect since perinatal mortality is increased.

Interactions—Clomiphene decreases uptake of radioactive estradiol by the uterus, pituitary, and hypothalamus.[44] Therefore, clomiphene may antagonize estrogen effects and decrease the responsiveness of tissues to estrogen.

Dosage—See Approach to Therapy.

HUMAN MENOPAUSAL GONADOTROPIN (Pergonal)

Induction of ovulation with human menopausal gonadotropin (HMG) is reserved for those who do not respond to clomiphene even with the addition of HCG. These patients generally are both hypogonadotropic and hypoestrogenic, but have ovaries capable of responding to gonadotropin stimulation. Only about 4% of patients requiring induction of ovulation will require HMG.[45] Since HMG is a combination of FSH and LH, this medication simulates the endogenous gonadotropin secretion necessary for follicular development and maturation. HCG is used sequentially with HMG to simulate the midcycle surge of luteinizing hormone necessary for ovulation.

Adverse Reactions—The most serious hazard is the hyperstimulation syndrome which includes ovarian enlargement, abdominal pain, ascites, and hydrothorax. The other major problem is the 20 to 25% rate of multiple pregnancies with the associated increased fetal death rate. Other reported reactions include nausea and vomiting, diarrhea, and fever.

Interactions—The actions of clomiphene citrate and HMG appear to be synergistic.[46] Estrogens and progestins decrease the effectiveness of HMG.[47,48] Also, suppressive doses of dexamethasone decrease the ovarian response to HMG.[49]

Dosage—Intravenous: One vial of HMG contains 75 IU of FSH and 75 IU of LH. See Approach to Therapy for the actual dosage schedule.

HUMAN CHORIONIC GONADOTROPIN (Antuitrin-S, A.P.L., Follutein)

HCG is a purified preparation of chorionic gonadotropin extracted from the urine of pregnant females. It is capable of simulating the surge of luteinizing hormone at midcycle, thereby inducing ovulation. In the male, it can stimulate androgen production by the Leydig cells of the testes. HCG is therefore used in sequence with HMG or clomiphene for the induction of ovulation. It is also indicated in the treatment of cryptorchidism and male hypogonadism secondary to pituitary failure.

Adverse Reactions—HCG can produce the ovarian hyperstimulation syndrome when used sequentially with HMG. Other side effects include fluid retention, headaches, and depression. In prepubertal males sexual precocity may occur. It is contraindicated in those with known prostatic carcinoma.

Dosage—Intramuscular: 10,000 USP units at midcycle in conjunction with clomiphene citrate or HMG.

REFERENCES

1. Anon: Estrogens and endometrial cancer. FDA Drug Bull 6:18–20, (February-March) 1976.
2. Meema S, Bunker ML, Meema EH: Preventative effect of estrogen on postmenopausal bone loss. Arch Intern Med 135:1436–1440, 1975.
3. Lindsay R, Aitken JM, Anderson JB, et al: Long-term prevention of postmenopausal osteoporosis by estrogen. Lancet 1:1038–1040, 1976.
4. Coronary Drug Project Research Group: Coronary Drug Project: Initial findings leading to modification of its research protocol. JAMA 214:1303–1313, 1970.
5. Coronary Drug Project Research Group: Coronary Drug Project: Findings leading to discontinuation of the 2.5 mg/day estrogen group. JAMA 226:652–657, 1973.
6. Rosenberg L, Armstrong B, Jick H: Myocardial infarction and estrogen therapy in postmenopausal women. N Engl J Med 294:1256–1259, 1976.
7. Kuchera LK: Postcoital contraception with diethylstilbesterol. JAMA 218:562–563, 1971.
8. Inman WH, Vessey MP: Investigation of deaths from pulmonary, coronary, and cerebral thrombosis and embolism in women of childbearing age. Br Med J 2:193–199, 1968.
9. Ziel HK, Finkle WD: Increased risk of endometrial carcinoma among users of conjugated estrogens. N Engl J Med 293:1167–1170, 1975.
10. Smith DC, Prentice R, Thompson DJ, et al: Association of exogenous estrogens and endometrial carcinoma. N Engl J Med 293:1164–1167, 1975.
11. Silverberg S, Makowski EL: Endometrial carcinoma in young women taking oral contraceptive agents. Obstet Gynecol 46:503–506, 1975.
12. Boston Collaborative Drug Surveillance Program: Surgically confirmed gallbladder disease, venous thromboembolism, and breast tumors in relation to postmenopausal estrogen therapy. N Engl J Med 270:15–19, 1974.
13. Edmondson HA, Henderson R, Benton B: Liver cell adenomas associated with the use of oral contraceptives. N Engl J Med 294:470–472, 1976.
14. Janevich DT, Piper JM, Glebatis DM: Oral contraceptives and congenital limb-reduction defects. N Engl J Med 291:697–700, 1974.
15. Nora JJ, Nora AH: Birth defects and oral contraceptives. Lancet 1:941–942, 1973.
16. Irigarry S, Paniagua M, Pineus G, et al: Effect of cyclic administration of certain

progestin-estrogen combinations on the 24 hour radioiodine thyroid uptake. J Clin Endocrinol Metab 26:6–10, 1966.
17. Hamolsky MW: Thyroid factors. In *Progress in Infertility,* 2nd edition. Edited by SJ Behman, RW Kistner. Boston, Little Brown and Co., 1975, p 571.
18. Koch-Weser J, Sellers EM: Drug interactions with coumadin anticoagulants. N Engl J Med 285:547–558, 1971.
19. Khurana RC: Estrogen-imipramine interaction. JAMA 222:702–703, 1972.
20. Theuer RC: Effect of oral contraceptive agents on vitamin and mineral needs: a review. J Reprod Med 8:13–19, 1972.
21. Shojania AM, Hornady GJ, Barnes PH: Effect of oral contraceptives on folate metabolism. Am J Obstet Gynecol 111:782–791, 1971.
22. MacDonald PC, Siiteri PK: The relationship between the extraglandular production of estrone and the occurrence of endometrial neoplasia. Gynecol Oncol 2:259–263, 1974.
23. Yen SSC, Martin PL, Burnier AM, et al: Circulating estradiol, estrone, and gonadotropin levels following the administration of orally active 17-beta estradiol in postmenopausal women. J Clin Endocrinol Metab 40:518–521, 1975.
24. Herbst A, Poskanzer S, Robboy L, et al: Prenatal exposure to stilbestrol, a prospective comparison of exposed female offspring with unexposed controls. N Engl J Med 292:334–339, 1975.
25. Schwallie PC: Experience with depo-provera as an injectable contraceptive. J Reprod Med 13:113–117, 1974.
26. Wilkins L, Jones HM, Holman GH, et al: Masculinization of the female fetus associated with non-adrenal female pseudohermaphrodism. J Clin Endocrinol Metab 18:559–585, 1958.
27. Johnson J, Austin KL, Jones GS, et al: Efficacy of 17 alpha-hydroxyprogesterone caproate in the prevention of premature labor. N Engl J Med 293:675–680, 1975.
28. Wentz WB: Effect of a progestational agent on endometrial hyperplasia and endometrial cancer. Obstet Gynecol 24:370–374, 1964.
29. Beck P: Effects of gonadal hormones and contraceptive steroids on glucose and insulin metabolism. In *Metabolic Effects of Gonadal Hormones and Contraceptive Steroids.* Edited by HA Salhanick, DM Kipnis, RL VanderWiele. New York, Plenum Press, 1969, p 97.
30. Heinonen OP, Slone D, Monson RR, et al: Cardiovascular birth defects and antenatal exposure to female sex hormones. N Engl J Med 296:67–70, 1977.
31. Nora JJ, Nora AH, Perinchief AG, et al: Congenital abnormalities and first trimester exposure to progestagen-oestrogen. Lancet 1:313–314, 1976.
32. Smith OW, Smith GV, Kistner RW: Actions of MER-25 and of clomiphene on the human ovary. JAMA 184:876–878, 1963.
33. MacGregor AH, Johnson JE, Bunde CA: Further clinical experience with clomiphene citrate. Fertil Steril 19:616–622, 1971.
34. Kistner RW: Use of clomiphene citrate, human chorionic gonadotropin and human menopausal gonadotropin for induction of ovulation in the human female. Fertil Steril 17:569–583, 1966.
35. Kase N, Mroulh A, Olson LE: Clomid therapy for anovulatory infertility. Am J Obstet Gynecol 98:1037–1042, 1967.
36. Merrell—National Laboratories, Product Information Booklet, 1971.
37. Southam AL, Janovski NA: Massive ovarian hyperstimulation with clomiphene citrate. JAMA 181:443–445, 1962.
38. Tsapoulis AD, Crooke AG: Comparison of clomiphene and human gonadotropin in failure of ovulation. Lancet 2:1321–1323, 1968.
39. Thompson CR, Hansen LM: Pergonal: a summary of clinical experience in the induction of ovulation and pregnancy. Fertil Steril 21:844–853, 1970.
40. Engel T, Jewelewicz R, Dyrenfurth I, et al: Ovarian hyperstimulation syndrome: report of a case with notes on pathogenesis and treatment. Am J Obstet Gynecol 112:1052–1060, 1972.
41. Taymor MD, Yussman MA, Gminski D: Estrogen monitoring in ovulatory induction. Fertil Steril 21:759–762, 1970.
42. Marshall JR, Wider JA: Results of human menopausal gonadotropin therapy for anovulatory infertility using a nonvariable treatment schedule: comparison with previous reports. Fertil Steril 22:19–25, 1971.

43. Hack M, Brish J, Sen DM, et al: Outcome of pregnancy after induced ovulation: follow-up of pregnancies and children born after gonadotropin therapy. JAMA 211:791–797, 1970.
44. Roy S, Greenblatt RB, Mahesh VB, et al: Clomiphene citrate: further observations on its use in the induction of ovulation in the human and on its mode of action. Fertil Steril 14:575–595, 1963.
45. Rakoff AE, Plaster EL, Goldfarb AF: Comparison of various therapies for treatment of anovulation. In *Gonadotropin Therapy in Female Infertility*. Edited by E Rosemberg. Amsterdam, Excerpta Medica, 1973.
46. Crooke AC, Hansotia MD, Bertrand PV: Joint action of clomiphene citrate and human pituitary gonadotropins. Lancet 1:587–588, 1969.
47. Marshall JR, Jacobson A, Cargille CM: Effects of estrogen on FSH, LH, and ovulatory response rate to gonadotropin therapy in women with normal sellae turcicae or following hypophysectomy. In *Gonadotropin Therapy in Female Infertility*. Edited by E Rosemberg. Amsterdam, Excerpta Medica, 1973.
48. Lunenfeld B, Sulimovici S, Raban E: Preliminary report on the mechanism of action of anti-ovulatory compounds. J Endocrinol 24:32, 1962.
49. Grodin JM, Doriaux DL, Nieschlag E, et al: Functional studies of ovarian responsiveness to human menopausal gonadotropins. In *Gonadotropin Therapy in Female Infertility*. Edited by E Rosemberg. Amsterdam, Excerpta Medica, 1973, p 150.

52. ORAL CONTRACEPTIVES

Victor A. Drill

Oral contraceptives are primarily used for the prevention of pregnancy and the regulation and planning of family size. Administration of these agents from day 5 through day 24 or 25 of the menstrual cycle (ie, for 20 or 21 days of the cycle), followed by a rest period of 7 days, is almost completely effective in preventing pregnancy. When the combination oral contraceptives (containing a progestin and an estrogen) are taken correctly throughout the month without omission of a daily dose, the pregnancy rate is about 0.1 or less per 100 women per year. Under conditions of widespread clinical use, when some women forget one or more tablets during the month, the pregnancy rate is about 0.7 cases per 100 women per year. The combination oral contraceptives are much more effective in preventing pregnancy than medicated creams, douches, intrauterine devices or other mechanical procedures. The sequential oral contraceptives are less effective than the combination products, but sequentials will not be discussed in this chapter since they have been withdrawn from clinical use. The effectiveness of a progestin given alone is also less than that of the combination oral contraceptives; the pregnancy rate is about 3 cases per 100 women per year.

PHARMACOLOGIC PROPERTIES

Mechanism of Action

The progestin and estrogen combination prevents ovulation by inhibiting the secretion of hypothalamic releasing hormone (LH-FSH-RH), thereby suppressing the release of pituitary gonadotropins; they may also act directly on the pituitary gland to inhibit the release of gonadotropins.[1-3] Ovulation is thereby prevented. The suppression of follicle-stimulating hormone and luteinizing hormone is enhanced by the administration of the estrogen and progestin together, thus allowing each to be used in a lower dose. Combination oral contraceptives also increase the viscosity of cervical mucus, inhibit ferning, alter the endometrium, and may affect tubal transport. Although these secondary actions may contribute to contraceptive effectiveness, the primary mode of action is prevention of ovulation.

The mechanism of daily progestin-alone contraception is not known, although its main effect is probably to alter the properties of cervical mucus, thereby inhibiting sperm penetration. Progestin alone can also disturb hypothalamic-pituitary-ovarian function, induce endometrial changes which may prevent implantation, and inhibit ovulation in some cases.[4,5]

Reproductive Organs

The effects of oral contraceptives on the reproductive organs are consistent with their hormonal properties. The combination oral contraceptives stimulate growth of the endometrium sufficient to induce a withdrawal bleeding at the end of the treatment cycle. The mean cycle length of treated women is close to 28 days. About 1 to 3% of women do not experience withdrawal bleeding during the seven medication-free days.[1] When the dose is inadequate, spotting and bleeding may occur. The frequency of spotting and bleeding is higher when lower doses are given. Changes in menstrual patterns, such as short cycles, unpredictable bleeding, or amenorrhea, occur with higher frequency in women using the progestin-alone preparation.[6–8]

The ovarian steroids secreted during an ovulatory cycle may produce breast discomfort, soreness, or enlargement, and similar effects occur during the use of oral contraceptives. Breast symptoms are generally mild, transient, and most common during the first cycle of therapy.[1] The frequency of galactorrhea one year postpartum is not increased by contraceptive steroids.[9,10]

Fertility After Discontinuation of Oral Contraceptives

When cyclic oral contraceptive medication is stopped, spontaneous menstrual cycles return rapidly in most patients and a normal fertility rate is obtained. When contraceptive procedures other than oral contraceptives were discontinued, 62% of the women became pregnant after 3 months and 79% after 6 months.[11] Fertility rates are similar when oral contraceptives are discontinued.[1,12–15] The pregnancy rate will never reach 100%, since even among women who have not used oral contraceptives about 6% will not be pregnant after two years of attempting to conceive.[11] Furthermore, the capacity to conceive decreases with age.[16]

Although cyclic function returns promptly in most women, the first spontaneous menses may occasionally be delayed for six to ten weeks after termination of therapy.[1] The patient's prior menstrual rhythm then returns. The duration of therapy does not influence return of ovulation. Almost all women ovulate by the sixth post-treatment cycle, although some may require one year or longer before spontaneous menses occur. The incidence of post-pill amenorrhea lasting longer than 6 months is reported as 1% and 0.2%, respectively.[17,18] The exact cause of the amenorrhea is unknown. Many such women had oligomenorrhea and other menstrual problems before starting treatment, and post-pill amenorrhea may represent recurrence of the pre-pill problems. Late onset of menarche, dieting, weight loss, and psychological factors contribute significantly to the amenorrhea.[19–23] If anovulation persists for more than a year and other pathology is ruled out, therapy with clomiphene will usually induce ovulation.

Benign Breast Lesions

Fibroadenomas are the most frequent benign breast tumors found in young women and therefore occur by chance in women taking oral contraceptives. Oral contraceptives do not increase the occurrence of fibroadenomas.[24–26] Retrospective case-control studies[27–30] and a hospital survey[31]reveal no association between oral contraceptives and fibroadenoma, fibrocystic disease or other benign diseases. The contraceptive steroids may reduce the hospitalization rate for fibrocystic disease and fibroadenomas.[32]

Mammary Cancer

Breast cancer was not observed in 428 women taking a sequential contraceptive for nearly five years[33] and in a prospective clinical study mammary carcinoma occurred in control groups but not in 139 women using oral contraceptives for 8 to 13 years.[34] Other clinical studies have reported no increase in the frequency of breast cancer associated with oral contraceptives,[15,25,35] and mammography revealed no increase in pathological findings during the use of these drugs.[36] Retrospective case-control studies[27,37] and a hospital survey[31] demonstrated neither an increased nor a decreased use of oral contraceptives in women with breast cancer. A partial risk was found in one study.[27]

Cervical Cancer

Oral contraceptives produce histological changes in the cervix similar to those seen during pregnancy.[38,39] Endocervical glandular hyperplasia (adenomatous hyperplasia), although benign, may be sufficiently atypical to be confused with early adenocarcinoma.[24] Many studies reveal no effect of oral contraceptives on the occurrence of abnormal Papanicolaou smears, cervical dysplasia, cervical cancer in situ, or invasive cancer.[26,34,40,41]

Endometrial Cancer

An association between endometrial cancer and estrogen use by menopausal and post-menopausal women has been reported.[42–44] Cases of adenocarcinoma of the endometrium have also been observed in users of oral contraceptives, primarily in women using the sequential preparation of dimethisterone and ethinyl estradiol.[45–49]

Thyroid Gland

Oral contraceptives do not affect thyroid function, but their estrogenic component increases serum concentrations of thyroxin-binding globulin, thus altering tests of thyroid-function which depend on protein binding. Protein-bound iodine (PBI) and butanol-extractable iodine (BEI) levels are elevated and the T_3 (triiodothyronine) uptake is decreased. The basal metabolic rate (BMR), cholesterol levels, ^{131}I uptake, and free thyroxin index (FTI) remain unchanged. Values of thyroid function tests return to pretreatment levels within two months after discontinuing therapy.[1,50,51]

Adrenal Gland

Pregnancy, estrogens, or the combination oral contraceptives increase plasma corticosteroid-binding globulin (transcortin) and thereby total plasma cortisol, but the amount of free or unbound cortisol is not changed.[52–54] Estrogens and oral contraceptives also decrease the response to metyrapone, but the response to bacterial pyrogen or ACTH is normal.[52,55,56]

Lactation

The 5- or 10-mg doses of oral contraceptives studied in the early 1960's inhibited lactation in many women.[1] The new combined oral contraceptives have no effect or a slight inhibitory effect on lactation, depending on parity, previous nursing history, and the indices used to evaluate lactation.[57] If the infant is allowed to nurse, oral contraceptives do not suppress the establishment of lactation.[58] Maintenance of lactation is lessened in some women, but several placebo-controlled studies show little or no effect of the estrogen-progestin combinations on lactation.[59,60] Progestins alone do not appear to affect lactation.[57] Following administration of labeled estrogens and progestins, small amounts of radioactivity can be detected in the milk of nursing mothers.[57]

Psychological Effects

Patients with a history of anxiety reactions may complain of irritability, tension, or depression during use of an oral contraceptive. Various factors may account for depression developing during oral contraceptive use,[61–63] and it is unlikely on a pharmacological basis that these steroids cause psychiatric symptoms.[63] Disturbance of tryptophan and pyridoxine metabolism, as well as favorable response to pyridoxine treatment of depression have been reported.[64]

Migraine

Migraine occurs in 5 to 10% of the population, and the relation of migraine headaches to oral contraceptive use is not established. These agents have been associated with intensification of migraine in some patients, have no effect in others, and possibly improve migraine in some individuals. It is reasonable that oral contraceptives be discontinued if migraine attacks begin concomitant with their use or show a marked increase in intensity or frequency during treatment.[65–67]

Ophthalmological Effects

Comparison with controls demonstrate that oral contraceptives do not affect the frequency of common ophthalmologic abnormalities.[68–70] Cases of optic neuropathy, retinal vascular occlusions, retinal vasculitis (Eales' disease), retinal edema, and pseudotumor cerebri have been observed in association with the use of oral contraceptives. Oral contraceptives should be discontinued if such neuro-ophthalmic disorders occur.

Blood Pressure

Cases of hypertension have been associated with the use of oral contraceptives, and various studies have evaluated the relationship of the contraceptives to blood pressure.[71–75] Some reports describe only slight changes in blood pressure, without development of hypertension. In other studies elevations of blood pressure above 150/90 have been recorded. Discontinuance of medication may be associated with a return of normal blood pressure. Comparison of oral contraceptives with a placebo has not shown a difference in blood pressure response,[76] and the administration of oral contraceptives to groups of women with hypertension did not increase blood pressure.[77] Combination oral contraceptives may increase plasma renin activity, renin substrate and blood angiotension II; a three-fold increase in angiotensin II elevated blood pressure an average of only 3.4 mm systolic and 1.5 diastolic.[78]

Carbohydrate and Lipid Metabolism

The estrogen-progestin contraceptives may retard glucose utilization and produce a compensatory increase in secretion of insulin.[79–81] The estrogen component is probably responsible for changes in glucose tolerance, but progestins may also affect carbohydrate metabolism. A peripheral anti-insulin effect of growth hormone may be involved, since the combination contraceptives increase the secretion of pituitary growth hormone.[82] Patients who are diabetic during pregnancy but not otherwise seem more vulnerable to developing an abnormal glucose tolerance. Other forms of contraception may be considered for these women. Adverse effects usually are not observed in controlled diabetic patients; however, the status of diabetics using oral contraceptives should be reviewed periodically.[83,84] Estrogens and oral contraceptives may increase the fasting serum triglyceride concentration, due primarily to the increased hepatic production of triglycerides.[85] In some women hypertriglyceridemia may be quite marked.

DRUG INTERACTIONS

Drugs that are potent inducers of hepatic microsomal enzymes may affect the metabolism of oral contraceptives and lessen their effectiveness. Breakthrough bleeding and pregnancy have been noted particularly in women using rifampin and oral contraceptives.[86] Cases of menstrual abnormalities and pregnancy have been reported in women taking oral contraceptives concurrently with barbiturates, anticonvulsants, or ampicillin.[87] Such interactions are more likely to be important with low estrogen preparations, and the occurrence of spotting or breakthrough bleeding in such situations may necessitate a higher dose of estrogen. Oral contraceptives may inhibit the hypoprothrombinemic action of the coumarin anticoagulants.[88]

ADVERSE REACTIONS AND TOXICITY

Various side effects and toxic reactions have been associated with the use of oral contraceptives, but in many cases cause-and-effect relationships have not been established. Subjective complaints in women using an intrauterine device and in those taking an oral contraceptive are similar in frequency.[89] Placebo responses may also be expected, and patients given a placebo oral contraceptive reported many side effects commonly associated with anovulant medication.[90] In double-blind, placebo-controlled studies, the incidence of side effects in the placebo group accounted for many symptoms present in the contraceptive treated groups.[76,91]

Approximately 10 million women in the United States presently take an oral contraceptive, and one may therefore expect chance associations with many diseases. However, physicians should be aware of the adverse effects and risks attributed to oral contraceptives, and consider these when planning an individual contraceptive program.

Miscellaneous Systemic Complaints

Nausea may occur in some women during the first and perhaps second and third cycles of treatment, and vomiting has been reported.[76,89,90] Symptoms such as abdominal fullness, pain, diarrhea, constipation, increase or decrease in appetite, increase or decrease in libido, malaise, tiredness, and insomnia, all have been associated with contraceptive use, but causal relationships are generally not established.

Hemopoietic System

Cases of megaloblastic anemia have been reported in users of oral contraceptives. Studies reporting a decreased absorption of dietary folate have not been confirmed.[92,93] Oral contraceptives have been observed to increase the plasma clearance of folic acid or urinary secretion of folates.[92,94] Most clinical studies have found normal red blood indices and normal serum folate levels during the use of oral contraceptive steroids,[92,94,95] and it is probable that the oral contraceptives do not cause folate deficiency anemia in the otherwise normal individual.[96,97]

Liver

A reversible sulfobromphthalein (BSP) retention of moderate degree, similar to that seen during pregnancy or after the administration of estrogens, may occur during use of oral contraceptives.[1] The retention is due to decreased transfer of BSP from liver cells to the bile, and tests which measure parenchymal cell functions are usually not altered. The administration of oral contraceptives to a small group of women with chronic liver disease did not alter liver function tests.[98] Liver function tests remained normal when oral contraceptives were given during the convalescent period of viral hepatitis,[99] and use of these compounds during acute viral hepatitis did not affect the severity of the acute illness or the frequency of sequelae.[100]

Patients with inherited defects of hepatic excretory function, such as familial recurrent jaundice or Dubin-Johnson syndrome, may experience a further reduction in hepatic excretory function and the occurrence of jaundice when oral contraceptives are given.[101,102] Also, women with a history of benign cholestatic jaundice of pregnancy (idiopathic or recurrent jaundice of pregnancy) or nulliparous women with a genetic disposition to the disease may develop cholestatic jaundice when given oral contraceptives. When the contraceptives are discontinued the pruritis and jaundice disappear, and the liver function tests return to normal without any residual effect on the liver.[103]

Hepatic adenomas and other benign hepatocellular tumors are relatively uncommon, but occur most frequently in women of childbearing age.[104] Cases of hepatic adenoma or focal nodular hyperplasia have been reported in association with the use of oral contraceptives.[105–107] Peliosis may accompany the adenoma or may be present independently. Rupture of the tumor may be a life-threatening complication.[105–107]

Gallbladder

An association between the occurrence of gallbladder disease and the use of estrogen in postmenopausal women or the use of oral contraceptives in women age 20 to 44 has been reported.[31,108] Administration of oral contraceptives increased cholesterol saturation and the percent of cholic acid in bile and decreased the proportion of chenodeoxycholic acid and lithocholic acid in bile.[109]

Thromboembolic Disease

Case-control retrospective epidemiologic studies[110–112] and a hospital survey[31] have reported an association between the use of oral contraceptives and the occurrence of peripheral venous thrombophlebitis and pulmonary embolism. In Great Britain,[110,111] the risk of morbidity and mortality was estimated to be increased about 6 to 8 times that of a pill nonuser. A retrospective case-control study in the United States[112] estimated that the risk of hospitalization for deep vein idiopathic thromboembolic disease was increased 4.4 times in women using oral contraceptives. Most prospective studies, however, have not shown that the use of oral contraceptives increases the incidence of disease.[15,113–116] Other relevant data demonstrate that the incidence of venous thrombosis is not increased during pregnancy when estrogen secretion is markedly increased.[113]

A retrospective case-control study[117,118] reported an association between the use of oral contraceptives and the occurrence of strokes, particularly thrombotic strokes, where risk was estimated to be increased 4.1 to 9.5 times. Other studies show no relationship between use of oral contraceptives and the occurrence of stroke.[119–121]

Another case-control study estimated the risk of myocardial infarction in users of oral contraceptives was increased 3 to 6 times.[122] The risk for mortality from infarction was estimated to be increased 2 to 3 times in women below the age of 40 and 4 to 5 times in women age 40 to 44.[123] A later study of 54 women age 40 to 44 who died from myocardial infarction did not show an association with the use of oral contraceptives,[124] but the authors combined the data with that of their previous study to calculate a reduced risk factor.

An association has been reported between the risk of postoperative thromboembolic disease and the use of oral contraceptives.[125,126] The theory of an association was not confirmed by a study of the occurrence of postoperative pulmonary embolism and death.[127]

In view of the association between oral contraceptive use and a number of thrombotic and thromboembolic phenomena, oral contraceptives should be discontinued immediately if signs and symptoms of thromboembolism or neurologic or neuro-ophthalmic disorders occur. Also, patients with a history of deep venous thrombosis, pulmonary embolism, or cerebral thrombosis, should be considered in a high-risk category, and it is prudent not to use oral contraceptives in this group.

Cutaneous System

Chloasma may occur in some women after administration of oral contraceptives.[1,128] It is perhaps the most common cutaneous side effect of oral contraceptives and usually disappears when oral contraceptives are discontinued. Hirsutism and acne have been reported in some women, although in some women acne has improved during use of the contraceptive steroids.[128]

Congenital Abnormalities

Retrospective case-control studies have reported an association between the use of a hormonal pregnancy test or oral contraceptives in early pregnancy and the occurrence of deformities such as neural tube defects,[129] abnormalities of the heart and great vessels,[130,131] limb reduction changes,[132] and multiple abnormalities that are designated VACTERL.[133] Subsequent retrospective studies[134,135] and other analyses[136–139] did not support these findings.

Pregnancy and Malformations

Prior use of oral contraceptives does not influence the frequency of spontaneous abortion, the gender of the offspring, or the frequency of congenital anomalies.[13,33,140–148] Measurement of the intelligence of the offspring at 5 to 8 years of age showed no change.[149] A case-control study revealed no association between the use of oral contraceptives and the occurrence of Down's syndrome.[150]

SUMMARY

The combination oral contraceptives are highly effective in preventing conception and provide, in most women, a regular menstrual pattern. Progestins administered alone are not as effective as the combination oral contraceptives in controlling fertility or in maintaining the endometrium. Various adverse effects have been associated with the use of oral contraceptives. Most of the reported side effects are minor in nature or represent placebo responses and usually disappear with continued use of the compounds. Physicians should be aware of the increased risk of various thromboembolic diseases and the cases of amenorrhea, hypertension and other changes which have been observed during the use of oral contraceptives. Several aspects of cancer and oral contraceptives are still being studied and patients receiving these compounds should be examined periodically.

PREPARATIONS

Table 1 lists the combination oral contraceptives available for use in the United States. For some of the products, the number of tablets in the dispensing package (20, 21 or 28) are specified in the trademark name; for the others this is given in parentheses. Packages containing 28 tablets provide 21 tablets of oral contraceptive plus 7 placebo tablets so that the patient need not count or record the number of days between each 21 day cycle of medication.

Two progestin-only preparations are available, namely, norethindrone 0.35 mg (Micronor, Nor.Q.D.) and norgestrel 0.075 mg (Ovrette). Tablets are taken each day without cyclic interruption.

Although the various progestins differ in potency, and therefore in the daily milligram dose employed, they are administered in approximately equipotent biological doses sufficient to aid (along with estrogen) in preventing ovulation, to stimulate and maintain the endometrium, and provide for a monthly withdrawal bleeding. Similarly, ethinyl estradiol probably has a higher estrogenic potency than mestranol, which is reflected in the dosage of the two estrogens in oral contraceptive combinations. Pills with a lower dose of estrogen (50 micrograms or less) are used in an attempt to decrease the risk of thrombosis, but both estrogen dose and potency must be evaluated.[151,152] Furthermore, the estrogen-to-progestin ratio must be considered as well as the dose and potency of each steroid.

TABLE 1 Composition of Combination Oral Contraceptives

Progestin and Dose		Estrogen and Dose		Trademark Name(s)	1978 Cost for One Cycle
Ethynodiol diacetate	1 mg	Mestranol	100 μg	Ovulen (20)	\$3.41/20
				Ovulen 21	\$3.41/21
				Ovulen 28	\$3.44/28
	1 mg	Ethinyl estradiol	50 μg	Demulen (21)	\$3.37/21
				Demulen 28	\$3.41/28
Norethindrone	10 mg	Mestranol	60 μg	Ortho-Novum 10 mg (20)	\$4.70/20
	2 mg	Mestranol	100 μg	Ortho-Novum 2 mg (21)	\$3.26/21
				Norinyl 2 mg (20)	\$2.72/20
	1 mg	Mestranol	80 μg	Ortho-Novum 1/80 21	\$2.95/21
				Ortho-Novum 1/80 28	\$2.95/28
				Norinyl 1 + 80 21-day	\$2.53/21
				Norinyl 1 + 80 28-day	\$2.53/28
	1 mg	Mestranol	50 μg	Ortho-Novum 1/50 21	\$2.95/21
				Ortho-Novum 1/50 28	\$2.95/28
				Norinyl 1 + 50 21-day	\$2.53/21
				Norinyl 1 + 50 28-day	\$2.53/28
	1 mg	Ethinyl estradiol	50 μg	Ovcon-50 (28)	\$2.49/21
	0.5 mg	Ethinyl estradiol	35 μg	Brevicon (21)	\$2.53/21
				Brevicon 28	\$2.53/28
				Modicon (21)	\$2.95/21
				Modicon 28	\$2.95/21

	0.4 mg	Ethinyl estradiol	35 μg	Ovcon-35 (28)	$2.49/28
Norethindrone acetate	2.5 mg	Ethinyl estradiol	50 μg	Norlestrin 2.5/50	$3.41/21
	1.5 mg	Ethinyl estradiol	30 μg	Loestrin 1.5/30 (28) Loestrin-21 1.5/30 Zorane 1.5/30 (28)	$2.77/28 $2.77/21 $3.38/28
	1 mg	Ethinyl estradiol	50 μg	Norlestrin 21 1/50 Norlestrin 28 1/50 Zorane 1/50 (28)	$3.29/21 $3.29/28 $3.28/28
	1 mg	Ethinyl estradiol	20 μg	Loestrin-21 1/20 Zorane 1/20 (28)	$3.29/21 $3.38/28
Norethynodrel	9.85 mg	Mestranol	150 μg	Enovid 10 mg	$15.76/50
	5 mg	Mestranol	75 μg	Enovid 5 mg (20)	$3.61/20
	2.5 mg	Mestranol	100 μg	Enovid-E (20) Enovid-E 21	$3.35/20 $3.35/21
Norgestrel	0.5 mg	Ethinyl estradiol	50 μg	Orval (21) Orval 28	$3.52/21 $3.52/28
	0.3 mg	Ethinyl estradiol	30 μg	Lo/Orval (21)	$3.52/21

Choice of Preparation

The initial choice of contraceptive preparation depends on such factors as prior menstrual history, premenstrual weight gain, and the occurrence of other premenstrual and menstrual symptoms. Clinically, Enovid-E is generally regarded as providing a more estrogen-dominant response, while Norlestrin 2.5 mg and Ovral produce a more progestin-dominant response. Other oral contraceptives listed in Table 1 fall somewhere in-between. Changing from one oral contraceptive to another is not necessarily simple, since dosage and ratio of component must be considered. For example, the occurence of hypomenorrhea may be related to progestin excess or estrogen deficiency and may be controlled by selecting a combination with a different ratio of ingredients or a different dose of an individual ingredient. Conversely, hypermenorrhea may be related to progestin deficiency or estrogen excess. Mid-cycle breakthrough bleeding commonly occurs with oral contraceptives that supply too low a dose of steroids. Mucorrhea may indicate estrogen excess but patients with hirsutism, acne, or premenstrual tension may adjust better to a more estrogenic combination. A lesser estrogenic effect and a greater progestin action may be of value in the patient with cyclic premenstrual weight gain or dysmenorrhea. Although a given oral contraceptive may be satisfactory for a large number of women, individual variation in response will exist and the subsequent change in the type or dosage of these hormonal combinations must be based on the individual patient response.

REFERENCES

1. Drill VA: *Oral Contraceptives.* New York, Blakiston, McGraw.Hill, 1966.
2. Becker H, Kleisl HP, Reuter A, et al: Die Beeinflussbarkeit der Gonadotropin-absonderung durch den synthetisierten LH-Releasing-Faktor unter der Medikation eines Ovulationsblockers. Klin Wochenschr 51:759–761, 1973.
3. McGuire JL, Bariso CD, Yuliano E, et al: Effects of low dose oral contraceptives containing norethindrone and ethinyl estradiol on serum levels of progesterone and pituitary gonadotropins. Contraception 11:329–338, 1975.
4. Roland M: Prevention of sperm migration into the uterine cavity by a microdose progestagen. Fertil Steril 21:211–216, 1970.
5. Moghissi KS, Syner FN, McBride LC: Contraceptive mechanism of microdose norethindrone. Obstet Gynecol 41:585–594, 1973.
6. Eckstein P, Whitby M, Fotherby K, et al: Clinical and laboratory findings in a trial of norgestrel, a low-dose progestogen-only contraceptive. Br Med J 3:195–200, 1972.
7. Larsson-Cohn U: Contraceptive treatment with low doses of gestagens. Acta Endocrinol 64(Supp 144):7–46, 1970.
8. Cohen MR, Lieberman JS: D-norgestrel: an estrogen-free, cyclic oral contraceptive. J Reprod Med 17:125–130, 1976.

9. Friedman S, Goldfien A: Breast secretions in normal women. Am J Obstet Gynecol 104:846–849, 1969.
10. Shevach AB, Spellacy WN: Galactorrhea and contraceptive practices. Obstet Gynecol 38:286–289, 1971.
11. Tietze C: Differential fecundity and effectiveness of contraception. Eugen Rev 50:231–237, 1959.
12. Mears E: Pregnancy following antifertility agents. Int J Fertil 13:340–345, 1968.
13. Peterson WF: Pregnancy following oral contraceptive therapy. Obstet Gynecol 34:363–367, 1969.
14. Westoff CF, Bumpass L, Ryder NB: Oral contraception, coital frequency, and the time required to conceive. Soc Biol 16:1–10, 1969.
15. Royal College of General Practitioners: *Oral Contraceptives and Health.* New York, Pitman, 1974.
16. Tietze C: Pregnancy rates and birth rates. Population Studies 16:31–37, 1962.
17. Shearman RP: Prolonged secondary amenorrhea after oral contraceptive therapy. Lancet 2:64–66, 1971.
18. Golditch IM: Postcontraceptive amenorrhea. Obstet Gynecol 39:903–908, 1972.
19. Furuhjelm M, Carlström K: Amenorrhea following use of combined oral contraceptives. Acta Obstet Gynecol Scand 52:373–379, 1973.
20. Fries H, Nillius SJ: Psychological factors, psychiatric illness and amenorrhea after oral contraceptive treatment. Acta Psychiatr Scand 49:653–668, 1973.
21. Fries H, Nillius SJ: Dieting, anorexia nervosa and amenorrhea after oral contraceptive treatment. Acta Psychiatr Scand 49:669–679, 1973.
22. Fries H, Nillius SJ, Pettersson F: Epidemiology of secondary amenorrhea. II. A retrospective evaluation of etiology with special regard to psychogenic factors and weight loss. Am J Obstet Gynecol 118:473–479, 1974.
23. Evrard JR, Buxton BH Jr, Erickson D: Amenorrhea following oral contraception. Am J Obstet Gynecol 124:88–91, 1976.
24. Drill VA: Oral contraceptives: relations to mammary cancer, benign breast lesions, and cervical cancer. Annu Rev Pharmacol 15:367–385, 1975.
25. Prechtel K, Seidel H: Brustdrüsenveränderungen nach Langzeitbehandlung mit sogenannten Ovulationshemmern. Verh Dtsch Ges Pathol 56:529–532, 1972.
26. Prechtel K: Ovulationshemmer und Brustdrüsenveränderungen bei Frauen im geschlechtsreifen Alter. Munch Med Wochenschr 111:2443–2447, 1969.
27. Fasal E, Paffenbarger RS: Oral contraceptives as related to cancer and benign lesions of the breast. J Natl Cancer Inst 55:767–773, 1975.
28. Vessey MP, Doll R, Sutton PM: Oral contraceptives and breast neoplasia: a retrospective study. Br Med J 3:719–724, 1972.
29. Sartwell PE, Arthes FG, Tonascia JA: Epidemiology of benign breast lesions: lack of association with oral contraceptive use. N Engl J Med 288:551–554, 1973.
30. Kelsey JL, Lindfors KK, White C: A case-control study of the epidemiology of benign breast diseases with reference to oral contraceptive use. Int J Epidemiol 3:333–340, 1974.
31. Boston Collaborative Drug Surveillance Program: Oral contraceptives and venous thromboembolic disease, surgically confirmed gallbladder disease, and breast tumors. Lancet 1:1399–1404, 1973.
32. Ory H, Cole P, McMahon B, et al: Oral contraceptives and reduced risk of benign breast diseases. N Engl J Med 294:419–422, 1976.
33. Goldzieher JW, Maas JM, Hines DC: Seven years of clinical experience with a sequential oral contraceptive. Int J Fertil 13:399–404, 1968.
34. Keifer WS, Scott JC: A clinical reappraisal of patients following long-term contraception. Am J Obstet Gynecol 122:446–458, 1975.
35. Fechner RE: Breast cancer during oral contraceptive therapy. Cancer 26:1204–1211, 1970.
36. Brezina K, Janisch H, Müller-Tyl E: Das Mammogramm unter Kontrazeptiva. Wien Klin Wochenschr 85:785–790, 1973.
37. Vessey MP, Doll R, Jones K: Oral contraceptives and breast cancer. Lancet 1:941–943, 1975.
38. Maqueo M, Azuela JC, Calderon JJ, et al: Morphology of the cervix in women treated with synthetic progestins. Am J Obstet Gynecol 96:994–998, 1966.
39. Carbia E, Rubio-Linares G, Alvarado-Duran A, et al: Histologic study of the uterine cervix

during oral contraception with ethynodiol diacetate and mestranol. Obstet Gynecol 35:381–388, 1970.
40. Drill VA: Effect of estrogens and progestins on the cervix uteri. J Toxicol Environ Health 1(Supp 1):193–204, 1976.
41. Sandmire HF, Austin SD, Bechtel RC: Carcinoma of the cervix in oral contraceptive steroid and IUD users and nonusers. Am J Obstet Gynecol 125:339–345, 1976.
42. Smith DC, Prentice R, Thompson DJ, et al: Association of exogenous estrogen and endometrial carcinoma. N Engl J Med 293:1164–1167, 1975.
43. Ziel HK, Finkle WD: Increased risk of endometrial carcinoma among users of conjugated estrogens. N Engl J Med 293:1167–1170, 1975.
44. Mack TM, Pike MC, Henderson BE, et al: Estrogens and endometrial cancer in a retirement community. N Engl J Med 294:1262–1267, 1976.
45. Lyon FA: The development of adenocarcinoma of the endometrium in young women receiving long-term sequential oral contraception. Am J Obstet Gynecol 123:299–301, 1975.
46. Silverberg SG, Makowski EL: Endometrial carcinoma in young women taking oral contraceptive agents. Obstet Gynecol 46:503–506, 1975.
47. Kelly HW, Miles PA, Buster JE, et al: Adenocarcinoma of the endometrium in women taking sequential oral contraceptives. Obstet Gynecol 47:200–202, 1976.
48. Lyon FA, Frisch MJ: Endometrial abnormalities occurring in young women on long-term sequential oral contraception. Obstet Gynecol 47:639–643, 1976.
49. Kaufman RH, Reeves KO, Dougherty CM: Severe atypical endometrial changes and sequential contraceptive use. JAMA 236:923–926, 1976.
50. Barsivala V, Virkar K: Thyroid functions of women taking oral contraceptives. Contraception 9:305–314, 1974.
51. Goolden AWG, Gartside JM, Sanderson C: Thyroid status in pregnancy and in women taking oral contraceptives. Lancet 1:12–15, 1967.
52. Drill VA: Some metabolic actions and possible toxic effects of hormonal contraceptives in animals and man. Acta Endocrinol 75(Supp 185):169–202, 1974.
53. Burke CW: Biologically active cortisol in plasma of oestrogen-treated and normal subjects. Br Med J 2:798–800, 1969.
54. Bulbrook RD, Hayward JL, Herian M, et al: Effect of steroidal contraceptives on levels of plasma androgen sulphates and cortisol. Lancet 1:628–631, 1973.
55. Ansari AH, Beck PR: Pituitary-adrenocortical effect of short- and long-term progestational therapy. Am J Obstet Gynecol 103:511–519, 1969.
56. Mestman JH, Anderson GV, Nelson DH: Adrenal-pituitary responsiveness during therapy with an oral contraceptive. Obstet Gynecol 31:378–386, 1968.
57. Chopra JG: Effect of steroid contraceptives on lactation. Am J Clin Nutr 25:1202–1214, 1972.
58. Semm K, Dittmar FW: Post partum ovulation: inhibition and milk yield. Curr Ther Res 8:48–51, 1966.
59. Kaern T: Effect of an oral contraceptive immediately post partum on initiation of lactation. Br Med J 3:644–645, 1967.
60. Kamal I, Hefnawi F, Ghoneim M, et al: Clinical, biochemical, and experimental studies on lactation. V. Clinical effects of steroids on the initiation of lactation. Am J Obstet Gynecol 108:655–658, 1970.
61. Bakker CB, Dightman CR: Side effects of contraceptives. Obstet Gynecol 28:373–379, 1966.
62. Murawski BJ, Sapir PE, Shulman N, et al: An investigation of mood states in women taking oral contraceptives. Fertil Steril 19:50–63, 1968.
63. Weissman MM, Slaby AE: Oral contraceptives and psychiatric disturbance: evidence from research. Br J Psychiatry 123:513–518, 1973.
64. Adams PW, Wynn V, Rose DP, et al: Effect of pyridoxine hydrochloride (vitamin B_6) upon depression associated with oral contraception. Lancet 1:897–904, 1973.
65. Diddle AW, Gardner WH, Williamson PJ: Oral contraceptive medications and headache. Am J Obstet Gynecol 105:507–511, 1969.
66. Larsson-Cohn U, Lundberg PO: Headache and treatment with oral contraceptives. Acta Neurol Scand 46:267–278, 1970.

67. Kudrow L: The relationship of headache frequency to hormone use in migraine. Headache 15:36–40, 1975.
68. Faust JM, Tyler ET: Ophthalmologic findings in patients using oral contraception. Fertil Steril 17:1–6, 1966.
69. Connell EB, Kelman CD: Eye examinations in patients taking oral contraceptives. Fertil Steril 20:67–74, 1969.
70. Andelman MB, Zackler J, Slutsky HL, et al: Family planning and public health. Int J Fertil 13:405–414, 1968.
71. Kunin CM, McCormack RC, Abernathy JR: Oral contraceptives and blood pressure. Arch Intern Med 123:362–365, 1969.
72. Clezy TM, Foy BN, Hodge RL, et al: Oral contraceptives and hypertension. An epidemiological survey. Br Heart J 34:1238–1243, 1972.
73. Spellacy WN, Birk SA: The effect of intrauterine devices, oral contraceptives, estrogens, and progestogens on blood pressure. Am J Obstet Gynecol 112:912–919, 1972.
74. Fisch IR, Freedman SH, Myatt AV: Oral contraceptives, pregnancy, and blood pressure. JAMA 222:1507–1510, 1972.
75. Weir RJ, Briggs E, Mack A, et al: Blood pressure in women taking oral contraceptives. Br Med J 1:533–535, 1974.
76. Goldzieher JW, Moses LE, Averkin E, et al: A placebo-controlled double-blind crossover investigation of the side effects attributed to oral contraceptives. Fertil Steril 22:609–623, 1971.
77. Spellacy WN, Birk SA: The effects of mechanical and steroid contraceptive methods on blood pressure in hypertensive women. Fertil Steril 25:467–470, 1974.
78. Cain MD, Walters WA, Catt KJ: Effects of oral contraceptive therapy on the renin-angiotensin system. J Clin Endocrinol Metab 33:671–676, 1971.
79. Spellacy WN: A review of carbohydrate metabolism and the oral contraceptives. Am J Obstet Gynecol 104:448–460, 1969.
80. Beck P: Contraceptive steroids: modifications of carbohydrate and lipid metabolism. Metabolism 22:841–855, 1973.
81. Kalkhoff RK: Effects of oral contraceptive agents on carbohydrate metabolism. J Steroid Biochem 6:949–956, 1975.
82. Davidson MB, Holzman GB: Role of growth hormone in the alteration of carbohydrate metabolism induced by oral contraceptive agents. J Clin Endocrinol Metab 36:246–255, 1973.
83. Beck P, Arnett DM, Alsever RN, et al: Effects of contraceptive steroids on arginine-stimulated glucagon and insulin secretion in women. II. Carbohydrate and lipid physiology in insulin-dependent diabetics. Metabolism 25:23–31, 1976.
84. Fuertes-de la Haba A, Vega-de Rodriguez G, Pelegrina I: Carbohydrate metabolism in long-term oral contraceptive users. Obstet Gynecol 37:220–224, 1971.
85. Beck P: Alterations of lipid metabolism by contraceptive steroids. J Steroid Biochem 6:957–959, 1975.
86. Skolnick JL, Stoler BS, Katz DB, et al: Rifampin, oral contraceptives, and pregnancy. JAMA 236:1382, 1976.
87. Roberton YR, Johnson ES: Interactions between oral contraceptives and other drugs: a review. Curr Med Res Opin 3:647–661, 1976.
88. Koch-Weser J, Sellers EM: Drug interactions with coumarin anticoagulants. N Engl J Med 285:487,498, 547–558, 1971.
89. Goldzieher JW: The incidence of side effects with oral or intrauterine contraceptives. Am J Obstet Gynecol 102:91–94, 1968.
90. Aznar-Ramos R, Giner-Velazquez J, Lara-Ricalde R, et al: Incidence of side effects with contraceptive placebo. Am J Obstet Gynecol 105:1144–1149, 1969.
91. Goldzieher JW, Moses LE, Averkin E, et al: Nervousness and depression attributed to oral contraceptives: a double-blind, placebo-controlled study. Am J Obstet Gynecol 111:1013–1020, 1971.
92. Stephens MEM, Craft I, Peters, TJ, et al: Oral contraceptives and folate metabolism. Clin Sci 42:405–414, 1972.
93. Shojania AM, Hornady GJ: Oral contraceptives and folate absorption. J Lab Clin Med 82:869–875, 1973.
94. Shojania AM: The effect of oral contraceptives on folate metabolism. III. Plasma clearance and urinary folate excretion. J Lab Clin Med 85:185–190, 1975.

95. McLean FW, Heine MW, Held B, et al: Relationship between the oral contraceptive and folic acid metabolism. Am J Obstet Gynecol 104:745–747, 1969.
96. Johnson GK, Geenen JE, Hensley GT, et al: Small intestinal disease, folate deficiency anemia, and oral contraceptive agents. Am J Dig Dis 18:185–190, 1973.
97. Paine CJ, Grafton WD, Dickson VL, et al: Oral contraceptives, serum folate, and hematologic status. JAMA 231:731–733, 1975.
98. Jenny S, Markoff N: Ovulationshemmer bei Lebererkrankungen. Schweiz Med Wochenschr 97:1502–1505, 1967.
99. Eisalo A, Konttinen A, Hietala O: Oral contraceptives after liver disease. Br Med J 3:561–562, 1971.
100. Schweitzer IL, Weiner JM, McPeak CM, et al: Oral contraceptives in acute viral hepatitis. JAMA 233:979–980, 1975.
101. Schinella RA: Jaundice with Dubin-Johnson-Sprinz syndrome precipitated by oral contraceptives. NY State J Med 72:2810–2813, 1972.
102. Cohen L, Lewis C, Arias IM: Pregnancy, oral contraceptives, and chronic familial jaundice with predominantly conjugated hyperbilirubinemia (Dubin-Johnson syndrome). Gastroenterology 62:1182–1190, 1972.
103. Drill VA: Benign cholestatic jaundice of pregnancy and benign cholestatic jaundice from oral contraceptives. Am J Obstet Gynecol 119:165–174, 1974.
104. Sörensen TIA, Baden H: Benign hepatocellular tumours. Scand J Gastroenterol 10:113–119, 1975.
105. McAvoy JM, Tompkins RK, Longmire WP Jr: Benign hepatic tumors and their association with oral contraceptives. Arch Surg 111:761–767, 1976.
106. Mays ET, Christopherson WM, Mahr MM, et al: Hepatic changes in young women ingesting contraceptive steroids. Hepatic hemorrhage and primary hepatic tumors. JAMA 235:730–732, 1976.
107. Edmondson HA, Henderson B, Benton B: Liver-cell adenomas associated with use of oral contraceptives. N Engl J Med 294:470–472, 1976.
108. Howat JMT, Jones CB, Schofield PE: Gall-stones and oral contraceptives. J Int Med Res 3:59–62, 1975.
109. Bennion LJ, Ginsberg RL, Garnick MB, et al: Effects of oral contraceptives on the gallbladder bile of normal women. N Engl J Med 294:189–192, 1976.
110. Vessey MP, Doll R: Investigation of relation between the use of oral contraceptives and thromboembolic disease. A further report. Br Med J 2:651–657, 1969.
111. Inman WHW, Vessey MP: Investigation of deaths from pulmonary, coronary and cerebral thrombosis and embolism in women of child-bearing age. Br Med J 2:193–199, 1968.
112. Sartwell PE, Masi AT, Arthes FG, et al: Thromboembolism and oral contraceptives: an epidemiologic case-control study. Am J Epidemiol 90:365–380, 1969.
113. Drill VA: Oral contraceptives and thromboembolic disease. I. Prospective and retrospective studies. JAMA 219:583–592, 1972.
114. Fuertes-de la Haba A, Curet JO, Pelegrina I, et al: Thrombophlebitis among oral and nonoral contraceptive users. Obstet Gynecol 38:259–263, 1971.
115. Grounds M: Anovulants: thrombosis and other associated changes. Med J Aust 2:440–446, 1974.
116. Goldzieher JW, Dozier TS: Oral contraceptives and thromboembolism: a reassessment. Am J Obstet Gynecol 123:878–914, 1975.
117. Collaborative Group for the Study of Stroke in Young Women: Oral contraception and increased risk of cerebral ischemia or thrombosis. N Engl J Med 288:871–878, 1973.
118. Collaborative Group for the Study of Stroke in Young Women: Oral contraceptives and stroke in young women. Associated risk factors. JAMA 231:718–722, 1975.
119. Illis L, Kocen RS, McDonald WI, et al: Oral contraceptives and cerebral arterial occlusion. Br Med J 2:1164–1166, 1965.
120. Jennett WB, Cross JN: Influence of pregnancy and oral contraception on the incidence of strokes in women of childbearing age. Lancet 1:1019–1023, 1967.
121. Schoenberg BS, Whisnant JP, Taylor WF, et al: Strokes in women of childbearing age. A population study. Neurology 20:181–189, 1970.
122. Mann JI, Vessey MP, Thorogood M, et al: Myocardial infarction in young women with special reference to oral contraceptive practice. Br Med J 2:241–245, 1975.
123. Mann JI, Inman WHW: Oral contraceptives and death from myocardial infarction. Br Med J 2:245–248, 1975.

124. Mann JI, Inman WHW, Thorogood M: Oral contraceptive use in older women and fatal myocardial infarction. Br Med J 2:445–447, 1976.
125. Vessey MP, Doll R, Fairbairn AS, et al: Postoperative thromboembolism and the use of oral contraceptives. Br Med J 3:123–126, 1970.
126. Greene GR, Sartwell PE: Oral contraceptive use in patients with thromboembolism following surgery, trauma, or infection. Am J Public Health 62:680–685, 1972.
127. Krauss V, Breitner J: Ovulationshemmer und postoperatives Lungenembolierisiko. Dtsch Med Wochenschr 96:176–177, 1971.
128. Prenen M, Ledoux-Corbusier M: Hormonal contraceptives and dermatology. Contraception 4:79–89, 1971.
129. Gal I: Risks and benefits of the use of hormonal pregnancy test tablets. Nature 240:241–242, 1972.
130. Nora JJ, Nora AH: Birth defects and oral contraceptives. Lancet 1:941–942, 1973.
131. Levy EP, Cohen A, Fraser FC: Hormone treatment during pregnancy and congenital heart defects. Lancet 1:611, 1973.
132. Janerich DT, Piper JM, Glebatis DM: Oral contraceptives and congenital limb-reduction defects. N Engl J Med 291:697–700, 1974.
133. Nora AH, Nora JJ: A syndrome of multiple congenital anomalies associated with teratogenic exposure. Arch Environ Health 30:17–21, 1975.
134. Mulvihill JJ, Mulvihill CG, Neill CA: Prenatal sex hormone exposure and cardiac defects in man. Teratology 9:A.30, 1974.
135. Yasuda M, Miller JR: Prenatal exposure to oral contraceptives and transposition of the great vessels in man. Teratology 12:239–244, 1975.
136. Mitchell SC, Sellmann AH, Westphal MC, et al: Etiologic correlates in a study of congenital heart disease in 56,109 births. Am J Cardiol 28:653–657, 1971.
137. Laurence M, Miller M, Vowles M, et al: Hormonal pregnancy tests and neural tube malformations. Nature 233:495–496, 1971.
138. David TJ, O'Callaghan SE: Birth defects and oral hormone preparations. Lancet 1:1236, 1974.
139. Oakley GP Jr, Flynt JW Jr: Hormonal pregnancy tests and congenital malformations. Lancet 2:256–257, 1973.
140. Macdonald RR: Norethynodrel and mestranol (Enavid) in the prevention of recurrent abortion. Lancet 2:362–365, 1965.
141. Rice-Wray E, Cervantes A, Gutierrez J, et al: Pregnancy and progeny after hormonal contraceptives—genetic studies. J Reprod Med 6:101–104, 1971.
142. Robinson SC: Pregnancy outcome following oral contraceptives. Am J Obstet Gynecol 109:354–358, 1971.
143. Royal College of General Practitioners' Oral Contraception Study: The outcome of pregnancy in former oral contraceptive users. Br J Obstet Gynaecol 83:608–616, 1976.
144. Behrman SJ: Choice of an oral contraceptive. Obstet Gynecol Digest 8:37–41, 1966.
145. Banks AL: Pregnancy and progeny. Int J Fertil 13:346–348, 1968.
146. Crawford JS, Davies P: Pre-pregnancy oral contraception and sex ratio among subsequent progeny. Lancet 2:453–454, 1973.
147. Rothman KJ, Liess J: Gender of offspring after oral contraceptive use. N Engl J Med 295:859–861, 1976.
148. Döring GK, Kauka E, Netzer A: Schwangerschaftsverlauf und Zustand der Kinder nach Anwendung von Ovulationshemmern. Gubertshilfe Frauenheilkd 36:57–61, 1976.
149. Fuertes-de la Haba A, Santiago G, Bangdiwala IS: Measured intelligence in offspring of oral and nonoral contraceptive users. Am J Obstet Gynecol 125:980–983, 1976.
150. Janerich DT, Flink EM, Keogh MD: Down's syndrome and oral contraceptive usage. Br J Obstet Gynaecol 83:617–620, 1976.
151. Inman WHW, Vessey MP, Westerholm B, et al: Thromboembolic disease and the steroidal content of oral contraceptives. Br Med J 2:203–209, 1970.
152. Drill VA: Oral contraceptives and thromboembolic disease. II. Estrogen content of oral contraceptives. JAMA 219:593–596, 1972.

53. THYROID HORMONES

Gilbert H. Daniels

The thyroid gland synthesizes thyroxine (tetraiodothyronine) and triiodothyronine on a large precursor molecule, thyroglobulin, under the control of pituitary thyroid stimulating hormone (TSH).[1] Proteolysis of the stored thyroglobulin releases thyroxine (T_4) and triiodothyronine (T_3) from the thyroid gland. Normally, up to 85% of circulating T_3 is derived from deiodination of T_4 by peripheral tissues rather than direct secretion by the thyroid gland.[2,3] T_4 and T_3 are tightly bound to serum proteins. The unbound hormones are metabolically active and exert negative feedback on the pituitary gland to shut off TSH secretion. Although exogenous administration of T_4 or T_3 leads to TSH suppression and shrinkage of the thyroid gland, an otherwise normal pituitary-thyroid axis always returns to normal function within six weeks of discontinuing these agents.[4]

The available thyroid hormone preparations contain L-thyroxine (T_4) and/or L-triiodothyronine (T_3 liothyronine). Thyroglobulin is also available; it is digested in the gastrointestinal tract to T_3 and T_4. Thyroid hormones are prescribed either for physiological replacement in hypothyroid individuals or in suppressive doses for diagnosis or therapy.[5] In practice, the dosages required for physiological replacement closely approximate those used for suppression.

DIAGNOSIS AND THERAPY OF HYPOTHYROIDISM

The symptoms of hypothyroidism are often nonspecific and may be easily missed. They include weight gain (marked obesity is unusual), dry skin, cold intolerance, decreased energy, apathy, depression, decreased mental acuity, constipation, muscle cramps, paresthesias, and meno-metrorrhagia. In general, therapy should await chemical confirmation of the diagnosis. Many patients who are treated for hypothyroidism do not have that diagnosis; therapy is often incorrectly started on the basis of one of the above complaints, without confirmatory data.

A low serum thyroxine concentration suggests the diagnosis of primary hypothyroidism. However, the earliest sign of a failing thyroid gland is an increase in the serum TSH concentration, even before the serum thyroxine falls to abnormally low levels (Table 1). TSH should be measured to confirm the diagnosis since other types of hypothyroidism, in which TSH concentrations are normal or depressed, require different therapy. Euthyroid patients with deficiency of the thyroid-binding proteins have a low serum concentration of total thyroxine, but normal levels of the metabolically-active free (unbound) hormone and of TSH. This condition can be diagnosed by measuring T_3 resin uptake (Table 1) which gives an inverse measure of the number of protein-binding sites for thyroxine. Primary hypothyroidism, in which the thyroid gland fails (TSH concentrations will be elevated), must be distinguished from secondary hypothyroidism, in which the pituitary or hypothalamus is at fault (TSH will be 'normal' or low). In secondary hypothyroidism, partial adrenal insufficiency usually coexists and cortisol therapy is mandatory before initiating thyroid hormone treatment (Table 1).

A diagnosis of hypothyroidism usually implies lifelong therapy. However, drug-induced hypothyroidism (eg, due to iodides, lithium, or thionamides) or the hypothyroid phase of subacute thyroiditis requires therapy only for the duration of the abnormality.

SUPPRESSION TESTING OR THERAPY

Suppression Test

Seven to ten days of suppressive dosages of thyroid hormone lead to at least a 50% reduction of the thyroid gland's capacity to concentrate and organify radioactive iodine as measured by the 24-hour radioactive iodine uptake. An autonomous thyroid gland (ie, one which is independent of TSH) is resistant to such therapy.

Suppressive Therapy

Diffuse and nodular nontoxic goiters are often amenable to suppressive therapy with thyroid hormone, particularly when the TSH concentration is somewhat elevated. If the goiter does not shrink, the thyroid gland may be autonomous and a suppression test can be carried out. In the presence of thyroid gland autonomy, thyroid hormone is best avoided. Thyroid hormone can be administered prophylactically together with thionamide therapy for hyperthy-

TABLE 1 Differential Diagnosis of Hypothyroidism and Low Serum Thyroxine

Diagnosis	Results of Diagnostic Tests			Therapy
	Serum Thyroxine Concentration	T_3 Resin Uptake	Serum TSH Concentration	
Primary Hypothyroidism	↓	↓	↑	Thyroid hormone
Secondary Hypothyroidism	↓	↓	"Normal" or ↓	Cortisol, then thyroid hormone
Thyroxine Binding Globulin Deficiency	↓	↑	Normal	None
Early Primary Hypothyroidism	Normal or slightly ↓	Normal or slightly ↓	↑	Thyroid hormone

roidism, to prevent goiter enlargement or the development of hypothyroidism (see Chapter 54, Antithyroid Agents). Cold thyroid nodules may decrease in size as pituitary TSH is suppressed, but they rarely disappear completely.

Well-differentiated thyroid carcinoma (papillary or follicular) is often TSH-dependent. Complete suppression of TSH by thyroid hormone is mandatory therapy in such patients, barring contra-indications.

An increased risk for developing thyroid carcinoma exists for at least 30 years after neck irradiation, whether the radiation is given in childhood for enlarged tonsils or thymus, or during the teenage years for acne. Prophylactic administration of thyroid hormone has been advocated in patients so treated, even in the absence of thyroid gland abnormalities. Although confirmatory data are lacking, thyroid cancer may be prevented by TSH suppression, or detected early by shrinking normal thyroid tissue, allowing abnormalities to be more easily palpated. This probably is a valid use for thyroid hormone therapy.

Thyroid hormones should not be prescribed for simple obesity in the absence of laboratory confirmation of hypothyroidism. These agents do not improve fertility in women who are not hypothyroid.

DRUG MONOGRAPHS

LEVOTHYROXINE SODIUM (Letter, Synthroid)

Levothyroxine (T_4) is my personal drug of choice for all conditions requiring long-term thyroid hormone replacement or suppressive therapy because of its smooth action and uniform potency. The cost of synthetic levothyroxine is now only slightly greater than the relatively crude thyroid extracts.

Absorption of T_4 after oral administration is about 50 to 75% complete,[6] and it apparently does not depend upon the patient's thyroid status.[7] The rather long elimination half-life (7 days) provides remarkably stable blood levels of thyroxine and prevents problems when one or more doses are inadvertently missed. The conversion of T_4 to T_3 by peripheral tissues closely mimics the normal physiological situation. The relatively slow rate of this conversion leads to a gradual onset of therapeutic effect in hypothyroid patients, a distinct advantage in those patients with underlying cardiac disease. Patients

TABLE 2 Preparations and Costs of Thyroid Hormones

GENERIC NAME	TRADEMARK NAME(S)	PREPARATIONS AND 1978 COSTS
Levothyroxine Sodium	Synthroid (Letter)	Tablets 0.025 mg—$1.75/100; 0.05 mg—$1.90/100; 0.1 mg—$2.04/100; 0.15 mg—$2.48/100; 0.2 mg—$2.76/100; 0.3 mg—$4.14/100 Injection (lyophilized powder) 0.5 mg—$9.59/vial
Thyroid USP	generic	Tablets 15 mg—$0.66–$1.00/100; 30 mg—$0.72–$1.20/100; 60 mg—$0.84–$1.61/100; 90 mg—$1.20/100; 120 mg—$0.95–$2.30/100; 180 mg—$2.30–$2.40/100
Thyroglobulin	Proloid	Tablets 15 mg—$1.15/100; 30 mg—$1.25/100; 60 mg—$1.50/100; 90 mg—$1.90/100; 120 mg—$2.70/100; 180 mg—$3.65/100; 300 mg—$4.65/100
Liothyronine Sodium (L-triiodothyronine sodium)	Cytomel	Tablets 5 μg—$1.80/100; 25 μg—$2.70/100; 50 μg—$4.10/100
Liotrix	Euthroid	Tablets "½" (containing levothyroxine sodium 30 mg and liothyronine sodium 7.5 mg)—$2.65/100; "1" (60/15 mg)—$3.30/100; "2" (120/30 mg)—$4.00/100; "3" (180/45 mg)—$4.75/100
	Thyrolar	Tablets "¼" (containing levothyroxine sodium 12.5 mg and liothyroxine sodium 3.1 mg)—$2.27/100; "½" (25/6.25 mg)—$2.27/100; "1" (50/12.5 mg)—$3.14/100; "2" (100/25 mg)—$3.80/100; "3" (150/37.5 mg)—$4.51/100; "5" (250/62.5 mg)—$5.46/100

who are euthyroid while taking L-thyroxine will have normal or slightly high serum T_4 concentrations.[8]

Although L-triiodothyronine (T_3, liothyronine) has traditionally been the agent of choice for suppression testing, a single 3 mg dosage of T_4 is equally effective and less toxic, and it circumvents the issue of patient compliance.[9,10]

Only small amounts of T_4 cross the placenta; it is not contraindicated in pregnancy.

Severe illness of any sort impairs the peripheral conversion of T_4 to T_3, both in normals and those on thyroxine replacement.[11] No untoward effects of this reduced T_3 concentration have been noted to date in athyreotic individuals maintained on L-thyroxine.

Adverse Reactions—Levothyroxine mimics the natural hormone in structure. Adverse effects are due to overdosage or too rapid correction of hypothyroidism, conditions that simulate the spontaneously-occurring hyperthyroid state. There are no well documented 'allergic' reactions to levothyroxine.

The possible symptoms of thyroid hormone excess include: weight loss with preserved appetite, anxiety, tremor, palpitations, increased frequency of bowel movements, shortness of breath, muscle weakness, oligomenorrhea, emotional lability and irritability, heat intolerance and difficulty in sleeping. Hypothyroid patients with underlying heart disease may develop or exacerbate angina, tachyarrhythmias, or congestive heart failure. As the sodium component of myxedema fluid is mobilized, pitting edema may appear. Symptoms may not appear for one to three or more weeks after a change in dosage.

Toxicity can be prevented by initiating therapy with very low dosages in those patients with known heart disease or severe hypothyroidism of long duration and in the elderly. In such patients at least 4 weeks should elapse before the dosage is increased. The concomitant use of beta adrenergic blocking agents such as propranolol may facilitate thyroxine replacement in patients with known angina, by decreasing the chronotropic effect of the thyroid hormone.

Adrenal crisis or insufficiency can be precipitated during the transition from hypo- to euthyroidism in patients with primary or secondary (hypothalamic-pituitary) hypothyroidism.[12] With established adrenal insufficiency and new hypothyroidism, the dosage of glucocorticoids must be increased when prescribing levothyroxine. With secondary hypothyroidism, hydrocortisone or one of its congeners must be started before initiation of levothyroxine replacement therapy.

Interactions—The absorption of levothyroxine is diminished by cholestyramine,[13] presumably by direct binding. If both drugs are to be prescribed, they should be administered four or more hours apart. The enterohepatic circulation of levothyroxine is probably impaired in malabsorption syndromes,[6] leading to increased requirements. Phenytoin and phenobarbital increase the hepatic biotransformation of levothyroxine, presumably by microsomal enzyme induction.[14–16] An increased requirement for T_4 in hypothyroid patients taking these drugs may be anticipated.

The rate of glucocorticoid biotransformation parallels thyroid activity,[17,18] requiring initiation of steroid therapy in secondary hypothyroidism and increases of steroid dosage in adrenal insufficiency prior to levothyroxine therapy.

The general metabolic state is depressed in hypothyroidism, and this causes increased sensitivity to many drugs.[19] As levothyroxine is administered to such patients, requirements for sedative, narcotics, and digoxin[20] may increase. One important exception is the anticoagulant warfarin. Hypothyroid patients are more resistant to the effects of warfarin and decreasing dosages are required with levothyroxine therapy.[21] The transition from hypo- to euthyroidism may result in deterioration of glucose tolerance and worsening diabetes in insulin-requiring diabetics.

Although phenytoin and aspirin displace the protein-bound (metabolically inactive) thyroxine, no acute hyperthyroid effects have been noted, even when the free thyroxine concentration acutely increases.[16] Increased concentrations of protein-bound thyroxine occur with the administration of estrogenic compounds and during pregnancy. Although increased requirements for thyroxine have not been clearly demonstrated in such patients, their thyroid status should be carefully reassessed.

Many prescriptions and proprietary medications, including antihistamines and sympathomimetic agents, carry the warning that they should not be used in patients with thyroid disease. Such prohibitions *do not* apply to patients on thyroid hormone therapy once they have become euthyroid.

Dosage—Individualization of initial dosage, final dosage, and rate of increase is mandatory. Although full replacement therapy is generally between 0.1 to 0.2 mg, there is no unequivocally correct dosage.[22,23] Some patients cannot tolerate as much as 0.1 mg and occasional individuals require more than 0.2 mg. If symptoms of hyperthyroidism develop, the dosage must be diminished. If a given dosage is not initially tolerated by a hypothyroid patient, it may be tolerated subsequently after a more gradual increase in therapy. The full benefit of a given dosage may not be reached for 4 to 8 or more weeks.[24]

(a) *Hypothyroidism.* Primary and secondary hypothyroidism must be clearly distinguished before initiating therapy.[25] The endpoint of therapy is usually determined by the clinical status of the patient. A reasonable chemical endpoint, in patients with primary hypothyroidism who have not had adverse effects, would be normalization or suppression of the initially elevated TSH level. Once the TSH has been suppressed there is generally no advantage in increasing the dosage, even if some symptoms (such as inability to lose weight) persist. In secondary hypothyroidism a reasonable chemical endpoint is normalization of the serum thyroxine concentration, usually in the high part of the normal range. Once a stable replacement dosage has been determined it usually does not need to be altered unless there is a change in the patient's status.

(1) *Mild hypothyroidism.* In patients without known heart disease, before age 50, begin therapy with 0.1 mg. Increase as necessary by 0.05 mg at 4 week intervals.

(2) *Severe hypothyroidism.* In the absence of known heart disease, begin with 0.05 mg. Increase dosage by 0.025 to 0.05 mg at 4 to 6 week intervals, the lower dosages and longer intervals reserved for the older patients.

(3) *Hypothyroidism with known angina or heart disease.* Begin with 0.025 mg. Increase by 0.025 mg at 4 to 6 week intervals. The final dosage is often less than that necessary for achieving the euthyroid state, in order to balance symptoms of hypothyroidism versus worsening heart disease. Propranolol may allow for somewhat higher dosage in patients with angina.

(4) *Myxedema coma.* Therapy in this situation remains quite controversial.[26,27] Dosage of thyroid hormone may not be critical if strict attention has been paid to fluid and electrolyte balance, ventilatory status, avoidance of central nervous system (CNS) depressant drugs, treatment of infection, and administration of hydrocortisone at dosages of 200 mg/day. Both high (500 to 700 μg intravenous bolus, followed by 100 μg per day intravenously) and low

(50 μg per day intravenously) dosages have been recommended, with and without concomitant L-triiodothyronine (liothyronine) therapy. A reasonable compromise in this often life-threatening emergency would be levothyroxine 100 μg per day intravenously as a single bolus with the addition of small amounts of T_3 (6.25 to 12.5 μg twice daily) by mouth or nasogastric tube.

(b) *Suppression.* (1) *Suppression test.* Levothyroxine, 3 mg orally 7 days before repeat radioactive iodine uptake is performed.

(2) *Suppressive therapy in euthyroid patients.* 'Full' replacement can often be initiated, 0.1 to 0.2 mg orally daily. The older the patient, the lower the initial dosage. If symptoms of toxicity develop dosage should be decreased by 0.05 mg. Dosages can be increased by 0.05 mg at 4-week intervals until the therapeutic effect is achieved or the serum TSH is suppressed, whichever occurs first.

In the absence of contraindications, the endpoint of therapy in patients with untreated or surgically removed, well-differentiated thyroid carcinoma (papillary or follicular) is complete TSH suppression, to prevent spread or regrowth. An undetectable serum TSH concentration 20 minutes after the administration of thyrotropin releasing hormone (200 μg by intravenous bolus) is ideal.[28] Such stringent criteria are not necessarily applied to patients being treated for goiter suppression or in prophylactic fashion. Here, an undetectable basal TSH usually suffices.

THYROID (USP)

Desiccated thyroid has long been the mainstay of thyroid hormone therapy because of its low cost. The extract of beef or pork thyroid contains variable amounts of thyroglobulin as well as free and covalently-bound T_4 and T_3. Standardization is generally by iodine content, which does not insure any biological potency. Some manufacturers perform bioassays of the material supplied, insuring relatively uniform potency. A recent survey of different products yielded a range from zero to 155% of expected potency.[29] In some cases the pills contain inert material (iodinated casein and other inactive ingredients); in others the pills have almost twice the desired potency. Furthermore, the variable T_4 versus T_3 content makes thyroid function testing somewhat confusing, with low or high concentrations of serum thyroxine being possible in clinically euthyroid patients.[30,31] Initiation of therapy using USP thyroid is not recommended for any patient.

Adverse Reactions—See levothyroxine monograph. Some patients develop hypersensitivity reactions to some component of the beef or pork products.

Interactions—See levothyroxine.

Dosage—Therapeutic considerations are the same as with levothyroxine. Full replacement therapy approximates 90 to 180 mg (1.5 to 3 grains). The equivalence between levothyroxine and USP thyroid varies depending on the particular preparation. However, levothyroxine, 0.2 mg, is roughly equivalent to 120 to 180 mg (2 to 3 grains) of USP thyroid.

Initial dosages are as low as 15 mg (0.25 grain) in hypothyroid patients with cardiac disease to 30 mg (0.5 grain) in elderly hypothyroid patients. With mild hypothyroidism 60 mg (1 grain) is a reasonable initial dosage. This dose should be adjusted by 15 to 30 mg (0.25 to 0.5 grain) increments at 4 to 6 week intervals.

THYROGLOBULIN (Proloid)

This purified extract of pig thyroid is similar to USP thyroid. Occasional batches have had extremely high T_3 contents.[30] There is no compelling reason to prescribe this agent. The adverse effects, interactions and dosage are those of USP thyroid.

LIOTHYRONINE SODIUM (Cytomel)

Liothyronine is the synthetic levorotatory isomer of triiodothyronine (T_3). T_3 is three to four times as potent as T_4[32] and is less extensively bound to serum proteins (99.8% vs 99.98% for T_4).[33] Therapy with T_3 results in low serum concentrations of thyroxine and variable concentrations of T_3 (elevated initially after administration, lower later in the day).[34] Accordingly, replacement therapy is often difficult to monitor. Rapid onset of toxic symptoms, including cardiovascular decompensation, more than outweighs the possible advantage of rapid dissipation of symptoms after discontinuation of T_3. In my experience patients are more frequently intolerant of this drug than T_4. The cost is quite high compared with levothyroxine or USP thyroid. Although better goiter suppression has been claimed, there is no evidence that T_3 is more beneficial than T_4 at equal degrees of TSH suppression. T_3 is virtually completely absorbed from the gastrointestinal tract.[35]

Presently, there are only three potential uses for liothyronine, none of which involve chronic therapy.

(1) *Suppression testing.*[36] A possible advantage of this agent comes from the additional information obtained by measuring the fall in serum thyroxine as well as the fall in radioactive iodine uptake during suppression testing. Monitoring of the elevated T_3 level assures patient compliance. The T_3 suppression test should not be used in elderly patients or those with known cardiac disease.

(2) *Thyroid cancer.* When patients with thyroid cancer are to be treated with therapeutic dosages of radioactive iodine, their thyroid hormone preparations are often discontinued to allow endogenous TSH to rise. It takes as long as 4 to 6 weeks off levothyroxine for the maximal rise in TSH because of the long elimination half-life of T_4, during which time the patient becomes hypothyroid. If the patient is switched to T_3 for a month before discontinuing the agent, the symptomatic time off therapy may be shortened to 2 to 3 weeks.

(3) *Myxedema coma.* The therapeutic onset and conversion of T_4 to T_3 are relatively slow. Although full therapy with T_3 is probably too dangerous in myxedema coma, small amounts of T_3 may be added to the regimen.

Adverse Reactions—See levothyroxine monograph. Cardiac toxicity is thought to be more likely because of the increased potency and rapid onset of action.

Dosage—T_3 is 3 to 4 times as potent as T_4. Full replacement dosage is about 50 to 75 μg per day. For maximum TSH suppression and minimum toxicity, the drug should be administered in three divided doses. It is not commercially available for parenteral administration.

(1) *Suppression test.* 25 μg orally three times a day for 8 to 10 days before repeat radioactive iodine uptake testing. T_3 is contraindicated in the elderly or those with heart disease.

(2) *Cancer patients.* 50 to 75 μg orally daily for one month prior to discontinuing thyroid hormone therapy for radioactive iodine administration.

(3) *Myxedema coma.* Consider the use of 6.25 to 12.5 μg two times a day orally or by nasogastric tube.

LIOTRIX (Euthyroid, Thyrolar)

This mixture, containing T_4 and T_3 in the ratio of 4:1, was designed to provide 'physiologic' replacement, before the peripheral conversion of T_4 to T_3 was understood.[37] The commercial preparations are expensive and contain a relative excess of T_3, leading to the same problems that occur with T_3 alone. A clear indication for these agents is not presently established.[38]

It is possible that hypothyroid patients with chronically impaired T_4 to T_3 conversion will be discovered, or those ill patients with impaired conversion of T_4 to T_3 may be shown to have symptomatic hypothyroidism. At that time the use of T_3, either singly or in combination, can be reassessed.

Interactions—See levothyroxine.

Dosage—Therapy is unnecessarily complicated by the availability of two liotrix preparations of different potency. Euthyroid 1 contains 60 μg of levothyroxine sodium and 15 μg of liothyronine sodium while Thyrolar 1 contains 50 μg and 12.5 μg, respectively. Full replacement is said to be between 1 and 3, although many patients will develop symptoms of hyperthyroidism on liotrix 3. Although liotrix 1 is said to be equivalent to one grain (60 mg) of USP thyroid, it is probably more potent.

REFERENCES

1. Daniels GH, Maloof F: Regulatory mechanisms of the pituitary thyroid axis. In *Pathophysiology: Altered Regulatory Mechanisms in Disease.* Edited by ED Frohlich. Philadelphia, JB Lippincott Co., 1976, p 341.
2. Surks MI, Schadlow AR, Stock JM, et al: Determination of iodothyronine absorption and conversion of L-thyroxine (T_4) to L-triiodothyronine (T_3) using turnover rate techniques. J Clin Invest 52:805–811, 1973.
3. Braverman LE, Ingbar SH, Sterling K: Conversion of thyroxine to triiodothyronine in athyreotic human subjects. J Clin Invest 49:855–864, 1970.
4. Vagenakis AG, Braverman LE, Azizi F, et al: Recovery of pituitary thyrotropic function after withdrawal of prolonged thyroid-suppression therapy. N Engl J Med 293:681–684, 1975.
5. Refetoff S: Thyroid hormone therapy. Med Clin North Am 59:1147–1162, 1975.
6. Hays MT: Absorption of oral thyroxine in man. J Clin Endocrinol 28:749–756, 1968.
7. Read DG, Hays MT, Hershman JM: Absorption of oral thyroxine in hypothyroid and normal man. J Clin Endocrinol 30:798–799, 1970.
8. Evered D, Young ET, Ormston BJ, et al: Treatment of hypothyroidism: a reappraisal of thyroxine therapy. Br Med J 3:131–134, 1973.
9. Wallack MS, Adelberg HM, Nicoloff JT: A thyroid suppression test using a single dose of L-thyroxine. N Engl J Med 283:402–405, 1970.
10. Wenzel KW, Meinhold H: Evidence of lower toxicity during thyroxine suppression after a single 3 mg L-thyroxine dose: comparison to the classical L-triiodothyronine test for thyroid suppressibility. J Clin Endocrinol 38:902–905, 1974.
11. Carter JN, Corcoran JM, Eastman CJ, et al: Effect of severe chronic illness on thyroid function. Lancet 2:971–974, 1974.
12. Means JH, Hertz S, Lerman J: The pituitary type of myxedema or Simmonds disease masquerading as myxedema. Trans Assoc Am Physicians 55:32–53, 1940.
13. Northcutt RC, Stiel JN, Hollifield JW, et al: The influence of cholestyramine on thyroxine absorption. JAMA 208:1857–1861, 1969.
14. Cavalieri RR, Sung LC, Becker CE: Effects of phenobarbital on thyroxine and triiodothyronine kinetics in Graves' disease. J Clin Endocrinol 37:308–316, 1973.
15. Hansen JM, Skorsted L, Lauridsen UB, et al: The effect of diphenylhydantoin on thyroid function. J Clin Endocrinol 39:785–789, 1974.

16. Larsen PR, Atkinson AJ, Wellman HN, et al: The effect of diphenylhydantoin on thyroxine metabolism in man. J Clin Invest 49:1266–1279, 1970.
17. Tomkins GM, McGuire JS: The effect of thyroid hormones on adrenal steroid metabolism. Ann NY Acad Sci 86:600–604, 1960.
18. Hellman L, Bradlow HL, Zunoff B, et al: The influence of thyroid hormone on hydrocortisone production and metabolism. J Clin Endocrinol 21:1231–1247, 1961.
19. Crooks J, Hedley AJ, MacNee C, et al: Changes in drug metabolizing ability in thyroid disease. Br J Pharmacol 49:156P–157P, 1975.
20. Doherty JE, Perkins WH: Digoxin metabolism in hypo- and hyperthyroidism. Ann Intern Med 64:489–507, 1966.
21. Bibliography: Drug interferences with clinical laboratory tests. Clin Chem 18:1160, 1972.
22. Stock JM, Surks MI, Oppenheimer JH: Replacement dosage of L-thyroxine in hypothyroidism. A re-evaluation. N Engl J Med 290:529–533, 1974.
23. Cotton GE, Gorman CA, Mayberry WE: Suppression of thyrotropin (h-TSH) in serums of patients with myxedema of varying etiology treated with thyroid hormones. N Engl J Med 285:529–533, 1971.
24. Maeda M, Kuzuya N, Masuyama Y, et al: Changes in serum triiodothyronine, thyroxine and thyrotropin during treatment with thyroxine in severe primary hypothyroidism. J Clin Endocrinol 43:10–17, 1976.
25. Hershman JM, Pittman JA: Utility of the radioimmunoassay of serum thyrotropin in man. Ann Intern Med 74:481–490, 1971.
26. Holvey DN, Goodner CJ, Nicoloff JT, et al: Treatment of myxedema coma with intravenous thyroxine. Arch Intern Med 113:89–96, 1964.
27. Green WL: Guideline for the treatment of myxedema. Med Clin North Am 52:431–450, 1968.
28. Pittman JA: Thyrotropin-releasing hormone. Adv Intern Med 19:303–325, 1974.
29. Mangieri CN, Lund MH: Potency of United States Pharmacopeia desiccated thyroid tablets as determined by the antigoitrogenic assay in rats. J Clin Endocrinol 30:102–104, 1970.
30. Pileggi VJ, Golub OJ, Lee ND: Determination of thyroxine and triiodothyronine in commercial preparation of desiccated thyroid and thyroid extract. J Clin Endocrinol 25:949–956, 1965.
31. Braverman LE, Ingbar SH: Anomalous effects of certain preparations of desiccated thyroid on serum protein bound iodine. N Engl J Med 270:439–442, 1964.
32. Gross J, Pitt-Rivers R: 3:5:3′-triiodothyronine. 2. Physiological activity. Biochem J 53:652–657, 1953.
33. Blackburn CM, McConahey WM, Keating FR, et al: Calorigenic effects of single IV doses of L-triiodothyronine and L-thyroxine in myxedematous patients. J Clin Invest 33:819–824, 1954.
34. Lieblich J, Utiger RD: Triiodothyronine radioimmunoassay. J Clin Invest 51:157–166, 1972.
35. Hays MT: Absorption of triiodothyronine in man. J Clin Endocrinol 30:675–679, 1970.
36. Burke G: The triiodothyronine suppression test. Am J Med 42:600–608, 1967.
37. Selenkow HA, Wool MS: A new synthetic thyroid hormone combination for clinical therapy. Ann Intern Med 67:90–99, 1969.
38. Smith RN, Taylor SA, Massey JC: Controlled clinical trial of combined triiodothyronine and thyroxine in the treatment of hypothyroidism. Br Med J 4:145–148, 1970.

54. ANTITHYROID AGENTS

Ivor M. D. Jackson and William E. Cobb

Hyperthyroidism is usually due to diffuse thyroid hyperplasia (Graves' disease), less often to one or more autonomous thyroid nodules (Plummer's disease), and occasionally to subacute or to 'silent' thyroiditis. Rare causes of hyperthyroidism include surreptitious ingestion of thyroid hormone, overproduction of thyroid stimulating hormone (TSH) by a pituitary adenoma, secretion of a TSH-like product from neoplastic tissue (eg, choriocarcinoma), and excess thyroid hormone secretion from toxic metastatic thyroid carcinoma or from ectopic thyroid tissue in an ovarian teratoma (struma ovarii). Possible therapeutic approaches include: reduction of circulating thyroid hormone levels by drugs that interfere with the synthesis, release or peripheral effects of thyroid hormone, radioactive iodine, and surgery. Precise guidelines for choice of a given modality are not established. This chapter outlines the properties and potential clinical role of antithyroid drugs in the treatment of hyperthyroidism. Table 1 describes drug therapy for specific indications.

DRUG MONOGRAPHS

THIONAMIDES

PROPYLTHIOURACIL
METHIMAZOLE (Tapazole)

Thionamides are the most important agents available for long-term control of thyrotoxicosis caused by a hyperfunctioning thyroid gland.[1-3] They prevent thyroid hormone synthesis by inhibiting the coupling of iodotyrosines, and possibly also by retarding the oxidation and organic binding of thyroid iodide. Propylthiouracil (PTU) and methimazole have short plasma half-lives[4] (less than 6 hours), but the relation of this to the optimal frequency of

TABLE 1 Drugs Used to Treat Hyperthyroidism According to Specific Indications

Indication	First Choice	Second Choice	Adjuncts
Graves' disease	(1a) propylthiouracil 100–150 mg every 8 hours *OR* (1b) methimazole 10–15 mg every 8 hours *AND/OR* (2) $Na^{131}I^{a}$ 3–10 mCi	(1) propranolol 10–40 mg four times a day	(1) propranolol 10–40 mg four times a day
To render euthyroid prior to thyroidectomy	(1) thionamides (dosage same as for Graves' disease)	(1) propanolol (dosage same as for Graves' disease)	(1) propanolol 10–40 mg four times a day (2) iodides 25–100 mg every 8 hours (1 or 2 drops of SSKI *or* 3 to 5 drops of strong iodine solution) *after* control of hyperthyroidism and for 1–2 weeks *prior* to surgery
Persistent or recurrent hyperthyroidism after surgery or $Na^{131}I$ treatment of Graves' disease	(1) thionamides (dosage same as for Graves' disease)	(1) iodides (may be used as the drug of First Choice, especially after treatment with $Na^{131}I$) *OR* (2) lithium 600–1200 mg daily in divided doses	(1) propranolol 10–40 mg four times a day

Thyroid storm	(1) propylthiouracil 200 mg every 4 hours on the first day *AND* (2) iodides (started 1 hour after first dose of propylthiouracil) 500 mg every 4 hours orally (10 drops of SSKI *or* 7.5 ml of strong iodine solution) *OR* 1–2 g of sodium iodide intravenously every 24 hours	(1) propanolol 1–5 mg intravenously every 4 hours *OR* (2) reserpine 2.5–5 mg intramuscularly every 8 hours	(1) propanolol 1–5 mg IV every 4 hours *OR* (2) reserpine 2.5–5 mg intramuscularly every 8 hours
Toxic multinodular goiter (or single toxic nodule[b])	(1) $Na^{131}I$ 15–25 mCi[a]	(1) thionamides (dosage same as for Graves' disease) (2) propranolol (dosage same as for Graves' disease)	(1) propranolol (dosage same as for Graves' disease)
Subacute thyroiditis	(1) propranolol 10–40 mg four times a day	(1) prednisone 10–40 four times a day	(1) aspirin 650 mg every 4–6 hours *OR* (2) prednisone 10–40 mg four times a day

TABLE 1 *(continued)*

INDICATION	FIRST CHOICE	SECOND CHOICE	ADJUNCTS
Neonatal Graves' Disease	(1) propylthiouracil 5–10 mg/kg/day in divided doses every 8 hours *AND* (2) iodides (started 1 hour after first dose of PTU) 8 mg every 8 hours orally (1 drop of strong iodine solution) *AND in severe cases* (3) prednisone 0.5 mg/kg every 6 hours		(1) propranolol 0.5 mg/kg every 6 hours
Other[c]			

Note: Initial dosage in parentheses; see text for maintenance dosage.

[a]Patients who are to receive therapeutic doses of $Na^{131}I$ should, in general, be first made euthyroid with antithyroid drugs *(see text).*

[b]Surgery may be preferred treatment for a single toxic nodule.

[c]The primary treatment of "other" causes of hyperthyroidism is directed at the underlying disorder. Thionamides may be of value in controlling hyperthyroidism which is dependent on active synthesis of hormone by thyroid tissue such as metastatic toxic thyroid carcinoma, TSH producing pituitary adenoma struma ovarii and choriocarcinoma. Propranolol may also be used to control manifestations of hyperthyroidism in these disorders and is probably the drug of choice in symptomatic hyperthyroidism due to iodide-induced or factitious thyrotoxicosis.

TABLE 2 Preparations and Costs of Antithyroid Agents

Generic Name	Trademark Name(s)	Preparations and 1978 Costs
Thionamides		
Propylthiouracil	generic	Tablets 50 mg—$1.06–$4.20/100
Methimazole	Tapazole	Tablets 5 mg—$2.75/100; 10 mg—$4.37/100
Iodine		
Potassium Iodide Solution, USP	generic	Solution—$7.50–$14.80/pint
Strong Iodine Solution, USP (Lugol's Solution)	generic	Solution—$2.00–$5.20/pint
Sodium Iodide	generic	Injection (solution) 100 mg/ml—$0.32–$0.96/10 ml
Sodium Iodide ^{131}I	Iodotope I-131	—
	Oriodid-I-131	—
	Theriodide-131	—
Andrenergic Antagonists		
Propranolol	Inderal	Tablets 10 mg—$4.10/100; 40 mg—$7.08/100; 80 mg—$11.32/100 Injection (solution) 1 mg/ml—$0.61/1-ml ampul
Reserpine	generic	Tablets 0.25 mg—$0.48–$1.25/100 Injection (solution) 2.5 mg/ml—$0.51/2-ml ampul
Miscellaneous		
Lithium Carbonate	Eskalith (Lithionate) (Lithane)	Capsules 300 mg—$3.00/100

administration is not clear. Some patients can be maintained on a once-daily dose,[5,6] suggesting that trapping of thionamides in the thyroid is more important than serum concentration in controlling hormone synthesis. Other patients require dosing every 6 to 8 hours for effective control of hyperthyroidism.

Thionamides are usually prescribed to control hyperthyroidism for a specified period of time in anticipation of a spontaneous remission of Graves' disease or prior to radioactive iodine or thyroidectomy. Prolonged use is feasible in patients with unremitting hyperthyroidism who either do not wish to be treated by or are unsuitable candidates for surgery or radioactive iodine.

Remission of Graves' disease after 12 to 24 months of treatment with thionamides is becoming less frequent, declining from 50 to 80% of cases in the early history of thionamide use to as low as 14% more recently.[7] This change has been related to a higher average dietary iodine content in recent years.[7] A long-term remission after stopping antithyroid therapy is seen more often in patients who initially present with a small goiter or triiodothyronine toxicosis.[8] The minimum duration of treatment required before assessing whether spontaneous remission has occurred is not clearly established. It has been generally accepted that the patient should be euthyroid for a minimum of one year on drugs before attempting to taper below maintenance levels, but a recent study of short-term antithyroid therapy (4 to 5 months total treatment time) has resulted in a remission rate which approximates that of the longer regimens.[8]

Initial drug treatment of thyrotoxicosis is required in all patients undergoing thyroidectomy. Propylthiouracil or methimazole may be used to render patients euthyroid and the pre-operative addition of iodide decreases thyroid vascularity. (See also the monographs on iodide and propranolol).

Thionamides may be administered prior to radioiodine therapy and thereby lower the risk of exacerbation of the thyrotoxic state due to radiation thyroiditis. Following radioiodine therapy, thionamides may be needed since two to six months is the average time required for definitive effect of radioiodine.

Thionamides are initially administered in high doses in the management of thyroid storm.[9] The first dose should be given prior to iodide administration to prevent intrathyroidal iodine accumulation. Propylthiouracil is theoretically more effective in thyroid storm because, unlike methimazole, it blocks the extrathyroidal conversion of thyroxine (T_4) to triiodothyronine (T_3).[10]

Thionamides readily cross the placenta and may cause fetal hypothyroidism,[11] but this is not likely to occur if the maintenance dose of propylthiouracil does not exceed 100 to 150 mg per day. Thionamides may be used by themselves[12] or prior to thyroidectomy in the management of maternal hyperthyroidism.[12–15] The concurrent administration of thyroid hormone has been suggested as a way to reduce the risk of thionamide-induced fetal hypothyroidism. This approach is unnecessary[13] and creates an additional risk to the fetus because it may increase the requirement for antithyroid drugs, and thionamides, but not thyroid hormone, readily cross the placenta. Breast feeding should be discouraged because thionamides are secreted in milk.[14]

Carbimazole, a carbethoxy derivative of methimazole, is the most widely used thionamide in Great Britain. It is converted to methimazole in the body, and its dosage and clinical indication are about the same as those of methimazole.

Adverse Reactions—Common minor reactions, such as altered taste sensation (dysgeusia) or mild hair loss, may be related primarily to the underlying disease. The appearance of skin rash suggests sensitivity and the offending drug should be discontinued. The most serious adverse reaction is agranulocytosis, which occurs with an overall incidence of 0.2 to 1.6%.[16,17] Physicians should anticipate its occurrence within the first two months of treatment and advise patients to report immediately any unexplained fever, sore throat and malaise. Screening blood counts is less reliable. Less frequently, autoimmune phenomena may occur. Arthralgias, vasculitis,[17,18] and 'lupus-like' syndromes, with or without positive serum levels of anti-nuclear antibody or lupus preparations, may[17] or may not[19] be dose-dependent. Hepatitis is more common with methimazole, and may be prolonged.[20] Chronic active hepatitis has been seen with propylthiouracil.[21] Paradoxically PTU has been shown to reverse the histologic changes of alcoholic hepatitis in the rat[22] and has been proposed as a possible treatment for this condition in man.[23] Propylthiouracil, but not methimazole, may rarely have a coumarin-like anticoagulant effect which usually, but not always, responds to vitamin K.[24] Rarely, aplastic anemia, pancytopenia, and hemolytic anemia occur. Methimazole has been associated with the development of scalp lesions, including aplasia cutis, in the offspring of mothers treated in pregnancy.[25]

Dosage—Oral: Adults, initially, propylthiouracil (100 to 150 mg) or methimazole (10 to 15 mg) every 6 hours for 6 to 8 weeks. In severe cases up to 1,200 mg of propylthiouracil (or 120 mg methimazole) daily may be required. Maintenance doses are variable, but the daily dose is usually one-third to two-thirds of the starting dose and is given at 6 to 12 hourly intervals. In some cases a single daily dose will suffice. In thyrotoxic crisis, 200 mg of propylthiouracil (or 20 mg of methimazole) is given every 4 hours during the first day. No commercial parenteral preparations are available. However, methimazole may be dissolved in normal saline and heat-sterilized for parenteral use.

IODINE

POTASSIUM IODIDE
SODIUM IODIDE
STRONG IODINE SOLUTION

Inorganic iodide is the most important therapeutic agent for the *emergency* treatment of thyrotoxicosis, and is especially valuable for thyrotoxic crisis,[9] in circumstances where an intravenous preparation is required for rapid control of thyrotoxicosis (eg, when emergency non-thyroid surgery is indicated) and for preoperative use to reduce the vascularity of the thyroid gland.[26] Iodine is usually ineffective by itself as the primary treatment of thyrotoxicosis,[27] since 'escape' may occur after 2 to 3 weeks. However, if the thyroid gland has previously been treated with ^{131}I, the thyrotoxicosis can be satisfactorily controlled by iodide alone.[28]

Adverse Reactions—Iodides may precipitate thyrotoxicosis when given to patients with nodular goiters,[29] or in euthyroid patients with autonomous thyroid function (eg, during remission of hyperthyroidism following a course of thionamides).[30] In patients with chronic thyroiditis, previous radioiodine therapy or thyroidectomy, iodides may induce hypothyroidism.[29]

Toxic reactions to iodine occur, especially with large doses. They include skin rashes, drug fever, sialadentitis, conjunctivitis, rhinitis, and conditions resembling polyarteritis such as thrombotic thrombocytopenic purpura and a leukemoid eosinophilia. If these reactions occur, the iodide should be stopped.[1]

Dosage—Oral: Adults and children, although 6 mg/day is reported to produce maximal inhibition of thyroid hormone release, the doses usually prescribed are much higher.[31] The usual dose is 1 or 2 drops of a saturated solution of potassium iodide [SSKI] (50 mg iodide per drop), three times a day. Alternatively, Strong Iodine Solution, USP, [Lugol's solution] (8.3 mg iodide per drop), in a dose of 3 to 5 drops, three times a day, may be used. *Intravenous:* sodium iodide, 1 to 2 g daily.

SODIUM IODIDE ^{131}I

^{131}I is effective treatment for hyperthyroidism caused by Graves' disease or toxic nodular goiter (single or multiple nodules).[32] Successful use has also been described in children,[33,34] but neither the carcinogenic potential nor the adverse effect of resultant hypothyroidism upon growth have been fully evaluated in follow-up studies. Therefore, the use of radioactive iodine in children is not fully acceptable primary therapy.[35]

Adverse Reactions—Although permanent cure of hyperthyroidism with one or more doses of ^{131}I is expected, the high incidence of subsequent hypothyroidism is a major drawback. Hypothyroidism may occur in the first (early) or subsequent (late) years, probably reflecting two separate mechanisms.[36] Early hypothyroidism is dose-dependent, its incidence being dramatically reduced by low dose schedule, while late hypothyroidism has approximately the same cumulative yearly incidence regardless of the dose used.[28,37] Serum thyroid stimulating hormone (TSH) is frequently elevated following treatment but normal levels generally rule out the risk of hypothyroidism developing during the next two years.[38] Theoretical considerations[39] have led to the alternative use of ^{125}I, but in the doses employed no significant alteration in the incidence of hypothyroidism has been noted.[40]

The occurrence of thyroid carcinoma is no greater with ^{131}I than with medical therapy or surgery.[41]

Radiation thyroiditis, manifested as a local discomfort, may occur shortly after a dose of radioiodine. It is usually transient and will respond to salicylates or, in severe cases, to corticosteroids. Exacerbation of thyrotoxicosis from radiation thyroiditis, which may occur 5 to 17 days after a dose of radioiodine, is a potentially serious complication, especially in the older patient with heart disease. Administration of an antithyroid drug for several weeks prior to radioiodine depletes glandular hormone stores and prevents an abrupt release of thyroid hormone should radiation thyroiditis occur.

It has been suggested that exophthalmos may be adversely effected by ^{131}I therapy.[42]

Dosage—Oral: Toxic nodule[43] or multinodular goiter: 15 to 25 millicuries (mCi), or more, for the initial dose. Diffuse toxic goiter: although goiter size, gland susceptibility and uptake of radioactive iodine are important theoretical variables in determining dose, the relative contributions of each is difficult to determine in practice.[28] We recommend an intermediate initial dose (5–10 mCi). Lower doses (2–5 mCi) produce early hypothyroidism less frequently, but repeated doses are needed more often.[44] High doses (12.5–15 mCi) and radioablative doses[45,46] may be used when the mass of functioning tissue is very large, or where recurrent hyperthyroidism would be more detrimental than ^{131}I-induced hypothyroidism. A decision to give additional ^{131}I should be deferred for a minimum of four to six months.[44] Patients with only mild residual hyperthyroidism can frequently be maintained on antithyroid medication (see section on thionamides and iodide) for a year or more before a decision is made.

ADRENERGIC ANTAGONISTS

PROPRANOLOL (Inderal)

Propranolol, by beta adrenergic antagonism,[47,48] inhibits the manifestations of thyrotoxicosis mediated through the sympathetic nervous system and, by a poorly understood effect on the peripheral degradation of thyroid hormone, lowers the serum level of triiodothyronine.[49,50] The latter effect may be accompanied by a small rise in serum thyroxine.[50] Propranolol results in rapid improvement of tachycardia, diaphoresis, restlessness, tremor, hyperreflexia, and pulse pressure in most patients with thyrotoxicosis, but may have minimal or no effect on lid lag, stare, and oxygen consumption.[47,48] The exophthalmos and pre-tibial myxedema of Graves' disease are not affected by propranolol. Specific syndromes occurring in the context of thyrotoxicosis such as proximal myopathy,[51] periodic paralysis[52] and hypercalcemia[53] may respond to propranolol prior to chemical control of hyperthyroidism.

Propranolol is used most frequently in conjunction with antithyroid drugs or radioactive iodine[54] for short-term rapid control of tachycardia, tremor, restlessness, and diaphoresis. Propranolol is probably less effective than thionamides when used as the only drug in the long-term management of Graves' disease but it may be considered as alternative therapy in patients allergic to these agents.[55] Propranolol may be useful in the preoperative management of patients undergoing thyroidectomy because it provides excellent control of thyrotoxicosis in a short period of time and, like iodides, decreases the vascularity of thyroid tissue.[56,57] Thyrotoxicosis in pregnancy can be effectively managed with propranolol alone, but such use is controversial; transplacental passage and stimulation of myometrial activity pose potential problems.[58]

Propranolol may be an extremely useful adjunct in thyroid storm.[59] Life-threatening arrhythmias often respond promptly after intravenous doses and extreme pyrexia may improve with propranolol although this response is less well established.

In the hyperthyroidism of acute or 'silent' thyroiditis, wherein thionamides or ^{131}I are inappropriate, propranolol is the treatment of choice for the symptoms of thyrotoxicosis.[50a]

Adverse Reactions—The major adverse effects and contraindications of propranolol are related to its beta adrenergic blocking property. Thus, myocardial depression and congestive heart failure, exacerbation of chronic lung disease or asthma and hypoglycemia in susceptible individuals (eg, diabetics receiving insulin or oral hypoglycemics) are potential complications.[48] Propranolol should be discontinued 48 hours prior to surgery[60b] except when it is the only medication given for pre-operative management of thyroidectomy. In this setting propranolol should be continued up to the morning of surgery. Propranolol should not be prescribed for patients receiving drugs which elevate circulating catecholamines such as monoamine oxidase inhibitors.

Dosage—Oral: Initially 10 mg four times daily. This may be increased to 80 mg four times daily. *Intravenous:* 1 to 5 mg every 4 hours (but not more than 1 mg per minute).

RESERPINE

Reserpine, a sympathetic antagonist, is very effective in thyrotoxic crisis. It may be used when sedation might be beneficial (eg, an agitated patient), or where propranolol is contraindicated (asthma, congestive heart failure, diabetes). Reserpine is more effective by the intramuscular than the oral route; this is due to extensive first-pass metabolism.

Adverse Reactions—These include hypotension, mental depression and aggravation of underlying peptic ulcer disease. See Chapter 25, Antihypertensive Agents, for a more detailed description.

Dosage—Oral: 0.25 mg every 8 hours. *Intramuscular:* 2.5 to 5 mg every 8 hours.

CORTICOSTEROIDS

A number of corticosteroid effects on thyroid function are useful in the treatment of thyrotoxicosis. Large doses alter the peripheral mono-deiodination of T_4 resulting in a lower level of serum T_3 and higher level of the metabolically inactive isomer, reverse T_3.[61,63] In thyrotoxic, but not in normal patients, pharmacologic doses lower serum T_4 acutely, suggesting that corticosteroids may block thyroid gland stimulation by pathologic stimulators but not TSH.[64] A possible, but not yet proven, effect of long-term steroid treatment in Graves' disease is suppression of thyroid immunostimulator synthesis.

Large doses of corticosteroids are important in the medical treatment of severe Graves' ophthalmopathy[65,66] and, in combination with other drugs, in the management of thyroid storm. Hyperpyrexia, hypotension, and raised serum T_4 and T_3 levels are features of thyroid storm which respond well to corticosteroids. Steroids may be the preferred treatment in other situations when a prompt reduction in thyroid hormone levels is needed and where propranolol may be contraindicated (eg, a patient with severe heart failure and thyrotoxicosis). Steroid therapy may also be beneficial in reducing the thyroid discomfort of subacute thyroiditis and in treating the thyrotoxicosis of this condition as well as that caused by other disorders causing 'hyperthyroiditis'.[60a] The effect on the thyrotoxicosis is due both to a direct effect on the thyroid gland and a peripheral effect on T_4 conversion to T_3.

Corticosteroids have been used alone[67] to induce remission of Graves' disease, but the high incidence of long-term adverse effects (see Chapter 49) militates against their use as primary therapy.

Dosage—Oral: Prednisone, 10 to 20 mg every 6 hours; dexamethasone, 1 to 2 mg every 6 hours. *Intravenous:* Hydrocortisone 400 mg or dexamethasone 8 mg daily by infusion or in divided doses.

MISCELLANEOUS AGENTS

LITHIUM CARBONATE

Lithium carbonate can inhibit thyroid hormone release similarly to iodides. Although control of thyrotoxicosis may be achieved in patients refractory to other agents,[68] thyroid 'escape' is frequent[69] and thionamides may be required concurrently. Thyrotoxicosis may, in fact, appear in patients already receiving lithium for manic-depressive illness.

Adverse Reactions—Adverse effects are common and dose-dependent. Serum levels must be monitored and kept between 0.5 and 1 mEq/liter. Higher levels may produce tremor, ataxia, dizziness, confusion, coma, anorexia, nausea, vomiting, diarrhea, cardiac arrhythmia and shock.

Dosage—Oral: 600 to 1200 mg daily in divided doses.

OTHER MISCELLANEOUS AGENTS

Guanethidine, a postganglionic sympathetic blocker, is occasionally used. Its major drawbacks are postural hypotension, diarrhea, and impairment of male sexual function. Potassium perchlorate, which blocks thyroid trapping of iodide, is no longer used since it causes an unacceptably high incidence of aplastic anemia and nephrotic syndrome. Phenobarbital, which enhances biliary excretion of thyroid hormones, may be used to increase the rate of peripheral thyroid hormone turnover.

Dosage—Oral: Guanethidine, 10 to 50 mg every 8 hours; potassium perchlorate, 200 mg every 6 hours; phenobarbital, 30 to 60 mg three times daily.

REFERENCES

1. Jackson IMD: Management of thyrotoxicosis. Am J Hosp Pharm 32:933–939, 1975.
2. Vanderlaan WP: Antithyroid drugs in practice. Mayo Clin Proc 47:962–965, 1972.
3. Haibach H, Avioli LV: Hyperthroidism in Graves' disease. Current trend in management and diagnosis. Arch Intern Med 136:725–731, 1976.
4. McMurray JF, Gilliland PF, Ratliff CR, et al: Pharmacodynamics of propylthiouracil in normal and hyperthyroid subjects after a single oral dose. J Clin Endocrinol Metab 41:362–364, 1975.
5. Greer MA, Meihoff WC, Studer H: Treatment of hyperthyroidism with a single daily dose of propylthiouracil. N Engl J Med 272:888–891, 1965.
6. Wise PH, Marion M, Pain RW: Single-dose 'block-replace' drug therapy in hyperthyroidism. Br Med J 4:143–145, 1973.
7. Wartofsky L: Low remission after therapy for Graves' disease. JAMA 226:1083–1088, 1973.
8. Greer MA, Kammer H, Bouma DJ: Short-term antithyroid drug therapy for the thyrotoxicosis of Graves' disease. N Engl J Med 297:173–176, 1977.
9. Mackin JF, Canary JJ, Pittman CS: Thyroid storm and its management. N Engl J Med 291:1396–1398, 1974.
10. Abuid J, Larsen PR: Triiodothyronine and thyroxine in hyperthyroidism. Comparison of the acute changes during therapy with antithyroid agents. J Clin Invest 54:201–208, 1974.
11. Werner SC (Moderator): Two panel discussions of hyperthyroidism. J Clin Endocrinol Metab 27:1637–1654, 1967.

12. Mestman JH, Manning PR, Hodgman J, et al: Hyperthyroidism and pregnancy. Arch Intern Med 134:434–439, 1974.
13. Herbst AL, Selenkow HA: Hyperthyroidism during pregnancy. N Engl J Med 273:627–633, 1965.
14. Worley RJ, Crosby WM: Hyperthyroidism during pregnancy. Am J Obstet Gynecol 119:150–155, 1975.
15. Prout TE: Thyroid disease in pregnancy. Am J Obstet Gynecol 122:669–676, 1975.
16. McGarack TH, Chevalley J: Untoward hematologic responses to the antithyroid compounds. Am J Med 17:36–41, 1954.
17. Wiberg JJ, Nuttall FQ: Methimazole toxicity from high doses. Ann Intern Med 77:414–416, 1972.
18. Amrhein JA, Kenny FM, Ross D: Granulocytopenia, lupus-like syndrome and other complications of propylthiouracil therapy. J Pediatr 76:54–64, 1970.
19. Hung W, August GP: A 'collagen-like' syndrome associated with antithyroid therapy. J Pediatr 82:852–854, 1973.
20. Fischer MG, Nayer HR, Miller A: Methimazole-induced jaundice. JAMA 223:1028–1029, 1973.
21. Fedotin MS, Lefer LG: Liver disease caused by propylthiouracil. Arch Intern Med 135:319–321, 1975.
22. Israel Y, Kalant H, Orrego H, et al: Experimental alcohol-induced hepatic necrosis: suppresion by propylthiouracil. Proc Nat Acad Sci 72:1137–1141, 1975.
23. Isselbacher KJ: Metabolic and hepatic effects of alcohol. N Engl J Med 296:612–616, 1977.
24. Gotta AW, Sullivan CA, Seaman J, et al: Prolonged intraoperative bleeding caused by propylthiouracil-induced hypoprothrombinemia. Anesthesiology 37:562–563, 1972.
25. Burrow GN: The thyroid in pregnancy. Med Clin North Am 59:1089,1098, 1975.
26. Wartofsky L, Ransil BJ, Ingbar SH: Inhibition of iodine by the release of thyroxine from the thyroid glands of patients with thyrotoxicosis. J Clin Invest 49:78,86, 1970.
27. Emerson CH, Anderson AJ, Howard WJ, et al: Serum thyroxine and triiodothyronine concentrations during iodine treatment of hyperthyroidism. J Clin Endocrinol Metab 40:33–36, 1975.
28. Cevallos JL, Hagen GA, Maloof F, et al: Low-dosage ^{131}I therapy of thyrotoxicosis (diffuse goiters). N Engl J Med 290:141–143, 1974.
29. Vagenakis AG, Braverman LE: Adverse effects of iodides on thyroid function. Med Clin North Am 59:1075–1088, 1975.
30. Ermans AM, Camus M: Modifications of thyroid function induced by chronic administration of iodine in the presence of 'autonomous' thyroid tissue. Acta Endocrinol 70:463–475, 1972.
31. DeGroot LJ, Stanbury JB: *The Thyroid and Its Diseases,* 4th edition. New York, John Wiley and Sons, 1975, p. 126.
32. Werner SC, Ingbar SH: *The Thyroid,* 3rd edition. New York, Harper and Row, 1971, pp 697–704.
33. Hayek A, Chapman E, Crawford JD: Long-term results of treatment of thyrotoxicosis in children and adolescents with radioactive iodine. N Engl J Med 283:949–953, 1970.
34. Safa AM, Schumacher OP, Rodriquez-Antunez A: Long-term follow-up results in children and adolescents treated with radioactive iodine (^{131}I) for hyperthyroidism. N Engl J Med 292:167–171, 1975.
35. Braverman LE: Consequences of thyroid radiation in children (editorial). N Engl J Med 292:204–205, 1975.
36. Malone JF, Cullen MJ: Two mechanisms for hypothyroidism after ^{131}I therapy. Lancet 2:73–75, 1976.
37. Glennon JA, Gordon ES, Sawin CT: Hypothyroidism after low-dose ^{131}I treatment of hyperthyroidism. Ann Intern Med 76:721–723, 1972.
38. Toft AD, Irvine WJ, Hunter WM, et al: Plasma TSH and serum T_4 levels in long-term follow-up of patients treated with ^{131}I for thyrotoxicosis. Br Med J 3:152–153, 1974.
39. McDougall IR, Greig WR, Gillespie FC: Radioactive iodine (^{125}I) therapy for thyrotoxicosis. N Engl J Med 285:1099–1104, 1971.
40. Bremner WF, McDougall IR, Greig WR: Results of treating 297 thyrotoxic patients with ^{125}I. Lancet 2:281–282, 1973.
41. Dobyns BM, Sheline GE, Workman JB, et al: Malignant and benign neoplasms of the

thyroid in patients treated for hyperthyroidism: a report of the Cooperative Thyrotoxicosis Therapy Follow-Up Study. J Clin Endocrinol Metab 38:976–998, 1974.
42. Kriss JP, Pleshakov V, Rosenblum AL, et al: Studies on the pathogenesis of the ophthalmopathy of Graves' disease. J Clin Endocrinol Metab 27:582–593, 1967.
43. Hamburger JI: Solitary autonomously functioning thyroid lesions. Diagnosis, clinical features and pathogenetic considerations. Am J Med 58:740–748, 1975.
44. Sterling K: Radioactive iodine therapy. Med Clin North Am 59:121–122, 1975.
45. Volpe R, Desbarats-Schonbaum ML, Schonbaum E, et al: The effect of radioablation of the thyroid gland in Graves' disease with high levels of long-acting thyroid stimulator (LATS). Am J Med 46:217–226, 1969.
46. Wise PH, Burnet RB, Ahmad A et al: Intentional radioiodine ablation in Graves' disease. Lancet 2:1231–1233, 1975.
47. Shanks RG, Hadden DR, Lowe DC, et al: Controlled trial of propranolol in thyrotoxicosis. Lancet 1:993–994, 1969.
48. Levey GS: The heart and hyperthyroidism. Use of beta-adrenergic blocking drugs. Med Clin North Am 59:1193–1201, 1975.
49. Verhoeven RP, Visser TJ, Docter R, et al: Plasma thyroxine, 3,3α,5-triiodothyronine and 3,3α,5α-triiodothyronine during β-adrenergic blockade in hyperthyroidism. J Clin Endocrinol Metab 44:1002–1005, 1977.
50. Harrower ADB, Fyffe JA, Horn DB, et al: Thyroxine and triiodothyronine levels in hyperthyroid patients during treatment with propranolol. Clin Endocrinol 7:41–44, 1977.
51. Pimstone N, Marine N, Pimstone B: Beta adrenergic blockade in thyrotoxic myopathy. Lancet 2:1219,1220, 1968.
52. Conway M, Seibel JA, Eaton RP, et al: Thyrotoxicosis and periodic paralysis: improvement with beta blockade. Ann Intern Med 81:332–336, 1974.
53. Rude RK, Oldham SB, Singer FR, et al: Treatment of thyrotoxic hypercalcemia with propranolol. N Engl J Med 294:431–433, 1976.
54. Hadden DR, Montgomery DAD, Shanks RG, et al: Propranolol and iodine-131 in the management of thyrotoxicosis. Lancet 2:852–854, 1968.
55. Mazzaferri EL, Reynolds JC, Young RL, et al: Propranolol as primary therapy for thyrotoxicosis. Results of a long-term prospective study. Arch Intern Med 136:50–56, 1976.
56. Lee TC, Coffey RJ, Mackin J, et al: The use of propranolol in the surgical treatment of thyrotoxic patients. Ann Surg 177:643–647, 1974.
57. Tuft AD, Irvine WJ, McIntosh D, et al: Propranolol in the treatment of thyrotoxicosis by subtotal thyroidectomy. J Clin Endocrinol Metab 43:1312–1316, 1976.
58. Bullock JL, Harris RE, Young R: Treatment of thyrotoxicosis during pregnancy with propranolol. Am J Obstet Gynecol 121:242–245, 1975.
59. Das G, Krieger M: Treatment of thyrotoxic storm with intravenous administration of propranolol. Ann Intern Med 70:985–988, 1969.
60a. Jackson IMD: Hyperthyroiditis—a diagnostic pitfall. N Engl J Med 293:661–662, 1975.
60b. Faulkner SL, Hopkins JT, Boerth RC, et al: Time required for complete recovery from chronic propranolol therapy. N Engl J Med 289:607–611, 1973.
61. Duick DS, Warren DW, Nicoloff JT, et al: Effect of single dose dexamethasone on the concentration of serum triiodothyronine in man. J Clin Endocrinol Metab 39:1151–1154, 1974.
62. Chopra IJ, Williams DE, Orgiazzi J, et al: Opposite effects of dexamethasone on serum concentrations of 3,3α,5α-triiodothyronine (reverse T_3) and 3,3α,5-triiodothyronine (T_3). J Clin Endocrinol Metab 41:911–920, 1975.
63. Burr WA, Ransden DB, Griffiths RS, et al: Effect of a single dose of dexamethasone on serum concentrations of thyroid hormones. Lancet 2:58–61, 1976.
64. Williams DE, Chopra IJ, Orgiazzi J, et al: Acute effects of corticosteroids on thyroid activity in Graves' disease. J Clin Endocrinol Metab 41:354–361, 1975.
65. Werner SC: Prednisone in emergency treatment of malignant exophthalmos. Lancet 1:1004–1007, 1966.
66. Ivy KH: Medical approach to opthalmopathy of Graves' disease. Mayo Clin Proc 47:980–985, 1972.

67. Werner SC, Platman SR: Remission of hyperthyroidism (Graves' disease) and altered pattern of serum thyroxine binding induced by prednisone. Lancet 2:751–756, 1966.
68. Lazarus JH, Richards AR, Addison GM, et al: Treatment of thyrotoxicosis with lithium carbonate. Lancet 2:1160–1162, 1974.
69. Temple R, Berman M, Robbins J, et al: The use of lithium in the treatment of thyrotoxicosis. J Clin Invest 51:2746–2756, 1972.

DRUGS USED IN RESPIRATORY AND ALLERGIC DISORDERS

55. ANTIASTHMATIC DRUGS

Miles Weinberger and Leslie Hendeles

According to the American Thoracic Society, 'Asthma is a disease characterized by an increased responsiveness of the trachea and bronchi to various stimuli manifested by widespread narrowing of the airways that changes in severity either spontaneously or as a result of therapy.' 'Hyperreactive airway disease' or 'reversible obstructive airway disease' are common abbreviated versions of this definition. Evaluation of an asthmatic patient first requires confirmation of the diagnosis with documentation that airway pathophysiology conforms to the above definition. The presenting symptoms can vary from the classical picture of wheezing and acute dyspnea to chronic cough indistinguishable from chronic bronchitis. Dyspnea, manifested by shortness of breath or tightness in the chest following exertion, is common and may be the only complaint. Viral respiratory infections are major precipitants of asthma in children,[1,2] and many asthmatic infants or children first develop cough and respiratory distress during a 'cold.'

Rational therapeutic decisions require not only confirmation of the diagnosis but also characterization of the disease pattern from a detailed history and appropriate physiological measurements of the airway obstruction (Figure 1). The combined use of historical information and pulmonary function measurements allows consideration of chronicity, severity, and bronchodilator responsiveness in establishing a rational scheme for pharmacotherapy (Figure 2).[3]

COMPREHENSIVE APPROACH TO THE MANAGEMENT OF ASTHMA

Acute Symptoms

Acute symptoms are best treated initially by prompt use of an inhaled sympathomimetic (Figure 2). In an emergency room,

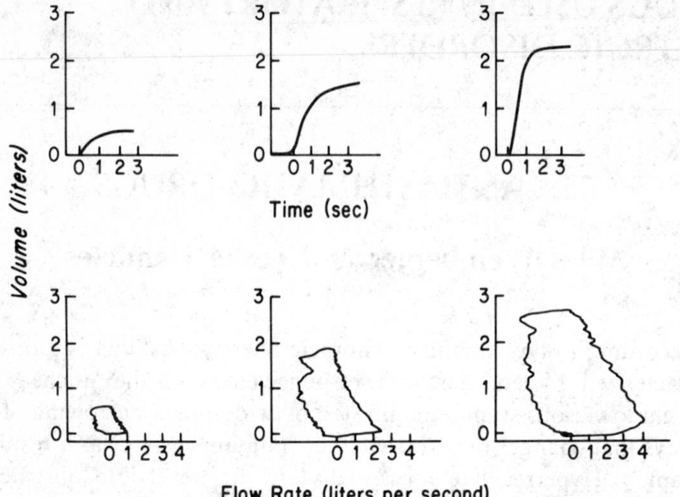

FIGURE 1. Time-volume (upper) and flow-volume (lower) spirometric tracings of a 12-year old boy with chronic asthma. The first tracings were after bronchodilator therapy at the time of his first visit. The second was performed after inhaled isoproterenol following 5 days of prednisone, 40 mg twice daily, and was associated with relief of asthmatic symptoms. Vital capacity, FEV_1, and flow rates all continued to improve and become normal after 5 more days of prednisone (third tracing). *Explanatory Note:* the time-volume tracing reflects the volume expired during a maximal forced expiration in relation to time. Airway obstruction is associated with slower air flow and incomplete emptying of the lungs during this maneuver. The flow-volume loop monitors and plots the flow rate during the same forced expiration. During expiration, a positive flow rate is indicated by a rapidly rising curve as expiration begins, rapid attainment of a peak flow rate, and a falling curve during the course of expiration until a zero flow rate again occurs at end expiration. Negative flow rates indicate inspiration.

injectable epinephrine or terbutaline may be substituted, but the goal of managing recurrent acute symptoms is to instruct the patient in home care where an inhaled sympathomimetic is generally more practical. Failure of an adequate response warrants rapid theophyllinization, ie, the administration of a loading dose of theophylline (5 to 7.5 mg/kg assuming no prior theophylline during the previous 24 hours), followed by continuous therapy designed to maintain serum theophylline concentrations of 10 to 20 μg/ml.[4] Repeat administration of an inhaled or parenteral sympathomimetic following the

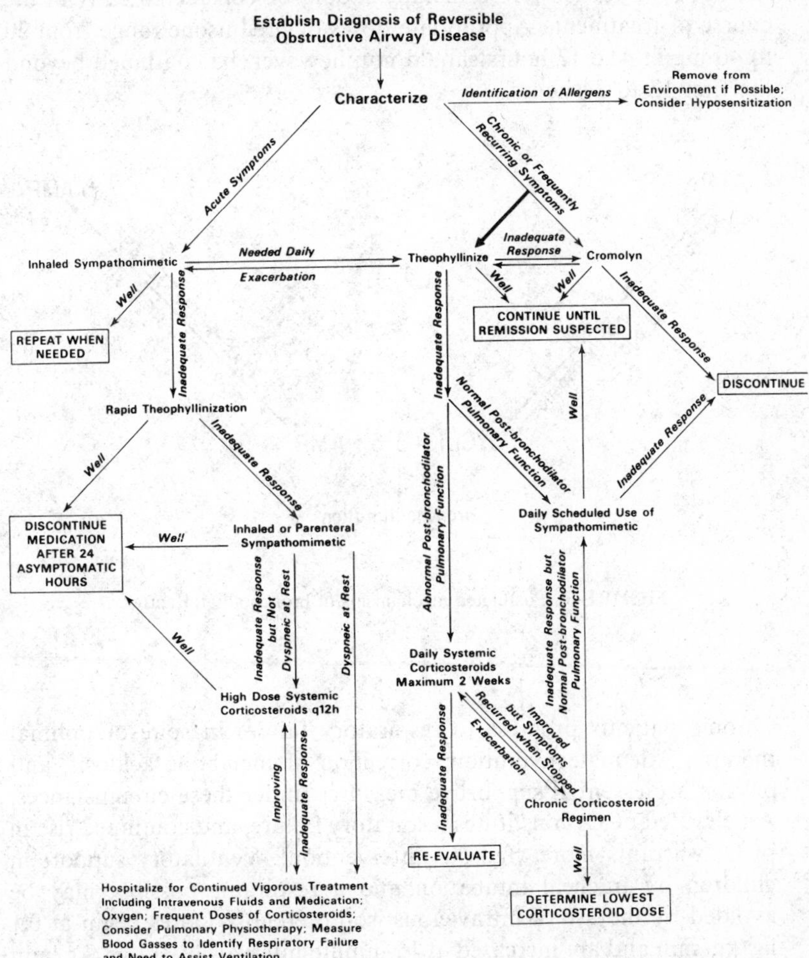

FIGURE 2. Outline of asthma management[3].

rapid theophyllinization is then indicated, since these bronchodilators may have additive effects (Figure 3). After bronchodilator responsiveness is rapidly evaluated, corticosteroids can be begun if signs and symptoms of active asthma remain after 1 to 2 hours. Since corticosteroids provide little clinical improvement for 8 to 12 hours, the need for corticosteroid therapy should be considered early in the course of treatment. Appropriate doses of prednisone range from 20 to 40 mg at 4 to 12 hours should not, however, be continued beyond the first 12 to 24 hours.

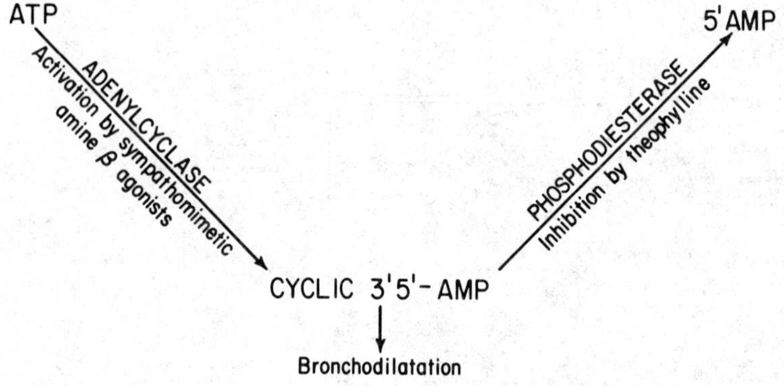

FIGURE 3. Postulated mechanisms of bronchodilator activity.

Some patients progress to respiratory failure in spite of optimal therapy. Adequate hydration, correction of metabolic acidosis, and oxygen are essential supportive measures under these circumstances. An elevated pCO_2 constitutes respiratory failure, and continued rise in pCO_2 warrants more vigorous intervention.[5] Ventilatory support in children by tracheal intubation and a respirator possibly may be avoided by the use of intravenous isoproterenol.[6] Doses begin at 0.1 μg/kg/min and are increased at 15-minute intervals by 0.1 μg/kg/min up to a maximum of 0.8 μg/kg/min. The electrocardiogram must be monitored for the development of arrhythmias or tachycardia exceeding 180 beats per minute; these adverse effects require prompt cessation of therapy or reduction of dosage. Intravenous isoproterenol therapy should only be employed in a well-equipped intensive care unit with personnel familiar with this treatment. Ventilatory assistance becomes necessary when other measures fail to reverse progressive hypercapnia.

Chronic Symptoms

A plan for suppression of chronic as well as acute disease becomes important when symptoms occur repeatedly or continually (Figure 2). Following initial relief of airway obstruction, theophyllinization is effective in suppressing further symptoms of chronic asthma.[7] Dosage should be started at 400 mg/day or 16 mg/kg/day, whichever is lower, and increased no more frequently than every third day until average therapeutic doses are reached, *if tolerated*.[8] These average doses are 900 mg/day or 13 mg/kg/day for adults (use the lower dose), 18 mg/kg/day for children 12 to 16 years old, 20 mg/kg/day for children 9 to 12 years old, and 24 mg/kg/day for children 6 months to 9 years old. Infants below 6 months of age have much lower dose requirements which are not well defined. More careful monitoring of serum theophylline is therefore warranted. Adverse effects necessitate omitting the next dose, then decreasing subsequent doses to the highest that was previously tolerated. At these doses, serum theophylline must then be measured to document whether the dose is appropriate or whether higher doses can be given safely.

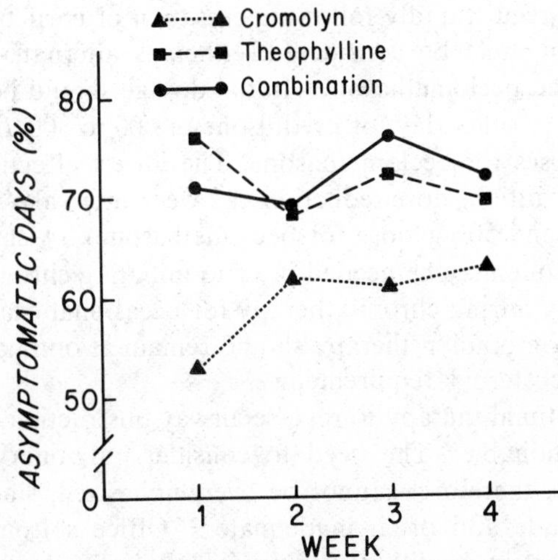

FIGURE 4. Asymptomatic days among 28 children with chronic asthma who received cromolyn (20 mg four times a day), theophylline in therapeutic doses (serum concentrations 10 to 20 μg/ml), and the two drugs together for four weeks each[7].

Some patients, such as young children and those with high dose requirements, may benefit from a reliable sustained-release preparation,[9,10] but only those products with reliable and complete absorption should be used.

An alternative to theophyllinization for initial therapy, although generally less effective, is cromolyn[7] (Figure 4). A few patients may not tolerate theophylline even in low dosage,[9] and clinical titration of theophylline dosage may be difficult. In the conventional dose of 20 mg four times a day, inhaled cromolyn may be effective without risk of acute toxicity (except for occasional allergic reactions[11]).

When symptoms are not fully controlled with theophylline, additional bronchodilator therapy may by indicated if pulmonary function testing demonstrates bronchodilator responsiveness to an inhaled or injected beta-agonist sympathomimetic. Bronchodilator-unresponsive airway obstruction that recurs during theophylline or cromolyn maintenance suggests the need for an additional short course of corticosteroids as described above. Repeated use of short courses (eg, less than 6 days) may be acceptable when exacerbations do not immediately follow cessation of corticosteroids, and they are required less frequently than once a month.

If symptoms recur rapidly following cessation of corticosteroids, a chronic regimen must be considered, either as alternate-day prednisone or inhaled beclomethasone. Initial dosage should be high, eg, 30 to 40 mg every other day for prednisone or 600 to 800 μg/day in 3 to 4 divided doses for beclomethasone. The lowest effective dose is determined by cautious dose reduction at 2 week intervals (5 mg/dose for prednisone and 50 μg/dose for beclomethasone). A short course of daily prednisone may be needed prior to initiating chronic therapy and additionally during chronic therapy for occasional exacerbation. Theophylline or cromolyn therapy should remain at optimal doses to minimize corticosteroid requirements.

Failure of optimal therapy to reverse airway obstruction makes the diagnosis questionable. The need to consider pulmonary function data in therapy, therefore, cannot be overemphasized, since clinical judgment is crude and often inadequate.[12] Office spirometry with simple equipment is readily available at reasonable cost.

Other therapeutic measures for asthma include consideration of environmental control and immunotherapy. In the asthmatic who chronically inhales tobacco smoke or is exposed to inhaled substances that result in bronchospasm, avoidance is more desirable than additional drugs. Immunotherapy (the injection of allergenic extracts to decrease sensitivity to inhaled allergens) is not proven to be effective *per se*[13] but may be rational when symptoms correlate well with the presence of inhaled allergens. Immunotherapy may be especially indicated when other symptoms of inhalant allergy, eg, allergic rhinitis and conjunctivitis, are present since these symptoms have been treated successfully with allergenic extracts in controlled studies.[14]

DRUG MONOGRAPHS

PARENTERAL SYMPATHOMIMETICS

Indications—Subcutaneous terbutaline or epinephrine is indicated for severe acute symptoms for patients in whom inhaled sympathomimetics are impractical or ineffective. They are particularly useful for severe dyspnea and in younger children and infants. Appropriately monitored intravenous isoproterenol may obviate mechanical ventilation in patients with respiratory failure.[5,6] Although not yet available in the United States, intravenous albuterol (salbutamol) appears as effective as single 1-hour infusions of aminophylline and may have fewer side effects in the initial treatment of patients with life-threatening asthma.[15]

Product Selection—At equal or higher doses, subcutaneous terbutaline may be somewhat more effective and longer-acting than epinephrine.[16] Terbutaline produces minor side effects (tremor) more frequently than epinephrine, but none are clinically serious. Terbutaline is much more costly than epinephrine (Table 1). In bronchospasm associated with anaphylactic reactions, however, epinephrine remains the agent of choice since it is both a bronchodilator as well as an alpha-adrenergic agonist necessary to reverse peripheral vascular collapse.

Aqueous suspensions of epinephrine (Sus-Phrine) appear to provide an initial dose of aqueous epinephrine and slowly release the remainder over several hours. However, the reliability of the releasing pattern is not adequately studied. Epinephrine in oil, also designed for sustained effect, is antiquated and should not be used. It requires intramuscular injection with a larger bore needle (terbutaline and Sus-Phrine are given subcutaneously), and it may cause sterile abscesses.

Adverse Reactions—Epinephrine stimulates alpha, $beta_1$ and $beta_2$ receptors, and produces transient hypertension, pallor, and urinary retention (in patients with benign prostatic hypertrophy). Tremors, palpitations, tachycardia, and, rarely, arrhythmias are potential adverse effects of beta stimulation. Central nervous system stimulation or headaches are common, and vomiting frequently follows administration to children. Tremors frequently follow subcutaneous administration of terbutaline. Although terbutaline has more selective $beta_2$ agonist effects at the 0.5 mg dose, it can considerably increase heart rate[16] and cardiac output.[17]

Intravenous isoproterenol will always produce a tachycardia (frequently with extrasystoles or other arrhythmias).

Drug Interactions—The bronchodilator efficacy of epinephrine may be decreased by systemic acidosis or concurrent use of propranolol. Bronchodilator response to epinephrine may be improved by correction of acidosis with sodium bicarbonate and treatment with theophylline and corticosteroids.[18]

Administration of epinephrine to patients taking chlorpromazine (Thorazine) or other alpha adrenergic blocking agents may produce a paradoxical hypotensive effect.[19] The alpha adrenergic effects of epinephrine may be accentuated by tricyclic antidepressants.[20]

Dosage, Preparations and Costs—See Table 1.

INHALED SYMPATHOMIMETICS

Indications—Aerosol sympathomimetics generally provide rapid and effective relief of asthmatic symptoms. They generally appear to be as effective as subcutaneous sympathomimetics but have fewer side effects and can be self-administered. The metered-dose inhaler is convenient, but administration may be difficult in the severely dyspneic patient or in a younger child. For these patients terbutaline can be more reliably administered if diluted in saline and given over a few minutes by an air-driven nebulizer (eg, Maximist, DeVilbiss). In contrast, administration by intermittent positive-pressure breathing (IPPB) equipment is discouraged, since it is of no additional value and incurs risks such as pneumothorax.

When used in recommended dosage and under supervision, inhaled sympathomimetics are extremely safe. The potential for overuse, however, with the subsequent possibility of paradoxical bronchoconstriction[21] and toxicity from both the drug and/or freon propellant,[22-25] warrants caution. Inhalants should be dispensed only by prescription, and not prescribed casually by emergency room or other physicians who cannot take full responsibility for ongoing clinical care. They should be used *only* as part of an overall program for asthma management. Inhalants can also be given prior to vigorous physical activity to prevent exercise-induced bronchospasm.[26,27]

Product Selection—Until albuterol (salbutamol) or terbutaline aerosol become available in the United States, metaproterenol remains the metered-dose inhaler of choice. It is equal to isoproterenol in peak intensity of effect with a more prolonged duration of action.[28] Terbutaline and albuterol are equal in peak intensity to isoproterenol and provide somewhat more prolonged bronchodilation than metaproterenol with no significant effect on the heart rate (when administered by this route).[29-31]

In infants, younger children, and others too dyspneic to effectively use the metaproterenol metered-dose inhaler, terbutaline can be administered by nebulizer; 1.0 mg of the injectable preparation is diluted with 2 ml of normal saline and nebulized by any adequate source of air or oxygen.

Adverse Reactions—Metaproterenol produces tachycardia more frequently than terbutaline or albuterol aerosols, but this rarely limits its use. Transient palpitations and tremors occur less commonly than by the oral route. Albuterol, metaproterenol, and terbutaline have thus far not produced the paradoxical 'locked lung' syndrome demonstrated with overusage of isoproterenol. Daily use of metaproterenol for 60 days, however, results in a decrease in the duration (but not intensity) of effect.[28]

Drug Interactions—Clinically important drug interactions have not been reported for inhaled metaproterenol, terbutaline or albuterol. Beta adrenergic blocking agents such as propranolol which may precipitate or aggravate bronchospasm might antagonize the bronchodilating effect of sympathomimetic aerosols.

Dosage—See Table 1.

Metaproterenol—1.3 mg (2 inhalations). Ambulatory patients should contact their physician if the 1.3 mg dose does not *completely* clear the symptoms, or if this dose must be repeated more than 2 times in any 24 hour period unless more frequent use has been prescribed previously.

TABLE 1 Dosage, Preparations, and Costs of Sympathomimetic Drugs

Generic Name	Trademark Name(s)	Dose: Adult	Dose: Pediatric	Frequency	Preparations and 1978 Costs
Parenteral—Subcutaneous					
Epinephrine Hydrochloride	Adrenalin Chloride			Every 20 minutes, 3 doses	Injection (solution) 1:1000 (1 mg/ml)—$0.19/1 ml ampul, $1.16/30 ml vial
Epinephrine	Sus-Phrine		0.01 ml/kg up to 0.25 mg	Do not repeat	Injection (aqueous suspension) 1:200 (5 mg/ml)—$1.19/0.5 ml ampul, $11.88/5 ml vial
Terbutaline Hydrochloride	Brethine (Bricanyl)			Every 30 minutes, 2 doses	Injection (solution) 1:1000 (1 mg/ml)—$0.82/1 ml ampul
Parenteral—Intravenous					
Isoproterenol Hydrochloride	Isuprel Hydrochloride	—	Begin with 0.1 μg/kg/min; increase by 0.1 μg/kg/min at 15-minute intervals until clinical response, heart rate greater than 180, or 0.8 μg/kg/min	Continuous infusion	Injection (solution) 1:5000 (0.2 mg/ml)—$0.79/1 ml ampul, $2.66/5 ml vial
Inhalation					
Metaproterenol Sulfate	Alupent (Metaprel)	2 inhalations (1.3 mg)	Same as adult	Every 2 to 4 hours[a]	Oral inhalation 0.65 mg/metered dose—$3.71/225 mg inhaler (300 doses)

Terbutaline	Brethine (Bricanyl)	0.9–1.0 mg diluted in 1.0 ml normal Saline; given in nebulizer	Same as adult	Every 2 to 4 hours[a]	(Inhaler not available but solution for injection may be used)
Oral					
Terbutaline	Brethine (Bricanyl)	2.5–5 mg	1.25–5 mg	4 times a day	Tablets 2.5 mg—$7.53/100; 5 mg—$10.05/100
Metaproterenol	Alupent (Metaprel)	20 mg	10–20 mg	4 times a day	Tablets 20 mg—$7.79/100. Syrup 10 mg/5 ml—$6.10/pt

[a]Some degree of tolerance, i.e., decreasing effect, may occur with continuous use of 4 times daily dosage; more frequent use is advised only for short periods when the patient is under medical supervision.

Terbutaline aerosol—0.25 to 0.5 mg may be administered every 2 to 4 hours as needed in hospitalized patients. Ambulatory patients should contact their physicians if inadequate response occurs or excessive frequency is required.

Preparations and Costs—See Table 1.

ORAL SYMPATHOMIMETICS

Indications—Ephedrine alone neither blocks exercise-induced bronchospasm[32] nor suppresses chronic asthmatic symptoms.[33,34] Thus, the role of such compounds in the management of chronic asthma is not well established. Like inhaled sympathomimetics, tolerance appears to occur with continued use.[35] Patients who have been optimally theophyllinized and still experience bronchospasm may thus benefit from the addition of daily oral sympathomimetic therapy. The delay in onset of action, however, makes them less desirable than the inhaled sympathomimetics for intermittent therapy of acute symptoms.

Product Selection—The newer agents all appear to have therapeutic advantages over ephedrine which is a weak bronchodilator.[36] Albuterol (not currently available in the United States) and terbutaline are equally effective and more potent than metaproterenol although the results of various studies are inconsistent.[37–39]

Adverse Reactions—Ephedrine can produce amphetamine-like central nervous system effects, increase blood pressure, and cause urinary retention in patients with benign prostatic hypertrophy. About one-third of patients experience tremors following oral administration of the more potent $beta_2$ agonists, terbutaline and albuterol.[37]

Drug Interactions—Ephedrine and theophylline exhibit synergistic toxicity; nausea, vomiting, nervousness, and headache occur with doses of the two drugs that are well tolerated individually.[34] This interaction has not been examined for the newer oral sympathomimetic agents. Monoamine oxidase inhibitors may potentiate the hypertensive effect of ephedrine.[40] This interaction has not been described for the newer agents that have minimal alpha adrenergic properties.

Dosage—To minimize tremors from oral terbutaline, the initial dose should be low, 1.25 to 2.5 mg every 8 hours, and gradually increased to 5 mg every 8 hours if tolerated; 7.5 mg every 8 hours in adults is more effective than 5 mg every 8 hours, but the frequency of side effects often outweighs the potential benefits.[38] Some patients develop tolerance to the tremors, but others require dose reduction or discontinuation. In those who cannot tolerate terbutaline, metaproterenol can be tried.

Preparations and Costs—See Table 1.

THEOPHYLLINE

Indications—Theophylline is used both for acute bronchodilation and chronic prophylaxis. The following summarizes recent findings pertinent to the rational clinical use of theophylline:

(1) Benefit and toxicity are related to theophylline serum concentration; 10 to 20 μg/ml is a conservative recommendation for the therapeutic range.[33,41–46]

(2) Theophylline dosage must be individualized to achieve serum levels in the therapeutic range because of individual pharmacokinetic variations.[8,9,42]

(3) Synergism for toxicity of theophylline and ephedrine has been demonstrated without significant additive therapeutic effect.[33,34]

(4) Addition of a basic compound such as ethylenediamine, choline (oxtriphylline), calcium salicylate, sodium glycinate, etc., increases theophylline solubility, probably by increasing the pH of the solution, but neither increases bioavailability nor decreases adverse effects.[47–49] The addition of alcohol has a similar effect though still without an increase in the rate or completeness of absorption.[50]

(5) Bioavailability of oral theophylline is excellent;[51] tablet dissolution appears to be the major rate limiting factor. Delayed-disintegration preparations may therefore yield erratic and decreased bioavailability.[10,52] However, this probably depends upon product design since sustained-release preparations with reliable and predictable absorption characteristics are available.[10]

(6) Rectal suppositories are poorly bioavailable.[52,53] Again, this probably is due to formulation rather than the administration site since rectal solutions are well absorbed.[53]

(7) Dyphylline is a stable derivative of theophylline (dihydroxypropyltheophylline) with a more rapid rate of disposition.[54] Its relative potency and toxicity are not defined and data do not currently justify its routine usage.

Product Selection—Parenteral theophylline is now available only under the irrational label of aminophylline U.S.P. This may contain anywhere from 78 to 85% theophylline with the remainder being ethylenediamine, an inactive ingredient. It is indicated *only* for intravenous and not for intramuscular use.

Theophylline solutions for oral administration are available in a variety of concentrations. Absorption is rapid and complete and appears unaffected by formulation or solubilizing agent. Thus, elixirs are therapeutically indistinguishable from other solutions. Taste is generally bad and individual preferences may be important in choosing specific products. Uncoated tablets are absorbed almost as rapidly as liquids. Both are suitable for acute therapy where the severity of symptoms does not justify parenteral medication.

A nonparenteral alternative to oral medication for acute therapy is the use of a rectal solution. Unlike suppositories, these are rapidly and completely absorbed.

Tablets or reliable sustained-release preparations are suitable for long-term therapy. Oral theophylline solutions may be used in small children, but the solid dosage form is less expensive and better tolerated if the child can swallow a pill or capsule (which many will quickly learn to do after they have tasted the liquid preparations). A recently released chewable tablet (Theophyl Chewable) may be preferred. An alternative for young children is the use of the beads from the inside of a *reliable* sustained-release capsule, administered as a sprinkling over a spoonful of soft food that can be swallowed without chewing; administration of the medication should be followed promptly by a drink to insure that the beads are all swallowed without disruption. Table 2 includes sustained-release products with acceptable bioavailability data. Other sustained-release products should not be used without adequate studies of the rate and completeness of absorption.

Adverse Reactions—The risk of toxicity increases progressively as serum concentrations exceed 20 μg/ml. At levels over 25 μg/ml, 75% of patients have some degree of toxicity such as nausea, headache, and insomnia and occasionally diarrhea and other minor complaints.[55] Serious toxicity, including cardiac arrhythmias, seizures, and death, have rarely been reported at serum concentrations under 40 μg/ml.[44,45] Even at these levels, some patients do not have obvious complaints. Less severe adverse effects do not necessarily precede seizure and death.

A few patients (about 2 to 3% of adults and 1% of children) do not tolerate theophylline at doses in the therapeutic range. Some will not tolerate theophylline at any dose. The limiting factor appears to be the caffeine-like side effects such as vague abdominal discomfort, insomnia, light-headedness, or the feeling of being 'spaced out'. A larger minority of patients will experience such effects transiently when therapy is initiated, particularly if therapy is not initiated at a sufficiently low dose. Most patients, however, become tolerant to these minor effects and are no longer bothered after a 1 to 3 week period. In a small number of individuals, low doses of phenobarbital or hydroxyzine have been used, with varying degrees of success, to ameliorate the side effects.

Drug Interactions—Theophylline and ephedrine have synergistic toxicity. Some measurable additive benefit for the combination can be observed when theophylline is used in lower doses, though the clinical importance of this is not clear.

The risk of theophylline toxicity is increased when administered with troleandomycin, a macrolide antibiotic.[56] The metabolic clearance of theophylline in the presence of 1 g/day of troleandomycin is decreased by 50%, resulting in serum concentrations that approximately double. Other macrolide antibiotics (eg, erythromycin) may similarly affect theophylline metabolism, although currently available data are limited.

Dosage—Acute therapy requires an initial loading dose of 1 mg/kg for each desired 2 μg/ml increase in serum theophylline concentration. If no theophylline has been administered in the previous 24 hours, 5 mg/kg of lean body weight by any rapidly absorbed route is a safe initial dosage with a 50% chance of exceeding 10 μg/ml and virtually no risk of exceeding 20 μg/ml. When essential, a second dose of 2.5 mg/kg may be tolerated within the next hour. Further doses should not be given immediately; a continuous infusion should instead be begun to maintain therapeutic serum concentrations (Table 3). The initial dose should be reduced if prior theophylline has been taken.

Chronic dosing requires individualization because of the wide range of clearances. The mean dose requirements have been determined for children and otherwise healthy adults with uncomplicated asthma (Figure 5). Requirements in adults, however, are also influenced by a variety of factors that may affect theophylline metabolism. Cigarette smoking[57] and unusually high protein diets[58] appear to increase theophylline metabolism, while heart failure and liver disease may decrease theophylline elimination.[45] When initiating chronic therapy, initial dosage should generally not exceed 16 mg/kg/day or 400 mg/day, whichever is smaller. Increases of 25% at approximately 3 day intervals can then be made until the appropriate age-specific maximum doses (see chronic therapy section of introduction) are reached (Figure 5) and no adverse effects occur.[59] Serum theophylline measurement should guide final dosage for optimal safety and efficacy.

Preparations and Costs—See Table 2.

CROMOLYN SODIUM (Aarane, Intal)

This drug, administered as an inhaled dry powder, represents a new approach to asthma management. It is neither a bronchodilator nor an anti-inflammatory agent and has no effects on acute symptoms of asthma. It does, however, act as a prophylactic agent and suppresses the symptoms of chronic asthma, probably by preventing or decreasing release of endogenous asthma-inducing chemical mediators. Cromolyn will block antigen-induced and, to a degree, exercise-induced bronchospasm.[60] Its efficacy, however, cannot be reliably predicted by the presence of inhalant allergy.[61]

Despite the unique mechanism of cromolyn, its actual potency is limited. Optimally administered theophylline is more effective than cromolyn in suppressing both exercise-induced bronchospasm[62] and the symptoms of chronic asthma.[7] In one collaborative study, both pulmonary function and freedom from asthmatic symptoms were greater with appropriate doses of theophylline than with recommended doses of cromolyn[7] (Figure 4). On the other hand, cromolyn is virtually nontoxic. Acute overdosage has not been reported and, other than a few allergic reactions, serious adverse effects appear rare.

Adverse Reactions—Chest tightness and coughing after inhalation occur in some patients though rarely of sufficient severity to limit therapy. These effects can sometimes be prevented by prior use of an inhaled sympathomimetic, and appears to be less frequent in patients already receiving theophylline. Occasional allergic reactions, manifested primarily by rash, are seen.[11] A suggestion of pulmonary infiltrates and eosinophilia have been reported. Renal toxicity has been reported in animals but not in humans.

Drug Interactions—None reported.

TABLE 2 Recommended Theophylline Preparations and Costs

Dosage Form	Trademark Name(s)	Anhydrous Theophylline Content	Alcohol Content	1978 Cost for 100 mg of Anhydrous Theophylline ($)
Tablet	Slo-Phyllin	100 mg		0.03
		200 mg		0.02
	Theophyl-225	225 mg		0.03
	Theolair	125 mg		0.05
		250 mg		0.04
Oral Liquid	Somophyllin-T	18 mg/ml	none	0.09
	Quibron Elixir[b]	10 mg/ml	15%	0.15
	Slo-Phyllin-GG[a,b]	5.3 mg/ml	none	0.14
	Theophyl-225 Elixir	7.5 mg/ml	5%	0.12
Sustained Release[c]	Slo-Phyllin Gyrocaps	60 mg		0.09
		125 mg		0.06
		250 mg		0.03
	Theo-Dur	100 mg		0.05
		200 mg		0.04
		300 mg		0.03
	Theophyl-SR	125 mg		0.05
		250 mg		0.03
Rectal Solution	Somophyllin	51 mg/ml		0.10
Intravenous Solution	(Aminophylline U.S.P.)	21 mg/ml		0.20

[a]Warning—These trademarked products are available in two or more preparations containing different concentrations of theophylline; only the most useful is listed. Prescriptions for these products should specify the theophylline concentration.

[b]Guaifenesin, included in this product, is not an active ingredient.

[c]Only those products with acceptable bioavailability data are listed.

Dosage—Children and adults—20 mg by inhalation four times daily. Larger or more frequent doses may provide additional benefit for a minority of patients. Cromolyn is administered by inhalation via a turbo-inhaler (Spinhaler) which punctures the cromolyn capsule and allows the powder to be aerosolized during inhalation. Multiple inhalations are generally necessary to empty the capsule.

Preparations and Costs—Intal capsules 20 mg—$10.70/60; Aarane capsules 20 mg—$10.74/60.

TABLE 3 Continuous Theophylline Dosage for Acutely Ill Patients Following an Initial Loading Dose

	INFUSION RATE (MG/KG/HR[a])
Children under 9 years	0.85
Children over 9 and otherwise healthy adults who smoke	0.75
Otherwise healthy nonsmoking adults	0.4
Cardiac decompensation or liver dysfunction	0.2

[a]These are guidlines for initial infusion rates of theophylline (aminophylline = theophylline/0.85). Final dosagae requirements may be higher or lower and should be guided by serum theophylline measurement.

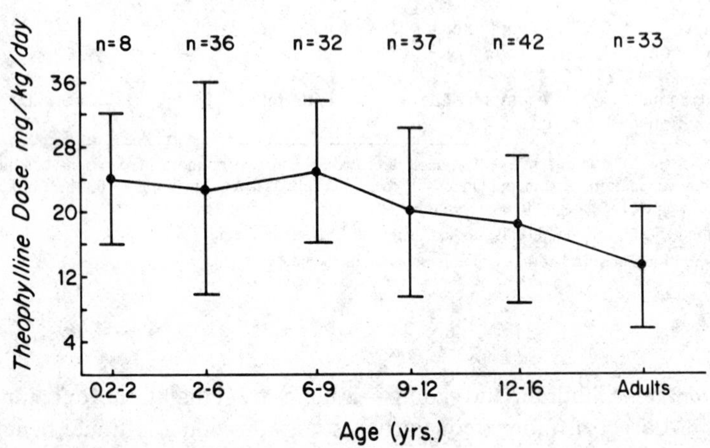

FIGURE 5. Theophylline dosage required to maintain therapeutic serum concentrations in 157 children and 33 adults with uncomplicated asthma receiving theophylline tablets or solution chronically[59].

CORTICOSTEROIDS

Indications—These are often the most potent drugs available for the treatment of asthma, but they also have potentially serious toxicity during long-term administration.

The mechanism of corticosteroid effects on asthma is not established. They do not affect the immediate response to antigen challenge (either by skin testing or inhalation)[63,64] nor do they inhibit exercise-induced bronchospasm[65] or other procedures for inducing experimental asthma, such as inhalation of methacholine or histamine. Clinically, however, corticosteroids stop production of the tenacious asthmatic mucous that is associated with cough and occasionally obstructs airways sufficiently to cause suffocation and death. It seems likely that the nonbronchospastic components of airway obstruction in asthma, mucosal edema and mucuous secretion, are manifestations of bronchial inflammation that are antagonized by corticosteroids. These drugs are most effective when used on a daily or multiple dose schedule. Fortunately, short-term corticosteroid use is virtually nontoxic even in very high doses. Thus, corticosteroids can freely be used for acute symptoms of asthma that are unresponsive to bronchodilators. Whether used acutely or for chronic therapy, however, bronchodilator therapy should be continued; corticosteroids thus are added and not substituted.

When corticosteroids are essential for control of asthma over extended periods of time, the mode of administration with the least risk of toxicity must be chosen. Even low daily doses, eg, 5 mg of prednisone daily, can suppress growth in children. Additionally, such doses may promote bone demineralization; long-term administration of steroids has been associated with vertebral compression fractures.

Appropriate corticosteroid administration schedules can minimize risk while maintaining benefit. Alternate day prednisone, even in relatively high doses, rarely results in clinically important toxicity[66–70] and, in fact, children with growth suppression from severe chronic asthma may have increased growth as a result of disease control. When used in low doses by inhalation, beclomethasone dipropionate and related medications not yet marketed in the United States (betamethasone valerate, triamcinolone acetonide, and others) represent a newer approach to relatively safe long-term suppressant therapy with corticosteroids.[71–73] Current data are insufficient to allow a rational choice between alternate day prednisone (in doses under 40 mg on alternate mornings) and beclomethasone (in doses under 800 μg/day).

Product Selection—Prednisone is rapidly converted *in vivo* to prednisolone, the active metabolite. Although both are commercially available, prednisone can be obtained in more varied dosage sizes in the United States and is less expensive. Bioavailability problems have been documented for some prednisone preparations; brand name and/or manufacturer should therefore be specified (Table 4). Methylprednisolone is about 1.2 times as potent as prednisone and prednisolone; this offers no particular advantage. These steroids are therapeutically equivalent and preferable to the naturally-occurring corticosteroids (cortisol and cortisone) because they have less sodium-retaining potential. Prednisone, prednisolone, and methylprednisolone are also preferable synthetic corticosteroids because their shorter duration of action decreases toxic potential during alternate-day chronic therapy. For acute symptoms, there is no therapeutic advantage to parenteral therapy, other than assurance of delivery.

Inhaled beclomethasone dipropionate is not indicated for acute symptoms, but is clearly preferable to any daily-dose oral corticosteroid for chronic therapy. The merits of this newer drug relative to alternate-day prednisone are not yet well defined. Beclomethasone is impractical for children too young to use the metered-dose inhaler properly.

Adverse Reactions—The long-term potential of excessive corticosteroid effect in children is substantial. Growth suppression, bone demineralization, muscle wasting, compression factures of vertebrae, posterior subcapsular cataracts, change in appearance due to redistribution of fat, and appetite stimulation all can occur[74] (Figure 6). These risks are reduced by alternate-day prednisone and daily use of inhaled beclomethasone, although their safety is dose-related. The risk of adrenal suppression increases as alternate-day prednisone doses exceed 40 mg and beclomethasone doses exceed 800 μg/day.

Drug Interactions—Corticosteroids may increase the sensitivity of beta adrenergic receptors in the lung and thereby enhance responsiveness to sympathomimetic bronchodilators.[18]

Additive adrenal suppressive effects may occur when inhaled beclomethasone and alternate-day prednisone are used simultaneously.

Dosage—For acute therapy, prednisone, prednisolone, or methyl-

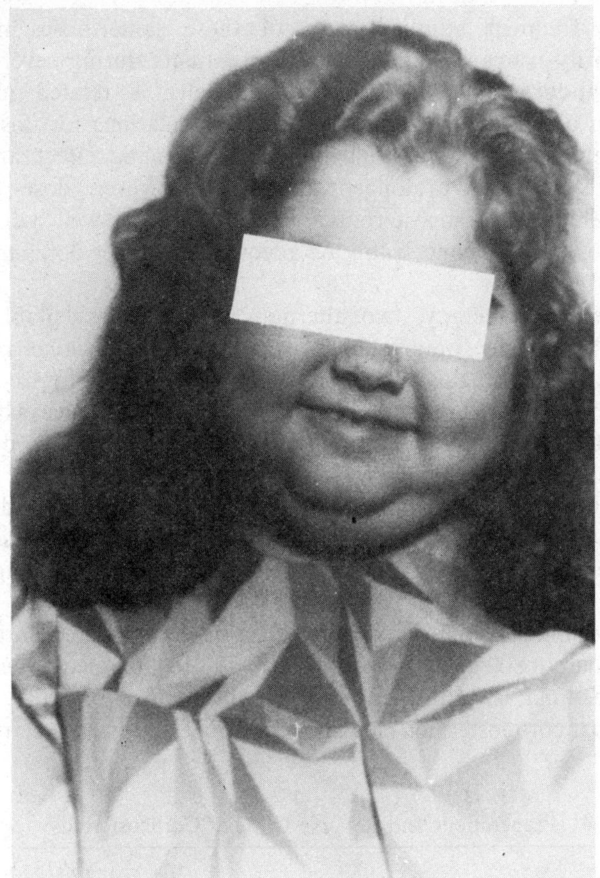

FIGURE 6. A 14-year old girl with asthma who received 40 mg of prednisone daily for 4 months.

prednisolone are given until the patient is free of active asthma. Five to ten days of therapy with the following empirically determined doses are usually sufficient:

Children under 1 year—10 mg twice daily
Children 1 to 4 years—20 mg twice daily
Children 5 to 11 years—30 mg twice daily
Children 12 and over—40 mg twice daily
Adults—40 mg twice daily

More frequent administration of these same doses may be temporarily warranted in hospitalized patients during severe acute exacerbations. Since corticosteroid toxicity is related more to duration of therapy than to dose, recommendations for dosage are arbitrarily high to assure maximal anti-asthmatic effect and thus minimize need for prolonged treatment. However, dose-response relationships for corticosteroids in asthma are not well defined (ie, lower doses might conceivably be adequate or higher doses might be more effective).

For chronic therapy, two alternatives provide acceptable risks:

(1) Prednisone, prednisolone, or methylprednisolone may be administered in single doses every 48 hours. After a short course of acute therapy with daily doses (see above) until active asthma is eliminated, alternate-day dosage is begun using 10 mg doses of prednisone or prednisolone for children under 1 year, 20 mg up to 3 years, 30 mg up to 6 years, and 40 mg for older children and adults. The lowest dose that controls the asthma should then be determined by lowering the dose by 5 mg at 2 to 4 week intervals so long as the disease is controlled.

(2) Beclomethasone dipropionate can be administered chronically in doses up to 800 μg/day by inhalation as 3 to 4 divided doses. After active asthma is controlled with a short course of daily oral or parenteral corticosteroids (see above), 800 μg/day can be started and

TABLE 4 Preparations and Relative Costs of Corticosteroids

Dosage Form	Generic Name	Trademark Name(s)	1978 Costs for 20 mg of Prednisone or Equivalent ($)
Tablet	Prednisone	Deltasone Orasone	0.08 0.07
	Prednisolone	Delta-Cortef	0.05 (5 mg)
	Methylprednisolone	Medrol	0.66 (16 mg)
Injection	Methylprednisolone Sodium Succinate	Solu-Medrol	1.92 (16 mg)
Aerosol	Beclomethasone diproprionate	Vanceril	0.32 (400 μg)

decreased by 150 to 200 μg/day increments at 2 to 4 week intervals until the lowest dose that controls asthmatic symptoms is established.

Preparations and Costs—See Table 4.

REFERENCES

1. McIntosh K, Ellis EF, Hoffman LS, et al: The association of viral and bacterial respiratory infections with exacerbations of wheezing in young asthmatic children. J Pediatr 82:578–590, 1973.
2. Minor TE, Dick EC, DeMeo HN, et al: Viruses as precipitants of asthmatic attacks in children. JAMA 227:290–298, 1974.
3. Weinberger M, Hendeles L: Pharmacotherapy of asthma. Am J Hosp Pharm 33:1071–1080, 1976.
4. Weinberger MM, Matthay R, Ginchansky E, et al: Intravenous aminophylline dosage: use of serum theophylline measurement for guidance. JAMA 235:2110–2113, 1976.
5. Cotton EK, Parry W: Treatment of status asthmaticus and respiratory failure. Pediatr Clin North Am 22:163–171- 1975.
6. Wood DW, Downes JJ, Scheinkopf H, et al: Intravenous isoproterenol in the management of respiratory failure in childhood status asthmaticus. J Allergy Clin Immunol 50:75–81, 1972.
7. Hambleton G, Weinberger M, Taylor J, et al: A collaborative study comparing the relative efficacy of cromolyn and theophylline in controlling the symptoms of chronic asthma. Lancet 1:381–385, 1977.
8. Weinberger M, Ginchansky E: Theophyllinization of the child with chronic asthma. In *Clinical Pharmacy and Clinical Pharmacology*. Edited by WA Gouveia, G Tognoni, E van der Kleijn. Amsterdam, North-Holland Publishing Company, 1976, pp 319–328.
9. Ginchansky E, Weinberger M: Relationship of theophylline clearance to oral dosage. J Pediatr 91:655–660, 1977.
10. Weinberger M, Hendeles L, Bighley L: The relation of formulation to absorption of oral theophylline. N Engl J Med 299:852–857, 1978.
11. Scheffer AL, Ross EP, Goetzl EJ: Immunologic components of hypersensitivity reactions to cromolyn sodium. N Engl J Med 293:1220–1224, 1975.
12. McFadden ER, Kiswer R, de Grout WJ: Acute bronchial asthma. Relations between clinical and physiologic manifestations. N Engl J Med 288:221–225, 1973.
13. Liechtenstein LM, Normas PS, Bruce CA, et al: Immunotherapy in extrinsic asthma. In *New Directions in Asthma*. Edited by M Stein. Park Ridge, Illinois, American College of Chest Physicians, 1975, pp 457–482.
14. Lichtenstein LM, Normas PS, Winkenwerder WL: A single year of immunotherapy for therapy for ragweed hay-fever. Immunologic and clinical studies. Ann Intern Med 75:663–671, 1971.
15. Williams SJ, Parrish RW, Seaton A: Comparison of intravenous aminophylline and salbutamol in severe asthma. Br Med J 4:685, 1975.
16. Schwartz HJ, Trautlein JJ, Goldstein AR: Acute effects of terbutaline and epinephrine on asthma. J Allergy Clin Immunol 58:516–522, 1976.
17. Amory DW, Burnham SC, Cheney FW Jr: Comparison of the cardiopulmonary effects of subcutaneously administered epinephrine and terbutaline in patients with reversible airway obstruction. Chest 67:279–286, 1975.
18. Ellul-Micallef R, Fenech FF: Effect of intravenous prednisolone in asthmatics with diminished adrenergic responsiveness. Lancet 2:1269–1271, 1975.
19. Sletten IW, Lang WJ, Brown ML, et al: Chronic chlorpromazine administration: some pharmacological and psychological effects in man. Clin Pharmacol Ther 6:575–586, 1965.
20. Boakes AJ, Laurence DR, Teoh PC, et al: Interactions between sympathomimetic amines and antidepressant agents in man. Br Med J 1:311, 1973.
21. Reisman RE: Asthma induced by adrenergic aerosols. J Allergy 46:162–177, 1970.
22. Stolley PD: Asthma mortality. Am Rev Respir Dis 105:883–890, 1972.
23. VanMetre TE: Adverse effects of inhalation of excessive amounts of nebulized isoproterenol in status asthmaticus. J Allergy 43:101–113, 1969.

24. Eisenstadt WS, Nicholas SS: The adverse effect of adrenergic aerosols in bronchial asthma. Ann Allergy 27:283–288, 1969.
25. Aviado DM: Toxicity of aerosols. J Clin Pharmacol 15:86–104, 1975.
26. Godfrey S, Konig P: Suppression of exercise-induced asthma by salbutamol, theophylline, atropine, cromolyn, and placebo in a group of asthmatic children. Pediatrics 56(Suppl):930–934, 1975.
27. Sly RM: Effect of β-adrenoreceptor stimulants on exercise-induced asthma. Pediatrics 56(Suppl):910–915, 1975.
28. Chervinsky P, Belinkoff S: Comparison of metaproterenol and isoproterenol aerosols: spirometric evaluation after two months therapy. Ann Allergy 27:611–616, 1969.
29. Gaddie J, Legge JS, Palmer KN: Aerosols of salbutamol, terbutaline, and isoprenaline-phenylephrine in asthma. Br J Dis Chest 67:215–220, 1973.
30. Chatterjee SS, Perry AE: Salbutamol: clinical application as pressure packed aerosol. Postgrad Med J 47(Suppl):53–55, (Mar) 1971.
31. Formgren H: Clinical comparison of inhaled terbutaline and orciprenaline in asthmatic patients. Scand J Respir Dis 51:203–211, 1970.
32. Blerman CW, Pierson WE, Shapiro GG: The pharmacological assessment of single drugs and drug combinations in exercise-induced asthma. Pediatrics 56(Suppl):919–926, 1975.
33. Weinberger MM, Bronsky EA: Evaluation of oral bronchodilator therapy in asthmatic children. J Pediatr 84:421–427, 1974.
34. Weinberger MM, Bronsky EA: Interaction of ephedrine and theophylline. Clin Pharmacol Ther 17:585–592, 1975.
35. Nelson HS, Raine D, Doner C, et al: Subsensitivity to the bronchodilator action of albuterol produced by chronic administration. Am Rev Resp Dis 116:871–878,1977.
36. Weinberger MM: Use of ephedrine in bronchodilator therapy. Pediatr Clin North Am 22:121–127, 1975.
37. Legge JS, Gaddie J, Palmer KN: Comparison of two oral selective β_2-adrenergic stimulant drugs in bronchial asthma. Br Med J 1:637–639, 1971.
38. Formgren H: A clinical comparison of the effect of oral terbutaline and orciprenaline. Scand J Respir Dis 51:195–202, 1970.
39. O'Donnell TV, Butler GM, Tocker MD: A comparison of orciprenaline and salbutamol administered orally in 12 adult asthmatic patients. Postgrad Med J 47(Suppl):115–118, (Mar) 1971.
40. Goldberg LI: Monoamine oxidase inhibitors. Adverse reactions and possible mechanisms. JAMA 190:456–462, 1964.
41. Turner-Warwick M: Study of theophylline plasma levels after oral administration of new theophylline compounds. Br Med J 2:67–69, 1957.
42. Jenne JW, Wyze MS, Rood FS, et al: Pharmacokinetics of theophylline. Application to adjustment of the clinical dose of aminophylline. Clin Pharmacol Ther 13:349–360, 1972.
43. Mitenko PA, Ogilvie RI: Rational intravenous doses of theophylline. N Engl J Med 289:600–603, 1973.
44. Zwillich CW, Sutton FD, Neff TA, et al: Theophylline-induced seizures in adults: correlation with serum concentrations. Ann Intern Med 82:784–787, 1975.
45. Hendeles L, Bighley L, Richardson RH, et al: Frequent toxicity from IV aminophylline infusions in critically ill patients. Drug Intel Clin Pharm 11:12–18, 1977.
46. Levy G, Koysooko R: Pharmacokinetics of the effect of theophylline on pulmonary functions in asthmatic children. J Pediatr 86:789–793, 1975.
47. Calesnick B, Munch JC, DiPalma JR: Bioassay of theophylline preparations using human subjects. Br Med J 2:33–35, 1960.
48. Waxler SH, Moy HB: A comparative study of theophylline preparations: digestive absorption. J Am Pharm Assoc 49:619–621, 1960.
49. Boswell R, McGinn JT: Blood levels produced by three oral theophylline-containing preparations: double-blind crossover study. NY State J Med 64:887–890, 1964.
50. Koysooko R, Ellis EF, Levy G: Effect of ethanol on theophylline absorption in humans. J Pharm Sci 64:299–301, 1975.
51. Hendeles L, Weinberger M, Bighley L: Absolute bioavailability of oral theophylline. Am J Hosp Pharm 34:525–527, 1977.
52. Waxler SH, Schack JA: Administration of aminophylline. JAMA 143:736–739, 1950.
53. Lillehei JP: Aminophylline: oral vs rectal administration. JAMA 205:530–533, 1968.

54. Simons FER, Simons KJ, Blerman CW: The pharmacokinetics of dihydroxypropyl-theophylline: a basis for rational therapy. J Allergy Clin Immunol 56:347–355, 1975.
55. Jacobs MH, Senior RM, Kessler G: Clinical experience with theophylline. Relationships between dosage, serum concentration, and toxicity. JAMA 235:1983–1986, 1976.
56. Weinberger M, Hudgel D, Spector D, et al: Inhibition of theophylline metabolism by troleandomycin. J Allergy Clin Immunol 59:228–231, 1977.
57. Hunt SN, Jusko WJ, Yurchak AM: Effect of smoking on theophylline disposition. Clin Pharmacol Ther 19:546–551, 1976.
58. Kappas A, Anderson KE, Conney AH, et al: Influence of dietary protein and carbohydrate on antipyrine and theophylline metabolism in man. Clin Pharmacol Ther 21:643–653, 1976.
59. Wyatt R, Weinberger M, Hendeles L: Oral theophylline dosage for the management of chronic asthma. J Pediatr 92:125–130, 1978.
60. Eggleston PA, Blerman CW, Pierson WE, et al: A double blind trial of the effect of cromolyn sodium on exercise-induced bronchospasm. J Allergy Clin Immunol 52:57–63, 1972.
61. Blumenthal MN, Schoenwetter WF, MacDonald FM, et al: Cromolyn in extrinsic and intrinsic asthma. J Allergy Clin Immunol 52:105–114, 1973.
62. Kiechel F, Pollack J, Cooper D, et al: Inhibition of exercise-induced bronchospasm by theophylline or cromolyn. Pediatrics 60:840–844, 1977.
63 Booij-Noord H, Orie NGM, deVries K: Immediate and late bronchial obstructive reactions to inhalation of house dust and protective effects of disodium cromoglycate and prednisone. J Allergy Clin Immunol 48:344–354, 1971.
64. Galant SP, Bullock J, Wong D, et al: The inhibitor effect of antiallergy drugs on allergen and histamine induced wheal and flare response. J Allergy Clin Immunol 51:11–21, 1973.
65. Konig P, Jaffe P, Godfrey S: Effect of corticosteroids on exercise-induced asthma. J Allergy Clin Immunol 54:14–19, 1974.
66. Harter JG, Novitch AM: Evaluation of steroid analogues in terms of suitability for alternate day steroid therapy. J Allergy 37:108–109, 1966.
67. Easton JG, Busser RJ, Neimlich EM: Effect of alternate-day steroid administration on adrenal function in allergic children. J Allergy Clin Immunol 48:355–360, 1971.
68. Falliers CJ, Chai H, Molk L, et al: Pulmonary and adrenal effects of alternate-day corticosteroid therapy. J Allergy Clin Immunol 49:156–166, 1972.
69. Morris HG, Neuman I, Ellis EF: Plasma steroid concentrations during alternate-day treatment with prednisone. J Allergy Clin Immunol 54:350–358, 1974.
70. Reimer LG, Morris HG, Ellis EF: Growth of asthmatic children during treatment with alternate-day steroids. J Allergy Clin Immunol 55:224–231, 1975.
71. Godfrey S: The place of a new aerosol steroid, beclomethasone dipropionate, in the management of childhood asthma. Pediatr Clin North Am 22:147–155, 1975.
72. Campbell IA, Somner AR, Angel JH, et al: Inhaled corticosteroids compared with oral prednisone in patients starting long-term corticosteroid therapy for asthma. Lancet 2:469–473, 1975.
73. Falliers CJ: Triamcinolone acetonide aerosols for asthma. I. Effective replacement of systemic corticosteroid therapy. J Allergy Clin Immunol 57:1–11, 1976.
74. Morris H: Corticosteroids in asthma. In *Annual Review of Allergy,* 1972. Edited by CA Frazier. Flushing, New York, Medical Publishing Co., 1973, pp 105–130.

56. NASAL DECONGESTANTS

Collin S. Karmody

Nasal decongestants reduce the volume of the nasal mucosa, thereby widening the air passages. They act by constricting blood vessels of the nasal mucosa, temporarily reducing the quantity of its secretions. Decongestants may be administered topically as drops, sprays, or vapors, or orally in solid or liquid form. The most widely used group of drugs are those with biochemical effects similar to norepinephrine. Their actions are partly due to stimulation of the release of norepinephrine and partly due to direct stimulation of the receptor sites. Because of their chemical structures and similarity, they are collectively known as sympathomimetic drugs.

SYMPATHOMIMETIC DRUGS

All sympathomimetic drugs cause vasoconstriction of blood vessels in the skin and mucosa, elevation of blood pressure, an increase in heart rate and cardiac output, dilation of the pupils, relaxation of some smooth muscles (eg, in the blood vessels of the skeletal muscles, bronchi, intestine, etc.), and stimulation of the central nervous system. The activity of an individual sympathomimetic agent will depend upon its relative affinity for the various target receptors.

NASAL DECONGESTANTS

Most of the nasal decongestants in common use are sympathomimetic drugs. Generally, topical use is preferable to systemic administration because these agents produce much more intense vasoconstriction when used topically. Intense vasoconstriction also results in reduced absorption of decongestants into the circulation. Therefore, negligible systemic effects occur following the topical use of nasal decongestants unless large quantities in high concentrations are used, in which case swallowing causes excessive absorption from the stomach.

Vasoconstriction from topically administered nasal decongestants lasts from two to six hours, depending on the agent and the concentration. Constriction is usually followed by a relaxation of the vessel wall and a period of dilation, resulting in rebound congestion which becomes more severe if use of the topical decongestant is prolonged. Thus topical nasal decongestants should be used for minimal periods and, where possible, should not be used for more than fourteen days. Apart from the sympathomimetic drugs, the only other agent that is used topically as a nasal decongestant is cocaine.

Some sympathomimetic drugs are effective as nasal decongestants when administered orally. The intensity of vasoconstriction in the nasal mucosa is less than with topical application and, therefore, the relief of nasal congestion is not as marked. Rebound congestion is not as important with oral nasal decongestants, but systemic effects are much more troublesome. Adverse effects include anxiety, dizziness, sleeplessness, and, in older patients, difficulty with voiding. Oral decongestants should be used with caution in patients with hypertension, heart disease, diabetes mellitus, hyperthyroidism, and prostatic hypertrophy. In addition, patients taking other drugs whose actions are similar to sympathomimetic amines, eg, the monoamine oxidase inhibitors, should not take nasal decongestants orally.

Most of the standard preparations for topical application are potentially dangerous to children, and their use should be avoided in the younger patient. A few preparations are made specifically for children and pediatric decongestant therapy should be confined to these drugs. Children tolerate oral decongestants in the usual pediatric doses very well without obvious systemic effects. As with adults, topical administration should be restricted to as short a period as is possible, preferably to under one week and almost never beyond fourteen days of regular daily usage. The lowest effective concentration should be prescribed.

DRUG MONOGRAPHS

NASAL DECONGESTANTS PRIMARILY USED TOPICALLY

PHENYLEPHRINE HYDROCHLORIDE (Neo-Synephrine Hydrochloride)

Phenylephrine is a safe and effective topical nasal decongestant.

Use of an 0.25% aerosol is effective for about four hours in patients with chronic rhinitis.[1] Objective measurements using rhinometry have shown a significant decongestion of the nasal passages at 60 and 180 minutes after application.[2] Phenylephrine also is useful as an orally administered decongestant. In double-blind studies oral doses of 5 to 25 mg of phenylephrine were more effective than a placebo. The time of onset of decongestion was 15 to 20 minutes, with a duration of 2 to 4 hours.[3]

Dosage—Oral: Adults, 10 mg every 4 hours, not exceeding 60 mg in 24 hours. *Children, 6 to 12 years,* 5 mg every 4 hours, not exceeding 30 mg in 24 hours.

Topical: Adults, 0.5% or 1% drops, 3 drops in each nostril every 4 to 6 hours. Alternatively the nasal spray may be used. *Children,* 0.125 or 0.25%, 2 drops in each nostril every 6 hours; the 0.25% spray may be used.

EPHEDRINE SULFATE

In concentrations of 0.5 to 1%, topically administered ephedrine produces prompt nasal decongestion which persists at maximal levels for up to one hour and declines to pretreatment levels at about the fourth hour. Ephedrine, therefore, is somewhat less effective as a topical nasal decongestant than other agents.[4]

Oral ephedrine has been used chiefly as a bronchodilator, but it is also effective as a nasal decongestant. One controlled study in patients with nasal obstruction demonstrated effective decongestion by 25 mg of orally administered ephedrine sulphate; the data for 8 to 12 mg doses were inconclusive.

Dosage—Oral: Adults, 8 to 12 mg every 4 hours, not exceeding 72 mg in 24 hours. *Children, 6 to 12 years,* 4 to 6 mg not more than every 4 hours and not exceeding 36 mg in 24 hours.

Topical: Adults, 0.5 to 3% solution, 3 to 4 drops every 6 to 8 hours. *Children, 6 to 12 years,* 0.25 to 0.5% solution, 3 to 4 drops every 8 hours.

NAPHAZOLINE HYDROCHLORIDE (Privine Hydrochloride)

Naphazoline hydrochloride is a useful topical decongestant, but it produces rebound congestion four to six hours after application.[5] Rebound congestion tends to perpetuate dependence,[6] and it is advised that naphazoline not be used for more than three days. In

TABLE 1 Preparations and Costs of Nasal Decongestants

Generic Name	Trademark Name(s)	Preparations and 1978 Costs
Decongestants Primarily Used Topically		
Phenylephrine Hydrochloride	Neo-Synephrine Hydrochloride	Drops 0.125%—$0.99/30 ml; 0.25%—$1.06/30 ml; 0.5%—$1.19/30 ml; 1%—$1.39/30 ml Spray 0.25%—$1.13/22.5 ml; 0.5 %—$1.35/22.5 ml
Ephedrine Sulfate	generic	Capsules 25mg—$0.98–$2.86/100; 50 mg—$1.45–$4.25/100 Syrup 20 mg/5 ml—$1.70–$3.89/pint Drops 3%—$1.61/30 ml
Naphazoline Hydrochloride	Privine Hydrochloride	Drops 0.05%—$0.92/30 ml Spray 0.05%—$1.08/20 ml
Oxymetazoline Hydrochloride	Afrin	Drops 0.025%—$1.54/20 ml; 0.05%—$1.81/20 ml Spray 0.05%—$0.37/3 ml, $1.44/15 ml
Xylometazoline Hydrochloride	Otrivin Hydrochloride	Drops 0.05%—$1.81/30 ml; 0.1%—$1.82/30 ml Spray 0.1%—$1.41/15 ml
Cocaine Cocaine Hydrochloride	generic generic	No manufactured dosage forms available; pharmacist must compound preparations
Propylhexedrine	Benzedrex	Inhaler 250 mg—$0.79/each
Oral Nasal Decongestants		
Phenylpropanolamine Hydrochloride	Propadrine Hydrochloride	Capsules 25 mg—$3.27/100; 50 mg—$4.64/100 Elixir 20 mg/5 ml—$3.23/pint
Pseudoephedrine Hydrochloride	Sudafed (D-Feda) (Novafed)	Tablets 30 mg—$2.85/100; 60 mg—$3.95/100 Syrup 30 mg/5 ml—$3.15/pint

concentrations of 0.05 to 0.1%, its topical use in children and infants has been associated with sedation, nervousness, and a rise in systolic blood pressure.[7] This agent is not recommended for children under six years of age.

Dosage—Topical: Adults, 0.05% solution, 2 to 3 drops or sprays.

OXYMETAZOLINE HYDROCHLORIDE (Afrin)

Oxymetazoline is an effective and relatively long-acting nasal decongestant. When used topically in a concentration of 0.5% this agent induces nasal vasomotor constriction that persists for five to six hours and gradually declines thereafter.[2] Rebound congestion is, therefore, somewhat lessened but is not completely eliminated. In a study of 33 children with allergic rhinitis, the use of 0.025% of oxymetazoline caused no demonstrable rebound congestion over a six-hour period.[8] Animal studies indicate that the rate of systemic absorption from nasal application is too slow to achieve systemic levels. Oxymetazoline is, therefore, comparatively safe when used topically. Oxymetazoline is effective and causes no adverse reactions in children when used in a 0.025% concentration.[9] The effect may last from nine to twelve hours. Even children, ages 2 to 6 years, have been treated without difficulties.

Dosage—Topical: Adults, 0.05%, 2 to 3 drops or sprays every 12 hours. *Children, 6 to 12 years,* 1 to 2 drops or sprays.

XYLOMETAZOLINE HYDROCHLORIDE (Otrivin Hydrochloride)

The decongestant action of topical xylometazoline persists for up to five hours. Solutions containing 0.05 and 0.1% are effective in children and infants when used three times daily. Rebound congestion is negligible when use is limited to short periods.[1] No cardiovascular changes were produced by nasal application of xylometazoline.

Dosage—Topical: Adults, two to three drops or sprays in each nostril of 0.1% solution every eight to ten hours. *Children, 2 to 12 years,* two to three drops or sprays in each nostril of 0.05% solution every eight to ten hours.

COCAINE
COCAINE HYDROCHLORIDE

Cocaine has been in clinical use for almost 100 years. It is an alkaloid, derived from the leaves of the shrub erythroxylon coca, which produces excellent anesthesia and vasoconstriction of the mucous membranes when applied topically. It is usually reserved for hospitalized patients with acute sinusitis. As a topical decongestant, cocaine is used in 2% solution; higher concentrations are not recommended. Applied topically, cocaine is rapidly absorbed from the nasal mucosa with detectable serum levels at 15 minutes and peak levels of its major metabolite 4 to 5 hours after application.[10] It is usually stated that the maximum safe dose for topical application is 200 to 300 mg,[11] but this is only an estimate. Toxic reactions, however, can occur with much smaller doses although many physicians use substantially larger quantities without problems.

Adverse Reactions—Cocaine reactions usually occur promptly after topical application. It is suggested that only a minimum quantity of cocaine be used, and that the patient be advised not to swallow the medication. Cocaine reactions generally are stimulatory in nature. The patient becomes restless, garrulous, and confused, with tachycardia, tachypnea, mydriasis and possibly hyperthermia. Abdominal pain, nausea, and vomiting may occur. Seizures and respiratory arrest characterize more serious adverse reactions.

Dosage—Topical: A 0.5 to 2% solution is applied as a spray or on a tampon.

INHALANTS

PROPYLHEXEDRINE (Benzedrex)

Propylhexedrine is primarily used in cases of mild nasal obstruction and rhinitis. Maximal reduction of nasal airway resistance occurs in 30 minutes and the overall duration of action is about two hours. Inhalants are not recommended for patients with acute or chronic sinusitis.

Adverse Reactions—In recommended doses, propylhexedrine has a wide margin of safety and is relatively free from toxic effects. Excessive doses produced no undesirable side effects in twenty patients with histories of severe angina.[12]

Use of oral propylhexedrine has not been extensive. In a dosage of 100 mg, there is mild systolic hypertension but no other systemic symptoms. Ingestion of 250 mg by one patient caused serious toxicity.[13] There have been two reports of psychotic behavior in patients with habitual ingestion of propylhexedrine.[14,15] Propylhexedrine is marketed outside of the United States as an anorexiant.

Dosage—Adults and children six years and older, two inhalations in each nostril at a maximum of every two hours. Inhalers are manufactured so that they deliver 0.4 to 0.5 mg of propylhexedrine per 800 ml of air. The inhalers retain effectiveness for about three months.

ORAL NASAL DECONGESTANTS

PHENYLPROPANOLAMINE HYDROCHLORIDE (Propadrine Hydrochloride)

The action of phenylpropanolamine is similar to ephedrine but with less stimulation of the central nervous system.[16] Three double-blind studies have compared phenylpropanolamine with a placebo and found it effective.[3,17,18] Subjective evaluation in adults have shown that phenylpropanolamine in doses of 50 mg every three hours is associated with minimal side effects.[19] This agent seems to cause less problems with bladder outlet obstruction than does ephedrine.[19] Phenylpropanolamine has been used successfully in children 2 to 15 years of age in doses of 6.25 to 25 mg four times daily and has relieved symptoms of nasal congestion with minimal incidence of side effects.[20] In doses of 50 mg four times daily in adults, there have been no adverse cardiovascular effects after five to forty days of treatment.[21] Isolated cases of patients with nervousness, headaches, etc. have been reported; these seem to be idiosyncratic. Phenylpropanolamine is a component of many cold preparations.

Dosage—Oral: Adults, 25 mg every 4 hours or 50 mg every 8 hours, not exceeding 150 mg in 24 hours. *Children, 6 to 12 years,* 12.5 mg every 4 hours or 25 mg every 8 hours, not exceeding 75 mg in 24 hours. *Children, 2 to 6 years,* 6.25 mg or less every 4 hours, not exceeding 37.5 mg in 24 hours.

PSEUDOEPHEDRINE HYDROCHLORIDE (D-Feda, Novafed, Sudafed)

Pseudoephedrine preparations are safe and effective as oral nasal decongestants when used in specified dosages. Pseudoephedrine and its salts may produce mild side effects such as drowsiness, insomnia, and headache in about 30% of patients.[22] Objective studies in patients with allergic rhinitis have shown pseudoephedrine to be better than a placebo.[22] This has been confirmed in children. In one study, however, there were no differences between the effect of pseudoephedrine and a placebo on nasal airways as measured by rhinometry.[3] In other studies, however, nasal resistance improved by 20% after 60 mg of pseudoephedrine orally.[23] Pseudoephedrine is frequently combined with antihistamines and/or bronchodilators.

Dosage—Oral: Adults, 60 mg every 4 hours, not exceeding 360 mg in 24 hours. *Children, 6 to 12 years,* 30 mg every 4 hours, not exceeding 180 mg in 24 hours. For children under 2 years old, pseudoephedrine should be used with caution.

REFERENCES

1. Harris HH: Comparative study of decongestive effectiveness of oxymetazoline hydrochloride in rhinitis. Eye Ear Nose Throat Dig 46:41–43, 1967.
2. Connell JR: Effectiveness of topical nasal decongestants. Ann Allergy 27:541–546, 1969.
3. Slodkl SJ, Montgomery CA: Clinical comparison of oxymetazoline and ephedrine in nasal decongestion. Curr Ther Res 7:19–22, 1965.
4. McLaurin JW, Chipman WF, Rosedale R Jr: Oral decongestants. A double-blind comparison study of the effectiveness of four sympathomimetic drugs: objective and subjective. Laryngoscope 81:54–67, 1961.
5. Mertins PS Jr: Excessive self medication with naphazoline hydrochloride ('Privine Hydrochloride'). JAMA 134:1175, 1947.
6. Putnam LE, Herwick RP: Privine dependence of two years duration. JAMA 130:702–703, 1946.
7. Gillespie JB: Poisoning from naphazoline (Privine) hydrochloride. J Pediatr 44:443–444, 1954.
8. Green M: Double-blind study of nasal decongestion with oxymetazoline and phenylephrine in asthmatic children with rhinitis. Rev Allergy 20:863–868, 1966.
9. Cohen BM, Duffy EP: Physiologic and clinical estimates of the relief of nasal flow obstruction in allergic rhinitis: effects of a topical decongestant (oxymetazoline). J Asthma Res 7:65–73, 1969.
10. Johns ME, Berman AR, Price JC, et al: Metabolism of intranasally applied cocaine. Ann Otol 86:342–347, 1977.
11. Adriani J, Zepernick R: Clinical effectiveness of drugs used for topical anesthesia. JAMA 188:711–718, 1964.
12. Burnett JB, Gundersen SM: The effect of volatile 1-cyclohexyl-2-methylaminopropane (Benzedrex Inhaler) on patients with coronary arteriosclerosis. N Engl J Med 246:449–450, 1952.
13. Marsden P, Sheldon J: Acute poisoning by propylhexedrine. Br Med J 1:730, 1972.
14. Anderson ED: Propylhexedrine (Benzedrex) psychosis. NZ Med J 71:302, 1972.
15. Johnson J, Johnson DAW: Propylhexedrine chewing and psychosis. Br Med J 3:529–530, 1972.
16. *AMA Drug Evaluations,* first edition. Chicago, American Medical Association, 1971, p 350.
17. Rodgers JM, Reilly EB, Bickerman HA: Physiologic and pharmacologic studies on nasal airway resistance (abstract). Clin Pharmacol Ther 14:146, 1977.
18. Dressler WE, Myers T, London SJ, et al: A system of rhinomanometry in the clinical evaluation of nasal decongestants. Ann Otol 86:310–317, 1977.
19. Boyer WE: The clinical use of phenylpropanolamine hydrochloride (Propadrine) in the treatment of allergic conditions. J Allergy 9:509–513, 1938.
20. Carter CH: Treatment of upper respiratory tract disorders in children: an evaluation of a new pediatric suspension. Curr Ther Res 8:648–654, 1965.
21. Black JH: The control of allergic manifestations by phenylpropanolamine (Propadrine) hydrochloride. Lancet 57:101–102, 1937.

22. Arbesman CE, Ehrenreich RJ: New drugs in the treatment of allergies. NY State J Med 61:219–229, 1961.
23. Empey DW, Bye C, Hodder M, et al: A double-blind crossover trial of pseudoephedrine and triprolidine alone and in combination for the treatment of allergic rhinitis. Ann Allergy 34:41–46, 1975.

57. EXPECTORANTS AND INHALANTS

Henry J. Pfeifer

Expectorants are used to facilitate removal of respiratory tract secretions. Currently available expectorants include orally ingested drugs as well as agents which are inhaled and act directly within the respiratory tract.

The most effective aid for facilitating removal of respiratory secretions is adequate hydration. Dehydration accompanies many disease states and should always be appropriately treated if present. Any condition which decreases the available water supply to respiratory fluid will increase its viscosity. Adequate systemic hydration should be the first mode of treatment for mildly thickened respiratory secretions, and water or saline administered by inhalation should be used in difficult cases. Inhalation mucolytics may be added to increase the efficacy of the inhaled water or saline, but should be considered only as adjunctive therapy; they are not replacements for hydration.

ORAL EXPECTORANTS

The use of drugs to facilitate removal of bronchial secretions has a long history in clinical medicine. Ipecac has been used orally as an expectorant for generations. The United States Dispensatory, 1895 states, 'Ipecacuanha is in large doses emetic, in smaller doses diaphoretic and expectorant, and in still smaller, stimulant to the stomach, exciting appetite and facilitating digestion.'[1]

Despite the overwhelming popularity of oral expectorants, the literature does not substantiate claims of therapeutic efficacy. Untoward effects of these drugs range from the innocuous to the overtly toxic. Although actual clinical benefit from these agents is doubtful, their action has been classified in most pharmacology texts as either 'direct' or 'reflex.' The direct-acting agents (eg, terpin hydrate) are those which theoretically affect the secretory cells of the respiratory tract by direct contact with these cells through secretion into the respiratory tract fluid. The indirect or reflex acting agents (eg, ipecac, guaifenesin) supposedly increase flow of fluid into the respiratory tract by irritation of the gastric mucosa or through stimulation of a higher emetic center, which in turn causes a general increase in both gastric and respiratory secretions.

Although oral expectorant therapy has been used for years, the use of these agents is primarily empirical. The pharmacological classifications of their actions are tenuous and misleading. Current knowledge of their effects suggests that they offer little therapeutic benefit at best, and that they should not be routinely prescribed in clinical practice.

INHALANTS

Hydration of the respiratory tract via inhalation provides the most effective direct means for aiding the removal of viscous bronchopulmonary secretions. Deep, efficient hydration of the respiratory tract can be achieved using techniques in routine clinical use. Water or normal saline alone will usually produce satisfactory results. Mucolytics serve as effective adjuncts to, but not replacements for, adequate hydration.

After a rational course of therapy has been prescribed, its success depends largely upon the talents of those who administer the care. The skill of respiratory and physical therapists are important determinants of response to therapy, and effort should be made where possible to coordinate the skills of those responsible for the patient's management.

DRUG MONOGRAPHS

EXPECTORANTS

GUAIFENESIN (Robitussin)

Guaifenesin (glyceryl guaiacolate) has been used as an oral expectorant for many years. Its use stems mainly from extrapolation of animal studies of Boyd and coworkers in the early 1940's,[2,3] who themselves questioned the value of this agent in humans.[4] Nevertheless, it is the most widely purchased oral expectorant and is available without prescription.

Few well-controlled studies of the expectorant activity of guaifenesin exist. It has been and continues to be frequently administered in combination with decongestants (eg, phenylephrine, pseudoephedrine), bronchodilators (eg, oxtriphylline, theophylline), and antitussives (eg, codeine, dextromethorphan) which probably accounts for beneficial effects attributed to guaifenesin in early studies.[5,6] Minor benefit not related to increased expectoration have been reported,[7,8] but any clinically significant benefit is doubtful. A comprehensive, well-controlled study of the expectorant effect of guaifenesin was conducted by Hirsch, et al.[9] This study consisted of three phases designed to measure both *in vitro* and *in vivo* effects of the drug upon sputum volume and consistency. No benefit over water in reducing sputum viscosity *in vitro* was observed, and daily doses of 800 and 1600 mg were found ineffective when compared to placebo in reducing sputum consistency, increasing sputum volume, or improving ventilatory function. Subjective improvement over 20 days of therapy was also investigated, and guaifenesin offered no improvement over placebo in easing expectoration.

Adverse Reactions—Fortunately, guaifenesin has a low order of toxicity, and adverse effects are infrequent. Data of the Boston Collaborative Drug Surveillance Program indicate that it is widely

TABLE 1 Preparations and Costs of Expectorants and Inhalants

Generic name	Trademark Name(s)	Preparations and 1978 Costs
Expectorants		
Guaifenesin	Robitussin Generics	Syrup 100 mg/5 ml—$0.92/4 oz, $1.67/8 oz
Inhalants		
Acetylcysteine	Mucomyst	Inhalation (sterile solution) 10%—$2.66/ 10 ml, $7.23/30 ml; 20%—$3.19/10 ml, $8.68/30 ml

used among hospitalized medical patients and that side effects are unusual.[10,11] The most common untoward effects are gastrointestinal disturbances. Among 2336 patients who received the drug, gastrointestinal disturbances were observed among 1.4%, and the overall adverse reaction rate was 1.7%.[11]

Guaifenesin has been reported to decrease platelet adhesiveness and to prolong activated-plasma clotting time without altering other coagulation parameters.[12–15] These effects have been observed both *in vitro* and *in vivo* but probably are clinically unimportant.

Interactions—Guaifenesin can interfere with the Undenfriend method for detecting 5-hydroxyindolacetic acid (5-HIAA) in urine, a diagnostic test for carcinoid tumors. The formation of a distinct purple color indicates a positive result. In those patients receiving guaifenesin, a red or pink endpoint may occur, which should not be interpreted as a positive result.[16,17] Due to its structural similarity to mephenesin and methocarbamol, guaifenesin may produce a false positive result in urine tests for vanilmandelic acid (VMA). Reports of guaifenesin causing false positive results in the guaiac test for occult blood[18] seem unfounded.[19,20]

IODIDES

Iodides are secreted into the saliva and respiratory tract fluid and are commonly classified as 'indirect' or 'reflex' acting expectorants. Toxicity resulting from iodide therapy is predictable and associated with serious risk. The efficacy of these agents is doubtful.

Iodides available for oral use include inorganic iodides such as potassium iodide and hydroiodic acid. An organic product, iodinated glycerol, which contains organically-bound iodide and no free iodine, is also available. Sodium iodide is available for intravenous administration.

Documentation of the value of iodides as expectorants is lacking. Studies describing beneficial effects generally refer to subjective improvements during adjunctive treatment of asthma. Although 'improvement' of asthma has been reported,[21] the relationship to any expectorant activity is unclear. Controlled studies of chronic-dose iodide therapy failed to demonstrate any significant changes in sputum viscosity,[22] and symptoms of iodine toxicity often accompanied therapy.[23]

Adjunctive drug therapy which would permit reduction in systemic steroid dosing has always been a primary goal in the pharmacotherapy of asthma, and iodides have been used with this objective. However, new, effective adjunctive medications for asthma management are now available (cromolyn sodium, beclomethasone dipropionate) and they often permit effective control of asthma with minimal risk. Newer methods for hydrating the respiratory tract, as well as effective inhalant mucolytics, are also available for use when needed. Thus, the use of iodides as an adjunct to asthma management or as an expectorant is outdated. Iodides are associated with severe risks which outweigh any potential benefit.

Adverse Reactions—Iodides can induce hypothyroidism and goiter, two well-documented and predictable consequences of iodide therapy that occur with both the organic and inorganic products.[21,24,25] Paradoxically, thyrotoxicosis may also be precipitated by iodide therapy, especially in those with pre-existing goiter,[26–29] and may persist after iodide therapy has been withdrawn.[26] Thyroid enlargement in the fetuses of pregnant women receiving iodides has been observed and has led to neonatal death.[30,31] Galina, et al[31] reported two neonatal deaths apparently caused by iodide therapy in pregnant women. Marked thyroid enlargement with compression of the trachea occurred.

Symptoms of iodide toxicity generally occur after chronic rather than short-term therapy.[11] Iodism can often complicate the clinical features of diseases for which it is prescribed. Early symptoms of iodism resemble the common cold, including sore throat and gums, salivation, irritation of the eyes and eyelids, frontal sinus headache, respiratory tract irritation, and glandular swelling in the head and neck.[32] Acneform lesions may appear to be aggravated in some individuals, especially adolescents.[21] Allergic reactions may occur as well and are potentially fatal. Dermatologic complications include iododerma and hair loss, and manifestations which may be delayed.[32–34]

Interactions—Iodides can interfere with several laboratory tests.[35,36] Increase of false-positive results in those receiving iodides may occur in the benzidine and guaiac tests for occult blood, and protein bound iodine. Inorganic iodides may also interfere with determination of 17-hydroxycorticosteroids and may decrease radioactive iodine uptake.

AMMONIUM CHLORIDE

Ammonium chloride is another widely-used agent with little substantiation of its expectorant action. At usual expectorant doses ammonium chloride is associated with few risks, but higher doses can produce systemic acidosis.

Few recent studies of ammonium chloride as an expectorant are available. One study[22] among adult patients failed to demonstrate any significant expectorant value of 500 mg administered four times daily for one week. Systemic acidosis is an important potential hazard and near-fatalities have followed large doses of the drug.[37,38]

Adverse Reactions—The use of ammonium chloride orally may induce nausea and vomiting. Systemic acidosis may result from high doses; lower doses can cause urinary acidification, which in turn can influence the pharmacologic activity of many drugs. Increased urinary excretion of weak bases and decreased excretion of weak acids occur in the presence of acid urine. The actions of methenamine and mercurial diuretics are potentiated, while those of carbonic anhydrase inhibitors can be antagonized. In addition, certain sulfonamides may crystallize more readily in acid urine. In all cases ammonium chloride should be administered with substantial amounts of water. It should be used with extreme caution in the presence of renal and hepatic disease.

Interactions—Ammonium and chloride ions may interfere with some common laboratory tests. Serum amylase and chloride may appear elevated, while serum potassium and total protein values may be decreased.[35]

INHALANTS

ACETYLCYSTEINE (Mucomyst)

Acetylcysteine reduces sputum viscosity both *in vitro*[39–42] and *in vivo*[43–53] and can be administered by inhalation or by direct instillation. Its value has been demonstrated over saline alone[43,45,48,50] and over other mucolytic drugs.[44,47] Although adverse reactions are rare, acetylcysteine is irritating and can cause bronchospasm in susceptible individuals.[50,51] Addition of an adrenergic bronchodilator is useful in preventing bronchospasm.

The mucolytic activity of acetylcysteine is attributed to a free sulfhydryl group which cleaves the disulfide bonds in mucous,[41] thereby reducing viscosity. Although acetylcysteine appears to be active in thinning both mucoid and mucopurulent sputum, the action on the mucoid component apparently accounts for its clinical efficacy.

Acetylcysteine can safely be administered by nebulization, particularly using intermittent positive-pressure breathing (IPPB) equipment to maximize aerosol dispersion. The use of IPPB has been under debate in recent years.[54,55] The choice of such therapy is a medical decision that must be weighed individually. Hand nebulizers are not recommended since the particle size generated is generally too large.

Mucoid impaction resulting from mucous plugs can produce atelectasis and subsequent total collapse of the lungs. Acetylcysteine can liquefy these plugs.[46,58] Nebulization through IPPB apparatus can be successful, but direct instillation is more effective and results in rapid liquefaction. Liquefied secretions must be removed rapidly by suction or other mechanical means. Postural drainage and chest physical therapy should be employed as required. Instillation will generally induce cough and possibly bronchospasm; the latter may be prevented by coadministration of a bronchodilator.

Both short- and long-term studies indicate that acetylcysteine is safe and not associated with cumulative toxicity.[48,49,51,59] In an early short-term study, no mucosal changes were seen in mucosal biopsies and resected lung specimens.[52] A recent, single-blind long-term study, in which six adult patients were observed for a period ranging from 5 to 54 weeks showed that daily use of 3 to 5 ml of 10% acetylcysteine together with 0.05% isoproterenol administered by IPPB nebulization was safe, efficacious and nontoxic.[49]

An unpleasant (rotten egg) odor is the chief complaint expressed by patients who receive acetylcysteine. Gargling or brushing the teeth after each therapy is often of benefit.

Because it is a reducing agent, acetylcysteine reacts with rubber and certain metals such as copper and iron. Modern equipment should not present any difficulty, but contact with these substances should be considered when choosing equipment.

Interactions—Most commonly used inhalant drugs are physically compatible with acetylcysteine, and can be mixed together just prior to use without significant loss of potency of either agent. Several antibiotics are physically incompatible with acetylcysteine. These include ampicillin, amphoterecin B, chlortetracycline, erythromycin, oxytetracycline and tetracycline.[56] Lawson and Saggars[57] report that penicillins, tetracycline and cephaloridine are pharmacologically inactivated by acetylcysteine. They also observed inactivation of acetylcysteine by oxygen, but the commercial product contains ethylene diamine tetracetic acid (EDTA) to prevent oxidation and subsequent inactivation of the drug. Chymotrypsin and trypsin are incompatible, but pancreatic dornase is compatible with acetylcysteine.[56]

Dosage—The usual dose of acetylcysteine is variable and must be individualized. Nebulization via IPPB of 3 to 5 ml of a 10% solution should be adequate in most cases. Increasing the volume of the 10% solution, or use of a 20% solution, may be indicated in more refractory cases. Direct instillation of a few ml of a 5 to 20% solution can be used with caution. Concomitant use of a bronchodilator is advisable, especially in asthmatics and those with other respiratory disorders which may predispose them to bronchospasm (see Chapter 55, Antiasthmatic Therapy).

DETERGENTS

Despite early claims of effectiveness,[60,61] surface-active agents such as tyloxapol (Alevaire) appear not to be superior to water or saline for liquefying sputum.[62–66] The benefit observed with these agents is probably due to simple hydration. Surfactants are no longer widely used and cannot be recommended.

REFERENCES

1. Wood HC, Remington JP, Sadtler SP: *United States Dispensatory,* 17th edition. Philadelphia, JB Lippincott Co., 1895, p 753.
2. Connell WF, Johnston GM, Boyd EM: On the expectorant action of resyl and other guaiacols. Can Med Assoc J 42:220–223, 1940.
3. Perry WF, Boyd EM: A method for studying expectorant action in animals by direct measurement of the output of respiratory tract fluids. J Pharmacol Exp Ther 72:65–77, 1941.
4. Boyd EM, Sheppard EP, Boyd CE: The pharmacological basis of the expectorant action of glyceryl guaiacolate. Appl Ther 9:55–59, 1967.
5. Cass LJ, Frederick WS: Comparative clinical effectiveness of cough medication. Am Practit Dig Treat 2:844–851, 1951.
6. Schwartz E, Levin L, Leibowitz H, et al: The use of antitussives in the management of bronchial asthma. Am Practit Dig Treat 7:585–588, 1956.
7. Chodosh S: Glyceryl guaiacolate: a controlled laboratory and clinical study. Am Rev Respir Dis 90:285–286, 1964.
8. Thomson ML, Pavia D, McNicol MW: A preliminary study of the effect of guaiphenesin on mucociliary clearance from the human lung. Thorax 28:742–747, 1973.
9. Hirsch SR, Viernes PF, Kory RC: The expectorant effect of glyceryl guaiacolate in patients with chronic bronchitis: a controlled *in vitro* and *in vivo* study. Chest 63:9–14, 1973.
10. Jick H, Miettinen OS, Shapiro S, et al: Comprehensive drug surveillance. JAMA 213:1455–1460, 1970.
11. Greenblatt DJ: Bronchodilators and expectorants. In *Drug Effects in Hospitalized Patients: Experiences of the Boston Collaborative Drug Surveillance Program, 1966–1975.* Edited by RR Miller, DJ Greenblatt. New York, John Wiley and Sons, 1976, pp 215–225.
12. Eastham RD, Griffiths EP: Reduction in platelet adhesiveness and prolongation of coagulation time of activated plasma by glyceryl guiacolate. Lancet 1:975–976, 1966.

13. Silverman JL, Wurzel HA: The comparative effects of glyceryl guaiacolate and adenosine on the inhibition of ADP-induced platelet aggregation. Am J Med Sci 254:491–498, 1967.
14. Silverman JL, Wurzel HA: The effect of glyceryl guaiacolate on platelet function and other coagulation factors *in vivo*. Am J Clin Pathol 51:35–40, 1969.
15. Duval DL, Didisheim P, Spittell JA, et al: Effects of monoamine oxidase inhibitors, glyceryl guaiacolate and ethanol on experimental arterial thrombosis. Mayo Clin Proc 45:579–585, 1970.
16. Sjoerdsma A: Clinical and laboratory features of malignant carcinoid. Arch Intern Med 102:936–938, 1958.
17. Ravel R: *Clinical Laboratory Methods,* 2nd edition. Chicago, Year Book Medical Publishers, Inc., 1973.
18. Law DH, Gregory DH: Gastrointestinal bleeding. In *Gastrointestinal Disease.* Edited by MH Sleisenger, JS Fordtran. Philadelphia, WB Saunders Co., 1973, pp 208–209.
19. Ogburn RM, Craner GE: Negative guaiac test after glyceryl guaiacolate. N Engl J Med 293:1267, 1975.
20. Brown JR, Self TH, Taylor WJ, et al: Guaifenesin effects on the guaiac test for occult blood. JAMA 236:1881, 1976.
21. Falliers CJ, McCann WP, Chai H, et al: Controlled study of iodotherapy for childhood asthma. J Allergy 38:183–192, 1966.
22. Simon SW, Harmon GA: A comparison of various expectorant drugs employing a new method for determining sputum viscosity. J Allergy 32:493–500, 1961.
23. Forbes J, Wise L: Expectorants and sputum viscosity. Lancet 1:767–770, 1957.
24. Murray IPC, Stewart RDH: Iodide goitre. Lancet 1:922–926, 1967.
25. Block SH: Goiter complicating therapy with iodinated glycerol. J Pediatr 83:84–85, 1973.
26. Vagenakis AG, Wang C, Burger A, et al: Iodide-induced thyrotoxicosis in Boston. N Engl J Med 287:523–527, 1972.
27. Anon: Iodide-induced thyrotoxicosis. Lancet 2:1072–1073, 1972.
28. Savoie JC, Massin JP, Thomopoulus P, et al: Iodide-induced thyrotoxicosis in apparently normal thyroid glands. J Endocrinol Metab 41:685–691, 1975.
29. Gutknecht DR: Asthma complicated by iodine-induced thyrotoxicosis. N Engl J Med 296:1236, 1977.
30. Carswell F, Kerr MM, Hutchinson JH: Congenital goitre and hypothyroidism produced by maternal ingestion of iodides. Lancet 1:1241–1243, 1970.
31. Galina MP, Avnet NL, Einhorn A: Iodides during pregnancy. N Engl J Med 267:1124–1127, 1962.
32. Baumgartner TG: Potassium iodide and iododerma. Am J Hosp Pharm 33:601–603, 1976.
33. Rosenberg FR, Einbinder J, Walzer RA, et al: Vegetating iododerma. Arch Dermatol 105:900–905, 1972.
34. Chapman RS, Main RA: Diffuse thinning of hair in iodide-induced hypothyroidism. Br J Dermatol 79:103–105, 1967.
35. Elking P, Kabat H: Drug induced modifications of laboratory test values. Am J Hosp Pharm 25:485–519, 1968.
36. Meyers FH, Jawetz E, Goldfein A: *Review of Medical Pharmacology,* 2nd edition. Los Altos, California, Lange Medical Publications, 1970.
37. Relman AS, Shelbourne PF, Talman A: Profound acidosis resulting from excessive ammonium chloride in previously healthy subjects. N Engl J Med 264:848–852, 1961.
38. Ticktin HE, Fazekas JF, Evans JM: Ammonia intoxication in a patient with congestive heart failure receiving ammonium chloride orally. N Engl J Med 255:905–907, 1957.
39. Kubica GP, Dye WE, Cohn ML, et al: Sputum digestion and decontamination with N-acetyl-L-cysteine-sodium hydroxide for culture of mycobacteria. Am Rev Respir Dis 87:775–779, 1963.
40. MacDonald J: Liquefication of sputum by N-acetyl-L-cysteine and dithiothreitol. Can J Med Technol 34:204–217, 1972.
41. Sheffner AL: The reduction *in vitro* in viscosity of mucoprotein solutions by a new mucolytic agent, N-acetyl-L-cysteine. Ann NY Acad Sci 106:298–310, 1963.
42. Sheffner AL, Medler EM, Jacobs LW, et al: The *in vitro* reduction in viscosity of human tracheobronchial secretions by acetylcysteine. Am Rev Respir Dis 90:721–729, 1964.
43. Hirsch SR, Kory RC: An evaluation of the effect of nebulized N-acetylcysteine on sputum consistency. J Allergy 39:265–273, 1967.

44. Hirsch SR, Viernes PF, Kory RC: Clinical and physiological evaluation of mucolytic agents nebulized with isoproterenol: 10% N-acetylcysteine versus 10% 2-mercaptoethane sulphonate. Thorax 25:737–743, 1970.
45. Kory RC, Hirsch SR, Giraldo J: Nebulization of N-acetylcysteine combined with a bronchodilator in patients with chronic bronchitis: a controlled study. Dis Chest 54:18–23, 1968.
46. Irwin RS, Thomas HM: Mucoid impaction of the bronchus: diagnosis and treatment. Am Rev Respir Dis 108:955–959, 1973.
47. Dietzsch H-J, Gottschalk B, Heyne K, et al: Cystic fibrosis: comparison of two mucolytic drugs for inhalation treatment (acetylcysteine and arginine hydrochloride). Pediatrics 55:96–100, 1975.
48. Grater WC, Cato A: Double-blind study of acetylcysteine-isoproterenol and saline-isoproterenol in non-hospitalized patients with asthma. Curr Ther Res 15:660–671, 1973.
49. Chodosh S, Baigelman W, Medici TC, et al: Long-term home use of acetylcysteine in chronic bronchitis. Curr Ther Res 17:319–334, 1975.
50. Denton R, Kwart H, Litt M: N-acetylcysteine in cystic fibrosis. Am Rev Respir Dis 95:643–651, 1967.
51. Webb WR: New mucolytic agents for sputum liquefaction. Postgrad Med 36:449–453, 1964.
52. Webb WR: Clinical evaluation of a new, effective mucolytic agent (N-acetyl-L-cysteine). Am Rev Respir Dis 86:115–116, 1962.
53. Shaw PB, Hurst GA, LeMaistre CA: Clinical evaluation of a new mucolytic agent (N-acetyl-L-cysteine). Am Rev Respir Dis 86:115, 1962.
54. Barach AL, Segal MS: The indiscriminate use of IPPB. JAMA 231:1141–1142, 1975.
55. Engel G: Problems associated with the use of drugs administered by intermittent positive pressure ventilation. Med J Aust 2:529–533, 1976.
56. Anon: Mucomyst (acetylcysteine): in vitro compatibility with other agents. Evansville, Indiana, Mead Johnson & Co., 1974.
57. Lawson D, Saggers BA: N.A.C. and antibiotics in cystic fibrosis. Br Med J 1:317, 1965.
58. Urschel HC, Paulson DL, Shaw RR: Mucoid impaction of the bronchi. Ann Thorac Surg 2:1–16, 1966.
59. Moser KM, Rhodes PG: Acute effects of aerosolized acetylcysteine upon spirometric measurements in subjects with and without obstructive pulmonary disease. Dis Chest 49:370–373, 1966.
60. Miller JB, Brown LL, Goldfarb PM, et al: Alevaire inhalation for eliminating secretions in asthma, sinusitis, bronchitis and bronchiectasis of adults: a preliminary report. Ann Allergy 12:611–626, 1954.
61. Tainter ML, Nachod FC, Bird JC: Alevaire as a mucolytic agent. N Engl J Med 253:764–767, 1955.
62. Lieberman J: The appropriate use of mucolytic agents. Am J Med 49:1–4, 1970.
63. Palmer KNV: The effect of an aerosol detergent in chronic bronchitis. Lancet 1:611–613, 1957.
64. Palmer KNV: Sputum liquefiers. Br J Dis Chest 60:177–181, 1966.
65. Hirsch SR, Kory RC, Hamilton LH: Evaluation of changes in sputum consistency with a new instrument. Am Rev Respir Dis 94:784–789, 1966.
66. Hirsch SR, Zastrow JE, Kory RC: Sputum liquefying agents: a comparison comparative in vitro evaluation. J Lab Clin Med 74:346–353, 1969.

58. ANTITUSSIVE AGENTS

John S. Urbanetti

Cough is an extremely important reflex that helps clear secretions from congested airways and protects those airways from accidental inhalation of foreign material. Failure of the cough reflex can lead to respiratory complications such as obstruction atelectasis and aspiration pneumonia. When suppression of cough seems desirable, antitussives may provide symptomatic relief, but they generally do not treat the underlying cause and may in fact delay or complicate therapy of the underlying disorder.

PHYSIOLOGY OF COUGH AND PHARMACOLOGIC ACTIONS OF ANTITUSSIVE AGENTS

Cough may be initiated as a reflex or voluntary action. The reflex consists of (a) a deep inspiration, followed by (b) a forceful expiratory effort against a closed glottus, followed about 0.2 seconds later by (c) sudden glottal opening, allowing subsequent forceful expiration. By this mechanism the peripheral airways are compressed and discharge their contents into more central airways. The turbulence of high gas flow and velocity in the central airways aids the cilia in airway clearance.[1,2] The cough reflex arc has several components, each of which may be separately affected by antitussive agents.

Peripheral receptors appear to be of two types. Mechanoreceptors are concentrated primarily at the carina and in the posterior tracheal wall. The number of these receptors, and hence the overall sensitivity to mechanical stimuli, decreases markedly as more peripheral lobar bronchi are reached.[3] The adaptability of these receptors to continuous mechanical stimulation has been one of the factors limiting experimental assessment of antitussives.[4]

Receptors responding primarily to chemical irritation are concentrated at the glottus and in increasing numbers more peripherally;[5,6]

this partly explains the glottal-spastic or bronchospastic response to various gaseous/chemical irritants.

Several agents (eg, caramiphen, benzonatate, diphenhydramine) are thought to act partly through a local anesthetic or receptor suppressive effect. However, only the topical or parenteral anesthetics (eg, lidocaine, tetracaine) are effective for short-term suppression of receptor sensitivity.[7]

Afferent nerve fibers travel centrally via the superior laryngeal nerve and vagus. Local abnormalities of the vagus or 'false' stimuli arriving from the auricular branch may precipitate cough.[8] Local anesthesia delivered directly to the vagus may abort cough caused by mechanical pressure.[4] No other chemotherapeutic agents are effective at this level.

Central integration and mediation of the cough reflex is thought to occur in a poorly defined portion of the pons.[5] No discrete 'cough center' has been demonstrated. Voluntary control of cough occurs at this level, possibly in a manner similar to centrally active antitussives (eg, codeine) which presumably affect the threshold of sensitivity to incoming stimuli.[4,6] Aberrent central stimuli at this level may be responsible for nervous or psychogenic cough. Overflow activity into the neighboring vomiting center may account for the frequent association of severe cough and vomiting.[9]

Efferent nerve fibers passing via vagal, spinal, and phrenic nerves are thought to be specifically affected by a few drugs (eg, oxolamine, ethyl dibunate), but supporting data are weak. Efferent nerves to the larynx are readily stimulated locally, perhaps playing a part in the self-perpetuating aspect of cough.[9]

Peripheral effector mechanisms (glottus, diaphragm, and accessory muscles) are incompletely studied. If the glottus is bypassed (eg, by tracheostomy), cough may continue to be effective[4] (though less so). Paralysis or weakened musculature readily leads to retained secretions and recurrent pulmonary infection.[10] No drugs effectively suppress cough at this level without producing a generalized paralysis.

ADJUNCTIVE ACTIONS OF ANTITUSSIVE AGENTS

In addition to interfering with the basic cough reflex, currently available drugs may have additional actions that can be useful in cough with associated pain or other complications.

Analgesia (eg, codeine, other narcotics) may be useful in cough associated with pain, particularly if the pain limits deep respiratory effort (potentially leading to atelectasis and/or pneumonia). Effective analgesia may require doses greater than those normally used for antitussive purposes.

Anesthetic effects are theoretically useful in cough due to excessive mechanical/chemical stimulation. Those few oral agents with experimentally demonstrated mild anesthetic effect (eg, caramiphen, benzonatate, diphenhydramine) have not had this effect clinically demonstrated. Other specific topical and parenteral anesthetics (eg, lidocaine, tetracaine) are effective both experimentally and clinically.

Antihistaminic effects (eg, diphenhydramine) might be useful in allergic cough but often are undesirable for reasons of inspissation of secretions and other atropine-like side effects (see Drug Monographs).

Secretion inhibition or augmentation theoretically may be useful in cough. Dextromethorphan[11] and codeine[12] have both been reported to decrease secretions, but clinical benefit from this action has not been reported.

Sedative effects (eg, codeine) are potentially useful in cough associated with anxiety. Codeine may act in part by subjective diminution of the severity of cough. Various hypnotics (eg, methaqualone, barbiturates)[13] have been suggested for this purpose; however, the complication rate and nonspecific effect of hypnotics render them undesirable for routine use in uncomplicated cough.[9]

METABOLISM OF ANTITUSSIVES

The metabolism of antitussives, with the exception of codeine, dextromethorphan (see Drug Monographs), and diphenhydramine,[14] has been poorly studied. Generally, they are rapidly absorbed in the fasting state, are primarily metabolized by the liver and excreted by the kidneys. Their metabolism may be increased by other drugs that induce microsomal enzymes, thereby leading to lower drug blood levels.[15] Hepatic or renal failure or immaturity of hepatic enzyme systems may lead to increased blood levels.[16,17] Older individuals may also demonstrate increased blood levels due to decreased metabolic rates.[18]

CHOICE OF AN ANTITUSSIVE

Selection of an antitussive requires:

(1) Assessment of the cough—its etiology, effectiveness and complications.

(2) Assessment of the antitussive—effectiveness, interactions, side effects (including those of other constituents in a cough mixture).

(3) Assessment of the antitussive results—evaluation of patient subjective/objective responses.

Cough is most effectively treated by investigation and removal of the underlying cause. Fortunately, cough usually is an acute and self-limited response to low-grade viral infection and will remit spontaneously with time.

Cough persisting for a week or more requires intensive investigation, occasionally with therapeutic trials, in order to evaluate its cause. Inhalation of allergens with resulting bronchospasm and cough may be alleviated with bronchodilators. Chronic postnasal drip in nonsmokers may respond to antihistamine drying or antibiotic therapy. Persistent cough after viral illness may be responsive to steroid therapy in individuals who have airway smooth muscle hyperactivity.

Sporadic reflexive cough rarely requires or benefits from therapy. Aside from short-term suppression for endoscopy, inhibition of the reflex may produce complications secondary to inadequate clearance of foreign or aspirated material.

Cough that is chronic or persistent should be carefully investigated (see Table 1). The dry, 'nonproductive' cough often seen during recovery from viral illness can be self-perpetuating and truly nonproductive as it interferes with a patient's normal lifestyle. Suppression is generally appropriate in this case. A 'productive' cough, however, should be suppressed only if major complications of cough appear (see Table 2). In such circumstances, nocturnal suppression only, or adjunctive use of bronchodilators or antibiotics, may be useful to prevent the complications of mucus plugging and atelectasis.

Assessment of the effectiveness of a particular antitussive is exceptionally difficult. The wide variety of cough types and etiologies may or may not respond to a particular agent. Day-to-day variation in cough frequency and severity and frequent discrepancy between subjective and objective assessment of cough lead to further problems with drug evaluation. Various experimental methods for cough production have been described in animal and human subject populations, but their relevance to pathologic cough is still unclear.[30,31]

Single-entity antitussives are listed in Table 3. Combination preparations containing codeine and dextromethorphan are described in Table 4.

TABLE 1 Causes of Persistent Cough

Upper Respiratory	Lower Respiratory
Infectious	
Viral and bacterial upper respiratory infections	Viral, bacterial, fungal, tubercular, mycoplasma infections of trachea, bronchus, parenchyma
Rhinitis	Parasites (pneumocystis, visceral larval migrans)
Pharyngitis	Bronchiectasis
Sinusitis	Lung abscess
Otitis	
Allergic	
Nasal polyps	Asthma
Allergic rhinitis	Allergic alveolitis
Environmental	
Abnormal ambient temperature, humidity	Pneumoconioses
Smoke, dust, fumes	
Prolonged use of nose drops	
Developmental/Neoplastic	
Tracheo-esophageal fistula	Mass legion compressing airway
Vascular ring	Congenital cysts
Cystic fibrosis	Sequestration of lung
Esophageal diverticulum	Diaphragmatic hernia
Vocal cord palsy	
Other	
Tympanic membrane irritation (hair, cerumen, foreign body)	Aspiration (foreign body)
Vagus nerve abnormalities	Congestive failure
Cough tic (psychogenic)	Drug/radiation induced pulmonary disease
	Pleural irritation
	Hemosiderosis
	Atelectasis

DEPENDENCE AND ABUSE POTENTIAL

Narcotics have significant dependence potential. Codeine is of least concern and can be confidently prescribed for short periods. Nonnarcotic antitussives (eg, dextromethorphan) have no demonstrated dependence liability and hence may be more useful in longer term cough suppression.

Abuse of narcotic antitussives has become a relatively minor problem since the institution of federal regulatory controls. Nonnarcotic antitussive abuse is reported but is sporadic; the alcohol

TABLE 2 Consequences of Cough

Consequence	Reference
Soft Tissues/Bone	
Rib fractures	19
Postoperative wound dehiscence	4
Ligament/muscle tears (eg, rectus)	20
Serum CPK elevation with muscle tears	21
Circulatory/Cardiac	
Atrioventricular block	22
Reduced cardiac output	4
Cough syncope	23
Malfunction of ventriculo-atrial shunts	24
Air embolism	4
Pulmonary	
Asthma/bronchospasm induction	25
Pulmonary interstitial and subcutaneous emphysema	4
Pneumothorax and pneumomediastinum	4
Tracheal occlusion with posterior wall invagination	26
Ventilation-perfusion abnormality with hypoxia	27
CNS/Other	
Venous rupture (nose, conjuctiva, rectum)	28, 29
Loss of sleep, fatigue, irritability	19
Urinary incontinence	4
Nausea and emesis	9

content of many preparations (up to 40%) is probably responsible for their abuse.

Overdosage of narcotic antitussives is rarely lethal. Most symptoms of overdosage readily respond to the use of narcotic antagonists (eg, naloxone).

PRECAUTIONS AND DRUG INTERACTIONS

Drug interactions have been reported only for codeine and dextromethorphan (see Drug Monographs). Generally, any centrally acting antitussive should be given cautiously with other centrally acting agents. Concurrent use with other narcotics, alcohol, hypnotics, or tranquilizers may produce excessive depression of respiration and other centrally controlled functions.

When antitussive combination preparations are used, the prescriber should be concerned with not only the antitussive agent but also the other components.

Sugars. Cough mixture vehicles may contain up to 85% w/v sucrose, providing up to 15 calories/5 ml. This may be of concern in very brittle diabetics and, in some rare instances, may exacerbate a dumping syndrome or induce an osmotic intestinal disorder.

Ethanol. Liquid antitussives may contain up to 40% w/v ethanol, hence providing up to 30 calories/5 ml. This caloric intake may be of concern in very brittle diabetics. The alcohol content may be of concern in former alcoholics or in concurrent administration with drugs that interact with ethanol or have additive central depressant effects. Such drugs include anticoagulants, oral hypoglycemics, disulfiram, and various sedatives and tranquilizers. Most other drugs that interact with alcohol do so only at doses higher than those achieved through normal antitussive use.[32]

Sympathomimetics. Various decongestants may be found in antitussive/cold remedies. These mixtures should be used cautiously, if at all, because: (1) they have a gluconeogenic action in very brittle diabetics, (2) they have alpha and beta adrenergic effects that may be dangerous in hypertension, hyperthyroidism, and coronary artery disease, (3) they may interact with monoamine oxidase inhibitors and cause hypertensive crises, and (4) they may antagonize the antihypertensive effects of guanethidine.[32] Sympathomimetics may be of some value in cough associated with allergic bronchospasm. In this circumstance, the doses and specificity of the agents found in most cough mixtures are lacking and a more specific agent should be utilized.

Antihistamines of various types are included in many antitussive/cold formulations to diminish excessive nasal secretions through their anticholinergic effect. This effect, perhaps desirable in allergic rhinitis, is counterproductive in the lower airways where drying of secretions could lead to mucus plugging, possibly complicating the course of patients with asthma or lower respiratory tract infection (see Drug Monographs).

Expectorants are frequently included in many antitussive/cold formulations to increase mucus production and thereby protect inflamed airway linings. There have been only rare adverse reactions reported with the various expectorants found in cough/cold preparations (see Chapter 57, Expectorants). These have generally been of a hypersensitivity nature. There are insufficient data to support the efficacy of most expectorants at the dosage levels normally utilized.

Finally, assessment of the results of cough suppression is of obvious importance, bearing in mind the observed discordance between the patient's subjective and objective responses. No drug will entirely suppress, short of paralysis, every cough. Failure to alleviate the cough should prompt further investigation of etiology. If cough 'breakthrough' should occur, slight dosage increments will often provide control. Substitution of another antitussive will generally not be of value unless the new compound has significant adjunctive effects (eg, sedative, bronchodilatory) not previously used.

CONCLUSIONS

Codeine given alone continues to be the antitussive of choice in most clinical circumstances because of its efficacy and relative safety. Dextromethorphan is an acceptable alternative when there is a concern about narcotic (codeine) dependence or abuse. Data are insufficient to recommend any other antitussive.

A large number of antitussive-containing mixtures are available, and the advantages and disadvantages of each ingredient should be individually weighed. Antihistamine-containing mixtures should be avoided since they may cause atropine-like dessication of secretions and possible secondary atelectasis.

DRUG MONOGRAPHS

NARCOTIC ANTITUSSIVES

CODEINE
CODEINE PHOSPHATE
CODEINE SULFATE

Well-controlled trials have demonstrated the efficacy of codeine in both experimental and pathologic cough under acute and chronic circumstances.[4,33] It is the reference standard in studies of other antitussive agents. Codeine also has mild analgesic[9] and sedative[34] actions in usual antitussive doses. These adjunctive actions may make codeine particularly useful in cough accompanied by pain or anxiety.

Dependence, Overdose, and Other Abuse—The dependence potential of codeine relative to other narcotics is low. High doses must be administered every few hours for extended periods, perhaps one month or more,[35,36] to establish physical dependence. The drug can support a pre-existing dependence on morphine,[37] and a few cases of physical dependence have been reported,[38] including narcotic with-

TABLE 3 Preparations and Costs of Single-Entity Antitussive Agents

GENERIC NAME	TRADEMARK NAME(S)	PREPARATIONS AND 1978 COSTS
Codeine Sulfate	generic	Tablets 15 mg—$4.65–$5.94/100; 30 mg—$6.24–$9.68/100
Benzonatate	Tessalon	Capsules 100 mg—$8.60/100
Chlophedianol	Ulo	Syrup 25 mg/5 ml—$5.28/12 oz
Levopropoxyphene Napsylate	Novrad	Capsules (equivalent of levopropoxyphene) 100 mg—$4.41/50 Suspension (equivalent of levopropoxyphene) 50 mg/5 ml—$1.79/120 ml
Noscapine	Tusscapine	Liquid 15 mg/5 ml—$1.80/120 ml

drawal in an infant born to a mother taking 360 to 500 mg daily for pain.[39] However, former narcotic addicts do not easily identify the drug as 'dope'[40] and the United States Public Health Service Addiction Research Center at Lexington, Kentucky regards codeine addiction sufficiently uncommon to be a virtual medical curiosity.[37]

Abuse of codeine-containing compounds has been reported sporadically and may relate more to the alcohol content of some codeine-containing preparations (up to 40%).

Overdosage leading to death has been reported with doses of 800 to 1,000 mg.[33,41] Overdosage is seen most frequently in children, and is of most concern in neonates in whom hepatic or renal immaturity or decreased urine output[17] may lead to cumulative effects with deep coma[42] or death.[17] Narcotic antagonists (eg, naloxone) are useful in treating overdosage.

Adverse Reactions—At the low doses commonly used for antitussive purposes (10 to 30 mg), adverse reactions occur rarely, perhaps no more frequently than with placebo.[9] The most common reactions are nausea, dizziness, sedation, anorexia, and headaches. Slightly higher doses of 60 to 100 mg may produce excitement, orthostatic hypotension, vertigo, and mydriasis. Still larger doses of 100 to 500 mg may produce abdominal pain or constipation.[4] Rare allergic reactions include dermatitis, hepatitis, thrombopenia, and anaphylaxis.[33,43]

TABLE 4 Antitussive Mixtures Containing Codeine or Dextromethorphan[a]

Product	Codeine or Dextromethorphan (mg/5 ml)	Sympathomimetic (mg/5 ml)	Expectorant (mg/5 ml)	Other (mg/5 ml)	1978 Cost
Codeine Preparations					
Broncho-Tussin Expectorant	10.8		Ammonium hypophosphite 80 Terpin hydrate 40 Potassium guaicolsulfonate 80	Alcohol 40% (Sugar free)	$1.43/120 ml
Calcidrine Syrup	8.4	Ephedrine HCl 4.2	Calcium iodide 152	Alcohol 6%	$2.27/120 ml
Cetro-Cirose Syrup	5		Ipecac fluid extract 0.01 ml Potassium guaiacolsulfonate 86 Sodium citrate 180 Citric acid 60	Glycerin 3 ml	$0.72/120 ml
Cheracol Syrup	11		Guaifenesin 15 Antimony potassium tartrate 0.9 Chloroform 16 mg	Alcohol 3% Extract of white pine and wild cherry bark	$2.44/120 ml
Copavin Tablets or Capsules	15	Papaverine HCL 15			Tablets—$4.22/40; Capsules—$11.44/100

Cosanyl Cough Syrup	10.95	Pseudoephedine HCl 30		Alcohol 6%	$1.76/120 ml
Cotussis Syrup	10		Terpin hydrate 20 Menthol 2.5 Chloroform 20	Alcohol 20%	$1.20/120 ml
Ephedrol with Codeine	10	Ma huang 660	Potassium guaiacolsulfonate 88 Squill 0.32 ml Tolu balsam and menthol	Alcohol 3%	$1.97/120 ml
Prunicodeine (Elixir)	10		Prunus Virginiana 265 Pinus strobus 175 Sanguinaria 44 Terpin hydrate 29	Alcohol 25% (Sugar free)	$1.85/120 ml
Robitussin A-C (Syrup)	10		Guaifenesin	Alcohol 3.5%	$2.20/120 ml
Terpin Hydrate with Codeine Elixir	10		Terpin hydrate Glycerin	Sweet orange peel	$1.70/120 ml
Dextromethorphan Preparations					
Cheracol D Cough Syrup	9.86		Guaifenesin 15 Antimony potassium tartrate 0.9	Alcohol 3% Extract of white pine and wild cherry bark	$1.54/120 ml
Cosanyl DM Cough Syrup	15	Pseudoephedrine 30		Alcohol 6%	$1.76/120 ml

TABLE 4 *(continued)*

Product	Codeine or Dextromethorphan (mg/5 ml)	Sympathomimetic (mg/5 ml)	Expectorant (mg/5 ml)	Other (mg/5 ml)	1978 Cost
Dorcol Pediatric Cough Syrup	7.5	Phenylpropanolamine HCl 8.75	Guaifenesin	Alcohol 5%	$1.48/120 ml
Ornacol Capsules	30	Phenylpropranolamine HCL 25		Alcohol 5%	$11.75/100
Liquid	15	Phenylpropranolamine HCl 12.5			$1.98/120 ml
Robitussin-DM					
DM Cough Calmers (tablets)	7.5		Guaifenesin 50		$0.88/16
DM Syrup	15		Guaifenesin 100	Alcohol 1.4%	$1.42/120 ml
CF Cough Formula	10	Phenylpropranol-amine HCl 12.5	Guaifenesin 50	Alcohol 1.4%	$1.45/120 ml
Romilar Children's Cough Syrup	7.5		Guaifenesin 25		$1.80/120 ml

Romilar III	5	Phenylpropranol-amine HCl 12.5	Guaifenesin	Alcohol 10%	$2.07/120 ml
2/G-DM Elixir	15		Guaifenesin 100	Alcohol 5% Corn derivative	$1.70/120 ml
Trind DM	7.5	Phenylephrine HCl 2.5	Guaifenesin 50	Alcohol 15% Acetaminophen 120	$1.90/120 ml
Unproco Caps	30		Guaifenesin 200		$12.50/100

[a]Mixtures containing antihistamines are specifically not recommended and are not included in this table.

Respiratory depression may be manifested by slight decreases in ventilation and respiratory flow rates in codeine users.[44] Some decrease in bronchial ciliary activity has been reported as well.[45] Neither of these effects seems clinically significant at usual antitussive dose levels.[46,47] Measurable respiratory depression, however, is seen with 60 mg doses[48] and significant depression occurs with 120 mg every few hours.[47] Thus, high doses are potentially hazardous for patients with respiratory insufficiency, particularly with carbon dioxide retention.

Metabolism—Codeine is well absorbed orally and has peak effects at one to two hours, with usual duration of four to six hours.[43,46] Codeine is metabolized mainly in the liver, and renal excretion of unchanged drug and metabolites is virtually complete within 24 hours. Small amounts may be found in maternal milk.[39] Biotransformation of codeine to morphine has been demonstrated, but this is probably not of clinical significance.[49] Metabolism may be speeded by hepatic enzyme induction or inhibited by age, hepatic failure, or neonatal hepatic enzyme immaturity,[15–18] occasionally leading to cumulative effects (see overdosage).

Dosage—Oral: Adults, 10 to 30 mg every four to six hours. Larger doses do not have proportionally increased effect. Minor cumulative effects may occur. *Children,* 1 to 1.5 mg/kg/day in six divided doses. Cumulative effects may occur especially if urine output is diminished.

Parenteral: 75% of the above doses may be used subcutaneously, intramuscularly or intravenously.

OTHER NARCOTICS

Hydrocodone, hydromorphone, methadone, morphine, and other narcotics are effective antitussive agents, but no objective clinical trials or well-controlled studies demonstrate their superiority over codeine. There is a greater incidence of side effects and increased likelihood of addiction with each of these drugs.[50,51] Consequently they should be used as antitussives only when major sedative and/or analgesic effect is desired.

NON-NARCOTIC ANTITUSSIVES

DEXTROMETHORPHAN HYDROBROMIDE (Romilar)

Dextromethorphan is a synthetic morphinan derivative that apparently acts centrally, similar to codeine.[52] Despite a paucity of well-controlled studies, several reported trials demonstrate effective control of both experimental and pathologic cough under acute and chronic circumstances.[53,54] Decrease in secretions[4] and a mild anti-inflammatory effect[55] have been reported; neither of these effects seems clinically significant. Unlike codeine, dextromethorphan has no demonstrable analgesic effect[56] and appears to suppress ciliary activity only in higher than normal dosage.[57]

Dependence, Overdosage, and Other Abuse—Despite derivation from a morphine-like substance, dextromethorphan (unlike the levorotatory methorphan) apparently does not have dependence or addiction liability.[58] Drug abuse has been recorded wherein cannabis-like effects are sought.[59,60] This phenomenon may be in part related to the alcohol in commercial formulations, since no physical dependence could be demonstrated upon abrupt withdrawal.[61] Overdosage produces dizziness, diplopia, headache, nausea, and vomiting.[58] Mild respiratory stimulation has been occasionally reported at normal antitussive dose ranges.[12] Although significant respiratory depression occurs with very large doses,[62] no deaths have been reported.[63]

Adverse Reactions—Adverse reactions are infrequent and generally mild, and include slight drowsiness, dizziness, headache, nausea, and vomiting; these remit after discontinuation of the drug.[64] Children from two months to 15 years of age exhibit variation in the reaction pattern.[65,66]

Metabolism—Dextromethorphan is rapidly absorbed orally, achieving peak plasma levels at 30 to 60 minutes after ingestion.[52] The drug is biotransformed in the liver, and the metabolites excreted by the kidney. Metabolism is primarily hepatic with excretion primarily renal. No specific data are available with respect to the effects of renal or hepatic failure.[43]

Drug Interactions—A fatal interaction with the monoamine oxidase inhibitor phenelzine has been recorded,[67] and this combination probably should be avoided. Dextromethorphan should be given cautiously with other central nervous system depressants.

Dosage—Oral: Adults, 10 to 20 mg every four to six hours (maximum 120 mg/day). Higher doses do not increase effectiveness but may prolong action to 10 to 12 hours; this may be useful for nocturnal cough control.

Children, 1 mg/kg daily in three to four divided doses.

Parenteral: Parenteral dosage is used by at least one center to improve tolerance to endotracheal tubes.[68]

ANTIHISTAMINES

Antihistamines are not properly classified as antitussives since their antihistaminic (anticholinergic) properties do not parallel their antitussive effects. Atropine, for example, has no measurable antitussive effect in dogs in doses up to 5 mg/kg. Only diphenhydramine has been advocated as a specific antitussive; it is included in several cough mixtures. However, it is no more effective than codeine and may cause unwanted sedation.[9,63,69,70]

Various antihistamines are included in cough/cold mixtures. They do not shorten duration of viral infection and are likely effective in diminishing rhinorrhea only in the early phases of a cold. Atropine-like drying of mucus may lead to mucus plugging and inspissation—of particular concern in patients with asthma or lower respiratory tract infection.[69,71]

Antihistamines, therefore, seem useful only for the symptomatic relief of cough associated with allergic rhinitis. Under all other circumstances, antihistamine-free cough preparations should be selected.

VOLATILE SUBSTANCES

Volatile oils have been incorporated into mouthwash, ointments, lozenges, and inhalants for their antitussive properties. Camphor, menthol, peppermint, eucalyptus, and thymol are most commonly used. Each has been considered safe within usual dosage ranges; however, none has been demonstrated clearly effective as an antitussive agent.

Abuse and Overdosage—Some volatile oil preparations have been abused by sniffing, but most toxicity has been reported with ingestion.[63] Camphor toxicity is manifested primarily by central nervous system stimulation; convulsions may occur when 2 g or more are given. As little as 0.7 g of camphor has been lethal for a child,[63] but up to 45 g has been tolerated.[72]

Menthol and peppermint oil toxicity is manifested by nausea, vomiting, abdominal pain, dizziness, staggering gait, slowed respiration, facial flushing, somnolence and coma. Fatalities have occurred with doses of 2 g.[72] Hypersensitivity may occur with repeated topical exposure.[63] Death through asphyxiation has been reported due to menthol-induced glottal spasm with administration of intranasal menthol drops in an infant.[73] Apparently two to five times the recommended dose for vaporizers may be used without substantially increasing irritating toxic effects.[63]

Eucalyptus oil may be fatal in doses of as little as 3.5 mg. Ingestion may produce nausea and vomiting, epigastric burning, vertigo, ataxia, muscle weakness and stupor. There are no reports of hypersensitivity. Approximately two to five times the recommended doses for vaporizers may be used without substantially increasing the irritating or toxic effects.[63]

Thymol oil is less toxic than menthol; 50 to 120 g is thought to be necessary to cause poisoning.[63]

ETHANOL

A single study of the effects of ethanol on experimentally produced cough shows that doses of one ml per kilogram (producing blood levels of 80 to 100 mg/100 ml) may effectively reduce cough.[74] This observation may partly explain the high incidence of aspiration and lung abscess in alcoholic populations. The lesser doses of alcohol ingested with normal use of cough/cold preparations have not been studied for their antitussive effects.

LOCAL ANESTHETICS

Topically administered lidocaine, tetracaine and other local anesthetics are effective cough suppressants for short periods. They are too difficult to administer and too short-acting to be useful for the general treatment of cough, but they are useful in endoscopic and radiologic studies of the airways. Absorption through mucus membranes may result in rapid attainment of potentially toxic levels.[7,75] In a rapid intravenous bolus dose of 150 to 200 mg lidocaine is effective as a cough suppressant for eight to nine minutes.[76] Emergency support for the control of toxic manifestations should be available.

OTHER DRUGS

A wide variety of other agents are available as over-the-counter or prescription antitussive drugs. Well-controlled clinical studies are often not available, and advantages over codeine or dextromethorphan have generally not been demonstrated.[9,19,53,77–79]

Benzonatate (Tessalon) is felt to be unique as an antitussive because of its combined central effect and peripheral inhibition of stretch receptors.[80] Clinical trials are few and generally poorly controlled. Some efficacy has been demonstrated in pathologic cough, but careful comparison with codeine is difficult due to the comparatively delayed onset and peak of action of benzonatate.[81,82] In doses of 100 mg oral benzonatate seems somewhat less effective than dextromethorphan;[83] however, in parenteral use, benzonatate appears to be effective in preparation for bronchoscopy or laryngoscopy.[84] Further study of this use is indicated.

Noscapine (Tusscapine) is an opium-derived alkaloid that has neither analgesic nor addictive properties.[85] Several clinical trials suggest equipotency with codeine; doses of 30 to 60 mg are used orally. Side effects, predominantly gastrointestinal, are seen in up to 30% of patients studied.[9] Further controlled trials are needed to determine the role of this drug in cough control.

Levopropoxyphene (Novrad) is a synthetic non-narcotic isomer of propoxyphene without analgesic properties. Several moderately well-controlled human studies in patients with pathologic cough demonstrate efficacy approaching that of dextromethorphan.[9,86,87] Doses of 50 to 100 mg are used for cough control, but one study noted a 40% incidence of side effects after one week of use at this level. There is no evidence that this drug is superior to codeine or dextromethorphan.

REFERENCES

1. Evans JN, Jaeger MJ: Mechanical aspects of coughing. Pneumonologie 152:253–257, 1975.
2. Ross BB, Gramiak R, Rahn H: Physical dynamics of the cough mechanism. J Appl Physiol 8:264–268, 1955.
3. Widdicombe JG: Receptors in the trachea and bronchi of the cat. J Physiol (London) 123:71–104, 1954.
4. Bucher K: Pathophysiology and pharmacology of cough. Pharmacol Rev 10:43–58, 1958.
5. Widdicombe JG: Respiratory reflexes. In *Handbook of Physiology,* Section 3, Respiration volume 1. Edited by H Rahn, WO Fenn. Washington, American Physiological Society, 1964, pp 606–609.
6. Widdicombe JG: Respiratory reflexes from the trachea and bronchi of the cat. J Physiol (Lond) 123:55–70, 1954.
7. Petty TL: *Pulmonary Diagnostic Techniques.* Philadelphia, Lea and Febiger, 1975, p 138.
8. Wolff AP, May M, Nuelle D: The tympanic membrane, a source of the cough reflex. JAMA 223:1269, 1973.
9. Eddy NB, Friebel H, Hahn KJ, et al: *Codeine and Its Alternates for Pain and Cough Relief.* Geneva, World Health Organization, 1970.
10. Swyer PR: Cough (editorial). Can Med Assoc J 75:524–525, 1956.
11. Boyd EM: Expectorants and respiratory tract fluid. Pharmacol Rev 6:521–542, 1954.
12. Bedell GN, Seebohm PM: Treatment of pulmonary emphysema. JAMA 169:1699–1702, 1959.

13. Tedeschi RE, Tedeschi DH, Hitchens JT, et al: A new antitussive method involving mechanical stimulation in unanesthetized dogs. J Pharmacol Exp Ther 126:338–344, 1959.
14. Glazko WA, Dill RM, Young TC, et al: Metabolic disposition of diphenhydramine. Clin Pharmacol Ther 16:1066–1076, 1974.
15. Ballinger B, Browning M, O'Malley K: Drug-metabolizing capacity in states of drug dependence and withdrawal. Br J Pharmacol 45:638–643, 1972.
16. Castleman B, Kibbee BU (editors): Case 67–1961. N Engl J Med 265:801–804, 1961.
17. Davis KK: Codeine intoxication in infancy. N Engl J Med 265:592–593, 1961.
18. O'Malley K, Crooks J, Duke E, et al: Effect of age and sex on human drug metabolism. Br Med J 3:607–609, 1971.
19. Chodosh, S, Segal MS: Chronic bronchitis. N Engl J Med 270:894–897, 1964.
20. Anderton RL: Rectus abdominal muscles pulled by coughing (letter). JAMA 222:486, 1972.
21. Schen RJ, Zurkowski S: Increased serum creatinine phosphokinase activity with violent coughing. N Engl J Med 289:328–329, 1973.
22. Irani F, Sanchis J: Inspiration- and cough-induced atrioventricular block. Can Med Assoc J 105:735–736, 1971.
23. Aaronson DW, Rovner RN, Patterson R: Cough syncope: case presentation and review. J Allergy 46:359–363, 1970.
24. Natelson SE, Molnar W: Malfunction of ventriculoatrial shunts caused by the circulatory dynamics of coughing. J Neurosurg 36:283–286, 1972.
25. Bookman R: Cough in allergic respiratory disease. Ann Allergy 29:367–371, 1971.
26. Herzog VH: Erschlaffung und exspiratorische Invagination des membranösen teils der intrathorakalen luftröhre und der hauptbronchien als ursache der asphyktischen anfälle beim asthma bronchiale und bei der chronischen asthmoiden bronchitis des lungenemphysems. Schweiz Med Wschr 84:217–221, 1954.
27. Jones JG, Clarke SW: Dynamics of cough. Br J Anaesth 42:280–285, 1970.
28. Banyai AL, Joannides M: Cough hazard. Chest 29:52–61, 1956.
29. Sharpey-Schafer EP: The mechanism of syncope after coughing. Br Med J 2:860–863, 1953.
30. Bickerman HA: Evaluation of antitussive drugs: clinical and challenge techniques. In *Principles and Techniques of Human Research and Therapeutics,* Vol. 9. Edited by FG McMahon. Mt. Kisco, NY, Futura Publishing Co., 1975, pp 113–115.
31. Woolf CR, Rosenberg A: Objective assessment of cough suppressants under clinical conditions using a tape recorder system. Thorax 19:125–130, 1964.
32. *Evaluations of Drug Interactions,* second edition. Washington, American Pharmaceutical Association, 1976, p 480.
33. von Oettingen WF: *Poisoning: A Guide to Clinical Diagnosis and Treatment,* second edition. Philadelphia, WB Saunders Co, 1958, p 309.
34. Gravenstein JS, Devloo RA, Beecher HK: Effect of antitussive agents on experimental and pathological cough in man. J Appl Physiol 7:119–139, 1954.
35. Seevers MH: Codeine cough syrups—a medical viewpoint. Presented at the Panel Session on 'Medical Aspects of Drug Abuse,' Seventh Annual Conference of International Narcotic Enforcement Officers Association, Montreal, August 24–28, 1966.
36. Himmelsbach CK: Part I. A review of the literature on codeine addiction. Public Health Rep 158(Suppl):1–67, 1940.
37. Brown CT: The addiction liability of codeine. Milit Med 129:1077–1080, 1964.
38. Fraser HF, Van Horn GD, Martin WR, et al: Methods for evaluating addiction liability. (A) 'Attitude' of opiate addicts toward opiate-like drugs. (B) A short-term 'direct' addiction test. J Pharmacol Exp Ther 133:371–387, 1961.
39. Van Leeuwen G, Guthrie R, Stange F: Narcotic withdrawal reaction in a new born infant due to codeine. Pediatrics 36:635–636, 1965.
40. Fraser HF, Isbel H: Human pharmacology and addictiveness of ethyl 1-(3-cyano-3,3-phenylpropyl)-4-phenyl-4-piperidine carboxylate hydrochloride (R-1132, diphenoxylate). Bull Nar 13:29–43, 1961.
41. Winek CL, Collom WD, Wecht CH: Codeine fatality from cough syrup. Clin Toxicol 3:97–100, 1970.
42. Garland J: Drugs and the newly born (editorial). N Engl J Med 271:373, 1964.
43. Medical Literature Department, Merck Sharp & Dohme Research Laboratories: Codeine and certain other analgesic and antitussive agents, a review. Rahway, NJ, Merck & Co, Inc, 1970, p 67.

44. Bellville JW, Seed JC: A comparison of the respiratory depressant effects of dextropropoxyphene and codeine in man. Clin Pharmacol Ther 9:428–434, 1968.
45. Chalmers RK, Cormier JF: Antitussives. In *Handbook of Non-Prescription Drugs*. Edited by LL Hawkins, GB Griffenhagen. Washington, American Pharmaceutical Association, 1973, pp 15–25.
46. Beaver WT: Mild analgesics: a review of their clinical pharmacology (Part II). Am J Med Sci 251:576–599, 1966.
47. Bellville JW, Escarraga LA, Wallenstein SL, et al: The respiratory effects of codeine and morphine in man. Clin Pharmacol Ther 9:435–441, 1968.
48. Bellville JW, Wallenstein, SL, Wald GH, et al: Effect of noscapine and codeine on the respiratory response to carbon dioxide. Anesthesiology 19:545–551, 1958.
49. Johannesson T: Morphine and codeine. The analgesic effect in tolerant and non-tolerant rats. Acta Pharmacol Toxicol 25(Suppl 3):3–83, 1967.
50. Lambert A: Therapeutics of drug habits. N Engl J Med 215:72–82, 1936.
51. Rosenwald RJ, Russell DH: Cough-syrup addiction. N Engl J Med 264:927, 1961.
52. Hahn VKJ, Friebel H: Wirkungen hustenhemmender pharmaka im zentralen anteil der hustenreflexbahn. Med Pharmacol Exp 14:87–97, 1966.
53. Stefko PL, Denzel J, Hickey I: Experimental investigation of nine antitussive drugs. J Pharm Sci 50:216–221, 1961.
54. Calesnick B, Christensen JA: Latency of cough response as a measure of antitussive agents. Clin Pharmacol Ther 8:374–379, 1967.
55. Randall LO, Selitto JJ: Anti-inflammatory effects of Romilar CF. J Am Pharm Assoc 47:313–314, 1958.
56. Winter CA, Flataker L: Antitussive compounds: testing methods and results. J Pharmacol Exp Ther 112:99–108, 1954.
57. Van Dongen K: The effect of narcotine, ticarda and Romilar on coughs and on the movements of the cilia in the air passages. Acta Physiol Pharmacol Neerl 4:500–507, 1956.
58. Isbell H, Fraser HF: Effects and addiction liabilities of the isomers of the 3-methyl ether of Dromoran. J Pharmacol Exp Ther 106:397–398, 1962.
59. Mansky P, Jasinski DR: Effects of dextromethorphan (D) in man. Pharmacologist 12:231, 1970.
60. Isbell H, Fraser HF: Actions and addiction liabilities of dromoran derivatives in man. J Pharmacol Exp Ther 107:524–530, 1953.
61. Degkwitz, R: Dextromethorphan (Romilar) als Ranschmittel. Nervenarzt 35:412–414, 1964.
62. Jacobziner H: The accidental chemical poisoning problem. Postgrad Med 22:283–298, (Sept) 1957.
63. Federal Register, Vol. 41, No. 176, Thursday, September 9, 1976, p 38340–38353.
64. Ralph N: Evaluation of a new cough suppressant. Am J Med Sci 227:297–303, 1954.
65. Carter CJ: A clinical evaluation of the effectiveness of Novrad and acetylsalicylic acid in children with cough. Am J Med Sci 245:105–109/713–717, 1963.
66. Reece CA, Cherry AC, Reece AT, et al: Tape recorder for evaluation of coughs in children, evaluation of antitussive agents. Am J Dis Child 112:124–128, 1966.
67. Rivers N, Horner B: Possible lethal reaction between Nardil and dextromethorphan. Can Med Assoc J 103:85, 1970.
68. Van Poznak A: Dextromethorphan for intubation (letter). Anesthesiology 37:662, 1972.
69. Tempero KF, Hunninghake DB: Antihistamines. Postgrad Med 48:149–154, (Aug) 1970.
70. Lilienfield LS, Rose JC, Princiotto, JV: Antitussive activity of diphenhydramine in chronic cough. Clin Pharmacol Ther 19:421–425, 1976.
71. Greenblatt DJ, Shader RI: Anticholinergics. N Engl J Med 288:1215–1219, 1973.
72. Gleason MN, Gosselin RE, Hodge HC, et al: *Clinical Toxicology of Commercial Products*. Third edition. Baltimore, Williams & Wilkins, 1969, pp 77–79.
73. Lesoine W: Dangers and complications in the use of preparations containing menthol. Hals-Nasen-Ohrenkranke 13:238–239, 1965.
74. Berkowitz H, Reichel J, Shim C: The effect of ethanol on the cough reflex. Clin Sci Mol Med 45:527–531, 1973.
75. Amikam B, Landa J, West J, et al: Bronchofiberscopic observations of the tracheobronchial tree during intubation. Am Rev Resp Dis 105:747–755, 1972.

76. Smith FR, Kundahl PC: Intravenously administered lidocaine as cough depressant during general anesthesia for bronchography. Chest 63:427–429, 1973.
77. Kautz HD: New and nonofficial remedies. JAMA 161:970, 1956.
78. Segal MS, Goldstein MM, Attinger EO: The use of noscapine (narcotine) as an antitussive agent. Dis Chest 32:305–309, 1957.
79. Darke CS, Snowden BA, Verel D, et al: Action of 'Tessalon' on the dyspnoea of patients with chronic lung disease. Br Med J 1:622–624, 1959.
80. Carter CH: A clinical evaluation of the effectiveness of Novrad and acetylsalicylic acid in children with cough. Am J Med Sci 245:713–717, 1963.
81. Simon SW: Symptomatic treatment of asthmatic bronchitis. J Am Geriatr Soc 8:107–111, 1960.
82. Chen JYP, Biller HF, Montgomery EG: Pharmacologic studies of a new antitussive, alpha (dimethylaminoethyl)-ortho-chlorobenzhydrol hydrochloride (SL-501, Bayer B-186). J Pharmacol Exp Ther 128:384–391, 1959.
83. Simon SW: The effectiveness of non-narcotic antitussive drugs. J Am Geriatr Soc 10:653–657, 1962.
84. Lineback M: Benzonatate as cough and gag reflex suppressive. Clin Med 69:1806–1808, 1962.
85. Expert Committee on Drugs Liable to Produce Addiction: Report. Technical Report Series, No. 95. Geneva, World Health Organization, March, 1955, pp 1–16.
86. Abruzzi WA: Clinical evaluation of levo propoxyphene, a new antitussive. J New Drugs 2:310–313, 1972.
87. Ernst CE, Jeffrey M: A new antitussive, levopropoxyphene. Ariz Med 19:221–225, (Oct) 1962.

59. ANTIHISTAMINES USEFUL IN ALLERGIC DISORDERS

David S. Pearlman

The development of antihistamines for anti-allergic therapy stemmed from the implication of histamine as a mediator of allergic reactions. Histamine, however, is only one of many chemical mediators involved in allergic reactions. Antihistamines are extremely useful in the treatment of some but not all allergic disorders.

PHARMACOLOGY

Antihistamines are diverse pharmacologic agents that inhibit the actions of histamine. Some but not all actions of histamine can be blocked by these agents. Recently, the existence of two histamine receptors has been established through the use of conventional antihistamines and a new generation of histamine antagonists.[1] These receptors have been designated H_1 and H_2, and antihistamines now are classified correspondingly as H_1- or H_2-receptor inhibitors. H_1-receptor activation is largely responsible for the histamine-induced tissue responses associated with allergic reactions. H_2-receptor activation is responsible for histamine-induced gastric acid secretion. Although H_2-receptors are also involved in some vascular and other responses to histaminic action and consequently may play a role in allergic inflammation,[2] the use of H_2-receptor inhibitors for anti-allergic therapy currently is entirely experimental. At present, the therapeutic usefulness of H_2-receptor inhibitors is confined to syndromes of gastric hyperacidity.[3]

Both H_1- and H_2-receptor inhibitors are specific and act by competitive inhibition at the respective receptor.[1,4] Antihistaminic compounds are varied in structure, but all have some structural similarity to histamine—specifically, an ethylamine configuration which is involved in histamine receptor activation. H_1-receptor

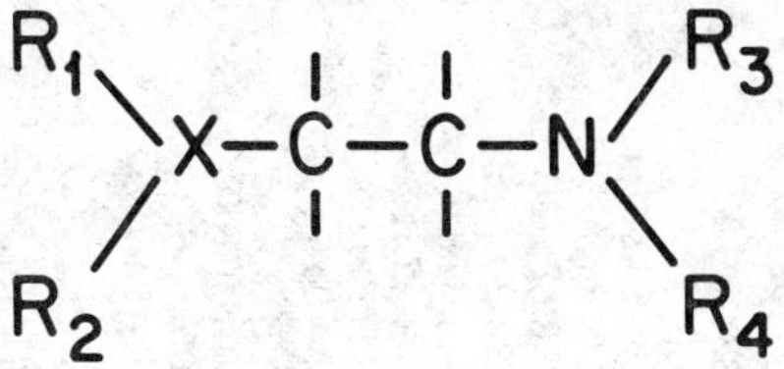

$$R_1R_2X\text{–}\overset{|}{\underset{|}{C}}\text{–}\overset{|}{\underset{|}{C}}\text{–}NR_3R_4$$

FIGURE 1. General structural formula for antihistamines (H_1-receptor inhibitors).

inhibitors generally have structures as in Figure 1, with R_1 and R_2 usually being ring configurations, and R_3 and R_4 most often methyl groups. H_2-receptor inhibitors tend to be smaller molecules, and they more closely resemble histamine itself.

H_1-receptor inhibitors are conventionally classified according to the substituent connecting to the ethylamine, and include alkylamines, ethanolamines, ethylenediamines, phenothiazines, and piperazines (Table 1). Tropines are an additional group having antihistaminic activity.[5] They resemble atropine in structure and possess greater anticholinergic properties than the antihistamines discussed above. Some antihistamines, such as cyproheptadine, are difficult to classify.

Because of the structural similarities between histamine and other biogenic amines (acetylcholine, 5-hydroxytryptamine, epinephrine, norepinephrine) most competitive antagonists have some cross-reactivity. Thus, some alpha-adrenergic inhibitors (eg, phentolamine),[6,7] and tricyclic antidepressants (eg, imipramine) also possess antihistaminic properties. On the other hand, antihistaminic compounds may possess weak anticholinergic activities.[6,8] Cyproheptadine is an effective inhibitor of both histamine and 5-hydroxytryptamine activity.[9]

Since competitive inhibitors are more effective if they reach the receptor site before the agonists, antihistamines are more useful if given before, rather than after, exposure to allergens. Furthermore, effective receptor concentrations of antihistamine are sometimes high. The achievement of such high local concentrations can be limited both by accessibility of the drug to the receptor site and by the side effects of 'high' concentrations. Finally, because antihistamines are competitive inhibitors, and many allergic reactions involve chemical mediators other than or in addition to histamine, antihistamines are less effective than so-called physiologic antagonists (eg, epinephrine) of these chemical mediators.

TABLE 1 Dosage, Preparations and Costs of Antihistamines

Generic Name	Trademark Name(s)	Suggested Oral Dosage (mg)[a] Children 1-6 years	Children 6-12 years[b]	Older Children and Adults	Preparations and 1978 Costs
Ethanolamines					
Diphenhydramine Hydrochloride	Benadryl	12.5 to 25	25 to 50	50	Capsules 25 mg—$3.09/100; 50 mg—$4.60/100 Elixir 12.5 mg/5 ml—$3.68/pt Injection (solution) 10 mg/ml—$1.64/10-ml vial, $3.86/30-ml vial; 50 mg/ml—$0.90/1-ml ampul, $5.99/10-ml vial
Carbinoxamine Maleate	Clistin	2 to 4	4 to 8	4 to 8	Tablets 4 mg—$3.31/100 Elixir 4 mg/5 ml—$4.06/pt
Doxylamine Succinate	Decapryn	3.12 to 6.25	6.25 to 12.5	12.5 to 25	Tablets 12.5 mg—$4.10/100; 25 mg—$5.60/100 Syrup 6.25 mg/5 ml—$4.75/pt
Alkylamines					
Chlorpheniramine Maleate	Chlor-Trimeton (Histaspan) (Teldrin)	0.5 to 2	3 to 4	4	Tablets 4 mg—$3.15/100 Tablets (timed-release) 8 mg—$5.87/100; 12 mg—$8.21/100 Syrup 2 mg/5 ml—$1.00/4 oz Injection (solution) 10 mg/ml—$0.38/1-ml ampul; 100 mg/ml—$1.96/2-ml vial

Brompheniramine Maleate	Dimetane	1 to 2	2 to 4	4 to 8	Tablets 4 mg—$2.70/100 Tablets (timed-release) 8 mg—$4.90/100; 12 mg—$6.80/100 Elixir 2 mg/5 ml—$4.00/pt Injection (solution) 10 mg/ml—$0.54/1-ml ampul
Dexchlorpheniramine Maleate	Polaramine	0.5 to 2	1 to 2	2	Tablets 2 mg—$3.40/100 Tablets (timed-release) 4 mg—$5.86/100; 6 mg—$8.39/100 Syrup 2 mg/5 ml—$3.94/pt
Triprolidine Hydrochloride	Actidil	1.25	1.25 to 2.5	2.5	Tablets 2.5 mg—$2.50/100 Syrup 1.25 mg/5 ml—$2.65/pt
Ethylenediamines					
Tripelennamine Citrate	Pyribenzamine Citrate	12.5 to 25 (doses expressed in terms of hydrochloride salt)	25 to 50	25 to 50	Elixir 37.5 (equivalent to 25 mg of hydrochloride salt)/5 ml—$3.35/pt
Tripelennamine Hydrochloride	Pyribenzamine Hydrochloride	12.5 to 25	25 to 50	25 to 50	Tablets 25 mg—$2.40/100; 50 mg—$3.35/100 Tablets (timed-release) 50 mg—$3.70/100; 100 mg—$6.50/100
Methapyrilene Hydrochloride	Histadyl	—	25	25 to 50	Capsules 25 mg—$2.82/100; 50 mg—$4.01/100 Injection (solution) 20 mg/ml—$1.33/10 ml vial

TABLE 1 *(continued)*

		Suggested Oral Dosage (mg)[a]			
		Children			
Generic Name	Trademark Name(s)	1-6 years	6-12 years[b]	Older Children and Adults	Preparations and 1978 Costs
Piperazines					
Hydroxyzine Hydrochloride	Atarax	5 to 10	10 to 20	10 to 100	Tablets 10 mg—\$8.05/100; 25 mg—\$11.82/100; 50 mg—\$14.42/100; 100 mg—\$16.93/100 Syrup 10 mg/5 ml—\$7.61/pt
Phenothiazines					
Trimeprazine Tartrate	Temaril	1.25 to 2.5	2.5	2.5	Capsules (timed-release) 5 mg—\$6.70/50 Tablets 2.5 mg—\$7.40/100 Syrup 2.5 mg/5 ml—\$2.50/4 oz
Miscellaneous					
Cyproheptadine Hydrochloride	Periactin Hydrochloride	1 to 2	2 to 3	2 to 4	Tablets 4 mg—\$8.73/100 Syrup 2 mg/5 ml—\$6.32/pt

[a] Suggested average starting dose, repeated approximately every six hours as necessary with non-timed-release preparations, every eight to twelve hours for timed-release preparations.

[b] As a rough rule, antihistamine dosage for children 6 to 12 years old is equivalent to the lower end of the adult dose recommendations.

H_1-receptor inhibitors can effectively inhibit histamine-induced vascular permeability, but the vasodilating effects of histamine are only partly inhibited by such agents. Histamine-induced bronchial constriction is effectively blocked, but antigen-induced bronchoconstriction, believed to be mediated in part by histamine, generally is not inhibited effectively. Histamine-induced pruritus is inhibited, but pruritus induced by proteases or by other agents is not.[10] Antihistamines also interfere with the erythematous flare induced by histamine, a response largely based on an axon reflex mechanism. Thus, antihistamines tend to be therapeutic in urticaria and in allergic rhinitis, but not in bronchial asthma (see below). In low concentrations, antihistamines can inhibit histamine release;[11] in high concentrations, however, they may induce histamine release.[12,13] Antihistamines can produce central nervous system stimulation or depression, possibly by mechanisms other than histamine antagonism.

Antihistamines are absorbed well orally and parenterally. The liver, and to a lesser extent, the kidneys, are responsible for metabolizing antihistamines, and the majority of antihistamines are eliminated by the kidneys as water-soluble metabolites. When given orally, some therapeutic effect generally can be expected within 30 to 60 minutes. Liquid and non-enteric-coated tablets usually exert an effect for 3 to 6 hours. The use of enteric-coated preparations can prolong the effect up to 8 to 12 hours. Antihistamines given parenterally have a more rapid onset of action. When given by the intravenous route, they should be administered over a period of a few minutes, since hypotension can result from too rapid administration.

Antihistamines can stimulate hepatic microsomal enzymes,[14–16] but few, if any, clinically important drug interactions resulting from this mechanism have been identified. Tolerance to the therapeutic effects of antihistamines is observed commonly, although the cause for this is not well established. When tolerance occurs, substitution of an alternative antihistamine may be effective; there is some rationale for selecting a replacement from a different chemical class.[17]

ADVERSE EFFECTS

The most frequently observed adverse effects include sedation or, occasionally, excitatory central nervous system effects, dryness of the mucous membranes (particularly a feeling of dryness of the mouth), and nausea, anorexia, or epigastric discomfort[18–21] (Table 2). Certain

TABLE 2 Adverse Effects Associated with the Use of Conventional Antihistamines (H_1-Receptor Inhibitors)[a]

1. Somnolence, drowsiness, lassitude, fatigue, weakness, depression, impaired judgment, incoordination, ataxia, hyporeflexia, delirium, coma

   Tinnitus, vertigo; diplopia, blurred vision, hyperreflexia, paresthesias, paralysis

   Convulsions, syncope, EEG abnormalities
2. Tachycardia, hypertension, hypotension, shock; ECG abnormalities
3. Fever, extreme hyperthermia
4. Loss of appetite[b], nausea, epigastric distress, vomiting, constipation, diarrhea
5. Dysuria, urinary frequency, urinary retention; renal failure
6. Dry mouth, nose, throat; cough
7. Leukopenia, agranulocytosis, haemolytic anaemia; impaired platelet function; hepatitis (phenothiazines)
8. Hypersensitivity, including photosensitivity (phenothiazines)

[a]From various sources; in particular, see references 17, 18, 19, 20.
[b]Cyproheptadine increases appetite.

adverse effects occur more or less frequently, depending on the chemical class to which the antihistamine belongs. For example, sedation tends to be more prominent among the ethanolamine antihistaminic drugs, whereas ethylenediamines as a group are less sedating but are associated with more gastrointestinal side effects. There is considerable variation within each class, however. Diphenhydramine commonly produces sedation, whereas other ethanolamines (such as carbinoxamine) are less sedating even than tripelennamine, an ethylenediamine.[5] The use of two or more antihistaminics in combination can result in synergism without increasing side effects.[22]

Leukopenia and agranulocytosis are uncommon complications of antihistamines and are completely reversible on discontinuation of the drug.[23] A rare complication of phenothiazine antihistamine therapy is blockade of alpha receptors and epinephrine reversal. Specifically, profound hypotension can result when epinephrine is administered to a patient who also is receiving a potent phenothiazine drug.[24] Paradoxically, hypersensitivity reactions, including photosensitivity, to antihistamines have been observed,[25] due either to the drug itself or to preservatives or fillers in the preparation. Antihistamines can interfere with skin testing for skin-sensitizing (reaginic or IgE) antibody but do not interfere with serologic tests for IgE antibody (eg, radioallergosorbent test or RAST). Generally, inhibition or interference is incomplete, but significant interference can persist for days after the drug is discontinued, particularly with the use of hydroxyzine.[26]

Teratogenic effects of piperazine antihistamines have been reported in animals; rarely if ever in humans.[27] Antihistamines are commonly used drugs in pregnancy[28] and have been only rarely implicated as teratogens,[29–31] but, as with all drugs, administration of these compounds during pregnancy requires careful risk-benefit analysis. Antihistamines used late in pregnancy have been rarely associated with interference of fetal platelet function[32] and the induction of jaundice in prematurely born infants.[33] These reports suggest that antihistamines cross the placental barrier, but there is little other direct evidence for transplacental transfer of antihistamines.[30] Excretion in breast milk occurs but the resulting concentrations are low.[34] Nevertheless, the possibility of a clinically significant effect on a nursing infant should be kept in mind.

Some tolerance to antihistaminic side effects as well as to their therapeutic effects can develop. In particular, sedative effects can diminish or disappear during chronic use.

INTERACTIONS

Caution is warranted when antihistamines are given with barbiturates, alcohol, tranquilizers, or other potential central nervous system depressants. Antihistamines also should be used with caution in disorders (such as glaucoma or prostatic hypertrophy) in which anticholinergic effects may be undesirable and in combination with other atropine-like agents and tricyclic antidepressants.

SELECTION AND USE OF ANTIHISTAMINES

Whenever possible, antihistamines should be used in anticipation of an allergic reaction. Thus, the individual who characteristically has allergic rhinitis or conjunctivitis at a neighbor's or relative's house is more likely to benefit from an antihistamine if taken an hour prior to the anticipated contact rather than after symptoms have begun to occur.

Whatever antihistamine is chosen, the patient should be forewarned of potential side effects, particularly sedation. In individuals with a history of high sensitivity to the soporific effects of antihistamines, selection of a drug with a relatively low sedating potential (eg, carbinoxamine) is desirable, starting with a low dosage.

For the treatment of an acute allergic reaction, a rapid but relatively short-acting antihistamine may be sufficient. On the other hand, for treatment of prolonged allergic symptoms, long-acting preparations are preferable. In general, the longer-acting preparations are desirable for treatment of perennial or seasonal allergic rhinitis, especially since they can be administered at bedtime for some residual action during the night and early morning hours.

The dosage of an antihistamine is as important as the selection of a particular antihistamine. Doses required for effective therapeutic action often are significantly higher (two to four-fold) than generally recommended by the drug manufacturers.[35] High doses should be achieved gradually, with the patient warned of potential side effects.

The main indication for the parenteral administration of antihistamines is acute severe allergic reactions, but the use of antihistamines is clearly secondary to the need for physiologic antagonists such as epinephrine.

Many combination preparations, containing sympathomimetic and/or anticholinergics in addition to antihistamines, are available for clinical use (Table 3). The clinical value of such preparations is generally not established. Topical antihistamines are potentially sensitizing and generally are not to be recommended.

Allergic Rhinitis and Conjunctivitis

Antihistamines are useful in the pharmacologic management of seasonal or perennial allergic rhinitis and conjunctivitis. They tend to be more effective in controlling pruritus, sneezing, and rhinorrhea, than in nasal obstruction.[20] In perennial allergic rhinitis, nasal congestion often is the most prominent symptom. The addition of sympathomimetics to antihistamines may be superior therapeutically to antihistamines alone, but this is largely unproven. In perennial allergic rhinitis, round-the-clock therapy generally is required for alleviation of moderate to severe symptoms, but symptoms may be adequately controlled (particularly early morning symptoms such as postnasal drip, hoarseness, sneezing or rhinorrhea) with long-acting medication only, taken just prior to retiring. Administration of an antihistamine is recommended one hour prior to anticipated development of symptoms. Antihistamines also may be helpful in controlling some of the rhinorrhea and nasal itching in nonallergic 'vasomotor' rhinitis, along with adrenergic decongestants. Topical antihistaminic preparations are available for use in acute allergic conjunctivitis, but systemic antihistaminics are preferable, especially when long-term therapy is necessary. Antihistamines are of little value in infectious rhinitis.[20,36]

Middle Ear Disease and Sinusitis

Serous otitis media and sinusitis occur in association with allergic rhinitis, although the bulk of these disorders occur in individuals without demonstrable 'allergy'. The use of antihistamines to prevent or minimize serous otitis media or sinusitis associated with allergic rhinitis makes theoretical sense, but there is little evidence of their effectiveness. There is no evidence that antihistaminic compounds are effective in the treatment of acute infectious otitis media or sinusitis.

Bronchial Asthma (Reactive Airway Disease)

Because histamine may play a role in asthma, antihistamines were expected to be effective in its treatment. However, except for an occasional patient,[37] the therapeutic value of antihistamines in asthma has been disappointing. In some patients, mild asthmatic symptoms may be aborted or diminished by the use of antihistamines, particularly when given for nighttime asthma in advance of asthmatic symptoms,[38,39] and pulmonary function sometimes can improve following antihistamine administration.[40] Antihistamines also can exert some suppressive effect on cough[20] which may intensify the pulmonary obstruction of asthma. On the other hand, antihistamines can induce bronchospasm.[41] Because some antihistamines have anticholinergic properties and may dry and thicken bronchial mucus secretions, it is frequently held that antihistamines should not be used for asthma. This impression, however, is not well substantiated.[42,43] Antihistamines can be helpful in controlling allergic upper respiratory symptoms which aggravate or possibly precipitate asthma in susceptible individuals.

TABLE 3 Dosage, Preparations, and Costs of Selected Antihistamine-Sympathomimetic Combination Preparations

Preparation	1978 Cost	Antihistamine(s)[a]	
Actified		triprolidine HCl	
tablets	$4.75/100	2.5 mg	
syrup	$4.30/pt	1.25 mg	
Co-Pyronil		methapyrilene HCl	pyrrobutamine phosphate
capsules	$7.64/100	25 mg	15 mg
pediatric capsules	$4.78/100	12.5 mg	7.5 mg
suspension	$9.13/pt	12.5 mg	7.5 mg
Deconamine		chlorpheniramine maleate	
capsules (timed-release)	$10.47/100	8 mg	
tablets	$5.34/100	4 mg	
elixir	$4.80/pt	2 mg	
Demazin		chlorpheniramine maleate	
tablets (timed-release)	$7.59/100	4 mg	
syrup	$1.18/4 oz	1 mg	
Dimetapp		brompheniramine maleate	
tablets (timed-release)	$9.00/100	12 mg	
elixir	$4.50/pt	4 mg	
Disophrol		dexbrompheniramine maleate	
tablets (timed-release)	$11.73/100	6 mg	
tablets	$6.05/100	2 mg	
Drixoral		dexbrompheniramine maleate	
tablets (timed-release)	$11.73/100	6 mg	
Naldecon		chlorpheniramine maleate	phenyltoloxamine citrate
tablets (timed-release)	$12.61/100	5 mg	15 mg
syrup	$7.24/pt	2.5 mg	7.5 mg
pediatric syrup	$6.73/pt	0.5 mg	2 mg
drops	$3.24/20 ml	0.5 mg	2 mg
Rondec		carbinoxamine maleate	
tablets	$7.91/100	4 mg	
chewable tablets	$6.79/60	4 mg	
syrup	$6.64/pt	4 mg	
drops	$3.08/20 ml	2 mg	

	Suggested Dosage[b]			
		Children		
Sympathomimetic(s)[a]	Infants	1 to 6 Years	6 to 12 Years	Older Children
pseudoephedrine HCl	—	—	1	1
60 mg	—	1	2	2
30 mg	—	1	2	2
cyclopentamine HCl				
12.5 mg	—	—	1	1 or 2
6.25 mg	—	—	1 or 2	—
6.25 mg	—	½ or 1	1 or 2	2
pseudoephedrine HCl				
120 mg	—	—	—	1
60 mg	—	—	½	1
30 mg	—	½	½ or 1	2
phenylephrine HCl				
20 mg	—	—	1	1 or 2
2.5 mg	—	½ to 2	2	2 or 3
phenylpropanolamine HCl phenylephrine HCl				
15 mg each	—	—	1	1
5 mg each	—	1	2	2
pseudoephedrine sulfate				
120 mg	—	—	—	1
60 mg	—	—	½ or 1	1 or 2
pseudoephedrine sulfate				
120 mg	—	—	—	1
phenyl-propanolamine HCl — phenylephrine HCl				
40 mg — 10 mg	—	—	1	1
20 mg — 5 mg	—	—	½	2
5 mg — 1.25 mg	—	1	2	—
5 mg — 1.25 mg	½ to 2 ml	—	—	—
pseudoephedrine HCl				
60 mg	—	—	1	1
60 mg	—	½	1	1
60 mg	—	½	1	1
25 mg	½ to 1 ml	—	—	—

TABLE 3 *(continued)*

PREPARATION	1978 COST	ANTIHISTAMINE(S)[a]
Triaminic		pyrilamine maleate pheniramine maleate
tablets (timed-release)	$9.69/100	25 mg each
pediatric tablets (timed-release)	$4.30/50	12.5 mg each
syrup	$4.49/pt	6.25 mg each
drops	$2.24/15 ml	10 mg each

[a]Amount of antihistamine or sympathomimetic listed for syrups, elixirs, and suspension is per 5 ml (1 teaspoonful); amount for drops is per 1 ml.

[b]Suggested average starting dose (closely resembles manufacturer's recommendations in most cases).

Cough

Antihistamines are incorporated in many cough mixtures, partly because of their antitussive effect; this effect is presumably due to the local anesthetic properties possessed by some antihistamines. Amelioration of cough also may be mediated through control of rhinitis and pharyngeal drainage which can trigger or aggravate coughing. Antihistaminic cough preparations may be useful in ameliorating mild cough, but rarely are effective in controlling severe cough.

Anaphylaxis

Antihistamines are at best only moderately effective inhibitors of some of the components of the anaphylactic reaction.[44] They are most useful in controlling the urticarial component and pruritus, and, to a lesser extent, angioedema.[44] If given early enough, they also may play a role in preventing the development of hypotension, but the ability of antihistamines to reverse severe manifestations of anaphylaxis, once they have occurred, is limited. Antihistamines are only adjunctive in the treatment of anaphylactic reactions, secondary to adrenergic agents. When employed for this purpose, initially, administration of a potent antihistaminic (eg, diphenhydramine 50 mg) intravenously or intramuscularly is advised. Subsequently, depending upon the clinical status of the patient, medication can be

	Suggested Dosage[b]			
		Children		
Sympathomimetic(s)[a]	Infants	1 to 6 Years	6 to 12 Years	Older Children
phenylpropranolamine HCl				
50 mg	—	—	—	1
25 mg	—	—	1	—
12.5 mg	—	½ or 1	2	—
20 mg	5 to 10 drops	—	—	—

Dosage frequency for syrups, tablets, and capsules (non-timed-release) is usually three times a day; timed-release tablets, every 8 to 12 hours. Dosage quantities listed are either number of tablets or capsules or teaspoonsful of liquid.

taken orally. Continued administration of antihistamines is advised round-the-clock for at least 48 hours after all symptoms have abated. Antihistamines may be helpful in the prevention of severe allergic reactions to contrast media and allergic transfusion reactions,[45,46] but this is not always true.

Urticaria and Angioedema

Antihistamines are of great use in the treatment of acute, and, to a lesser extent, chronic urticaria. Among the most effective agents are diphenhydramine, cyproheptadine, and hydroxyzine. The latter is especially useful in controlling chronic urticaria and pruritus.[47] In some patients with cold urticaria, cyproheptadine is more effective than other antihistamines.[48] When used to treat urticaria and angioedema, antihistamines should be employed round-the-clock until symptoms abate completely. Conventional antihistamines are of little value in the treatment of hereditary angioedema.

Eczema and Other Forms of Dermatitis

Antihistamines are useful in relieving the pruritus of atopic dermatitis and other forms of eczema, including contact dermatitis, but they have little or no effect on the underlying disease. The antipruritic effects of antihistamines are independent of their sedative effects. However, since itching tends to be most intense at night, potent antihistamines with prominent sedative effects (eg, diphenhydramine, hydroxyzine) may be of particular value for nocturnal symptoms. The most effective antipruritic in eczematoid dermatoses is the control of the inflammatory condition itself. Antihistamines may be helpful in ameliorating histamine-induced pruritus, but pruritus induced by other chemical mediators are not effectively relieved.[10] Topical antihistamines *should not* be employed because of their sensitizing potential.[49]

Other Allergic Conditions

Antihistamines are of use in the treatment of serum sickness, particularly the urticaria and angioedema. The effectiveness of antihistamines in so-called allergic migraine and in gastrointestinal disturbances attributed to allergic reactivity is unclear, but antihistamines have been claimed to afford relief in some patients.

TREATMENT OF ANTIHISTAMINE TOXICITY

Side effects associated with antihistamines are described above. The most important effects of antihistamine overdosage relate to the central nervous system.[21] In the young child, hallucinations, general excitement, ataxia, athetosis, and convulsions may occur. Signs may resemble atropine poisoning, with fixed dilated pupils, a flushed face, and fever.[50] Vision may be blurred, coma may ensue, and cardiorespiratory collapse and death can occur. In adults, there tends to be less excitation and more central nervous system depression.

In addition to discontinuation of antihistaminic drugs, treatment in general is supportive. Analeptics should not be used but means for mechanical ventilation should be at hand for use if necessary. If convulsions occur, short-acting anticonvulsants should be employed. Hemodialysis can be considered in cases of gross antihistamine overdosage.

REFERENCES

1. Black JW, Duncan WAM, Durant GJ, et al: Definition and antagonism of H_2-receptors. Nature 236:385–390, 1972.
2. Eyre P, Wells PW: Histamine H_2-receptors modulate systemic anaphylaxis: a dual cardiovascular action of histamine in calves. Br J Pharmacol 49:364–367, 1973.
3. Celestin LR, Harvey V, Saunders JHB, et al: Treatment of duodenal ulcer by metiamide. A multicentre trial. Lancet 2:779–781, 1975.

4. Ariëns EJ, Simonis AM, van Rossum JM: Drug-receptor interaction: action of one or more drugs with one receptor system. In *Molecular Pharmacology: The Mode of Action of Biologically Active Compounds* (Medicinal Chemistry Series, Vol. 1). Edited by EJ Ariëns. New York, Academic Press, 1974, pp 119–286.
5. Wilhelm RE: The newer anti-allergic agents. Med Clin North Am 45:887–906, 1961.
6. Winder CV, Kaiser ME, Anderson MM, et al: Myotropic spasmolytic, histaminolytic, and atropine-like actions of some derivatives of dimethylaminoethyl benzhydryl ether hydrochloride (Benadryl). J Pharmacol Exp Ther 87:121–131, 1946.
7. Nickerson M, Collier B: Drugs inhibiting adrenergic nerves and structures innervated by them. In *The Pharmacological Basis of Therapeutics,* 5th edition. Edited by LS Goodman, A Gilman. New York, Macmillan, 1975, pp 533–564.
8. Loew ER: The pharmacology of Benadryl and the specificity of antihistamine drugs. Ann NY Acad Sci 50:1142–1160, 1950.
9. Stone CA, Wenger HC, Ludden CT, et al: Antiserotonin-antihistaminic properties of cyproheptadine. J Pharmacol Exp Ther 131:73–94, 1961.
10. Hägermark Ö: Influence of antihistamines, sedatives, and aspirin on experimental itch. Acta Derm Venereol 53:363–368, 1973.
11. Lichtenstein LM, Gillespie E: Inhibition of histamine release by histamine is controlled by an H_2-receptor. Nature 244:287–288, 1973.
12. Arunlakshana O: Histamine release by antihistamines. J Physiol 119:47–48P, 1953.
13. Mota I, Dias de Silva W: The anti-anaphylactic and histamine releasing properties of the antihistaminics. Their effects on the mast cells. Br J Pharmacol Chemother 15:396–404, 1960.
14. Conney AH, Schneidman K, Jacobson J, et al: Drug induced changes in steroid metabolism. Ann NY Acad Sci 123:98–107, 1965.
15. Kuntzman R: Drugs and enzyme induction. Annu Rev Pharmacol 9:21–36, 1969.
16. Hansten PD: *Drug Interactions,* 2nd edition. Philadelphia, Lea and Febiger, 1973.
17. Grayson LD, Shair HM: Atopic dermatitis. III. The correct choice of antihistaminic agents. Ann Allergy 21:168–170, 1963.
18. Arbesman CE: The pharmacology, physiology, and clinical evaluation of the new antihistaminic drugs (Pyribenzamine and Benadryl). NY State J Med 47:1775–1781, 1947.
19. Loveless MH, Dworin M: Allergy and antihistamine therapy. A review. Bull NY Acad Med 25:473–487, 1949.
20. Feinberg SM, Malkiel S, Feinberg AR: *The Antihistamines: Their Clinical Application.* Chicago, Yearbook, 1950.
21. Wyngaarden JB, Seevers MH: The toxic effects of antihistaminic drugs. JAMA 145:277–282, 1951.
22. Naranjo P, Banda de Naranjo E: Studies of the combined action of some antihistaminic agents. Ann Allergy 11:699–716, 1953.
23. Blanton WB, Owens MEB Jr: Granulocytopenia due probably to 'pyribenzamine'. JAMA 134:454–455, 1947.
24. Legge DA, Tiede JJ, Peters GA, et al: Death from tension pneumothorax and chlorpromazine cardiorespiratory collapse as separate complications of asthma. Ann Allergy 27:23–29, 1969.
25. Cahn MM, Levy EJ: Ultraviolet light factor in chlorpromazine dermatitis. Arch Dermatol 75:38–40, 1975.
26. Cook TJ, MacQueen DM, Wittig HJ, et al: Degree and duration of skin test suppression and side effects with antihistamines. J Allergy Clin Immunol 51:71–77, 1973.
27. Cahen RL: Evaluation of teratogenicity of drugs. Clin Pharmacol Ther 5:480–514, 1964.
28. Hill R: Drugs ingested by pregnant women. Clin Pharmacol Ther 14:654–659, 1973.
29. Cohlon SQ: The teratogenicity of drugs in man. Pharmacol Physicians 3:1–5, 1969.
30. Martin EW, Alexander SF, Farage DJ, et al: *Hazards of Medicine*. Philadelphia, Lippincott, 1971, pp 216–320.
31. Mellin GW: Drugs in the first trimester of pregnancy and the fetal life of Homo sapiens. Am J Obstet Gynecol 90:1169–1180, 1964.
32. Pockedly C, Ente G: Adverse hematologic effects of drugs. Pediatr Clin North Am 19:1095–1111, 1972.
33. Done AK: Developmental pharmacology. Clin Pharmacol Ther 5:432–479, 1964.

34. Knowles JA: Excretion of drugs in milk—a review. J Pediatr 66:1068–1082, 1965.
35. Hyde JS, Floro LD: Theophylline and chlorpheniramine in childhood asthma. Dose requirements for children 6 to 12 years (therapeutic orphans) and young adults 13 to 18 years of age receiving cromolyn sodium prophylaxis. Ann Allergy 32:73–79, 1974.
36. Lorriman G, Martin WJ: Trial of Antistin in the common cold. Br Med J 2:430–431, 1950.
37. Farr RS, Spector SL: Medical management of reversible obstructive airway disease. In *Recent Advances in Asthma Therapy*. Edited by RS Farr, E Middleton Jr, and SL Spector. Miami, Symposia Specialists Medical Books, 1976, pp 39–53.
38. Herxheimer H: Aleudrine and anthisan in bronchial spasm. Lancet 1:667–671, 1948.
39. Herxheimer H: Antihistamines in bronchial asthma. Br Med J 2:901–905, 1949.
40. Simonsson BG: Effect of Multergan on ventilatory capacities in patients with generalized airways obstruction. Acta Allergol 19:305–310, 1964.
41. Hawkins DF: Bronchoconstrictor and bronchodilator actions of antihistaminic drugs. Br J Pharmacol Chemother 10:230–239, 1955.
42. Drug Committee of the American College of Allergists: An investigation of the possible disadvantages of antihistamines in allergic asthma. Ann Allergy 30:95–97, 1972.
43. Karlin JM: The use of antihistamines in asthma. Ann Allergy 30:342–347, 1972.
44. Feinberg SM, Friedlaender S: Histamine antagonists. IV. Pyridil-N' benzyl-N-demethylethylenediamine (Pyribenzamine) in symptomatic treatment of allergic manifestations. Am J Med Sci 213:58–60, 1947.
45. Wilhelm RE, Nutting HM, Devlin HB, et al: Antihistamines in allergic and pyrogenic transfusion reactions. JAMA 158:529–531, 1955.
46. Zweiman B, Mishkin MM, Hildreth EA: An approach to the performance of contrast studies in contrast material-reactive persons. Ann Intern Med 83:159–162, 1975.
47. Feinberg AR, Pruzansky JJ, Feinberg SM, et al: Hydroxyzine (Atarax) in chronic urticaria and in allergic manifestations. J Allergy 29:358–361, 1958.
48. Wanderer AA, Ellis EF: Treatment of cold urticaria with cyproheptadine. J Allergy Clin Immunol 48:366–371, 1971.
49. Fisher AA: Antihistamine dermatitis. Cutis 18:329–366, 1976.
50. Greenblatt DJ, Shader RI: Anticholinergics. N Engl J Med 288:1215–1219, 1973.

DRUGS USED TO TREAT NEUROMUSCULAR DISORDERS

60. ANTIPARKINSONISM AGENTS

Richard T. Scheife and Michael M. Cohen

Parkinson's disease is a major cause of disability among the elderly. The frequency of Parkinson's disease, although not known precisely, is probably around 100 to 150 per 100,000 with an annual incidence of about 20 new cases per 100,000. The clinical tetrad of akinesia (poverty of spontaneous movement, mask-like facies), rigidity of muscular tone, tremor in repose (usually a rhythmic, 3 to 5 cycle per second tremor present at rest, exacerbated by stress and completely absent during sleep) and aberrations of postural control (flexed stance, difficulty in turning, and the characteristic festinating, hurried gait) are readily recognized by most clinicians.

The exact etiology of Parkinson's disease is not established. Hence, most cases of parkinsonism are termed idiopathic. The complete parkinsonian syndrome has been observed in patients following certain forms of encephalitis (post-encephalitic parkinsonism), most notably after the influenza pandemic of 1918–1919. A similar symptom complex, that is particularly resistant to treatment, can occur following carbon monoxide or manganese toxicity. A modified and generally reversible form of parkinsonism often occurs in patients being treated with agents that deplete intraneuronal stores of dopamine (eg, reserpine, tetrabenazine) or agents that block access of dopamine to its receptor (eg, butyrophenones, thioxanthines, many of the phenothiazines, other neuroleptic agents).

The underlying abnormality in Parkinson's disease appears to be a degeneration of dopaminergic neurons in the extrapyramidal tracts of the central nervous system,[1–5] and more specifically the degeneration of melanin-containing neurons, including both dopaminergic and specific noradrenergic neurons as well as other pigmented neurons of the brain stem.[6] While it appears clear that deficiency of central dopamine occupies the dominant role in the pathogenesis of Parkinson's disease, there is abundant evidence that other neurotransmitters (norepinephrine, histamine, serotonin, gamma-aminobutyric acid) at least modify the symptoms of parkinsonism. Within the central nervous system, there exists a *check-and-balance* reciprocal relationship between dopamine and acetylcholine. In Parkinson's disease there is a relative deficiency of dopamine leading to dominance of the reciprocal cholinergic system. Indeed, the symptoms of the disease appear to correlate roughly with either dopaminergic deficiency or cholinergic dominance.

The current pharmacological management of Parkinson's disease is primarily limited to manipulations within the dopamine-acetylcholine system. Manipulation of other putative neurotransmitters has been largely unrewarding. The possible exception to this is the employment of antihistamines or bromocriptine[7] to modify the histamine-serotonin system.[3,4]

It is now clear that currently available antiparkinsonian drugs provide only symptomatic benefit. They alter neither the clinical nor the histologic progression of the underlying disease process.[4,8] These agents do, however, grant most patients a temporary and sometimes prolonged remission or attenuation of symptomatology, thus allowing a more productive, meaningful life. Proper treatment may also prolong survival.[5,8] The price of successful treatment is exacted in the form of a demanding, constantly changing medication regimen, numerous side effects associated with the various medications, and the eventual imposition of periodic, dyskinetic movements. These drawbacks are serious but almost always preferred by parkinsonian patients over the disability associated with the untreated disease.

Several therapeutic approaches are possible in the pharmacologic management of Parkinson's disease. These include (1) increasing the synthesis of brain dopamine by administration of dopamine precursors; (2) direct stimulation of central dopamine receptors; (3) blocking or decreasing the central cholinergic dominance; (4) blocking the reuptake and/or stimulating the release of dopamine at the synaptic cleft; or (5) blocking or decreasing the catabolism of dopamine. These approaches are discussed below. Detailed reviews of the neuropharmacology and neurochemistry of parkinsonism are available elsewhere.[2,3,9–12]

DRUG MONOGRAPHS

AGENTS THAT INCREASE THE SYNTHESIS OF BRAIN DOPAMINE

LEVODOPA (Dopar, Larodopa)
LEVODOPA-BENSERAZIDE (Madopar)
LEVODOPA-CARBIDOPA (Sinemet)

Levodopa, with or without a peripheral dopa-decarboxylase inhibitor, is presently the drug of choice in the management of the majority of patients with idiopathic and post-encephalitic Parkinson's disease.[4,5,8,12,13] Levodopa has no place in the treatment of neuroleptic-induced parkinsonism, since the receptor blockade that the neuroleptics induce is equally effective against endogenous as well as exogenous dopamine.[3,5,10] Antihistamines and anticholinergic agents appear to be the drugs of choice in neuroleptic-induced extrapyramidal syndromes (see below).

Levodopa, the amino acid precursor of dopamine, crosses the blood-brain barrier, whereas dopamine itself does not.[5,14] Levodopa is then metabolized to dopamine by L-aromatic acid (dopa) decarboxylase, an enzyme of ubiquitous distribution. Dopa decarboxylase also mediates this transformation peripherally, resulting in large quantities of circulating dopamine, as well as its immediate metabolites, norepinephrine and epinephrine. These catecholamines all possess potent peripheral effects (cardiac arrhythmias, severe nausea, and vomiting) and severely limit the dose of levodopa that can be administered. By selectively inhibiting the peripheral decarboxylation of levodopa without affecting central dopa decarboxylase, carbidopa and benserazide maximize the percentage of levodopa reaching the brain and minimize peripheral side effects;[12] benserazide is not yet available in the United States. With the introduction of a levodopa-carbidopa combination (Sinemet) in the United States, most clinicians have observed a significant decrease in the incidence and severity of nausea and vomiting,[12,15–17] as well as a consistent decrease in the amount of levodopa required to achieve the level of control previously attained with levodopa alone. Most patients require only 20 to 25% of their former dose of levodopa.[12,16,18] Other advantages to combination therapy include a smoother, more rapid induction phase (days versus weeks for levodopa alone) and, at maximum tolerated doses, patients appear clinically better.[12,15,17] The only real disadvantage to combination therapy is the more rapid and perhaps slightly more frequent appearance of abnormal, involuntary movements (dyskinesias). It may be that many of these patients were never able to achieve sufficient intracerebral levels of dopamine to reveal these dyskinesias before nausea, vomiting, or other peripheral side effects intervened.[3,10,12] There may also be an increase in the incidence of centrally-mediated orthostatic hypotension in Sinemet users (see adverse reactions section).

Occasionally, patients who have been well controlled by levodopa for a number of years will suddenly assume a state of akinesia, masked facies, and stooped posture. This state may rapidly alternate with a phase of dyskinetic movements. This so-called 'on-off' phenomenon can occur within seconds, persist for minutes or hours, and then remit for variable periods of time.[19] It is usually observed only after prolonged levodopa therapy, is most common in patients with advanced disease, and is not observed in untreated patients.[9,19] It may occur less often with combination levodopa-carbidopa therapy[12,20] and in patients treated with long-acting, direct dopaminergic agonists (eg, bromocriptine),[21] but this issue is not entirely settled. A number of therapeutic maneuvers can be attempted in an effort to ameliorate the on-off phenomenon: increasing or decreasing the levodopa dose, decreasing the dosing interval, temporarily discontinuing the levodopa, adding adjunctive medication (ie, anticholinergics, amantadine, bromocriptine), placing the patient on a low protein diet (other aromatic amino acids may compete in the small bowel as well as centrally for a common carrier mechanism), or by the use of long-acting levodopa preparations.[9,19,20,22] The on-off phenomenon may be due to loss of dopamine storage capability of the remaining central dopaminergic neurons, thus accounting for the exaggerated initial response to exogenous dopamine (the 'on' portion) followed by an abbreviated duration of action (the 'off' portion).[9,19,23]

Prolonged dopamine deficiency and its attendant neuronal degeneration appears to decrease responsiveness to exogenous levodopa. Symptoms of Parkinson's disease usually do not progress during the first two years of levodopa therapy, and patients with long-standing, untreated disease are consistently among the poorest responders to levodopa therapy.[3,5] Accordingly, levodopa therapy should probably be initiated early in the course of the disease rather than withheld until the symptoms become severe.

Adverse Reactions—Patients seldom benefit from levodopa therapy without also experiencing some undesirable effects, many of which have already been discussed (dyskinesias, cardiac arrhythmias, the on-off syndrome, and gastrointestinal symptoms). Other commonly encountered side effects include neuropsychiatric disturbances (hypomania, dementia, hallucinations) and postural hypotension, with or without syncopal episodes.[4,5] Postural hypotension may seem to be 'paradoxical', since levodopa metabolism yields pressor amines (dopamine, norepinephrine and epinephrine). However, the peripheral activity of these metabolites appears to be overshadowed by the central hypotensive activity of dopamine and norepinephrine.[24,25] Postural hypotension occurs with both levodopa and levodopa-carbidopa, with perhaps a slightly higher incidence associated with the combination.[12,24,26] In a parkinsonian patient who is deriving marked benefit from levodopa therapy, but is experiencing severe and persistent orthostatic hypotension, treatment with oral fludrocortisone acetate, 0.05 to 0.2 mg daily may reduce the degree of hypotension,[24] provided there is no medical contraindication to its use. Alternatively, oral ephedrine, 25 mg three times daily and/or elastic stockings are often beneficial in reducing or abolishing orthostatic hypotension.

A single case of levodopa-induced thrombocytopenia, presumably of immunologic origin, has been reported.[27]

Drug Interactions—Phenytoin, when administered to patients who are well controlled on levodopa, appears to diminish the therapeutic effects of the levodopa. The mechanism is unclear.[28] Reserpine and the neuroleptics should generally not be given to patients being treated with levodopa,[18] as they may deplete interneuronal dopamine stores or effect a blockade of the dopaminergic receptor. Methyldopa is an agent that exhibits a weak blocking effect on dopa decarboxylase but, unlike carbidopa, it appears to work centrally as well as peripherally in therapeutic doses. As a result, its effects on levodopa are quite unpredictable; antagonism,[18,29] as well as synergism[18,30] have been reported. Pyridoxine, a coenzyme for dopa decarboxylase, can cause a significant increase in the peripheral metabolism of levodopa. This effect is negligible with combination therapy.[12,31] The monoamine oxidase inhibitors can significantly interact with levodopa, as discussed below.

Contraindications—Levodopa should be used with extreme caution, if at all, in patients with angina pectoris or severe cardiovascular occlusive disease, since moderate to severe hypotension may aggravate ischemia or even precipitate myocardial infarction. Similarly, it should be avoided in patients with transient cerebral ischemic attacks. Levodopa is relatively contraindicated in patients with a history of major affective disorders and in patients with a history of or predisposition to malignant melanoma, since levodopa is both a precursor to melanin and a stimulant to growth hormone release.[4-6,32,33] Levodopa is also relatively contraindicated in patients with a history of hemolytic anemia or glucose 6-phosphate dehydrogenase deficiency.[4]

Dosage—Combination therapy (Sinemet) has essentially replaced treatment with levodopa alone. Therefore, treatment with levodopa alone is not discussed; extensive reviews on this topic have been published elsewhere.[4,5]

Induction Phase: Parkinsonian patients not previously treated with levodopa should be started on combination therapy (Sinemet). Sinemet is available in a fixed ratio of 1:10 (carbidopa:levodopa), either 10/100 mg or 25/250 mg. Carbidopa in a dose of 70–100 mg/day will effectively inhibit the majority of peripheral dopa decarboxylase. Higher doses have no apparent utility or toxicity.[12] The usual starting dosage is one 10/100 mg tablet three times daily. Dosage is increased by one tablet every day or every other day until six tablets per day are reached. Above this dosage 25/250 mg tablets can be used. Further titration can be done with either 10/100 mg tablets or levodopa alone. One of the advantages of combination therapy is said to be the ease of administration; many patients reportedly do well on thrice daily dosing while still avoiding the moderate fluctuations in performance throughout the day that are common with levodopa alone. In our experience dosing every 3 or 4 hours provides a more uniform response than dosing 3 or 4 times daily.

If a patient is currently receiving an excellent response from levodopa without appreciable side effects, then nothing is gained by switching to Sinemet. If, however, the response is less than 'maximal' and the patient is continually inconvenienced by side effects, transfer can be accomplished without interruption. The usual daily schedule should be completed, omitting the evening doses of levodopa. The next morning Sinemet may be started at approximately 20 to 25% of the former levodopa dosage.

Maintenance Phase: Once the patient has received a 'maximal' benefit or involuntary movements (dyskinesias) appear, the maintenance dosage has been achieved. However, many minor adjustments in the dosage regimen may be needed to conform to diurnal fluctuations or a new range of activities in a previously disabled patient. Eventually, an increased frequency of these variations in performance may occur,[34] and they may take the form of good periods (usually in the morning and early evening) alternating with bad periods (usually in the afternoon and late evening), good periods alternating with dyskinesias, or even bad periods alternating with dyskinesias. Often these fluctuations are amenable to schedule alterations but the last of the above may indicate excessive overdosage.

AGENTS THAT DIRECTLY STIMULATE CENTRAL DOPAMINERGIC RECEPTORS

BROMOCRIPTINE MESYLATE (Parlodel)
N-PROPYLNORAPORPHINE
LERGOTRILE
PIRIBEDIL

With the exception of bromocriptine none of these drugs have been approved for marketing in the United States. However, several drugs that act by directly stimulating the dopamine receptors are currently undergoing clinical trials and probably will be marketed in the near future. The rationale for the use of direct dopamine agenists is clear: the efficacy of levodopa depends on the ability of the remaining central dopaminergic neurons to decarboxylate levodopa to dopamine, whereas a direct-acting drug would act independently of neuronal degeneration.

There are currently four drugs which are postulated to act predominantly at the dopamine receptor. The most promising is bromocriptine, an ergot derivative. Early trials were most encouraging.[35,36] Recently completed trials in the United States have shown that bromocriptine: (1) may be nearly as effective as levodopa with similar side effects,[37,38] (2) may be especially efficacious against tremor,[37–39] (3) is effective in severely affected patients when levodopa is not,[38,40] (4) is an effective adjunctive agent when given in combination with levodopa or levodopa-carbidopa,[39] (5) appears to have no active metabolites, and (6) has a significantly longer half-life than levodopa (6 to 8 hours versus 2 to 4 hours).[21,38,39,41] Bromocriptine's extended duration of action results in less dramatic swings

TABLE 1 Preparations and Costs of Antiparkinsonism Drugs (Other than Anticholinergic Agents)

Generic Name	Trademark Name(s)	Preparations and 1978 Costs
Levodopa	Dopar	Capsules 100 mg—$2.82/100; 250 mg—$4.50/100; 500 mg—$7.80/100
	Larodopa	Capsules or tablets 100 mg—$3.21/100; 250 mg—$5.18/100; 500 mg—$8.96/100
Carbidopa 10 mg and Levodopa 100 mg	Sinemet 10/100	Tablets—$13.02/100
Carbidopa 25 mg and Levodopa 250 mg	Sinemet 25/250	Tablets—$21.68/100
Amantadine Hydrochloride	Symmetrel	Capsules 100 mg—$16.60/100

of performance and has been employed with some degree of success in the treatment of the 'on-off' syndrome.[19,21]

Apomorphine, a semisynthetic derivative of morphine, has been utilized experimentally with good results. However, it has a rather short duration of action, possesses rather marked intrinsic emetic properties, and can cause a significant degree of azotemia.[41] Recently, Cotzias and co-workers[41] have employed an apomorphine analog, N-propylnoraporphine, with favorable initial results, most notably a decrease in the severity of the azotemia.

Lergotrile, another ergot alkaloid and presumed dopamine receptor stimulating agent, appears to be primarily effective in alleviating tremor[42] with little improvement observed in the other clinical manifestations of Parkinson's disease. Another agent, piribedil (ET-495), initially appeared to have the same therapeutic limitations as lergotrile, but piribedil in fact can produce significant improvement when used adjunctively with levodopa.[43]

The side effects that have been observed with all of these experimental agents are qualitatively similar to those of levodopa[36] with the exception of pedal edema and erythema, a burning discomfort in the eyes, diplopia, and perhaps a slightly higher incidence of extrasystoles which has been observed during high dose (100 mg per day) bromocriptine therapy.[36,38]

AGENTS THAT BLOCK OR DECREASE CHOLINERGIC DOMINANCE—ANTICHOLINERGIC THERAPY

The anticholinergics are among the oldest preparations employed in the treatment of Parkinson's disease. Tincture of belladonna has been used for well over 100 years. Since the 1940's, many synthetic anticholinergic compounds have become available that have relatively greater central as opposed to peripheral action (see Table 2).

In general, anticholinergics produce only a modest improvement in parkinsonian symptomatology, most commonly a decrease in the rigidity and akinesia with a lesser effect upon the tremor.[4] Their limited therapeutic effects are consistent with the limited role of cholinergic dominance in the pathogenesis of Parkinson's disease. Additionally, maximal doses of the anticholinergic agents are severely limited by their peripheral (blurring of vision, dry mouth, constipation, urinary retention) and central (ataxia, hallucinations, dysarthria, memory impairment, somnolence) side effects.[4,13] Anticholinergic agents have the additional capacity to inhibit the reuptake and storage of dopamine at the central dopamine receptors, thereby prolonging the action of dopamine.[4,44]

In spite of their marked limitations, anticholinergics still have certain indications in the management of Parkinson's disease. First, they may be used in mild cases where the severity of the disease does not warrant the risks or demands of levodopa therapy. Second, they may be used adjunctively in those patients who tolerate or respond to levodopa poorly or not at all. Third, they are probably the drugs of choice in the treatment of neuroleptic-induced Parkinson's disease since, in contrast to other forms of parkinsonism, the neuroleptic-induced syndrome usually responds dramatically to modest doses of the anticholinergics, especially benztropine or diphenhydramine.[4]

With the possible exceptions of elderly patients (who are generally less tolerant to anticholinergic side effects) and neuroleptic-induced parkinsonism, both of which appear to respond more favorably to treatment with one of the antihistamines, there is little reason except personal preference or individual tolerance to choose one agent over another.[4,8]

TABLE 2 Dosage, Preparations, and Costs of Anticholinergic Agents Used in Parkinson's Disease

Generic Name	Usual Dose	Preparations and 1978 Costs
Naturally Occurring Alkaloids		
Atropine	100 to 250 μg 4 times daily	Tablets 300 μg—\$1.06/100; 400 μg—\$1.13/100; 600 μg—\$1.00/100
Scopolamine (Hyoscine)	300 to 1000 μg 3 to 4 times daily	Tablets 400μg—\$1.34/100; 600 μg—\$1.53/100
Synthetic Anticholinergics		
Trihexyphenidyl (Artane, Tremin, Pipanol)	2 to 4 mg 3 times daily	Tablets 2 mg—\$2.58/100; 5 mg—\$5.11/100
Procyclidine (Kemadrin)	2.5 to 10 mg 3 times daily	Tablets 2 mg—\$1.80/100; 5 mg—\$3.25/100
Biperiden (Akineton)	2 mg 3 to 4 times daily	Tablets 2 mg—\$6.36/100
Cycrimine (Pagitane)	2.5 to 5 mg 3 times daily	Tablets 1.25 mg—\$2.37/100; 2.5 mg—\$3.75/100
Antihistamines		
Diphenhydramine (Benadryl)	25 to 50 mg 3 to 4 times daily	Capsules 25 mg—\$3.09/100; 50 mg—\$4.60/100
Orphenadrine (Disipal, Norflex)	50 to 100 mg 3 times daily	Tablets 50 mg—\$6.90/100
Chlorphenoxamine (Phenoxene)	50 mg 3 times daily	Tablets 50 mg—\$10.73/100
Synthetic Anticholinergic-Antihistamines		
Benztropine (Cogentin)	1 to 4 mg 2 times daily	Tablets 0.5 mg—\$3.85/100; 1 mg—\$4.39/100; 2 mg—\$5.55/100
Phenothiazines		
Promethazine (Phenergan, Remsed)	6.25 to 25 mg 1 to 3 times daily	Tablets 12.5 mg—\$5.27/100; 25 mg—\$9.30/100; 50 mg—\$14.30/100
Ethopropazine (Parsidol, Profenamine)	10 to 100 mg 4 times daily	Tablets 10 mg—\$1.30/100; 50 mg—\$4.10/100; 100 mg—\$6.05/100

AGENTS THAT STIMULATE THE RELEASE OR BLOCK THE REUPTAKE OF DOPAMINE

AMANTADINE HYDROCHLORIDE (SYMMETREL)

Amphetamine may produce a mild degree of benefit if the prominent symptom is akinesia, but it can exacerbate tremor and should be used judiciously.[45,46] Methylphenidate and phenmetrazine appear to be similarly effective.

The tricyclic antidepressants inhibit presynaptic reuptake of norepinephrine, serotonin, and epinephrine. They do not similarly inhibit reuptake of dopamine.[4,47,48] These agents do possess some antiparkinsonian effects, probably attributable to their mild anticholinergic properties. They may be useful in the treatment of the depression that often accompanies Parkinson's disease.

Amantadine has a clinically significant antiparkinsonian effect in approximately 60% of patients, and may be additionally effective in the presence of levodopa.[49] Since amantadine appears to increase the release of dopamine and to decrease its reuptake,[46] patients who respond to amantadine (indicating that their dopamine receptors are still capable of responding to dopamine) generally respond to treatment with levodopa. Conversely, patients who respond poorly to amantadine usually exhibit little if any response to levodopa.[3] Amantadine may provide additional benefit to a levodopa responder and should be considered whenever maximal benefit cannot be achieved with levodopa alone. Amantadine is commonly given as 200 mg daily in two equal doses. Its effectiveness may decline over a period of two or three months but, as with many of the antiparkinsonian agents, a brief respite from therapy may allow prolonged benefit. Several investigators have advocated the use of amantadine in the treatment of neuroleptic-induced Parkinson's disease.[50]

Adverse Reactions—In contrast to levodopa and the anticholinergic agents, amantadine is relatively free from serious side effects. When side effects do occur, they are usually mild, transient, and reversible.[51–53] Perhaps one of the most disturbing side effects is livedo reticularis, which commonly presents as a diffuse, reddish-blue mottling of the skin, occasionally with mild pedal edema. It usually occurs on the lower extremities but can also be seen on the arms. Increased peripheral release of catecholamines causing peripheral vasoconstriction, expressing itself as cutaneous discoloration is postulated to account for this syndrome.[51] The reported incidence of livedo reticularis varies widely,[53,54] it is relatively benign, completely reversible, and usually does not require discontinuation of the amantadine. Other infrequently reported side effects include insomnia, dysarthria, drowsiness, affective changes, and rarely, convulsions.

AGENTS THAT DECREASE DOPAMINE CATABOLISM

The only medications marketed at present with this capability are the monoamine oxidase (MAO) inhibitors. These agents should never be used in conjunction with levodopa; in addition to inhibiting the catabolism of levodopa, the MAO inhibitors also inhibit the catabolism of the levodopa metabolites (dopamine, norepinephrine and epinephrine), all of which are potent pressor agents.[18,55] This could predispose the patient to a hypertensive crisis.[12]

REFERENCES

1. Barbeau A: The pathogenesis of Parkinson's disease: a new hypothesis. Can Med Assoc J 87:802–807, 1962.
2. Cooper JR, Bloom FE, Roth RH: *The Biochemical Basis of Neuropharmacology*. New York, Oxford University Press, 1974.
3. Klawans HL: *The Pharmacology of Extrapyramidal Movement Disorders*. Basle, Karger, 1973, pp 98–105.
4. Yahr MD: The treatment of parkinsonism. Med Clin North Am 57:1377–1392, 1972.
5. Yahr MD: Levodopa. Ann Intern Med 83:677–682, 1975.
6. Parkes JD, Debono AG, Marsden CD: Growth-hormone response in Parkinson's disease (editorial). Lancet 1:483–484, 1976.
7. Hutt CS, Snider SR, Fahn S: Interaction between bromocriptine and levodopa. Neurology 27:505–510, 1977.
8. Sweet RD, McDowell FH: Five years treatment of Parkinson's disease with levodopa. Ann Intern Med 83:456–463, 1975.
9. Cohen MM, Scheife RT: Pharmacotherapy of Parkinson's disease. Am J Hosp Pharm 34:531–538, 1977.
10. Marsden CD: The neuropharmacology of abnormal involuntary movement disorders (the dyskinesias). In *Modern Trends in Neurology*, Volume 6. Edited by D Williams. London, Butterworths, 1975, pp 141–166.
11. Moskowitz MA, Wurtman RJ: Catecholamines and neurologic diseases. N Engl J Med 293:274–280, 332–338, 1975.
12. Pinder RM, Brogden RN, Sawyer RP, et al: Levodopa and decarboxylase inhibitors: A review of their clinical pharmacology and use in the treatment of parkinsonism. Drugs 11:329–377, 1976.
13. Selby G: Treatment of parkinsonism. Drugs 11:61–70, 1976.
14. Cotzias GC, van Woert MH, Schiffer LM: Aromatic amino acids and modification of parkinsonism. N Engl J Med 276:374–379, 1967.
15. Marsden CD, Parker JD, Rees JE: A year's comparison of treatment of patients with Parkinson's disease with levodopa combined with carbidopa versus treatment with levodopa alone. Lancet 2:1459–1462, 1973.
16. Markham CH, Diamond SG, Treciokas LJ: Carbidopa in Parkinson disease and in nausea and vomiting of levodopa. Arch Neurol 31:128–133, 1974.

17. Mones RJ: Evaluation of alpha-methyldopa and alpha-methyldopa hydrazine with L-dopa therapy. NY State J Med 1:47–51, 1974.
18. Bianchine JR, Sunyapridakul L: Individualization of levodopa therapy. Med Clin North Am 58:1071–1081, 1974.
19. Marsden CD, Parkes JD: 'On-off' effects in patients with Parkinson's disease on chronic levodopa therapy. Lancet 1:292–296, 1976.
20. Sweet RD, McDowell FH, Wasterlain CG, et al: Treatment of 'on-off effect' with a dopa decarboxylase inhibitor. Arch Neurol 32:560–563, 1975.
21. Kartzinel R, Calne DB: Studies with bromocriptine, Part 1: On-off phenomena. Neurology 26:508–510, 1976.
22. Gilligan B, Hancock R: Enteric-coated L-dopa (prodopa). Med J Aust 2:824–826, 1975.
23. Duvoisin RC: Variations in the 'on-off' phenomenon. In *Advances in Neurology*, Volume 5. Edited by FH McDowell, A Barbeau. New York, Raven Press, 1974, pp 339–340.
24. Hoehn MM: Levodopa-induced postural hypotension: treatment with fludrocortisone. Arch Neurol 32:50–51, 1975.
25. Tarsy D, Parkes JD, Marsden CD: Clonidine in Parkinson disease. Arch Neurol 32:134–136, 1975.
26. Reid JL, Calne DB: Cardiovascular effects of levodopa in Parkinsonism. In *Advances in Neurology*, Volume 3. Edited by D Calne. New York, Raven Press, 1973, pp 223–232.
27. Wanamaker WM, Wanamaker SJ, Celesia GG, et al: Thrombocytopenia associated with long-term levodopa therapy. JAMA 235:2217–2219, 1976.
28. Menoez JS, Cotzias GC, Mena I, et al: Diphenylhydantoin: blocking of levodopa effects. Arch Neurol 32:44–46, 1975.
29. Kofman O: Treatment of Parkinson's disease with L-dopa: a current appraisal. Can Med Assoc J 104:483–487, 1971.
30. Sweet RD, Lee JE, McDowell FH: Methyldopa as an adjunct to levodopa treatment of Parkinson's disease. Clin Pharmacol Ther 13:23–27, 1972.
31. Mars H: Levodopa, carbidopa, and pyridoxine in Parkinson disease. Arch Neurol 30:444–447, 1974.
32. Weldon VV, Gupta SK, Klingensmith G, et al: Evaluation of growth hormone release in children using L-dopa and arginine in combination. J Pediatr 87:540-544, 1975.
33. Rayfield EJ, George DT, Eichner HL, et al: L-dopa stimulation of glucagon in man. N Engl J Med 293:589–590, 1975.
34. Barbeau A: The clinical physiology of side effects in long-term L-dopa therapy. In *Advances in Neurology*, Volume 5. Edited by FH McDowell, A Barbeau. New York, Raven Press, 1974, pp 347–365.
35. DeBono AG, Donaldson I, Marsden CD: Bromocryptine in parkinsonism. Lancet 2:987–988, 1975.
36. Teychenne PF, Leigh PN, Reid JL, et al: Idiopathic parkinsonism treated with bromocryptine. Lancet 2:473–476, 1975.
37. Kartzinel R, Perlow M, Techenne P, et al: Treatment of parkinsonism: bromocryptine, carbidopa/levodopa, and levodopa compared in a double-blind study. Presented at the American Academy of Neurology, Toronto, April 1976.
38. Kartzinel R, Shoulson I, Calne DB: Studies with bromocryptine. Part 2. Neurology 26:511–513, 1976.
39. Lieberman A, Zolfaghari M, Boal D, et al: The antiparkinsonian efficacy of bromocryptine. Neurology 26:405–409, 1976.
40. Lieberman A, Kuppersmith M, Vogel B, et al: Treatment of Parkinson's disease with bromocryptine. Presented at the American Academy of Neurology, Toronto, April 1976.
41. Cotzias GC, Papvasiliou IS, Tolosa ES, et al: Treatment of Parkinson's disease with aporphines. N Engl J Med 294:567–572, 1976.
42. Lieberman A, Miyamoto T, Battista A, et al: Studies on the antiparkinsonian efficacy of lergotrile. Neurology 25:459–462, 1975.
43. Feigenson J, Sweet R, McDowell F: Piribedil: its synergistic effect in multi-drug regimens for parkinsonism. Neurology 26:430–433, 1976.
44. Coyle JT, Snyder SN: Antiparkinsonian drugs: inhibition of dopamine uptake in the corpus striatum as a possible mechanism of action. Science 166:899–901, 1969.
45. Birkmayer W: The alpha-methyl-p-tyrosine effect in extrapyramidal disorders. Wien Klin Wschr 81:10–14, 1969.

46. Moore KE, Thornburg JE: Drug-induced dopaminergic supersensitivity. In *Advances in Neurology,* Volume 9. Edited by DB Calne, A Barbeau. New York, Raven Press, 1975, pp 93–104.
47. Glowinski J: Metabolism of catecholamines in brain and antidepressant drugs. 5th Int Congr Neuropsychopharmacol, 1966, pp 44–51.
48. Ross SB, Renyi AL: Inhibition of the uptake of tritiated catecholamines by antidepressant and related agents. Eur J Pharmacol 2:181–186, 1967.
49. Fahn S, Isgree WP: Long-term evaluation of amantadine and levodopa combination in parkinsonism by double-blind cross-over analyses. Neurology 25:695–700, 1975.
50. DiMascio A, Bernardo DL, Greenblatt DJ, et al: A controlled trial of amantadine in drug-induced extrapyramidal disorders. Arch Gen Psychiatry 33:599–602, 1976.
51. Pearce LA, Waterbury LD, Green HO: Amantadine hydrochloride: alteration in peripheral circulation. Neurology 24:46–48, 1974.
52. Franz DN: Drugs for Parkinson's disease. In *The Pharmacological Basis of Therapeutics,* 4th Edition. Edited by LS Goodman, A Gilman. New York, Macmillan, 1975, pp 227–244.
53. Schwab RS, Poskanzer DC, England AC, et al: Amantadine in Parkinson's disease; review of more than two years' experience. JAMA 222:792–795, 1972.
54. Vollum DI, Parkes JD, Doyle D: Livedo reticularis during amantadine treatment. Br Med J 2:627–628, 1971.
55. Friend DG, Bell WR, Kline NS: The action of L-dihydroxyphenylalanine in patients receiving nialamide. Clin Pharmacol Ther 6:362–366, 1965.

61. AGENTS USED IN MYASTHENIA GRAVIS

John R. Hills and Richard T. Scheife

Myasthenia gravis is a disease that is characterized by weakness and abnormal fatigueability of skeletal muscle. Weakness is more profound after exercise and improves with rest or with the administration of inhibitors of acetylcholinesterase (cholinomimetic agents). Muscle involvement is seldom generalized. In many patients, weakness involves only one or two muscle groups, and even in patients with generalized myasthenia, all muscle groups are not affected to a similar degree.[1] The primary abnormality in myasthenia gravis is a reduction in the number of acetylcholine receptors at the myoneural junction due to an autoimmune reaction.[2–13] This results in decreased neuromuscular transmission and weakness.

Myasthenia gravis occurs at all ages, but the highest incidence is during the third decade of life.[14] Overall, females are affected twice as often as males, but this ratio is subject to variation when age is considered.[1,14,15]

Neonatal myasthenia gravis is a transient form of myasthenia that occurs in 12 to 20% of children born to myasthenic mothers. It is caused by the transplacental transfer of myasthenia immunoglobulin (IgG) from the mother to the child.[13,15–17] Antibodies to acetylcholine receptors have been demonstrated in a mother and her two children born with neonatal myasthenia.[4] Weakness is present at birth or within the first three days of life often requiring anticholinesterase treatment. The weakness lasts for a few days to several weeks, then spontaneously remits.[15,17] Further treatment is not necessary.[18]

The onset of myasthenia gravis in adults is usually subacute and is frequently precipitated by an infection. Once manifest, the disease may advance irregularly, remain static for prolonged periods of time, or spontaneously remit.[14] Partial or complete remissions occur in approximately 50% of patients, usually within the first few years.[14] Other patients become so incapacitated that the disease becomes life-threatening. Death is most often due to respiratory failure.[14]

The muscles innervated by the cranial nerves, the so-called 'bulbar' musculature, are the most frequently affected. In patients with severe, longstanding myasthenia, it is very uncommon to observe generalized muscular weakness without concomitant bulbar musculature involvement.[14] Intermittent diplopia or ptosis are often the initial symptoms. The pupils, however, are spared.[14] Facial, pharyngeal and laryngeal muscles are involved in over 70% of myasthenic patients. In severe, generalized myasthenia, weakness tends to be more proximal than distal.[14]

DIAGNOSIS OF MYASTHENIA GRAVIS

The simplest diagnostic procedure is to have the patient perform some repetitive motor activity with the involved muscle groups, eg, deep-knee bends, repeated eye closures, counting to 100, repeated gripping, possibly with a dynamometer. Rapid fatigue and weakness is diagnostic.[14,19]

In doubtful cases the diagnosis can usually be established by parenteral administration of edrophonium (Tensilon), an ultra-short acting inhibitor of acetylcholinesterase, which will transiently increase muscle strength in myasthenic patients. Guidelines for the 'Tensilon test' are as follows:[1,17]

1. If possible, all other drugs should be discontinued for at least 8 to 24 hours prior to the test.
2. A 'keep open' intravenous infusion should be started with 5% dextrose in water or normal saline to facilitate the administration of all test solutions as well as any emergency or antidotal drugs.
3. A labeled syringe containing atropine 0.4 mg should always be available. The atropine may be used to block the muscarinic side effects of edrophonium if they become overly bothersome. Muscarinic side effects most commonly observed include increased salivation, diaphoresis, abdominal cramping, nausea, and vomiting. Side effects that are uncommonly observed but may be life-threatening include bronchoconstriction, severe hypotension, bradycardia, and cardiac arrest. There is some debate as to whether all patients should routinely receive atropine prior to the edrophonium test to protect against muscarinic side effects. In patients over 50 years of age, we routinely give atropine 0.4 mg unless it is specifically contraindicated; the atropine is given two minutes before the

edrophonium to protect against possible bradycardia and hypotension. In other patients we believe prophylactic atropine is rarely warranted.

4. A placebo (eg, normal saline) should be injected prior to the edrophonium to identify 'placebo reactors.'

5. For the actual test, 10 mg of edrophonium (10 mg/ml) is drawn up into a syringe and labeled. Then 0.2 ml (2 mg) is given intravenously as a test dose to determine if the patient is a 'hyper-responder' to edrophonium. If there is no response within 45 seconds, the remaining 0.8 ml (8 mg) is rapidly injected.

6. The patient is observed for objective changes in the strength of the tested muscles, improvement in ptosis, the ability to talk longer before the onset of 'nasal speech,' etc. A positive test consists of not only an increase in muscle strength but also an increase in endurance. These effects are short-lived, lasting only 5 to 10 minutes after the injection. Rarely, a patient may experience a markedly prolonged effect of the edrophonium, sometimes lasting as long as 1 to 2 hours.[8] The extraocular muscles often respond poorly to cholinesterase inhibitors and diplopia may be quite resistant to edrophonium as well as the other longer acting cholinesterase inhibitors.

The edrophonium test can also evaluate the appropriateness of a dosage change of a long-acting cholinesterase inhibitor, such as pyridostigmine (Mestinon) or neostigmine (Prostigmin). One hour after the last dose of the long-acting inhibitor (ie, approximately at its peak effect), 2 mg of edrophonium is injected intravenously. If the patient clearly improves after the edrophonium, subsequent oral doses of pyridostigmine or neostigmine should be increased by ¼ to ½ tablet, since more inhibition of cholinesterase probably will be beneficial. If the patient becomes weaker, subsequent oral doses of pyridostigmine or neostigmine should be similarly decreased, since the patient is probably receiving too much inhibitor. If there is no appreciable change, the current dose is appropriate.[1,17]

The regional curare test is another diagnostic procedure. A small dose of d-tubocurare is injected in a single limb, and the effects of the curare are confined to the limb by use of a blood pressure cuff or a tourniquet.[20,21] Myasthenic patients are 10 to 100 times more sensitive than normal subjects to the neuromuscular blocking effects of curare and other neuromuscular blocking agents (eg, pancuronium, gallamine).[13,17] Therefore, a profound muscular weakness occurs if the patient has myasthenia. In the past, curare was administered

TABLE 1 Preparations and Costs of Cholinesterase Inhibitors Used in Myasthenia Gravis

Generic Name	Trademark Name(s)	Preparations and 1978 Costs
Pyridostigmine Bromide	Mestinon	Tablets 60 mg—$4.08/100 Tablets (timed-release) 180 mg—$9.65/100 Syrup 60 mg/5ml—$3.99/pint Injection (solution) 5 mg/ml—$8.76/2-ml ampul
Neostigmine Bromide	Prostigmin Bromide	Tablets 15 mg—$4.36/100
Neostigmine Methylsulfate	Prostigmin Methylsulfate	Injection (solution) 0.25 mg/ml–$0.21/1-ml ampul; 0.5 mg/ml–$0.27/1-ml ampul; $2.15/10-ml vial; 1 mg/ml–$2.85/10-ml ampul
Ambenonium Chloride	Mytelase Chloride	Capsules 10 mg—$6.14/100
Edrophonium Chloride	Tensilon	Injection (solution) 10 mg/ml—$0.52/1-ml ampul, $2.53/10-ml vial

systemically in diagnosis. This proved too dangerous because of frequent respiratory paralysis.

Some clinicians employ electrophysiologic tests. Under standard conditions of supramaximal stimulation of motor nerves, a progressive decrease in the amplitude of the evoked response is observed in 95% of myasthenic patients who have three or more muscles adequately evaluated.[13] Another electrophysiologic phenomenon that is characteristic of myasthenia is 'post-activation exhaustion.' Details of this test are provided elsewhere.[17]

Measurement of anti-receptor antibody titers may useful in diagnosis.[4,11] These antibodies are not found in normal subjects but occur in approximately 90% of patients.

TREATMENT OF MYASTHENIA GRAVIS

Pharmacotherapy of myasthenia gravis has two main objectives: (1) direct enhancement of cholinergic transmission, most often accomplished by the use of agents that inhibit the enzymatic degradation of acetylcholinesterase, and (2) repair or reversal of the underlying immunological flaw (immunotherapy).

Cholinesterase Inhibitors

The cholinesterase inhibitors (also referred to as anticholinesterase drugs and cholinomimetic agents) have been used in the treatment of myasthenia gravis for almost 40 years, and they are still in widespread use. However, prednisone, thymectomy, and other immunosuppressive procedures are now considered primary therapy in the majority of myasthenic patients. The cholinesterase inhibitors are most often used as adjunctive agents and are recommended as the primary form of therapy only in patients with mild or purely ocular myasthenia.[15,22,23] They do not inhibit or reverse the basic immunologic flaw and may actually induce further damage to acetylcholine receptors.[9,13,15,24–26]

Anticholinesterase drugs inhibit or inactivate acetylcholinesterase, the enzyme responsible for terminating the action of acetylcholine. As a result, acetylcholine released from presynaptic sites can remain bound to acetylcholine receptors for a greater period of time. Acetylcholine not yet bound to the receptors may remain in the synaptic cleft longer, increasing the probability that it will eventually interact with a receptor. In either case, enhanced cholinergic transmission results.[1,17]

The most commonly used cholinesterase inhibitors are pyridostigmine bromide (Mestinon) and neostigmine bromide (Prostigmin). Pyridostigmine has a smoother, more prolonged duration of action and possibly fewer gastrointestinal side effects than neostigmine. However, patients may find that pyridostigmine does not provide as marked a 'boost' as neostigmine.[1] This boost may be important just before an anticipated activity or a meal. Ambenonium chloride (Mytelase) is not routinely used, but it may be of value in the myasthenic patient who is intolerant of bromides.[1] In this regard, Mestinon is available as the chloride salt, upon special request from the manufacturer, Roche Laboratories. Edrophonium chloride (Tensilon) is an ultra-short acting cholinesterase inhibitor that is used primarily in the diagnosis of myasthenia (see above). Because of its rapid onset and short duration, the cholinomimetic effects of edrophonium are accurately titratable. Thus, it may be useful in the acute treatment of myasthenic crisis.[1] Preparations and costs of cholinesterase inhibitors marketed in the United States are given in Table 1.

All of the cholinesterase inhibitors currently employed in the treatment of myasthenia are quaternary ammonium compounds. At therapeutic doses, they exhibit poor oral absorption and do not cross the blood-brain barrier. They are metabolized by plasma esterases and hepatic microsomal enzymes. The resultant metabolites are excreted, with varying fractions of free drug, in the urine.[27]

Guidelines for the Use of Cholinesterase Inhibitors. The titration of cholinesterase inhibitors in a particular myasthenic patient is an empiric and dynamic exercise that defies the 'cookbook' approach. The following guidelines should, however, permit optimal therapeutic results with a minimum of toxicity. Pyridostigmine is discussed as a representative drug.

(1) Initiate therapy with low doses. Do not try to achieve maximal strength with the initial dosage regimen. In adults, a typical oral starting dose is 30 to 60 mg of pyridostigmine three times daily. In children, 7 mg/kg of body weight or 200 mg/M^2 body surface area per day is the usual oral starting dose, divided into three equal doses.[27]

(2) Patients should be counseled to keep an accurate diary documenting the times of dosing, periods of peak effect, periods of worsening, and any adverse effects. From this diary, the results of gradual increases or decreases in the magnitude and frequency of the doses can be accurately assessed. In many patients, optimum control is achieved only when the drug is administered every three or four hours. The usual adult daily dose of oral pyridostigmine ranges widely—from 60 mg to more than 1,500 mg, with an average of 600 mg.[27]

(3) Requirements for cholinesterase inhibitor medications may change abruptly due to intercurrent infection or emotional or physical stress. Dosage alterations may have to be made continuously to maintain an acceptable level of control. Many patients exhibit a wide range of medication requirements during the day—more for eating and exercise and less for resting, reading or watching television. While most patients find that a 3- to 4-hour dosage interval is optimal, few patients maintain maximal control from the same dose of the drug every 3 to 4 hours. For example, to maintain optimal control, a patient may require 30 mg of pyridostigmine upon arising at 6 AM, 40 mg at 9 AM, 60 mg at noon (to assist with chewing and swallowing

lunch), 30 mg at 3 PM, 90 mg at 6 PM (to assist with dinner and a period of evening exercise) and 30 mg at 9 PM.

(4) Although the manufacturer states that Mestinon Timespan Tablets (180 mg) may be used on a once- or twice-a-day schedule in adults, we do not feel that these tablets provide reliable coverage; they probably should be used only as a bedtime dose for patients who experience symptomatic night-time or early morning weakness.[27]

(5) Pyridostigmine syrup (60 mg/5 ml) may be used for patients who require very exacting dosage titration, and those patients who have difficulty swallowing tablets. If necessary, it can be administered through a nasogastric tube.[27]

(6) Some myasthenic patients on long-term inhibitor therapy become progressively refractory to the effects of the drug. The exact mechanism of this is unknown, but responsiveness can usually be restored by decreasing or discontinuing the cholinesterase inhibitor for several days.[27] These respites from therapy should be undertaken only with adequate medical supervision.

(7) Myasthenic patients who fail to respond to one agent will rarely benefit by the substitution of another.[1,27]

(8) In response to an increase or decrease in dosage, patients may exhibit increasing strength in one group of muscles, indicating relative underdosage and a need to increase medication, while showing decreasing strength in other muscle groups, indicating relative overdosage and a need to decrease the medication. The dosage must be chosen for satisfactory response of the more important muscles (eg, respiratory status), often at the expense of less than optimal strength in other, less critical muscles.[1] It is uncommon to achieve complete restoration of strength while being treated with cholinesterase inhibitors alone.[13,27]

(9) The equivalent parenteral dose of both pyridostigmine and neostigmine is approximately 1/30th of the oral dose.[27,28]

Toxicity of Cholinesterase Inhibitors. Toxicity is usually mild but can be severe. Muscarinic and nicotinic side effects are common, and at higher doses, the central nervous system may be involved (Table 2). Patients most often complain of the muscarinic effects. These side effects may be controlled with judicious use of Lomotil or atropine. Atropine-like anticholinergic agents selectively block the muscarinic receptor without compromising neuromuscular transmission at nicotinic receptors.[28] The administration of cholinesterase inhibitors with food or milk may decrease their muscarinic effects by slowing the absorption of the drug and reducing serum peaks.[27] The routine use of oral atropine to block the muscarinic side effects of cholinesterase inhibitors may be of symptomatic benefit in a few patients, but it is dangerous in others. By reducing the annoying but benign muscarinic side effects, the patient is deprived of a valuable monitoring system; progressive weakness and respiratory failure may occur without warning in the overdosed patient.[1,17]

TABLE 2 Adverse Effects of Cholinesterase Inhibitors

Muscarinic Effects
Secretory—increased salivation, lacrimation, sweating, bronchial secretions
Smooth muscle—abdominal cramps, nausea, vomiting, diarrhea, miosis of the pupils, bronchoconstriction
Cardiovascular—bradycardia, hypotension, cardiac arrest
Nicotinic Effects
Skeletal muscle weakness, fasciculations
Central Nervous System Effects
Confusion, ataxia, slurred speech, areflexia, respiratory depression, convulsions, coma

Nicotinic side effects are more serious. They often present as increased muscular weakness that may be difficult to differentiate from myasthenic weakness. The increase in weakness may be interpreted as a need to increase, rather than decrease, the medication. The edrophonium test is often helpful in differentiating nicotinic toxicity from myasthenic weakness.

In patients suspected of inhibitor overdose, respiratory status is of major concern. Pulmonary function must be scrupulously monitored whenever a patient's drug regimen is changed. The respiratory status of the patient may be influenced by at least four separate mechanisms: (1) acetylcholine-induced bronchoconstriction (muscarinic effect), (2) increased bronchial secretions (muscarinic), (3) respiratory muscular weakness or paralysis (nicotinic), and (4) depression of the central respiratory centers. The latter is usually seen only in cases of profound intoxication or in cases of poisoning with cholinesterase inhibitors that readily traverse the blood-brain barrier (eg, physostigmine, parathione).[1,28] Atropine will effectively antagonize muscarinic side effects; 1 mg is given intravenously every hour until atropinization occurs and then repeated as needed. The remaining toxic effects are best treated conservatively with support of ventilation.[1,28]

Adrenal Corticosteroids

Numerous studies have demonstrated the efficacy of carefully controlled steroid therapy in the treatment of myasthenia gravis.[1,8,13,15,17,23,29] Sixty-three to 100% of the patients achieve good to excellent results with an acceptably low incidence of serious side effects.[8,22,23,29] Increased muscle weakness occurring early in treatment has been significantly reduced and, with some treatment regimens, largely eliminated. Steroid therapy must be continued indefinitely. Essentially all patients relapse after withdrawal of steroids.[8,13]

Antacids and/or cimetidine, replacement potassium therapy (80 to 120 mEq daily), and low-sodium, low-carbohydrate, high-protein diets are important ancillary measures in long-term corticosteroid treatment.[1,8,17]

The rationale for using corticosteroids in myasthenia gravis is based on their immunosuppressive activity. The major defect in neuromuscular transmission in myasthenia is caused by an immunological interaction at the post-synaptic acetylcholine receptor which is at least partially repaired by immunosuppressive doses of corticosteroids.[12,13,15,30] Steroids also exert a direct, positive, short-term effect on neuromuscular transmission, which may account for the early improvement sometimes observed with steroid therapy.[3,13,29]

Two regimens are of proven efficacy in the treatment of myasthenia; each has advantages and disadvantages. One begins with low doses of prednisone on a daily or alternate day schedule, gradually progresses to high doses on a daily or alternate day schedule, and finally reaches maintenance on large single doses given every other day. This approach has the advantage of minimizing the number and severity of 'early worsening' episodes and is useful in 'brittle' myasthenics. The disadvantage is the length of time required to achieve maximal dose and optimal benefit. A typical regimen starts with 25 mg of prednisone every other day. The dose is increased by 12.5 mg every third dose (every sixth day) to maximum improvement or to a maximum dose of 100 mg every other day. 'Off-day' deterioration is treated with a 5 to 10 mg 'booster' dose on the off-day, with an equivalent decrease in the on-day dose.[29] Others have recommended variations of this approach.[8,13,15]

The second regimen starts with high doses of prednisone on a daily or alternate day schedule; if a daily schedule is followed, the patient is quickly switched to alternate day therapy. This approach has the advantages of rapid improvement and minimum time spent in adjusting steroid dosage and the disadvantage of more frequent early worsening of myasthenia. A typical dosage regimen begins with 50 to 100 mg of prednisone daily until the patient is stabilized. Then the patient is switched to alternate day therapy while maintaining the same total maintenance dose. Variations of this regimen have been advocated by several authors.[1,13,17,22,23]

When an optimal response is achieved and no exacerbations have occurred for 2 to 8 months, most clinicians attempt to decrease the maintenance dose gradually. In a stabilized patient, the alternate day prednisone dose is reduced by 5 mg per month until the patient reaches a maintenance dose of 80 mg every other day. At this point, the dose is tapered more slowly (eg, 2.5 mg per month).[17] The median minimal maintenance dose is approximately 70 mg of prednisone every other day.[17] Myasthenic weakness will increase, often dramatically, if the prednisone is tapered too rapidly. To regain control in such a patient often requires the employment of prednisone doses considerably greater than the dose that previously gave control.[13]

Patients who eventually respond almost always do so within the first 1 to 4 months, usually showing distinct improvement within the first 1 to 6 weeks.[8,17] Vital capacity, ptosis, eye movements, and limb strength often improve first; diplopia and dysphagia are commonly the last to respond.[17]

Anticholinesterase drugs should be continued when steroid therapy is started. As the prednisone becomes effective, the requirement for these, and tolerance of them, lessen. The dose should be titrated to the optimal levels. This requires scrupulous monitoring for signs and symptoms of inhibitor overdosage and frequent dosage adjustments.[8,13,22,23,29]

Patients of both sexes and all ages may respond well to steroids. Males over 40 or 50 years of age respond particularly well.[8,13,15,17] Older women do not respond as frequently as older males.[8,13,15,17] Young male myasthenic patients, including juveniles, respond unpredictably. Those patients who do respond tend to do so dramatically. We feel that most young male myasthenic patients should be given a 3 month trial of steroids to assess their usefulness in each case.[15,17] Young female myasthenic patients, including juveniles, have not responded as well as others. Fortunately, this group of patients respond optimally to thymectomy.[17] Response to prednisone is not correlated with severity or duration of the disease; only to sex and age of the patient.[13,17]

Toxicity of Adrenal Corticosteroids. The side effects observed in myasthenic patients treated with steroids are similar to those seen in other patients treated with long-term, high-dose steroid therapy (see Chapter 49, Adrenal Corticosteroids). These side effects include Cushingoid facies, duodenal and gastric ulcer, sodium retention, hypokalemia, cataracts,[13,17,22] osteoporosis,[13,17,22,29] aseptic necrosis of the femoral head,[22] chemical diabetes,[13,17] and hypertension.[13,17] These effects are rarely severe enough to warrant discontinuation of therapy. Side effects are largely dose-dependent and are nearly always reduced when the steroids are given on a single-dose, alternate day schedule.

Thymectomy

Surgical resection of the thymus gland (thymectomy) has become an accepted approach to therapy in selected myasthenic patients.[1,11,13,17,22,23,31] While young female myasthenics appear to respond especially well to thymectomy,[17] thymic pathology appears to be predictive of outcome. In one study,[1] 92% of patients whose thymus glands revealed no germinal centers exhibited marked to moderate improvement following thymectomy. The presence of germinal centers reduced the improvement rate to 66%. Patients with thymoma have only a 25% response rate. While thymectomy has been shown to be a most valuable therapeutic tool in many cases of myasthenia, a major drawback is that its therapeutic benefits may be delayed, extending at times to five or more years after surgery. In one study,[1] 50% of the patients who experienced a remission following thymectomy did so after a delay of two or more years.

Other Immunosuppressive Measures

Immunosuppressive agents other than steroids have been advocated in the treatment of severe myasthenia gravis unresponsive to more conventional measures. Azathioprine or 6-mercaptopurine have been of benefit in 80 to 89% of myasthenic patients, often after failure on

TABLE 3 Drugs That May Aggravate Myasthenia Gravis

Drug	Proposed Mechanism of Action	Clinical Significance in Myasthenia Gravis	Comment	Reference
Antibiotics Aminoglycosides Polymyxins Bacitracin Colistin Clindamycin Lincomycin	Inhibit presynpatic release of acetylcholine and depress motor endplate sensitivity to acetylcholine	++	Effect reversible with intravenous calcium	17,34,35
Nondepolarizing (Competitive) Neuromuscular Blockers Curare Pancuronium Gallamine	Compete with acetylcholine for the cholinergic receptor site	++++	Myasthenics highly sensitive; effects reversible with cholinesterase inhibitors	1,17,36
Depolarizing (Noncompetitive) Neuromuscular Blockers Succinylcholine Decamethonium	Acetylcholine-like postsynaptic depolarization	++++	Effects not readily reversible	36

Membrane Stabilizers				
Propranolol Anesthetics (ether, haloethane, cycloproprane, fluroxene, methoxyflurane, enflurane) Antiarrhythmics (procainamide, quinidine)	"Stabilization" of postsynaptic membrane	++ to +++	Synergistic with competitive neuromuscular blockers	1,17,36,37
Anticonvulsants				
Phenytoin Trimethandione Magnesium salts	Stabilize pre- and postmyoneural junction	?	Interactions reported only anecdotally	1,17,38,39
Antimalarials				
Quinine	Stabilization of postsynaptic membrane	++	Occasional myasthenics are very sensitive	1,17
Lactate	Reduction of acetylcholine release due to hypocalcemia	+ to ++		17
Diuretics	Effects probably attributable to hypokalemia	+		40

steroids or steroids plus thymectomy.[11,13,16,32] The potential for serious side effects (bone marrow depression, increased incidence of neoplasia, increased risk of infection) is substantial.

Depletion of serum immunoglobins by thoracic duct drainage[32] or plasmaphoresis[11] has been employed successfully in a small number of patients. While transient benefit, intrinsic hazard, and cost[33] preclude routine use, these interventions may be of significant benefit in the treatment of severe myasthenic crisis, when rapid resolution of the patient's symptoms may be lifesaving.[13]

DRUG-INDUCED MYASTHENIA GRAVIS

A significant number of drugs can induce or enhance neuromuscular blockade (Table 3). Most of these agents present a threat only to a patient with an already compromised neuromuscular junction, but several can induce skeletal muscle weakness in normal subjects. These include curare, pancuronium and succinylcholine. These agents should be avoided or used with extreme caution in patients with myasthenia gravis.

REFERENCES

1. Dahl DS: The management of myasthenia gravis. Drug Therapy 1:21–29, 1976.
2. Kao I, Drachman DB: Thymic muscle cells bear acetylcholine receptors: possible relation to myasthenia gravis. Science 195:74–75, 1977.
3. Leeuwin RS, Wolters E: Effect of corticosteroids on sciatic nerve-tibialis anterior muscle of rats treated with hemicholinium-3. Neurology 27:171–177, 1977.
4. Lindstrom JM, Seybold ME, Lennon VA, et al: Antibody to acetylcholine receptor in myasthenia gravis. Neurology 26:1054–1059, 1976.
5. Fulpius BW, Zurn AD, Granato DA, et al: Acetylcholine receptor and myasthenia gravis. Ann NY Acad Sci 274:116–129, 1976.
6. Drachman DB, Kao I, Pestronk A, et al: Myasthenia gravis as a receptor disorder. Ann NY Acad Sci 274:226–234, 1976.
7. Birnbaum G, Tsairis P: Suppressor lymphocytes in myasthenia gravis and effect of adult thymectomy. Ann NY Acad Sci 274:527–535, 1976.
8. Engel WK: Myasthenia gravis, corticosteroids, anticholinesterases. Ann NY Acad Sci 274:623–630, 1976.
9. Check W: A revamped view of myasthenia gravis. JAMA 238:1338–1343, 1977.
10. Engel AG, Lindstrom JM, Lambert EH, et al: Ultrastructural localization of the acetylcholine receptor in myasthenia gravis and in its experimental model. Neurology 27:307–315, 1977.
11. Dau PC, Lindstrom JM, Cassel CK, et al: Plasmaphoresis and immunosuppressive drug therapy in myasthenia gravis. N Engl J Med 297:1134–1140, 1977.
12. Engel AG, Lambert EH, Howard FM: Immune complexes (IgG and C_3) at the motor end-plate in myasthenia gravis. Mayo Clin Proc 52:267–280, 1977.
13. Drachman DB: Myasthenia gravis. N Engl J Med 298:136–142, 186–193, 1978.
14. Adams RD: Episodic muscular weakness. In *Harrison's Principles of Internal Medicine,* 8th edition. Edited by GW Thorn, RD Adams, E Braunwald, et al. New York, McGraw-Hill Company, 1977, pp 1996–1999.
15. Engel WK: New prednisone regimen in myasthenia gravis. JAMA 237:635–636, 1977.

16. Mertens HG, Balzereit F, Leipert M: The treatment of severe myasthenia gravis with immunosuppressive agents. Eur Neurol 2:321–339, 1969.
17. Engel WK, Festoff BW, Pattern BM, et al: Myasthenia gravis: NIH conference. Ann Intern Med 81:225–246, 1974.
18. Namba T, Brown SB, Grob D: Neonatal myasthenia gravis: report of two cases and review of the literature. Pediatrics 45:488–504, 1970.
19. Fullerton DT, Munsat TL: Pseudo-myasthenia gravis: a conversion reaction. J Nerv Ment Dis 142:78–86, 1966.
20. Foldes FF, Klonymus DH, Maisel W, et al: A new curare test for the diagnosis of myasthenia gravis. JAMA 203:649–653, 1968.
21. Horowitz SH, Genkins G, Kornfeld P, et al: Electrophysiologic diagnosis of myasthenia gravis and the regional curare test. Neurology 26:410–417, 1976.
22. Mann JD, Johns TR, Campa JF, et al: Long-term prednisone followed by thymectomy in myasthenia gravis. Ann NY Acad Sci 274:608–622, 1976.
23. Mann JD, Johns TR, Campa JF: Long-term administration of corticosteroids in myasthenia gravis. Neurology 26:729–740, 1976.
24. Cohan SL, Dretchen KL, Neal A: Malabsorption of pyridostigmine in patients with myasthenia gravis. Neurology 27:299–301, 1977.
25. Dawson DM: Human disease transferred to mice: myasthenia gravis. N Engl J Med 296:168–169, 1977.
26. Engel AG, Lambert EH, Santa T: Study of long-term anticholinesterase therapy—effect on neuromuscular transmission and on motor end-plate time structure. Neurology 23:1273–1281, 1973.
27. Parasympathomimetic agents (12:04). In *The American Hospital Formulary Service*. Edited by MJ Reilly, JA Kepler. Washington, American Society of Hospital Pharmacists, 1977.
28. Koelle GB: Anticholinesterase agents. In *The Pharmacological Basis of Therapeutics,* 5th edition. Edited by LS Goodman, A Gilman. New York, MacMillan Company, 1975, pp 445–466.
29. Seybold ME, Drachman DB: Gradually increasing doses of prednisone in myasthenia gravis. N Engl J Med 290:81–84, 1974.
30. Drachman DB, Angus CW, Adams RN, et al: Myasthenic antibodies cross-link acetylcholine receptors to accelerate degradation. N Engl J Med 298:1116–1122, 1978.
31. Sarnat HB, McGarry JD, Lewis JE: Effective treatment of infantile myasthenia gravis by combined prednisone and thymectomy. Neurology 27:550–553, 1977.
32. Matell G, Bergstrom K, Franksson C, et al: Effects of some immunosuppressive procedures on myasthenia gravis. Ann NY Acad Sci 274:659–676, 1976.
33. Keesey J: Caution on plasmaphoresis for myasthenia gravis. N Engl J Med 298:1029, 1978.
34. Barza M, Scheife RT: Antimicrobial spectrum, pharmacology, and therapeutic use of antibiotics. IV. The aminoglycosides. Am J Hosp Pharm 34:723–737, 1977.
35. Fogdall RP, Miller RD: Prolongation of a pancuronium-induced neuromuscular blockade by clindamycin. Anesthesiology 41:407–408, 1974.
36. Koelle GB: Neuromuscular blocking agents. In *The Pharmacological Basis of Therapeutics,* 5th edition. Edited by LS Goodman, A Gilman. New York, MacMillan Company, 1975, pp 575–588.
37. Usubiaga JE: Neuromuscular effects of beta-adrenergic blockers and their interaction with skeletal muscle relaxants. Anesthesiology 29:484–492, 1968.
38. Brumlik J, Jacobs RS: Myasthenia gravis associated with diphenylhydantoin therapy for epilepsy. Can J Neurol Sci 1:127–129, 1974.
39. Streib EW: Adverse effects of magnesium salt cathartics in a patient with myasthenic syndrome (Lambert-Eaton's syndrome). Ann Neurol 2:175–176, 1977.
40. Gessa GL, Ferrari W: Influence of chlorothiazide, hydrochlorothiazide, and acetazolamide on neuromuscular transmission in mammals. Arch Int Pharmacodyn Ther 144:258–268, 1963.

GASTROINTESTINAL AGENTS

62. ANTISPASMODICS

George L. Arnold and Andrew G. Plaut

Anticholinergic antispasmodic agents have a limited role as adjunctive therapy in the management of peptic ulcer disease.[1] They may be useful in reducing the abdominal pain associated with the irritable bowel syndrome.[2,3] Antispasmodics are competitive antagonists of acetylcholine, which is released at the endings of the parasympathetic nerves supplying the gastrointestinal tract. The few controlled studies show that these drugs cause a mean reduction of basal acid output of about 50%. They also reduce maximal acid output by 15 to 50%. A recent study of food stimulated gastric acid secretion in duodenal ulcer patients demonstrated a mean of 29% inhibition over a 3 hour period when 15 mg of propantheline was administered with the meal. Contrary to popular belief and previous studies, higher doses of this agent failed to increase the degree of inhibition of acid secretion.[4]

Evidence from clinical trials do not establish their efficacy in promoting ulcer healing and preventing complications or reoccurrences.[5] Most authors agree that to be effective anticholinergics must be given every six hours.

Many synthetic anticholinergic agents are currently available, twenty-one of which were classified by the Food and Drug Administration as 'effective for use as adjunctive therapy in the treatment of peptic ulcer'.[6] Most of the favorable published experience has been with glycopyrrolate (Robinul), propantheline bromide (Pro-Banthine), poldine methylsulfate (Nacton), oxyphencyclimine hydrochloride (Daricon), methantheline bromide (Banthine), and methscopolamine bromide (Pamine). Although some of these agents may produce a greater degree of inhibition of gastric secretion with fewer disturbing side effects, the evidence on this point is inconclusive. Therefore, if an anticholinergic is used at all, we recommend either belladonna tincture or propantheline bromide, the two most widely employed agents.

TABLE 1 Preparations and Costs of Single-Entity Antispasmodics

GENERIC NAME	TRADEMARK NAME(S)	PREPARATIONS AND 1978 COSTS
Belladonna Tincture	generic	Tincture—$0.16–0.26/30 ml
Propantheline Bromide	Pro-Banthine	Tablets 15 mg—$8.33/100
Anisotropine Methylbromide	Valpin-50	Tablets 50 mg—$9.35/100
Dicyclomine Hydrochloride	Bentyl	Capsules 10 mg—$5.60/100 Tablets 20 mg—$8.00/100
Glycopyrrolate	Roninul Robinul Forte	Tablets 1 mg—$3.85/100 Tablets 2 mg—$6.40/100
Hexocyclium Methylsulfate	Tral	Tablets 25 mg—$7.24/100 Tablets (long-acting) 50 mg—$7.16/50; 75 mg—$10.97/50
Methantheline Bromide	Banthine	Tablets 50 mg—$7.50/100
Methscopolamine Bromide	Pamine	Tablets 2.5 mg—$7.16/100
Oxyphencyclimine Hydrochloride	Daricon	Tablets 10 mg—$6.54/100
Oxyphenonium Bromide	Antrenyl Bromide	Tablets 5 mg—$5.50/100
Tridihexethyl Chloride	Pathilon	Tablets 25mg—$7.40/100 Capsules (long-acting) 75 mg—$5.60/30

Anticholinergics are available alone (Table 1) and in combination with sedatives (eg, Butibel, Combid, Donnatal, Librax). It is unlikely that these fixed dosage combinations will be optimal for more than a few patients, and they are, therefore, not recommended.

Anticholinergics may be useful in the following settings[5]: (1) In severe or persistent ulcer pain at night, when side effects of the drug may be better tolerated. The combined use of cimetidine and an anticholinergic has been shown to produce an additive effect and may be more useful for this indication than either agent alone. (2) When true peptic ulcers are healing slowly. (3) In patients with a high rate of ulcer reoccurrence. (4) For patients who tolerate antacids poorly, as a means of reducing their dosage (cimetidine alone would be more effective for this indication). (5) Irritable bowel syndrome, especially for those patients in whom abdominal pain is the dominant symptom. They should be used with great caution, and in some cases may be contraindicated, in patients with reflux esophagitis, achalasia, partial gastric outlet obstruction, paralytic ileus, intestinal obstruction, narrow angle glaucoma, and prostatism.

In general, the vast majority of patients with peptic ulcer probably do not require anticholinergic agents.

DRUG INTERACTIONS

When propantheline is taken concurrently with slowly dissolving digoxin tablets, it may cause increased serum digoxin levels; this presumably reflects more complete absorption of the cardiac glycoside as intestinal motility is slowed.[7,8] This effect has not been demonstrated in patients receiving rapidly dissolving digoxin tablets, liquid digoxin preparations, or digitoxin.

ADVERSE REACTIONS

The most common unwanted effects are dry mouth, blurred vision, photophobia, constipation, urinary hesitancy, nervousness, dizziness, nausea, vomiting, headache, loss of taste, and gastric retention.

DOSAGE

Oral: Adults, tincture of belladona: 12 to 15 drops in one-half glass of water 1 hour before meals and at bedtime. Propantheline bromide (Pro-Banthine): 15 mg three times a day with meals and 30 mg at bedtime.

REFERENCES

1. Littman A, Pine BH: Antacids and anticholinergic drugs. Ann Intern Med 82:544–551, 1975.
2. Ivey KJ: Are anticholinergics of use in the irritable colon syndrome. Gastroenterology 68:1300–1307, 1975.
3. Drossman DA, Powell DW, Sessions JT: The irritable bowel syndrome. Gastroenterology 73:811–822, 1977.
4. Feldman M, Richardson CT, Peterson WL, et al: Effect of low-dose propantheline on food stimulated gastric acid secretion. N Engl J Med 297:1427–1430, 1977.
5. Ivey KJ: Anticholinergics: Do they work in peptic ulcer? Gastroenterology 68:154–166, 1975.
6. Certain anticholinergic drugs. Federal Register. Vol 36 (118):18, 1971.
7. Manninen V, Melin J, Apajalhati A, et al: Altered absorption of digoxin in patients given propantheline and metoclopramide. Lancet 1:398–399, 1973.
8. Manninen V, Apajalhati A, Simonen H, et al: Effect of propantheline and metoclopramide on absorption of digoxin. Lancet 1:1118–1119, 1973.

63. ANTACIDS

Martin G. Kistin and Richard A. Norton

Antacids are agents that neutralize or remove acid from the gastric contents and decrease peptic activity. They are useful in the treatment of hyperchlorhydria, peptic ulcer, and reflux esophagitis. Pepsin is maximally active between pH 1.5 and 2. At higher pH values pepsin becomes progressively less active until it becomes irreversibly inactivated (above pH 7.5).[1,2]

It is now generally believed that gastric acid and pepsin contribute to the formation of peptic ulcers. Recently it has been suggested that some peptic ulcer patients have normal gastric acid secretion, yet still have damage to the gastric mucosa which allows the diffusion of hydrogen ions.[3–7]

The therapeutic effect of antacids in ulcer disease is unclear. Three studies support the view that antacids do not improve healing but merely relieve pain.[8–10] Investigators in other large studies have concluded that antacids promote healing.[11–13] All of these studies are inadequately controlled, and none are double-blind.

Assuming that antacids promote healing, it is not known whether it is sufficient to neutralize gastric acid partially with relatively small quantities of antacid, or whether it is necessary to suppress or inactivate pepsin with larger quantities. Raising stomach pH from 1.3 to 2 decreases gastric acid by 80% but increases pepsin activity four-fold.[14,15] The optimal antacid dose therefore is controversial. If gastric pH is raised to 4.5, pepsin becomes inactive, and healing of an ulcer can be presumed to proceed.

For constant buffering, antacids must be given by hourly drip infusion of large doses. On an empty stomach the buffering effect of various antacids lasts from 5 to 60 minutes. It is believed that antacids given 1 hour after a meal buffer gastric contents for up to 3 hours.[16] However, this has not been universally found.[17] A currently popular regimen uses 30 to 60 ml of liquid antacid one hour after meals and at bedtime. This regimen theoretically provides about 15 hours of buffering per day.

Fordtran has published a guide to the buffering capacity of antacids and antacid mixtures by brand name.[18] Great difficulty was encountered in attempting to predict with accuracy the relative antacid potency of commercial antacids from product labels, because the amounts of different components are often not specified and because of varying solubility of aluminum and magnesium salts, depending on the specific manufacturing process. In general, compounds containing magnesium hydroxide, calcium carbonate and sodium bicarbonate had higher neutralization capacity than compounds containing aluminum hydroxide.

Other differences among antacids include their sodium content, laxative or cathartic effects, and amount of absorption of the cation moiety. Absorbable antacids (eg, sodium bicarbonate) can produce metabolic alkalosis because of bicarbonate absorption. 'Nonabsorbable' antacids (eg, calcium carbonate) contain insoluble cations. Some antacid mixtures may combine a fast and a slow, long-acting agent, but most mixtures are designed to combine a laxative (magnesium containing) agent with a constipating (aluminum or calcium containing) agent. Individual patient response is unpredictable, and agents causing diarrhea in one patient may constipate another. Although the effects on bowel habits may be cancelled out by these mixtures, other side effects like hypermagnesemia, phosphate depletion and water retention are not diminished and may be additive. Many patients make their own 'mixtures' by alternating laxatives when constipation or diarrhea occurs.

The sodium content of the antacid preparations varies greatly and many contain enough sodium to be of concern in patients with hypertension, heart disease, renal failure, or cirrhosis.[19–21]

DRUG MONOGRAPHS

SODIUM BICARBONATE

Sodium bicarbonate is a highly soluble antacid which reacts immediately with hydrochloric acid. Although its onset is rapid and its neutralizing capacity is high, its duration of action is very short. For every equivalent of acid neutralized, the body receives an equivalent of bicarbonate. Excess sodium bicarbonate is emptied rapidly into the small intestine where it is absorbed.

Adverse Reactions—Sodium bicarbonate is not recommended for long-term use because of its short duration of action and its alkalosis-producing properties. Although alkalosis is not usually a problem in relatively healthy patients,[22–24] sodium bicarbonate may cause volume expansion, hypertension, and edema in patients with renal insufficiency, hypertension or congestive heart failure.[25]

Dosage—300 mg to 2 g per dose.

CALCIUM CARBONATE

Calcium carbonate is a non-absorbable antacid. It combines with hydrochloric acid to form soluble calcium chloride. In the small intestine most of the calcium chloride is reconverted to insoluble calcium carbonate or calcium phosphate.

Calcium carbonate is potent and inexpensive. It has a rapid onset of action. Since calcium carbonate is emptied from the stomach more slowly than sodium bicarbonate its antacid action is more prolonged.

Calcium-containing antacids cause a paradoxical increase in acid production. The mechanism of this effect is not clear. Although hypercalcemia can cause increased gastrin secretion with resultant increase in acid secretion, the acid rebound phenomenon is not related to gastrin and occurs in the absence of detectable hypercalcemia.[26–28]

The amount of calcium absorbed is variable and seems to be a function of the amount of gastric acid present.[29]

Adverse Reactions—Adverse effects include a chalky taste, constipation, acid rebound, hypercalcemia and the milk-alkali syndrome.[30] Tetracycline absorption is reduced by simultaneous administration of calcium ions.

Dosage—2 g per dose, not to exceed 8 g per day.[16,31]

ALUMINUM HYDROXIDE (Amphojel)

Aluminum hydroxide is a slow-acting, low-potency, 'non-absorbable' antacid. It reacts with hydrochloric acid in the stomach to form aluminum chloride. In the small intestine aluminum chloride reacts to form insoluble aluminum salts. Therefore, there is very little aluminum absorption. However, in some studies 17 to 31% of dietary aluminum was excreted in the urine, and aluminum was found deposited in bones and lungs.[32,33]

Aluminum phosphate is one of the insoluble salts precipitated in the small intestine, and phosphate absorption is reduced by aluminum therapy.[34,35] This action provides a basis for lowering serum phosphate levels in patients with calcinosis universalis,[36] and in chronic renal disease.[37,38] It is also a potential hazard in causing phosphorous depletion.

Adverse Reactions—Aluminum is constipating and may be poorly tolerated. Aluminum toxicity has been reported in uremic rats fed a soluble aluminum preparation or if aluminum is injected intravenously. Toxicity was manifested as lethargy, periorbital bleeding, anorexia, and death.[39] Recently it has been suggested that the phenomenon of hemodialysis encephalopathy in man may be related to aluminum toxicity.[40]

Interactions—Aluminum hydroxide reduces the absorption of tetracycline, isoniazid, chlorpromazine, aminosalicyclic acid and possibly of iron and atropine.[35,41,42] The antacid should be administered an hour or more after these other drugs.

Dosage—600 mg per dose.

MAGNESIUM HYDROXIDE

Magnesium hydroxide (Milk of Magnesia) is a potent antacid which is emptied slowly from the stomach, prolonging its antacid action. There is little effect on acid-base balance. About 5 to 15% of the ingested magnesium is absorbed, and this is readily excreted in the urine if kidney function is normal.[43]

Adverse Reactions—A major difficulty with the use of this agent alone is its marked laxative effect. It is rarely used without an aluminum or calcium-containing compound. In patients with renal disease, magnesium retention may result from the chronic use of magnesium salts and can cause neurological, neuromuscular and cardiovascular impairment.[43]

Interactions—Chlorpromazine or tetracycline should be given an hour or more before magnesium-containing medications to ensure adequate absorption.

Dosage—5 to 30 ml per dose.

MAGALDRATE (Riopan)

Magaldrate is a chemical combination of magnesium and aluminum hydroxides. It neutralizes gastric acid in two stages, the magnesium portion more rapidly and the aluminum more slowly.

Acid is buffered more consistently than by mixtures (see below). The sodium content is very low, making this compound the drug of choice where a patient must be on a restricted intake of sodium.[20,21]

Adverse Reactions—Magaldrate shares with aluminum hydroxide and with magnesium hydroxide the difficulties listed above.

Dosage—400 to 800 mg; 5 to 10 ml of suspension or 1 to 2 tablets.

ANTACID MIXTURES

Mixtures have been developed to balance the constipating effect of an aluminum salt with the laxative effect of a magnesium salt, while still offering the excellent acid neutralizing effect of the latter. The total capacity for neutralizing acid is roughly the sum of the capacities of the constituents, but the pH value at which buffering occurs may be shifted downward. This shift seems to be of relatively little significance clinically.

TABLE 1 Characteristics of Antacid Mixtures (Suspensions)

	Capacity[b] Components[a]	Neutralizing Capacity (mEq/15 ml)	1978 Cost per 40 mEq ($)
Aludrox	1,2	42	0.08
Camalox	1,2,5	54	0.06
Creamalin	1,2	39	0.08
Di-Gel	1,2,3	37	0.07
Gelusil	1,4	20	0.13
Gelusil-M	1,2,4	34	0.09
Maalox	1,2	39	0.07
Mylanta	1,2,3	36	0.08
Mylanta II	1,2,3	62	0.07
WinGel	1,2	34	0.07

[a]1-Aluminum hydroxide, 2-magnesium hydroxide, 3-simethicone, 4-magnesium trisilicate, 5-calcium carbonate.

[b]Neutralizing capacity in mEq is based on Fordtran's method [31].

TABLE 2 Preparations and Costs of Antacids

GENERIC NAME	TRADEMARK NAME(S)	PREPARATIONS AND 1978 COSTS
Single-Entity Antacids		
Aluminum hydroxide	Amphojel	Suspension 320 mg/5 ml—$1.83/12 oz Tablets 300 mg—$1.42/100; 600 mg—$2.22/100
Calcium carbonate	Dicarbosil	Tablets 500 mg—$5.30/500
	generic	Tablets 600 mg—$2.06/100
Magaldrate	Riopan	Suspension 80 mg/ml—$2.17/12 oz Tablets 400 mg—$2.57/100
Magnesium hydroxide (Milk of Magnesia)	generic	Suspension—$3.60/16 oz Tablets 300 mg—$0.75/100; 600 mg—$0.85/100
Sodium bicarbonate	generic	Tablets 300 mg—$0.61–$1.28/100; 600 mg—$0.68–$1.52/100
Antacid Mixtures[a]		
	Aludrox	Suspension—$1.83/12 oz Tablets—$2.16/100
	Camalox	Suspension—$1.93/12 oz Tablets—$1.56/50
	Creamalin	Suspension—$2.59/pt Tablets—$1.97/50
	Di-Gel	Suspension—$1.60/12 oz
	Gelusil	Suspension—$1.53/12 oz Tablets—1.68/100
	Gelusil-M	Suspension—1.80/12 oz Tablets—$1.95/100
	Maalox	Suspension—$1.73/12 oz No. 1 tablets—$1.74/100 No. 2 tablets—$1.63/50
	Mylanta	Suspension—$1.66/12 oz Tablets—$1.60/100
	Mylanta II	Suspension—$2.57/12 oz Tablets—$1.79/60
	WinGel	Suspension—$1.45/12 oz Tablets—$1.59/100

[a]For the composition of antacid mixtures and their cost per 40 mEq of neutralizing capacity see Table 1.

The taste of various antacid mixtures was studied in 100 different subjects by Schneider and Roach using a double-blind technique similar to wine tasting.[44] Of the 19 mixtures tested, the most pleasant, in order of preference were: Marblen, Titralac, Kudrox, Mylanta II, Camalox, Silain-Gel, and Aludrox.

Table 1 is adopted from Green, et al.[45]

Adverse Reactions—Diarrhea may result from administration of any of these mixtures, as well as phosphorus depletion, hypermagnesemia (in renal insufficiency) and increased fluid retention. An antacid mixture should not be given with or immediately before tetracycline because of interference with absorption.

Dosage—See Table 1.

REFERENCES

1. Turner MD: Pepsinogen and pepsins. Gut 9:134–138, 1968.
2. Samloff IM: Pepsinogens, pepsins, and pepsin inhibitors. Gastroenterology 60:586–604, 1971.
3. Piper DW, Heap TR: Medical management of peptic ulcer with reference to antiulcer agents in other gastro-intestinal disease. Drugs 3:366–403, 1972.
4. Rhodes J: Etiology of gastric ulcer. Gastroenterology 63:171–181, 1972.
5. Birnbaum D: Peptic ulcer and the central nervous system—etiology and management. Clin Gastroenterol 2:245–257, 1973.
6. Scratchard T: Gastric secretory mechanisms and peptic ulcer. Clin Gastroenterol 2:259–274, 1973.
7. Wormsley KG: The pathophysiology of duodenal ulceration. Gut 15:59–81, 1974.
8. Doll R, Price AV, Pygott F, et al: Continuous intragastric milk drip in the treatment of uncomplicated gastric ulcer. Lancet 1:70–73, 1956.
9. Baume PE, Hunt JH: Failure of potent antacid therapy to hasten healing in chronic gastric ulcers. Aust Ann Med 18:113–116, 1969.
10. Hermann RP, Piper DW: Factors influencing the healing rate of chronic gastric ulcer. Am J Dig Dis 18:1–6, 1973.
11. Rosett NE, Knox FH Jr, Stephenson SL Jr: Peptic ulcer: medical cure by efficient gastric acid neutralization. Ann Intern Med 36:98–109, 1952.
12. Rosett NE, Kashgarian M: Peptic ulcer: medical cure of ambulatory patients by efficient gastric acid neutralization. J Tenn State Med Assoc 61:798–801, 1968.
13. Veterans Administration Gastric Ulcer Study Group: The Veterans Administration cooperative study on gastric ulcer. Gastroenterology 61:567–654, 1971.
14. Fordtran JS, Walsh JH: Gastric acid secretion rate and buffer content of the stomach after eating. Results in normal patients and in patients with duodenal ulcer. J Clin Invest 52:645–657, 1973.
15. Piper DW, Fenton B: The absorption of pepsin. Am J Dig Dis 6:134–141, 1961.
16. Fordtran JS, Morawski SG, Richardson CT: *In vivo* and *in vitro* evaluation of liquid postcibal gastric acidity and peptic activity. N Engl J Med 274:921–927, 1966.
17. Powell RL, Westlake WJ, Longaker ED, et al: A clinical evaluation of a new concentrated antacid. I. Effects on gastric pH. J Clin Pharmacol 11:288–295, 1971.
18. Fordtran JS, Morawski SG, Richardson CT: In vivo and in vitro evaluation of liquid antacids. N Engl J Med 288:923–928, 1973.
19. *Handbook of Nonprescription Drugs*. Edited by GB Griffenhagen, LL Hawkins. Washington, American Pharmaceutical Association, 1973.
20. Bleifer KH, Belsky JL, Bliefer DJ: Sodium content of four antacids. N Engl J Med 261:604–605, 1959.
21. Rimer DG, Frankland M: Sodium content of antacids. JAMA 173:995–997, 1960.

22. Kirsner JB, Palmer WL: Alkalosis complicating the Sippy treatment of peptic ulcer. Arch Intern Med 69:789–807, 1942.
23. Kirsner JB, Palmer WL: Studies on the effect of massive quantities of sodium bicarbonate on the acid-base equilibrium and renal function. Report of a case with remarkable tolerance. Ann Intern Med 18:100–104, 1943.
24. Van Goidsenhoven GM-T, Gray OV, Price AV, et al: The effect of prolonged administration of large doses of sodium bicarbonate in man. Clin Sci 13:383–401, 1954.
25. Edwards CC: Proposal establishing a monograph for OTC antacid products. Fed Register 38:8714–8724, 1973.
26. Fordtran JS: Acid rebound. N Engl J Med 279:900–905, 1968.
27. Texter EC Jr, Laureta MC, Martin GA: Absence of acid rebound with two gram doses of calcium carbonate. Clin Res 19:72, 1971.
28. Barreras RD: Acid secretion after calcium carbonate in patients with duodenal ulcer. N Engl J Med 282:1402–1405, 1970.
29. Ivanovich P, Fellows H, Rich C: The absorption of calcium carbonate. Ann Intern Med 66:917–923, 1967.
30. McMillan DE, Freeman RB: The milk-alkali syndrome: a study of the acute disorder with comments on the development of the chronic condition. Medicine 44:485–501, 1965.
31. Fordtran JS: Comparison of antacids for peptic ulcer. N Engl J Med 275:1316, 1966.
32. Schroeder HA, Nason AP: Trace-element analysis in clinical chemistry. Clin Chem 17:461–474, 1971.
33. Thurston H, Gilmore GR, Swales JD: Aluminum retention and toxicity in chronic renal failure. Lancet 1:881–883, 1972.
34. Fauley GB, Freeman DS, Ivy AC, et al: Aluminum phosphate in the therapy of peptic ulcer. Arch Intern Med 67:563–578, 1941.
35. Lotz M, Zisman E, Bartter FC: Evidence for a phosphorous-depletion syndrome in man. N Engl J Med 278:409–414, 1968.
36. Nassim JR, Connolly CK: Treatment of calcinosis universalis with aluminum hydroxide. Arch Dis Child 45:118–121, 1970.
37. Pendras JP, Erickson RV: Hemodialysis: a successful therapy for chronic uremia. Ann Intern Med 64:293–311, 1966.
38. Goldsmith RS, Furzifer J, Johnson WJ, et al: Control of secondary hyperparathyroidism during long-term hemodialysis. Am J Med 50:692–699, 1971.
39. Berlyne GM, Yagil R, Benari J, et al: Aluminum toxicity in rats. Lancet 1:564–567, 1972.
40. Alfrey AC, LeGendre GR, Kaehny WD: The dialysis encephalopathy syndrome. Possible aluminum toxicity. N Engl J Med 294:184–188, 1976.
41. Chin TF, Lach JL: Drug diffusion and bioavailability: tetracycline metallic chelation. Am J Hosp Pharm 32:625–629, 1975.
42. Hurwitz A, Schlozman DL: Effects of antacids on gastrointestinal absorption of isoniazid in rat and man. Am Rev Respir Dis 109:41–47, 1974.
43. Randall RE, Cohen MD, Spray CC, et al: Hypermagnesemia in renal failure: etiology and toxic manifestations. Ann Intern Med 61:73–88, 1964.
44. Schneider RP, Roach AC: An antacid tasting: the relative palability of 19 liquid antacids. South Med J 69:1312–1313, 1976.
45. Green FW, Norton RA, Kaplan MM: Pharmacology and clinical use of antacids. J Maine Med Assoc 66:110–114, 117, (Apr) 1975.

64. ANTIDIARRHEAL AGENTS

George L. Arnold and Andrew G. Plaut

Antidiarrheal agents are primarily useful in the symptomatic management of short-term, self-limited, diarrheal illnesses. They play a lesser role in the treatment of more chronic conditions such as inflammatory bowel disease, post-vagotomy diarrhea, and high-output ileostomies. They are of little benefit, and have some potential hazards in acute, severe (often infectious) diarrheal states. Despite the availability of more than 100 over-the-counter products, including popular preparations such as Donnagel (a mixture of anticholinergics with kaolin and pectin) and Parepectolin (kaolin, pectin, and a small amount of paregoric), there are few controlled trials and little objective data to guide their usage. Clinical experience indicates that Kaopectate should be used for only mild diarrheal problems. Diphenoxylate or loperamide are next logical choices for more pronounced diarrhea because of their ease of administration and relative efficacy. Paregoric and opium tincture should be reserved for refractory diarrhea.

DRUG MONOGRAPHS

DIPHENOXYLATE HYDROCHLORIDE WITH ATROPINE SULFATE (Lomotil)

Diphenoxylate is a meperidine congener used exclusively in the treatment of diarrhea. Available in combination with atropine sulfate as Lomotil (atropine added to prevent abuse), it is currently the most useful drug for diarrhea when more addictive opiates are undesirable.[1] It possesses low analgesic activity and is free of parasympatholytic and dependence potential when used in the recommended dosage. Like other opiates, it acts primarily by inhibiting peristalsis. It must be used with caution, however, in acute diarrheal illnesses, since there

TABLE 1 Preparations and Costs of Antidiarrheal Agents

GENERIC NAME	TRADEMARK NAME(S)	PREPARATIONS AND 1978 COSTS
Diphenoxylate Hydrochloride with Atropine Sulfate	Lomotil	Tablets (diphenoxylate hydrochloride 2.5 mg, atropine sulfate 0.025 mg)—$11.66/100 Liquid (diphenoxylate hydrochloride 2.5 mg, atropine sulfate 0.025 mg/5 ml)—$3.45/2 oz
Loperamide	Imodium	Capsules 2 mg—$17.40/100
Opium Tincture	generic	Tincture—$5.65–$8.45/120 ml
Paregoric	generic	Tincture—$1.88–$3.48/pint
Kaolin with Pectin	Kaopectate	Suspension—$1.23/8 oz

is no evidence that decreasing motility reduces the loss of fluid and electrolytes into the inflamed bowel, and thus the drug may aggravate preexisting dehydration and electrolyte imbalance. In shigellosis, Lomotil prolongs fever and delays the clearance of infecting organisms from the stool.[2,3] In patients with acute ulcerative colitis and amebic colitis, Lomotil and other opiates may precipitate toxic megacolon[4–6] and thus should be used with extreme caution, if at all, in these conditions. Lomotil should be used with caution in patients with advanced liver disease since it may precipitate hepatic coma. Lomotil is contraindicated in children[7] because of the risks of unrecognized volume depletion.

Adverse Reactions—Dry mouth, flushing, urinary retention, hyperthermia, sedation, paralytic ileus, respiratory depression, nausea and vomiting, and, rarely, physical dependence have been reported.

Dosage—Up to 5 mg (2 tablets) every 6 hours until diarrhea is controlled. Dosage reduction is then usually possible, with a single tablet often effective, given every 6 hours.

LOPERAMIDE HYDROCHLORIDE (Imodium)

Loperamide hydrochloride, a new synthetic antidiarrheal agent similar in structure to diphenoxylate, has recently become available in the United States. *In vitro* studies suggest that it has a direct antiperistaltic action on intestinal nerve endings or intramural ganglia or both.[8] Double-blind controlled studies have demonstrated its efficacy in a number of diarrheal states including chronic inflammatory bowel disease, diarrhea associated with ileorectal anastomoses and high output ileostomies.[9,10] A large randomized double-blind study in acute diarrhea of many causes carried out by the European manufacturer showed a significantly better response than diphenoxylate over a three day period.[11] Daily administration for periods up to 18 months has resulted in no loss of effectiveness or appearance of significant toxicity.[10] Although no cases of toxic megacolon have been reported in association with loperamide therapy, it should not be administered to patients acutely ill with inflammatory bowel disease. Physical dependence has not been described in man but is theoretically possible. Its safety has not been established for use in children, pregnant women, or nursing mothers.[12]

Adverse Reactions—Constipation, drowsiness, abdominal cramping, nausea, vomiting, skin rash, dry mouth.

Dosage—4 mg initially followed by 2 mg after each unformed stool, up to 16 mg per day. Maintenance dose is usually 4 to 8 mg/day.

OPIUM TINCTURE

This hydroalcoholic solution containing 10% opium (representing 1% morphine) is an effective antidiarrheal agent and is useful in conditions that are likely to be of short duration. In the dosage recommended, it is active against diarrhea while providing little analgesia. Opiates act by reducing propulsive contractions in large and small bowel, but they increase bowel tone and augment anal sphincter tone as well. A central depression of the defecation reflex also occurs. As with other opiates, deodorized tincture of opium should be avoided in acute ulcerative colitis, shigellosis, amebic colitis, and advanced liver disease.

Adverse Reactions—Nausea, vomiting, constipation, mental confusion, rare allergic phenomena, and dependence have been observed.

Dosage—0.5 to 1.5 ml three or four times daily.

PAREGORIC

Paregoric (camphorated opium tincture) is a hydroalcoholic opium alkaloid preparation with benzoic acid, camphor and anise oil. It has traditionally been used for diarrhea in children and offers no advantage in the therapy of diarrhea over other opiate preparations.

Adverse Reactions—Same as for other opiates.

Dosage—4 to 8 ml after each loose stool or four times daily.

KAOPECTATE

Kaopectate is useful in the treatment of mild diarrhea. It is a mixture of 20% kaolin, hydrated aluminum silicate (an adsorbent), and 1% pectin, a purified carbohydrate product obtained from citrus fruit or apples. Its mechanism of action is probably through adsorption of water.

Dosage—30 to 90 ml four times daily or as needed.

REFERENCES

1. Barowsky H, Schwartz SA: Method for evaluating diphenoxylate hydrochloride: Comparison of its antidiarrheal effect with that of camphorated tincture of opium. JAMA 180:1058–1061, 1962.
2. DuPont HL, Hornick RB: Adverse effect of Lomotil therapy in shigellosis. JAMA 226:1525–1528, 1973.
3. Morbidity and Mortality Weekly Report. 24:358, 1975.
4. Garrett JM, Saver WG, Moertel CG: Colonic motility in ulcerative colitis after opiate administration. Gastroenterology 53:93–100, 1967.
5. Wruble LD, Duckworth JK, Duke DD, et al: Toxic dilatation of the colon in a case of amebiasis. N Engl J Med 275:926–928, 1966.
6. Pittman FE: Adverse effects of Lomotil. Gastroenterology 67:408–410, 1974.
7. Anon: Lomotil for diarrhea in children. Med Lett Drugs Ther 17:104, 1975.
8. Van Nueten JM, Janssen PAJ, Fontaine J: Loperamide (RI8553), a novel type of antidiarrheal agent. Part 3: *In vitro* studies on the peristaltic-reflex and other experiments on isolated tissues. Arzneim Forsch 24:1641–1645, 1974.
9. Tytgat GN, Huibregtse K, Dagevos J, et al: Effect of loperamide on fecal output and composition in well-established ileostomy and ileorectal anastomosis. Am J Dig Dis 22:669–676, 1977.
10. Galambos JT, Hersh T, Schroder S, et al: Loperamide: A new antidiarrheal agent in the treatment of chronic diarrhea. Gastroenterology 70:1026–1029, 1976.
11. Dom J, Leyman R, Schuermans V, et al: Loperamide (RI8553), a novel type of antidiarrheal agent. Arzneim Forsch 24:1660–1665, 1974.
12. Anon: Loperamide for diarrhea. Med Lett Drugs Ther 19:73–75, 1977.

65. LAXATIVES

Daniel S. Matloff and Karim A. Fawaz

Constipation sporadically occurs in nearly all individuals. In attempting to regulate what is perceived to be irregular bowel movements, a large segment of the population often uses laxatives. Over $130 million worth of laxatives are purchased yearly in the United States.

Laxatives may be categorized as follows: (1) osmotically-active agents; (2) mucosal irritants; (3) lubricants; (4) bulk-increasing agents; and (5) stool softeners. Effective laxatives result in increased fecal water excretion secondary to altered intestinal fluid and electrolyte transport.[1] This water and electrolyte accumulation can occur in either the small or large intestine. Combinations of active ion secretion, altered intestinal motility, increased mucosal permeability, and mucosal damage all contribute to altered fluid and electrolyte movement. The traditional classification of laxatives, although conceptually useful, does not reflect this basic underlying mechanism of laxative action.

Numerous laxative drugs are on the market, including many multiple-ingredient preparations. This chapter will deal only with effective agents that are both readily available and clinically useful.

DRUG MONOGRAPHS

OSMOTICALLY-ACTIVE AGENTS

GLYCERIN SUPPOSITORIES
MAGNESIUM CITRATE SOLUTION
MAGNESIUM SULFATE [Epsom Salt]
MILK OF MAGNESIA [Magnesium Hydroxide]

SODIUM PHOSPHATE AND SODIUM BIPHOSPHATE
(Fleet's Enema and Fleet's Phospho-Soda)
SORBITOL SOLUTION

These effective drugs promote defecation by retaining water in the intestinal lumen through osmotic forces. They may also act by stimulating the release of cholecystokinin.[2-4] All the magnesium salts are equally effective in promoting evacuation of the bowel. They should be used with extreme caution in patients with renal impairment since 20% or more of the magnesium cation may be absorbed systemically. Sufficient water should be ingested with each dose to prevent intravascular volume depletion. Sorbitol is primarily used in conjunction with the anion exchange resin, sodium polystyrene sulfonate (Kayexelate), to treat hyperkalemia.

Drug Interactions—Simultaneous administration of magnesium ions with either tetracycline or phenothiazine compounds may diminish gastrointestinal absorption of these agents.[5,6]

Dosage—Oral: Adults, Magnesium sulfate, 30 ml of a 50% solution; magnesium citrate solution, 200 ml; milk of magnesia, 15 to 30 ml; Fleet's Enema, $4^1/_2$ oz. pre-filled bottle; Fleet's Phospho-Soda, 20 ml mixed with water; sorbitol 20% solution, 100 to 200 ml. *Rectal:* Glycerin suppositories, one rectally.

MUCOSAL IRRITANTS

BISACODYL (Dulcolax)
CASCARA SAGRADA
CASTOR OIL
PHENOLPHTHALEIN
SENNA PREPARATIONS

These agents act by increasing motility of the intestine through an irritant action on the bowel.[7] Castor oil stimulates the small bowel, usually within three hours; it should not be given at bedtime. The other mucosal irritants mainly influence the large bowel and take about six to eight hours to act. These agents are often used in conjunction with an osmotically active agent as a cleansing preparation prior to or after x-ray studies.

Adverse Reactions—An excessive laxative effect is the most common side effect. Prolonged abuse may cause a characteristic radiographic appearance, the so-called cathartic colon.[8] Prolonged

TABLE 1 Preparations and Costs of Laxatives

GENERIC NAME	TRADEMARK NAME(S)	PREPARATIONS AND 1978 COSTS
Osmotically Active Agents		
Magnesium Sulfate [Epsom Salt]	generic	Powder—\$0.37–\$0.63/4 oz
Magnesium Citrate Solution	generic	Solution—\$0.32–\$1.09/10 oz
Milk of Magnesia	generic	Suspension—\$0.62–\$1.45/pint
Sodium Phosphate and Sodium Biphosphate	Fleet's Enema	Solution (sodium phosphate 6 g and sodium biphosphate 16 g)—\$0.39/4½ oz
	Fleet's Phospho-Soda	Sodium (sodium phosphate 18 g and sodium biphosphate 48 g)—\$0.35/2½ oz
Sorbitol Solution 70%	generic	Solution—\$2.00–\$3.25/pint
Glycerin Suppositories	generic	Suppositories (Adult)—\$0.31–\$0.88/12 Suppositories (Children)—\$0.31–\$0.88/12
Mucosal Irritants		
Bisacodyl	Dulcolax	Tablets (enteric-coated) 5 mg—\$1.60/24 Suppositories 10 mg—\$0.73/2, \$1.43/4
Cascara Sagrada Aromatic Fluidextract	generic	Fluidextract—\$2.94–\$5.87/pint
Castor Oil	generic	Oil—\$0.19–\$0.58/30 ml, \$0.28–\$0.69/60 ml
Phenolphthalein	Phenolax	Wafers 64.8 mg—\$1.31/100
Senna	Senokot	Tablets—\$2.34/50 Syrup—\$1.43/2 oz
Bulk-Increasing Agents		
Methylcellulose	generic	Tablets 500 mg—\$1.80–\$3.83/500
Psyllium Hydrophilic Mucilloid	Metamucil	Noneffervescent powder—\$1.87/7 oz, \$3.12/14 oz Effervescent powder (Instant Mix)—\$1.70/16 packets, \$2.95/30 packets

TABLE 1 *(continued)*

GENERIC NAME	TRADEMARK NAME(S)	PREPARATIONS AND 1978 COSTS
Stool Softeners		
Dioctyl Calcium Sulfosuccinate	Surfak	Capsules 50 mg—\$2.60/30; 240 mg—\$3.40/30
Dioctyl Sodium Sulfosuccinate	Colace	Capsules 50 mg—\$2.15/30; 100 mg—\$2.58/30 Liquid 10 mg/ml—\$1.92/30 ml Syrup 4 mg/ml—\$2.75/8 oz

use of the anthracene laxatives—cascara or senna—may cause a characteristic sigmoidoscopic picture of melanosis coli.[9] Of all the laxatives, the anthracene derivatives are the most abused by the public.[10,11]

Dosage—Oral: Adults, Castor oil, 15 to 60 ml; phenolphthalein, 100 mg daily (available in many proprietary preparations); cascara sagrada aromatic fluid extract, 5 ml (often taken with 30 ml of milk of magnesia); bisacodyl, 10 to 15 mg per day; senna concentrate (Senokot), 2 to 4 tablets two times daily, 2 to 3 teaspoonfuls syrup one or two times daily. *Children,* Castor oil, 5 to 15 ml; bisacodyl, 5 to 10 mg per day. *Rectal: Adults,* Bisacodyl, 10 mg suppository.

LUBRICANTS

MINERAL OIL

This mixture of liquid hydrocarbons, obtained from petroleum, promotes bowel movement by retarding water reabsorption; there is no stimulation of peristalsis.

Adverse Reactions—Adverse effects include lipoid pneumonia, secondary to aspiration, and interference with absorption of fat soluble vitamins.[12,13] Many patients object to the oily consistency of this tasteless preparation. Pruritis ani and anal leakage can be annoying side effects during short-term use. Mineral oil is combined with phenolphthalein in some multiple-ingredient preparations.

Drug Interactions—The effect of warfarin may be potentiated due to interference with vitamin K absorption.

Dosage—Oral: Adults, 15 to 45 ml.

BULK-INCREASING AGENTS

BRAN
METHYLCELLULOSE
PSYLLIUM HYDROPHILIC MUCILLOID (Metamucil)

These agents increase nonabsorbable bulk, resulting in a soft, well-hydrated stool.[14] They are often used to promote soft feces and easy defecation in patients who should avoid straining at stool, such as postoperative patients and the elderly.[15] Sufficient water intake is needed to prevent possible intestinal or esophageal obstruction in patients with narrowed lumens due to various disorders. They have no other serious adverse effects or interactions. The fiber content of the diet has recently been implicated in the pathogenesis of certain colonic disorders, particularly carcinoma and diverticular disorders.[16,17] These disorders seem to have a lower incidence in geographic areas where a higher fiber (and, hence, higher residue) diet is common, such as Africa.

Dosage—Oral: Psyllium hydrophilic mucilloid (Metamucil), 4 to 10 g in a glass of water, one to three times per day; methylcellulose, *Adults,* 1 g one to four times daily; *Children,* 500 mg two to three times daily; bran, as crude form or processed in cereal, amount determined by patient experience.

STOOL SOFTENERS

DIOCTYL CALCIUM SULFOSUCCINATE (Surfak)
DIOCTYL SODIUM SULFOSUCCINATE (Colace)

These agents have a detergent action that increases the water content of stool, and hence, its softness.[18] They produce their effect in 24 to 48 hours and are commonly used in patients who should have or desire a moderately soft, formed stool.[19] There are no adverse effects or known interactions, but alterations in drug absorption have been suggested in some studies.

Dosage—Dioctyl sodium sulfosuccinate (Colace), *Adults,* 50 to 200 mg per day in single or divided doses; *Children,* 10 to 40 mg per day; dioctyl calcium sulfosuccinate (Surfak), *Adults,* 240 mg per day; *Children,* 50 to 150 mg per day.

REFERENCES

1. Binder HJ, Donowitz M: A new look at laxative action. Gastroenterology 69:1001–1005, 1975.
2. Harvey RF, Read AE: Effects of oral magnesium sulphate on colonic motility. Gut 14:425, 1973.
3. Harvey RF, Read AE: Mode of action of the saline purgatives. Am Heart J 89:810–813, 1975.
4. Harvey RF, Read AE: Saline purgatives act by releasing cholecystokinin. Lancet 2:185–187, 1973.
5. Kunin CM, Finland F: Clinical pharmacology of the tetracycline antibiotics. Clin Pharmacol Ther 2:51–69, 1961.
6. Forrest FM, Forrest IS, Serra MT: Modification of chlorpromazine metabolism by some other drugs frequently administered to psychiatric patients. Biol Psychiatry 2:53–58, 1970.
7. Travell J: Pharmacology of stimulant laxatives. Ann NY Acad Sci 58:416–425, 1954.
8. Urso FP, Urso MJ, Lee CH: The cathartic colon: pathological findings and radiological/pathological correlation. Radiology 116:557–559, 1975
9. Wittoesch JH, Jackman RJ, McDonald JR: Melanosis coli: general review and a study of 887 cases. Dis Colon Rectum 1:172–180, 1958.
10. Gossain YV, Werk EE: Surreptitious laxation and hypokalemia. Ann Intern Med 76:761, 1972.
11. Cummings JH, Sladen GE, James OFW, et al: Laxative-induced diarrhoea: a continuing clinical problem. Br Med J 1:537–541, 1974.
12. Becker GL: Laxatives and dietary fiber. Med Lett Drugs Ther 15:98–100, 1973.
13. Rosenow EC: The spectrum of drug-induced pulmonary disease. Ann Intern Med 77:977–991, 1972.
14. Tainter ML, Buchanan OH: Quantitative comparisons of colloidal laxatives. Ann NY Acad Sci 58:438–454, 1954.
15. Rafsky HA, Hoing LJ: Changes in the colonic function and use of laxatives in the aged. Ann NY Acad Sci 58:513–519, 1954.
16. Bodribb ASM, Humphreys DM: Diverticular disease: three studies. Br Med J 1:424–430, 1976.
17. Vaisrub S: Fiber feeding—fad or finger of fate? (editorial). JAMA 235:182–183, 1976.
18. Donowitz M, Binder HJ: Effect of dioctyl sodium sulfosuccinate on colonic fluid and electrolyte movement. Gastroenterology 69:941–950, 1975.
19. Schoenfeld RC: Management of postpartum constipation with dicotyl sodium sulfosuccinate. Am J Obstet Gynecol 74:1114–1115, 1974.

66. ANTIEMETICS

Stephen E. Sallan and Carol Cronin

Nausea, the feeling of the imminent need to vomit, and vomiting, the forceful expulsion of the gastric contents, generally are mild, self-limiting symptoms associated with numerous organic and psychiatric diseases. On the other hand, the effects of vomiting can be devastating: dehydration, post-operative wound dehiscence, refusal to accept cancer therapy, psychological depression. Literature on the antiemetics dates primarily from the 1950's and 1960's, and many physicians continue to prescribe one or two 'standards' learned during training and reinforced by pharmaceutical advertising.

Although the control of nausea and vomiting is achieved best by treatment of the underlying disease, symptomatic therapy may be indicated in some situations. Understanding of the physiology and clinical etiology of vomiting and the pharmacology of antiemetic drugs facilitates selection of an appropriate agent. When vomiting can be anticipated, as with motion sickness or cancer chemotherapy, prophylaxis usually is more effective than post facto treatment. The optimal drug must have a relatively specific and rapid effect and be free from adverse side effects.

PHYSIOLOGY OF VOMITING

Vomiting is controlled by two functionally distinct medullary centers: the vomiting center and the chemoreceptor trigger zone (CTZ).[1] The actual act of vomiting is integrated by the vomiting center of the lateral reticular formation of the medulla. Located among loci controlling the functional aspects of vomiting (salivation, spasmodic respiratory movements, forced inspiration), this center functions as a coordinating mechanism. The vomiting center is excited directly by: (1) afferent impulses from the walls of the gut and heart via the vagus nerves and sympathetic nervous system; (2) higher cortical centers such as the labyrinthine apparatus; (3) the midbrain when hypoxia is present, as in increased intracranial pressure; (4) psychological stimuli such as taste, sight or smell; and (5) the CTZ. Important efferent pathways from the vomiting center include phrenic nerves to the diaphragm, spinal nerves to the abdominal musculature, and visceral efferent nerves to the stomach and esophagus.

A second and distinct medullary center, the CTZ, is located in the floor of the fourth ventricle. The CTZ can be activated by drugs such as apomorphine, cardiac glycosides, cancer chemotherapeutic agents, and presumably by other toxins and infectious agents. However, the CTZ is not an autonomous chemosensitive vomiting center, and thus is intrinsically incapable of initiating emesis without mediation of its efferent impulses through the medullary vomiting center.

Experimental evidence suggests that impulses elicited by motion stimulate the vestibular apparatus and traverse the cerebellum and the CTZ en route to the vomiting center. Ablation of the CTZ in some animals results in a decrease in the vomiting induced by vestibular stimuli, and suggests that non-chemical emetic stimuli may be chemically mediated via the CTZ.[1] Classic experiments in animals accordingly suggested two major types of emetic agents: (1) drugs such as copper sulfate that, when administered intragastrically, directly stimulate the vagus nerve and sympathetic nervous system resulting in afferent stimuli to the vomiting center; and (2) drugs such as apomorphine that, when administered intravenously, stimulate the CTZ which then funnels afferent stimuli to the vomiting center.

CLINICAL CLASSIFICATION OF VOMITING

Causes of vomiting include: (1) acute abdominal emergencies (inflammation or obstruction of a viscus); (2) central nervous system disorders resulting in increased intracranial pressure (inflammation, neoplasms, or anoxia); (3) infections; (4) cardiac diseases such as inferior wall infarction and congestive heart failure (the former causing nausea and vomiting by direct afferent stimuli to the vomiting center, the latter presumably secondary to hepatic congestion); (5) labyrinthine disorders such as Menière's disease; (6) endocrine abnormalities such as diabetic acidosis, adrenal insufficiency and morning sickness of pregnancy; (7) radiotherapy; and (8) drug-induced, such as that associated with cancer chemotherapy, post-operative vomiting, and cardiac glycosides, usually in toxic doses.

PHARMACOLOGY OF ANTIEMETIC DRUGS

The antiemetic drugs can be classified into three general groups: phenothiazines, antihistamines, and others.

Phenothiazines

In usual therapeutic doses, many of the phenothiazines exert a depressant effect on the CTZ and may also directly influence the vomiting center.[2] These agents act on both the central and autonomic nervous systems and do not produce significant cortical depression. They are widely distributed throughout the body, cross the placental barrier, and are 90% protein bound. Metabolism is primarily by the liver, with metabolic products being excreted in the urine, bile, and feces. The phenothiazines are usually non-addicting.

Specific adverse effects generally are associated with the chemical class of each phenothiazine. Those of the aliphatic type (eg, chlorpromazine [Thorazine]) are associated with a high incidence of orthostatic hypotension, sedation, prolongation of the sedative effects of narcotics and barbiturates, and blood dyscrasias. On the other hand, the piperazine type (eg, prochlorperazine [Compazine], perphenazine [Trilafon] and thiethylperazine [Torecan]) have an increased incidence of extrapyramidal reactions, whereas their sedative and hypotensive effects are less pronounced.

The phenothiazines, especially those of the piperazine class, are the antiemetics of choice as adjuncts to cancer chemotherapy, radiation therapy, and postoperative nausea and vomiting (Table 1). With the possible exceptions of promethazine (Phenergan) and thiethylperazine (Torecan),[3] they are ineffective in the prevention of motion sickness and the treatment of Menière's disease. The phenothiazines are best utilized in the control of nausea and vomiting of short duration, since with prolonged use the incidence of most of their adverse effects increases.

Haloperidol, a phenothiazine-like drug, may be one of the more effective antiemetics.[4,5] Its exact mechanism of antiemetic action is unknown, although it is thought to depress the CTZ. The antiemetic dose of haloperidol is low compared to its tranquilizing dose, thus alleviating many adverse effects.[6]

TABLE 1 Antiemetics of Choice

Cause of Vomiting	First Choice	Second Choice
Drug-Induced	Thiethylperazine[a] (Torecan)	Perphenazine[a] (Trilafon)
Radiation Sickness	Thiethylperazine	Perphenazine
Motion Sickness	TTS-Scopolamine	Dimenhydrinate (Dramamine)
Postoperative	Thiethylperazine	Haloperidol (Haldol)
Menière's Disease	Meclizine (Antivert, Bonine)	Dimenhydrinate
Pregnancy	—[b]	—[b]

[a]For patients allergic to phenothiazines, we suggest the use of haloperidol or delta-9-tetrahydrocannabinol.

[b]All antiemetics are contraindicated in pregnancy. If symptoms are severe, use Bendectin.

Antihistamines

Many antihistamines have antiemetic properties, but there is no correlation between antihistaminic potency of a drug and its ability to prevent motion sickness.[7] Both dimenhydrinate (Dramamine) and diphenhydramine (Benadryl) are effective antiemetics[8,9] that appear to act by blockade of labyrinthine impulses.[10] Neither antagonizes apomorphine-induced emesis.[11] Other antihistamines include meclizine (Antivert, Bonine), cyclizine (Marezine), and hydroxyzine (Atarax, Vistaril); there is no conclusive evidence regarding the effectiveness of hydroxyzine in comparison to the other two agents. Both meclizine and cyclizine are teratogenic in animals at high doses,[12] and hydroxyzine is structurally related to both of them. However, in a prospective study of 20,500 pregnancies, there was no indication that meclizine or cyclizine were associated with teratogenicity in humans.[13]

Trimethobenzamide (Tigan) is an ethanolamine antihistamine that acts primarily on the CTZ.[14] Reports of its effectiveness as an antiemetic are variable, ranging from very good[15] to no better than placebo.[16,17] Its efficacy appears to be inversely proportional to the intensity of the emetic stimulus.[18]

Other Drugs

Benzquinamide (Emete-Con), a benzquinolizine derivative structurally unrelated to the phenothiazines or antihistamines,[19] acts by depression of the CTZ.[20,21] In studies of postoperative patients, benzquinamide was as effective as prochlorperazine.[22] In other studies of general medical patients, benzquinamide has been shown to be superior to the phenothiazines in the control of nausea and vomiting.[21] The degree of somnolence associated with benzquinamide is equal to that of phenothiazines;[22] there have been no reported hypotension or extrapyramidal reactions. Therefore, benzquinamide appears to be an effective non-phenothiazine antiemetic.

The barbiturates pentobarbital (Nembutal) and secobarbital (Seconal) historically have been used as antiemetics. They are effective only in doses causing somnolence. The presumed mode of action is related to generalized central nervous system depression,[23] which may result in aspiration when used to control vomiting. They have no specific antiemetic effect.[24]

Scopolamine, an anticholinergic agent, acts primarily by reducing the excitability of the labyrinthine receptors and by depressing conduction in the vestibular cerebellar pathway. It is especially effective in the prevention of motion sickness,[25] but side effects (dry mouth, mydriasis and central nervous system confusion) limit its usefulness.[3] Sophisticated new delivery systems such as the Transdermal Therapeutic System-Scopolamine have permitted the safe delivery of markedly reduced, yet pharmacologically active, doses of scopolamine while obviating its adverse side effects.[26]

Bendectin, until 1976 a combination of three agents and now a combination of two (pyridoxine and doxylamine), is claimed to be more active than placebo in the control of vomiting. The mechanism of its antiemetic effect is unclear.

Delta-9-tetrahydrocannabinol is more effective than placebo in the control of nausea and vomiting associated with cancer chemotherapeutic agents,[27] but the pharmacology of this antiemetic effect is poorly understood. Delta-9-tetrahydrocannabinol may be a general central nervous system depressant, although many patients experience an antiemetic effect without associated somnolence.

CHOICE OF AN ANTIEMETIC

Since most nausea and vomiting are self-limited, the prescriber must first decide whether to use an antiemetic. Many factors influence such a decision; ultimately, the benefits must outweigh the hazards of treatment. The relative safety of most antiemetic agents and the distress of the symptoms are such that antiemetics are generally indicated. In some situations, such as pregnancy, where unnecessary drugs are contraindicated, a placebo might be considered. Since anxiety is common to all causes of vomiting, placebo effects frequently can be observed.[28,29] Because controlled studies indicating the efficacy of antiemetics in children are few in number, conservative measures such as sipping coke syrup and sucking ice may suffice.

Indications for prophylactic use of antiemetics include prevention of drug or radiation-induced vomiting, motion sickness, and vomiting associated with anesthesia when the patient is known to have such a history.[30]

Drug-Induced Vomiting

Most emetic drugs act by stimulation of the CTZ. Drug-induced nausea and vomiting is associated with individual drug toxicity and/or overdose. Drugs most commonly associated with vomiting include the opiates (eg, morphine, merperidine), cardiac glycosides (digitalis, especially at toxic doses), cancer chemotherapeutic agents (eg, cyclophosphamide, doxorubicin, nitrogen mustard), general anesthetics, as well as acute and post-alcoholic states. The antiemetics of choice in the treatment of these disorders are the phenothiazines and haloperidol. Whenever drug-induced vomiting can be anticipated, prophylaxis is more effective than subsequent control. Clinical studies suggest that vomiting associated with cancer chemotherapeutic agents can be prevented by the use of phenothiazines,[24,31] delta-9-tetrahydrocannabinol,[27] and TTS-Scopolamine.[32]

Radiation Sickness

Although the pathogenesis of nausea and vomiting associated with radiation therapy has not been definitively established, animal experiments demonstrate that ablation of the CTZ decreases vomiting in irradiated dogs.[33] The total dose of radiation, number of fractions, and portal of treatment all influence the extent of vomiting. Patients receiving upper abdominal radiation most commonly experience nausea and vomiting.[34] Control has been variable, depending in part on the severity of symptoms. The agents found to be most effective in controlling these symptoms are the phenothiazines, specifically thiethylperazine and perphenazine.

Motion Sickness

Motion sickness results from accelerated forces on the endolymph of the semi-circular canals in the inner ear giving rise to excitability impulses in the region of the vestibular apparatus.[10,35] The nausea and vomiting of motion sickness are more easily prevented than treated. Prior to the advent of transdermal systems, central nervous system side effects precluded general use of scopolamine; however, with the transdermal system, scopolamine (TTS-Scopolamine) is the drug of choice.[25] Antihistamines, including dimenhydrinate, diphenhydramine, meclizine, and cyclizine, are also effective in the prevention of motion sickness.[8,9,36] One study comparing antihistamines to a phenothiazine (thiethylperazine) found the latter to be superior.[35] Promethazine also has proven efficacy in prevention of motion sickness, but excessive sedation and postural hypotension diminish its usefulness.

Vomiting of Pregnancy

Vomiting associated with pregnancy is manifested in morning sickness, hyperemesis gravidarum, hydatidiform mole, twin pregnancy, hydramnios, preeclampsia, and onset of labor.[37] Morning sickness occurs in the majority of pregnancies, usually between the 6th and 14th week, and has been attributed to both psychological and endocrine changes, especially increases in progesterone. Other causes of vomiting, such as gastroenteritis, pyelonephritis, and uremia, must be considered in the differential diagnosis of vomiting during pregnancy.

Many drugs taken during the first three months of pregnancy are teratogenic and/or may cause fetal injury. Therefore, unless an antiemetic is absolutely required, it should not be used. Teratogenicity in animals may not be predictive of teratogenicity in man. Meclizine and cyclizine have teratogenic effects in animals when given in high doses.[10] However, a large prospective study of human pregnancies showed these same drugs were not associated with teratogenicity.[13] This study also demonstrated the absence of teratogenic effects in patients who had received phenothiazines, whereas trimethobenzamide (Tigan) suggested an excess of severe congenital anomalies.

The safest management of nausea in pregnancy is small, frequent feedings. Should this prove ineffective, antihistamines, Bendectin and phenothiazines (although they have not been approved for use in pregnancy) have been used. Phenothiazines used late in pregnancy may result in neonatal hyperbilirubinemia.

Postoperative Vomiting

Postoperative vomiting often results from anesthetic agents but may also be secondary to other factors, including distension or traction of a viscus, stimulation of the vagus nerve, hypoxia, sex, age, and psychological set. Thus, emetic stimuli may be transmitted either via the CTZ or directly to the vomiting center. Among the more successful antiemetic agents are thiethylperazine,[38] haloperidol,[4] and benzquinamide.[22] The routine use of preoperative analgesics, especially opiates, may result in increased excitability of the medullary threshold for vomiting. However, improved anesthetic agents and techniques have obviated the need for routine prophylactic preoperative antiemetics for most surgical procedures.

Other Causes of Vomiting

Other emetic stimuli must be considered when evaluating causes of vomiting. For example, vomiting caused by infections, toxins, and uremia is presumably blood-borne, CTZ-mediated, and optimally controlled by (1) treating the underlying disorder, and (2) using drugs affecting the CTZ. Thus, the phenothiazines are the antiemetics of choice in these disorders.

Menière's disease, a disorder of labyrinthine function, consists of recurrent aural vertigo accompanied by tinnitus and deafness. Bed rest is often sufficient treatment for mild attacks; however, when symptomatology is protracted, antihistamines have proven effective in reducing the severity and frequency of attacks.[39] Effective antihistamines include meclizine, dimenhydrinate and cyclizine.

DRUG MONOGRAPHS

CHLORPROMAZINE (Thorazine)
CHLORPROMAZINE HYDROCHLORIDE (Thorazine Hydrochloride)

PERPHENAZINE (Trilafon)
PROCHLORPERAZINE EDISYLATE (Compazine Edisylate)
PROCHLORPERAZINE MALEATE (Compazine Maleate)
THIETHYLPERAZINE MALATE (Torecan Malate)
THIETHYLPERAZINE MALEATE (Torecan Maleate)

The phenothiazines, by suppressing the CTZ, are the antiemetics of choice in many patients who are vomiting.[24] However, two less commonly known phenothiazines, perphenazine (Trilafon) and thiethylperazine (Torecan) have greater antiemetic activity than traditionally employed drugs such as prochlorperazine (Compazine) and chlorpromazine (Thorazine). Animal studies have shown perphenazine to be 24 times more active than chlorpromazine and 8 times more active than prochlorperazine in preventing apomorphine-induced emesis.[40] It has been suggested that the increased antiemetic activity of perphenazine may be due to its greater affinity to and its tighter binding with receptors in the CTZ.[41]

Thiethylperazine decreases the severity of symptoms as well as the incidence of nausea and vomiting;[38] it does not potentiate narcotics, prolong post-anesthetic sleep time, or produce the hypotension that is associated with many other phenothiazines.[38] Thiethylperazine may influence the vomiting center as well as the CTZ.[30]

These agents should be used cautiously in patients with severe liver disease and seizure disorders and in elderly patients.

Adverse Reactions—Extrapyramidal reactions (tremor, muscle rigidity, oculogyric crises) may occur with the effective antiemetic phenothiazines,[42] whereas sedation and orthostatic hypotension are relatively less common.[43] Skin reactions (urticaria, photosensitivity), jaundice, dry mouth, and rarely blood dyscrasias may also occur.

Drug Interactions—Among the many interactions are those with guanethidine (blockade of antihypertensive effect); morphine (potentiates sedation); meperidine (increases respiratory depression); barbiturates and other central nervous system depressants including alcohol (potentiation resulting in increased sedative effect or prolonged post-anesthetic sleep time); levodopa (decreases uptake and effectiveness); anticonvulsants (lowers seizure threshold); procarbazine (potentiation of behavioral abnormalities). See Chapter 35, Antipsychotic Agents, for a complete discussion of interactions.

Dosage—Adults, perphenazine, *intramuscular*, 5mg; *oral* 4 mg every 6 hours. Thiethylperazine, *intramuscular*, 10 mg; *oral*, 10 mg every 8 hours. Pediatric dosage has not been established.

TABLE 2 Preparations and Costs of Recommended Antiemetics

Generic Name	Trademark Name(s)	Preparations and 1978 Costs
Phenothiazines		
Perphenazine	Trilafon	Tablets 2 mg—$3.25/50; 4 mg—$4.46/50 Solution 16 mg/5 ml—$4.24/4 oz Injection (solution) 5 mg/ml—$0.60/1-ml ampul
Thiethylperazine Maleate	Torecan	Injection (solution) 5 mg/ml—$0.85/2-ml ampul
Thiethylperazine Maleate	Torecan Maleate	Tablets 10 mg—$8.27/100 Suppositories 10 mg—$3.99/12
Haloperidol	Haldol	Tablets 0.5 mg—$7.06/100; 1 mg—$10.10/100; 2 mg—$15.16/100 Solution 2 mg/ml—$4.14/15 ml, $17.44/120 ml Injection (solution) 5 mg/ml—$0.99/1-ml ampul
Antihistamines		
Dimenhydrinate	Dramamine	Tablets 50 mg—$6.32/100 Liquid 12.5 mg/4 ml—$5.44/pint Injection (solution) 50 mg/ml—$0.65/1-ml ampul, $1.94/5 ml Suppositories 100 mg—$2.96/12
Meclizine Hydrochloride	Antivert	Tablets 12.5 mg—$6.07/100; 25 mg—$10.24/100 Tablets (chewable) 25 mg—$10.23/100
	Bonine	Tablets (chewable) 25 mg—$10.24/100
Other		
Benzquinamide Hydrochloride	Emete-Con	Injection (powder) 50 mg—$1.74/vial

DIMENHYDRINATE (Dramamine)

Dimenhydrinate is a nonphenothiazine antihistamine which works on the peripheral vestibular structure.[7] It is an effective agent in both motion sickness and Menière's disease[7] and is ineffective in post-operative nausea and vomiting.[23] It has been shown to be more effective than diphenhydramine (Benadryl),[3] which suggests that antiemetic efficacy is not related to antihistaminic potency.[7]

Adverse Reactions—Sedation, mild anticholinergic effects, and rarely, blood dyscrasias may occur.

Drug Interactions—Antihistamines may be additive with barbiturates and other central nervous system depressants. Antihistamines are known to induce hepatic microsomal enzymes, and concurrent use with anticoagulants may be questioned; however, no adverse effects have been reported.

Dosage—Oral: Adults, 50 to 100 mg thirty minutes prior to departure. Repeat before meals. If given intravenously, solution should be diluted with saline.

HALOPERIDOL (Haldol)

Haloperidol is an effective antiemetic in the treatment of postoperative nausea and vomiting[4] and may be useful in patients receiving radiation therapy and cancer chemotherapy.[6] A butyrophenone derivative pharmacologically related to the piperazine class of phenothiazines, haloperidol is an effective antiemetic at relatively low doses, thus causing fewer side effects than phenothiazines.[4,6] The absence of hypotension and other side effects make it a drug of choice for elderly or debilitated patients.[44] Animal studies have shown haloperidol to be 40 times more potent as an antiemetic and its duration of action four times longer than chlorpromazine.[45] In a study of 62 postoperative patients receiving haloperidol 1 mg, the incidence of vomiting was relieved in 83% versus 29% in the placebo patients.[4] The Federal Drug Administration has not approved the use of haloperidol as an antiemetic.

Adverse Reactions—Most adverse reactions occur when haloperidol is used at higher, tranquilizing doses, rather than the relatively low antiemetic doses. Bradycardia has been reported at doses of 2 to 4 mg,[45] and extrapyramidal reactions, sedation, hypotension and anticholinergic effects may occur. Usage in children and in pregnancy has not been established.

Drug Interactions—Haloperidol is additive with or may potentiate other central nervous system depressants, enhances analgesics, potentiates the sedative effect of alcohol, and may decrease convulsive thresholds of anticonvulsant drugs.

Dosage—Oral: Adults, 0.5 to 1.0 mg every eight hours. *Intramuscular: Adults,* 1 mg. Pediatric dosage has not been established.

TRANSDERMAL THERAPEUTIC SYSTEM-SCOPOLAMINE

Scopolamine is one of the most effective drugs currently available for both prevention and treatment of nausea and vomiting.[46] Use of the traditional dosage forms of scopolamine, however, is accompanied by unwanted pharmacological effects. Thus, the drug has not been extensively used, although it has been available since 1885. The Transdermal Therapeutic System-Scopolamine (TTS-Scopolamine) provides a novel method for the systemic administration of scopolamine that minimizes unwanted pharmacological effects. The system comprises small flexible membranes that adhere comfortably to the skin. Following placement behind the ear, the drug is absorbed through the skin into the bloodstream and is distributed throughout the body. The system provides controlled administration of drug at a predetermined rate for up to three days.[47]

TTS-Scopolamine has been shown an effective agent in prevention of motion sickness.[48,49] and preliminary evidence suggests a use in controlling the nausea and vomiting associated with administration of cancer chemotherapeutic agents and surgery.

Adverse Reactions—Dry mouth and drowsiness may occur. Considerably larger doses of drug than those delivered from the TTS-Scopolamine have been reported to cause restlessness, giddiness, or confusion; no such adverse reactions have been reported during development and clinical testing of TTS-Scopolamine.

Drug Interactions—Scopolamine may interact with other centrally active agents. Individuals should be advised against excessive drinking of alcoholic beverages while wearing the TTS-Scopolamine.

Dosage—Adults: apply 1 or 2 2.5 cm^2 Transiderm System(s) to clean, dry skin in the post-auricular area several hours before antiemetic protection is required. *Children:* if less than 100 pounds body weight, apply a 1.6 cm^2 Transiderm System; if greater than 100 pounds apply a 2.5 cm^2 Transiderm System.

REFERENCES

1. Wang SC, Borison HL: A new concept of organization of the central emetic mechanism: recent studies on the sites of action of apomorphine, copper sulfate and cardiac glycosides. Gastroenterology 22:1–12, 1952.
2. Wang SC, Amals W, Merritt H: Neural mechanism of emesis and antiemesis. Scientific Exhibit, World Congress of Gastroenterology, Washington, D.C., May, 1958.
3. Wood CD, Kennedy RS, Graybiel A: Review of antimotion sickness drugs from 1954–1964. Aerosp Med 36:1–4, 1965.
4. Barton M, Libonanti M, Cohen P: The use of haloperidol for treatment of postoperative nausea and vomiting—a double-blind placebo-controlled trial. Anesthesiology 42:508–512, 1975.

5. Sheilds K, Ballinger C, Hathaway B: Antiemetic effectiveness of haloperidol in human volunteers challenged with apomorphine. Anesth Analg 50:1017–1027, 1971.
6. Christman R, Weinstein R, Larose J: Low-dose haloperidol as antiemetic treatment in gastrointestinal disorders: a double-blind study. Curr Ther Res 16:1171-1176, 1974.
7. Chinn HI, Smith PK: Motion sickness. Pharmacol Rev 7:33–82, 1955.
8. Gay LN, Carliner PE: The prevention and treatment of motion sickness. Bull Johns Hopkins Hosp 84:470–487, 1949.
9. Nickerson M: Dramamine. Science 111:312–313, 1950.
10. Jaju BP, Wang SC: Effects of diphenhydramine and dimenhydrinate on vestibular neuronal activity of cat: a search for the locus of their antimotion sickness action. J Pharmacol Exp Ther 176:718–723, 1971.
11. Wyant GM: A comparative study of eleven antiemetic drugs in dogs. Can Anesth Soc J 9:399–407, 1962.
12. Sadusk JF, Palmisano PA: Teratogenic effect of meclizine, cyclizine and chlorcyclizine. JAMA 194:987–989, 1965.
13. Milkovich L, VandenBerg B: An evaluation of the teratogenicity of certain antinauseant drugs. Am J Obstet Gynecol 125:244–248, 1976.
14. Schallek W, Heise GA, Keith EC, et al: Antiemetic activity of 4-(2-dimethylaminoethoxy)-N-(3,4,5-trimetho xybenzoyl) benzylamine hydrochloride. J Pharmacol Exp Ther 126:270–277, 1959.
15. Kolodny L: A controlled study of trimethobenzamide, a specific antiemetic. Am J Med Sci 239:682–688, 1960.
16. Bardfield P: A controlled double-blind study of trimethobenzamide, prochlorperazine and placebo. JAMA 196:796–798, 1966.
17. Dobkin A, Evers W, Israel J: Double-blind evaluation of metoclopramide, trimethobenzamide and a placebo as postanesthetic antiemetics following methoxyflurane anaesthesia. Can Anaesth Soc J 15:80–91, 1968.
18. Wolfson B, Torres-Kay M, Foldes F: Investigation of the usefulness of trimethobenzamide for the prevention of postoperative nausea and vomiting. Anesth Analg 41:172–177, 1962.
19. Pitts N: A clinical pharmacological evaluation of benzquinamide, a new antiemetic agent. Curr Ther Res 11:325–337, 1969.
20. Klien R, Graves C, Kim Y, et al: Inhibition of apomorphine-induced vomiting by benzquinamide. Clin Pharmacol Ther 11:530–537, 1970.
21. Medoff J: A double-blind evaluation of the antiemetic efficacy of benzquinamide. Curr Ther Res 12:706–710, 1970.
22. Finn H, Urban B, Thomas J, et al: Antiemetic efficacy of benzquinamide. NY State J Med 71:651–653, 1971.
23. Knapp MM, Beecher HK: Postanesthetic nausea, vomiting and retching. JAMA 160:376–385, 1956.
24. Moertel C, Reitmeier R: Controlled clinical studies of orally administered antiemetic drugs. Gastroenterology 57:262–268, 1969.
25. Brand JJ, Calfuhorn WP, Gould AH, et al: Hyoscine and cyclizine as motion sickness remedies. Br J Pharmacol Chemother 30:463–469, 1967.
26. Shaw JE, Schmitt LG, McCauley ME, et al: Transdermally administered scopolamine for prevention of motion sickness in a vertical oscillator. Clin Pharmacol Ther 21:117, 1977.
27. Sallan S, Zinberg N, Frei E III: Antiemetic effects of delta-9-tetrahydorcannabinol in patients receiving cancer chemotherapy. N Engl J Med 293:795–797, 1975.
28. Burwell JA, Wolfson B, Perryman CR, et al: The use of trimethobenzamide (Tigan) for the treatment of radiation-induced nausea and emesis. Am J Roentgenol Radium Ther Nucl Med 86:752–756, 1961.
29. Parsons J, Webster J, Dowd J: Evaluation of placebo effect in the treatment of radiation sickness. Acta Radiol 56:129–140, 1961.
30. Codiga V: A new antiemetic for the treatment of nausea and vomiting associated with roentgen therapy. Int Rec Med 174:375–379, 1961.
31. Moertel C, Reitermeier R, Gage R: A controlled clinical evaluation of antiemetic drugs. JAMA 186:116–118, 1963.
32. Sawicka J, Sallan S: Transdermal therapeutic system-scopolamine (TS): Prevention of vomiting associated with cancer chemotherapy. Presented at American Society of Clinical Oncology Meeting, Denver, Colorado, May 17, 1977.

33. Chinn HI, Wang SC: Locus of antiemetic action following irradiation. Proc Soc Exp Biol Med 85:472–474, 1954.
34. Kurohara S, Goerge F, Levitt S, et al: Factors concerned with 'Clinical Radiation Nausea.' Radiology 86:262–265, 1966.
35. Bradford W: Preliminary report of trials of antimotion sickness drugs. Med Serv J Can 21:310–315, 1965.
36. Trumbull R, Chinn R, Maag C, et al: Effect of certain drugs on the incidence of seasickness. Clin Pharmacol Ther 1:280–283, 1960.
37. Midwinter A: Vomiting in pregnancy. J Obstet Gynecol Br Commonw 206:743–750, 1971.
38. Purkis I: The action of thiethylperazine, a new antiemetic, compared with perphenazine, trimethobenzamide and a placebo in the suppression of post anaesthetic nausea and vomiting. Can Anesth Soc J 12:595–607, 1965.
39. Cohen B, DeJong JMB: Meclizine and placebo in treating vertigo of vestibular origin. Arch Neurol 27:129–135, 1972.
40. Rosenkilde H, Govier WM: A comparison of some phenothiazine derivatives in inhibiting apomorphine induced emesis. J Pharmacol Exp Ther 120:375–378, 1957.
41. Wang SC: Perphenazine, a potent and effective antiemetic. J Pharmacol Exp Ther 123:306–310, 1958.
42. Braly B, Moore D: The use of intramuscular perphenazine to control postoperative vomiting. Am J Surg 102:120–123, 1961.
43. Ernst E, Snyder A: Perphenazine in nausea and vomiting, and anxiety states. Pa Med J 61:355–359, 1958.
44. Robbins E, Nagel J: Haloperidol parenterally for the treatment of vomiting and nausea from gastrointestinal disorders in a group of geriatric patients: double-blind, placebo-controlled study. J Am Geriatr Soc 23:38–41, 1975.
45. Tornetta F: Double-blind evaluation of haloperidol for antiemetic activity. Anesth Analg 51:964–967, 1972.
46. Shaw JE, Bayne W, Schmitt LG: Clinical pharmacology of scopolamine. Clin Pharmacol Ther 19:115, 1976.
47. Shaw JE, Chandrasekaran SK, Campbell PS, et al: New procedures for evaluating cutaneous administration. In *Cutaneous Toxicity*. Edited by VA Drill, P Lazar. New York, Academic Press, 1977, pp 83–95.
48. Graybiel A, Knepton J, Shaw HE: Prevention of experimental motion sickness by scopolamine absorbed through the skin. Aviat Space Environ Med 47:1096–1100, 1976.
49. Shaw JE, Schmitt LG, McCauley ME, et al: Transdermally administered scopolamine for prevention of motion sickness in a vertical oscillator. Clin Pharmacol Ther 21:117, 1977.

67. MISCELLANEOUS DRUGS USED IN GASTROINTESTINAL DISORDERS

George L. Arnold, Karim A Fawaz, Marshall M. Kaplan, Martin G. Kistin, Daniel S. Matloff, Leo A. Millette, Richard A. Norton, Edward S. Orris, James F. Patterson, Andrew G. Plaut, and James S. Singer

AZATHIOPRINE (Imuran)
AZATHIOPRINE SODIUM (Imuran Sodium)

Azathioprine, an imidazole derivative of 6-mercaptopurine (6-MP), is absorbed by the small intestine and then metabolized to 6-MP. It is a purine analog and interferes with the synthesis of nucleic acids and the formation of essential sulfhydryl groups. Azathioprine is primarily used in relatively high doses as an immunosuppressive agent after renal transplantation, as well as in lower doses for Crohn's disease, ulcerative colitis, chronic active hepatitis, primary biliary cirrhosis and systemic lupus erythematosus.[1] The clinical effect of these doses may be due to antiinflammatory rather than immunosuppressive effects.

Early studies in Crohn's disease of the large and small bowel suggested that azathioprine was effective in patients with active disease and enterocutaneous fistulae.[2–4] In two controlled trials, however, azathioprine was not effective in the treatment of active Crohn's disease,[5,6] although there was a subset of patients who seemed to respond dramatically to the drug. Therapeutic effects required at least two weeks of administration. In two additional controlled studies on patients with stable disease, azathioprine had a steroid-sparing effect and was useful in maintaining remissions after reduction of total prednisone dose.[7,8]

Controlled studies demonstrate no beneficial effect of azathioprine in active ulcerative colitis.[7,8] It does not maintain remission after prednisone withdrawal,[9] but may allow a reduction in prednisone dose without increasing the relapse rate.[10] In chronic active hepatitis the addition of 50 mg of azathioprine to 10 mg of prednisone is as effective as higher doses of prednisone in maintaining remission.[11] Azathioprine has no effect on outcome in primary biliary cirrhosis.[12]

Adverse Reactions—Severe and irreversible bone marrow depression is the most serious complication. This usually occurs with doses greater than 3 to 5 mg/kg/day, and has not been reported with doses less than 2 mg/kg/day.[2,10]

An allergic response to azathioprine (chills, fever and arthralgias) sometimes occur after 5 to 21 days of therapy.[4,6] Symptoms subside with discontinuation of the drug. Chromosomal abnormalities and azospermia have been reported, but there is no evidence of congenital malformation occurring in the offspring of treated parents.[7,13]

Azathioprine increases the incidence of neoplasms in renal transplant patients.[13]

Other reactions include rash, drug fever, alopecia, pancreatitis, arthralgias, steatorrhea, hepatotoxicity, and an increased risk of infections.

Dosage—Oral or Intravenous: 1.5 mg/kg/day in one dose.

Edward S. Orris and James F. Patterson

CHENODEOXYCHOLIC ACID

Chenodeoxycholic acid, a normal constituent of human bile, causes slow dissolution of radioluscent (cholesterol) gallstones when taken orally.[14–18] The drug decreases hepatic cholesterol output, and increases both the size of the bile salt pool and the extent of cholesterol solubility.[19] However, gallstones are likely to form again or increase in size once chenodeoxycholic acid therapy is stopped, and, therefore, life-long therapy may be necessary.[17] Adverse reactions consist mainly of diarrhea and abdominal cramping; both are relieved by dosage reduction.[20] One metabolite, lithocholic acid, is hepatotoxic in animals, but in man it is detoxified biochemically, and only transient elevation of serum transaminases and nonspecific liver biopsy abnormalities have been noted. The potential exists for passage of partially dissolved calculi into the bile ducts. Obstructive jaundice, acute cholecystitis and biliary colic can occur but are infrequent.[14,15] No other serious adverse effects have been observed in patients treated for up to 4 years. Chenodeoxycholic acid is presently available only for investigational use.

George L. Arnold and Andrew G. Plaut

TABLE 1 Preparations and Costs of Miscellaneous Gastrointestinal Drugs[a]

GENERIC NAME	TRADEMARK NAME(S)	PREPARATIONS AND 1978 COSTS
Azathioprine	Imuran	Tablets 50 mg—$15.10/100
Azathioprine Sodium	Imuran	Injection (lyophilized powder) 100 mg—$6.00/vial
Cholestyramine Resin	Questran	Powder—$12.80/378-g can, $16.87/50 4-g packets
Cimetidine	Tagamet	Tablets 300 mg—$23.50/100 Injection 150 mg/ml—$1.76/ 2-ml vial
Corticotropin (ACTH)	Acthar (Cortrophin Gel)	Injection (lyophilized powder) 25 USP units—$2.65/vial 40 USP units—$4.08/vial Injection (repository gel) 40 USP units/ml—$2.59/ 5-ml vial 80 USP units/ml—$5.17/ 5-ml vial
Hydrocortisone	Cortenema	Retention enema 100 mg/60 ml—$1.65/unit
Methylprednisolone Acetate	Medrol Enpak	Retention enema 40 mg/unit—$16.18/unit
Pancreatin	Panteric (Viokase)	Capsules 325 mg—$6.18/100 Tablets (enteric-coated) 325 mg—$4.69/100 Granules—$11.23/4 oz
Pancrelipase	Cotazym	Capsules—$6.00/100 Powder (regular)—$27.50/250 packets Powder (flavored)—$26.95/100 packets
D-penicillamine	Cuprimine	Capsules 250 mg—$22.88/100
Simethicone	Mylicon (Silain)	Oral Drops 40 mg/0.6 ml—$3.55/30 ml Tablets 40 mg—$3.73/100; 80 mg—$4.96/100
Sulfasalazine (salicylazosulfapyridine)	Azulfidine	Tablets 500 mg—$5.82/100
Neomycin Sulfate	generic	Tablets 500 mg—$7.95–$30.72/100

TABLE 1 *(continued)*

GENERIC NAME	TRADEMARK NAME(S)	PREPARATIONS AND 1978 COSTS
Paromomycin Sulfate	Humatin	Capsules 250 mg—$10.45/16 Syrup 125 mg/5 ml—$3.92/60 ml
Lactulose	Cephulac	Syrup—$7.85/500 ml
Levodopa	Dopar (Larodopa)	Capsules 100 mg—$2.82/100; 250 mg—$4.50/100; 500 mg—$7.80/100
Betazole Hydrochloride	Histalog	Injection (solution) 50 mg/ml—$0.86/1-ml ampul
Glucagon	generic	Injection (powder) 1 mg—$7.18/vial
Pentagastrin	Peptavlon	Injection (solution) 0.25 mg/ml—$2.28/2-ml ampul
D-xylose	generic	Powder—$5.90/25 g

[a]Oral and parenteral dosage forms of adrenal corticosteroids are not listed in this table but may be found in Table 6 of Chapter 49, Adrenal Corticosteroids.

CHOLESTYRAMINE RESIN (Cuemid, Questran)

Cholestyramine resin is a chloride salt of a basic anion exchange resin that has a strong affinity for bile salts in the intestine. It exchanges a chloride ion for an ionized bile salt molecule which is then excreted in the feces. Cholestyramine in effect produces a 'medical bile fistula.'

A major indication for cholestyramine is in relieving pruritus due to cholestatic jaundice, provided there is not complete bile duct obstruction. By removing bile salts from the enterohepatic circulation, cholestyramine eventually decreases the bile salt concentration in the skin which, when excessive, probably causes the pruritus of obstructive jaundice.

Cholestyramine is also useful in the treatment of diarrhea due to increased concentration of bile salts in the colon; patients with ileectomy or regional enteritis are often candidates for such therapy.[21,22] It may also be useful in postgastrectomy patients with diarrhea where no other treatable cause is determined.[23] Cholestyramine has been used to treat clindamycin-induced pseudomembranous colitis.[24] Its effectiveness in this disorder, as well as in postoperative alkaline reflux gastritis requires further study.[25,26]

Adverse Reactions—The main untoward effects include nausea and constipation.

Interactions—Long-term administration can result in a deficiency of folic acid[27] and of the fat soluble vitamins A, D, E, and K. These should be added to the diet and given at night so they are not bound by the cholestyramine. In addition, since cholestyramine can bind a number of other drugs such as chlorothiazide, phenylbutazone, phenobarbital, anticoagulants, thyroxin, and digitalis preparations, it is best to keep the interval as long as possible between the administration of cholestyramine and any other medication.

Dosage—The starting dose is 12 g per day (4 g, 3 times daily with meals). Dosage ranges from 12 to 32 g. In pruritus of cholestatic jaundice, it usually takes 2 to 4 days after starting cholestyramine before the itching is relieved, but as long as 5 to 10 days may be required. Since the resin acts by mixing with the bile, it has to be taken with meals. Because bile salts accumulate in the gallbladder overnight and empty during the morning meal, the breakfast dose may be the most effective; thus, higher doses at breakfast may enhance efficacy.

James S. Singer and Marshall M. Kaplan

CIMETIDINE (Tagamet)

Cimetidine is one of a new class of drugs, the H_2 antihistamines, that are useful agents for the treatment of some acid-peptic disorders. Cimetidine is as effective, if not more effective, than intensive antacids in duodenal ulcer and is superior in Zollinger-Ellison syndrome. It also appears to be superior to antacids in gastric ulcer, esophageal reflux, and upper gastrointestinal bleeding due to acid-peptic disease; in addition it is more convenient to use which may improve patient compliance.

The H_2 antihistamines should not be confused with older antihistamines (eg, diphenhydramine, chlorpheniramine) that are used to treat allergies and cold symptoms; these agents are now referred to as 'H_1 antihistamines.' The effects of the H_2 antihistamines are largely, though not entirely, limited to the gastrointestinal tract. They inhibit gastric acid secretion stimulated not only by histamine, but also by insulin, pentagastrin, food, caffeine, and the physiological vagal reflex.[28] The H_1 antihistamines, by contrast, have more systemic effects and few actions on the gastrointestinal tract.

Cimetidine is primarily absorbed from the upper part of the small intestine, with peak blood levels occurring in 30 to 90 minutes. Onset of action occurs within the first 30 minutes and maximal inhibition of gastric acid secretion occurs at two hours. The duration of action is 7 to 8 hours.[29] Given before meals, cimetidine produces earlier and higher blood levels, but when it is taken after food, blood levels are highest at the time when the buffer capacity of the food is waning.[30] Cimetidine is rapidly excreted from the body, primarily in the urine.

Duodenal Ulcer. Results from many studies show that healing rates with cimetidine are usually between 60 to 80% after 4 to 6 weeks of therapy. The healing rates in the control (placebo, as needed antacids, or intensive antacids) vary but are consistently lower than the healing rates with cimetidine; the differences are frequently statistically significant. Pain and antacid requirements were also substantially reduced.[31,32]

Gastric Ulcer. Cimetidine alone appears to be as effective as intensive antacids, while the combination of cimetidine and antacids gives a slightly better response.[33]

Zollinger-Ellison (ZE) Syndrome. Chronic therapy for six months or longer gives excellent control of symptoms and resolution of upper gastrointestinal lesions. Patients with ZE syndrome can be managed medically and gain little from the added risk of gastrectomy. Cimetidine is particularly useful for elderly patients and those who have undergone previous gastric surgery in whom operative mortality is high.[34]

Other Conditions. The administration of cimetidine provides rapid symptomatic relief of esophagitis, with improvement or complete healing of lesions in most patients.[35] Cimetidine is as effective in controlling bleeding from hemorrhagic gastritis as other medical measures and is more convenient to use than the large volumes of antacids currently recommended. Cimetidine also is useful in the prophylaxis and treatment of bleeding in patients with severe liver damage.[36,37]

Adverse Reactions—In short- and long-term animal studies, cimetidine has not produced any serious adverse effects.[38] In short-term human studies, only minor adverse effects (rash, diarrhea, muscle pain) have been reported. The serum creatinine concentration has risen in some patients, but the rise was not progressive and occurred without evidence of renal deterioration.[39] No hematological abnormalities have been seen. Rises in transaminase concentrations have been as common in controls as in patients taking cimetidine.[40] A few men (mostly on high-dose regimens) have developed tender gynecomastia after several months therapy, but with no other hormonal or sexual dysfunction.[41] The long-term human toxicity of cimetidine is unknown.

Dosage—Oral: Adults, 200 to 300 mg orally four times daily with or immediately after meals and at bedtime for three to six weeks. Initially, the patient may want to take antacids to control pain. Discontinuation of treatment or use of only a bedtime dose to control nocturnal hypersecretion should be tried when healing has been demonstrated by endoscopy or x-rays.

Intravenous: Adults, for a bolus injection, 300 mg is diluted to 20 ml in normal saline or dextrose 5% solution and injected over a two-minute period four times a day. For an intermittent intravenous injection, 300 mg is diluted in 100 ml of an intravenous solution and infused over 15 minutes four times a day. The dosage should be adjusted to maintain an intragastric pH greater than 5 when this is possible. When signs of bleeding have been absent for 48 hours, oral administration should be substituted.

Children, 20 to 40 mg/kg in divided doses has been given orally or intravenously. Clinical experience in children is limited.

Leo A. Millette

CORTICOSTEROIDS

Adrenal corticosteroids are useful in the treatment of certain gastrointestinal disorders because of their antiinflammatory effect. The naturally occurring hormone (hydrocortisone) and the synthetic analogues (prednisone, methylprednisolone, dexamethasone) all have equal antiinflammatory action when given in equivalent doses. Corticotropin (ACTH) is also utilized in the treatment of inflammatory bowel disease.

Oral Administration of Corticosteroids. Oral corticosteroids are indicated in the treatment of patients with mild to moderate inflammatory bowel disease (ulcerative colitis and Crohn's disease) who have not responded to, or are unable to tolerate, sulfasalazine. Oral corticosteroids are also used in severely ill patients after they have responded to parenteral corticosteroids.

Corticosteroids given orally or intravenously alone, or in combination with steroid enemas, are more effective in the treatment of acute attacks of ulcerative colitis than sulfasalazine.[42,43] In additional well-controlled studies, however, oral corticosteroids in small doses (15 mg of prednisone per day) are ineffective in maintaining remissions and preventing relapses.[44,45] When oral corticosteroids are ineffective or the patient has severe disease including toxic megacolon, corticosteroids should be given intravenously.[46,47]

In Crohn's disease of the large and small bowel there are no controlled studies utilizing corticosteroids but two articles suggest that they are of benefit.[48,49] The general feeling is that patients with Crohn's disease should be treated in the same manner as patients with ulcerative colitis.

Corticosteroids do not appear to be beneficial in alcoholic hepatitis,[50] and are not routinely utilized in this disorder. In acute severe viral hepatitis, prednisone was found to be detrimental and associated with a higher mortality rate than placebo.[51]

Prednisone alone, or in combination with azathioprine, is the mainstay of treatment in chronic active hepatitis. It improves survival and promotes clinical, biochemical, and histologic remissions.[11]

Rectal Administration of Corticosteroids. Corticosteroid retention enemas and rectally-instilled foam preparations are used to provide a local mucosal antiinflammatory action in patients with acute ulcerative colitis. The effect is not entirely a local one, since as much as 50% of the steroid dose may be absorbed.[52] Corticosteroid enemas are used in mild to moderate ulcerative colitis, particularly colitis of the left side of the colon. They may be utilized alone or with sulfasalazine to avoid the need for oral steroids. Corticosteroid enemas alone are effective in acute ulcerative proctitis,[53,54] as well as in selected cases of diffuse ulcerative colitis.[55] With more extensive disease, however, the chance of a beneficial response is decreased. Truelove[47] has recommended that corticosteroid enemas be added to the treatment regimen of patients with severe ulcerative colitis.[47]

There are no data concerning use of corticosteroid enemas in Crohn's disease of the colon, but they may be useful when the disease is limited to the distal colon.

Corticotropin. Corticotropin (ACTH) stimulates the synthesis and release of naturally-occurring adrenal cortical hormones, including aldosterone and a number of weak androgenic substances. Initial studies of ACTH versus cortisone in acute ulcerative colitis suggested that ACTH might be effective in inducing remission, especially in those with a relapse.[43,44] However, in these studies ACTH was given parenterally (40 units/day) while cortisone was given by mouth and at lower equivalent doses. ACTH was associated with more frequent side effects. In a recent study of equivalent parenteral doses of ACTH and hydrocortisone, the two were equally beneficial in acute ulcerative and Crohn's disease of the colon, although prior corticosteroid therapy might have decreased the response to ACTH.[56] Since some patients do in fact respond to one mode of therapy and not the other, ACTH can be tried in patients refractory to parenteral corticosteroids.

Adverse Reactions—The side effects of corticosteroids include: menstrual irregularities, acne, Cushingnoid changes, electrolyte disturbances, metabolic alkalosis, hypokalemia, hyperglycemia, glucosuria, posterior subcapsular cataracts, glaucoma, behavioral changes and psychosis, osteoporosis, myopathy, edema, activation of tuberculosis, and pancreatitis. Corticosteroid therapy is thought to increase the risk of peptic ulcers, although a recent review suggests that this may not be true.[57]

Withdrawal of corticosteroids is associated with adrenal insufficiency, pseudotumor cerebri, and the corticosteroid withdrawal syndrome, which is characterized by fever, malaise, myalgia, and arthralgias.

Corticotropin preparations have occasionally caused hypersensitivity reactions ranging from fever to anaphylaxis and death. The major toxicity of ACTH is attributable to the release of adrenocortical hormones; there is a greater incidence of acne, sodium retention, and hypokalemic metabolic alkalosis.

There is no evidence that prior treatment with corticosteroids adversely influences the outcome of surgical treatment for ulcerative colitis.[58]

Dosage—Prednisone (or an equivalent corticosteroid), 40 to 60 mg per day in 3 divided doses, is recommended for patients with mild to moderate disease refractory to other forms of therapy. Once the bowel symptoms have improved, the dose may be initially decreased in 5 to 10 mg decrements every 1 to 3 weeks. Sulfasalazine should be added to the regimen to allow more rapid withdrawal of prednisone while preventing relapses. Below 30 mg a day, the corticosteroid dose should be reduced in 5 and then 2.5 mg decrements. Many physicians administer antacids during corticosteroid therapy with the hope of preventing peptic ulcer disease. Alternate day therapy (a single dose every 48 hours) has been used to avoid adrenal suppression and to reduce side effects, but is not uniformly effective in controlling these diseases.

When corticosteroids are used in chronic active hepatitis, a similar program is used. Liver function tests and symptoms are monitored as steroids are withdrawn. Azathioprine is often used in conjunction with corticosteroids to allow reduced steroid dosage.

Hydrocortisone sodium succinate, 100 mg intravenously every 6 to 8 hours, is used for patients with severe disease or toxic megacolon, and in those unable to take oral medications or who fail to respond to alternative therapy. When a response has been obtained, the dose may be reduced and treatment continued with oral corticosteroids.

Methylprednisolone sodium succinate, 20 to 25 mg every 6 to 8 hours intravenously, can substitute for hydrocortisone sodium succinate.

The enemas should be tapered gradually to an every-other-day maintenance regimen as symptoms are brought under control. At this point the enemas may be withdrawn and the patient continued on a maintenance dose of sulfasalazine.

The recommended dose of ACTH for severe or refractory inflammatory bowel disease is 40 units intravenously over 8 to 12 hours twice a day. When the patient has responded to therapy, corticosteroids are given orally in place of ACTH.

Edward S. Orris and James F. Patterson

PANCREATIN (Panteric, Viokase)
PANCRELIPASE (Cotazym)

Porcine pancreatic extracts are useful for decreasing malabsorption in patients with pancreatic exocrine insufficiency and steatorrhea due to various pancreatic disorders. In many patients with pancreatic insufficiency and coexisting diabetes, the absorption of food can be stabilized using these drugs, thereby avoiding wide fluctuations in insulin requirements.[59] Pancreatin and pancrelipase are porcine pancreatic extracts standardized for amylase, trypsin, and lipase activity. Recent *in vitro* and *in vivo* studies in humans have demonstrated a wide range of enzyme activity among the available preparations.[60] Panteric, Viokase, Ilozyme, and Cotazym were among the most active products. It has also been shown that most of the pancreatic enzyme activity is destroyed by gastric acid. In some cases coadministration of bicarbonate or antacids to raise intraduodenal pH makes these agents more effective.[61] Recent data show that cimetidine administered with meals is the most potent currently available means of enhancing the activity of pancreatic extracts. Pancreatic extracts are probably most effective when given with meals but dosing should be individualized.[62]

Adverse Reactions—Allergic reactions occur rarely. Precipitation of gouty attacks, due to the high purine content of these agents, has been described.[63]

Dosage—Oral: Adults, pancreatin preparations: 6 to 18 tablets daily in divided doses hourly or with meals. Pancrelipase: 6 to 18 tablets daily in divided doses.

George L. Arnold and Andrew G. Plaut

D-PENICILLAMINE (Cuprimine)

D-penicillamine is an amino acid degradation product of penicillin, possessing no antibacterial activity. Rather, it is useful as a chelating agent of heavy metals including copper, iron, mercury, and lead. D-penicillamine is the drug of choice for hepatolenticular degeneration (Wilson's disease).[64]

Wilson's disease is an inherited (autosomal recessive) defect in the transport and storage of copper that leads to copper deposition in body tissues, particularly liver, brain and kidneys. D-penicillamine is an effective and relatively safe and convenient drug for arresting and reversing the disease. Since Wilson's disease can progress rapidly, treatment should be instituted as soon as possible after baseline serum copper, ceruloplasmin, urinary copper excretion, complete blood count, platelet count, and renal and liver function tests are obtained.

D-penicillamine is effective in the treatment of cystinuria. It also may be useful for rheumatoid arthritis[65] and heavy metal poisoning, although not FDA-approved for these indications. Other proposed uses include scleroderma,[66] chronic active hepatitis, and primary biliary cirrhosis, but evidence of efficacy in these diseases is not established.

Adverse Reactions—The most common adverse reactions involve the skin, bone marrow, and kidney. Urticaria, erythematous and maculopapular rashes, leukopenia, and thrombocytopenia have been reported. These reactions usually occur early in the course of therapy, and can be managed by halving the dosage and instituting an antihistamine. If this is unsuccessful, the D-penicillamine may be discontinued for 2 weeks and then restarted at one half the dose, along with 20 mg of prednisone.

More severe complications generally occur later in the course of treatment, and include granulocytosis, nephrotic syndrome,[67] Goodpasture's syndrome,[68] and a lupus-like syndrome.[69] If such reactions occur, D-penicillamine should be discontinued until the patient recovers. Treatment may then be reinstituted with specially-prepared 25 mg tablets (D-penicillamine usually comes in 250 mg tablets). Beginning with 25 mg, the dosage can be doubled weekly. Prednisone may accompany this treatment program.

Excess intake of D-penicillamine can cause gastritis with abdominal pain, nausea, and vomiting. These symtoms are dose-related and will remit with dosage reduction.

D-penicillamine also is a pyridoxine antimetabolite but is much less so than L-penicillamine. Pyridoxine (50 mg weekly) can be given to avoid the possibility of pyridoxine deficiency.

Dosage—An average starting dose is 0.02 g/kg orally in 4 divided doses (30 min before meals and at bedtime). For most individuals, the dose ranges from 750 to 1500 mg daily. Dosage should be based on urinary copper excretion, aiming for a cupriuresis of 2000 μg daily. Dosage may be slowly increased to a maximum of 2.5 g if necessary to achieve adequate copper excretion. As body stores of copper are depleted the urinary copper excretion will also decrease. Therefore, reduction in copper excretion alone does not necessarily indicate a requirement for increased dosage.

Once clinical remission is achieved, and the serum transaminases, copper, and ceruloplasmin levels have returned to normal, the maintenance dose should be lowered by 50% if possible. Since the basic defect in copper storage persists, treatment in Wilson's disease is life-long. The patient should be followed closely with serum copper, ceruloplasmin, urinary copper excretion and transaminases. If there is any change in these tests, treatment at full dosage should be reinstituted.

James S. Singer and Marshall M. Kaplan

SIMETHICONE (Mylicon, Silain)

Simethicone is a mixture of liquid dimethylpolysiloxanes with antifoaming and water-repellent properties. It causes gas bubbles to coalesce by changing their surface tension. Simethicone is marketed alone and in combination with antacids, antispasmodics, sedatives, and digestants as an adjunct in the treatment of conditions in which gas is a problem—flatulence, functional gastric bloating, and postoperative gaseous distention.

Simethicone is useful in upper gastrointestinal tract endoscopy to remove foam that can obscure the field of vision. It has also been used to reduce gas shadows in radiography.

In two studies simethicone was effective in reducing postoperative abdominal pain and in hastening the spontaneous passage of gas.[70,71]

Although there have been two studies from the Department of Medical Research of Plough, Inc. (makers of Di-Gel, a simethicone-containing product) supporting the efficacy of simethicone as an antiflatulent,[72,73] most consultants to the *Medical Letter* feel that there is no convincing evidence that simethicone or any of the combination preparations containing simethicone is effective in the treatment of gas associated with functional disorders of the gastrointestinal tract.[74]

Simethicone is believed to be physiologically inert and without toxicity.

Dosage—Oral: For endoscopy, approximately 20 mg in 20 ml of water. The manufacturer's suggested adult dosage is 160 to 320 mg daily in divided doses.

Martin G. Kistin and Richard A. Norton

SULFASALAZINE (Azulfidine, Rorasul)

Sulfasalazine[75,76] is the new official name for salicylazosulfapyridine. When given orally, a small part of the dose is absorbed in the small intestine. The remainder reaches the colon where bacteria cleave an azo bond and liberate sulfapyridine (SP) and 5-aminosalicylic acid (5-ASA). The mechanism of action of sulfasalazine and its metabolites is unclear; the beneficial clinical response and toxicity may be correlated with sulfapyridine blood levels. There is little evidence for an antibacterial role of sulfasalazine.

Sulfasalazine is the treatment of choice for mild to moderate ulcerative colitis and proctitis.[77,78] A dose of 4 to 6 grams per day is more effective than placebo in controlling symptoms in most cases. After remission has occurred, a maintenance dose of 2 g of sulfasalazine per day for three years or more will significantly reduce the relapse rate.[78–80] In severe ulcerative colitis sulfasalazine may be given after an initial response to corticosteroids to facilitate corticosteroid withdrawal.

The role of sulfasalazine in treatment of Crohn's disease of the small bowel and colon is less clear. Most clinicians believe that sulfasalazine is effective in mild to moderate disease and should be utilized in ulcerative colitis. A controlled trial in Crohn's disease suggested that sulfasalazine was beneficial in patients who had not had surgery.[81]

Adverse Reactions—In a recent series[82] 21% of patients developed one or more adverse effects. The majority of patients with symptoms were taking more than 4 grams a day, were slow acetylators, and had sulfapyridine levels greater than 50 μg/ml. With reduction of the dose or discontinuation and slow reintroduction, therapy could be continued without further side effects. There appear to be two major groups of reactions. The first is dose-related and includes nausea, vomiting, fever, headache, 'cyanosis',[82] rash, arthralgias, and transient reticulocytosis. The second group is more severe and is caused by hypersensitivity. It includes fever, rash, bronchospasm, pulmonary eosinophilia, and fibrosing alveolitis.[83,84] Hepatotoxicity, peripheral neuropathy, pancreatitis, Stevens-Johnson syndrome, crystalluria, nephrotic syndrome, and toxic epidermal necrolysis have been reported. Hemolytic anemia, leukopenia, agranulocytosis and thrombocytopenia have also occurred.

Sulfasalazine is contraindicated in patients with hypersensitivity to sulfanomides and salicylates, and in patients with severe drug allergies. It should be avoided in patients with porphyria and glucose 6-phosphate dehydrogenase deficiency.

Interactions—Salicylate is an effective chelator of ferrous iron. The simultaneous administration of ferrous sulfate and sulfasalazine decreases levels of sulfasalazine.[75] Folic acid malabsorption is common with inflammatory bowel disease. The addition of sulfasalazine further decreases the absorption of folic acid, whereas SP and 5-ASA do not.[85]

Dosage—Oral: Adults, acute disease: 2 to 6 g per day in 4 divided doses. It is advisable to begin with 0.5 to 1.0 g a day and increase the dose gradually over a few days until a maintenance dose is reached. After remission is achieved a daily dose of 2 g is advised. *Children,* 40 to 60 mg/kg/day in 4 divided doses with 30 mg/kg/day in 4 divided doses for maintenance.

Edward S. Orris and James F. Patterson

AGENTS FOR TREATMENT OF HEPATIC ENCEPHALOPATHY

Although the pathogenesis of hepatic encephalopathy is incompletely understood, the objective of therapy is still the reduction of ammonia production and absorption from the gastrointestinal tract.[86,87] Treatment with adrenergic precursors is also being advocated.

NEOMYCIN SULFATE
PAROMOMYCIN SULFATE (Humatin)

These nonabsorbable antibiotics act by bowel sterilization to decrease the urease-producing bacterial bowel flora, thereby decreasing the production of ammonia, amines, and other toxic substances. Along with protein restriction, avoidance of sedatives, and the correction of electrolyte imbalances, these drugs are the mainstay of the treatment of portal-systemic encephalopathy. Neomycin has several well-known adverse effects including diarrhea, malabsorption, ototoxicity, and nephrotoxicity,[88,89] of which the latter two are attributable to the 1 to 3% absorption by the gut of oral neomycin.[90] In patients with renal impairment, neomycin blood levels should be periodically determined. These drugs also may be used for preoperative bowel sterilization, in conjunction with mechanical cleansing.

Dosage—Oral: Adults, neomycin sulfate, 4 to 6 g per day in divided doses; paromomycin sulfate, 4 g per day in divided doses. *Rectal: Adults,* 1 g in enema given once or twice.

LACTULOSE (Cephulac)

Lactulose is a synthetic sugar of the disaccharide group containing one molecule of galactose and one molecule of fructose. This sugar is neither metabolized nor absorbed by the proximal small bowel. Its major site of action is in the ileum and colon where it is degraded by the bacterial flora. Possible mechanisms of action include reduction in stool pH with subsequent reduction in the net absorption of ammonia and other toxic nitrogenous substances from the gut, and a direct cathartic effect due to osmotic factors. Lactulose can in fact be used as a mild laxative for chronic constipation.[91–93]

The adverse effects of lactulose are minor and consist of nausea, bloating, cramps, diarrhea, and occasional anorexia. It is contraindicated in patients with galactosemia. Combination treatment with lactulose and neomycin is controversial. Since lactulose requires bacterial degradation and neomycin inhibits bacterial growth, their combination might be self-defeating. However, several studies demonstrate synergism, presumably resulting from neomycin's incomplete sterilization of the gut, thereby leaving fermentative organisms to degrade lactulose.[94]

Dosage—For hepatic encephalopathy, 30 to 50 ml three times per day orally or by retention enema; for chronic constipation, 10 to 20 ml per day.

LEVODOPA

An antiparkinsonian drug, levodopa has a limited role in the treatment of hepatic encephalopathy. Biogenic amines, released by colonic bacterial action and not detoxified by the normal hepatic mechanisms, may accumulate in the central nervous system of patients with hepatic encephalopathy and function as false neurotransmitters.[95] Since levodopa is a precursor of the true neurotransmitters—dopamine and norephinephrine—it has been used as a competitive inhibitor of the false neurotransmitters.[96] Clinical effects of levodopa in hepatic encephalopathy, however, are variable, and it is not currently a first-line drug for this disorder (see Chapter 60 for adverse reactions and interactions).

Dosage—Oral: Adults, 1 to 4 g per day.

Daniel S. Matloff and Karim A. Fawaz

AGENTS USED IN THE DIAGNOSIS OF GASTROINTESTINAL DISORDERS

BETAZOLE HYDROCHLORIDE (Histalog)

Betazole (3-beta-aminoethylpyrazole) is an isomer of histamine with preferential effects on gastric secretion.[97] It possesses characteristic actions of histamine on gastric acid secretion, smooth muscle and blood pressure, but unlike histamine, the effects on acid secretion predominate.[98,99]

Betazole in a dose of 2 mg/kg subcutaneously gives a slightly greater peak acid output than 50 μg/kg of histamine, but there is highly significant correlation between the secretory response produced by the two agents.[100]

There are many side effects with both histamine and betazole.[98,99]

These include pain at the site of injection, dizziness, nausea, palpitations, abdominal cramps, headache, flushing, hypotension, and shock. The incidence of betazole-induced hypotension is approximately 2.5% when doses of 2 mg/kg are used.[99] Most patients experience pain at the injection site and a flushed sensation without other side effects. The incidence of side effects seems to be dose-dependent.[101]

Since peak acid effect occurs during the second postinjection hour,[102] gastric secretions must be collected for at least two hours.

Dosage—Subcutaneous: Adults, 1.5 mg/kg in a single injection.

GLUCAGON

Glucagon, a polypeptide hormone secreted by the alpha islet cells of the pancreas, inhibits gastrointestinal motility in man and animals.[103–105] This effect has been used in radiology for hypotonic duodenography[106,107] and to facilitate endoscopic retrograde cholangiopancreatography. Recently glucagon has begun to replace anticholinergic agents for hypotonic examination of the colon.[108,109] Barium enema examinations performed with glucagon appear to result in less subjective discomfort and a more relaxed colon, with no significant change in vital signs or electrocardiogram.[110]

In 'physiologic' doses, glucagon stimulates glycogenolysis in the liver and causes elevated blood levels of glucose. However, in the lower, 'nonphysiologic' doses used in radiology, glycogenolysis is not clinically important. Occasionally, nausea is noted shortly after injection and persists for 1 to 2 minutes.

Dosage—For endoscopic retrograde cholangiopancreatography, 0.2 mg is given intravenously and repeated as necessary. For hypotonic duodenography with barium enema, 0.2 to 2 mg is given intravenously.

PENTAGASTRIN (Peptavlon)

Pentagastrin, a synthetic pentapeptide, is an alternative to histamine or betazole for gastric secretory testing. Pentagastrin increases secretion of gastric acid, pepsin, and intrinsic factor. Given as a continuous infusion or as an intramuscular or subcutaneous injection, pentagastrin produces peak rates of gastric acid secretion similar to those produced by histamine, betazole or gastrin II.[111,112] Duration of action is short, with a serum half-life of ten minutes.[113] Pentagastrin is now the agent of choice in gastric secretory testing.

Adverse effects are generally mild and include nausea, dizziness, faintness, flushing, warmth, abdominal cramps, and hypotension. The incidence of side effects is lower than with histamine or betazole.[111]

Dosage—6 μg/Kg subcutaneously.

D-XYLOSE

D-xylose, a 5-carbon monosaccharide, is used to evaluate malabsorption.[114,115] It is a simple sugar absorbed primarily by passive diffusion in the proximal small bowel. Providing the test is done properly (see below), an abnormal test indicates either disease of the proximal jejunum, or proximal small bowel bacterial overgrowth. Administration of antibiotics will correct the test to normal in the latter situation.

False positive test might occur in the following situations: 1) vomiting of the D-xylose; 2) inadequate or delayed gastric emptying; 3) inadequate hydration; 4) intrinsic renal disease; and 5) presence of massive ascites. The mean normal excretory values decrease with age.

For the D-xylose test, 25 g is given orally in the fasting state. Either a 5 hour urine sample and/or a 2 hour serum sample is obtained. Excretion of 4.5 grams or more in a 5 hour urine is normal, less than 3 grams is abnormal, and between 3.0 and 4.5 grams is equivocal. A normal 2 hour plasma level is over 32.5 mg/100 ml.

Adverse reactions include mild abdominal cramps and diarrhea.

Martin G. Kistin and Richard A. Norton

REFERENCES

1. Steinberg AP, Platz PH, Wolff SM, et al: Cytotoxic drugs in treatment of nonmalignant diseases. Ann Intern Med 76:619–642, 1972.
2. Drucker WR, Feejeebhay KN: Azathioprine: an adjunct to surgical treatment for granulomatous enteritis. Ann Surg 172:618–626, 1970.
3. Brooke BN, Javett SL, Davison OA: Further experiencing with azathioprine for Crohn's disease. Lancet 2:1050–1053, 1970.
4. Patterson JF, Norton RA, Schwartz RS: Azathioprine treatment of ulcerative colitis, granulomatous colitis and regional enteritis. Am J Dig Dis 16:327–332, 1971.
5. Rhodes J, Bainton D, Peck P, et al: Controlled trial of azathioprine in Crohn's disease. Lancet 2:1273–1276, 1971.
6. Klein M, Binder HJ, Mitchell M, et al: Treatment of Crohn's disease with azathioprine: a controlled evaluation. Gastroenterology 66:916–922, 1974.
7. Willoughby JMT, Kumas PJ, Beckett J, et al: Controlled trial of azathioprine in Crohn's disease. Lancet 2:944–947, 1971.
8. Rosenberg JL, Levin B, Wall AJ, et al: A controlled trial of azathioprine in Crohn's disease. Am J Dig Dis 20:721–726, 1975.
9. Jewell DP, Trulove SC: Azathioprine in ulcerative colitis: final report on controlled therapeutic trial. Br Med J 4:627–630, 1974.

10. Rosenberg JL, Wall AJ, Levin B, et al: A controlled trial of azathioprine in the management of chronic ulcerative colitis. Gastroenterology 69:96–99, 1975.
11. Summerskill WHJ, Korman MG, Ammon HV, et al: Prednisone for chronic active liver disease: dose titration, standard dose, and combination with azathioprine compared. Gut 16:876–883, 1975.
12. Heathcote L, Ross A, Sherlock S, et al: A prospective controlled trial of azathioprine in primary biliary cirrhosis. Gastroenterology 70:656–660, 1976.
13. Roseman M, Bertino JR: Azathioprine. Ann Intern Med 79:694–700, 1973.
14. Bell DG, Dowling RH, Whitney B: Gallstone dissolution in man using chenodeoxycholic acid. Lancet 2:1213–1216, 1972.
15. Coyne MJ, Bonorris GG, Chung A, et al: Treatment of gallstones with chenodeoxycholic acid and phenobarbital. N Engl J Med 292:604–607, 1975.
16. Danzinger RG, Hofmann AF, Schoenfield LJ, et al: Dissolution of cholesterol gallstones by chenodeoxycholic acid. N Engl J Med 286:1–8, 1972.
17. Iser JH, Dowling RH, Mok HYI, et al: Chenodeoxycholic acid treatment of gallstones. N Engl J Med 293:378–383, 1975.
18. Thistle JL, Hofmann AF: Efficacy and specificity of chenodeoxycholic acid therapy for dissolving gallstones. N Engl J Med 289:655–659, 1973.
19. LaRusso NF, Hoffman NE, Hofmann AF, et al: Effect of primary bile acid ingestion on bile acid metabolism and biliary lipid secretion in gallstone patients. Gastroenterology 69:1301–1314, 1975.
20. Mok HYI, Dowling RH, Bell GD: Effect of different doses of chenodeoxycholic acid on bile.lipid composition and on frequency of side-effects in patients with gallstones. Lancet 2:253–257, 1974.
21. Hardison WGM, Rosenberg IH: Bile salt deficiency in steatorrhea following resection of the ileum and proximal colon. N Engl J Med 277:337–342, 1967.
22. VanDiest BW, Fordtran JS, Morawshi SG, et al: Bile salt and micellar fat concentration in proximal small bowel contents of ileectomy patients. J Clin Invest 47:1314–1324, 1968.
23. Condon JR, Robinson V, Suleman MI, et al: The cause and treatment of post vagotomy diarrhea. Br J Surg 62:309–312, 1975.
24. Burbige E, Milligan E: Pseudomembraneous colitis. Association with antibiotics and therapy with cholestyramine. JAMA 231:1157–1158, 1975.
25. Bushkin FL, Wickborn G, DeFord J, et al: Postoperative alkaline reflux gastritis. Surg Gynecol Obstet 138:933–939, 1974.
26. Scudamore H, Eckstam E, Fencil W, et al: Bile reflux gastritis. Am J Gastroenterol 60:9–21, 1973.
27. West RJ, Lloyd JK: Use of cholestyramine in treatment of children with familial hypercholesterolemia. Arch Dis Child 48:370–374, 1973.
28. Schoon IM, Olbe L: Effect of cimetidine on cholinergic reflex stimulation of gastric acid secretion in duodenal ulcer patients. In *Cimetidine: Second International Symposium on Histamine Hd2.Receptor Antagonist*. Edited by WL Burland, MA Simkins. Amsterdam, Excerpta Medica, 1977, pp 207-216.
29. Burland WL, Duncan WA, Hessello T, et al: Pharmacological evaluation of cimetidine, a new histamine H_2 receptor antagonist, in healthy man. Br J Clin Pharmacol 2:481–486, 1975.
30. Richardson CT, Walsh JH, Hicks MI: The effect of cimetidine, a new histamine H_2-receptor antagonist, on meal-stimulated acid secretion, serum gastrin, and gastric empyting in patients with duodenal ulcers. Gastroenterology 71:19–23, 1976.
31. Haggie SJ, Earmont DC, Wyllie JH: Treatment of duodenal ulcer with cimetidine. Lancet 1:983–984, 1976.
32. Bodemar G, Norlander B, Walan A: Cimetidine in the treatment of active peptic ulcer disease. In *Cimetidine: Second International Symposium on Histamine H_2.Receptor Antagonist*. Edited by WL Burland, MA Simkins. Amsterdam, Excerpta Medica, 1977, pp 224–239.
33. Bader JP, Morin T, Bernier JJ, et al: Treatment of gastric ulcer by cimetidine: a multicenter trial. In *Cimetidine: Second International Symposium on Histamine H_2.Receptor Antagonist*. Edited by WL Burkland, MA Simkins. Amsterdam, Excerpta Medica, 1977, pp 287–292.

34. McCarthy DM: Long-term therapy of Zollinger-Ellison syndrome with H_2-histamine receptor blocking agents (Abstract). Gastroenterology 72(5, part 2):1162, 1977.
35. McCluskie RA, Bardhan KD, Saul DM, et al: Cimetidine in the treatment of esophagitis. In *Cimetidine: Second International Symposium on Histamine H_2-Receptor Antagonist*. Edited by WL Burland, MA Simkins. Amsterdam, Excerpta Medica, 1977, pp 297–305.
36. Dykes PW, Kang JY, Hoare A, et al: Treatment of upper gastrointestinal hemorrhage with cimetidine. In *Cimetidine: Second International Symposium on Histamine H_2-Receptor Antagonist*. Edited by WL Burland, MA Simkins. Amsterdam, Excerpta Medica, 1977, pp 337–344.
37. Bailey RJ, MacDougall BRD, Williams R: A controlled trial of H_2-receptor antagonists in prophylaxis of bleeding from gastrointestinal erosion in fulminant hepatic failure (Abstract). Gut 17:389, 1976.
38. Brimlecombe RW, Duncan WA, Durant GJ, et al: Cimetidine, a non-thiourea H_2 receptor-antagonist. J Int Med Res 3:86–92, 1975.
39. Haggie SJ, Fremont DC, Wyllie JH: Treatment of duodenal ulcer with cimetidine. Lancet 1:983–984, 1976.
40. Blackwood WS, Maudgal DP, Pickard RG, et al: Cimetidine in duodenal ulcer: controlled trial. Lancet 2:194–195, 1976.
41. Hall WH: Breast changes in males on cimetidine (letter). N Engl J Med 295:841, 1976.
42. Truelove SC, Watkinson G, Draper G: Comparison of corticosteroids and sulphasalazine therapy in ulcerative colitis. Br Med J 2:1708–1711, 1962.
43. Kirsner JB, Sklar M, Palmer WL: The use of ACTH, cortisone, hydrocortisone and related compounds in the management of ulcerative colitis. Am J Med 22:264–274, 1957.
44. Truelove SC, Witts LJ: Cortisone and corticotropin in ulcerative colitis. Br Med J 1:387–394, 1959.
45. Lennard.Jones JE, Misiewicz JJ, Connell AM, et al: Prednisone as maintenance therapy for ulcerative colitis in remission. Lancet 1:188–189, 1965.
46. Gardner RC: Pharmacotherapy of inflammatory bowel disease. Am J Hosp Pharm 33:831–838, 1976.
47. Truelove SC, Jewell DP: Intensive intravenous regimen for severe attacks of ulcerative colitis. Lancet 1:1067–1070, 1974.
48. Jones H, Lennard-Jones JE: Corticosteroids and corticotropin in the treatment of Crohn's disease. Gut 7:181–187, 1966.
49. Sparberg M, Kirsner JB: Long-term corticosteroid therapy for regional enteritis: an analysis of 58 courses in 54 patients. Am J Dig Dis 11:865–880, 1966.
50. Campra JL, Hamlin EM, Kirshbaum RJ, et al: Prednisone therapy of acute alcoholic hepatitis. Ann Intern Med 79:625–631, 1973.
51. Gregory PB, Knauer CM, Kempson RL, et al: Steroid therapy in severe viral hepatitis. N Engl J Med 294:681–687, 1976.
52. Powell-Tuck J, Lennard-Jones JE, May CS, et al: Plasma prednisolone levels after administration of prednisolone-21-phosphate as a retention enema in colitis. Br Med J 1:193–195, 1976.
53. Farmer RG, Schumaker OP: Treatment of ulcerative colitis with hydrocortisone enemas. Dis Colon Rectum 13:355–361, 1970.
54. Truelove SC: Treatment of ulcerative colitis with local hydrocortisone hemisuccinate sodium: a report on a controlled therapeutic trial. Br Med J 2:1072–1077, 1958.
55. Brown CH, Merlo M: Topical steroid therapy for ulcerative colitis: report of 50 cases. Am J Gastroenterol 36:343–354, 1961.
56. Kaplan HP, Portnoy B, Binder HJ, et al: A controlled trial of intravenous adrenocorticotropic hormone and hydrocortisone in the treatment of acute ulcerative colitis. Gastroenterology 69:91–95, 1975.
57. Conn HO, Blitzer BL: Nonassociation of adrenocorticosteroid therapy and peptic ulcer. N Engl J Med 294:473–479, 1976.
58. Jalan KN, Prescott RJ, Smith AN, et al: Influence of corticosteroids in the results of surgical treatment for ulcerative colitis. N Engl J Med 282:588–592, 1971.
59. Littman A, Hanscom DH: Pancreatic extracts. N Engl J Med 281:201–204, 1969.
60. Graham DY: Enzyme replacement therapy of exocrine pancreatic insufficiency in man. N Engl J Med 296:1314–1317, 1977.

61. Regan PT, Malagelada JR, DiMagno EP, et al: Fate and efficacy of oral enzymes in pancreatic insufficiency: Effects of neutralizing antacids, cimetidine and enteric coating. Gastroenterology 72:A-95/1118, 1977.
62. DiMagno EP, Malagelada JR, Go VLW, et al: Fate of orally ingested enzymes in pancreatic insufficiency. N Engl J Med 296:1318–1322, 1977.
63. Stapleton FB, Kennedy J, Nousia-Arvanitakis S, et al: Hyperuricosuria due to high-dose pancreatic extract therapy in cystic fibrosis. N Engl J Med 295:246–248, 1976.
64. Walshe JM: Penicillamine, a new oral therapy for Wilson's disease. Am J Med 21:487–495, 1956.
65. Multicenter Trial Group: Controlled trial of D-penicillamine in severe rheumatoid arthritis. Lancet 1:278–280, 1973.
66. Harris ED Jr, Sjoerdsma A: Effect of penicillamine on human collagen and its possible application to the treatment of scleroderma. Lancet 2:996–1001, 1966.
67. Sternlieb I: Penicillamine and the nephrotic syndromes. JAMA 198:1311–1312, 1966.
68. Sternlieb I, Bennett B, Scheinberg H: D-penicillamine induced Goodpasture's syndrome in Wilson's disease. Ann Intern Med 82:673–676, 1975.
69. Harpey JP, Caille B, Moulias R, et al: Lupus-like syndrome induced by D-penicillamine in Wilson's disease. Lancet 1:292, 1971.
70. Gibstein A, Cooper JJ, Wisot AL, et al: Prevention of postoperative abdominal distention and discomfort with simethicone. Obstet Gynecol 38:386–389, 1971.
71. Danhof IE, Stavola JJ: Accelerated transit of intestinal gas with simethicone. Obstet Gynecol 44:148–154, 1974.
72. Bernstein JE, Schwartz SR: An evaluation of the effectiveness of simethicone in acute upper gastrointestinal distress. Curr Ther Res 16:617–620, 1974.
73. Bernstein JE, Kasich AM: A double-blind trial of simethicone in functional disease of the upper gastrointestinal tract. J Clin Pharmacol 14:617–623, 1974.
74. Anonymous: Simethicone for discomfort caused by gastrointestinal gas. Med Lett Drugs Ther 17:80, 1975.
75. Goldman P, Peppercorn MA: Sulfasalazine. N Engl J Med 293:2–23, 1975.
76. Das KM, Sternlieb I: Salicylazosulfapyridine in inflammatory bowel disease. Am J Dig Dis 20:971–976, 1975.
77. Baron JH, Connell AM, Lennard-Jones JE, et al: Sulphasalazine and salicylazoralphadimidine in ulcerative colitis. Lancet 1:1094–1096, 1962.
78. Dick AP, Grayson MJ, Carpenter RG, et al: Controlled trial of sulphasalazine in the treatment of ulcerative colitis. Gut 5:437–442, 1964.
79. Misiewicz JJ, Lennard-Jones JE, Connell AM: Controlled trial of sulphasalazine in maintenance therapy for ulcerative colitis. Lancet 1:185–188, 1965.
80. Dissanayake AS, Truelove SC: A controlled therapeutic trial of long-term maintenance treatment of ulcerative colitis with sulphasalazine (Salaxopyrin). Gut 14:923–926, 1973.
81. Anthanisin P, Barany F, Folkenborg O, et al: The clinical effect of salazosulphapyridine in Crohn's disease. Scand J Gastroenterol 9:549–554, 1974.
82. Das KM, Eastwood MA, McManus JPA: Adverse reactions during salicylazosulfapyridine therapy and the relation with drug metabolism and acetylator phenotype. N Engl J Med 289:491–495, 1973.
83. Editorial: Sulphasalazine induced lung disease. Lancet 2:504–505, 1974.
84. Davies D, MacFarlane A: Fibrosing alveolitis and treatment with sulphasalazine. Gut 15:185–188, 1974.
85. Franklin JL, Rosenberg IH: Impaired folic acid absorption in inflammatory bowel disease: effects of salicylazosulfapyridine. Gastroenterology 64:517–525, 1973.
86. Schenker S, Breen KJ, Hoyumpa AM: Hepatic encephalopathy: current status. Gastroenterology 66:121–151, 1974.
87. Fischer JE: Hepatic coma in cirrhosis, portal hypertension, and following portacaval shunt. Arch Surg 108:325–336, 1974.
88. Breen KJ, Bryant RE, Levinson JD, et al: Neomycin absorption in man: studies of oral and enema administration and effect of intestinal sterilization. Ann Intern Med 76:211–218, 1972.
89. Berk DP, Chalmers T: Deafness complicating antibiotic therapy of hepatic encephalopathy. Ann Intern Med 73:393–396, 1970.

90. Kunin CM, Chalmers TC, Leevy CM, et al: Absorption of orally-administered neomycin and kanamycin. N Engl J Med 262:380–385, 1966.
91. Avery GS, Davies EF, Brogden RN: Lactulose: a review of its therapeutic and pharmacological properties with particular reference to ammonia metabolism and its mode of action in portal systemic encephalopathy. Drugs 4:7–48, 1972.
92. Fessel JM, Conn HO: Lactulose in the treatment of acute hepatic encephalopathy. Am J Med Sci 266:103–110, 1973.
93. Kersh ES, Rikin H: Lactulose enemas. Ann Intern Med 78:81–84, 1973.
94. Conn HO: Interactions of lactulose and neomycin. Drugs 4:4–6, 1972.
95. Fisher JE, Baldessarini RJ: False neurotransmitter and hepatic failure. Lancet 1:75–79, 1971.
96. Parkes JD, Sharpstone P, Williams R: Levodopa in hepatic coma. Lancet 2:1341–1343, 1970.
97. Rosiere CE, Grossman MI: An analog of histamine that stimulates gastric acid secretion without other actions of histamine. Science 113:651, 1951.
98. Blum NI, Mayoral LG, Kalser MH: Augmented gastric analysis: a word of caution. JAMA 191:339–341, 1965.
99. Goldenberg J, Cummins AJ, Gompertz MJ: A clinical evaluation of the maximal Histalog test. Am J Dig Dis 12:468–474, 1967.
100. Isenberg JI, Brooks AM, Grossman MI: Pentagastrin versus betazole as stimulant of gastric secretion: comparative study in man. JAMA 206:2897–2898, 1968.
101. Laudano OM, Roncoroni EL: Determination of the dose of Histalog that provokes maximal gastric secretory response. Gastroenterology 49:372–374, 1965.
102. Ward S, Gillespie IE, Passaro EP, et al: Comparison of Histalog and histamine as stimulants for maximal gastric secretion in human subjects and in dogs. Gastroenterology 44:620–626, 1963.
103. Stunkard AF, VanItallie TB, Reis BB: The mechanism of satiety: effect of glucagon on gastric hunger contractions in man. Proc Soc Exp Biol Med 89:258–261, 1955.
104. Kock NG, Darle N, Dotevall G: Inhibition of intestinal motility in man by glucagon given intraportally. Gastroenterology 53:88–92, 1967.
105. Necheles H, Sporn J, Walker L: Effect of glucagon on gastrointestinal motility. Am J Gastroenterol 45:34–39, 1966.
106. Miller RE, Chernish SM, Rosenak BD, et al: Hypotonic duodenography with glucagon. Radiology 108:35–42, 1973.
107. Miller RE, Chernish SM, Skulas J, et al: Hypotonic roentgenography with glucagon. Am J Roentgenol 121:264–274, 1974.
108. Gohel VK, Dalinka MK, Coren GS: Hypotonic examination of the colon with glucagon. Radiology 115:1–4, 1975.
109. Meeroff JC, Jorgens J, Isenberg JI: The effect of glucagon on barium-enema examination. Radiology 115:5–7, 1975.
110. Harned RK, Stelling CB, Williams S, et al: Glucagon and barium enema examinations: a controlled clinical trial. Am J Roentgenol 126:981–984, 1976.
111. Multicentre Pilot Study: Pentagastrin as a stimulant of maximal gastric acid response in man. Lancet 1:291–295, 1967.
112. Jepson K, Duthie HL, Fawcett AN, et al: Acid and pepsin response to gastrin. I. Pentagastrin, tetragastrin, histamine, and pentagastrin snuff. Lancet 2:139–141, 1968.
113. Merchant FJ, Bombeck CT, Pissidis A, et al: Hepatic destruction of synthetic gastrin pentapeptide. J Natl Med Assoc 64:246–249, 1972.
114. Wilson FA, Dietschy JM: Differential diagnostic approach to clinical problems of malabsorption. Gastroenterology 61:911–931, 1971.
115. Christiansen PA, Kirsner JB, Ablaza J: D-xylose and its use in the diagnosis of malabsorptive states. Am J Med 27:443–453, 1959.

INDEX

Some diseases and other drug indications have been indexed, but the majority of index entries are for drugs. Individual drug names or drug category names are main headings; indications and interactions with other drugs are subheadings. Trademark names are capitalized; generic names are not. Trademark name entries generally refer to drug monographs only; the generic name should be used for complete page references. A (C) follows names for drug combinations. Bold face page numbers refer to drug monographs or other major discussions of a drug.

B

E

F

G

M

N